MAGILL'S
MEDICAL GUIDE

MAGILL'S

MEDICAL GUIDE

Second Revised Edition

Volume III
Paramedics — Zoonoses
Index

Medical Consultants

Karen E. Kalumuck, Ph.D.
The Exploratorium, San Francisco

Nancy A. Piotrowski, Ph.D.
University of California, Berkeley

Connie Rizzo, M.D.
Pace University

Project Editor
Tracy Irons-Georges

SALEM PRESS, INC.
Pasadena, California   Hackensack, New Jersey

Editor in Chief: Dawn P. Dawson
Project Editor: Tracy Irons-Georges
Research Supervisor: Jeffry Jensen
Photograph Editor: Philip Bader
Production Editor: Joyce I. Buchea
Page Design: James Hutson
Layout: William Zimmerman
Cover Design: Moritz Design

Illustrations: Hans & Cassady, Inc., Westerville, Ohio

Magill's Medical Guide: Health and Illness, 1995
Supplement, 1996
Magill's Medical Guide, revised edition, 1998
Second revised edition, 2002

∞ The paper used in these volumes conforms to the American National Standard for Permanence of Paper for Printed Library Materials, Z39.48-1992 (R1997).

Note to Readers
The material presented in *Magill's Medical Guide, Second Revised Edition*, is intended for broad informational and educational purposes. Readers who suspect that they suffer from any of the physical or psychological disorders, diseases, or conditions described in this set should contact a physician without delay; this work should not be used as a substitute for professional medical diagnosis or treatment. This set is not to be considered definitive on the covered topics, and readers should remember that the field of health care is characterized by a diversity of medical opinions and constant expansion in knowledge and understanding.

Library of Congress Cataloging-in-Publication Data
Magill's medical guide / medical consultants, Karen E. Kalumuck, Nancy A. Piotrowski, Connie Rizzo ; project editor, Tracy Irons-Georges.
    p. : cm.
Includes bibliographical references and index.
    1. Medicine—Encyclopedias. I. Kalumuck, Karen E. II. Piotrowski, Nancy A. III Rizzo, Connie. IV. Irons-Georges, Tracy.
RC41.M34   2001
610′.3—dc21
ISBN 1-58765-003-7 (set)   2001041169
ISBN 1-58765-006-1 (vol. 3)   CIP

First Printing

PRINTED IN THE UNITED STATES OF AMERICA

CONTENTS

MAGILL'S
MEDICAL GUIDE

Paramedics

Specialty

Anatomy or system affected: All

Specialties and related fields: Cardiology, critical care, emergency medicine, geriatrics and gerontology, pulmonary medicine

Definition: Trained professional emergency medical technicians (EMTs) who provide sophisticated advanced life support in the field, especially intravenous therapy, cardiac monitoring, drug administration, cardiac defibrillation, and advanced airway management.

Key terms:

abandonment: the failure of an emergency medical technician to continue emergency medical treatment

advanced life support (ALS): procedures such as intravenous therapy, pharmacology, cardiac monitoring, and defibrillation

basic life support (BLS): simple emergency lifesaving procedures that can aid a person in respiratory or circulatory failure

cardiopulmonary resuscitation (CPR): the artificial establishment of circulation of the blood and movement of air into and out of the lungs in a pulseless, nonbreathing patient

certification: the formal notice of certain privileges and abilities after completion of certain training and testing

defibrillation: the termination of atrial or ventricular fibrillation (irregular heart muscle contractions), with restoration of the normal rhythm

emergency medical services (EMS): the combined efforts of several professionals and agencies to provide prehospital emergency care to the sick and injured

intravenous therapy: the introduction of medication into a vein with a special needle

intubation: the introduction of a tube into a body cavity, as into the larynx

negligence: failure to perform an important or necessary technique, or the performance of such a technique in a careless or unskilled manner so as to cause further injury

Science and Profession

The emergency medical technician-paramedic (EMT-P) provides hospital emergency care in the field under medical command authority to acutely ill and/or injured patients and then transports those patients to the hospital by ambulance or other appropriate vehicle.

The clinical knowledge possessed by the EMT-P includes the following systems and areas: the cardiovascular system, including the recognition of arrhythmias, myocardial ischemia, and congestive heart failure; the respiratory system, including acute airway obstruction, pneumothorax, chronic obstructive pulmonary disease (COPD), and respiratory distress; trauma to the head, neck, chest, spine, abdomen, pelvis, and extremities; medical emergencies, including acute abdominal infections, diabetes mellitus, and allergic reactions; the central nervous system, including strokes, seizures, and alterations in levels of consciousness; obstetrical emergencies such as eclampsia; pediatric cases, including croup, epiglottitis, dehydration, child abuse, and care of the newborn; psychiatric emergencies, including problems with individuals who are suicidal, assaultive, destructive, resistant, anxious, confused, amnesiac, or paranoid; drug-related problems, including alcoholism, drug addiction, or overdoses; sexual assault and abuse; and various special situations, such as carbon monoxide and other noxious inhalations, poisoning, near drownings, overexposure to heat and cold, electrocution, burns, and exposure to hazardous materials.

The EMT-P must be able to fulfill many roles. First, paramedics must recognize a medical emergency, assess the situation, manage emergency care, and, if needed, extricate the patient. They must also coordinate their efforts with those of other agencies that may be involved in the care and transport of the patient. Paramedics should establish a good rapport with patients and their significant others in order to decrease their state of anxiety.

The next step is to assign priorities to emergency treatment data for the designated medical control authority. Emergency treatment priorities must be assigned in cases where the medical direction is interrupted by communication failure or in cases of immediate, life-threatening conditions. Paramedics must record and communicate pertinent information to the designated medical command authority.

Meanwhile, they must initiate and continue emergency medical care under medical control, including the recognition of presenting conditions and the initiation of appropriate treatments. Such conditions include traumatic and medical emergencies, airway and ventilation problems, cardiac arrhythmias or standstill, and psychological crises. Paramedics must also assess the response of patients to treatment, modifying the medical therapy as directed by the medical control authority. EMT-Ps exercise personal judgment; provide such emergency medical care as has been specifically authorized in advance; direct and coordinate the transport of the patient by selecting the best available methods in concert with the medical command authority; record, in writing, the details related to the patient's emergency care and the incident; and direct the maintenance and preparation of emergency care equipment and supplies.

EMT-Ps must have a good working knowledge of human anatomy and must be familiar with its topographical language. Even though paramedics are not expected to diagnose every injury or illness, they can aid emergency department personnel by conveying correct information using medical terminology. Such information is gathered after examination of a patient at the scene of an accident or sudden illness.

The most important function of the paramedic is to identify and treat any life-threatening conditions first and then to assess the patient carefully for other complaints or findings that may require emergency treatment or transportation to a hospital setting. Paramedics must distinguish between signs (measured information such as pulse, respiration, and temperature) and symptoms (patient complaints). They must be able to take complete patient histories, document all medications, and transfer this information to medical control.

The vital role of the respiratory system is stressed in all paramedical training courses. The function of the respiratory system is to provide the body with oxygen and to eliminate carbon dioxide. Paramedics must fully understand the breathing process, including gas exchange and the role and anatomic position of the air passages and lungs. They must understand the mechanics of breathing—how the diaphragm and intercostal muscles contract and relax during inspiration and expiration—and must realize that breathing is controlled by the brain's response to levels of carbon dioxide and oxygen present in the arterial blood. Of special concern to the paramedic is the patient with COPD, who needs specialized oxygen support and careful watching.

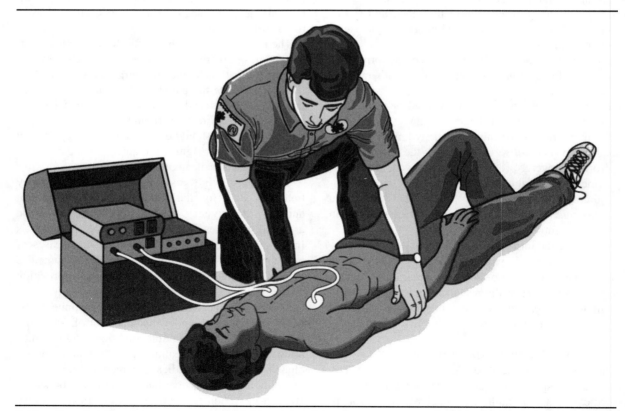

Paramedics administer emergency care in the field to sick or injured patients; among their primary tools are portable monitoring devices, such as an electrocardiograph (ECG or EKG) machine to check the electrical activity of the heart.

Basic life support (BLS), formerly called cardio-pulmonary resuscitation (CPR), is a series of emergency lifesaving procedures that are carried out in order to treat respiratory arrest, cardiac arrest, or both. CPR is a method of providing artificial ventilation and circulation. Its effectiveness depends on the prompt recognition of respiratory and/or cardiac arrest and the immediate start of treatment. Very often, the paramedic is able to defibrillate the patient immediately after cardiac arrest and restart the heart. Knowledge of how to provide BLS to the laryngectomy patient is part of paramedic education; in such cases, ventilation is often given via a stoma (opening) in the neck of the patient. Basic life support procedures must be modified for infants and children, since their respiration and pulse rates are higher than those of adults and require more rapid delivery of ventilatory and cardiac assistance.

Although breathing and heart rate are the primary interests of the paramedic, serious bleeding can also be life-threatening. Hence, paramedics must be well versed in blood circulation routes, control of bleeding, and the pressure points that can help in the control of serious hemorrhage. Serious bleeding often brings on a type of shock that is termed hypovolemic (meaning low blood volume). Paramedics must be alert to signs of impending shock and deal with this condition as soon as possible. Medical antishock trousers (MAST) are often used by paramedics to auto-transfuse volumes of blood from the patient's lower extremities to the heart, lungs, and brain. These trousers are also used to control severe hemorrhage or the complications of pelvic fractures. The paramedic must be aware of the contraindications to the use of these devices as well; for example, persons with head injuries should not have the MAST device applied to them.

Paramedics need to identify the many types of shock. Anaphylactic shock is caused by an unusual or exaggerated allergic reaction of a person to a foreign protein. Psychogenic shock (fainting) is often self-correcting. Septic shock is caused by severe bacterial infections, while metabolic shock may arise from severe, untreated illnesses. Cardiogenic shock arises from an underlying cardiac condition and inefficient blood flow. In each case, the paramedic must be alert to the signs of each type of shock and be prepared to treat it, either with drugs delivered under medical control or with equipment present on the paramedic ambulance.

The more common types of injuries encountered by the paramedic are soft tissue injuries, caused by falls or accidents. The skin is the largest single organ of the body. It protects the body from the environment, regulates the body temperature, and transmits information from the environment to the brain. Soft tissue injuries can cause breaks in the skin, leaving the body vulnerable to infection and bleeding. Paramedic training includes treatment for massive traumatic wounds, such as gunshot or knife wounds.

Dealing with fractures is another part of paramedic training. While most fractures are not life-threatening, they can be painful and bring on patient shock; hence, paramedics need to deal with them quickly. Knowledge of the body's musculoskeletal system is vital to the performance of a paramedic.

Head injuries are a very challenging part of paramedic treatment, since the scalp contains many blood vessels and bleeding from head injuries is often profuse. The more serious head injury is often bloodless externally, but internal bleeding brings on pressure buildup in the skull and sudden coma. Such injuries are life-threatening and often require rapid treatment and transport.

Other medical emergencies include strokes (cerebrovascular accidents), diabetic coma or insulin shock, acute abdominal infections, or seizures. Prompt recognition and treatment by the paramedic are essential. Finally, treating the pediatric patient can be one of the most difficult emergencies, but saving a child's life or rescuing a child from permanent, disabling injury is very rewarding. The broad range of knowledge required of paramedics makes them a very special part of the health care team.

DIAGNOSTIC AND TREATMENT TECHNIQUES

Three technologies that distinguish the paramedic from the basic EMT are intravenous therapy, advanced airway management, and defibrillation.

Intravenous (IV) therapy may be an important procedure during the resuscitation of a patient who is suffering from hypovolemia, burn injury, blood loss, heat stroke, shock, electrolyte imbalance, or many other medical and surgical conditions. IV therapy is also important in providing an avenue of medication delivery in many medical situations, such as cardiac arrest, seizures, and asthma attacks. IV therapy is an invasive procedure that requires extensive training in its use in order for the paramedic to maintain the necessary skill level. In addition, paramedics must be aware of the indication for the use of IV therapy, the maintenance of such therapy, and possible complications.

Infusion is the introduction of fluid other than blood or blood products into the vascular system. This technique is used to establish and maintain direct access to the circulation or to provide fluids in order to maintain an adequate circulating blood volume. Fluids used for IVs are often referred to as electrolyte solutions because the chemical compounds that they contain are electrolytes. The most common electrolyte solutions used are sodium chloride solutions; for example, NS is a normal saline solution containing 0.9 percent sodium chloride. Occasionally, paramedics use plasma expanders or colloids, including Dextran. A common intravenous fluid is D5W, which is a 5 percent dextrose solution. The procedure for starting an IV includes preparing the solution, selecting the proper catheter size, selecting and preparing the site, and performing the venipuncture. Local complications to IV therapy may include some pain from the needle stick, hematoma formation at failed IV sites, infection, accidental arterial puncture, nerve damage, and thrombophlebitis. Environmental complications include cold climates, which cause IV solutions to freeze, and the danger of a needle stick to medical personnel during disposal. Proper precautions and periodic retraining keep paramedics up-to-date in their skills.

Advanced airway management means placing a cylindrical tube into the patient's airway to maintain an open passage, to prevent aspiration of foreign bodies and stomach contents, and to allow the delivery of oxygen-enriched air. Three types of devices are employed in advanced airway management to achieve these objectives: the endotracheal tube (ENT), the esophageal obturator airway (EOA), and the pharyngeotracheal airway. The use of any of these devices by paramedics requires the consent of a medical director and adherence to written protocols. These devices require skill and instruction for proper insertion and use.

The ENT is placed through a patient's mouth or nose and directly through the larynx between the vocal cords. The tube may be placed blindly through the vocal cords using sounds of labored respirations as a guide, or it may be placed by feel through the cords. After placement, a soft balloon cuff near the end of the tube is then inflated with approximately 10 cubic centimeters of air to seal the trachea and anchor the tube, so that air can be blown directly into the lungs. The ENT prevents aspiration and gastric distension. It facilitates airway suctioning and enables the delivery of high volumes of oxygen at higher-than-normal pressures. In addition, certain medications may be given down the tube. ENT placement and use are difficult skills to master, requiring considerable practice and expert initial instruction. Direct visualization of the vocal cords is an important skill to have in order to prevent tracheal damage. If intubation takes too long, the resulting delay in oxygenation may lead to brain damage. Thus, constant monitoring of lung sounds is needed to ensure that the tube stays in place.

The EOA has been in use since 1973 to facilitate airway management in cardiopulmonary resuscitation. The EOA is a plastic, semirigid tube 34 centimeters long and 13 millimeters in diameter. The lower end of the tube is smooth, rounded, and closed. The upper one-third of the EOA is designed to function as an airway. It has sixteen holes in its wall at the junction of the middle and upper sections; when properly inserted, these holes will lie at the level of the pharynx and provide free passage of oxygen-enriched air to the lungs. The lower two-thirds of the EOA should lie in the esophagus. The balloon surrounding the end of the tube is normally inflated to block the esophagus and prevent the regurgitation of stomach contents backward into the airway. The face mask that comes with the EOA is designed to fit snugly about the patient's nose and mouth and must provide a tight seal. The EOA is used only for short-term airway management. It should be removed when the unconscious patient awakens and is able to protect the airway or when ENT placement has been performed over the EOA. At the time that the balloon is deflated and the EOA is removed, there is a high risk of vomiting and/or regurgitation of gastric contents. The EOA is not to be used on patients who are awake, on small children, or on patients with known esophageal disease.

The pharyngeotracheal airway is designed to provide lung ventilation when placed in either the trachea or the esophagus. This device is designed to be inserted blindly into the oropharynx and esophagus by paramedics who have received training and are authorized to use it. A pharyngeotracheal airway is contraindicated in conscious or semiconscious patients with a gag reflex. It should not be used with children under the age of fourteen or with adults under five feet tall.

With the use of any of these airway devices, the

patient may regain consciousness while intubated. Such patients will usually gag, choke, and grasp at the device in an attempt to remove it, often resulting in injury to the airway. The patient's hands must be immediately restrained while the airway device is removed.

Defibrillation is the delivery of an electric current through a person's chest wall and heart for the purpose of ending ventricular fibrillation. The device used for this procedure is called a defibrillator; it is typically a portable, battery-powered instrument that is used to record cardiac rhythm and to generate and deliver an electrical charge. Defibrillation can be a lifesaving measure in the treatment of sudden cardiac arrest in which the heart is in an arrhythmia known as ventricular fibrillation or ventricular tachycardia (VT). These two conditions occur when cardiac muscle becomes oxygen deficient or is injured or dies, causing the electrical system of the heart to be disturbed. Sometimes, the injured area of the heart begins to fire off uncoordinated electrical impulses. These irregular impulses can initiate abnormal beats called premature ventricular contractions (PVCs). If several of the PVCs occur close together, they produce the rhythm called ventricular tachycardia. If VT does not spontaneously convert back to a normal heart rhythm, it rapidly degenerates into ventricular fibrillation. The heart in VT beats faster and faster until its oxygen supply is depleted, at which point tissue injury begins and electrical impulses become completely uncoordinated and are fired at random.

If a defibrillator is applied to the patient and an electrical shock is given to the heart during the time of ventricular fibrillation, there is a good chance of restoring more normal electrical activity. This electrical countershock is thought to depolarize the cardiac muscle and conducting tissues instantaneously, thus resetting the electrical energies to the depolarized state. The patient's heart can then begin its normal conduction and contractions without having to contend with randomly generated electrical impulses. The electrical current delivered by defibrillators is measured in units called joules. In most protocols, the first shock is 200 joules, the second is between 200 and 300 joules, and the third and subsequent shocks are at the full 360 joule level. Paramedics using defibrillators need frequent continuing education in order to emphasize the practical skills of proper attachment of the electrodes, proper device operation, and recognition of cardiac arrhythmias.

PERSPECTIVE AND PROSPECTS

Emergency medical services (EMS) in the United States had its beginnings in 1966. In that year, the Committees on Trauma and Shock of the National Academy of Sciences National Research Council jointly published "Accidental Death and Disability: The Neglected Disease of Modern Society." This joint report brought public attention to the inadequate emergency medical care being provided to the injured and sick in many parts of the United States. Two federal agencies initiated reform measures: The Department of Transportation (DOT) initiated the Highway Safety Act in 1966, and the Department of Health, Education, and Welfare enacted the Emergency Medical Services Act in 1973. Both created funding sources to develop prehospital emergency care in an effort to eliminate the majority of prehospital deaths. Local EMS systems were established in the early 1970's. In the 1980's, practitioners took a hard look at what had been done in the past, and the focus changed from establishing EMS systems to developing educational programs to provide consistent levels of quality care to the sick and injured.

The EMS system is made up of various components that work together to provide the sick and injured with the best possible emergency care in the shortest possible time. The EMS system represents the combined efforts of the first responder, the EMT with basic life support skills, the EMT-paramedic with advanced life support skills, emergency department personnel, physicians, allied health personnel, hospital administrators, EMS system administrators, and the overseeing governmental agencies.

Emergency medical technology is an exciting field of study. Few areas offer more direct application of theory and skills. All the information received in an EMT class will be important when it comes to saving lives and lessening human suffering. Emergency medical technology combines theoretical information, practical skills, and common sense. Above all, the EMS person dealing with a patient must possess great compassion and understanding.

The certification of an EMT-paramedic is formal notice of certain privileges and abilities after the completion of specific training and testing. The possession of a certificate obligates the individual to conform to the standard of care of other certified emergency medical care personnel. Nearly every state exempts emergency medical care from the licensure requirements of the Medical Practices Act for non-medical personnel. (Because many emergency medical care procedures may be construed by the public to be the performance of a medical act, the EMT must be protected legally in those situations.) The need for prehospital care providers is ongoing, and recruiting people to enter this field continues to be a challenge to the agencies that oversee this work.

—*Jane A. Slezak, Ph.D.*

See also Arrhythmias; Burns and scalds; Choking; Critical care; Critical care, pediatric; Electrocardiography (ECG or EKG); Emergency medicine; Fracture and dislocation; Heart attack; Heat exhaustion and heat stroke; Respiration; Resuscitation; Shock; Strokes; Tracheostomy; Wounds.

FOR FURTHER INFORMATION:
Copass, Michael K., Mickey S. Eisenberg, and Steven C. Macdonald. *The Paramedic Manual.* 2d ed. Philadelphia: W. B. Saunders, 1987. This volume in the Saunders Blue Books series examines the function of the emergency medical technician and the paramedic, addressing the skills and knowledge that are required of these individuals. An index is provided.

Grant, Harvey D., et al. *Brady Emergency Care.* Rev. 7th ed. Englewood Cliffs, N.J.: Brady Prentice Hall Education, Career & Technology, 1995. A well-written basic text for emergency medical technicians.

Heckman, James D., ed. *Emergency Care and Transportation of the Sick and Injured.* 5th ed. Park Ridge, Ill.: American Academy of Orthopaedic Surgeons, 1992. A text covering both basic and advanced life support procedures for the EMT and the EMT-paramedic. Contains many illustrative diagrams.

Shapiro, Paul D., and Mary B. Shapiro. *Paramedic: The True Story of a New York Paramedic's Battles with Life and Death.* New York: Bantam Books, 1991. Paul Shapiro recounts his experiences in the field as a paramedic. A valuable firsthand account of the profession.

Tangherlini, Timothy R. *Talking Trauma: Paramedics and Their Stories.* Jackson: University Press of Mississippi, 1998. Tangherlini, a folklorist, reports the stories told by Alameda County (California) paramedics and explores what roles the stories play in their self-conceptions and their relations with colleagues and supervisors.

Ziga, Rosemary. "Keeping Pace." *Emergency* 23 (February, 1991): 41-43. A journal article pertaining to an automatic implantable cardioverter defibrillator as a method of countershock to victims of sudden cardiac arrest.

PARANOIA
DISEASE/DISORDER
ANATOMY OR SYSTEM AFFECTED: Psychic-emotional system

SPECIALTIES AND RELATED FIELDS: Psychiatry, psychology

DEFINITION: Pervasive distrust and suspiciousness of others and a tendency to interpret others' motives as malevolent.

CAUSES AND SYMPTOMS
Paranoia is characterized by suspiciousness, heightened self-awareness, self-reference, projection of one's ideas onto others, expectations of persecution, and blaming of others for one's difficulties. Conversely, though paranoia can be problematic, it can also be adaptive. In threatening or dangerous situations, paranoia might instigate proactive protective behavior, allowing an individual to negotiate a situation without harm. Thus, paranoia must be assessed in context for it to be understood fully.

Paranoia can be experienced at varying levels of intensity in both normal and highly disordered individuals. As a medical problem, paranoia may take the face of a symptom, personality problem, or chronic mental disorder. As a symptom, it may be evidenced as a fleeting problem; an individual might have paranoid feelings that dissipate in a relatively brief period of time once an acute medical or situational problem is rectified.

As a personality problem, paranoia creates significant impairment and distress as a result of inflexible, maladaptive, and persistent use of paranoid coping strategies. Paranoid individuals often have preoccupations about loyalties, overinterpret situations, maintain expectations of exploitation or deceit, rarely confide in others, bear grudges, perceive attacks that are not apparent to others, and maintain unjustified suspicions about their relationship partner's potential for betrayal. They are prone to angry outbursts, aloof, and controlling, and they may demonstrate a tendency toward vengeful fantasies or actual revenge.

Finally, paranoia may be evidenced as a chronic mental disorder, most notably as the paranoid type of schizophrenia. In paranoid schizophrenia, there is a tendency toward delusions (faulty beliefs involving misinterpretations of events) and auditory hallucinations. Additionally, everyday behavior, speech, and emotional responsiveness are not as disturbed as in other variants of schizophrenia. Typically, these individuals are seen by others as anxious, angry, and aloof. Their delusions usually reflect fears of persecution or hopes for greatness, resulting in jealousies, odd religious beliefs (such as persecution by God, thinking they are Jesus Christ), or preoccupations with their own health (such as the fear of being poisoned or of having a medical disorder of mysterious origin).

Paranoia may best be understood as being determined by a combination of biological, psychological, and environmental factors. It is likely, for example, that certain basic psychological tendencies must be present for an individual to display paranoid feelings and behavior when under stress, as opposed to other feelings such as depression. Additionally, it is likely that certain physical predispositions must be present for stressors to provoke a psychophysiological response.

Biologically, there are myriad physical and mental health conditions that may trigger acute and more chronic paranoid reactions. High levels of situational stress, drug intoxication (such as with amphetamines or marijuana), drug withdrawal, depression, head injuries, organic brain syndromes, pernicious anemia, B vitamin deficiencies, and Klinefelter syndrome may be related to acute paranoia. Similarly, certain cancers, insidious organic brain syndromes, and hyperparathyroidism have been related to recurrent or chronic episodes of paranoia.

In terms of the etiology of chronic paranoid conditions, such as paranoid schizophrenia and paranoid personality disorder, no clear causes have been identified. Some evidence points to a genetic component; the results of studies on twins and the greater prevalence of these disorders in some families support this view. More psychological theories highlight the family environment and emotional expression, childhood abuse, and stress. In general, these theories point to conditions contributing toward making a person feel insecure, tense, hungry for recognition, and hypervigilant. Additionally, the impact of social, cultural, and economic conditions contributing to the expression of paranoia is important. Paranoia cannot be interpreted out of context. Biological, psychological,

and environmental factors must be considered in the development and maintenance of paranoia.

TREATMENT AND THERAPY

Three major types of therapies are available to treat paranoia: pharmacotherapies, community-based therapies, and cognitive-behavioral therapies. For acute paranoia problems and the management of more chronic, schizophrenia-related paranoia, pharmacotherapy (the use of drugs) is the treatment of choice. Drugs that serve to tranquilize the individual and reduce disorganized thinking, such as phenothiazines and other neuroleptics, are commonly used. With elderly people who cannot tolerate such drugs, electroconvulsive therapy (ECT) has been used for treatment.

Community-based treatment, such as day treatment or inpatient treatment, is also useful for treating chronic paranoid conditions. Developing corrective and instructional social experiences, decreasing situational stress, and helping individuals to feel safe in a treatment environment are primary goals.

Finally, cognitive-behavioral therapies focused on identifying irrational beliefs contributing to paranoia-related problems have demonstrated some utility. Skillful therapists help to identify maladaptive thinking while unearthing concerns but not agreeing with the individual's delusional ideas.

PERSPECTIVE AND PROSPECTS

Certain life phases and social and cultural contexts influence behaviors that could be labeled as paranoid. Membership in certain minority or ethnic groups, immigrant or political refugee status, and, more generally, language and other cultural barriers may account for behavior that appears to be guarded or paranoid. As such, one can make few assumptions about paranoia without a thorough assessment.

Clinically significant paranoia is notable across cultures, with prevalence rates at any point in time ranging from 0.5 to 2.5 percent of the population. It is a problem manifested by diverse etiological courses requiring equally diverse treatments. Increased knowledge about the relationship among paranoia, depression and other mood disorders, schizophrenia, and the increased prevalence of paranoid disorders in some families will be critical. As the general population ages, a better understanding of more acute paranoid disorders related to medical problems will also be necessary. Better understanding will facilitate the development of more effective pharmacological and nonpharmacological treatments that can be tolerated by the elderly and others suffering from compromising medical problems.

—*Nancy A. Piotrowski, Ph.D.*

See also Anxiety; Delusions; Hallucinations; Posttraumatic stress disorder; Psychiatric disorders; Psychiatry; Psychiatry, child and adolescent; Psychiatry, geriatric; Psychoanalysis; Schizophrenia; Shock therapy; Stress.

FOR FURTHER INFORMATION:

McKay, Matthew, Peter D. Rogers, and Judith McKay. *When Anger Hurts: Quieting the Storm Within.* Oakland, Calif.: New Harbinger, 1989. This book is easy to follow and helpful for those patients who have recognized that they have trouble controlling their anger. The material and instruction presented here is straight to the point and very helpful.

Munro, Alistair. *Delusional Disorder: Paranoia and Related Illnesses.* New York: Cambridge University Press, 1999. Discusses the various subtypes of delusional disorders, such as the somatic, jealousy, erotomanic, persecutory/litigious, and grandiose subtypes. Also discusses treatments.

Robbins, Michael. *Experiences of Schizophrenia: An Integration of the Personal, Scientific, and Therapeutic.* New York: Guilford Press, 1993. Discusses such topics as the psychological system, the family system, society and culture, and the treatment of schizophrenia and includes a number of case studies.

Siegel, Ronald K. *Whispers: The Voices of Paranoia.* New York: Crown, 1994. In a mesmerizing journey into mental illness, the author captures the suspicion, terror, and rage that possess the minds of paranoids.

PARAPLEGIA

DISEASE/DISORDER

ANATOMY OR SYSTEM AFFECTED: Legs, muscles, musculoskeletal system, nerves, nervous system, spine

SPECIALTIES AND RELATED FIELDS: Neurology, physical therapy

DEFINITION: Paraplegia is partial or complete paralysis of both legs caused by spinal cord damage in the back; this damage may result from accidents, spinal cord tumors, or birth defects. If the spinal cord is completely severed, total paralysis of the legs will result, as well as dysfunction of the rectum and bladder. Lesser damage may only affect the legs. If the damage is minimal, there is a chance of recovery. Physical therapy and retraining are advised as soon as possible, and the use of special equipment will assist with the problems of incontinence and mobility.

—*Jason Georges and Tracy Irons-Georges*

See also Hemiplegia; Nervous system; Neuralgia, neuritis, and neuropathy; Neurology; Neurology, pediatric; Paralysis; Physical rehabilitation; Quadriplegia; Spinal cord disorders; Spine, vertebrae, and disks.

FOR FURTHER INFORMATION:

Carey, Joseph, ed. *Brain Facts: A Primer on the Brain and Nervous System.* Washington, D.C.: Society for Neuroscience, 1990.

Jenkins, David B. *Hollinshead's Functional Anatomy of the Limbs and Back.* Rev. 7th ed. Philadelphia: W. B. Saunders, 1998.

Kandel, Eric R., James H. Schwartz, and Thomas M. Jessell, eds. *Principles of Neural Science.* 2d ed. New York: Elsevier, 1991.

PARASITIC DISEASES

DISEASE/DISORDER

ANATOMY OR SYSTEM AFFECTED: All

SPECIALTIES AND RELATED FIELDS: Environmental health, epidemiology, family practice, internal medicine, public health, virology

DEFINITION: Diseases borne by parasites, or organisms that live within other, "host" organisms; parasites travel to their hosts via vectors which may include fleas, mosquitoes, rats, and other animals.

KEY TERMS:

commensalism: a relationship in which one symbiont, the commensal, benefits from a host symbiont, but the host neither benefits nor is harmed by the commensal

host: a living plant or animal harboring or affording subsistence to a parasite

hyperparasitism: a relationship in which parasites act as hosts to other parasites

mutualism: a relationship between symbionts in which both members benefit from the association

parasitism: a relationship in which one symbiont, a parasite, harms its host symbiont or in some way lives at the expense of the host

phoresis: when two symbionts "travel together" but neither is physiologically dependent on the other

symbiont: any organism involved in a symbiotic relationship with another organism

Common Human Parasites

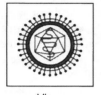
Virus

Bacterium

Amoeba

Fungus

Head louse

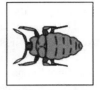
Bedbug

Cat flea

Tick

Mosquito

Roundworm

Hookworm

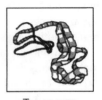
Tapeworm

Any organism that, temporarily or permanently, lives on or in another organism for the purpose of procuring food is considered a parasite; these parasites may cause infection in their human hosts.

symbiosis: a relationship in which two symbionts live in close association with each other; commonly, one symbiont lives in or on the body of the other

TYPES OF PARASITES

Parasites are organisms that take up residence, temporarily or permanently, on or within other living organisms for the purpose of procuring food. They include plants such as bacteria and fungi; animals such as protozoa, helminths (worms), and arthropods; and forms such as spirochetes and microscopic viruses.

The study of parasitism is a study of symbiosis. Symbiosis occurs when two organisms, known as symbionts, live in close association with each other, usually with one organism living in or on the body of the other. Such a living arrangement is called a symbiotic relationship. In a symbiotic relationship, the symbionts are usually, but not always, of different species, and the relationship need not be beneficial or damaging to either organism.

Often, two symbionts will exist together merely as traveling companions. Such a symbiotic relationship is called phoresis. In such cases, neither partner is physiologically dependent on the other, but the smaller of the two organisms has simply attached itself for the ride. Examples of phoresis are bacteria carried on the legs of a cockroach and fungus spores on the feet of ants and beetles.

If a situation exists in which both symbionts benefit from an association, the partnership is referred to as a mutual relationship. In most cases, mutualism is obligatory because both symbionts have evolved to a point at which they are physiologically dependent on each other and the survival of both symbionts requires a continuous interrelationship. Such a relationship exists between termites and the protozoan fauna that live in their guts. Termites are unable to digest cellulose fibers, because their bodies cannot produce the proper enzyme, but protozoa that live in a termite's gut synthesize the ingested cellulose fibers and excrete a fermented product that nourishes the host termite. The protozoa benefit by living in a stable, secure environment, with a constant supply of food, and the termite is supplied with sustenance.

Another form of mutualism that is not obligatory is called cleaning symbiosis. In this instance, certain animals, called cleaners, remove other parasites, injured tissues, fungi, or invading organisms from a cooperating host. Examples of cleaning relationships include birds that groom the skins of rhinoceroses and the mouths of crocodiles, and tiny shrimp that remove parasites from the body surfaces of fish.

When one symbiont benefits from its relationship

with its host but the host neither benefits nor is harmed, the condition is called commensalism. Examples of commensals are pilot fish and remoras, which attach themselves to turtles or other fish, using their hosts as transportation and scavenging food left over when the hosts eat; in no way, however, do they harm their hosts or rob them of food. Another example of commensalism exists between humans and the amoeba *Entamoeba gingivalis*. This amoeba lives in the human mouth, feeding on bacteria, food particles, and dead epithelial cells, but it never harms its human host. The amoeba is transmitted from person to person by direct contact and cannot exist outside the human mouth.

When one member of a symbiotic relationship actually harms its host or in some way lives at the expense of the host, it is then a parasite. The word "parasite" is derived for the Greek *parasitos*, which means "one who eats at another's table" or "one who lives at another's expense." A parasite may harm its host by causing a mechanical injury, such as boring a hole into it; by eating, digesting, or absorbing portions of the host's tissue; by poisoning the host with toxic metabolic products; or by robbing the host of nutrition. It has been found that most parasites inflict a combination of these conditions.

The majority of parasites are obligate parasites—that is, they must spend at least a portion of their lives as parasites to survive and complete their life cycles. Most of these obligate parasites have free-living stages outside their hosts in which they exist in protective cysts or eggs. Certain symbionts are referred to as facultative parasites, which means that the organism is not normally parasitic, but if the proper situation arises, it becomes a parasite. The most common facultative parasites are those that are accidentally eaten or enter a host through a wound or body orifice. One facultative parasite whose infection of humans is almost always fatal is the amoeba *Naegleria*, which is responsible for amebic meningitis. Many obligate parasites are also hyperparasites. Hyperparasitism exists when parasites play host to other parasites; for example, the malaria-causing parasite *Plasmodia* is carried in mosquitoes, and juvenile tapeworms live in fleas.

Parasites that live their entire adult lives within or on their hosts are called permanent parasites. Other parasites, such as mosquitoes and ticks, are called temporary parasites because they feed on their hosts and then leave. Temporary parasites are actually micropredators that prey on different hosts, or on the same host at different times, as the need for nourishment arises. There are many parallels between parasitism and predation in that both parasites and predators live at the expense of their hosts or prey. Parasites, however, do not normally kill their hosts, because to do so results in their own death. It is the mark of a well-adapted parasite to produce as few pathological conditions in the host as possible.

Despite the knowledge that parasites are a major cause of disease, it is wrong to assume that an animal hosting a parasite must ultimately be in danger. The healthiest human or wild animal is probably harboring some type of parasite, and while the host and parasite may live for years without interfering in each other's existence, at any given time, the healthy host can fall victim to a disease brought on by the parasite, or some change in the host may destroy the parasite.

Whether the host reacts to its symbiotic partner with indifference, annoyance, or illness is the result of many factors. The most important is how many parasites are being hosted. A single hookworm takes approximately 0.5 milliliter of blood per day from its host. This is about the same amount of blood lost when one pricks oneself with a needle. This amount of blood loss is so low that the host will never miss it and, in most instances, will not even know that the parasite is there. If a host harbors five hundred hookworms, however, the blood loss per day becomes 250 milliliters, approximately one half pint, and the result is physically devastating to the host.

CAUSES AND SYMPTOMS

Medical parasitology is the study of human diseases caused by parasitic infection. It is commonly limited to the study of parasitic worms (helminths) and protozoa. The science places nonprotozoan parasites in separate disciplines, such as virology, rickettsiology, and bacteriology. The branches of parasitology known as medical entomology and medical arthropodology deal with insects and noninsect arthropods that serve as hosts and transport agents for parasites, as well as with the noxious effects of these pests. The medical study of parasitic fungi (molds and yeasts) that cause human disease is called mycology.

Throughout history, human welfare has suffered greatly because of parasites. Fleas and bacteria killed one-third of the human population of Europe during the seventeenth century, and malaria, schistosomiasis, and African sleeping sickness have killed additional countless millions. Despite successful medical campaigns against yellow fever, malaria, and hookworm infections worldwide, parasitic diseases in combination with nutritional deficiencies are the primary killers of humans. Medical research suggests that parasitic infections are so widespread that if all the known varieties were evenly distributed among the human population, each living person would have at least one.

Most serious parasitic infections occur in tropical, less modernized regions of the world, and because most of the planet's industrially developed and affluent populations live in temperate regions, many people are unaware of the magnitude of the problem. On an annual basis, 60 million deaths occur worldwide from all causes; of these deaths, half are children under five years of age. Fifty percent of these, 15 million child deaths per year, are directly attributable to a combination of malnutrition and intestinal parasitic infection. It must be noted that less than 15 percent of the world's present population is served by adequate clean water supplies and sewage disposal programs, and that almost all intestinal parasitic infections are the result of ingesting food or water contaminated with human feces.

The transmission of parasitic diseases involves three factors: the source of the infection, the mode of transmission, and the presence of a susceptible host. The combined effect of these factors determines the dispersibility and prevalence of a parasite at a given time and place, thus regulating the incidence of a parasitic disease in a population. Because of host specificity, other humans are the chief source of most human parasitic diseases. The various manifestations of any human parasitic disease are a result of the particular species of parasite involved, its mode of transport, the immunological status of the host, the presence or absence of hosts, and the pattern of exposure.

Humans transmit parasitic diseases to one another through the intestinal tract, nose and mouth, skin and tissue, genitourinary tract, and blood. It is fecal discharge, however, that offers the most convenient and common means for a parasite or its ova and larvae to leave its host, since the majority of parasites inhabit the gastrointestinal tract. For this reason, the proper disposal of fecal material becomes the most important method of preventing the spread of parasitic disease. Since most parasites inhabit the intestinal tract, food and water are also important means of transmitting parasitic infections. The infective organism may

be present in contaminated drinking water, in animal and fish flesh used as food, in human feces used as fertilizer, or on the hands of food handlers.

Arthropods are one of the main sources of parasitic diseases in humans. Arthropods act as both mechanical carriers of and intermediate hosts to many diseases—bacterial, viral, rickettsial, and parasitic—which they transmit to humans. In most tropical countries, basic preventive medicine for many devastating parasitic diseases depends on the control or eradication of insects and arachnids.

There are four major groups of parasites that most often invade human hosts: nematodes, trematodes, cestodes, and protozoa. Most nematodes, or roundworms, are free-living, and nematodes are found in almost every terrestrial and aquatic environment. Most are harmless to humans, but some parasitic nematodes invade the human intestinal tract and cause widespread debilitating diseases. The most prevalent intestinal nematodes are *Ascaris lumbricoides*, which infects the small intestine and affects more than a billion people; the whipworm *Trichuris trichiura*, which infects the colon and is carried by an estimated 500 million individuals; the human hookworms *Necator americanus* and *Ancylostoma duodenale*, which suck blood from the human small intestine and cause major debilitation among undernourished people; and *Enterobius vermicularis*, the human pinworm, which infects the large intestine and is common among millions of urban dwellers because it is easily transmitted from perianal tissue to hand to mouth.

Nonintestinal, tissue-infecting nematodes are spread most often by hyperparasitic bloodsucking insects such as mosquitoes, biting flies, and midges. The most common tissue-infecting nematode is *Trichinella spiralis*, the pork or trichina worm, which is the agent of trichinosis. Other important parasitic nematodes include *Onchocerca volvulus*, which is transmitted by blackflies in tropical regions and causes blindness, and the mosquito-transmitted filarial worms that are responsible for elephantiasis.

Trematodes, or flatworms, are commonly called flukes. Flukes vary greatly in size, form, and host living location, but all of them initially develop in freshwater snails. The human intestinal fluke, the oriental liver fluke, and the human lung fluke are all transmitted to humans by the ingestion of raw or undercooked aquatic vegetables, fish, or crustaceans. An important group of trematodes consists of the blood flukes of the genus *Schistosoma*, which enter the body through skin/water contact and are responsible for schistoso-miasis.

Cestodes, commonly called tapeworms, are parasitic flatworms that parasitize almost all vertebrates, and as many as eight species are found in humans. The two most common cestodes—*Taenia saginata*, the beef tapeworm, and *Taenia solium*, the pork tapeworm—are transmitted to humans by infected beef or pork products obtained from livestock that grazed in fields contaminated by human feces, or by contaminated water. The resulting disease, cysticercosis, which is potentially lethal, develops mostly in the brain, eye, and muscle tissue. Another animal-transmitted cestode is the dog tapeworm, *Echinococcus granulosus*, which dogs ingest by eating contaminated sheep viscera and then pass on to humans, who ingest the parasite's eggs after petting or handling an infected dog. The human infestation of *E. granulosus* results in hydatid disease. Probably the most dramatic of the cestode parasites is the gigantic tapeworm *Diphyllobothrium latum*, which may reach lengths of 10 meters and a width of 2 centimeters. This tapeworm is transmitted to humans by the ingestion of raw or undercooked fish. This tapeworm, like most cestodes, can be effectively treated and killed by drugs, but if the worm merely breaks, leaving the head and anterior segments attached, it can regenerate its original body length in less than four months.

Protozoa that can infect human hosts are found in the intestinal tract, various tissues and organs, and the bloodstream. Of the many varieties of protozoa that can live in the human intestinal tract, only *Entamoeba histolytica* causes serious disease. This parasite, which is ingested in water contaminated by human feces, is responsible for the disease amebiasis, also known as amebic dysentery. A less serious, though common, waterborne intestinal protozoan is *Giardia lamblia*, which causes giardiasis, a common diarrheal infection among campers who ingest water fouled by animal waste.

Another group of protozoa parasites specializes in infecting the human skin, bloodstream, brain, and viscera. *Trypanosoma brucei*, carried by the African tsetse fly, causes the blood disease trypanosomiasis (African sleeping sickness). In Latin America, infection by the protozoa *Trypanosoma cruzi* results when the liquid feces of the reduviid bug is rubbed or scratched into the skin; it causes Chagas' disease, which produces often fatal lesions of the heart and brain. Members of the protozoan genus *Leishmania* are transmitted by

midges and sandflies, and their parasitic infestation manifests in long-lasting dermal lesions and ulcers; the destruction of nasal mucous, cartilage, and pharyngeal tissues; or in the disease kala-azar, resulting in the destruction of bone marrow, lymph nodes, and liver and spleen tissue.

Two other types of protozoa are parasitic to humans. The first is the ciliate protozoa, which are mostly free-living, and of which only a single species, *Balantidium coli*, is parasitic in humans. This species is responsible for balantidiasis, an ulcerative disease. The second is the sporozoans, all of which are parasitic. Many species of sporozoans are harmful to humans, the most important being *Plasmodium*, the agent of malaria. The sporozoan parasite *Toxoplasma gondii*, the agent of toxoplasmosis, is responsible for encephalomyelitis and chorioretinitis in infants and children and is thought to infect as much as 20 percent of the world's population. *Pneumocystis*, a major cause of death among persons with acquired immunodeficiency syndrome (AIDS), was formerly considered a result of sporozoan infection but is now thought to be fungal.

PERSPECTIVE AND PROSPECTS

Because of their size, the large parasitic worms were among the first parasites to be noted and studied as possible causes of disease. The Ebers papyrus, written about 1600 B.C.E., contains some of the earliest records of the presence of parasitic worms in humans. In early Egypt, trichinosis, cysticercosis, and salmonellosis were all likely to be acquired from pigs. This knowledge is reflected in the law of Moses, later reinforced in the Koran, which forbids the eating of "unclean swine" or the touching of their dead carcasses—a clear indication that people knew of the relationship between parasitic worms and human disease. Persian, Greek, and Roman physicians were also familiar with various parasitic worms, and many of their early medical writings describe the removal of worm-induced cysts. The Arabic physician and philosopher Avicenna (979-1037 C.E.) was the first to separate parasitic worms into classifications: long, small, flat, and round.

The modern study of parasites began in 1379 with the discovery of the liver fluke, *Fasciola hepatica*, in sheep. During the eighteenth century, many parasitic worms and arthropods were described, but progress was slow prior to the invention and widespread use of the microscope. The microscope made possible the study of small protozoan parasites and allowed for detailed anatomic and lifecycle studies of larger parasites.

In 1835, *Trichinella spiralis*, the parasite responsible for the disease trichinosis, was described, and quickly thereafter knowledge concerning the parasitic worms of humans began to accumulate. Many new species were discovered, prominent among which were the hookworm and the blood fluke.

Between 1836 and 1901, the first protozoan parasites of humans were recognized and described; among the most important of these were the parasites responsible for giardiasis, gingivitis, vaginitis, trichomoniasis, kala-azar, and Gambian trypanosomiasis (sleeping sickness).

Although arthropods had been recognized as parasites since early times, their role in transporting other parasites and in spreading disease was not noted until 1869, when the larval stages of the dog tapeworm were found in the dog louse. Further investigations led to the identification in 1893 of ticks as the transmitting agents of Texas fever in cattle. By 1909, parasitologists had observed the development of the malarial parasite in mosquitoes, proved the transmission of yellow fever by the mosquito *Aedes aegypti*, and had linked the tsetse fly to African sleeping sickness, the tick to African relapsing fever, the reduviid bug to Chagas' disease, and the body louse to the transmission of typhoid fever.

—*Randall L. Milstein, Ph.D.*

See also Arthropod-borne diseases; Bacterial infections; Bacteriology; Bites and stings; Diarrhea and dysentery; Elephantiasis; Encephalitis; Fungal infections; Giardiasis; Leishmaniasis; Lice, mites, and ticks; Lyme disease; Malaria; Microbiology; Pinworm; Protozoan diseases; Roundworm; Schistosomiasis; Shigellosis; Sleeping sickness; Tapeworm; Toxoplasmosis; Trichinosis; Tropical medicine; Typhoid fever and typhus; Viral infections; Worms; Yellow fever.

FOR FURTHER INFORMATION:

Despommier, Dickson D., Robert W. Gwadz, and Peter J. Hotex. *Parasitic Diseases*. 4th ed. New York: Springer-Verlag, 2000. This source provides a list of parasitic diseases of current concern to public health professionals. It also describes the assessment of and treatment options for a variety of these diseases.

Klein, Aaron E. *The Parasites We Humans Harbor.* New York: Elsevier/Nelson Books, 1981. An overview of common human-infecting parasites written for the general reader. The text is nontechnical, easy to follow, and presents numerous examples.

Noble, Elmer R., and Glenn A. Noble. *Parasitology: The Biology of Animal Parasites*. 5th ed. Philadelphia: Lea & Febiger, 1982. A graduate-level textbook on parasites that infect animals. The comprehensive and highly technical text deals with the biological, environmental, and pathological aspects of parasites.

Roberts, Larry S., and John Janovy, Jr., eds. *Gerald D. Schmidt and Larry S. Roberts' Foundations of Parasitology*. Rev. 6th ed. Boston: McGraw-Hill, 2000. A graduate-level textbook covering all aspects of parasitology. The text is highly technical and intended for the informed reader. The book is well illustrated, but sensitive readers may be disturbed by many of the case study photographs.

PARATHYROIDECTOMY
PROCEDURE
ANATOMY OR SYSTEM AFFECTED: Endocrine system, glands, neck
SPECIALTIES AND RELATED FIELDS: Endocrinology, general surgery
DEFINITION: The removal of all or part of the parathyroid gland.

INDICATIONS AND PROCEDURES
The parathyroid glands are four structures attached to the rear of the thyroid gland, which is found in the neck. Their main function is the secretion of parathyroid hormone (PTH), a protein which regulates the concentration of blood calcium. Abnormalities in proper calcium concentration can lead to bone demineralization, neuromuscular problems, or renal (kidney) damage.

Parathyroidectomy is occasionally warranted under conditions of hyperparathyroidism: the excess secretion of PTH. Hyperparathyroidism most commonly results in excess resorption of bone calcium, causing skeletal pain or loss of height. The demineralization may also lead to fractures of the spine or long bones, which may be accompanied by extreme muscle weakness and frequent urination. Since the patient may be asymptomatic, diagnosis is most commonly made on the determination of excess serum and urine calcium. X rays may also indicate bone abnormalities resulting from the resorption of calcium. The condition itself may be caused by hyperplastic (overactive or enlarged) glands, or in less common circumstances (2 percent of cases), hyperparathyroidism may result from a parathyroid adenoma (a benign tumor).

Asymptomatic patients, or patients with only mildly elevated blood calcium, may not need treatment. Should symptoms become more severe, surgical procedures may be necessary, generally involving the removal of excess parathyroid tissue. If the hyperplasia involves all four parathyroid glands, three of the glands are usually removed, with resection of the fourth. If the cause of the PTH elevation is an adenoma, it is necessary to remove the tumor surgically.

Uses and Complications

Since the primary symptom of hyperparathyroidism is excess blood calcium, the removal of excess tissue may suddenly reduce calcium levels to normal. The rapid fall of calcium may cause a transient tetany, but otherwise recovery from such surgery parallels any other surgical procedure. PTH and calcium levels must continue to be monitored postoperatively. If parathyroidectomy results in excessively low PTH levels, it may be necessary to provide lifelong diet supplements of calcium and vitamin D.

—*Richard Adler, Ph.D.*

See also Endocrine disorders; Endocrinology; Glands; Hormones; Hyperparathyroidism and hypoparathyroidism; Thyroid disorders; Thyroid gland; Thyroidectomy; Tumor removal; Tumors.

For Further Information:

Gardner, David, and Francis Greenspan. *Basic and Clinical Endocrinology.* East Norwalk, Conn.: Appleton & Lange, 2000.

Neal, J. Matthew. *Basic Endocrinology: An Interactive Approach.* Oxford, England: Blackwell Science, 1999.

Paloyan, Edward, Ann M. Lawrence, and Francis H. Straus. *Hyperparathyroidism.* New York: Grune & Stratton, 1973.

Parsons, John A., ed. *Endocrinology of Calcium Metabolism.* New York: Raven Press, 1982.

Parkinson's disease
Disease/disorder

Anatomy or system affected: Cells, muscles, musculoskeletal system, nerves, nervous system

Specialties and related fields: Geriatrics and gerontology, internal medicine, neurology, physical therapy

Definition: A progressive neurological disease characterized by tremor, slow movement, and muscle rigidity and typically seen only in those over the age of forty.

Key terms:

anticholinergic: referring to drugs that oppose the action of acetylcholine in nerve impulse transmission

basal ganglia: brain portions called the corpus striatum, thalamus, substantia nigra, and globus pallidus; processing centers for movement information

bradykinesia: the slowness of motion associated with Parkinson's disease

dopamine: a substance which serves as a neurotransmitter in certain brain cells; it is deficient in Parkinson's disease

dopamine agonist: a chemical that mimics the effects of dopamine in the brain

electroencephalogram (EEG): a graphic recording of the electrical activity of the brain, as recorded by an electroencephalograph

idiopathic disease: a disease of unknown origin

L-dopa (L-dihydroxyphenylalanine or levodopa): an amino acid that is the parent compound for dopamine; used to treat Parkinson's disease

neurotransmitter: a chemical messenger that mediates nerve impulse passage between neurons

substantia nigra: the black-pigmented basal ganglion that deteriorates in Parkinson's disease

Causes and Symptoms

In 1817, James Parkinson, a British physician, wrote a description of six patients suffering from a slowly progressing disease characterized by "involuntary tremulous motion, with lessened muscular power in parts not in action even when supported, with a propensity to bend their trunks forward from a walking to a running pace." Throughout the modern world, this disease—which Parkinson named shaking palsy—is called parkinsonism or Parkinson's disease in his honor.

Parkinsonism, also called paralysis agitans, is now defined as a medical condition characterized by a combination of symptoms including involuntary shaking (tremor) of the limbs at rest, stiffness of the muscles (rigidity), slowed or reduced ability to move the limbs and facial muscles (bradykinesia), and general muscular weakness. Worldwide, its occurrence is estimated at between 1.5 and 3 people per 1,000. In people over the age of fifty, this number increases to nearly 1 per 100, with the first appearance of symptoms usually occurring after the age of forty. The disease occurs in similar proportions in populations that eat such widely different diets that no particular food has been implicated as causative.

The most-often-used clinical scale that describes the extent of severity of parkinsonism is that of Melvin Yahr and his associates, which is divided into five stages. In stage 1, mild tremor or rigidity is seen on one side of the body. In stage 2, tremor, rigidity, and bradykinesia occur on both sides of the body, without any loss of balance. In stage 3, added to the symptoms of stage 2, come balance difficulty, loss of posture control, and hunching over. With stage 4, the extent of the functional disability increases, but some independent function is still possible. Such severe symptoms occur in stage 5 that patients are confined to bed or to wheelchairs. Thanks to modern therapy, relatively few patients progress beyond stage 3.

The body site of Parkinson's disease is clear, but most cases are idiopathic, meaning that although their site of action is known, the basic cause is not. Unlike several other neurologic diseases, Parkinson's disease does not appear to be inherited, because studies of identical twins have shown that in most cases only one twin is afflicted. In addition, the disease is about equally distributed among men and women.

The symptoms begin slowly, most often presenting as stage 1 tremor. After this, the progression to stage 3 usually takes five to ten years. This progression appears to be caused by the deterioration of several of the four brain structures called basal ganglia (the corpus striatum, thalamus, substantia nigra, and globus pallidus), which is related to depletion of the neurotransmitter dopamine. Dopamine depletion is most extreme in the normally dark-pigmented substantia nigra, which is often colorless in the autopsied brains of parkinsonism patients.

Some drugs and disease conditions produce parkinsonism that is indistinguishable from that occurring in their absence, and they have provided clues about the disease. These include certain widely used tranquilizers, such as haloperidol and chlorpromazine (Thorazine); the common heart drug reserpine; small cardiovascular strokes and brain tumors; some forms of viral encephalitis; and a drug called MPTP, first identified as a contaminant of designer heroins sold as street drugs. Therapeutic, drug-based parkinsonism symptoms do not appear to be causes of permanent parkinsonism because they diminish and slowly disappear after discontinuation of the causative drugs.

Parkinsonism

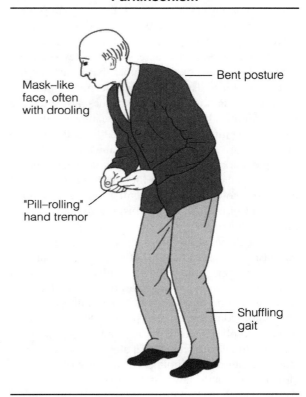

Parkinsonism, which often attacks older people, is characterized by debilitating symptoms that become more severe as the disease progresses.

Many have been linked, however, to decreased dopamine levels. Similarly, many stroke-related symptoms appear to be caused by drug therapy that diminished brain dopamine content. The effects of tumors have also offered helpful data because their location can better identify the brain areas associated with the disease. For example, information of this sort first linked the substantia nigra and corpus striatum to Parkinson's disease. In addition, viral encephalitis is still suspected by many of being an important causative factor. Belief in its involvement arose, however, from a 1918-1925 epidemic that damaged the basal ganglia, and contemporary parkinsonism as a result of encephalitis is very rare. Finally, discovery of the MPTP connection has yielded a useful model for parkinsonism related to psychoactive drugs that cause it.

Tremor is the most conspicuous parkinsonism symptom. Despite the fact that it is usually the least disabling aspect of the disease, tremor is so embarrassing that it is usually the phenomenon that brings patients to a physician for initial diagnosis. In stage 1 of Parkinson's disease, tremor appears only when afflicted people are very fatigued. Later in the course of the disease, it becomes increasingly widespread and continual. It is interesting to note that tremor ceases when a parkinsonism patient is asleep.

Although Parkinson's disease does not alter the mental abilities of afflicted persons, it eventually impairs their ability to carry out skilled tasks that require rapid, repetitive movement and manual dexterity. For example, Parkinson's disease very often causes handwriting to deteriorate to an illegible scrawl, makes it impossible to fasten a shirt's collar buttons or a brassiere, and turns shaving or brushing the teeth into a difficult chore.

Bradykinesia is the most incapacitating aspect of Parkinson's disease because it impairs communication by characteristic gestures; results in an awkward gait, with failure to swing the arms normally when walking; and produces the masklike, immobile facial expression common to later stages. Other symptoms include drooling, caused by problems with swallowing, and the development of a slow, muffled speech. Both are caused by diminished mobility of the muscles of the mouth, jaws, and throat.

The nature of Parkinson's disease is best understood after considering nerve impulse transmission between the cells of nervous tissue (neurons) and the arrangement and interactive function of the brain and nerves.

Nerve impulse transport between neurons is an electrochemical process which generates the weak electric current that makes up the impulse. The impulse leaves each neuron via an outgoing extension, called an axon, passes across a tiny synaptic gap that separates the axon from the next neuron in line, and then enters an incoming extension (dendrite) of that cell. This process is repeated many times in order to transmit a nervous impulse to its site of action. The cell bodies of neurons constitute the impulse-causing gray matter, and axons and dendrites (white matter) may be viewed as their connecting wires (nerve fibers). Nerve impulse passage across the synaptic gaps between neurons is mediated by chemical messengers called neurotransmitters, such as dopamine.

The brain and nerves—the central nervous system— are a complex arrangement of neurons designed to enable an organism to respond in a coordinated way to external stimuli. The brain may be viewed as the central computer in the system. Its most sophisticated structure is the cerebrum, which controls the higher mental functions. Underneath the cerebrum are the cerebellum and the brain stem, which connects both the cerebrum and the cerebellum to the spinal cord. This cord, a meter-long trunk of nerve fibers, carries nerve impulses between the brain and the peripheral nerves that control muscles and other body tissues. Most important to Parkinson's disease are the motor nerves, which control body motions. This control involves a portion of the cerebrum that deals with skilled motor patterns; the cerebellum, which controls posture and balance; and the basal ganglia, which are processing centers for movement information.

Particularly important to Parkinson's disease are the substantia nigra and the corpus striatum. Discovery of a functional interface between dopamine and parkinsonism began when it was found that this neurotransmitter was associated with the substantia nigra and connected the substantia nigra and the corpus striatum. Next, it was discovered that temporary parkinsonism mediated by reserpine was associated with dopamine depletion and that the brains of parkinsonism patients contained very little dopamine in the substantia nigra. Soon, it was confirmed that dopamine controlled movement in an inhibitory fashion that arose in the substantia nigra and occurred in the corpus striatum. From these observations, it has been inferred that bradykinesia results from the damage of the dopamine-containing nerve tissue that connects the substantia nigra to the corpus striatum. It is also suggested that decreased function of these fibers—and lack of their inhibitory action because of dopamine—allows excess, undesired nerve impulses to cause both the tremor and the rigidity seen in Parkinson's disease.

TREATMENT AND THERAPY

Parkinson's disease is most often identified by physical evidence (such as tremor and bradykinesia), coupled with a careful study of the medical history of the patient being evaluated. In all but a few cases, no information can be obtained via the three powerful tools useful in many other neurologic exams: The complex X-ray method, computed tomography (CT) scanning, is informative only when stroke or tumor is involved; magnetic resonance imaging (MRI) gives no more information than do CT scans; and electroencephalograms (EEGs) do not show abnormal electrical discharge such as that observed in brains of epileptics.

In practice, however, many physicians carry out CT scans, MRI, and EEGs and count their negative results into a diagnostic positive for Parkinson's disease.

Once Parkinson's disease is diagnosed, three main methods exist for handling it: chemotherapy, surgery, and physical therapy. All these methods—alone or in combination—are intended for symptom reversal because there is no cure for the disease. It is usually recommended that none of these methods be started until parkinsonism interferes seriously with a patient's work or daily life. Chemotherapy is the preponderant parkinsonism treatment mode in most cases. Many different medications are used, such as anticholinergics, L-dopa (levodopa), dopamine agonists, and antidepressants.

The anticholinergics were the first drugs used for parkinsonism, and they are still the medications most likely to be prescribed for mild cases. Often, they are used in mixed chemotherapy in severe cases. The first anticholinergic drug used, in the 1890's, was scopolamine, initially isolated from *Datura stramonium* (jimsonweed). Other anticholinergics include atropine and the antihistamine diphenhydramine (Benadryl). These drugs operate by interfering with the action of acetylcholine, a neurotransmitter involved in nerve impulse transport. High doses of anticholinergic drugs produce many side effects, including confusion, slurred speech, blurred vision, and constipation because of the wide influence of cholinergic nerves on body operation. This is why anticholinergics are usually used in early stages of Parkinson's disease, when they can be administered at low doses. The low doses used in various mixed chemotherapy regimens minimize anticholinergic side effects.

L-dopa, the amino acid that is made into dopamine by the body, is used as a treatment because it causes the brain to make more dopamine. Dopamine itself is not used because a blood-brain barrier prevents brain dopamine uptake from the blood. The blood-brain barrier does not stop L-dopa uptake, and its administration reverses parkinsonism symptoms dramatically. Therefore, it has become the mainstay of modern chemotherapy for the disease.

A difficulty associated with use of L-dopa is that the biochemical mechanism that converts it to brain dopamine also occurs outside the brain. When this happens in patients given high doses of L-dopa, body (nonbrain) dopamine levels rise. This dopamine and the chemicals into which it transforms outside the brain cause such side effects as nausea, fainting, flushing, confusion, and the involuntary muscular movements called dyskinesia. To minimize these unwanted—and sometimes irreversible—side effects, modern L-dopa therapy combines the drug with its chemical cousin, carbidopa. Carbidopa prevents the conversion of L-dopa to dopamine. Because it cannot cross the blood-brain barrier, carbidopa has no effect on the brain's conversion of L-dopa to dopamine.

Another chemotherapeutic tactic for treating Parkinson's disease is the use of drugs called dopamine agonists. These chemicals mimic dopamine action, reacting with the brain's receptors that produce dopamine effects in the corpus striatum and other sites. The best-known dopamine agonist is bromocriptine

In the News: Parkinson's Disease Genes

Recent research has identified genes associated with familial forms of Parkinson's disease. One of these genes, a-synuclein, is a protein that is associated with the neuronal synapse and is believed to play a significant role in neuronal plasticity. A-synuclein was previously associated with Alzheimer's disease as the nonamyloid component of Alzheimer's amyloid plaques (NAC peptide), and it is a component of the Lewy inclusion bodies found in the Parkinson's-associated Lewy body dementia. Mutations in another gene, Parkin, were found to underlie the development of juvenile onset Parkinson's disease. Parkin is believed to play a role in cellular protein degradation by interacting with ubiquitin, a protein that targets other proteins for degradation. A mutation in the ubiquitin-carboxy-terminal hydrolase-L1 (UCH-L1), gene has also been associated with familial Parkinson's disease. It has been postulated that this mutation may impair the activity of UCH-L1, leading to the abnormal accumulation and aggregation of proteins within nerve cells. It is hoped that the identification of these genes will lead to the elucidation of the pathogenic mechanisms underlying nonfamilial (sporadic) Parkinson's disease.

—*Robert L. Martone*

(Parlodel). It is about 50 percent as effective as L-dopa at reversing Parkinson's disease, but it produces a longer-lasting action. Because bromocriptine often causes nausea, confusion, and delirium in patients, it is usually used at low doses, in mixed therapy with carbidopa. The mixed therapy has the advantage of decreasing any possible L-dopa dyskinesia without causing the bromocriptine side effects. Another dopamine agonist is pergolide.

Antidepressants are also part of therapy for Parkinson's disease because some of the medications used cause depression as a side effect. In addition, it is not uncommon for those afflicted with Parkinson's disease to become depressed as they lose control of their motor functions. This is probably the case because, as noted by James Parkinson, "the senses and intellect are unimpaired" in such patients. Tricyclic antidepressants such as amitriptyline are useful, and their calming action also yields very useful sedatives. A wide variety of other drugs, for example, the antihypertensive propranolol and the tranquilizer diazepam (Valium); vitamins; and special diets are also used in individual cases as parts of, or adjuncts to, mixed chemotherapy.

Surgical treatment of Parkinson's disease was once attempted quite often, but it became relatively rare by the 1970's, after modern chemotherapy was developed. Since then, its utilization occurs when CT scanning or MRI indicates the presence of a tumor or brain damage caused by a severe trauma. Contemporary surgical techniques, developed in the 1980's, involve the injection of cells from fetal adrenal or brain into the brains of parkinsonism patients. This endeavor seems to be a promising one.

Two final topics worth mentioning are psychotherapy and physical therapy. Part of their purpose is to cure the depression that often accompanies severe Parkinson's disease. Psychotherapy can provide emotional support to help many patients rebuild their lives; refer patients to other available support efforts; and provide irreplaceable experience with psychoactive therapeutic drugs that may be needed to handle depression. Physical therapy can help patients to overcome some motor effects of the disease, not only improving the lifestyle possible for them but also elevating morale and curing depression.

PERSPECTIVE AND PROSPECTS

Treatment of Parkinson's disease has evolved tremendously, particularly since the late 1960's, when wide use of L-dopa began. At that time, most physicians were astounded to observe that its use converted many bedridden and wheelchair-bound stage 5 patients to much more functional, mobile states. A temporary setback occurred when severe L-dopa side effects were observed at high doses.

The discovery of carbidopa and related inhibitors of nonbrain dopamine decarboxylase ended this problem and produced a new generation of parkinsonism chemotherapy. Patients could take L-dopa at lower concentrations, which minimized its side effects, because diminished nonbrain L-dopa conversion to dopamine left more L-dopa available to enter the brain. In addition, carbidopa was the forerunner of a group of dopamine agonists that became candidates for independent use or use in mixed therapy. Perhaps stimulated by this type of discovery, wide examination of the entire arsenal of potentially valuable pharmaceuticals led to the discovery that many other types of drugs (for example, tranquilizers, inhibitors of the bodily destruction of dopamine, or hypertension drugs), and even vitamins and diet could be utilized in the fight to control parkinsonism symptoms. In addition, new drugs were discovered.

Discovery that psychiatric help and physical therapy can ease the depression observed in many afflicted people and help to control parkinsonism's inroads has also been of great value. Perhaps even more exciting have been reports that the injection of human fetal cells into the brains of those afflicted with Parkinson's disease may be able to reverse the disease. It is too soon, however, to judge the results of this procedure, and this technique raises the moral issue of the suitability of using fetal tissues in this way.

—Sanford S. Singer, Ph.D.;
updated by John Alan Ross, Ph.D.

See also Brain; Brain disorders; Encephalitis; Fetal tissue transplantation; Motor neuron diseases; Muscles; Nervous system; Neurology; Palsy; Paralysis; Trembling and shaking.

FOR FURTHER INFORMATION:

Barnhart, Edward R., ed. *Physician's Desk Reference.* 47th ed. Oradell, N.J.: Medical Economics Data, 1993. An atlas of prescription drugs. Includes a listing of the drugs used against Parkinson's disease, their manufacturers, their useful dose ranges, their metabolism and toxicology, and their contraindications. This valuable reference for physicians and patients is found in most public libraries.

Berkow, Robert, and Andrew J. Fletcher, eds. *The Merck Manual of Diagnosis and Therapy.* 17th ed. Rahway, N.J.: Merck Sharp & Dohme Research Laboratories, 1999. Offers a brief but valuable exposition of the characteristics, etiology, diagnosis, and treatment of Parkinson's disease. Information on related topics is also included.

Carroll, David L. *Living with Parkinson's: A Guide for the Patient and Caregiver.* New York: Harper-Collins, 1992. This book is based on methods used by the Brookdale Center on Aging. The main topic issues include an explanation and identification of Parkinson's disease, the medications and surgery used to treat it, the value of exercise, and advice on everyday living with the disease.

Duvoisin, Roger C. *Parkinson's Disease: A Guide for Patient and Family.* Rev. 2d ed. New York: Raven Press, 1998. Covers many topics related to Parkinson's disease in depth. Issues include the exposition of symptoms and principles of parkinsonism treatment; anticholinergic drugs, L-dopa, and dopamine agonists; corrective surgery; diet and exercise; historical perspectives; and support organizations.

Grimes, J. David, Peggy A. Gray, and Kelly A. Grimes. *Parkinson's Disease: One Step at a Time.* Ottawa, Canada: Parkinson's Society of Ottawa-Carleton, 1989. This slim book contains a wealth of information on Parkinson's disease. Offers an overview of symptoms, disability rating scales, causes, and types; drug treatments and other therapy; tips for overcoming problems associated with Parkinson's disease; and bibliographic references.

Hutton, J. Thomas, and Raye L. Dippel. *Caring for the Parkinson Patient.* Buffalo, N.Y.: Prometheus Books, 1989. Contains considerable information on Parkinson's disease. Articles include diagnosis and treatment, research, neural transplantation techniques, nursing care, physical therapy, psychiatric aspects, and family and community support.

Krause, J. K., and Joseph Jankovic. "Surgical Treatment of Parkinson's Disease." *American Family Physician* 54, no. 5 (1996): 1621-1629. An excellent article that succinctly explains recent pathophysiological mechanisms in neurosurgery, neuroradiology, and neurophysiology, particularly the use of functional stereotactic surgery for advanced Parkinson's disease.

Stern, Gerald, and Andrew Lees. *Parkinson's Disease: The Facts.* New York: Oxford University Press, 1986. This brief but technical book presents useful information on Parkinson's disease. Explains the history of the disease, its causes and symptoms, chemical and surgical treatments, life as a parkinsonism patient, and expected advances in research.

PATHOLOGY

SPECIALTY

ANATOMY OR SYSTEM AFFECTED: All

SPECIALTIES AND RELATED FIELDS: Biochemistry, cytology, forensic medicine, histology, microbiology, oncology

DEFINITION: The science that studies the changes to cells, tissues, and organs that result from the processes leading to diseases and disorders.

KEY TERMS:

autopsy: the dissection and examination of a human body after death

congenital: referring to a condition present at birth; it may result from an inherited trait or damage before birth

disease: an abnormal condition of the body, with characteristic symptoms associated with it

etiology: the cause of a disease or disorder

homeostasis: the maintenance of a stable internal environment needed for the proper functioning of the body's cells

metabolism: the collective term for the chemical activities of the body's cells

SCIENCE AND PROFESSION

The science of pathology seeks to identify accurately the etiology of a disease and its development in the human body, which in turn leads to other studies focused on the diagnosis, treatment, and prevention of the disease.

A pathologist may be a medical doctor or hold a doctoral degree in a related field such as cell biology or microbiology. He or she may be employed in one of several different types of work, such as research, clinical, surgical, and forensic pathology. The human body is a complex structure and, as in all living organisms, its basic unit of function is the cell. Similar cells are organized into tissues, tissues form organs, and organs are grouped into systems. All systems in the body must work together to maintain homeostasis. If this internal stability is changed too drastically, a disease results. In order to understand a disease thoroughly—and ultimately to diagnose, prevent, or treat it—its pathogenesis must be understood. This term includes the cause of the disease, its method of damaging the body, and the changes resulting from its presence. A specific disease may have many causes, and its symptoms and severity may vary in different patients. Nevertheless, it is convenient to place a disease into one of seven groups based on its primary cause or manifestation in the body: genetic defects, infections, immune disorders, nutritional disorders, traumas, toxins, and cancers.

Genetic disorders are those caused by a defect in one or more genes. Genes, which are found on chromosomes, are duplicated and passed from one generation to another. Each gene is responsible for directing the manufacture of a protein. Every protein has a characteristic three-dimensional structure, on which its function depends. If a mutation occurs in a gene, the protein may function poorly or not at all. Although the pathogenesis of a genetic disease may involve devastating effects in the body, its origin may be traced to the function of a single protein. A person with hemophilia may bleed to death because of a lack of the gene for blood-clotting protein. In sickle-cell disease, hemoglobin molecules are abnormal, which results in abnormal red blood cells and difficulty in transporting oxygen throughout the body. Changes in gene function occur throughout a person's life. Many degenerative changes associated with aging are believed to be caused by aging genes and the subsequent loss of cell, tissue, and organ function.

Infections are those diseases that are caused by other organisms, usually microorganisms such as viruses, bacteria, protozoa, or fungi. Such organisms, called pathogens, are parasitic on body tissues or fluids. The damage from pathogens may be direct, resulting from tissue destruction, or may be caused by the toxins that they produce. *Entamoeba histolytica*, for example, is a protozoan that is ingested in contaminated water or food. It begins feeding on the tissues of the intestine and may cause ulcerlike lesions in the intestinal wall. *Clostridium botulinum* is the bacterial species that causes botulism. Its deadly effects are attributable not to tissue destruction but to its production of a poison that attacks the nervous system.

Immune disorders include immune deficiencies, autoimmune diseases, and allergies. The body's immunity involves a complex system of checks and balances to protect against invasion by foreign cells or substances. It is the main defense against infectious diseases. When a person's immune system is not functioning properly, the body is unable to fight off infections. Some individuals are born with immune deficiencies. Others may acquire the deficiency later in life through the use of immunosuppressive drugs to prevent rejection of an organ transplant or because of an infectious disease such as acquired immunodeficiency syndrome (AIDS). Regardless of the primary cause of the immune deficiency, the patient may die as a result of an infection that would be considered harmless in the general population. Another group of immune disorders includes the autoimmune diseases. In these disorders, the immune system begins to make antibodies against the body's own tissues. For example, joint tissue is destroyed in rheumatoid arthritis, and nerve tissue is destroyed in multiple sclerosis. Allergies represent a third group of immune disorders. An allergic response is an overreaction to a substance that would ordinarily be considered harmless by the body. During this reaction, a chemical called histamine is released that causes such changes as rashes and upper respiratory symptoms. In more severe reactions, asthma or circulatory system collapse may occur.

Nutritional disorders include dietary deficiencies, excesses, and imbalances. Vitamins and minerals are needed to take part in certain chemical reactions in the body. In vitamin deficiencies, these reactions are blocked. For example, vitamin A is needed for the proper functioning of the nerve endings in the eye that are responsible for seeing black and white and in dim light; thus, a person with a vitamin A deficiency may develop night blindness. Proteins, carbohydrates, and fats must be ingested in sufficient amounts to supply energy and raw materials to build body tissue. Excessive consumption, however, is associated with such conditions as obesity, diabetes, and heart disease.

Trauma generally refers to injury done to the body by an external force, such as in an automobile accident. The damage to the body may be relatively minor but still have serious effects. Damage to a blood vessel may cause hemorrhaging and subsequent loss of blood. Injury to the brain or spinal cord may result in paralysis or loss of other body function. Physicians also use the word "trauma" to mean any occurrence that damages the body or organs. High fever, for example, may be said to cause trauma to the brain. Extreme emotions may also have effects on the body.

Toxins are poisons that may originate from the surroundings of an individual and be absorbed through the skin or inhaled. A person can be overcome by carbon monoxide from a defective furnace or automobile heater, for example. Toxins may also be ingested in water or food. Drug overdoses or accidental ingestion of household chemicals will also cause toxic reactions. Medical ecology is a field of medicine that concerns itself with the long-term toxic effects of chemicals released into the environment from plastics or other materials associated with modern life.

Cancers arise when the cell division process becomes abnormal. Ordinarily, cells in the body divide at a limited rate that is characteristic of a particular tissue. When cells divide rapidly in an uncontrolled manner and metastasize (spread) to other parts of the body, the condition is termed a malignancy or cancer. Cancers are grouped according to the type of tissue from which they develop. Carcinomas arise from epithelial tissue such as skin. Sarcomas arise from connective tissue such as bone or muscle. Leukemias result from abnormal and rapid reproduction of white blood cells in the bone marrow. Lymphomas are cancers of the lymphatic tissues, such as the lymph nodes or spleen. The severity of the cancer and the chances for recovery depend on the extent of the cancer when first diagnosed, the type of tissue or location involved, the speed at which the cells are dividing, and whether the cancer has spread to other areas of the body.

While it is convenient to place pathologies into separate groups, in reality their causes and effects overlap. An individual who is malnourished may have a weakened immune system and be vulnerable to infectious diseases. The immune system attacks not only foreign cells from outside the body but abnormal cells arising within the body as well, such as cancer. Thus, patients with AIDS often develop cancer. Some individuals are at increased risk for cancer because of genetic factors called oncogenes. If these individuals smoke or eat unwisely, they may develop cancer, while others with the same inherited risk who adopt a prudent lifestyle do not. It is important for researchers and physicians to understand these complex pathological relationships so that they can diagnose and treat such conditions.

DIAGNOSTIC AND TREATMENT TECHNIQUES

A pathologist must be familiar with the typical test values associated with body functions and with the microscopic appearance of healthy cells and tissues in order to be able to differentiate correctly a normal condition from a pathological one. This body of knowledge has involved the collection of tissues and the measurement of values gleaned from years of medical treatment and research. Although based on large populations, these values may be misleading. For example, the amounts of blood cholesterol were measured in Americans, and the average level of cholesterol was labeled "normal." In reality, this value has been shown to be unhealthy and linked to heart disease.

Research pathology concentrates on the basic study of diseases or disorders. This type of study usually focuses on the cellular and biochemical aspects of a disease. Information is exchanged with other researchers in an effort to gain a complete understanding of the etiology of a disease and the mechanisms by which it damages the body. Laboratory experiments may be performed to determine if the condition can be stopped or at least slowed.

Other pathologists are more closely associated with patient treatment. A clinical pathologist is involved in the diagnosis of disease through study of body fluids, secretions, and excretions. Such a person must be knowledgeable in hematology (blood), microbiology, and chemistry. A surgical pathologist is responsible for testing samples of cells and tissues excised during surgery. In such a procedure, called a biopsy, a small section of tissue is taken from the affected area and sent to the laboratory. The pathologist then examines the sample using a microscope and determines whether the tissue is normal or whether it indicates the presence of cancer or some other disease state.

At one time, it was necessary to perform what was known as exploratory surgery if laboratory tests and X rays did not lead to a diagnosis. Less invasive, and safer, techniques have been developed to eliminate that need. Fiber-optic methods involve the use of light shining through a flexible tube containing glass fibers. The flexible tube can be inserted through a body opening or through a small incision, allowing the physician to see internal cavities and determine if any visible abnormalities are present or to perform a biopsy. In some cases, the condition can be corrected without further surgery.

Many other tools and techniques are available to clinical and surgical pathologists. Some abnormalities can be observed directly, such as a rash or external tumor. Microscopes are used to detect changes that are too minute to be seen by the naked eye. Another tool used to diagnose disease or disorders is the medical X ray, which can determine the presence of a broken bone, kidney stones, or dense tumors. Soft tissues are not so easily visualized using normal X-ray techniques. Ingestion of an opaque substance such as barium may help to delineate the outline of a structure such as the esophagus or intestine. Other medical imaging procedures, such as ultrasound, magnetic resonance imaging (MRI), and computed tomography (CT) scans, allow even more detailed visualization of body structures.

An autopsy pathologist examines the body after death. In a hospital setting, the purpose of an autopsy is usually to confirm or determine the natural cause of death. Even when the cause is known, an autopsy may be requested, since information obtained in this way may lead to better understanding of the pathological processes that resulted in death and suggest possible ways of preventing deaths in the future.

A forensic pathologist, also called a coroner or medical examiner, is an autopsy pathologist who works closely with the police and criminal justice officials. This relationship is especially important if there are suspicious circumstances surrounding the death or the discovery of the body, in order to determine whether the death has resulted from an intentional poisoning or a violent act. In some cases, a coroner must also attempt to identify the body. Such abnormalities in the body as scars, healed fractures, and dental cavities can aid in this effort. Samples of cells may be used for DNA fingerprinting, a comparison of genetic material from the deceased to that of someone believed to be a close relative, in an attempt to verify identification. If it is determined that a murder has occurred, the pathologist contributes to the investigation by determining such facts as the cause and time of death. Special care must be taken during any autopsy since the information may be used as legal evidence.

The correct diagnosis and identification of the etiology of a disease are essential to providing insight into possible treatments. Pathologists also play a key role in determining the mode of transmission. The following historical examples illustrate this application of pathology.

In the 1930's, it was discovered that the urine of some retarded children had a peculiar odor. Analysis of the urine showed the presence of an abnormal chemical that damaged the nervous system, resulting in mental deficiencies. In turn, the chemical was found

to result from a failure of the body to make an enzyme necessary to break down the amino acid phenylalanine as a result of a genetic defect, termed phenylketonuria (PKU). Simple blood and urine tests can determine the presence of this defect at birth. While this disease cannot be cured, those with PKU can be placed on a special diet low in phenylalanine, and so avoid the buildup of the amino acid and its resulting damage. In this genetic disease and others, once the precise mechanism of damage is found, efforts can be made to identify the presence of the gene and then to lessen its effects.

In July, 1976, more than 5,000 members of the American Legion attended a convention in Philadelphia. Within two weeks of returning home, 170 of them became ill and 29 of these died. Laboratory tests and autopsies identified the process that caused death as severe pneumonia accompanied by high fever, but could not determine its origin. Although a pathogen was suspected, none could be found through microscopic examination of tissues or culture studies. Attention turned to the hotel and its air conditioning system in an attempt to determine if some toxin had spread through the air ducts, but no such substance was found. Several months later, a pathologist at the Centers for Disease Control in Atlanta was examining lung tissue sections taken from chick embryos and discovered the bacteria that had caused the illness, now known as Legionnaires' disease. Further tests showed it to be sensitive to the antibiotic erythromycin. When subsequent cases occurred, prompt diagnosis of the disease allowed the correct treatment to be given. Its presence in water tanks associated with large air conditioning systems has led to preventive measures.

In 1981, the first cases of AIDS were identified. While the mode of transmission was discovered fairly quickly, it was not until 1986 that the human immunodeficiency virus (HIV) was identified. The pathogenesis of this disease begins with the infection of white blood cells, called helper T cells, that are an essential link between the identification of an invading pathogen and the production of antibodies by other cells called B cells. At first, the body begins to make antibodies against the virus as it would any other infectious disease. Then, over a period of several years, an increasing number of T cells are infected and destroyed. Eventually, the body loses the ability to make the antibodies necessary to fight all infectious diseases and to destroy cancer cells. After further study of the virus, researchers were able to discover a chemical, azidothymidine, or AZT (now called zidovudine), that could interfere with a key enzyme needed by the virus to reproduce. Although it cannot cure the disease, the drug can slow its effects. AIDS research efforts are not aimed solely at attempts to kill the virus: By studying its pathogenesis, the means may be found to counteract the effects of the disease on the body's immune system.

PERSPECTIVE AND PROSPECTS

In the early days of medicine, knowledge of pathology was limited to what could be observed directly through the human senses. Treatments were empirical, a matter of trying different drugs or procedures until one was found that worked. Most basic knowledge of human anatomy and physiology was lacking. Often, human autopsies were not permitted because of religious and cultural practices.

A culture's beliefs about disease influence medical practice. From the time of the ancient Greeks until the rise of modern medicine, various theories were accepted. Some believed that disease had supernatural origins. The term "influenza," for example, came from the belief that the disease was caused by the influence of the stars. Others believed that the body's functions were dependent on fluids in the body, called humors. Thus, a healthy person was in a good humor. Bleeding was used to release the bad humors that were causing the disease.

By the seventeenth century, dissection of cadavers was practiced to identify completely the normal and abnormal gross anatomy of the human body. The microscope was developed and used to study human tissues. In the late nineteenth century, it was shown that microorganisms could cause disease, which in turn led to specific tactics aimed at prevention and treatment. With knowledge of the infectious process and the development of anesthesia, surgery became more widespread. This trend, in turn, increased the knowledge of disease processes in tissues and organs.

In the twentieth century, more sophisticated techniques were developed to focus on processes at the cellular level. The electron microscope allowed researchers to visualize structures within cells. Other research showed that series of chemical reactions, called metabolic pathways, are necessary for proper cell function. The comparison of these pathways in normal cells with those in abnormal cells enabled researchers to understand the pathogenic effect of toxins and many genetic diseases. The use of computers in medical analysis has increased the precision of laboratory tests and has permitted the detection of abnormal chemicals in smaller amounts than were possible before.

In 1990, an ambitious effort called the Human Genome Project officially began. The first phase of this effort involves mapping the human genome—that is, identifying and locating all the genes that are found on the forty-six human chromosomes. One of the techniques employed in this project is to compare the chromosomes of individuals known to have genetic diseases with those who do not, and so identify the abnormal gene. Identification of oncogenes (cancer-causing genes), or genes linked to such diseases as diabetes mellitus and heart disease may alert individuals at high risk in time for them to get regular diagnostic tests or to change their lifestyles. Knowledge gained by taking the study of disease to the genetic level will ultimately lead to more effective treatments and prevention for these and other pathological conditions.

—*Edith K. Wallace, Ph.D.*

See also Autopsy; Bacteriology; Biopsy; Blood testing; Cancer; Cytology; Cytopathology; Dermatopathology; Disease; Electroencephalography (EEG); Endoscopy; Epidemiology; Forensic pathology; Genetics and inheritance; Gram staining; Hematology; Hematology, pediatric; Histology; Homeopathy; Immunization and vaccination; Immunopathology; Inflammation; Invasive tests; Laboratory tests; Malignancy and metastasis; Microbiology; Microscopy; Mutation; Noninvasive tests; Oncology; Physical examination; Prion diseases; Serology; Toxicology; Urinalysis; Veterinary medicine.

FOR FURTHER INFORMATION:

Baden, Michael M. *Unnatural Death: Confessions of a Medical Examiner.* New York: Random House, 1989. Written by a forensic pathologist for the general public. Baden reviews famous cases and those with which he was involved. There are chapters on identification of the body, determination of the time and cause of death, and other aspects of forensic pathology.

Crowley, Leonard V. *Introduction to Human Disease.* 5th ed. Boston: Jones and Bartlett, 2001. This volume in the Jones and Bartlett series in health sciences discusses the causes, both known and theoretical, of disease. Includes a bibliography and an index.

Jensen, Marcus M., and Donald N. Wright. *Introduction to Microbiology for the Health Sciences.* 4th ed. Englewood Cliffs, N.J.: Prentice Hall, 1997. This introductory college textbook provides an overview of pathogenic species and the prevention and treatment of infectious disease. Four chapters are devoted to the immune system and immune disorders.

Shtasel, Philip. *Medical Tests and Diagnostic Procedures: A Patient's Guide to Just What the Doctor Ordered.* New York: Harper & Row, 1990. Written for people with nonmedical backgrounds. Describes sixteen medical specialties. The last five chapters describe laboratory tests and other diagnostic techniques. A glossary is included.

Wills, Christopher. *Exons, Introns, and Talking Genes.* New York: Basic Books, 1991. Outlines the procedures needed to map chromosomes, identify abnormal genes, and discover the proteins that these genes make or fail to make. Special emphasis is given to cancer, inherited diseases, possibilities for gene therapy, and implications for the future.

PEDIATRICS
SPECIALTY

ANATOMY OR SYSTEM AFFECTED: All

SPECIALTIES AND RELATED FIELDS: Family practice, genetics, neonatology, nursing, perinatology, pulmonary medicine, urology

DEFINITION: The field of medicine devoted to the care of children at birth and through childhood, puberty, and adolescence.

KEY TERMS:

acute: referring to a short and sharp disease process

chronic: referring to a lingering disease process

congenital: inborn, inherited

full-term: referring to a gestation period of a full nine months

premature: referring to a birth that is less than full term

puberty: the time of hormonal change when a child begins the physical process of becoming an adult

SCIENCE AND PROFESSION

The practice of pediatrics begins with birth. Most babies are born healthy and require only routine medical attention. Many hospitals, however, have a neonatology unit for babies who are born prematurely, who have disease conditions or birth defects, or who weigh less than 5.5 pounds (even though they may be full-term babies). All these infants may require short-term or prolonged care by pediatricians in the neonatology unit.

The problems of premature babies usually center on the fact that they have not fully developed physically, although other factors may also be involved, such as the health and age of the mother, undernourishment during pregnancy, lack of prenatal care, anemia, abnormalities in the mother's genital organs, and infectious disease. A past record of infertility, stillbirths, abortions, and other premature births may indicate that a pregnancy will not go to full term.

Low birth weight in both premature and full-term babies is directly related to the incidence of disease and congenital defects and may be indicative of a low intelligence quotient (IQ). Between 50 and 75 percent of babies weighing under 3 pounds, 5 ounces are mentally retarded or have defects in vision or hearing.

Because the lungs are among the organs that develop late in pregnancy, many premature infants are unable to breathe on their own. Some premature babies are born before they have developed the sucking reflex, so they cannot feed on their own.

Hundreds of congenital diseases can be present in the neonate. Some are apparent at birth; some become evident in later years. Some may be life-threatening to the infant or become life-threatening in later years. Others may be harmless.

The child may be born with an infection passed on from the mother, such as rubella (German measles) or human immunodeficiency virus (HIV), the virus that causes acquired immunodeficiency syndrome (AIDS). Rubella may also infect the child in the womb, causing severe physical deformities, heart defects, mental retardation, deafness, and other conditions.

Among the most prevalent congenital birth defects is cleft lip, which occurs when the upper lip does not fuse together, leaving a visible gap that can extend from the lip to the nose. Cleft palate occurs when the gap reaches into the roof of the mouth.

Various abnormalities may be present in the hands and feet of neonates. These can be caused by congenital defects or by medications given to the pregnant mother. Arms, legs, fingers, and toes may fail to develop fully or may be missing entirely. Some children are born with extra fingers or toes. In some children, fingers or toes may be webbed or fused together. Clubfoot is relatively common. In this condition, the foot is twisted, usually downward and inward.

Many congenital heart defects can afflict the child,

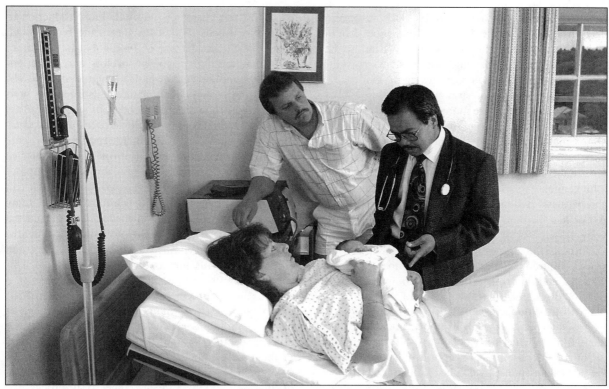

It is customary for pediatricians to visit newborns in the hospital in the days following delivery. (Digital Stock)

including septal defects (openings in the septum, the wall that separates the right and left sides of the heart), the transposition of blood vessels, the constriction of blood vessels, and valve disorders.

Congenital disorders of the central nervous system include spina bifida, hydrocephalus, cerebral palsy, and Down syndrome. Spina bifida is a condition in which part of a vertebra (a bone in the spinal column) fails to fuse. As a result, nerves of the spinal cord may protrude through the spinal column. This condition varies considerably in severity; mild forms can cause no significant problems, while severe forms can be crippling or life-threatening. In hydrocephalus, sometimes called "water on the brain," fluid accumulates in the infant's cranium, causing the head to enlarge and putting great pressure on the brain. This disorder, too, can be life-threatening.

Cerebral palsy is caused by damage to brain cells that control motor function in the body. This damage can occur before, during, or after birth. It may or may not be accompanied by mental retardation. Many children with cerebral palsy appear to be retarded because they have difficulty speaking, but, in fact, their intelligence may be normal or above normal. Down syndrome is one of the most common congenital birth defects, affecting 1 in 600 to 800 infants. It is caused by an extra chromosome passed on to the child. The distinct physical characteristics of Down syndrome include a small body, a small and rounded head, oval ears, and an enlarged tongue. Mortality is high in the first year of life because of infection or other disease.

Cystic fibrosis is one of the most serious congenital diseases of Caucasian children. Because the lungs of children with this disease cannot expel mucus efficiently, it thickens and collects, clogging air passages. The mucus also becomes a breeding ground for bacteria and infection. Other parts of the body, such as the pancreas, the digestive system, and sweat glands, can also be impaired. A common congenital disorder among African American children is sickle-cell disease. It causes deformities in red blood cells that clog blood vessels, impair circulation, and increase the susceptibility to infection.

One of the major problems of infancy is sudden infant death syndrome (SIDS), in which a baby that is perfectly healthy, or only slightly ill, is discovered dead in its crib. The incidence is high—about 1 in every 500 births—and the effects are devastating. The cause is not known. The child usually shows no symptoms of disease, and autopsies reveal no evidence of smothering, choking, or strangulation.

Infectious diseases are more prevalent in childhood than in later years. Among the major diseases of children (and often adults) throughout the centuries have been smallpox, malaria, diphtheria, typhus, typhoid fever, tuberculosis, measles, mumps, rubella, varicella (chickenpox), scarlet fever, pneumonia, meningitis, and pertussis (whooping cough). In more recent years, AIDS has become another significant threat to the young.

Certain skin diseases are common in infants and young children, such as diaper rash, impetigo, neonatal acne, and seborrheic dermatitis, among a wide variety of disorders. Fungal diseases of the skin occur often in the young, usually because of close contact with other youngsters. For example, tinea pedis (athlete's foot), tinea cruris (jock itch), and tinea corporis (a fungal infection that occurs on nonhairy areas of the body), are spread by contact with an infected playmate or by the touching of surfaces that harbor the organism. Similarly, parasitic diseases such as head lice, body lice, crabs, or scabies are easily spread among playmates. Some skin conditions are congenital. Between 20 and 40 percent of infants are born with, or soon develop, skin lesions called hemangiomas. They may be barely perceptible or quite unsightly; they generally resolve by the age of seven.

One form of diabetes mellitus arises in childhood, insulin-dependent diabetes mellitus (IDDM) or Type I. In the healthy individual, the pancreas produces insulin, a hormone that is responsible for the metabolism of blood sugar, or glucose. In some children, the pancreas loses the ability to produce insulin, causing blood sugar to rise. When this happens, a cascade of events causes harmful effects throughout the body. In the short term, these symptoms include rapid breathing, rapid heartbeat, extreme thirst, vomiting, fever, chemical imbalances in the blood, and coma. In the long term, diabetes mellitus contributes to heart disease, atherosclerosis, kidney damage, blindness, gangrene, and a host of other conditions.

Cancer can afflict children. One of the most serious forms is acute lymphocytic leukemia. Its peak incidence is between three and five years of age, although it can also occur later in life. Leukemic conditions are characterized by the overproduction of white blood cells (leukocytes). In acute lymphocytic leukemia, the production of lymphoblasts, immature cells that ordinarily would develop into infection-fighting lymphocytes, is greatly increased. This abnormal proliferation of immature cells interferes with the normal production of blood cells, increasing the child's susceptibility to infection. Before current treatment modalities, the prognosis for children with acute lymphocytic leukemia was death within four or five months after diagnosis.

In addition to the wide range of diseases that can beset the infant and growing child, there are many other problems of childhood that the parent and the pediatrician must face. These problems may involve physical and behavioral development, nutrition, and relationships with parents and other children.

Both parents and pediatricians must be alert to a child's rate of growth and mental development. Failure to gain weight in infancy may indicate a range of physical problems, such as gastrointestinal, endocrine, and other internal disorders. In three-quarters of these cases, however, the cause is not a physical disorder. The child may simply be underfed because of the mother's negligence. The vital process of bonding between mother and child may not have taken place; the child is not held close and cuddled, is not shown affection, and thus feels unwanted and unloved. This is seen often in babies who are reared in institutions where the nursing staff does not have time to caress and comfort infants individually.

Similarly, later in childhood, failure to grow at a normal rate can be caused by malnutrition or psychological factors. It could also be attributable to a deficiency in a hormone that is the body's natural regulator of growth. If this hormone is not released in adequate supply, the child's growth is stunted. An excess of this hormone may cause the child to grow too rapidly. Failure to grow normally may also indicate an underlying disease condition, such as heart dysfunction and malabsorption problems, in which the child does not get the necessary nutrition from food.

The parent and pediatrician must also ensure that the child is developing acceptably in other areas. Speech and language skills, teething, bone development, walking and other motor skills, toilet habits, sleep patterns, eye development, and hearing have to be evaluated regularly.

Profound mental retardation is usually evident early in life, but mild to moderate retardation may not

Doctor Visits by Children and Teenagers Each Year in the United States		
Year	Under 5	5 to 17
1986	6.3	3.3
1987	6.7	3.3
1988	7.0	3.4
1989	6.7	3.5
1990	6.9	3.2
1991	7.1	3.4
1992	6.9	3.5
1993	7.2	3.6
1994	6.8	3.5

Source: Statistical Abstract of the United States 1997. Washington, D.C.: GPO, 1997.

be apparent until the child starts school. Slowness in learning may be indicative of mental retardation, but this judgment should be carefully weighed because the real reason may be impaired hearing or vision or an underlying disease condition.

The battery of diseases and other disorders that may beset a child remains more or less constant throughout childhood. At puberty, however, hormonal changes begin that trigger new disease threats and vast psychological upheaval. As early as eight years of age in girls and after ten or eleven years of age in boys, the body begins a prolonged metamorphosis that changes the child into an adult. Hormones that were released in minimal amounts course throughout the body in great quantities.

In boys, the sex hormones are called androgens. Chief among them is testosterone, which is secreted primarily by the testicles. It causes the sexual organs to mature and promotes the growth of hair in the genital area and armpits and on the chest. Testosterone also enlarges the larynx (voicebox), causing the voice to deepen.

Girls also produce some testosterone, but estrogens and other female sex hormones are the major hormones involved in puberty. They cause the sexual organs to mature, the hips to enlarge and become rounded, hair to grow in the genital area and armpits, the breasts to enlarge, and menstruation to begin.

Many disease conditions can arise in association with the hormonal changes that occur during puberty, such as breast abnormalities and genital infections. Far and away the most significant medical disorder at this time, however, is acne. Acne is a direct result of the rise in testosterone that occurs during puberty. About 85 percent of teenagers experience some degree of acne, and about 12 percent of these will develop severe, deep acne, a serious condition that can leave lifelong scars.

Important psychological changes also occur during puberty. The personality can be altered as the developing child begins to crave independence. Ties to the family weaken, and the teenager becomes closer to his or her peer group. Sexual feelings can be strong and difficult to repress. In modern Western society, this is usually the time when the teenager may begin to experiment with tobacco, alcohol, drugs, or other means of achieving a "high," although in some groups the use of these substances begins much earlier. Drug and substance abuse is a major problem throughout the society, but it is particularly devastating among young people.

Sexual license among teenagers is widespread in Western cultures and has also become a significant medical problem. The incidence of sexually transmitted diseases (STDs) is higher among teenagers than any other group. Teenage pregnancy is one of the most challenging issues in modern society.

The pregnant teenage girl is usually from a disadvantaged background. She often receives little or no prenatal care. The fetus is not properly nourished and may be damaged because the mother smoked, drank alcohol, and/or took drugs throughout the pregnancy. The child is often born prematurely, with all the physical problems that premature birth involves. Hospital care of these infants is extremely costly, as is the maintenance of the mother and child if the baby survives.

Another important issue of teenage sexuality is the rapid spread of AIDS, both as a sexually transmitted disease and as an infection passed from mother to baby.

DIAGNOSTIC AND TREATMENT TECHNIQUES
Pediatrics is one of the widest-ranging medical specialties, embracing virtually all major medical disciplines. Some pediatricians are generalists, and others specialize in certain disease areas, such as heart disease, kidney disease, liver disease, or skin problems.

Doctors and nurses specializing in neonatology have become increasingly important. They have radically improved the survival rates of premature and low-weight babies. In neonatal care of the premature, the infant may have to be helped to breathe, fed through tubes, and otherwise maintained to allow it to develop.

Infectious diseases passed from the mother to the newborn child are a particular challenge. In some cases, appropriate antibiotics can be given. In others, such as with babies born with HIV, support measures and medications that help prevent the progress of the disease are the only procedures available.

Many birth defects and deformities can be repaired or at least ameliorated. Disorders such as cleft lip or palate, deformities of the skeletal system, heart defects, and other physical abnormalities can often be remedied by surgery. Certain structural malformations may require prosthetic devices and/or physical therapy.

The treatment of spina bifida depends on the seriousness of the condition; surgery may be required. With hydrocephalus, medication may be helpful, but most often a permanent shunt is implanted to drain fluids from the cranium. Before this technique was developed, the prognosis for babies with hydrocephalus was poor: More than half died, and a great many suffered from mental retardation and physical impairment. Today, 70 percent or more live through infancy. Of these, about 40 percent have normal intelligence; the others are mentally retarded and may also have serious physical impairment.

There are no cures for cerebral palsy, but various procedures can improve the child's quality of life, exercise and counseling among them. Neither is there a cure for Down syndrome. If retardation is profound, the child may have to be institutionalized. When a child with Down syndrome can be cared for at home in a loving family, his or her life can be improved.

SIDS continues to be a significant problem both in hospitals and in the home. There is no explanation for it, although many medical teams have given it priority in their research.

Managing the infectious diseases of childhood is one of the major concerns of pediatricians. They are often called on to treat infections, for which they have a wide variety of antibiotics and other agents. The pediatrician also seeks to prevent infectious diseases through immunization. Medical authorities now recommend routine vaccination of all children in the United States against diphtheria, tetanus, pertussis,

measles, mumps, rubella, poliomyelitis, pneumococcal pneumonia, *Hemophilus influenzae*, and hepatitis B. Vaccines are also available against rabies, influenza, cholera, typhoid fever, plague, and yellow fever; these vaccines can be given to the child if there is a danger of infection. Vaccines for diphtheria, tetanus, and pertussis are generally given together in a combination called DTP. Measles, mumps, and rubella vaccines are also given together as MMR. Repeated doses of some vaccines are necessary to ensure and maintain immunity.

Skin disorders of childhood, including the acne of teenagers, are usually treated successfully at home with over-the-counter remedies. As with any disease, however, a severe skin disorder requires the attention of a physician.

Patients with diabetes mellitus, Type I, are dependent on insulin throughout life. It is necessary for the pediatrician or attending nurse to teach both the parent and the patient how to inject insulin regularly, often several times a day. Furthermore, patients must monitor their blood and urine constantly to determine blood sugar levels. They must also adhere to stringent dietary regulations. This regimen of diet, insulin, and constant monitoring is often difficult for the child to learn and accept, but strict adherence is vital if the patient is to fare well and avoid the wide range of complications associated with diabetes.

Other serious conditions are now considered to be treatable. Modern pharmacology has greatly improved the prognosis of children with leukemia. Similarly, many children with growth disorders can be helped by treatments of growth hormone.

Medications and other treatment modalities for the mental disorders of childhood have improved in recent years. Mentally retarded children can often be taught to care for themselves, and some even grow up to live independently. Children with behavioral problems may be helped by pediatricians specializing in child psychology or psychiatry. Many medications are available to help young as well as mature victims of anxiety, depression, schizophrenia, paranoia, and other mental disorders.

The problems of sexuality, sexually transmitted diseases, and pregnancy among teenagers have provoked a nationwide response in the United States among medical and sociological professionals. Massive "safe sex" programs have been launched, and clinics specializing in counseling for teenage girls are in operation to stem the rise in teenage pregnancies.

PERSPECTIVE AND PROSPECTS

Pediatrics affects virtually every member of society. Diseases that once raged through populations of all ages are now being controlled through the mass immunization of children. Some diseases of childhood are not yet controllable by vaccines, but research in this area is being conducted.

Childhood health is directly related to economics. Middle-class and upper-class children have ready access to professional care for any problems that may arise. The medical and psychological needs of disadvantaged children, however, especially those who live in inner cities, are often neglected. Many of these children are not being immunized fully and remain susceptible to diseases that are no longer a problem among the middle and upper classes.

In an effort to improve the medical care of disadvantaged children, some vaccines are being made available at low or no cost to inner-city families. Programs educate parents and teachers about the need for a child to receive the full dosage of vaccine. Computerized records allow authorities to keep track of the immunization status of individual children and to alert their parents when a follow-up inoculation is due.

The psychological problems of inner-city children are at least as serious as the diseases that threaten them. They may live in a universe of violence, deprivation, drug addiction, lack of a stable family environment, and lack of opportunities for advancement. This environment fosters widespread asocial behavior. Some of these children become amoral and apathetic, not knowing—or caring—about right or wrong.

These children are one of the most significant societal challenges facing the United States. The pediatrician can help by becoming involved in massive medical, psychological, and sociological outreach programs to help inner cities and improve the lot of children there.

—*C. Richard Falcon*

See also Apgar score; Cardiology, pediatric; Childhood infectious diseases; Circumcision, male; Cognitive development; Critical care, pediatric; Dentistry, pediatric; Dermatology, pediatric; Developmental stages; Emergency medicine, pediatric; Endocrinology, pediatric; Family practice; Gastroenterology, pediatric; Genetic diseases; Growth; Hematology, pediatric; Motor skill development; Neonatology; Nephrology, pediatric; Neurology, pediatric; Optometry, pediatric; Orthopedics, pediatric; Perinatology; Psychiatry, child and adolescent; Puberty and adoles-

cence; Pulmonary medicine, pediatric; Safety issues for children; Surgery, pediatric; Urology, pediatric; Well-baby examinations.

FOR FURTHER INFORMATION:

Hoekelman, Robert, ed. *The New American Encyclopedia of Children's Health*. New York: New American Library/Dutton, 1991. This text concentrates on pediatric conditions. A useful reference for the quick identification of diseases and their treatments.

Larson, David E., ed. *Mayo Clinic Family Health Book*. 2d ed. New York: William Morrow, 1996. The chapters on childhood diseases are admirably thorough and clear, and the sections on childhood physical and psychological development are exemplary.

Taubman, Bruce. *Your Child's Symptoms*. New York: Simon & Schuster, 1992. Taubman, a doctor, catalogs the diseases of childhood and their symptoms.

Wagman, Richard J., ed. *The New Complete Medical and Health Encyclopedia*. 4 vols. Chicago: J. G. Ferguson, 2000. This set is a good general source of medical knowledge for the layperson. The listings under children's diseases are concise and thorough.

PELVIC INFLAMMATORY DISEASE (PID)
DISEASE/DISORDER

ANATOMY OR SYSTEM AFFECTED: Genitals, reproductive system, uterus

SPECIALTIES AND RELATED FIELDS: Bacteriology, gynecology, urology, virology

DEFINITION: PID is an infection of female reproductive organs that causes inflammation of the Fallopian tubes; it is contagious if attributable to a sexually transmitted organism. The symptoms include pain in the lower abdomen, abnormal vaginal bleeding, foul-smelling vaginal discharge, painful sexual intercourse, painful urination, fever, and chills. PID is caused by a virus or bacterial infection, such as chlamydia, gonorrhea, or mycoplasma. The use of an intrauterine contraceptive device (IUD) is known to increase the risk of contracting the disease. If it is left untreated, complications may occur, resulting in blood poisoning, scarring, infertility, and even death. A full course of antibiotics must be taken to prevent long-term PID.

—*Jason Georges and Tracy Irons-Georges*

See also Antibiotics; Bacterial infections; Chlamydia; Contraception; Genital disorders, female;

Gonorrhea; Gynecology; Infertility in females; Reproductive system; Sexually transmitted diseases; Viral infections.

FOR FURTHER INFORMATION:

Boston Women's Health Book Collective. *Our Bodies, Ourselves for the New Century.* New York: Simon & Schuster, 1998.

Carlson, Karen J., Stephanie A. Eisenstat, and Terra Ziporyn. *The Harvard Guide to Women's Health.* Cambridge, Mass.: Harvard University Press, 1996.

Gray, Mary Jane, and Florence Haseltine. *The Woman's Guide to Good Health.* Yonkers, N.Y.: Consumer Reports Books, 1991.

Novotny, P. P. *What Women Should Know About Chronic Infections and Sexually Transmitted Diseases.* New York: Dell, 1991.

PENILE IMPLANT SURGERY

PROCEDURE

ANATOMY OR SYSTEM AFFECTED: Genitals, reproductive system

SPECIALTIES AND RELATED FIELDS: General surgery, psychiatry, urology

DEFINITION: The surgical placement of a prosthetic device inside the penis to make it rigid enough for penetration.

KEY TERMS:

corpora cavernosa: two parallel erectile cylinders on the upper side of penis that are filled with blood during a natural erection

corpus spongiosum: a third cylinder in the penis below the corpora cavernosa; the urethra passes through it and the glans penis forms the front end of the cylinder

erection: a complex phenomenon involving nerves, blood vessels, and the mind that leads to the entrapment of blood in the penis, making it rigid

glans penis: the head of the penis

impotence: the lack of sustained erection that is rigid enough for penetration in sexual intercourse

urethra: the channel through which urine and seminal fluid are passed; it starts at the bladder neck, goes through the shaft of the penis, and ends at the glans penis

INDICATIONS AND PROCEDURES

Penile implant surgery is performed when all other, nonsurgical means of treating impotence have been exhausted or are not suitable for the patient. A thorough workup must be performed to diagnose the cause of the impotence, which can be psychogenic or organic. The term "psychogenic" is used when there are no anatomical, hormonal, or physiological problems with the patient's erectile mechanism; instead, the problem is in the patient's mind. Organic causes include poor blood flow to the penis, the inability of the erectile cylinders to trap blood in the penis (venous leak), or a problem with the nerves, which is seen in diabetic patients. Impotence may also result from a hormonal disturbance.

Penile implant surgery is only performed if the underlying cause is organic; it is never performed for psychogenic impotence. The organic cause can be determined with certain tests, including an analysis of blood chemistry and hormone levels, as well as a test for the presence of erection during sleep. Finally, the physician may perform an invasive test in which a drug is injected into the penis so that the erectile response can be observed. Usually, less aggressive, nonsurgical treatments are tried first. If they fail, then penile implant surgery is considered.

There are two types of implants: One is semirigid and malleable, and the other is inflatable. Semirigid rods, the earliest type of penile prostheses, are inserted in each corpora cavernosa in the penis. The advantages of this type are a simple surgical technique, lack of mechanical failure, and low cost. The disad-

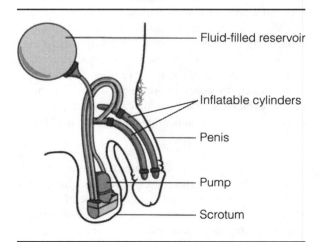

Fluid-filled reservoir

Inflatable cylinders

Penis

Pump

Scrotum

A penile implant is an artificial device, usually consisting of inflatable cylinders and a pump, that can simulate an erection in men who suffer from impotence that has a biological (rather than a psychological) cause. When the patient squeezes the pump in the scrotum, fluid from an implanted reservoir fills the cylinders.

vantages include poor cosmetic results because of a permanently rigid penis, which is difficult to conceal, and extrusion of the penile implant. The malleable prosthesis is like a semirigid one except that it can be bent in the middle, so that concealment is not as difficult. Lifting the prosthesis upward makes it rigid. The design of these prostheses is based on a central wire with multiple springs that cause the penis to become erect when the prosthesis is pulled upward and the springs come in position so that they support one another.

The second group of penile prostheses are inflatable. These multicomponent prostheses contain two cylinders that fit in the corpora cavernosa. The fluid from a reservoir is pumped into the cylinders to achieve an erection. After the prosthesis has been used, the fluid is pumped back into the reservoir, and the penis becomes flaccid. There are two types of inflatable prosthesis: one in which the pump and the fluid reservoir are combined (two-component type) and one in which the pump is separate from the reservoir (three-component type). The advantage of this type of penile prosthesis is that it more closely mimics a natural erection, in which the penis not only elongates but also expands in diameter. In addition, the penis is closer to a normal shape when in the flaccid state. The disadvantages are significantly higher cost, the chance of mechanical failure in the connections and tubing, and the chance of leakage of fluid from the reservoir or the cylinders. The total time of the operation is slightly more for inflatable penile prostheses than semirigid and malleable prostheses.

The surgical approaches for the placement of a penile prosthesis are the same for semirigid, malleable, and inflatable types. In the infrapubic approach, the patient is placed on his back. An incision is made at the junction where the penis meets the body, just above the penis in the lower part of the abdominal wall. After the skin and fatty tissues are cut, the corpora cavernosa are exposed. While carefully protecting the nerve responsible for sensation in the penis, the surgeon opens and dilates the corpora cavernosa. The lengths of the corpora are measured, appropriate-length artificial cylinders are inserted, and the corpora are closed.

In the case of semirigid and malleable prostheses, the operation ends after the skin is closed. In the case of an inflatable penile prosthesis, however, two extra steps are taken. A place is created for the pump and

reservoir. In a two-component inflatable penile prosthesis, a pocket is created for the combined pump and reservoir just underneath the skin of the scrotum, in an area that is easily accessible to the patient. In a three-component penile prosthesis, a pocket is created in the scrotum for the pump and a space is created for the reservoir in the lower part of abdomen, above the pubic bone and in front of the bladder. The reservoir is connected to the pump, and in this fashion the placement of the prosthesis is completed. An appropriate amount of fluid is left in the reservoir based on the length of the cylinders. The penile prosthesis is evaluated for proper function and cosmetic appearance, and the incision is closed.

Uses and Complications

In the immediate postoperative phase, the cylinder of the inflatable penile prosthesis is left totally deflated so that a scar forms around the pump and reservoir that will allow the normal function of the prosthesis in the future. After two weeks, the cylinders are cycled: The patient inflates his penile prosthesis for thirty to sixty minutes every day and then deflates it. In about six weeks, the pain should have subsided significantly so that the patient is ready to use his penile prosthesis for sexual intercourse. Close monitoring ensures that no infection develops, and the patient is asked to report to the doctor immediately if there is any redness or swelling in the area, which are signs of an impending infection. If an infection occurs, it is initially treated aggressively with antibiotics. If antibiotic therapy does not work, the penile prosthesis may have to be removed.

The complications associated with penile implants include infection, mechanical failure (resulting in the loss of pump or reservoir function), and inadvertent inflation of an inflatable penile prosthesis when the patient sits or stands up. In certain cases, the penile prosthesis can also migrate forward or backward. It can even perforate the corpora cavernosa and extrude through the penis, an emergency situation which needs to be corrected immediately. There is a remote possibility of gangrene of the penis if infection and extrusion take place simultaneously.

Perspective and Prospects

Penile implant surgery is an excellent procedure for patients who have problems with impotence, in that it allows them to achieve an erection rigid enough for penetration. This surgery is more applicable in younger patients who have become impotent, either because of diabetes mellitus or after surgical treatment of prostate or rectal cancer, which can lead to damage of the nerves responsible for erection. An older age is not a contraindication for penile prosthesis, however, if the patient is in good physical condition and wants a penile prosthesis. In all cases, it is important that surgery be performed only after significant counseling with the patient, who should understand all the benefits and risks.

The technology involved in penile implant surgery has evolved since the 1970's, starting from a simple, rigid prosthesis and leading to an inflatable, multicomponent prosthesis. The incidence of mechanical failure in the multicomponent inflatable prosthesis is constantly decreasing, and some companies that manufacture this type now offer a lifetime warranty.

—*Saeed Akhter, M.D.*

See also Diabetes mellitus; Genital disorders, male; Prostate cancer; Psychiatry; Reproductive system; Sex change surgery; Sexual dysfunction; Testicular surgery; Urology.

FOR FURTHER INFORMATION:

Dinsmore, Wallace, and Philip Kell. *Erectile Dysfunction*. London: Royal Society of Medicine, 2000.

Goldstein, Irwin, and Robert Krane. "Diagnosis and Therapy of Erectile Dysfunction." In *Campbell's Urology*, edited by Patrick C. Walsh et al. 7th ed. 3 vols. Philadelphia: W. B. Saunders, 1998.

Tanagho, Emil A., Tom F. Lue, and R. Dale McClure, eds. *Contemporary Management of Impotence and Infertility*. Baltimore: Williams & Wilkins, 1988.

PEPTIC ULCERS. *See* ULCERS.

PERINATOLOGY
SPECIALTY
ANATOMY OR SYSTEM AFFECTED: All

SPECIALTIES AND RELATED FIELDS: Embryology, neonatology, obstetrics, pediatrics

DEFINITION: The branch of medicine dealing with the fetus and infant during the perinatal period (from the twenty-eighth week of gestation to the twenty-eighth day after birth).

KEY TERMS:

amniotic fluid: fluid within the amniotic cavity produced by the amnion during the early embryonic period (two to eight weeks) and later by the lungs and kidneys

cesarean section: an incision made through the abdominal and uterine walls for the delivery of a fetus

fetus: the unborn offspring in the postembryonic period, from nine weeks after fertilization until birth

infant: a young child from birth to twelve months of age

ischemia: a local anemia or area of diminished or insufficient blood supply as a result of mechanical obstruction of the blood supply (commonly narrowing of an artery)

placenta: a fetomaternal organ that joins mother and offspring; it secretes endocrine hormones and selectively exchanges soluble, blood-borne substances through its interior structures

Rh: a human blood factor, originally identified in rhesus monkeys, that can be either positive (present) or negative (absent)

SCIENCE AND PROFESSION
Practitioners of perinatal medicine and nursing receive education in both obstetrics and pediatrics. They then complete additional training specifically related to the perinatal period. The emphasis of perinatology is on a time period rather than on a specific organ system. The principal event of the perinatal period is birth. Prior to delivery, the perinatologist is concerned with the physiological status and well-being of both mother and fetus. Immediately after delivery, the perinatologist strives to maximize the newborn's chances for survival.

DIAGNOSTIC AND TREATMENT TECHNIQUES
Prior to the birth, several diagnostic procedures are commonly employed by the perinatologist: ultrasonography, the measurement of fetal activity, and the evaluation of fetal lung maturity. Ultrasonography uses sound waves to create images. Sound waves are transmitted from a transducer that has been placed on the skin. Waves that are sent into the body reflect off internal tissues and structures, and the reflections are received by a microphone. Sound travels through tissues with different densities at different rates, which are characteristic for each tissue. Computers interpret the reflected sounds and convert them into an image which can be viewed. The images must be interpreted or read by someone with specialized training, usually a radiologist. Ultrasound does not involve radiation; thus it is not harmful to the fetus. Because sound waves are longer than radiation, the image generated is not as clear as that obtained with electromagnetic

waves: a computed tomography (CT) scan or a conventional radiograph.

The measurement of fetal activity is important in evaluating fetal health. Fetal movement is normal; the earliest movement felt by the mother is called quickening. The diminution or cessation of fetal movement is indicative of fetal distress. Accordingly, movement is monitored by reports from the mother, palpation by the perinatologist, and ultrasound: Mothers report movements, individuals examining pregnant women can apply their hands to the abdomen and feel fetal movements, and ultrasonography can show breathing and other movements in real time using continuous video records of fetal movements.

Fetal lung maturity is assessed by measuring the relative amounts of lecithin and sphingomyelin in amniotic fluid. The concentration of lecithin increases late in fetal development, while sphingomyelin decreases. A lecithin-sphingomyelin ratio which is greater than two indicates sufficient fetal lung maturity to ensure survival after birth.

Labor and delivery are the primary events of the perinatal period. Factors that can lead to difficulties include abnormalities of the placenta and prematurity. The placenta can be abnormally located (placenta previa) or can separate prematurely (placenta abruptio). Normally, the placenta is located on the lateral wall of the uterus. Placenta previa is defined as a placenta located in the lower portion of the uterus. The placenta is compressed by the fetus during passage through the birth canal. This compression compromises the blood supply to the fetus, which causes ischemia and can lead to brain or other tissue damage or to death. This condition is usually managed by a cesarean section. Placenta abruptio refers to a normal placenta that separates prior to fetal delivery. This condition is potentially life-threatening to both mother and fetus; immediate hospitalization is indicated.

Prematurity is defined as delivery before the fetus is able to survive without unusual support. Premature infants are placed in incubators. A lack of body fat in the infant leads to difficulty in maintaining a normal body temperature; special heating is provided to offset the problem. Lung immaturity may require mechanical assistance from a respirator. An immature immune system makes premature infants especially susceptible to infections; strict isolation precautions and prophylactic antibiotic therapy address this problem.

Many factors contribute to increasing the risks normally associated with pregnancy and delivery: maternal size and age; drug, tobacco, or alcohol use; infection; medical conditions such as diabetes mellitus and hypertension; and multiple gestations. A woman with a small pelvic opening may be unable to deliver her child normally. The solution is a cesarean section. The risk of genetic abnormalities increases with advancing maternal (and, to a lesser degree, paternal) age. Counseling prior to conception is indicated. Once an older woman becomes pregnant, amniotic fluid should be obtained to test for genetic abnormalities. The degree of surveillance is dependent on maternal age: The recommended frequency of medical checks by a physician increases with increased maternal age. Alcohol intake during pregnancy can result in an infant who is both developmentally and mentally retarded; smoking during pregnancy frequently leads to an infant with a low birth weight. Drug usage during pregnancy can lead to anatomic or mental impairment. Avoiding the use of all substances is the easiest way to eliminate problems completely; *any* drug should be used only under the guidance of a physician. Some viral infections such as German measles (rubella) early in pregnancy can cause birth defects. Immunization prior to conception will avoid these problems.

Diabetes mellitus can cause abnormally large intrauterine growth and babies (frequently more than 10 pounds and referred to as macrosomic) who are too large for normal delivery. Diabetes commonly develops during pregnancy, so-called gestational diabetes. Medical monitoring to detect diabetes early is prudent. Appropriate medical management of preexisting diabetes minimizes problems associated with pregnancy. A macrosomic infant must be delivered with a cesarean section. Hypertension can also develop during pregnancy. Like diabetes, it can compromise both mother and fetus. Appropriate and aggressive medical management, sometimes including complete bed rest, is needed to control high blood pressure during pregnancy. Multiple gestations strain the supply of maternal nutrients to the developing fetuses. Because space is limited, multiple fetuses are usually smaller than normal at birth.

Erythroblastosis fetalis, also known as Rh incompatibility, can complicate pregnancy. It can occur only with an Rh-positive father and an Rh-negative mother, and it affects the blood supply of a fetus. The treatment includes the identification of both maternal and paternal blood types and the administration of pooled gamma globulin to the mother at twenty-six weeks of gestation and again immediately after birth. An affected infant may require blood transfusions; in a severe case, transfusions may be needed during pregnancy.

PERSPECTIVE AND PROSPECTS

Management of a pregnancy requires specialized skills. As the number of risk factors related to either mother or fetus increases, the problems associated with pregnancy also increase. The care of a pregnant woman and her fetus requires input from many individuals with specialized training. Consequently, perinatology is very much a team effort. Together, the team members can ensure a safe journey through the perinatal period for a pregnant woman and a healthy transition to life outside of the womb for a newborn infant.

—*L. Fleming Fallon, Jr., M.D., Ph.D., M.P.H.*

See also Amniocentesis; Birth defects; Breast-feeding; Cesarean section; Childbirth; Childbirth complications; Chorionic villus sampling; Embryology; Fetal alcohol syndrome; Hematology, pediatric; Neonatology; Neurology, pediatric; Nursing; Obstetrics; Pediatrics; Pregnancy and gestation; Premature birth; Shunts; Umbilical cord.

FOR FURTHER INFORMATION:

Creasy, Robert K., and Robert Resnik, eds. *Maternal-Fetal Medicine: Principles and Practice*. 4th ed. Philadelphia: W. B. Saunders, 1999. This standard textbook covers the perinatal period in great depth. The chapters are written by experts. A layperson will probably require a dictionary to understand the technical terminology completely.

PERIODONTAL SURGERY

PROCEDURE

ANATOMY OR SYSTEM AFFECTED: Gums, mouth, teeth

SPECIALTIES AND RELATED FIELDS: Dentistry, general surgery, orthodontics

DEFINITION: Any surgical procedure involving tissues or bone associated with support of the teeth.

INDICATIONS AND PROCEDURES

Periodontal disease is the most common cause of tooth loss among persons middle-aged or older. Most periodontal problems originate as dental caries, or cavities, the decay and destruction of teeth by bacteria. While most common periodontal difficulties can be prevented or solved through regular visits to the dentist, if decay is untreated it may lead to serious dental problems. At their worst, periodontal problems may require surgery as part of the treatment.

If decay develops within the root area, a pus-filled abscess may develop. The first indication is an ache or throbbing in the area of the tooth. The gum may be tender and swollen. If the abscess begins to spread, local lymph nodes in the neck may become swollen, as well as that portion of the face. Without proper treatment, the abscess may damage the jawbone or even result in blood poisoning.

The abscess may be eliminated through a root canal procedure, in which the pus is drained and the canal cleaned and filled. If the infection has spread into underlying tissue, however, more general surgery may be required. In a procedure called an apicoectomy, both the root and the bone that covers the root may be drilled away by the oral surgeon. Antibiotics may also be administered to eliminate the infection completely.

USES AND COMPLICATIONS

Most periodontal problems begin with dental caries and gingivitis, an inflammation of the tissue of the gums by bacteria that are associated with the formation of caries. If these conditions are not treated by a dentist in their early stages, they may progress to more serious problems. In addition to the danger of abscess formation, pockets of infection may develop under the gums. Gingivectomy, a minor surgical procedure in which such sites of infection are removed, can usually treat cases that are not advanced.

In most instances, proper oral hygiene is sufficient to prevent problems. When necessary, surgical procedures can treat more advanced cases successfully. Complications are rare and are usually associated with bacteria that are able to survive in isolated crypts. Such sites offer threats of abscess formation. For this reason, the dentist or oral surgeon will monitor the results of the periodontal procedure for some months afterward.

—*Richard Adler, Ph.D.*

See also Abscess drainage; Abscesses; Cavities; Dental diseases; Dentistry; Endodontic disease; Gingivitis; Periodontitis; Root canal treatment; Teeth; Tooth extraction; Toothache.

FOR FURTHER INFORMATION:

Anderson, Pauline C., and Martha R. Burkard. *The Dental Assistant*. 6th ed. Albany, N.Y.: Delmar, 1995.

Renner, Robert. *An Introduction to Dental Anatomy and Esthetics*. Chicago: Quintessence, 1985.

Ring, Malvin E. *Dentistry: An Illustrated History*. Reprint. New York: Harry N. Abrams, 1992.

Ward, Brian R. *Dental Care*. New York: Franklin Watts, 1986.

PERIODONTITIS
DISEASE/DISORDER

ANATOMY OR SYSTEM AFFECTED: Bones, gums, mouth, musculoskeletal system, teeth

SPECIALTIES AND RELATED FIELDS: Dentistry

DEFINITION: Caused by poor dental hygiene and accumulation of plaque, periodontitis is the inflammation and infection of the gums, which may cause loss of the supporting bone and eventually lead to tooth loss. Symptoms include halitosis (bad breath), loosening of teeth in the sockets, and aching teeth and gums when cold, hot, or sweet foods are eaten. If an abscess develops, tenderness, swelling, pain, and fever may also occur. Good oral hygiene and regular visits to the dentist for teeth cleaning can both treat and prevent periodontitis. Avoiding sweet snacks can also assist in preventing plaque formation.

—Jason Georges and Tracy Irons-Georges
See also Abscess drainage; Abscesses; Cavities; Dental diseases; Dentistry; Endodontic disease; Gingivitis; Halitosis; Periodontal surgery; Teeth; Tooth extraction; Toothache.

FOR FURTHER INFORMATION:

Smith, Rebecca W. *The Columbia University School of Dental and Oral Surgery's Guide to Family Dental Care*. New York: W. W. Norton, 1997.

Ward, Brian R. *Dental Care*. New York: Franklin Watts, 1986.

Woodall, Irene R., ed. *Comprehensive Dental Hygiene Care*. 4th ed. St. Louis: C. V. Mosby, 1993.

PERISTALSIS
BIOLOGY

ANATOMY OR SYSTEM AFFECTED: Abdomen, gastrointestinal system, intestines, stomach

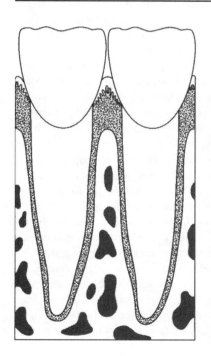
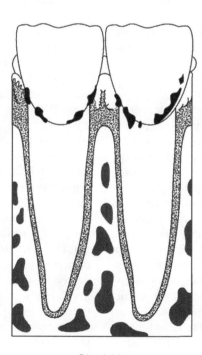
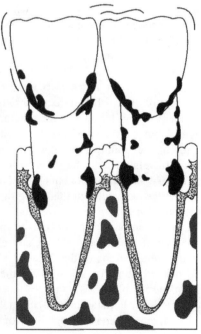

Normal   Gingivitis   Periodontitis

Periodontitis begins with poor oral hygiene; if unchecked, it leads to gingivitis, inflammation and infection of the gums, erosion of supporting bone, and tooth loss.

SPECIALTIES AND RELATED FIELDS: Gastroenterology, internal medicine

DEFINITION: A series of muscular contractions that sweep along the gastrointestinal tract, causing a localized narrowing that pushes food and waste material from the mouth to the anus for excretion.

KEY TERMS:

digestion: the mechanical and chemical process of breaking down food into small units called molecules, which are then absorbed into the bloodstream

distal: away from the point of origin; for example, the distal esophagus is the end toward the stomach

gastrointestinal motility: the spontaneous movement of the gastrointestinal tract; for example, it includes peristalsis but not chewing

gastrointestinal tract: the digestive tract; a tubelike series of organs which includes the mouth, pharynx, esophagus, stomach, small intestine, large intestine, and anus

involuntary muscle contractions: muscle contractions that occur unconsciously, such as those of the intestines

proximal: toward the origin; for example, the proximal esophagus is the end toward the throat

smooth muscle: muscle which, when viewed under a microscope, does not have striations, which are stripes seen in skeletal muscle cells; smooth muscle contracts involuntarily

STRUCTURE AND FUNCTIONS

The gastrointestinal (GI) tract is a muscular tube about 10 meters long. It includes the mouth, pharynx, esophagus, stomach, the small and large intestine, and anus. The channel running through this tube is the lumen. Food travels through the GI tract to be broken down into very small components called molecules. Food molecules pass through the lining of the GI tract into the bloodstream, a process called absorption. Waste material that is not absorbed is eliminated as feces.

Since digestion, absorption, and elimination occur in different regions of the GI tract, the contents must be pushed aborally, meaning in the direction away from the mouth. This occurs by means of peristaltic contractions. Peristaltic contractions begin with a localized, circumferential narrowing of the lumen. From the outside of the organ, it would look as if someone had put a tight, invisible ring around the tract, causing a localized constriction. This constriction sweeps along the digestive tract, pushing the contents aborally. Peristaltic contractions require four major components: the muscular wall of the GI tract, nerve cells in the walls of the GI tract, nervous connections with the brain, and a relay system in the brain. These work together so that the contractions are coordinated on all sides of the lumen, progressing aborally.

Most of the GI tract is lined with smooth muscle, which is controlled by a part of the nervous system that does not require any conscious effort for its function. The wall of the digestive tract contains two layers of muscle. The inner layer consists of several cell layers of muscle cells arranged concentrically. In the outer layer, the cells are arranged longitudinally. When the inner layer of cells is stimulated by nerves, it contracts, producing a narrowing of the lumen that pushes material aborally. When the outer layer of cells contracts, it produces shortening of the long axis of the GI tract, causing an increase in the diameter of the lumen. This enlargement is especially important in the esophagus, which must sometimes accommodate large pieces of food.

There are two networks of nerve cells in the wall of the GI tract. The important network that affects peristalsis is called the myenteric plexus, located between the circular and longitudinal layers of muscle cells. It contains nerve cells that receive impulses from nerves coming from the brain and transmit impulses to the muscle cells. This plexus probably has multiple functions; one is to help ensure that peristaltic contractions occur in the proper direction. It also enables peristalsis to begin after local distension of the esophagus. If a large piece of food is stuck in the esophagus, peristaltic contractions begin pushing the food down into the stomach.

Nervous connections between the esophagus and the brain influence peristalsis. Some neurons carry sensory information from the esophagus to the brain; this information is important for the brain to be able to sense discomfort in the esophagus. Other neurons carry information from the brain to the esophagus that can modulate the contraction strength and speed of peristalsis. A relay system in the brain stem is involved in the process of swallowing and may also play a role in controlling peristalsis. It is not yet clear to what degree peristalsis is governed by the brain as compared with the smooth muscle cells or the myenteric plexus.

Peristaltic contractions are measured by means of an instrument called a manometer, which can be advanced into organs such as the esophagus. It monitors increases in intraluminal pressure (pressure inside the

GI tract) caused by contractions. A tracing is obtained which plots pressure versus time. Different tracings are obtained for different regions of the esophagus. Thus in a recording of peristalsis, tracings of the proximal esophagus would show a transient increase in pressure, followed by an increase in pressure in the middle and then the lower esophagus.

Peristaltic contractions differ in the various regions of the GI tract and serve different purposes. In the esophagus, where peristalsis serves to propel food from the pharynx into the stomach, the main type of activity is called primary peristalsis. Initiated by swallowing, it propels material down toward the stomach. Primary peristaltic contractions can push a solid mass of food down the esophagus in about six seconds. With the aid of gravity, liquids do not need peristaltic contractions, pouring down the esophagus in one second. Between the lower end of the esophagus and the stomach is a narrowed region called the lower esophageal sphincter (LES). This is an area of muscular circular fibers that normally keep the junction between the esophagus and stomach closed. When food

The Action of Peristalsis

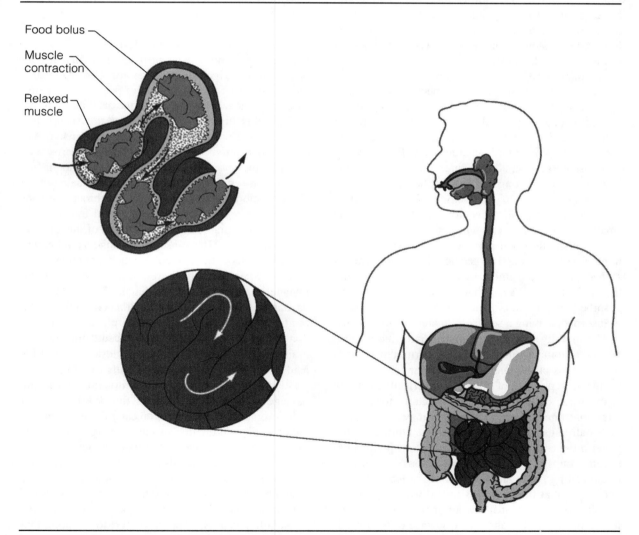

Food bolus

Muscle contraction

Relaxed muscle

Peristalsis, the means by which food is moved through the intestines, consists of a constant series of contractions and relaxations of the intestinal walls.

or liquids reach the lower esophagus, the LES relaxes, allowing them to pass into the stomach.

There are two main motility patterns in the stomach and small intestine: fasting and fed patterns. In the fasting pattern, there are long periods of relaxation that alternate with periods of intense, repeated peristaltic contractions. These contraction waves migrate along the stomach toward the small intestine. When viewed on a manometry tracing, they are called migrating motor complexes (MMCs). In the fed pattern, the motility response varies depending on the content of the meal. Solid meals cause different effects in different parts of the stomach. The proximal stomach is mainly for storing food after eating and for emptying stomach contents. After eating solids, the proximal stomach relaxes to accommodate the food. Later it slowly contracts, emptying the material toward the small intestine.

The distal stomach functions are mixing food with stomach acid and enzymes and mechanically grinding solids into smaller pieces. Solids and liquids are also propelled by peristaltic contractions toward the pylorus, a narrow region separating the stomach from the small intestine. Only material that is finely ground will pass into the small intestine. The small intestine is about 5 meters long and moves the material coming from the stomach, called chyme, toward the large intestine. During the transit of chyme through the small intestine, water and nutrients are absorbed. Enzymes digest the food particles in chyme down into minute particles called molecules. Molecules are absorbed through the lining of the small intestine into the bloodstream. Wastes that cannot be digested and absorbed pass to the large intestine, where more fluid is absorbed, leaving a semisolid material called feces.

The motility pattern of the small intestine is similar to the stomach during fasting: Intermittent periods of peristalsis push material down toward the large intestine. The purpose of this fasting peristaltic activity is to sweep cellular debris and bacteria toward the large intestine. Otherwise, bacteria may overgrow in the small intestine and cause diarrhea. During the fed pattern, there are no prolonged quiescent periods between groups of peristaltic contractions as there are in the fasting state. The function of the fed state is to make sure that the chyme is mixed well with digestive enzymes and that it has an opportunity to come into contact with the absorptive surface of the intestinal wall. Like the rest of the GI tract, small intestinal motility is subject to the brain's control. If a person is placed in a dangerous situation, the brain will send signals to decrease intestinal motility, which is no longer a priority.

In the large intestine, or colon, peristalsis slowly moves feces toward the rectum for elimination. The slow movement enables most of its water to be absorbed into the bloodstream. In the proximal large intestine, liquid feces are moved back and forth by contractions, eventually moving distally. Eventually, this material becomes more solid, moving intermittently toward the rectum. This intermittent peristalsis is called mass movement. It fluctuates during the day, increasing in frequency after meals. As the feces distend the rectum, a reflex occurs which stimulates passage of stool to the outside.

DISORDERS AND DISEASES

Peristalsis may not always progress normally: It may be absent, too vigorous, or uncoordinated. An example of a disorder involving lack of peristalsis is a disease called achalasia. Achalasia means "failure to relax." In this disease, the LES does not relax, thus impairing the passage of food into the stomach. Another characteristic of the disorder is aperistalsis, which is the absence of peristalsis of the esophagus. A common symptom of achalasia is dysphagia, which is a sensation of food sticking in the throat. Another symptom is regurgitation of undigested food, during or just after eating; thus, many victims of this disease will lose weight. The cause of achalasia is unknown. There is a reduction of cells called ganglion cells, which are nerve cells that are normally present in the myenteric plexus of the esophagus. There may also be damage to the cell bodies of nerve cells in the brain that innervate the myenteric plexus. It may be that the damaged ganglion cells cause damage to the brain cells, or vice versa. A neural lesion in the LES leads to a sphincter muscle that fails to relax appropriately, which in turn leads to an obstruction in the passage of food. One result is that the esophageal body eventually becomes chronically dilated. Another factor leading to dilation of the esophagus is the loss of ganglion cells in the wall of its body, which results in the absence of peristalsis.

Achalasia usually begins during middle age. The predominant symptom is dysphagia, which always occurs with solids and frequently occurs with liquids. Eating often causes chest discomfort to the point that people with achalasia lose weight because they avoid eating. Although regurgitation of undigested foods commonly occurs shortly after eating, it may occur hours later, especially when the patient lies down at night. Food contents may be regurgitated and inhaled, leading to nighttime coughing spells.

On manometry, the peristaltic waves normally seen after an act of swallowing are absent. Instead, there may be some low-pressure contractions appearing simultaneously in all parts of the esophagus. Their lack of orderly progression prevents the contractions from propelling food down the esophagus. The pressure in the lumen of the esophagus in the region of the LES may be elevated; often the LES is so tight that it is difficult to advance the manometry catheter through it. The LES also fails to relax normally after swallowing.

Treatment of achalasia rarely results in a return of peristalsis, but it may provide relief for the obstruction caused by a tight LES. Some drugs can relax the LES, but success with these is variable. Often, stretching of the LES with instruments called dilators is performed. The best dilator is a long instrument with an inflatable balloon at the tip. The dilator is advanced into the esophagus and through the LES. The balloon tip is positioned so that when the balloon is inflated, it stretches the LES. The LES needs to be stretched to the point of tearing the circular muscle in order to achieve a long-term reduction in LES pressure. This procedure is risky and may be complicated by the development of a large tear, creating a hole in the wall of the esophagus called a perforation.

Surgical cutting of the LES, called an esophagomyotomy, is more effective than dilation. The more reduction in LES tone that occurs, however, the more likely it is that the person will suffer from reflux of stomach acid. Although the stomach's lining is normally resistant to the irritating effects of acid, the esophagus may become irritated when exposed to chronic acid reflux. A common symptom of this reflux is heartburn, which is a sensation of hot material rising into the esophagus.

An example of a too vigorous peristalsis is esophageal spasm. There are a few different manometric patterns to esophageal spasm, the most consistent being one of intense contractions of the esophagus that do not sweep along its length and occur at the same time at different regions of the esophagus. During manometry, the esophagi of those patients with spasms are often very sensitive to stimulation with certain drugs, resulting in increased strength, or amplitude, of the contractions. Not only is there an exaggerated

motor response in esophageal spasm, but there may be an abnormal sensory component to the disorder as well. For example, loud noises or stressful mental tasks may cause an increase in the amplitude of contraction waves. Esophageal spasms tend to occur in middle age. The most common symptom is intermittent dysphagia that is variable in severity. It is not progressive and does not result in weight loss. Chest pain is a frequent complaint and may mimic that of a heart attack. The diagnosis of esophageal spasm often requires manometry. Another useful diagnostic test is to attempt to re-create symptoms of spasm. For example, a drug known to cause smooth muscle contraction is administered. If symptoms similar to the presenting chest pain complaints are re-created, then it is presumed that the pain was attributable to esophageal spasm. Various medications that relax smooth muscle have been used to treat these spasms, with moderate success. Once the medications are stopped, however, the symptoms recur.

Peristalsis requires both an intact myenteric plexus and well-coordinated connections with the central nervous system. Diabetics commonly suffer from neuropathy, a condition which damages various nerve cells in the body. This neuropathy is thought to be responsible for their various gastrointestinal motility disturbances. About 75 percent of diabetics can be shown to have esophageal peristaltic disturbances— up to one-third of diabetics suffer from dysphagia— although they are commonly not felt. Using manometry, an absence of coordinated peristaltic activity is usually found. Diabetics may have tertiary contractions, which are noncoordinated, nonpropulsive contractions of the wall of the esophagus.

Stomach, or gastric, motility is abnormal in about 25 percent of diabetics, resulting in disordered gastric emptying. Emptying of liquids may be normal, but emptying of solids is commonly delayed. There is commonly absence of MMCs, which results in a decrease in the ability of the stomach to grind food. There may also be spasms of the distal stomach, causing obstructions for materials that would normally flow out of the stomach and into the small intestine. Another gastric disturbance is gastroparesis, a decreased ability to relax in order to accommodate a large meal. Thus diabetics often have difficulty finishing an entire meal. They may also suffer from nausea, bloating, and vomiting after meals. Treatment of gastroparesis includes reduction of blood sugars if they are elevated. This may be accomplished by reducing food intake (if previously excessive) or increasing the dose of insulin. Medications called prokinetic drugs may increase gastric motor activity; examples include metoclopramide, dromperidone, and cisapride.

The neuropathy suffered by diabetics may damage the nerves that normally stimulate intestinal reabsorption of fluid; this results in diarrhea, which affects 10 percent of diabetics. Other diabetics suffer from constipation, which may be caused by impaired peristaltic activity of the colon.

PERSPECTIVE AND PROSPECTS

In 1674, the first case of what was probably achalasia was reported by Sir Thomas Willis. He called the disorder "cardiospasm." In 1937, F. C. Lendrum proposed that cardiospasm was attributable to incomplete relaxation of the LES, and he changed the condition's name to "achalasia," which means "failure to relax." The leaps and bounds in studying peristalsis occurred in the twentieth century. In 1927, E. Jacobson reported on an association between esophageal spasm and strong emotion; gastroenterologists continue to note a correlation between spastic disorders of the GI tract and anxiety. In 1938, E. M. Jones reported an experimental reproduction of esophageal spastic pain by the inflation of small balloons in the esophagus. The development of esophageal manometric techniques began to blossom in the 1970's. These techniques have allowed a much more thorough understanding of gastrointestinal motility, which enables the development of better drugs to alter it. Therapeutic advances in treating disorders such as achalasia have been made, most markedly starting in the 1940's, when A. M. Olsen performed pneumatic dilations of the esophagus.

One of the most practical advances for disorders involving decreased peristalsis is in the development of prokinetic drugs—drugs that increase gastrointestinal motility. Metoclopramide was the first to be developed, and it is still in use. Cisapride may prove to be effective, especially because its effects do not wear off with chronic use, as do those of metoclopramide.

Perhaps the most important advances in research into gastrointestinal motility are in studying the signals for smooth muscle contraction, such as which chemicals (neurotransmitters) are released by the nerve endings where they join up with nerve cells in the myenteric plexus or with the smooth muscle cells. More than fifteen hormones and neurotransmitters are

known to affect gastrointestinal motility. Once their specific functions are better understood, researchers can try to develop drugs that mimic their effects, depending on whether an increase or a decrease in motility is desired.

In the United States, some motility disorders are very prevalent, such as irritable bowel syndrome (IBS). This disorder involves symptoms such as abdominal distension, abdominal pain relieved by bowel movements, bowel movements that become more frequent during pain episodes, constipation, or loose stools. IBS accounts for almost as many working days lost because of illness as the common cold. It is the most common cause for referral to a gastroenterologist, accounting for 20 to 50 percent of their referrals. Surveys in the general population have shown that approximately 15 percent of Americans have symptoms to justify a diagnosis of irritable bowel syndrome.

Most disorders of peristalsis are not deadly, but they can cause much discomfort. With better understanding of the neurology of the gut, as well as the acceptance of a model for understanding the disorders that includes attention to psychological and sociological effects on the GI tract, medicine will be able to better decrease the suffering that occurs with these disorders.

—*Marc H. Walters, M.D.*

See also Colitis; Constipation; Crohn's disease; Diabetes mellitus; Diarrhea and dysentery; Digestion; Gastroenterology; Gastroenterology, pediatric; Gastrointestinal disorders; Gastrointestinal system; Intestinal disorders; Intestines; Irritable bowel syndrome (IBS); Obstruction.

FOR FURTHER INFORMATION:

American Medical Association. *Drug Evaluations Annual 1993*. Chicago: Author, 1993. This text, updated annually, contains practical information on prokinetic agents, including those not yet available in the United States as of 1993. Also contains information on most other prescribed drugs.

Feldman, Mark, Marvin H. Sleisenger, and Bruce F. Scharschmidt, eds. *Sleisenger and Fordtran's Gastrointestinal and Liver Disease: Pathophysiology, Diagnosis, Management*. 6th ed. 2 vols. Philadelphia: W. B. Saunders, 1998. One of the best comprehensive textbooks on gastrointestinal diseases and physiology. Dozens of journal articles are referenced at the end of each chapter.

Ganong, William F. *Review of Medical Physiology.* 19th ed. Stamford, Conn.: Appleton and Lange, 1999. This paperback includes a valuable section emphasizing control of gastrointestinal motility. A classic work.

Tortora, Gerard J., and Sandra R. Grabowski. *Principles of Anatomy and Physiology.* 9th ed. New York: John Wiley & Sons, 2000. Contains outstanding discussions of human anatomy and physiology.

Vantrappen, G., and J. Hellemans. "Treatment of Achalasia and Related Motor Disorders." *Gastroenterology* 79 (July, 1980): 144-154. This article mentions that medications are of little value in treating achalasia and then discusses surgery and dilation as treatments for achalasia.

PERITONITIS
DISEASE/DISORDER

ANATOMY OR SYSTEM AFFECTED: Abdomen

SPECIALTIES AND RELATED FIELDS: Emergency medicine, gynecology, internal medicine

DEFINITION: Peritonitis is a serious infection or inflammation of the peritoneum, the membrane lining the abdominal cavity. Most cases result from the rupture or perforation of one of the abdominal organs or from the spread of infection from an infected organ. Other causes include injury to the abdominal wall by a knife or bullet, pelvic inflammatory disease (PID), or the rupture of an ectopic pregnancy. The symptoms of peritonitis include abdominal pain, chills, fever, dizziness, rapid heartbeat, and low blood pressure. Possible complications include shock, blood poisoning, intestinal obstruction, and death. Peritonitis is curable with early diagnosis and treatment.

—Jason Georges and Tracy Irons-Georges
See also Abdomen; Abdominal disorders; Ectopic pregnancy; Gastrointestinal disorders; Gastrointestinal system; Infection; Intestinal disorders; Intestines; Pelvic inflammatory disease (PID).

FOR FURTHER INFORMATION:
Augustin, Rolf. *Peritonitis in CAPD.* New York: Karger, 1987.
Disease Prevention/Health Promotion: The Facts. Palo Alto, Calif.: Bull, 1988.
Fry, Donald W. *Peritonitis.* Mount Kisco, N.Y.: Futura, 1993.
Mitsuoka, Tomotari. *Intestinal Bacteria and Health.*

Translated by Syoko Watanabe. Tokyo: Harcourt Brace Jovanovich, 1978.
Phillips, S. F. *Diarrhea: Infectious and Other Causes.* Washington, D.C.: National Digestive Diseases Information Clearinghouse, U.S. Dept. of Health and Human Services, Public Health Service, National Institutes of Health, 1985.

PERTUSSIS. *See* WHOOPING COUGH.

PET SCANNING. *See* POSITRON EMISSION TOMOGRAPHY (PET) SCANNING.

PHARMACOLOGY
SPECIALTY

ANATOMY OR SYSTEM AFFECTED: Blood, brain, cells, immune system, nervous system, psychic-emotional system

SPECIALTIES AND RELATED FIELDS: Anesthesiology, biochemistry, cytology, endocrinology, family practice, microbiology, oncology, preventive medicine, public health, toxicology

DEFINITION: The science or knowledge of chemicals that affect biological processes.

KEY TERMS:
pharmacist: a person with a license to dispense or sell drugs prescribed by a medical practitioner, such as a dentist, physician, or veterinarian
pharmacognosy: the preparation of medicinal agents from natural sources
pharmacologist: a scientist who studies pharmacology
therapeutics: the use of chemicals in the diagnosis, prevention, or treatment of disease
toxicology: the study of the effects of toxins (poisons) and their antidotes

SCIENCE AND PROFESSION
The science of pharmacology includes the history, source, physical and chemical properties, and biochemical and physiological effects of therapeutic chemicals, diagnostic chemicals, toxins, and related substances.

"Drug" is a noun in common usage, but it has complex meanings, some of which are almost mystical. "Drug" or "medicine" is often used today to indicate a therapeutic substance usually obtained from a pharmacy or drugstore. "Drug" also is used to indicate an illegal substance used for mood-altering effects. Historically, people made their own drugs from materials found naturally in plants, animals, and minerals; some people continue to do so. The term "drug" in this article will focus on the meaning as it is understood by scientists called pharmacologists. Any chemical can be thought of as a drug by a pharmacologist: A drug is simply a chemical that produces a change in a biological process.

Water and oxygen can be thought of as drugs, as can foods and poisons. "Drug," therefore, is a word to indicate an idea, concept, or perception about a chemical. When the chemical, such as oxygen, is causing a change in a biological process, then the chemical is acting as a drug. If the same chemical is causing a change in some other kind of system—for example, causing an iron rod to rust—then the chemical is not acting as a drug. Drugs may be found in nature or made using human skills. There is no difference between a chemical that comes from nature (such as water, a sugar, or a protein) and one that comes from a factory. Most of the chemicals used today as drugs are made by humans.

The biological process that is being changed by a drug may be one occurring in a sick person. Many drugs are used therapeutically—that is, to treat diseases—but pharmacologists do not limit drugs to therapeutic chemicals. They are interested in drug effects on any biological process, even healthy ones occurring in plants and microorganisms, as well as those in animals and humans.

All drugs, even therapeutic drugs, will have several effects on biological processes. Some of these effects are seen only at high concentrations. Unwanted effects, especially if they are injurious, are called adverse effects. A serious adverse effect, especially if it requires special medical treatment, may be considered a toxic reaction, or poisoning. Any chemical that produces an injurious effect, one that is detrimental to a biological process, is called a toxin. The severity of the toxic effect is based on the concentration of the toxic substance. Toxic substances in the environment are called pollutants.

The idea of a drug concentration is very important. "Concentration" refers to the number of chemical molecules in a specified volume (such as a teaspoonful, an ounce, or a milliliter) of liquid or gas. Concentration is related to dosage and to the intensity of a drug's effect on a biological process.

Concentration and the related concept of dilution are easy to understand. Two spoonfuls of sugar in a glass of water form a more concentrated solution of sugar-water than one spoonful. The more concentrated sugar-water will taste sweeter. Since taste is a biological process caused by a chemical, the chemical (sugar) can be thought of as a drug. The concentration of the chemical affects the biological process. There is a limit, however, to the sweetness of a solution. At some point, more sugar added to the solution will not increase the sensation of sweetness. Adding more sugar may result in a "toxic" reaction of nausea and even vomiting.

There are also different kinds of sugars. When one says that some are sweeter than others, one means that sweeter sugars will be just as sweet at very dilute concentrations as less-sweet sugars at very high concentrations. Thus the first kind of sugar is said to be more potent than the second, even though the second can be just as sweet at high concentrations. Some sugars, however, will not taste very sweet regardless of the concentration. This example illustrates principles that are shared by many drugs. It is important to understand that taking a double dose of a drug will not necessarily produce a double effect. It is also important to understand that a tiny dose of one drug can have the same, or even stronger, biological effect than a large dose of a similar drug.

Most therapeutic drugs act directly on special parts of cells within the body called receptors. A receptor is part of the cell structure, just as a hand is part of human anatomy. A receptor for a specific drug is always located at the same place within a cell, just as the hand is always located at the end of an arm. Yet there are different kinds of receptors, just as people have both hands and feet, found at various locations in cells. Many receptors are found on the cell surface; others are found inside cells. Some receptors are found only on certain types of cells.

Each type of receptor has a specific function, just as hands and feet have specific functions. When a drug "fits" a receptor, like a ball or a glove fits a hand, the receptor starts the biological process for which the drug is known. Different kinds of drugs can fit a single type of receptor, which explains why different drugs (for example, aspirin and acetaminophen) can have similar effects (relieve pain). Furthermore, one drug may be able to act on several different types of receptors. A receptor, however, can have only one biological response to all the drugs that act on it.

A drug acting on receptors in cells of one organ can affect distant organs. For example, a drug acting on brain cells may cause the nerves acting on blood vessels to increase blood pressure, which can change the heartbeat. The effect of a drug on receptors is usually temporary and should be reversible. In most cases in which a drug works through a receptor, the receptor releases the drug after the two have come together. If this release does not occur, the receptor is said to be blocked. The blockage of a receptor can be therapeutically beneficial, but it may sometimes lead to an adverse reaction.

In humans and animals, most drugs travel in the bloodstream to reach cell receptors. The drug enters the bloodstream after being applied to a body surface or after being swallowed, inhaled, or injected. The effect of the drug is eventually diminished because the body dilutes the drug, chemically alters it (so that it no longer has a pharmacological effect), and eliminates it. Chemical alteration of drugs usually occurs in the liver by a process called biotransformation. Elimination of most drugs, or their biotransformed relatives, usually occurs through the urine but may sometimes occur through secretions (sweat, tears, or breast milk), feces, or even exhaled gases.

DIAGNOSTIC AND TREATMENT TECHNIQUES

Three examples of the use of therapeutic chemicals in the field of pharmacology are anesthesia, cardiac-enhancing drugs, and drugs that fight infections. These examples demonstrate the use of various classes of drugs and provide insight to the variety of drug action.

Anesthetics are chemical painkillers. They are very important drugs because most diseases are accompanied by pain. Often, the first objective of a patient is to get relief from the pain, even though the anesthetic may do nothing to cure the disease. Pain is a sensation felt in the brain, not at the site of injury. Special nerves at the site of injury send a signal (nerve impulse) to the brain, where it is interpreted as pain occurring at a specific location in the body. Mild pain and severe pain are detected by different kinds of nociceptive (pain) nerves. As pain increases in severity, the brain not only perceives and interprets the pain but also sends out special autonomic signals.

Autonomic signals from the brain serve an extremely important function: They control body functions that do not require conscious thought, such as sweating, heart rate, blood pressure, digestion, and eye focus. Autonomic signals coordinate these functions and change them in response to conditions outside the body. When the body is threatened, such as when a person is frightened, autonomic signals prepare the body to fight or to flee the threatening situa-

tion. The pain of surgery causes the brain to send autonomic signals to put the body in a defensive state, resulting in sweating and increased heart rate, breathing, and blood pressure. Additionally, all the muscles of the body will become tense. This defensive state is undesirable during surgery.

Drugs used to relieve pain without causing unconsciousness are called analgesics. Mild pain can usually be controlled with an analgesic such as aspirin. More severe pain may require an opioid analgesic such as morphine. Sometimes, the term "narcotic" is used as a synonym for opioid analgesics, but that term is often used in a legal context to indicate any chemical that can cause dependence (addiction). An analgesic changes the way in which the brain interprets a nociceptive stimulus. The most severe pain, such as that during surgery, is controlled by an anesthetic. An anesthetic may act at a specific site, such as on the nerves of a tooth; a local anesthetic such as novocaine blocks the transmission of the nociceptive stimulus to the brain. Other anesthetics, required for major surgery, cause a loss of consciousness; these are called general anesthetics. As with all therapeutic drugs, the action of an anesthetic is reversible.

A general anesthetic should perform several functions: It should alter the brain's interpretation of pain, cause a temporary amnesia that prevents remembrance of the nociceptive sensation, produce autonomic stability, and cause muscle relaxation. This is much to ask of a single drug. Therefore, general anesthesia is achieved by using several drugs, each capable of accomplishing one or more of the goals.

A general anesthetic agent usually works on nerve cells to provide pain relief and amnesia. These general functions are provided by both kinds of general anesthetics, those that are inhaled and those that are injected. Other drugs are used to control autonomic signals and to provide for muscle relaxation. When the surgery is completed, the patient returns to consciousness as the anesthetic agents are removed from the nerves. This is done by biotransformation and by excretion. Pain immediately after surgery will be controlled by an opioid analgesic. When the pain diminishes as healing progresses, it becomes milder and can be controlled with a nonopioid analgesic.

Drugs are also important in helping people recover from a myocardial infarction (heart attack). The heart is a pump that supplies blood to all cells of the body. Blood carries oxygen and nutrients to the cells and removes waste materials from them. The heart is a living muscle composed of cells, and blood vessels must supply each cell of the muscle. If a blood vessel in the heart becomes suddenly blocked, then the cells served by that blood vessel become starved and die. This is a heart attack. If only a small portion of the heart is injured, the person can survive the attack, especially if drugs are given that strengthen the heart.

An important class of drugs used to strengthen the heart is composed of the cardiac glycosides, such as digitalis. These drugs act to improve the ability of the heart cells to use calcium efficiently. Calcium is essential to maintaining a normal heartbeat. Because a heart attack is painful, it causes defensive autonomic response from the brain. It is important to use analgesics to relieve the pain and other drugs to control the autonomic response. Another important therapy is to provide more oxygen to the heart. This is done directly, by administering oxygen, but it is also done by using drugs that can remove the blockage from the blood vessel. Since the blockage usually occurs when a blood clot forms in a damaged blood vessel, drugs that dissolve clots can sometimes open the blocked vessel and restore the flow of oxygen-rich blood to the starved cells. A person recovering from a heart attack will sometimes be given drugs to prevent another blockage. Some drugs prevent fatty deposits from forming in the vessels, while others act to slow down clot formation.

Drugs used to treat infection are designed to kill cells. Infection is caused by foreign microbes attacking the body. The microbes may be viruses, bacteria, fungi, or even parasitic worms. Antimicrobial drugs (antibiotics) are given to the infected person to destroy the foreign cells without damaging the patient's own cells. Therefore, the drug must be selectively toxic to the foreign cells. Few drugs are perfectly selective, however, and most have some toxic effects on the patient as well.

There are many ways to develop a selectively toxic drug, but selectivity usually depends on a unique feature of the invading foreign cells, such as the cell walls of bacteria. Human cells are surrounded by cell membranes. Bacteria have cell membranes as well, but they also have cell walls outside of these membranes. If the bacterial cell wall is damaged, then the bacterium becomes weakened and can be killed by the body's defense mechanisms. Penicillin is an antimicrobial drug that damages the cell walls of many bacteria. Penicillin has very few adverse effects on the infected person, because human cells do not have

cell walls. (Unfortunately, some people develop an allergic reaction to penicillin.)

PERSPECTIVE AND PROSPECTS

In the prehistoric world, priests were called upon to intercede for persons suffering from disease and pain. As humans gained experience and developed a means of sharing that experience, especially through written records, it was noticed that certain components of the diet could reliably inflict or relieve pain; these were the first drugs. Similar effects could be obtained by inhaling natural materials or applying them to the skin through rubbing or injection. Such activities were thought to involve supernatural powers, however, and authority to use these drugs was still relegated to members of the priesthood, namely witch doctors.

Writings about the medicinal properties of natural materials can be found in Chinese, Egyptian, Greek, Indian, and Sumerian manuscripts, some of which are thought to be six thousand years old. The Ebers Papyrus of Egypt (1550 B.C.E.) contains more than eight hundred prescriptions using seven hundred drugs. It was known that some drugs were cathartics, some were diuretics, and others were purgatives, soporifics, or poisons. Yet factual knowledge about why these actions occurred was lacking, in large measure because knowledge of body function and chemistry was lacking. In this absence, people speculated that drug action was due to "essential properties" of the drug, such as warmth or wetness.

Only with the European Renaissance in the early sixteenth century was the domination of religion over intellectual inquiry challenged effectively. The scientific method was applied to questions about the natural world, both physical and living. In 1543, Andreas Vesalius published the first complete description of human anatomy. In the early seventeenth century, William Harvey discovered the circulation of blood, and Antoni van Leeuwenhoek discovered living cells with his microscope. In the eighteenth century, the chemistry of oxygen was established by Carl Scheele, Joseph Priestley, and Antoine Lavoisier, and by the end of the century, chemical methods were becoming available to separate pure drugs from crude natural concoctions. In 1806, Friedrich W. Serturner purified morphine from the opium poppy, and in 1856, Friedrich Wöhler isolated cocaine from coca. Also of great intellectual and economic significance was the 1828 synthesis by Wöhler of urea, the first of many chemicals which heretofore had been available only from living organisms. Hormones, general anesthetics, and the bacterial cause of infectious diseases were discovered.

Until the twentieth century, drugs were discovered empirically; they existed in nature and needed to be "found." The knowledge gained during the nineteenth century about how drugs worked enabled pharmacologists of the twentieth century to "design" drugs not found in nature. For example, Paul Ehrlich, a German scientist, announced in 1910 that he had successfully combined a dye that stains bacteria with the poison arsenic to create an antibacterial drug, arsphenamine (Salvarsan), that is highly effective in treating syphilis. In a similar way, the antibacterial sulfonamide chemicals were developed in the 1930's.

It was soon recognized that the powerful effect of pure drugs (in contrast to potions made from natural materials) had the potential to harm as well as to help, to kill or to cure. The safe use of these drugs required special knowledge, so government agencies were established in the twentieth century to regulate drug manufacture and distribution. The original Pure Food and Drug Act, passed by the United States Congress in 1906, imposed quality controls on drug manufacturers. In 1927, Congress created the Food, Drug, and Insecticide Administration (FDIA), to enforce the 1906 law. Until 1914, any drug could be obtained without a prescription; this was changed by the Harrison Narcotic Act. Further limitations on the sale of drugs to the general public came with the Food, Drug, and Cosmetic Act of 1938 and the Durham-Humphrey Amendment of 1951. The Controlled Substance Act of 1970 superseded the Harrison Narcotic Act.

With the passage of time, enforcement responsibilities were changed. The FDIA became the Food and Drug Administration (FDA) in 1931 and was transferred from the Department of Agriculture to what is now the Department of Health and Human Services. The Drug Enforcement Administration for controlled substances was established within the Justice Department.

At the end of the twentieth century, drugs were available to alter personality, to cure some types of cancer, to influence the reproductive system, and to control the body's response to foreign materials such as transplanted organs. Many of these drugs were designed using powerful computers. Drugs were available to alter plant and animal ecosystems. The use of these drugs, such as the pesticide DDT and the war-time defoliant Agent Orange, had devastating effects on humans and the environment that required remedial action. Drugs were even being developed to alter cellular genetics.

—Armand M. Karow, Ph.D.

See also Acid-base chemistry; Aging: Extended care; Anesthesia; Anesthesiology; Antibiotics; Anti-inflammatory drugs; Bacteriology; Catheterization; Chemotherapy; Clinical trials; Critical care; Critical care, pediatric; Digestion; Drug resistance; Emergency medicine; Enzyme therapy; Enzymes; Estrogen replacement therapy; Fluids and electrolytes; Food and Drug Administration (FDA); Food biochemistry; Genetic engineering; Geriatrics and gerontology; Glycolysis; Herbal medicine; Homeopathy; Hormone replacement therapy; Hormones; Laboratory tests; Melatonin; Metabolism; Microbiology; Narcotics; Oncology; Pain management; Pharmacy; Psychiatry; Psychiatry, child and adolescent; Psychiatry, geriatric; Rheumatology; Sports medicine; Steroids; Terminally ill: Extended care; Thrombolytic therapy and TPA; Toxicology; Tropical medicine; Veterinary medicine.

FOR FURTHER INFORMATION:

Barnhart, Edward R., ed. *Physician's Desk Reference.* 47th ed. Oradell, N.J.: Medical Economics Books, 1993. This widely available book is a compilation of the information that drug manufacturers must legally provide to physicians and pharmacists. Manufacturers pay the publishers to include their products.

Griffith, H. Winter. *Complete Guide to Prescription and Non-Prescription Drugs.* New York: Putnam, 1999. Compiled by a highly experienced physician, this paperback book provides the layperson with useful and authoritative descriptions of more than seven hundred generic drugs. These drugs are cross-indexed by drug classes and brand names.

Hardman, Joel G., and Lee E. Limbird, eds. *Goodman and Gilman's The Pharmacological Basis of Therapeutics.* 9th ed. New York: Pergamon Press, 1996. The premier authoritative reference on the pharmacology of therapeutic drugs in humans. It is written for scientists and medical specialists, but the diligent layperson can learn much from it.

Temin, Peter. *Taking Your Medicine.* Cambridge, Mass.: Harvard University Press, 1980. This scholarly book traces the history of drug regulation in the United States to 1980. Discusses policy formation and the roles of physicians, drug providers, and the government.

Winter, Ruth. *A Consumer's Dictionary of Household, Yard, and Office Chemicals.* New York: Crown, 1992. The author, a highly regarded science writer, catalogs alphabetically several thousand common chemicals, their intended use and potential hazards. Provides a helpful discussion of how to treat the toxic effects of these chemicals.

PHARMACY

SPECIALTY

ANATOMY OR SYSTEM AFFECTED: Blood, brain, cells, nervous system, psychic-emotional system

SPECIALTIES AND RELATED FIELDS: Anesthesiology, biochemistry, cytology, endocrinology, family practice, microbiology, oncology, pharmacology, preventive medicine, public health, toxicology

DEFINITION: The art or profession of preparing and dispensing drugs and medicine.

KEY TERMS:

apothecary: a pharmacist or druggist

compound: to mix or combine; to make by combining parts of elements

dispense: to prepare and distribute (as with medicines or prescriptions)

medicine: the science and art of diagnosing, treating, curing, and preventing disease, relieving pain, and improving and preserving health; any drug or other substance used in treating disease, healing, or relieving pain

pharmaceutical: of or relating to pharmacy; a medicinal drug

pharmaceutical care: the responsible provision of drug therapy to improve a patient's quality of life

SCIENCE AND PROFESSION

Traditionally, pharmacy was confined to the distribution and dispensation of medications, but modern pharmacists have become recognized drug experts. The concept of pharmaceutical care promises to change pharmacy practice for the public's benefit.

Pharmacy has always been primarily a retail practice. In the early days of the profession, physicians would often choose not to prepare medications for their patients and instead would refer them to apothecaries. These practitioners received the prescriptions and then prepared and dispensed them to patients. A patient who was familiar with the symptoms of the ailment might choose to return to the apothecary to seek another course of this medication. Recognizing that many problems responded well to standardized medicinal formulas, many apothecary shops expanded into ready-made products to accommodate patients when they chose to seek care from the pharmacist rather than from the physician. A similar situation exists in modern times with over-the-counter medications (those available without a prescription).

Until the 1970's, few changes occurred in the basic practice description of pharmacy. Physicians continued to devote themselves to the diagnosis and treatment of patients, and pharmacists continued to concentrate on pharmaceutical products. By this time, most of the collection and preparation phases of developing medications were done by the emerging pharmaceutical manufacturers. Most medications arrived at the pharmacy in a ready-to-dispense form such as a tablet, capsule, elixir, syrup, suppository, or ointment. This trend has progressed to the point that fewer than 1 percent of prescriptions require compounding.

Most people have some understanding of pharmacy and pharmacists, usually through visits to the local drugstore. In this setting, pharmacists practice what is known as retail or community pharmacy practice. For many customers, it is not clear whether the pharmacist is a businessperson or a health care professional; the pharmacist is actually both. On the one hand, a pharmacy often sells merchandise that many people associate with a variety store, such as pens, greeting cards, gift items, and photographic film. Yet a pharmacy also has a license to sell something no variety store can: prescriptions—such as antibiotics for an ear infection, pain medication for a broken arm, or high blood pressure medication to help prevent a stroke or heart attack.

Contemporary retail pharmacists operate and manage complex businesses. Pharmacists in this setting have additional challenges, such as personnel management, the organizational structure of the pharmacy, and the general focus of the business. Unrecognized activities may involve location analysis and selection, obtaining loans to purchase and operate the business, and store design. The pharmacist must evaluate a computer system for dispensing medicine, inventory control, reordering stock, and interfacing with insurance company computers for payment.

Not all retail pharmacy activity occurs in a community-based store. Many companies have founded large conglomerates called chain pharmacies. Occa-

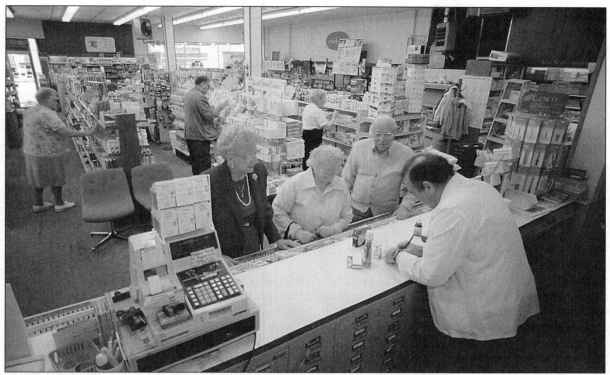

Pharmacists inform patients of drug interactions and precautions both verbally and through informational packaging. (Digital Stock)

sionally, these may resemble independent community stores, but they share common ownership. Most people are familiar with typical chain pharmacies within supermarkets and discount stores.

Other practice sites of pharmacy are associated with the use of numerous, highly complex medications. Typically, this practice setting is a hospital. The medications used in a hospital cannot be given to the patient for self-administration. Such medications include intramuscular or intravenous injections, implantable drug reservoirs, beads containing drugs, or medications requiring close observation of the patient. Hospital practice places a unique demand on the pharmacist to be a resource for drug information. Also, specialized pharmacists may become members of health care teams in which the pharmacist provides a service to improve patient care rather than supplying a product.

During the 1980's, the insurance industry in the United States reformed payment methods for hospitals, trying to reduce the time that a patient remains in the hospital. The goal was to minimize cost by allowing the patient to recover at home. This policy reduced expensive payments to hospitals and shifted

the expense to less costly home health care. Pharmacy's ability to provide sophisticated medications in this setting allows the patient to stay at home and has created a growing segment of practice for some pharmacists.

Pharmacists are not limited to the practice types or settings mentioned above. Large pharmaceutical manufacturing firms have typically been a fertile source for their employment. They provide positions in sales, marketing, management, and product development and manufacturing. Sometimes, pharmacists direct clinical research efforts, while others perform quality assurance activities or market research or may hold executive positions in upper management.

One career track with tremendous significance to the profession is pharmacy education. The educational process in pharmacy has seen many changes. The European apothecary used an apprenticeship system with no requirement for formal education. Modern pharmacists are well educated, often having more than 150 college credit hours at graduation. After graduation, many students will choose further study for an advanced degree. These degrees may focus on management (master of business administration or master of hospital pharmacy) or more academic areas (master of science or doctor of philosophy). Other pharmacists may choose postgraduate clinical studies (doctor of pharmacy). Traditionally, after completion of their advanced degree, most pharmacists join faculties at Colleges of Pharmacy. Others are recruited by institutional and corporate employers, who find that this training provides employees with skills that are beneficial to company operations.

The pharmacy student must complete an extensive application process to gain entry into a College of Pharmacy. In addition to good grades, applicants usually must score well on the Pharmacy College Admission Test (PCAT), although this test is not required by all schools. A favorable score gives the applicant a good idea of the level of preparation and skills that schools are seeking. An excellent workbook to help prepare for this test is *Pharmacy College Admissions Test (PCAT)* (2d ed., 1991), by Dick R. Gourley. It reviews sample test questions and discusses general information regarding pharmacy education. The work also contains a list of Colleges of Pharmacy to help the applicant decide where to apply.

Generally, an applicant must have a minimum of sixty-five hours of prepharmacy education. In the United States, required courses include English composition, general and organic chemistry, general biology (or botany and zoology), college physics, college algebra and trigonometry, principles of accounting, American history, principles of economics, and electives in the humanities and behavioral or social sciences.

An emerging area of pharmacy practice is the provision of clinical services. The clinical pharmacist is a high-level consultant and expert on drug therapy and related issues. Many of these persons conduct daily patient rounds with physicians and other health care providers. These clinical specialists review medication orders for their appropriateness, verify proper doses, inform nurses of special issues when giving the medication, recommend laboratory tests and other monitoring procedures, and assess the outcome of treatment with the physician.

Once, most clinical specialists were associated with general internal medicine services. Then the need for clinical pharmacy services in other areas became apparent. To serve these patients properly, pharmacists established specialty practices. Recognized specialty areas in pharmacy include pediatrics, geriatrics, nutri-

tion, drug information, ambulatory care, critical care, family practice, surgery, cardiology, oncology, nuclear medicine, mental health, and pharmacokinetics, a specialty unique to pharmacists. The latter discipline evaluates what happens to a medication when it enters the body. These practitioners help to choose the best dose of a medication in order to optimize clinical outcomes.

The increasing demands for enhanced services and the growing complexity of the tasks required to provide clinical services identified a need for further training. Many pharmacy specialists undergo residency training to provide this additional proficiency. In the United States, the Board of Pharmaceutical Specialities established credentials to allow pharmacists to become board certified within many of these specialty areas. Nonspecialized residency training is available in general hospital pharmacy practice. The hospital is becoming a complicated practice site requiring unique knowledge; this type of training addresses the practice needs of those pharmacists in hospital practice.

A lesser-known area of practice for pharmacists is clinical research. The pharmacist may serve as the principal investigator or research coordinator for another investigator. The research may address an unknown question about a drug already on the market, evaluate a new treatment, or gather information about drug-related problems. In the United States, clinical research usually serves as background material required by the Food and Drug Administration before it allows a pharmaceutical manufacturer to sell a new medication. Results from research are published in various medical and pharmacy journals so that interested professionals have rapid access to this new information and apply it to patient care.

DIAGNOSTIC AND TREATMENT TECHNIQUES
In the United States, the movement toward all Colleges of Pharmacy awarding an entry-level doctor of pharmacy (Pharm.D.) degree is allowing the entire profession of pharmacy to expand beyond the traditional roles of dispensing medications, compounding medications, storing and purchasing medications, and advising patients and other health care providers about drugs.

The ideas leading to this evolutionary spark are probably best described by Jack Robbins in *Pharmacy: A Profession in Search of a Role* (1979). He describes the challenges to the profession and the desires of the professionals within pharmacy practice. The changes in pharmacy practice since the 1960's, when Pharm.D. degrees were first awarded, have resulted in the development and acceptance of pharmaceutical care. Under this philosophy, the pharmacist has a responsibility to the patient to ensure that the most rational course of therapy is applied and that a positive outcome is fostered at all times.

Pharmaceutical care involves four major functions: curing disease, eliminating or reducing a patient's symptomatology, arresting or slowing a disease process, and preventing a disease or its symptomatology. A pharmacist works with other professionals in designing, carrying out, and monitoring a therapeutic plan that will produce specific therapeutic outcomes for the patient. These activities involve three major functions: identifying potential and actual drug-related problems, resolving drug-related problems, and preventing potential drug-related problems. This concept was conceived in the late 1980's by the nationally noted pharmacy educators Charles D. Hepler and Linda H. Strand. Hepler and Strand recognized that pharmaceutical care is applied in three distinct levels: primary (outpatient and community pharmacies); secondary, (acute care hospitals, skilled nursing facilities, home health care, and specialized care programs, such as oncology and pain control); and tertiary (inpatient critical care and teaching medical centers). Each level of practice demands specialized services from the pharmacist.

The specifics of pharmaceutical care have been described by noted pharmacists William E. Smith and Katherine Benderev. They state that it is the sum of all pharmaceutical services (clinical and nonclinical) that are required and received by a patient. The provision of pharmaceutical care means that the pharmacist is responsible for a patient's achievement of the desired clinical outcome secondary to the use of medications. Inherent in this idea are the basic functions of the pharmacist common to all levels of care: to develop and use a patient medication profile; to interpret, question, clarify, verify, and validate all drug-related orders; to provide a safe and efficient drug-dispensing system; to monitor drug therapy for safety, efficacy, and desired clinical outcome; to screen for drug allergies, drug interactions, and concomitant drug use; to detect and report drug allergies and adverse reactions; to recommend initial or alternative drug therapies; to respond to drug information requests from physicians, nurses, and patients; to teach health care providers and patients about drug use; to obtain medication histories by interviewing patients; to assist in the selection of the drugs of choice and dosage forms; to conduct drug-use evaluations in order to gauge the appropriateness of drug use and the achievement of desired therapeutic outcomes; and to apply pharmaceutical principles for selected drug therapies.

Pharmacy practice in the retail setting (independent community and chain stores) primarily stresses filling prescriptions, but many activities behind the scenes are also helping the patient. Besides buying safe and reasonably priced products, the pharmacist maintains a patient profile, which includes data about other medications the patient may be taking, allergies, and other relevant patient information. The pharmacist uses the system to screen for drug interactions, to avoid potential allergic reactions, and to ensure that the patient receives proper doses of the medication.

Traditionally, patient education by pharmacists has consisted of a brief discussion augmented by precaution labels on the prescription bottle. Pharmacists and other health care professionals have since recognized the importance of more thorough patient education in achieving optimal results using medications. Pharmacists will adapt this information to the needs of the patient. Their methods include one-on-one counseling, audiovisual programs, preprinted or computer-generated handouts, and other specific information sources. Some retail pharmacists use their computer systems to send refill reminders, allowing pharmacists to assist physicians in their efforts to ensure that people with chronic problems are treated adequately. Hospital-based pharmacists may implement detailed discharge counseling for patients returning home in order to review treatment plans or answer questions about medications unfamiliar to the patient.

Many pharmacists offer a very valuable service in nursing homes and long-term care facilities. Here the pharmacist evaluates the patient's medication regimen for problems. Elderly patients often use six or more medications, making them more prone to dangerous drug interactions. Moreover, these elderly persons may have many illnesses, making them more sensitive to the adverse effects of medications. Pharmacists assess whether chronic conditions are being controlled, whether medications are being given and are stored properly, and whether efforts to ensure the patient's safety are adequate. The latter activity may include recommendations to stop the use of a medication because of side effects, drug interactions, or toxicity. Also, the pharmacist may recommend laboratory tests to monitor drug therapy.

An area where pharmacy practice is expanding is hospital practice. In the United States in the 1960's, the pharmaceutical manufacturing process began to see radical growth, with both the numbers and the complexity of medications increasing steadily. Hospitalized patients place unique demands on pharmacists for specialized services. These pharmacists maintain their control and responsibility for dispensing medication, yet their role has extended into being part of the drug decision-making process. A simple example is a change in the traditional role of controlling medication inventory. The hospital pharmacist will establish and use a formulary, a list of medications approved for use in the hospital. Formularies control medication costs by preventing the purchase of unneeded products and by placing restrictions on the use of expensive or dangerous medications. The pharmacist helps make complex decisions, such as determining the proper doses of highly toxic medications. Since hospitalized patients are very ill, watching for potential allergic reactions and side effects is very important. For cases in which treatment decisions are unclear, the pharmacist may help the physician in selecting a treatment.

Often, hospitalized patients require special methods for the administration of medication. Pharmacists need to be knowledgeable about intramuscular and intravenous routes of administration. Intravenous medications may require complex mixing and preparation. These products must remain sterile (no bacteria can be present) and may have special storage or handling requirements. Frequently, intravenous medication is given over a fixed amount of time; therefore, the pharmacist must be familiar with the infusion pumps that regulate the amount of solution over a given period. Many medications also require specialized tubing called catheters for administration. One can readily see that the pharmacist plays a central role in addressing any special needs of patients requiring complex medications.

All these activities require the pharmacist to work closely with other professionals in the hospital. Frequently, the pharmacist will work with nurses to ensure proper administration and timing of doses or to monitor the patient for side effects. Laboratory personnel need to understand that medications may effect certain laboratory tests. In addition, laboratory technicians may draw blood from the patient to check the concentrations of many types of medication. Proper timing of the sample collection is very important in making changes to the patient's drug therapy.

PERSPECTIVE AND PROSPECTS

Pharmacy is a unique profession whose origins can be traced back to 3000 B.C.E. in the age of ancient Babylonia-Assyria, Egypt, and Greece. Early pharmacists tended to concentrate on the identification, collection, and preparation of materials for use in the medicinal drugs, or pharmaceuticals, of the period. Yet, commonly, the line separating medical practitioners and pharmacists was thin. Early pharmacists and physicians were equally regarded as healers, meaning either could make a diagnosis or prescribe and prepare a treatment. In Europe, the term "apothecary" was coined to define pharmaceutical activities of the era. These conditions persisted until around 1240 C.E., when the Holy Roman Emperor Frederick II issued an edict to separate the professions. Pharmacy became responsible for the preparation and dispensation of medications, and medicine became responsible for the diagnosis and treatment of the patient.

No professional practice is without change. Pharmacy practice evolved from the gathering, extraction, and preparation phase of the apothecary to the contemporary role of medication distribution. Now, with the complexity of drug therapy increasing rapidly as new medications enter the market, physicians are becoming increasingly dependent on pharmacists to keep them informed of this rapid expansion in knowledge. Moreover, pharmacists have become more active in dealing with patients and their physicians. Pharmaceutical care is a natural extension of this evolution, in which the pharmacist's role becomes more patient-centered rather than focusing on a product. The tenets of pharmaceutical care promise to become deeply ingrained in the practice of pharmacy, replacing the dated idea that the profession of pharmacy is limited to dispensing medications.

—*Charles C. Marsh, Pharm.D.*

See also Acid-base chemistry; Aging: Extended care; Antibiotics; Chemotherapy; Critical care; Critical care, pediatric; Digestion; Drug resistance; Emergency medicine; Enzyme therapy; Enzymes; Estrogen replacement therapy; Fluids and electrolytes; Food biochemistry; Genetic engineering; Geriatrics and gerontology; Glycolysis; Herbal medicine; Homeopathy; Hormone replacement therapy; Hormones; Melatonin; Metabolism; Narcotics; Pain management; Pharmacology; Sports medicine; Steroids; Terminally ill: Extended care; Toxicology; Veterinary medicine.

FOR FURTHER INFORMATION:

Ansel, H. C., and N. G. Popovich. *Pharmaceutical Dosage Forms and Drug Delivery Systems.* 7th ed. Philadelphia: Lea & Febiger, 1999. This general text discusses the traditional aspects of pharmaceutical product compounding and preparation (pharmaceutics).

Brown, Thomas R. *Handbook of Institutional Pharmacy Practice.* 3d ed. Bethesda, Md.: American Society of Hospital Pharmacists, 1992. Focuses on hospital pharmacy practice. The authors describe administrative and management topics, drug information activities, the research and education roles of pharmacists, and special issues, such as consulting in nursing homes.

Effective Pharmacy Management. 6th ed. Kansas City, Mo.: Marion Merrell Dow, 1990. This excellent publication is provided as a professional service by a pharmaceutical manufacturer. It provides information primarily on careers in retail pharmacy, giving the reader information about starting and managing a drugstore.

Gable, Fred. *Opportunities in Pharmacy Careers.* Lincolnwood, Ill.: VGM Career Horizons, 1990. This reference work provides the reader with a review of career tracks and the multiple practice sites available for pharmacists.

Generali, Joyce A., and Michele A. Danish, eds. *Pharmacy: 985 Questions and Answers.* 11th ed. Stamford, Conn.: Appleton and Lange, 1997. This is a source of practical answers to commonly asked questions about pharmacy. May be useful for consumers and for beginning pharmacy students.

Gourley, Dick R. *Pharmacy College Admission Test (PCAT).* 2d ed. New York: Prentice Hall, 1991. The author reviews pharmacy practice and education, job opportunities, and licensure and practice regulations. A practice test is provided.

PHARYNGITIS
DISEASE/DISORDER

ANATOMY OR SYSTEM AFFECTED: Respiratory system, throat

SPECIALTIES AND RELATED FIELDS: Family practice, internal medicine, otorhinolaryngology

DEFINITION: Pharyngitis is the inflammation or infection of the throat caused by infection from bacteria, viruses, or fungi. Symptoms may include a sore throat, difficulty in swallowing, fever, swollen glands in the neck, a red or grayish throat, and generalized aching. Chronic pharyngitis can be caused by smoking or by postnasal drip associated with allergies or other diseases or infections of the nose. The risk of developing pharyngitis also increases with illness, fatigue, diabetes mellitus, immune deficiencies, excess alcohol consumption, oral sex, and general epidemics. Gargles may be used to relieve throat pain; cool mist humidifiers can relieve dry, tight throats; and moist, warm compresses can alleviate swollen and tender glands. Recovery can be spontaneous or assisted with antibiotics or antifungal drugs.

—Jason Georges and Tracy Irons-Georges
See also Allergies; Nasopharyngeal disorders; Otorhinolaryngology; Sore throat.

FOR FURTHER INFORMATION:

Goldstein, Mark N. "Office Evaluation and Management of the Sore Throat." *Otolaryngologic Clinics of North America* 25 (August, 1992): 837-842.

Scott, Andrew. *Pirates of the Cell.* Oxford, England: Basil Blackwell, 1985.

Wagman, Richard J., ed. *The Complete Illustrated Book of Better Health.* Chicago: J. G. Ferguson, 1986.

PHENYLKETONURIA (PKU)
DISEASE/DISORDER

ALSO KNOWN AS: Phenylalaninemia, phenylpyruvic oligophrenia, Følling's disease

ANATOMY OR SYSTEM AFFECTED: Blood, brain, liver, nervous system

SPECIALTIES AND RELATED FIELDS: Biochemistry, embryology, epidemiology, genetics, neonatology, neurology, nutrition, pediatrics

DEFINITION: A genetic disorder caused by a deficiency of the liver enzyme phenylalanine hydroxylase.

KEY TERMS:

phenylalanine: an essential amino acid

phenylalanine hydroxylase: a liver enzyme that catalyzes the conversion of phenylalanine to tyrosine

tetrahydrobiopterin: a cofactor for the conversion of phenylalanine to tyrosine

CAUSES AND SYMPTOMS

Phenylketonuria (PKU) is a genetic disorder, occurring in about 1 in 10,000 births, that disrupts the metabolism of the amino acid phenylalanine. The disorder is caused by a deficiency of phenylalanine hydroxylase, a liver enzyme that catalyzes the conversion of phenylalanine to tyrosine. Since normal phenylalanine metabolism is blocked, the amino acid accumulates in blood and tissues, resulting in progressive, irreversible mental retardation and neurological abnormalities. Most forms of PKU are caused by a mutation—more than two hundred mutations are now characterized—in the gene for phenylalanine hydroxylase. A small percentage of infants with PKU have a variant form of the condition, known as malignant PKU. This disorder is caused by a defect in the synthesis or metabolism of tetrahydrobiopterin, a cofactor for the conversion of phenylalanine to tyrosine, or in other enzymes along the pathway. Without treatment, malignant PKU causes a progressive, lethal deterioration of the central nervous system.

Infants with classic and malignant PKU appear normal; however, if untreated, the condition severely impairs normal brain development and growth after a few months of age, causing mental retardation, seizures, eczema, and neurological and behavioral problems. Affected infants have plasma phenylalanine levels ten to sixty times above normal, along with normal or reduced tyrosine levels and high concentrations of the metabolite phenylpyruvic acid in their urine.

Newborns are screened routinely for PKU within the first three weeks of life, usually by using whole blood obtained from a heel prick. Elevated phenylpyruvic acid levels also can be detected in urine of infants with PKU after adding a few drops of 10 percent ferric chloride, resulting in a deep green color. Newborns often have transient PKU—elevated phenylalanine and phenylpyruvic acid levels in the first few weeks of life that normalizes—so classic PKU should be distinguished from transient conditions. Elevated phenylalanine levels that persist beyond a few weeks of life, accompanied by normal or low tyrosine levels, usually indicate an inborn error of metabolism. Malignant PKU is usually diagnosed by detecting biopterin metabolites in urine or showing that tetrahydrobiopterin supplementation restores normal phenylalanine and tyrosine levels.

Babies of mothers with PKU are at high risk of brain damage, impaired growth, and malformations of the heart and other organs. Managing maternal phenylalanine levels at near normal concentrations appears to be crucial to preventing these cognitive and neurological defects.

The clinical basis for the damaging effects of PKU on the brain is unclear. Elevated phenylalanine levels may interfere with brain myelination or neuronal migration during development. In addition, PKU decreases the levels of the neurotransmitters dopamine and serotonin, which may be the basis for its neurological effects.

TREATMENT AND THERAPY

The detrimental effects of PKU can largely be controlled by maintaining phenylalanine levels in the normal range through a strict low-phenylalanine diet. This complex diet, often supplemented with tyrosine, prevents the buildup of phenylalanine and its metabolites in body tissues. Children whose phenylalanine levels are regularly monitored and managed can achieve normal intelligence and development. In infants with malignant PKU, tetrahydrobiopterin or cofactor supplements are required to control phenylalanine levels successfully.

Treatment for PKU must begin at a very early age, before the first three months of life, and usually continue through adulthood, or else some degree of mental retardation or neurological abnormalities is expected. Screening newborns for PKU before three weeks of age is mandated in all fifty U.S. states. Strict control of phenylalanine levels also is indicated for pregnant women with PKU because their babies are at high risk for severe brain damage.

The successful treatment of PKU depends on managing phenylalanine levels. However, the diet is complex and challenging to sustain over many years. Since phenylalanine is an essential amino acid, found in virtually all proteins, maintaining adequate nutrition is nearly impossible on a low-phenylalanine diet. The treatment requires rigorous protein restriction and the substitution of most natural proteins in meat, fish, eggs, and dairy products. Phenylalanine intake must not be too restricted, however, or else phenylalanine deficiency can occur.

In some cases, dietary treatment for PKU can be discontinued or made less restrictive as children age, without causing severe effects. In many cases, however, the ill effects of the disorder carry into adulthood unless dietary management is continued over the long term. Untreated adolescents and adults may exhibit behavioral or neurological problems, difficulty concentrating, poor visual-motor coordination, and a low intelligence quotient (IQ).

PERSPECTIVE AND PROSPECTS

Phenylketonuria was the first inborn error of metabolism shown to affect the brain. This genetic disorder was discovered in the 1930's by Ivar Asbjørn Følling. Since its discovery, PKU has been controlled successfully by rigorous newborn screening programs and careful dietary management of phenylalanine levels in pregnant women and in children with the disease. Newer research has focused on improving medical formulations for low-phenylalanine diets and amino acid supplementation for children and adults.

In the 1980's, clinical trials examined the use of dialysis-like procedures that allowed the rapid breakdown of phenylalanine in the blood. The treatment applies to pregnant women with PKU or those with severely elevated phenylalanine levels resulting from stress or illness. In the 1990's, PKU became the focus of gene therapy research. Animal models of PKU have been successfully treated by introducing normal phenylalanine hydroxylase deoxyribonucleic acid (DNA) into the liver cells of mice. Since the underlying genetic defects are known in most cases of PKU, gene therapy appears a likely research focus for long-term treatment.

—*Linda Hart, M.S., M.A.*

See also Digestion; Enzymes; Genetic diseases; Mental retardation; Neonatology; Nervous system; Neurology, pediatric; Nutrition; Screening.

FOR FURTHER INFORMATION:

Behrman, Richard E., and Robert M. Kliegman, eds. *Nelson Essentials of Pediatrics*. 3d ed. Philadelphia: W. B. Saunders, 1998. This is a great text for medical students rotating through pediatrics. It has thorough explanations of diseases and treatments.

Dworkin, Paul H., ed. *Pediatrics*. 4th ed. Baltimore: Williams & Wilkins, 2000. This text offers helpful examination questions for determining diagnosis. Includes bibliographical references and an index.

Lloyd, June K., and Charles R. Scriver. *Genetic and Metabolic Disease in Pediatrics*. London: Butterworths, 1985. Discusses metabolic and hereditary diseases in infancy and childhood. Includes bibliographical references and an index.

PHLEBITIS
DISEASE/DISORDER

ANATOMY OR SYSTEM AFFECTED: Blood vessels, circulatory system

SPECIALTIES AND RELATED FIELDS: General surgery, internal medicine, vascular medicine

DEFINITION: The inflammation of a vein, often seen in conjunction with blood clots within the deep and superficial veins outside the heart.

KEY TERMS:

embolus: a detached blood clot that may travel through the venous system to lodge in other major veins, such as a pulmonary embolus, which may cause blockage of the major blood vessels within the lungs

endothelial damage: disruption of the cellular lining of a blood vessel such as a vein; part of Virchow's triad

hypercoagulability: an increase in the ability of blood to clot or to change from a liquid state to a solid one; coagulation of blood is dependent upon activation of clotting agents within the body

stasis: stagnation of blood or the failure of blood to flow; venous stasis may be the result of obstructions to outflow from the veins

superficial thrombophlebitis: inflammation and clotting of the veins of the arms and/or legs that lie just beneath the surface of the skin and drain into the deep veins of the limbs

venous thrombosis: formation of a blood clot within the veins of the body

CAUSES AND SYMPTOMS

Phlebitis, meaning the inflammation of a vein, is a general term used to describe the presence of blood clots, or thrombi, in the veins of the body outside the heart. Blood clots because of the formation of clotting agents, such as fibrin. When blood clots within the body, there are three principal factors involved: damage to the venous endothelium, the cells that form the lining of the vein; venous stasis, or failure of the blood to flow; and hypercoagulability, or an increase in clotting factors in the blood. These three features associated with phlebitic episodes—endothelial damage, stasis, and hypercoagulability—are referred to as Virchow's triad (named for Rudolf Virchow, who in 1846 described the characteristics of thrombus formation in the deep veins of the lower extremities).

Patients with phlebitis will complain of swelling, tenderness, and inflammation of the affected limb. If the clot has formed in the veins just beneath the surface of the skin, they may feel a hard, cordlike structure in the segment of the vein that is filled with a thrombus. If the blood clot has not attached firmly to the wall of the vein, it may break loose and travel in the bloodstream to enter the vessels within the lung.

These traveling clots are known as emboli and, depending on their size, they may either dissolve in the pulmonary vessels of the lung or block major vessels, preventing blood flow to that part of the lung. It has been shown that there is a greater risk of pulmonary embolism if the venous clots are formed in the leg veins above the knee than if phlebitis occurs in the calf veins.

In order to understand the factors that predispose the blood to clot within the body, it is necessary to understand the anatomy of the venous system and the mechanisms by which blood flows through the veins. Approximately 75 percent of the body's blood is found in the venous system, which is divided into three parts: the superficial veins, the deep veins, and the perforating, or communicating, veins. The superficial veins of the extremities are large, thick-walled, muscular structures that lie just beneath the skin. The deep veins are thin-walled and less muscular than the superficial veins. In the extremities, these deep veins are named after the arteries that they accompany. Blood is transported from the superficial to the deep veins by the communicating veins, or perforators. Thin, leaflike, bicuspid valves are found in most veins of the body, even in venules as small as 0.15 millimeter in diameter. These valves can open readily to allow blood to pass as it moves from the superficial to the deep veins on its return trip to the heart and can close rapidly to prevent blood flow from moving in the reverse direction. There are more valves in the veins of the calf than there are in the thigh veins, and no valves are found in the common iliac veins of the pelvis or in the inferior vena cava (the deep vein that transports blood through the abdomen).

The venous system must perform four important body functions. First, the veins must return blood that has been pumped through the arteries back to the heart. Additionally, the veins must be able to expand and contract so that they can regulate the increases and decreases in blood volume in the body. They must be responsive to the transport of blood during exercise and, along with the capillaries, play a major role in regulating body temperature.

Veins have the unique feature of being able to change their shape and size in order to respond to changes in pressure from within the vein (caused by increased fluid volume in the body) and to pressure from outside the vein (from tissue fluids and changes in pressure that occur as a result of gravity and the weight of the column of blood in the veins when one is standing or sitting up). As an example, when a hand is hanging at the side of the body, the veins on the back of the hand are full and visible because the veins are full of blood and the internal venous pressure is greater than the pressure from outside the vein. If the hand is raised over the head, the veins collapse because of the changes in internal venous pressure, gravitational and hydrostatic pressure, the pressures on the outside of the vein.

Blood is pumped under pressure by the heart to the arteries in order to supply nutrients and oxygen to the tissues. In contrast, the heart has little influence on moving blood through the low-pressure veins of the body on its return trip. Blood is returned from the extremities to the heart and lungs by contraction of the calf muscles during exercise and by changes in the intra-abdominal and intrathoracic pressures that occur with respiration. For example, with a limb at rest, blood will flow toward the heart from the superficial

Phlebitis

Thrombi: red and tender, hard along vein line

A phlebitic leg with thrombi of the surface veins.

system to the deep veins via the perforating veins as a result of the changes in abdominal and thoracic pressures that occur with breathing. With exercise, the calf muscles may exert more than 200 millimeters of mercury (mmHg) pressure on the large, saclike veins, the sinusoids in the sole, and the gastrocnemius veins of the calf, causing blood to move rapidly out of the foot and calf.

If the valves are incompetent such that the leaflets fail to meet when the valve closes, the column of forward-moving blood cannot be maintained in the segments of the veins between the valve sites. In this case, when one stops exercising, blood will flow backward toward the feet through the damaged valves, resulting in increased venous pressure at ankle level.

As one inhales, the diaphragm descends, compressing the inferior vena cava and stopping the flow of blood from the legs. With exhalation, the diaphragm rises and venous flow will continue toward the heart in a competent venous system. It is interesting that flow in the arms is under the control of intrathoracic, rather than intra-abdominal, pressure changes. Thus, with inhalation, the flow of blood from the arms increases as the pressure within the chest cavity is reduced. Upon exhalation, venous flow from the arms is impeded (which is in contrast to the respiratory effects that influence venous return from the legs).

As long as blood continues to circulate, the likelihood of clotting is reduced. There are, however, several risk factors that may cause changes in blood flow, damage to the vein wall, or hypercoagulability of the blood—the three features involved in venous thrombosis.

Venous thrombosis may occur as a result of obstructions to venous outflow from the limb. For example, taking a long trip by car, train, or airplane may require sitting for many hours without the freedom to walk around and exercise the calf muscles. Because the calf muscle pump is inactive, blood will pool in the veins of the legs. This failure of blood to flow, or venous stasis, places the individual at increased risk for clotting of blood in the calf veins. Similarly, patients who are prescribed bedrest because of accidents, pregnancy, or critical illnesses and those patients who undergo long surgical operations are at risk for forming thrombi in the leg veins because of venous stasis and, as a result of the thrombosis, are also at risk for pulmonary embolism.

The incidence of phlebitis increases linearly with age. This fact is thought to reflect an increase in the

diameter of the veins and the venous sinusoids within the calf muscles as a result of loss of elastic tissue in the vein walls. As the vein diameter increases, venous flow becomes sluggish. As an individual grows older, the muscle mass in the thigh and calf decreases and the calf muscle pump becomes less effective at moving venous blood toward the heart. This pooling of blood places elderly patients at risk for phlebitic episodes.

In the modern health care setting, the most common cause of phlebitis has been injury to the vein wall by intravenous catheters or by the infusion of drugs that cause inflammation of the venous endothelium. If a catheter is left in place for an extended period of time, infection may occur within the vein along its course, causing inflammation of the vein wall, venous stasis, and eventual thrombosis of the vein.

Inflammation of the vein may also occur as a result of venography, an invasive procedure used to determine if thrombi are present in the deep or superficial veins of patients. With this test, contrast dyes are injected into the veins to delineate the blood-flow patterns and venous anatomy and to define the segments of the vein where clots are present and are obstructing blood flow. Approximately 3 percent of patients have thrombi form in their veins following this diagnostic procedure. Approximately 8 percent of these patients will require hospitalization for treatment of postvenographic phlebitis.

Women who are taking oral contraceptives containing the hormone estrogen are thought to be at increased risk for phlebitis because of the decrease in the muscular tone of the vein wall and subsequent decrease in velocity of blood flow in the veins that results from the use of these drugs. Estrogen compounds may increase the surface adhesiveness of platelets, the blood cells that are responsible for clotting, causing them to stick together and form large clots that can block the veins. Additionally, estrogen compounds may influence chemicals within the blood that affect its ability to clot. Specifically, it is thought that these hormonal compounds affect clotting factors II, VII, VIII, and X and also cause a decrease in antithrombin III, a chemical which influences the production of thrombin, the principal factor controlling the formation of thrombi.

The influence of estrogen on the body's ability to control the production of appropriate levels of clotting factors is also noted during pregnancy and in the postpartum period. Phlebitis is diagnosed three to six times more frequently in women in the first four months following delivery than it is in women who have not become pregnant, as a result of estrogen-induced hypercoagulability of the blood. It is also interesting to note that women who deliver their babies by cesarean section are at increased risk for thrombophlebitis because of venous stasis occurring during the prolonged surgical procedure.

TREATMENT AND THERAPY

The symptoms of phlebitis—unilateral limb swelling, local inflammation, tenderness, and pain—may be associated with other medical conditions. Because there are no specific signs that are used to diagnose deep or superficial venous thrombosis, physicians misdiagnose phlebitis in approximately 50 percent of cases. As noted above, venography, once thought to be the standard for the identification of venous thrombosis, may actually predispose the patient to phlebitis. Noninvasive diagnostic techniques have been developed to demonstrate the presence, location, extent, and severity of the thrombotic process.

It has been shown that chemicals found naturally in the endothelial cells that line the veins can lyse, or dissolve, small clots. The veins of the calf have more lytic potential than the veins of the thigh and pelvis. In exercise, the compression of the calf muscles on the veins causes this material to be forced into the venous blood, thus helping to dissolve small thrombi.

Acute thrombosis of the deep veins above the knee usually requires hospitalization and infusion of heparin, a drug which can dissolve the blood clot, into the vein. If left untreated, clots in this location may continue to propagate toward the large pelvic veins or the inferior vena cava, or pieces of a thrombus, called emboli, may break off the clot and travel through the vena cava to enter the pulmonary circulation of the lungs. In many cases, pulmonary embolism is life-threatening.

Patients with clots in the deep veins of the legs are instructed to stay in bed with the leg elevated to prevent venous pooling, and moist heat is applied to the leg to promote local circulation of blood. Patients will continue to take anticoagulant drugs for several months following hospitalization to ensure that fresh clots do not form in the veins, and they are instructed to wear elastic compression stockings to promote venous circulation.

It has been shown that clots will resolve completely in approximately 70 percent of patients receiving anticoagulant therapy. The remainder of patients will continue to have obstructions of their veins because of a clot that did not lyse, and as a result of the phlebitic episode, the venous valves will become incompetent. These patients will continue to be at risk for phlebitis and frequently express complaints of having tired, aching, heavy legs. If damage to the valves is severe, venous pressure at ankle level is increased, and blood may be forced out of the veins into the surrounding tissues, causing ulcers to form.

When clots are formed in the veins of the calf, patients are requested to exercise in order to promote compression of the deep and superficial veins by the calf muscles. Such exercise encourages the release of the natural venous lytic agents and the circulation of venous blood. Small clots dissolve naturally, and there is less likelihood of a clot remaining in the veins or of the calf vein valves being severely damaged. If patients cannot exercise, they are given bedrest and treated in the same manner as those patients who have clots in the veins above the knee.

Thrombosis of the superficial veins, frequently called thrombophlebitis, is most often treated with hot compresses and elevation of the leg to relieve the local venous inflammation. Care must be taken to ensure that the clot does not continue to extend toward the segment of superficial vein where it joins the deep venous system, because the patient would then be at risk for pulmonary embolism.

Attempts have been made to bypass segments of a thrombosed vein surgically and to transplant new valves in venous segments that have become incompetent as a result of postphlebitic valve damage. Such procedures, however, have been unrewarding. Anticoagulant and lytic therapies begun early in the thrombotic process appear to offer the best results with the least long-term sequellae for phlebitic patients.

PERSPECTIVE AND PROSPECTS

It has been estimated that approximately two million people are affected by phlebitis each year in the United States and that there are approximately 200,000 deaths per year as a result of venous thrombosis. Autopsy data suggest that 1 to 2 percent of phlebitic patients will die from pulmonary embolism each year.

—*Marsha M. Neumyer*

See also Arteriosclerosis; Blood and blood disorders; Bypass surgery; Circulation; Embolism; Surgery, general; Thrombosis and thrombus; Varicose veins; Vascular medicine; Vascular system; Venous insufficiency.

FOR FURTHER INFORMATION:

Nicolaides, Andrew N., ed. *Thromboembolism: Etiology, Advances in Prevention, and Management.* Baltimore: University Park Press, 1975. This text provides an overview of venous disorders and the thrombotic process. Although dated, it continues to serve as a classic work on the fundamental concepts involved in thromboembolism.

Reader's Digest. *ABC's of the Human Body: A Family Answer Book.* Pleasantville, N.Y.: Reader's Digest Association, 1987. A concise, informative volume for home use. Contains descriptive, fascinating facts about everyday health problems.

Rutherford, Robert B., ed. *Vascular Surgery.* 5th ed. Philadelphia: W. B. Saunders, 2000. Written by one of the leaders in the field of vascular medicine, this is the clinician's textbook on vascular disorders and surgical approaches. This reference is the standard for knowledge in the field of vascular disease, diagnostic procedures, and management.

PHOBIAS

DISEASE/DISORDER

ANATOMY OR SYSTEM AFFECTED: Psychic-emotional system

SPECIALTIES AND RELATED FIELDS: Psychiatry, psychology

DEFINITION: Excessive fears of certain objects, people, places, or situations.

CAUSES AND SYMPTOMS

Phobias can induce a state of anxiety or panic, often debilitating sufferers, restricting them from full freedom of action, career progress, or sociability. For example, a heterosexual person who fears talking with the opposite sex will have problems dating and progressing socially.

Fear serves an important and necessary function in life. It keeps one from putting a hand in a flame or walking into oncoming traffic. The fear of death and the unknown is commonplace; it causes many to dislike, even dread, passing by cemeteries, even though there is no logical reason. While many forms of fear are normal, if they occur out of context, in socially unacceptable manners, too severely, or uncontrollably then the diagnosis is a phobia.

Many different phobias have been cited in the literature and have specific terms in dictionaries, constructed by prefixing the word "phobia" with Greek or Latin terms (such as acrophobia or claustrophobia). While their enumeration is an interesting pastime, phobias are serious conditions and should be treated by professional psychologists.

Phobias are caused by perceived dangerous experiences, both real and imagined. Sometimes, it is gradual: A worker may develop anxiety reactions to a boss over several weeks. Likewise, a single moment of terror can cause a lifetime of avoidance: A dog attack can generate cynophobia (fear of dogs) in a child. Children are especially susceptible to phobias, most of which are caused by fear of injury. The death of a close relative is difficult for children to understand and requires a delicate, sensitive, and honest explanation. Questions and expressions of feelings (often resentment) by the child should be encouraged and discussed. It is repression, unanswered questions, lack of supportive people, and guilt feelings that can lead to morbid attitudes and fantasies, by which phobias develop. Experiences in the past and associated fears remain dormant, to recur and be relived.

Anticipatory fears can also cause phobias. Driving trainees and beginning drivers often have phobic reactions, dreading possible accidents. Students, often the best or most conscientious ones, may spend sleepless nights worrying about the next day's examination. They fear experiences that may never occur, irrationally magnifying the consequences of their performance to one of absolute success or utter doom. Concentration produces positive results (that is, good grades), but obsession may cause paralyzing fear and pressure, even suicide. Several other theories exist regarding the cause of phobias.

Phobias can be classified into three primary groupings: simple phobias, social phobias, and agoraphobia. Simple phobias are directed toward specific things, animals, phenomena, or situations. Rodents, cats, dogs, and birds are common objects of fear. A swooping gull or pigeon may cause panic. Insects, spiders, and bugs can provoke revulsion. Many cultures have a fear of snakes. A phobia exists, for example, when a house is inspected several times each day for snakes; a phobic person may vacate a rural home for an urban dwelling in order to avoid them. Blood, diseased people, or hospital patients have caused fainting. Some vegetarians dread meat because of traumatic observations of slaughter. Fear of heights, water, enclosed spaces, and open spaces involves imagined dangers of falling, drowning, feeling trapped, and being lost in oblivion, respectively. These feelings are coupled with a fear of loss of control and harming oneself by entering a dangerous situation. Sometimes, a specific piece of music, building, or person triggers reactions; the initial trauma or conditioning events are not easily remembered or recognized as such.

Social phobias are fears of being watched or judged by others in social settings. For example, in a restaurant, phobics may eat in rigid, restrictive motions to avoid embarrassments. They may avoid soups, making noises with utensils, or food that requires gnawing for fear of being observed or drawing attention. Many students fear giving speeches because of the humiliation and ridicule resulting from mistakes. Stage fright, dating anxiety, and fear of unemployment, divorce, or other forms of failure are also phobic conditions produced by social goals and expectations. The desire to please others can exact a terrible toll in worry, fear, and sleepless nights.

Agoraphobia is a flight reaction caused by the fear of places and predicaments outside a sphere of safety. This sphere may be home, a familiar person (often a parent), a bed, or a bedroom. Patients retreat from life and remain at home, safe from the outside world and its anticipated perils. They may look out the window and fear the demands and expectations placed on them. They are prisoners of insecurity and doubt, avoiding the responsibilities, risks, and requirements of living. Many children are afraid of school, and some feign illness to remain safely in bed. Facing the responsibilities of maturation causes similar reactions.

TREATMENT AND THERAPY

Different schools of psychology espouse different approaches to the treatment of phobias, but central themes involve controlled exposure to the object of fear. Common core fears include fear of dying, fear of going crazy, fear of losing control, fear of failure, and fear of rejection.

The most effective approach to treating these disorders is a cognitive-behavioral strategy. With this approach, dysfunctional thinking is identified and changed through collaborative efforts between the patient and therapist. Additional dysfunctional behavior is identified and changed through processes involving conditioning and reinforcement.

Through an initial minimal exposure to the feared object or situation, discussion, and then progressively greater controlled contact, patients experience some stress at each stage but not at a level sufficient to cause a relapse. They will proceed to become desensitized to the object in phases. Therapists may serve as role models at first, demonstrating the steps that patients need to complete, or they may provide positive feedback and guidance. In either case, the role of the patient is active, and gradual exposure occurs. In the process, patients learn to adapt to stress and become more capable of dealing with life.

Other supervised therapies exist, some involving hypnosis, psychoanalysis, drugs, and reasoning out of one's fears. In dealing with phobics, it must be recognized that anyone can have a phobia. Patience, understanding, supportiveness, and professional help are needed. Telling someone simply to "snap out of it" increases stress and guilt.

—John Panos Najarian, Ph.D.;
updated by Nancy A. Piotrowski, Ph.D.

See also Anxiety; Bonding; Death and dying; Depression; Emotions: Biomedical causes and effects; Neurosis; Nightmares; Post-traumatic stress disorder; Psychiatric disorders; Psychiatry; Psychiatry, child and adolescent; Psychiatry, geriatric; Psychoanalysis; Psychosomatic disorders; Separation anxiety; Stress; Stress reduction; Toilet training.

FOR FURTHER INFORMATION:

Bourne, Edmond J. *The Anxiety and Phobia Workbook.* Oakland, Calif.: New Harbinger, 1995. This is an excellent self-help book for problems related to anxiety. It may also be helpful for family members seeking to understand anxiety better or to support those affected by anxiety.

Marks, I. M. *Fears, Phobias, and Rituals.* New York: Oxford University Press, 1987. This book draws on fields as diverse as biochemistry, physiology, pharmacology, psychology, psychiatry, and ethology, to form a fascinating synthesis of information on the nature of fear and of panic and anxiety disorders.

Stewart, Gail B. *Phobias.* San Diego, Calif.: Lucent Books, 2001. Discusses phobias, especially as they relate to children. Includes bibliographical references and an index.

Zane, Manuel, and Harry Milt. *Your Phobia: Understanding Your Fears Through Contextual Therapy.* Washington, D.C.: American Psychiatric Press, 1984. Introduces an effective method for treating any type of phobia and enjoy living again.

PHYSICAL EXAMINATION

PROCEDURE

ANATOMY OR SYSTEM AFFECTED: All

SPECIALTIES AND RELATED FIELDS: All

DEFINITION: A step in the diagnostic process in which the physician makes general observations about the patient and examines structures of the patient's body through touching (palpation), tapping (percussion), and listening, usually with the aid of a stethoscope (auscultation).

KEY TERMS:

auscultation: active listening, usually with the aid of a stethoscope, to sounds generated by the body

inflammation: irritation caused by such things as infection, injury, allergy, or toxins; symptoms include redness, swelling, warmth, pain, and drainage

organ system: structures of the body, in close proximity or distanced from one another, which together perform a function or functions

palpation: application of the hands, or touching, to determine the size, texture, consistency, and location of body structures

percussion: gentle tapping on the examiner's finger, which has been positioned on the patient; a hollow sound is heard over air-filled structures, while a dull thud is heard over solid areas or liquid-filled structures

sign: objective evidence of disease; a finding noted by the physician during the course of the physical examination

symptom: subjective evidence of disease, provided by the patient

INDICATIONS AND PROCEDURES

Physical diagnosis—the principles, practices, and traditions that form the foundation of the modern physical examination—has rightly been called an art. Usually taught during the first two years of medical training, the basic skills of observation, auscultation, palpation, and percussion are later augmented by hands-on experience with actual patients. For many students, this acquisition of physical diagnostic skills marks the point when they begin to feel like "real" doctors. Observation techniques may be overt or subtle, as a patient may have difficulty maintaining usual behavior if consciously aware of scrutiny. An examiner may even find it necessary to distract the patient in order to allow accurate assessment.

Auscultation, from the Latin *auscultare* ("to listen"), is generally performed with the aid of a stetho-scope. Normal bodily functions generate sounds, the presence or absence of which may provide clues to health or illness. Palpation, from the Latin *palpare* ("to touch softly"), involves the application of the examiner's hands to the patient's body. This touching conveys information about the size, texture, consistency, temperature, and tenderness of physical structures. This person-to-person contact can also exert an important calming or reassuring effect on the patient. Percussion, from the Latin *percussio* ("striking"), entails a gentle tapping on the examiner's finger, which has been placed on the patient. A resonant return is noted over hollow, air-filled structures. In contrast, solid or fluid-filled structures produce a dull fullness. A simple demonstration of this technique can be performed by partially filling a bucket with water. By tapping on the outside and noting the variations in sound, it is possible to estimate the fluid level without looking inside the bucket.

To some extent, the widespread use of sophisticated diagnostic imaging technologies has decreased the emphasis on physical examination skills in actual practice. This trend is unfortunate, because it lessens face-to-face contact between the patient and physician and may thus prove unsatisfying for both. It would be misleading, though, to view technological discoveries as competing only with the physical examination. Over the years, the usefulness of physical diagnosis has been enhanced by the availability of simple tools and elegant instruments that augment the examiner's biological senses. Common examples include the stethoscope, the oto-ophthalmoscope (a handheld halogen light source with interchangeable optics, used to view the inside of the eyes and ears), the reflex hammer, and the tuning fork. Indeed, the line separating physical diagnosis from other diagnostic procedures has been blurred as more portable devices find their way into the hands of the practicing physician.

During the physical examination, diagnostic techniques are applied in an interaction between the examiner and the patient at a unique moment in time. As such, the outcome depends on the skills of the individual examiner and on the patient's manifest physical characteristics. Changes in physical state over time are common; variation in physical examination findings over time is not unexpected. For example, heart murmurs, which are sounds generated by the heart, are graded on a scale from I/VI (one over six), designating a very faint murmur, to VI/VI (six over six), designating a murmur loud enough to be heard even without a stethoscope at a distance away from the patient. It is not uncommon for physicians, even cardiologists, who specialize in the heart, to disagree on the description of a murmur. In addition, a murmur itself can get louder or softer, or even disappear entirely with advancing age, exercise, pregnancy, or other factors. Physical diagnosis is an imprecise science. Medical educators have attempted to address this imprecision by modifying traditional instructional methods.

The physical examination should be considered within the larger context of medical information gathering. Customarily, it follows the collection of historical information about the patient's immediate and past health statuses. Like a road map, the history guides the scope and focus of the subsequent examination. This marriage of history taking and physical examination is colloquially referred to as the "H and P." Though not as often recommended as in the past, the annual complete (or "head-to-foot") physical examination may come to mind when this topic is discussed. More commonly, a physical examination is directed and focused on particular regions or organ systems.

In the general screening examination of an apparently healthy subject, a systematic survey is undertaken, following an assessment of structural and/or functional relationships. A structural division would involve examination of all the organ systems contained in or adjacent to a particular body part (for example, the foot), such as the bones, muscles, nerve supply, blood vessels, and skin. A functional examination of the cardiovascular organ system would include the heart, neck, lungs, abdomen, skin, and extremities, because manifestations of cardiovascular disease may be present in locations physically remote from the heart itself. A patient complaining of a specific problem undergoes a detailed examination of the organ systems or body structures most likely to be affected.

The sequential performance of a physical examination incorporates both structural and functional strategies. Though most examiners follow a similar framework, individual differences in physicians and patients result in a wide variety of acceptable pat-

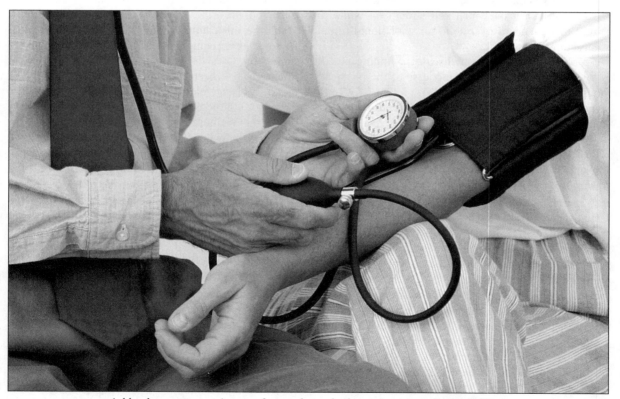

A blood pressure test is one of several standard examination tools. (PhotoDisc)

terns. Ideally, the process begins when the patient first arrives. Clues to a patient's overall level of independent function, such as mobility, dexterity, and speech patterns, may be noted. As the medical history is taken, the patient's level of alertness, as well as orientation to time, place, and self, often becomes apparent. The complete examination generally begins with the head, including the face and scalp. A survey of the skin surfaces may be accomplished with the patient completely naked, or it may be divided into discrete segments to be checked as the examination proceeds. Inspection of the eyes, ears, nose, and throat follow. Next, the neck, chest, and back are surveyed. A breast examination may be done at this time. After evaluation of the heart and lungs, the patient is asked to lie down for the abdominal examination. Genital organs may be checked at this time or may be deferred until a later part of the session. The neurologic inspection usually follows and entails the integration of findings from earlier parts of the examination with maneuvers specific to the neurological examination. In the mental status portion of the neurologic examination, formal evaluation of memory, orientation, speech patterns, and thought processes takes place. The musculoskeletal examination likewise integrates earlier findings with a detailed focus on bone and joint development and function. Finally, the extremities are checked. Upon completion of the history and physical, the diagnosis may be readily apparent or further evaluation may be needed.

Pertinent findings, whether normal or abnormal, are documented in the medical record and may be supplemented by diagrams or photographs if necessary. Depending on the purpose of the examination, these may be entered on a separate preprinted form with check-off spaces or simply noted in the chart. Computer technology allows the storage and retrieval of this information in a patient database file.

USES AND COMPLICATIONS

The application of physical examination techniques may be illustrated by considering three distinct cases: a child's school physical, a routine gynecologic examination with a Papanicolaou (Pap) smear test, and the evaluation of a sprained ankle. Each has a unique purpose dictating the breadth and detail of the techniques employed. In the school physical, the purpose of the examination is to screen a symptom-free individual for signs of previously unrecognized medical conditions; thus, the survey is broad. The annual

gynecologic examination with a Pap smear is more focused—screening for cervical cancer and other gynecologic illness, including sexually transmitted diseases— and will focus on the reproductive system. The evaluation of the sprained ankle is done to assess damage to an identified body part following a specific injury, and it will entail a detailed inspection of the affected area. How these underlying considerations influence the methods employed are apparent as each case is considered.

A child's school physical examination is preceded by a broad historical investigation of the individual's birth details, immunization status, social interactions, growth and development, and daily activity. Height and weight are measured and plotted on a growth chart to facilitate comparison with expected normal values for children of the same age and sex. In many cases, the actual numbers are of less importance than the trend relating repeated measurements. Vision and hearing screening are employed to identify defects that could interfere with school performance.

Vital signs—temperature, pulse, blood pressure, and breathing—are determined. Temperature is usually determined orally, though rectal or axillary (armpit) locations may be used. Although 37 degrees Celsius (98.6 degrees Fahrenheit) is often quoted as normal, a range of body temperatures can be found in healthy patients. Pulse rate is measured by palpation of the radial artery in the wrist. Circumstances may dictate performing this measurement in other locations, such as the carotid artery in the neck or the femoral artery in the groin. Most patients will have a pulse between sixty and one hundred beats per minute. Higher or lower numbers are common and may be related to athletic conditioning, medications, or illness.

Blood pressure is determined with the aid of a stethoscope and a sphygmomanometer (blood pressure cuff) and is expressed in millimeters of mercury. After pumping the cuff to a high pressure, the examiner slowly deflates the cuff while listening for the sounds of blood flow, usually in the brachial artery above the elbow. The onset and end of these sounds indicate the systolic and diastolic blood pressure measurements. A measurement of 120/80 (systolic over diastolic) is often considered normal, but acceptable blood pressures will vary among individuals. In this case, the normal blood pressure for a child is lower than for an adult. Breathing rate is checked by observation and varies, depending on age and medical conditions, from approximately twelve to forty

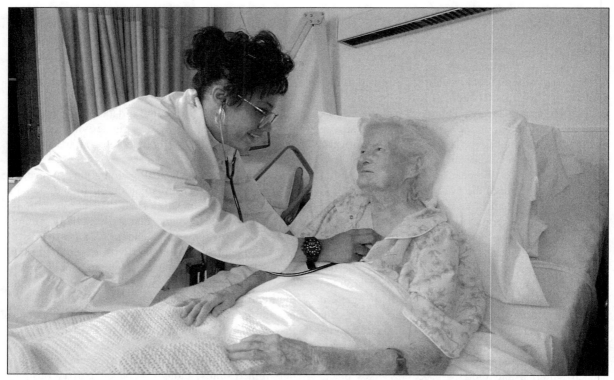

A physician uses a stethoscope to check a patient's airways. Such hands-on evaluation is important in diagnosis. (Digital Stock)

breaths per minute. Infants and children have higher rates than adults.

Following the determination of vital signs, a general physical survey is performed. The head is inspected to confirm normal shape and absence of injury. Eye movements and response to light are noted, along with any inflammation. The ears, nose, and throat are checked for signs of inflammation or scarring. A puff of air may be used to test the mobility of the eardrum. Palpation of the neck may reveal enlargement of the thyroid gland or lymph nodes. The chest is observed for abnormalities, and auscultation of the lungs is performed to monitor air flow during breathing. The cardiac examination will focus on possible murmurs, sounds generated by turbulent blood flow. Since many murmurs are harmless, and many children will have a murmur noted at some point, careful auscultation is needed to define the nature of heart sounds. If a murmur is heard, the patient may be asked to perform certain maneuvers, such as standing up quickly or taking a deep breath and straining. These actions may cause the murmur to change in a way that allows recognition of its underlying cause.

Next, the abdomen is observed for symmetry and distension. By palpation, the examiner may discover enlargement of the liver or spleen. Percussion over the liver area may confirm enlargement of that organ. Auscultation of the sounds produced by the bowels may provide clues to increased or decreased intestinal function. An external genital examination is appropriate for boys and girls. Proper descent of the testicles into the scrotum should be ascertained for boys, while menstrual complaints may dictate an internal examination for girls. Scoliosis (curvature of the spine) or other abnormalities in neurological or musculoskeletal development may be found. Examination of the skin surface is especially important in children; in addition to birthmarks, signs of child abuse may be visible and require evaluation. The length of time needed for the entire screening process will vary. If the child is already known to the examiner and has been seen recently for other reasons, the examination itself may be brief. The presence of abnormal findings may require a lengthy, detailed evaluation.

An annual gynecologic examination and Pap smear is preceded by a directed gathering of the patient's medical and family history, focusing on the reproductive system. This completed, the patient is asked to lie on her back, with her feet apart in foot rests that extend from the table. Examination of the female genital tract begins with a survey of the external structures, the clitoris, labia, and vaginal opening. A discharge or surface lesions such as sores or warts may arouse suspicion of sexually transmitted disease. Since many women have some discharge normally, however, laboratory tests are often needed to establish the diagnosis of infection. To examine the internal structures of the vagina, the examiner uses a speculum, a metal or plastic instrument about five inches long and shaped like a duck's bill. A hinge in the back allows it to be opened after insertion into the vagina, permitting inspection of the cervix and the vaginal walls with the help of a bright light. At this time, the Pap smear is taken from the cervix, usually with a small brush and wooden spatula. After removal of the speculum, the bimanual (literally, "two hands") examination is done. Gloved, lubricated fingers are inserted into the vagina, while the other hand presses down from the outside of the abdomen. For many women, this is the most uncomfortable part of the examination, though sensitivity by the examiner can lessen the discomfort. The cervix, uterus, Fallopian tubes, ovaries, and bladder may be palpated. A rectovaginal examination is performed by placing one finger in the vagina and another finger of the same hand in the rectum. This allows palpation of the space between the vagina and the rectum, as well as of the rectum itself. A breast examination may be performed during the office visit. Although most women focus on lumps, other potential signs of breast cancer, such as bleeding from the nipple, a persistent rash around the nipple, skin dimpling, or retraction (turning in) of the nipple, are noted. Because breast cancer is most common in upper and outer quadrants of the breasts and may spread to lymph nodes in the armpit, palpation of these areas is prudent.

In the examination of an apparent ankle sprain, the presence of an abnormality is a given, and the evaluation is geared to the documentation of the extent of the injury to the ankle itself and to adjacent structures. Initial observation may reveal that the patient has obvious pain while walking into the examining area. Swelling and redness may be prominent. Palpation of the leg and ankle will likely elicit tenderness over the damaged ligaments, especially with movement. Intact circulation can be confirmed by placing the fingers over the arteries of the foot and noting strong pulses. Instability of the joint itself may be discovered by applying pressure in various directions. The possibility of nerve damage is assessed by testing sensation and the strength in the foot. Though this examination is directed toward a relatively limited area of the body, it may require considerable time because of the depth of detail involved.

PERSPECTIVE AND PROSPECTS

The modern physical examination is the product of a gradual evolution rather than of a single discovery or invention. Though certain individuals are credited with the adoption of particular physical diagnostic techniques, the interpretation of bodily characteristics as indicators of health status has ancient roots that predate Hippocrates, who was born in 460 B.C.E. on the island of Cos in Greece. From the Middle Ages until the 1700's, physical examination focused on the pulse, which was accorded much diagnostic significance, and the feces. The scientific foundations of current practices were uncovered in Europe during the late 1700's and early 1800's. René Laënnec (1781-1826), a French physician, is generally acknowledged as the originator of the stethoscope, which greatly enhanced the power of auscultation. Compared to modern instruments, it was crude, consisting of a straight rigid tube which was placed between the patient's body and the physician's ear. The use of percussion as a diagnostic technique is credited to Leopold Auenbrugger and Jean-Nicolas Corvisart des Marets, contemporaries of Laënnec. Since that time, many physicians have contributed to the body of knowledge that supports physical diagnosis, and texts on the subject are filled with descriptions of maneuvers and findings that bear their names: Sir William Osler, Moritz H. Romberg, Joseph F. Babinski, William Heberden, Antonio M. Valsalva, Franz Chvostek, and so on.

Though the patient's history and physical examination have excellent diagnostic power, the adoption of advanced imaging techniques may lead to less reliance on physical diagnostic techniques. Thus, traditional hands-on examination risks falling by the wayside. Reasons for adopting new medical technologies in its place are many and controversial. Like other skills, physical diagnosis requires ongoing use if the practitioner is to remain sharp. Physical examinations can be imprecise, with disagreement among competent examiners regarding the presence or absence of findings. In contrast, electromechanical systems may provide more consistent information, though the interpretation of this information is still subjective. It is easy to forget that laboratory or radiological findings by themselves have very limited usefulness. It is not unusual for test reports to note, "Clinical correlation is advised." In other words, test results must be interpreted in the light of the information that has been gathered about the patient through the history and the physical examination. The performance of a detailed evaluation can be time consuming for the physician and the patient, especially when compared to requesting a test. Pressured by patient expectations or liability concerns, physicians may be reluctant to rely on the physical examination alone in lieu of a battery of confirmatory or exploratory scans or blood tests.

The consequences of this shift are likely to change the way in which the patient views the physician and the way in which the physician approaches the patient. Traditionally, the healing role has been intimately associated with the face-to-face meeting of doctor and patient, exemplified by the laying on of hands. From the patient's perspective, the concept of the personal physician, the familiar voice and touch of the healer who displays ongoing concern and compassion, should not be discounted. This therapeutic relationship will be compromised if physicians become mere brokers for imaging and testing services. With such an arrangement, there would be no reason for the doctor and patient even to see each other. Additionally, important diagnostic information may present itself in a manner that cannot be detected by a scan, such as a subtle clue in the patient's mannerisms or body language. Even a human examiner may have difficulty analyzing such vague information, but impressions can nevertheless contribute to the clinical evaluation. This suggests that the physical examination will continue to hold an important place in the physician's array of diagnostic tools.

—*Louis B. Jacques, M.D.*

See also Apgar score; Education, medical; Noninvasive tests; Nursing; Physician assistants; Screening; Well-baby examinations.

FOR FURTHER INFORMATION:

Kra, Siegfried J., ed. *Physical Diagnosis*. New York: Medical Examination, 1987. This textbook, replete with photographs and illustrations, is an excellent review of the subject for the reader desiring an indepth look at principles and techniques of physical diagnosis.

Shorter, Edward. *Bedside Manners*. New York: Simon & Schuster, 1985. The author describes the development of modern medicine in English-speaking cultures. A wealth of background information is provided for readers interested in the historical development of the positive and negative characteristics of the current health care system.

Siraisi, Nancy G. *Medieval and Early Renaissance Medicine*. Chicago: University of Chicago Press, 1990. This scholarly but reader-friendly work describes the rise of Western medicine from its Mediterranean and Asian roots. Chapters 4 and 5 shed light on primitive diagnostic and treatment methods.

Sochurek, Howard. *Medicine's New Vision*. Easton, Pa.: Mack, 1988. This overview of modern imaging techniques provides concise descriptions, clinical vignettes, and excellent photographs. A basic understanding of these techniques will help the reader appreciate their benefits and limitations, as well as how they supplement physical diagnosis.

Swartz, Mark H. *Textbook of Physical Diagnosis: History and Examination*. 3d ed. Philadelphia: W. B. Saunders, 1998. The author covers the taking of medical histories, physical examination, and diagnosis. Includes a bibliography and an index.

PHYSICAL REHABILITATION
SPECIALTY

ANATOMY OR SYSTEM AFFECTED: Bones, hips, joints, knees, legs, ligaments, muscles, musculoskeletal system, nerves, nervous system, spine, tendons

SPECIALTIES AND RELATED FIELDS: Exercise physiology, orthopedics, osteopathic medicine, physical therapy, sports medicine

DEFINITION: The discipline devoted to the restoration of normal bodily function, primarily of the muscles and skeleton.

KEY TERMS:

atrophy: a wasting away; a diminution in the size of a cell, tissue, organ, or part

cutaneous: pertaining to the skin

edema: the accumulation of an excessive amount of fluid in cells or tissues

electromyography: an electrodiagnostic technique for recording the extracellular activity (action and evoked potentials) of skeletal muscles at rest, during voluntary contractions, and during electrical stimulation

gangrene: necrosis (tissue death) caused by the obstruction of the blood supply; may be localized in a small area or may involve an entire extremity

goniometry: the measurement of angles, particularly those for the range of motion of a joint

ischemia: a local anemia or area of diminished or insufficient blood supply caused by mechanical obstruction of the blood supply (commonly, narrowing of an artery)

musculoskeletal: pertaining to or comprising the skeleton and the muscles

physiatry: the branch of medicine dealing with the prevention, diagnosis, and treatment of disease or injury and the rehabilitation from resultant impairments and disabilities; uses physical agents such as light, heat, cold, water, electricity, therapeutic exercise, mechanical apparatus, and pharmaceutical agents

rehabilitation: the restoration of normal form and function after injury or illness; the restoration of the ill or injured patient to optimal functional level in the home and community in relation to physical, psychosocial, vocational, and recreational activity

vascular: relating to or containing blood vessels

SCIENCE AND PROFESSION

Physical rehabilitation has been defined as a scientific discipline that uses physical agents such as light, heat, water, electricity, and mechanical agents in the management and rehabilitation of pathophysiological conditions resulting from disease or injury. Rehabilitation involves the treatment and training of patients with the goal of maximizing their potential for normal living physically, psychologically, socially, and vocationally.

Historical records indicate that the Chinese used rubbing as a therapeutic measure as early as 3000 B.C.E. Hippocrates also advocated rubbing in writings dated from 460 B.C.E.; it was used by subsequent Roman civilizations. The Roman poet Homer wrote about hydrotherapy as a cure for Hector. Immersion in the Nile and Ganges rivers as an aid to healing has been practiced for centuries. Peter Henry Ling developed and published a scientific basis for therapeutic massage in 1812. Modern physical therapy was established in 1917 with the creation of the Division of Special Hospitals and Physical Reconstruction. This effort was directed at persons injured in World War I and included educational and vocational training programs.

Physical rehabilitation is known for its work in restoring function to traumatized limbs. Practitioners in the field work with persons of all ages: with children to overcome birth defects, with adults to restore muscular function lost from strokes, with the elderly to maintain as much of normal functioning as possible in the face of advancing age, and with postoperative patients to accelerate healing and a return to normal activities. In addition, emphasis is placed on preventing and treating athletic injuries—prevention through the teaching of exercises to strengthen specific body parts and treatment through the restoration of normal bodily movements.

Prevention is defined as the avoidance of sickness, disability, or injury. There are three types or levels of prevention: primary, secondary, and tertiary. Primary prevention refers to complete avoidance before any problem has developed. A good example of primary prevention is being immunized for a specific disease. Secondary prevention refers to attempts to limit the extent of a disease, disability, or pathological process. A convenient illustration of secondary prevention is an individual who quits smoking. Some damage may have been done to the lungs and other organs, but it is curtailed when an individual stops smoking. The extent of recovery for lost function depends on the degree of damage incurred before the cessation of the activity. Tertiary prevention refers to attempts to recover functions or abilities that have been lost or severely compromised. Physical rehabilitation is a form of tertiary prevention: Attempts are made to restore normality that has been lost as a result of an accident, disease process, or injury.

Physical rehabilitation employs individuals with a variety of training. Physiatrists are physicians who have specialized training in physical medicine and rehabilitation. They are usually the leaders of rehabilitation teams and direct many of the activities of other personnel.

Physiatrists supervise the assessment of injured patients and actually conduct invasive tests such as electromyography. Physical therapists are specialists with some graduate-level training; in the United States, the scope of their activities is regulated by individual states and may vary from state to state. Typically, they operate alone but under the supervision or direction of a physiatrist, although in some states they are able to practice independently. Physical therapists carry out the treatment plan devised by a physiatrist and apply the therapeutic modalities. Speech and occupational therapists have specialized training in assisting patients in these particular areas. Speech therapists concentrate on overcoming language and speech difficulties, while occupational therapists specialize in providing injured persons with skills and training for new jobs. Therapy aides assist specialists in completing some of the more routine aspects of rehabilitation. Their education ranges from one to four years of training after high school.

DIAGNOSTIC AND TREATMENT TECHNIQUES
Individuals must be assessed prior to receiving physical rehabilitation. The assessment process begins with a complete history and physical examination. Subsequently, specific tests may be needed. Two common assessment tools are goniometry and electromyography. Goniometry refers to the measurement of joint motion. It is done by measuring angles of movement and is reported in degrees of arc. Electromyography is a technique that is used to evaluate the functioning of muscle units. Electrodes are placed in muscle groups. The nerve that controls the muscle is electrically stimulated, and the resultant muscle reaction is measured. Electromyography yields information concerning both the strength of muscle contractions and the speed of conduction along the nerve. These data help to pinpoint the basis of many muscular problems. As with all testing, patient-derived values are compared to standard norms to estimate pathology or lost function.

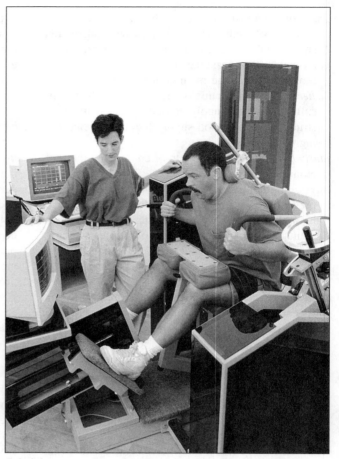

Rehabilitation may involve the use of high-tech equipment to control movements and to monitor results. (PhotoDisc)

Other aspects of an injured patient are also assessed: speech and language, psychological makeup, and vocation. Speech and language are needed for communication. Strokes or other injuries can interfere with the ability to communicate. Depending on where they occur in the brain, strokes can have different effects; these must be identified. Language ability requires both neurological integrity and muscular control. Any deficit in either component can impair speech. A primary goal of rehabilitation is communication proficiency (both speech and language), which is a prerequisite for success in many jobs.

Psychological makeup is assessed to pinpoint personality problems that could impede normal interactions with the world or success in a job. Individuals requiring assistance in this area are referred to other professionals for specialized help. Vocational

assessment is important because individuals sustaining strokes or serious injuries are frequently unable to return to their original jobs. When a vocational recommendation has been made for a patient, a specific course of rehabilitation is created.

There are four main therapeutic modalities used in physical rehabilitation: heat, diathermy, cold, and hydrotherapy. The primary reason for using heat is to raise the temperature in a specific area, usually the site of a wound. Heat increases the rate of cellular metabolism, thus increasing blood flow. Heat also has a sedative effect, relaxing the body part. Tissue repair occurs more rapidly with increased metabolism and circulation. Stress on the injured area is reduced, allowing tissue repair to proceed unimpeded. The net effect is to speed healing.

Heat is supplied by several methods. Compresses of cloth immersed in heated water have been used for centuries. Confining the heated water in a container provides heat in a dry form. Electric heating pads are more convenient because they can supply dry heat at a constant temperature for an unlimited length of time. Melted paraffin is occasionally used to concentrate heat in a specific location; this substance must be applied by a professional under controlled conditions. These modalities supply heat to the surface of skin; it penetrates passively, diminishing in intensity with increasing distance from the surface.

Infrared lamps provide heat that can penetrate to greater depths than heat sources applied to the surface of skin. Additional advantages include dryness and being able to position the body to be heated in any position. Because of its ability to penetrate, infrared light must be limited in exposure to avoid burns. It can also cause excessive drying of skin surfaces. Heat can also be supplied convectively, most often by immersion in warmed water. The stream of water can be directed at particular body parts, providing both heat and stimulation.

Diathermy is defined as deep heating. Deep tissues are heated because superficial heating produces only a few mild physiologic reactions. The problem is to avoid burning superficial tissues while heating deep structures. Three main methods are used to achieve this desired effect: shortwave, ultrasound, and microwave. In all three methods, energy is transferred and finally converted into heat when it reaches deep tissues. With shortwave, energy is transferred into deeper tissues by high-frequency current. Ultrasound uses high-frequency acoustic vibrations that penetrate into deep tissues. Microwave uses electromagnetic radiation to heat deeper tissues. Diathermy exploits all the advantages of heat: locally elevated temperatures, increased circulation, and decreased sensitivity of nerve fibers, which increases the threshold of pain. Diathermy is most useful in treating relatively deep muscular injuries. It cannot be used safely with sensory impairment because burning can occur, nor can it be used in joints that have been replaced with prostheses.

Cold creates physiological effects that are opposite to those of heat. Cooling decreases tissue metabolism. The application of cold slows blood circulation, which, in turn, tends to reduce tissue swelling caused by edema. Cold is more penetrating than heat. Too much cold, however, can become a problem. Cooling a large surface area of skin or lowering the core temperature of a body induces shivering, which causes the production of heat.

Cooling affects the nervous system. With cooling, the first cutaneous sense to be lost is light touch. Motor power is lost next. Pain and gross pressure are eventually lost with a sufficiently long application of cold. When ice is applied, an individual subjectively experiences an appreciation of the cooling, followed by a sense of burning or aching and, eventually, by cutaneous anesthesia. The total time needed to induce cutaneous anesthesia is between five and seven minutes. Cooled underlying muscle fibers lose some of their power; thus people are temporarily but noticeably weaker after cold is applied. The cooling of connective tissues around joints may diminish the ease and precision of movement.

Local cooling is used to reduce the unrestricted flow of fluid and blood into tissues after they have been traumatized. Cold reduces pain, both superficial and deep, and reduces reflex spasticity of muscles. Cold tends to preserve and extend the viability of tissues that have inadequate circulation, thus retarding the development of gangrene in an ischemic body part, which is most commonly seen in limbs.

There are reasons not to apply cold. Occasionally, individuals react to cold by abruptly increasing their arterial pressure. People who suffer from Raynaud's disease usually do not tolerate very well cold applied to their fingers or toes. The stiffness associated with rheumatoid arthritis is usually aggravated by cooling. Prolonged or excessive cooling can lead to frostbite. People who have experienced clinical hypothermia are must less tolerant of cold than those who have not had such an experience.

Several common methods exist for achieving therapeutic cooling: immersion, cold packs, cryokinetics, and a combination of local cooling and remote heating. Immersion is usually begun in cold water to which ice is steadily added. Total immersion is usually limited to ten or twenty minutes. The affected portion of the body is submerged in the chilled water. Cooling to a temperature above that of ice water may reduce muscular spasticity. Cold packs are often made by wrapping ice in a wet towel or plastic bag and applying it to the skin. Frozen cold packs should not be applied directly to the skin because they can cause locally severe tissue damage.

Cryokinetics is a procedure that combines cooling and exercise. Cooling is first accomplished by means of immersion or rubbing the skin over the affected part of the body with ice for five to seven minutes, so-called ice massage. The cooling produces a mild anesthesia which allows the individual to exercise the cooled body portion actively without pain. This method is considered to be particularly effective in recent acute muscle strains. The simultaneous application of heat and cold is sometimes effective. Heating an uninvolved portion of the body maintains the core temperature, which inhibits shivering, while cold applied to the injured portion of the body reduces pain. In theory, this arrangement allows cold to be applied for longer periods of time than would otherwise be possible. Because it is difficult to control heating and cooling simultaneously, however, this technique is not frequently used.

Hydrotherapy is the external application of water for therapeutic purposes. The water temperature can range from cold to hot. With immersion, water pro-

vides buoyancy, which relieves pressure on weight-bearing portions of the body. Water also provides resistance that is used in treating patients with motor weakness. Buoyancy alters the effect of exercises done in water by allowing a severely injured person to move; this provides psychological benefit and hope that the motion can eventually be done out of water. Brief application of cold has a tonic or stimulating effect, increasing blood pressure and the respiratory rate and stimulating shivering. Mild hot water provides sedation to irritated sensory and motor nerves, thus relieving pain caused by cramps and spasms in muscles. It also reduces stress, calming agitated or excited persons. The most common method of hydrotherapy is a whirlpool bath, which combines buoyancy, heat, and mechanical stimulation to the affected body part.

Massage and movement are key components of applied physical rehabilitation. Massage is the systematic and scientific manipulation of body tissues; massage is best performed by the hands. Massage has a sedative effect when constantly and steadily applied, and it leads to a decrease in muscular tension. Combined with heat or cold, the resulting relaxation facilitates the movement of injured body parts. Mechanically, massage stimulates the circulatory system, enhancing blood flow. The applied force of massage is effective in stretching muscle groups and breaking the adhesions between individual muscle fibers which limit motion. This same action mobilizes fluid and promotes its elimination. Massage does not develop muscle strength, however, and should not be used as a substitute for active exercise.

Therapeutic exercise is defined as the performance of movement to correct an impairment, improve musculoskeletal function, or maintain a state of well-being. Movement is the key: The energy to accomplish the movement can be supplied passively by a therapist or actively by an individual. Muscles are stretched with passive movement or contracted during the process of active flexion or contraction. Individuals with injuries that involve the nervous system may lose the function of any muscles supplied by the injured nerves. These muscles must be moved passively in

A devastating trauma such as the loss of a limb requires intense physical therapy to help the body adapt. (Digital Stock)

order to avoid loss of muscle mass and function as a result of disuse atrophy. Muscles respond to stimulation. Thus, exercises are designed to strengthen injured muscles. Parts in adjacent body structures must be stabilized to maximize the benefit derived from exercise. Prolonged moderate stretching is more beneficial than momentary vigorous stretching. Movements and stretching should be within the pain tolerance of the patient in order to avoid injury to blood vessels.

PERSPECTIVE AND PROSPECTS

Physical rehabilitation operates within a larger context of health care provision. The need for primary prevention is addressed by teaching correct methods for strengthening muscle groups to athletes and recreational fitness practitioners. Classes on first aid measures for treating common musculoskeletal injuries are taught by rehabilitation specialists such as physicians, therapists, and nurses. These classes are offered in schools and communities throughout the year. Physicians practicing occupational medicine also advocate primary prevention of musculoskeletal injuries associated with the work site. These professionals analyze working environments and recommend ways to restructure particular job tasks in order to reduce the chances of injury.

Secondary prevention is provided in office and hospital settings by professionals who treat injuries such as sprains, strains, and fractures. Care for acute injuries is usually accompanied by instruction in prevention in the hope that patients will avoid similar problems in the future. In the working environment, injured workers are provided with appropriate treatment and therapy and returned to work in an expeditious manner that is consistent with standards of proper care. This approach is usually best for all concerned, especially the injured worker. Such a case illustrates the many facets of rehabilitation. Normal physical functioning is returned with conventional therapy. Self-esteem is bolstered with return to meaningful work and previous income-earning capacity. Economically, the employer also benefits by having a trained and experienced worker on the job rather than having a skilled individual on disability and a less capable replacement worker on the job, both receiving payment.

Tertiary prevention involves the traditional rehabilitation activities that begin after treatment for a massive injury or chronic disease process. Frequently, such rehabilitation only returns a portion of lost func-

tions. Nevertheless, this treatment has value, improving self-esteem and the quality of life for an injured person. It underscores, however, the greater importance of the avoidance and prevention of injuries.

Health can be viewed as being on a continuum. One end is defined by death, the final termination of health. All life constitutes the rest of the spectrum. Health is frequently defined as the absence of disease or infirmity. This definition is appealing in its simplicity but is difficult to use because it is based on the absence rather than the presence of something. The question of where good health ends and impaired health begins is probably highly individual and open for debate. The division point between good and bad or acceptable and unacceptable health status, however, does provide a useful beginning for the activities encompassed by physical rehabilitation. The recovery of lost or impaired function is the domain of this field. This goal is also consistent with the definition of tertiary prevention. Rehabilitation and prevention are complementary opposites. Together, they span the entire spectrum of health.

—*L. Fleming Fallon, Jr., M.D., Ph.D., M.P.H.*

See also Aging, extended care; Allied health; Amputation; Bionics and biotechnology; Birth defects; Cardiac rehabilitation; Chiropractic; Exercise physiology; Healing; Heart attack; Hydrotherapy; Muscles; Nursing; Occupational health; Orthopedic surgery; Orthopedics; Orthopedics, pediatric; Osteopathic medicine; Speech disorders; Sports medicine; Strokes.

FOR FURTHER INFORMATION:

Braddom, Randall L., ed. *Physical Medicine and Rehabilitation*. Philadelphia: W. B. Saunders, 1996. Discusses physical therapy and medical rehabilitation. Includes a bibliography and an index.

DeLisa, Joel A., ed. *Rehabilitation Medicine: Principles and Practice*. 3d ed. Philadelphia: J. B. Lippincott, 1998. This standard textbook provides a comprehensive overview of rehabilitation. It is written for professionals but is accessible to laypeople. The subject entries are written by experts in their fields.

Fletcher, Gerald F., ed. *Rehabilitation Medicine*. Philadelphia: Lea & Febiger, 1992. An introduction to the subject of rehabilitation written for professional audiences. The writing is consistent and of high quality. The illustrations are unusually good.

Garrison, Susan J. *Handbook of Physical Medicine and Rehabilitation Basics*. Philadelphia: J. B. Lippincott, 1993. This text provides a good overview of the subject. Because it is written for students, it should be understandable to most readers. As an introduction to rehabilitation, it is well written.

Kottke, Frederic J., and Justus F. Lehmann, eds. *Krusen's Handbook of Physical Medicine and Rehabilitation.* 4th ed. Philadelphia: W. B. Saunders, 1990. A classic in the field, written by experts for professionals. The work is encyclopedic and comprehensive. A knowledge of physiology is useful for the general reader.

Sinaki, Mehrsheed, ed. *Basic Clinical Rehabilitation Medicine.* 2d ed. St. Louis: C. V. Mosby, 1993. An introductory textbook for students in the field. Well written, has good illustrations, and should be readily understood by laypeople.

PHYSICIAN ASSISTANTS

SPECIALTY

ANATOMY OR SYSTEM AFFECTED: All

SPECIALTIES AND RELATED FIELDS: Emergency care, family practice, general surgery, geriatrics and gerontology, internal medicine, neonatology, nursing, public health

DEFINITION: Health care providers who work under the supervision of licensed physicians and who are trained to perform physical examinations, diagnose illnesses, interpret laboratory tests, set fractures, and assist in surgeries.

KEY TERMS:

American Academy of Physician Assistants (AAPA): a professional society founded in 1968 to promote the role of PAs in providing high-quality, cost-effective health care

Association of Physician Assistant Programs (APAP): a consortium of educational institutions that offer accredited PA programs, providing academic guidance and standards for member schools

fee-for-service (FFS): the traditional way of paying for medical care by billing patients when services are rendered (in contrast to the practices of health maintenance organizations)

geriatrics: the branch of medicine dealing with problems and diseases of aging

health maintenance organization (HMO): a group of general practitioners, specialists, and allied health professionals who provide medical services to subscribers paying a regular maintenance fee

pediatrics: the branch of medicine dealing with the development and diseases of children

primary care: general medical services provided in family practice, internal medicine, pediatrics, geriatrics, obstetrics, and emergency care (in contrast to specialists, such as urology or cardiac surgery)

SCIENCE AND PROFESSION

The training of physician assistants was initiated at the Duke University Medical Center in 1965. There was a persistent shortage of qualified nurses for hospitals in the area. At the same time, the thousands of medical corpsmen who were discharged annually from the military services were unable to convert their skills into civilian occupations. Four Navy veterans with medical experience, all men, were enrolled in a trial program to give them additional training. A new curriculum was developed on a week-by-week basis, using the educational resources of the medical school. The men were graduated after two years and found their professional niche as assistants to licensed physicians.

The program at Duke served as a model that spread quickly to other medical institutions. Start-up funds became available from government agencies such as the Veterans Administration, the Office of Economic Opportunity, and the Public Health Service. By 1972, there were twenty-six training programs in operation in the United States. Two years later, the number had grown to fifty-three. New professional organizations were formed to evaluate and accredit the educational programs and to develop certification examinations for the individual graduates. In 1992, fifty-seven accredited PA programs were available at medical schools and teaching hospitals and through the armed forces.

The American Academy of Physician Assistants (AAPA) has adopted the following official definition for "physician assistant":

> Physician Assistants (PAs) practice medicine with supervision by licensed physicians. As members of the health care team, PAs provide a broad range of medical services that would otherwise be provided by physicians. It is the obligation of each team of Physician/ PA to ensure that the PA's scope of practice is identified; that delegation of medical tasks is appropriate to the PA's level of competence; that the relationship of, and access to, the supervising physician is defined; and that a process of performance evaluation is established. Adequate and responsible supervision of the PA contributes to both high quality patient care and continued professional growth.

The status of PAs as subordinates to M.D.'s is clearly delineated in this job description.

In 1993, there were more than 27,000 PAs in the United States, about 40 percent of them women. Each year, PA training programs produce approximately 1,700 new graduates. Most states require PAs to pass a national certifying examination before they can begin to practice. The examination is open only to graduates of accredited programs. To maintain certification, PAs must complete one hundred hours of continuing medical education every two years and take a recertification exam every six years. These requirements are intended to ensure the continued competency of PAs as qualified medical professionals.

The typical PA student has a bachelor's degree and four years of health care experience prior to admission into the program. About half of the entering students previously were either nurses, emergency medical technicians (EMTs), medics in the military, or emergency room technicians. There is strong competition to enter PA programs, with five applicants turned down for every student accepted.

The training program for PAs normally lasts two years. It is like a shortened version of the medical school curriculum for M.D.'s. The first year is composed of classroom and laboratory courses in anatomy, physiology, microbiology, and other basic sciences. Also, introductory instruction is given in pediatrics, obstetrics, general surgery, internal medicine, and emergency care. PAs often are in the same classes with medical students.

Second-year PA students are assigned to clinical rotations, seeing and treating patients under the supervision of a physician. The emphasis is on family practice and other primary care. They receive a variety of practical experience by working in an individual physician's office, a nursing home, a hospital, a rural clinic, a large group practice, or an emergency room. Some PAs learn to assist in major surgery and to provide preoperative and postoperative care.

After graduation, PAs practice in almost all types of health care settings. The demand for their services is increasing rapidly. National statistics show that there are approximately six jobs for every new graduate. The U.S. Department of Labor projected that PA employment would grow by 44 percent (about 12,000 new positions) between the years 1990 and 2005.

The majority of all PAs (57 percent) practice in primary care, where the shortage of qualified medical personnel is most severe. Rural clinics, small towns, and inner-city hospitals have a particularly difficult time recruiting M.D.'s for staff vacancies, so PAs are finding ready acceptance to fill the gap.

The median, net income of M.D.'s in general family practice is about $100,000 per year. PAs earn about half that much. In contrast, M.D.'s who work in radiology, surgery, anesthesiology, gynecology, and other specialties have about double the median income of general practitioners. It becomes clear that a strong economic incentive exists for physicians to become specialists, leaving vacancies in primary care for PAs.

The high cost of health care in the United States compared with other developed, industrial countries became a major political issue during the 1990's. In the United States, the ratio of M.D. specialists to general practitioners is 68 percent to 32 percent, whereas in Western Europe the ratio is roughly 50/50. Critics both within and outside the medical profession have pointed to this imbalance in the United States as a major factor that raises the cost of and limits broad access to health care. The problem worsened drastically during the 1980's. The number of new medical school graduates entering general practice declined from 36 percent to only 14 percent in ten years. The United States is producing an oversupply of specialists while the shortage of primary care doctors worsens.

An outspoken editorial published in 1993 in *The Journal of the American Medical Association* addressed the issue of how to deal with an impending crisis in primary care. One recommendation was to increase the supply of PAs, nurse practitioners, chiropractors, and other nonphysician providers. These individuals would participate as team members alongside physicians in an integrated, cost-effective health care setting. Another suggestion to reduce total health care costs was to place more emphasis on preventive medicine. PAs have acquired a good reputation for advising patients about how to adopt healthier lifestyles, whereas the busy M.D.'s may not want to spend extra time counseling patients after treatment has been completed.

Another proposal to deal with the primary care shortage would be to require a period of mandatory national health service for all medical school graduates. Such a policy could be justified by considering the substantial federal tax money that supports medical education. The U.S. Congress would have to enact appropriate legislation. The experience of working on the staff of a community health facility would broaden the training of physicians, even

1814 • Physician Assistants

if they go into specialty practice afterward.

If legislation were passed to provide guaranteed access to health care for everyone, the availability of medically trained personnel would be severely strained. It is clear that PAs and other intermediate-level health care providers would be essential to carry out such an ambitious program.

DIAGNOSTIC AND TREATMENT TECHNIQUES

After completing a two-year accredited training program and passing the certification examination, PAs are qualified to perform approximately 80 percent of the routine duties most commonly done by physicians. PAs can give general physical examinations; diagnose illnesses; determine treatments; give injections, immunizations, and catheterizations; interpret laboratory tests; suture wounds; set fractures; deal with medical emergencies; and assist in surgical operations. In a majority of states (thirty-five), PAs can write prescriptions for medication.

PAs are not independent medical practitioners. By law or regulation, all PAs must have a licensed physician to supervise and be responsible for their work. It is not necessary, however, for the physician and the PA to be located in the same building or even in the same town. In rural communities, for example, state law generally allows such supervision to occur via telephone.

Suppose that a small town is being served by a clinic with three physicians, one of whom is about to retire. There are several smaller towns nearby with no medical service at all, and the nearest hospital is 40 miles away. The Chamber of Commerce and other civic groups start a vigorous fund-raising and advertising campaign to find a replacement for the retiring doctor, but with no success. Finally, one of the doctors contacts the state medical school to inquire about the possibility of hiring a PA.

From the point of view of the doctor, a PA can take care of routine school and employment physical examinations, minor acute illnesses, baby checkups, and so forth, so that the doctor can focus on more complex problems. The PA can also relieve the doctor by making rounds at the community nursing home. The PA would be expected to share in call duty on nights and weekends. The doctor could take time off for occasional vacations, medical meetings, or family obligations. To help the underserved nearby towns, a satellite clinic could be set up that would be staffed by the PA perhaps half a day each week.

From the point of view of the PA, medical practice in a small town brings some special rewards. The PA is accorded a position of prestige as a member of the small, professional community that includes teachers and lawyers. This situation is in strong contrast to urban health care, where the PA is a minor figure among hundreds of doctors and other hospital personnel. Furthermore, rural PAs are likely to see a wider variety of medical problems and, after establishing rapport with their supervising physician, are able to exercise more independent judgment about diagnosis and treatment.

It will take some time for a PA to become accepted in a small town. The doctor must emphasize the team concept of medical care, of which the PA is a valued member. The supervisory role of the M.D. needs to be clearly and formally established. The majority of PAs, for example, are insured by a rider on the physician's malpractice policy. To fit into the social environment, PAs have stated that it helps if they themselves grew up in a small town and if they are married. A large number of PAs have successfully found their medical role as primary care providers in rural communities.

A very different role is filled by PAs serving as surgical assistants in a hospital. With specialized training, they can act as assistants during surgery as well as provide preoperative and postoperative care.

When a surgery patient is admitted, surgical PAs can be assigned to write up the medical history and give an entrance physical examination. They can evaluate preoperative laboratory tests and inform the surgeon of any potential complications. They can spend time with the patient and family members to explain the intended procedure and to answer their questions.

During surgery, PAs can assist the surgeon with clamping and tying as needed. They should be familiar with various patient monitoring devices and should inform the surgeon if problems arise. After surgery, the PA can accompany the patient to the recovery room or intensive care unit (ICU).

During the patient's recuperation time in the hospital, PAs will make regular rounds. They can prescribe medications, change dressings, and generally free the surgeon from the more routine tasks of daily patient care. They can write the discharge orders, which then have to be reviewed and approved by the supervising surgeon.

Surgical PAs have become accepted as assistants in almost all kinds of surgery. For example, they can specialize in orthopedics, kidney transplantation, heart surgery, urology, and skin grafts for burn victims. They must receive appropriate on-the-job training with clinical instruction from their supervising physician to prepare for such surgical specialties.

Health maintenance organizations (HMOs) are another area of employment for a large number of PAs. HMOs are becoming a popular, cost-effective alternative to the traditional fee-for-service (FFS) method of paying for health care. HMOs are prepaid health plans that provide medical, surgical, and hospital benefits to their members. Such a plan is usually offered as a fringe benefit of employment, with the company paying all or part of the monthly fee. When medical services are needed, the patient must come to doctors who are part of the HMO.

When PAs are hired by an HMO, they work under a supervising physician. PAs can examine patients, make a provisional diagnosis, initiate treatment, or refer a case to an appropriate specialist. In a primary care office, the majority of routine problems—a runny nose, infected wounds, or prenatal counseling—can be handled by the PA with little help. Access to staff doctors for consultation, however, is readily available.

From the viewpoint of the PA, working for an HMO brings increased job security. If the supervising physician happens to leave, the job of the PA continues. In a solo office, by contrast, when the physician leaves the PA has to look for a new position. Another advantage of HMO employment is the opportunity for professional growth through interactions with other health care staff members. Also, some PAs particularly like the diversity of experience at an HMO in providing primary care to all age groups, from infants to the elderly.

HMO administrators have reported that acceptance of PAs by patients generally has been good. Pamphlets are made available to explain the educational background of PAs, their subordinate status to physicians, and legal limitations on their level of responsibility. Malpractice suits against PAs have been relatively rare. Patients who insist on seeing an M.D. can be accommodated, but surveys have shown an equal degree of patient satisfaction with M.D. and PA services.

Depending on their individual interests and skills, PAs have established themselves in a wide variety of other health care settings. They can be found in geriatric practice, prison health programs, trauma centers, infant critical care units, and military hospitals or on American Indian reservations. Some PAs have gone into administration or public health management. New professional opportunities for PAs continue to evolve as their special contributions to health care are increasingly recognized.

PERSPECTIVE AND PROSPECTS

The concept of the physician assistant was created in the 1960's in response to a shortage of nurses and other health care workers. At that time, nurses were almost always women. Medical corpsmen in the armed forces were all men who wanted a new civilian designation to distinguish them clearly from the nursing profession. With a relatively short training program, they were envisioned as physician's helpers, always working under M.D. supervision. The role of women in the workplace has changed greatly since the 1960's; consequently the PA profession is no longer dominated by men.

By the 1990's, holding down medical costs had become a national priority. In the United States, about 14 percent of the gross national product is expended on health care, whereas comparable industrialized nations are able to provide broader coverage for their citizens at considerably lower expense. The role of PAs in providing cost-effective medical services is widely recognized. Other issues besides cost, however, need to be addressed.

A personnel crisis has arisen in the United States because of the relatively small fraction of physicians who choose to work in primary care and family medicine. By the 1990's, only about one-third of the country's nearly 500,000 M.D.'s were general practitioners, with the rest becoming specialists. Such an imbalance results in a lack of access to medical services, especially in rural areas and among the urban poor. A shift in the medical workforce from specialization to primary care is needed to help these underserved groups.

Another issue in the cost and allocation of health care is the growing number of elderly people. Certain illnesses such as Alzheimer's disease, heart disease, and strokes are particular problems of aging. Cataract surgery of the eye is performed largely on older people and is the biggest single line-item expense in the Medicare program. The American Association of Retired Persons (AARP) has made the funding of long-term care facilities a major priority.

The training of doctors has been criticized for overemphasizing the treatment of illnesses while neglecting preventive measures. For example, few physicians take a course in nutrition. The harmful consequences of smoking, alcohol consumption, lack of exercise, and poor diet are clearly established. If the medical profession would provide counseling about better health habits to patients, eventually the cost of treatment could be decreased. Such counseling would not require the expensive time of an M.D., who has gone through lengthy medical school and internship programs. It can be provided by a PA who has authoritative information and good communication skills.

Physician assistants, nurses, physical therapists, nurse practitioners, midwives, medical technologists, and other allied health professionals are all part of the total health care team, with different areas of responsibility. One commentator has stated that no one hires an electrical engineer to change a light bulb; similarly, it is not economical to use M.D.'s for routine care that can be supplied by others. The role of PAs is an expanding one.

—*Hans G. Graetzer, Ph.D.*

See also Allied health; Anatomy; Education, medical; Emergency medicine; Family practice; Hospitals; Internal medicine; Laboratory tests; Nutrition; Obstetrics; Pediatrics; Physical examination; Physiology; Preventive medicine; Surgery, general.

For Further Information:

Anderson, Susan M. *Selected Annotated Bibliography of the Physician Assistant Profession.* 4th ed. Arlington, Va.: Association of Physician Assistant Programs, 1993. An updating of earlier editions. Books, magazine articles, government documents, and monographs are included in this bibliography. A comprehensive resource for finding information on all aspects of the profession.

Arenofsky, Janice. "For a Healthy Prognosis: Examine a Career as a PA or CRNA." *Career World* 21 (January, 1993): 26-30. Career opportunities for the physician's assistant (PA) and the certified registered nurse anesthetist (CRNA) are described. Provides information about educational requirements, salaries, typical duties, and professional status relative to other health care providers.

Ballweg, Ruth, Sherry Stolberg, and Edward M. Sullivan, eds. *Physician Assistant: A Guide to Clinical Practice.* 2d ed. Philadelphia: W. B. Saunders, 1999. Discusses clinical competence standards among physician assistants. Includes a bibliography and an index.

Carter, Reginald D., and Henry B. Perry, eds. *Alternatives in Health Care Delivery: Emerging Roles for Physician Assistants.* St. Louis: Warren G. Green, 1984. A collection of fifty short essays dealing with all aspects of the physician assistant profession. Contributing authors discuss training programs, certification, employment opportunities, and national priorities in health care.

Lundberg, George D., and Richard D. Lamm. "Solving Our Primary Care Crisis by Retraining Specialists to Gain Specific Primary Care Competencies." *The Journal of the American Medical Association* 270 (July 21, 1993): 380-381. The authors are the editor of *JAMA* and a former governor of Colorado, respectively. This strongly worded editorial advocates major reforms in the U.S. health care system in order to correct the oversupply of specialists and the shortfall of primary care providers.

Workman, James. "Marcus Welby, PA." *The Washington Monthly* 24 (January/February, 1992): 26-30. The author cites examples in which doctors have tried to restrict the role of PAs in medical practice. The article argues that PAs can provide wider access and lower-cost services.

Physiology
Biology

Anatomy or system affected: All

Specialties and related fields: All

Definition: The branch of biology dealing with the structures and functions of various systems in living organisms.

Key terms:

extracellular fluid: the internal environment of the human body that surrounds the cells; the fluid contains ions, gases, and the nutrients needed by cells for proper functioning and is constantly circulated throughout the body by the blood and into tissues by diffusion

homeostasis: the maintenance of a constant internal environment; the systems of the body work together to maintain a constant temperature, pH, oxygen availability, water content, ion concentrations, and so on

negative feedback: a homeostatic control system designed to respond to a stress by returning body conditions to normal physiologic levels

pH: a measure of the acidity or alkalinity of a solution; equal to the negative logarithm of the hydrogen ion concentration (as measured in moles per liter)

positive feedback: when a stimulus causes more of the same to occur; can be useful in some instances, such as with blood clotting and uterine contractions during childbirth

scientific method: a method of scientific investigation of a problem through observation, the formation of a hypothesis (a possible explanation to a problem), experimentation, and the reevaluation of data

THE FUNDAMENTALS OF PHYSIOLOGY

Physiology is a branch of science that applies to all living things. The goal of the physiologist is to understand the mechanisms leading to the proper functioning of organisms such as bacteria, plants, animals, and humans. Physiology is an important aspect of many of the medical sciences. In immunology, researchers seek to understand the functioning of the immune system. Cardiovascular scientists study the workings of the heart. Knowledge of the normal physiologic functioning of an organism is important in identifying the diseases that cause a deviation from the normal state.

Essential to the discovery of new data is the application of the scientific method of research. The first step in this method is observation. This involves examining a particular system or organism of interest, such as the transport of nutrients in a plant stem or the flow of air into the lungs of an animal, and initially observing a specific event or phenomenon. Asking why and how the event occurs leads to the next step—forming a hypothesis, or scientific question. A hypothesis is a possible explanation of the observation, which can be tested further to see if it is true. Testing, or experimentation, is the third step in the scientific method. The experiment involves setting up a controlled situation that directly tests the hypothesis in order to determine the cause-and-effect relationship between the hypothesis and the initial observation. As the experiment is conducted, the investigator makes further observations of the system's functioning and collects these findings as data. Following data collection and analysis comes the fourth step, making conclusions. The conclusion may or may not support the researcher's original hypothesis. To confirm the results further, more testing is often done. If, upon additional testing, similar conclusions are reached, the researcher may move on to the final step of the scientific method: publication. The experimental design, results, and conclusions are written down in a paper that is then submitted to a scientific jour-

nal. Publication permits other researchers to be informed of and evaluate the experiment and possibly to use the results to further their own research endeavors.

Applying this scientific method to the human model, it becomes apparent that the physiological conditions of the human body are in a state of dynamic equilibrium. While variables such as pH, ion and nutrient concentrations, and water content are constantly changing, they never differ significantly from their optimum level, unless the body is in a state of disease. Sensors, an integrating center, and effectors are important contributors to the regulation of these variables. Sensors are located throughout the body and are designed to monitor specific physiologic conditions. For example, baroreceptors monitor arterial blood pressure, chemoreceptors monitor the concentrations of hydrogen ions and carbon dioxide in the extracellular fluid, and thermoreceptors monitor body temperature. The conditions of the body are then transmitted via nerve impulses to a particular integrating center located in the brain, spinal cord, or endocrine glands. The integrating center interprets the nerve impulses and determines if a response is required. To respond to a particular condition, the integrating center activates certain effectors. An effector is usually a muscle or a gland that, when activated, performs a specific function to return the body to normal physiologic conditions.

Extracellular fluid is also important in the maintenance of the above-mentioned variables. Two basic types of fluid compose about 60 percent of the human body. Two-thirds of the body's fluid is intracellular fluid (cytoplasm) and is found inside of cells. The other one-third of the fluid is extracellular fluid and is located in the spaces between cells (interstitial fluid), in blood vessels (plasma), and in the lymphatic vessels (lymph). This fluid is constantly circulated throughout the human body in the blood and lymphatic vessels. The ions, gases, and nutrients in the fluid can easily diffuse out of the capillaries and into the adjacent cells, where they can be utilized in normal cell activities. Because the estimated 100 trillion cells of the body are exposed to basically the same composition of extracellular fluid, it has been termed the body's internal environment.

The extracellular fluid is the medium of exchange of biologically important molecules and materials. Their concentration and availability is under the control of various organs and systems. For example, the kidneys play an important role in regulating the water content, ion and waste concentrations, and acid-base balance of the extracellular fluid. The gastrointestinal tract is responsible for digesting and making food available for absorption into the bloodstream. The liver maintains the normal glucose concentration in the blood through processes that store glucose, remove glucose from storage, or produce new glucose from other nutrients. The lungs aspirate to provide adequate oxygen and carbon dioxide exchange in the blood. An important job of the physiologist is to discover the mechanisms used by these and other organs to perform their respective functions.

HOMEOSTATIS AND FEEDBACK SYSTEMS

Each of the aforementioned variables has an optimum physiologic range over which the body can function normally. The systems of the body work together in an attempt to keep the body's internal environment within these normal ranges. This process is called homeostasis. Stress placed on the body—whether from the outside environment (heat, cold) or from within (disease, emotional reactions)—can lead to fluctuations in the internal environment. Significant deviations from the normal can lead to a state of disease in the body. To prevent these types of changes, the body has incorporated a number of control devices that are governed by the nervous and endocrine systems. The nervous system is constantly evaluating the state of the body and is able to detect when something is awry. When the body strays too far from its balanced condition, it responds in one of two ways. First, it may send nervous impulses to the proper organs that counteract the stress and return it toward its original state. Second, it may activate the endocrine system to release its chemical messengers or hormones that will bring the body back into balance.

The nervous and endocrine systems are also important components in the feedback systems that regulate the body's internal environment. The two basic types of feedback systems are called negative feedback and positive feedback. Negative feedback is a homeostatic control mechanism that responds to a stress-related change by returning a condition to its normal range. For example, an increase in the blood glucose level induces specific steps that reduce the glucose to its normal level. Positive feedback is designed to amplify the response given to a certain stress. For example, during childbirth, uterine contractions intensify as a result of a positive feedback

system, thus enabling the birth of a baby. The majority of the feedback systems in the human body are negative, since in most instances (with a few, specific exceptions) a positive system is detrimental to the body.

Negative feedback. Often, several systems work together to monitor and regulate a particular physiologic condition. An excellent example of this can be seen in the negative feedback regulation of the mean arterial blood pressure. Baroreceptors are the monitoring devices for arterial pressure. They are composed of nerve endings located in the arterial wall of specific blood vessels, such as in the arch of the aorta and the neck area where the common carotid artery divides into the internal and external carotid arteries. Baroreceptors respond to the stretching of the arterial wall. These arteries undergo greater-than-normal stretching during times of high blood pressure and are more relaxed in times of low blood pressure.

Baroreceptors are constantly informing the brain of the status of the mean arterial pressure by sending out nervous impulses to the cardiovascular control center, located in the medulla of the brain. When the body is subject to stress that causes the blood pressure to rise, the elastic arterial walls experience an increase in the amount that they are stretched. The baroreceptors, being stretch receptors, respond to this change by increasing their output of nervous impulses to the brain. In contrast, a drop in blood pressure decreases arterial wall stretching, causing the baroreceptors to send out fewer impulses to the brain.

The nervous impulses from the baroreceptors travel to the cardiovascular control center in the brain via afferent neurons. The cardiovascular control center is a network of neurons that receive and integrate nervous impulses from a variety of other control centers. The cardiovascular control center is connected to the heart by both sympathetic and parasympathetic nerves and to the blood vessels primarily by sympathetic nerves. An increase in the rate of impulses from the baroreceptors (in response to an increase in arterial pressure) results in an increase in the amount of parasympathetic stimulation and a decrease in sympathetic stimulation. On the contrary, a decrease in the rate of impulses from the baroreceptors (in response to a decrease in arterial pressure) results in a decrease in the amount of parasympathetic stimulation and an increase in sympathetic stimulation.

To understand the significance of the stimulation of parasympathetic-versus-sympathetic nervous stimulation, a brief comment must be made as to the organization of the nervous system. The central nervous system (CNS) is made up of the brain, the brain stem, and the spinal cord. The peripheral nervous system (PNS) comprises the nerves that go into and leave the brain stem and spinal cord. The peripheral nervous system is further divided into a somatic portion and an autonomic portion. The somatic nervous system's sensory receptors transmit impulses to the CNS, which then sends impulses through motor neurons to the skeletal muscles. The autonomic nervous system monitors the condition of the internal organs via sensory nerves to the CNS and responds via motor nerves to glands and involuntary muscles. The parasympathetic and sympathetic nerves are the two types of motor nerves that make up the autonomic nervous system. In general, sympathetic nerves initiate the body's fight-or-flight response to stressful situations. Parasympathetic nerves are responsible for more vegetative functions, such as the ingestion and digestion of food.

The combinations of particular nerve activations and deactivations have particular effects on the state of the heart and peripheral blood vessels. As stated above, an increase in mean arterial pressure, as detected by the baroreceptors, invokes a response that increases parasympathetic stimulation of the heart and decreases sympathetic stimulation of the heart and blood vessels. This response serves to reduce the heart rate and the contractility of the heart, thus reducing cardiac output. In addition, blood vessels in the skin and muscles are allowed to dilate, reducing the total peripheral resistance of the blood. The direct relationship of the mean arterial pressure (MAP) to the cardiac output (CO) and total peripheral resistance (TPR) is represented by the formula "MAP = CO × TPR." It can be observed that decreasing both CO and TPR results in a decrease in the MAP. This occurs to the point at which the MAP returns to its normal range. If the applied stress decreases the MAP as detected by the baroreceptors, parasympathetic stimulation decreases and sympathetic stimulation increases. This causes an increase in CO and an increase in TPR, resulting in an overall increase in mean arterial pressure.

Positive feedback. An example of positive feedback regulation can be seen in the process of childbirth. Weak, periodic uterine contractions begin during the third trimester of a human pregnancy. As the pregnancy progresses and the time comes for delivery of the baby, these contractions become stronger and increase in frequency. Such contractions are necessary for the expulsion of the baby and the placenta from the mother.

Contractions of the uterine muscles begin at the top, or apex, of the uterus and move down toward its base, at the location of the cervix. These contractions force the head of the baby onto the cervix and stretch it open in a process termed cervical dilation. Cervical stretching sends nerve impulses to the hypothalamus in the brain, which then stimulates the posterior pituitary gland to release the hormone oxytocin. Oxytocin makes the uterine contractions stronger and more rhythmic. Continued stretching of the cervix leads to an increase in the amount of oxytocin released by the pituitary. This positive feedback cycle continues until the baby is born, at which point the pressure on the cervix is removed and it can relax.

PERSPECTIVE AND PROSPECTS

Physiology began more than 2,000 years ago during the time of the ancient Greeks. The well-known philosopher Aristotle (384-322 B.C.E.) was also a physiologist who made biological observations and described the blood vessels as part of a system with the heart at its center. He also believed that the heart was a furnace that heated the blood and that it was the body's seat of intellect. In the city of Alexandria, Herophilus (335-280 B.C.E.) believed that the seat of intellect was the brain, not the heart. He studied arteries and veins and determined that arteries have thicker walls. Erasistratus (310-240 B.C.E.) began his training under Herophilus. He believed that arteries served as air vessels and that the veins carried the blood, which was made in the liver from food. Several hundred years later, Galen (129-c. 199 C.E.) conducted an experiment that showed that blood, not air, flowed through arteries. Though some of his other ideas were later disproved, he left behind a considerable number of writings on physiology, medicine, and philosophy.

Galen's ideas were taught for many hundreds of years until the Renaissance. During this time, physiologists made important discoveries and observations that challenged the findings of Galen. Andreas Vesalius (1514-1564) was trained as a doctor and became a professor of surgery and anatomy at a medical school in what is now Italy. Vesalius' style of teaching was to dissect a cadaver as he lectured, and he included anatomical drawings in his written texts. He wrote what has become known as the first modern anatomy textbook, *De Humanis Corporis Fabrica* (the structure of the human body), published in 1543.

A few decades later, William Harvey (1578-1657) was born in England and later trained as a doctor. He also did some lecturing and wrote a study of circulation, *De Motu Cordis et Sanguinis in Animalibus* (on the motion of the heart and of blood in animals), published in 1628. Harvey viewed the heart as a pump that contracted to expel blood and discovered that the blood moved in a circular path in the body. He believed that the blood traveled from the right ventricle to the lungs and then to the left ventricle, not directly from the right to the left ventricle. He also theorized that air stayed in the lungs and did not move to the heart to meet the blood.

Joseph Priestley (1733-1804), an English chemist, investigated the processes of combustion and breathing. Priestley's experiments used a bell jar, a candle, a green plant, and a mouse. He observed that a candle placed under a bell jar went out, but could later be lit after a green plant was placed under the jar for several days. He also observed that a mouse placed under the jar died after some time. When placed under the jar with a green plant, however, the mouse lived for a longer period of time.

Using an early microscope, Robert Hooke (1635-1703) studied a piece of cork and coined the term "cells" for he compartments that he observed. Two hundred years later, German biologists Matthias Schleiden (1804-1881) and Theodor Schwann (1810-1882) proposed their cell theory. Their theory encompassed some of the essential ideas in biology and physiology, including that all organisms are made of cells which have similar metabolic processes and chemical components, that an organism's functions result from different cells working together, and that all cells have their origin in preexisting cells.

The invention of the thermometer allowed scientists to gain further insights into human physiology. With this investigation came the discovery that the human body maintains a relatively constant internal body temperature, despite changes in the temperature of its environment. The French physiologist Claude Bernard (1813-1878) used the words "milieu intérieur" to describe this constant internal environment of the human body. American physiologist Walter Cannon (1871-1945) later coined the term "homeostasis" to describe this condition.

Essential to investigations and discoveries that advance the field of physiology is the ever-changing nature of technology. Early research was conducted simply with observations of the unaided eye. Later discoveries developed glass lenses to form a light microscope which magnified images up to 1,000 times and opened up a world of tissues and cells that were previously indiscernible. Newer technology lead to the formation of the electron microscope, which provided magnification of specimens greater than 100,000 times and revealed the intricacies of subcellular structures.

Technology has advanced to the growth of living cells and tissues in laboratory dishes. Cell culture allows the investigator to change or regulate the environment of the biological material and to determine the effect of such alterations on growth and reproduction. Techniques such as cytochemistry, autoradiography, and immunochemistry have been developed to stain or localize certain regulatory molecules or cellular structures, enabling the scientist to quantify their effects on cell physiology. Cell fractionation has been developed to separate cells into their various components or organelles, thus providing a way that a specific organelle can be studied in isolation. Genetic engineering is a powerful technology that allows the researcher to manipulate and alter the genes of cells that control their functions. All these techniques are frequently used in physiology research and are powerful forces that have expanded scientific understanding.

—*John L. Rittenhouse and Roman J. Miller, Ph.D.*

See also Anatomy; Cells; Cytology; Endocrinology; Exercise physiology; Fluids and electrolytes; Hormones; Kinesiology; Nervous system; Neurology; Systems and organs.

FOR FURTHER INFORMATION:

Fox, Stuart I. *Human Physiology.* 6th ed. Dubuque, Iowa: Wm. C. Brown, 1999. The author presents a simplified, yet highly accurate account of human medical physiology that is profusely illustrated with color photographs, line drawings, and abundant tables. Applications of physiological principles are frequently highlighted. Appropriate for high school students and for the general public.

Ganong, William F. *Review of Medical Physiology.* 19th ed. Stamford, Conn.: Appleton and Lange, 1999. The author attempts to detail the concepts of medical physiology in a succinct but coherent fashion. This book is designed to refresh the memory of the reader regarding specific details of physiology.

Guyton, Arthur C., and John E. Hall. *Textbook of Medical Physiology*. 10th ed. Philadelphia: W. B. Saunders, 2000. Guyton's textbook has been the recognized authoritative work on medical physiology for several decades. Specific details of physiological systems are clearly described in understandable terms for the reader.

Prosser, C. Ladd, ed. *Environmental and Metabolic Animal Physiology*. New York: Wiley-Liss, 1991. The author approaches physiology by comparing how specific systems differ among various animal organisms such as humans, rodents, and fish. Much of the experimentation in physiology is initially done with animals and then applied to humans.

Rhoades, Rodney, and Richard Pflanzer. *Human Physiology*. 3d ed. Fort Worth, Tex.: W. B. Saunders College, 1996. This college-level textbook clearly explains classic physiological systems in humans. Specific chapters deal with different body systems. Chapters open with an outline of the topics that follow and conclude with a summary of the more important concepts.

Tortora, Gerard J. *Introduction to the Human Body*. 5th ed. New York: HarperCollins, 2000. A simplified description of human physiology that is readily understood by most readers who have minimal prior knowledge of physiology. Profusely illustrated, this book surveys human physiology in a system-to-system fashion. Readable, accurate, and informative.

PID. *See* PELVIC INFLAMMATORY DISEASE (PID).

PIGEON TOES
DISEASE/DISORDER

ALSO KNOWN AS: In-toeing
ANATOMY OR SYSTEM AFFECTED: Bones, feet, legs, musculoskeletal system
SPECIALTIES AND RELATED FIELDS: Family practice, orthopedics, pediatrics, podiatry
DEFINITION: Pigeon toes is the most common childhood foot problem, affecting 15 percent of all children. It involves a minor abnormality in the leg or foot that causes the child's foot and toes to point inward. There are three causes of in-toeing in healthy babies: metatarsus adductus (a curve in the foot), internal tibial torsion (a twist in the tibia), and excessive femoral anteversion (a twist in the thigh bone). Most cases of pigeon toes are out-

grown and require no treatment. Occasionally, repetitive stretching exercises are prescribed to be done at home. If the exercises do not work, in rare occasions, surgery may be recommended.
—*Earl R. Andresen, Ph.D.*
See also Bones and the skeleton; Foot disorders; Lower extremities; Orthopedic surgery; Orthopedics; Orthopedics, pediatric.

FOR FURTHER INFORMATION:
Goldberg, Kathy E. *The Skeleton: Fantastic Framework*. Washington, D.C.: U.S. News Books, 1982.
Marieb, Elaine N. *Human Anatomy and Physiology*. 5th ed. Redwood City, Calif.: Benjamin/Cummings, 2000.
Seeley, Rod R., Trent D. Stephens, and Philip Tate. *Anatomy and Physiology*. 5th ed. Boston: McGraw-Hill, 2000.
Tortora, Gerard J., and Sandra R. Grabowski. *Principles of Anatomy and Physiology*. 9th ed. New York: John Wiley & Sons, 2000.

PIGMENTATION
BIOLOGY
ANATOMY OR SYSTEM AFFECTED: Eyes, hair, skin
SPECIALTIES AND RELATED FIELDS: Dermatology, environmental health
DEFINITION: The coloration of human skin and eyes based on the presence and amount of five different pigments; the most important of these pigments, melanin, protects the body from ultraviolet radiation.
KEY TERMS:
dermis: the layer of skin underneath the epidermis that contains hemoglobin and oxyhemoglobin
epidermis: the outer layer of the skin that contains melanocytes, which produce melanin
hypodermis: the layer of fat under the dermis that contains carotene
melanin: a protein that darkens the color of the skin and protects against ultraviolet radiation
melanoma: cancer of the melanocytes, the cells that produce melanin
ultraviolet radiation: radiation that is potentially damaging to the skin; it is not visible to humans

STRUCTURE AND FUNCTIONS
One of the most apparent human characteristics is the color of a person's skin. Five pigments play major roles: melanin, melanoid, carotene, hemoglobin, and

oxyhemoglobin. Melanin occurs in the greatest variation and is the most important of the five; in large amounts, it can mask the effects of the other pigments.

Melanocytes are cells that convert tyrosine, an amino acid, into the black pigment called melanin. The rate of production is controlled by a hormone called melanocyte-stimulating hormone (MSH), which is released by the anterior pituitary gland. About a thousand melanocytes occur on each square millimeter of the body (with the exception of the head and the forearms, which have twice as many). Interestingly, all human races vary greatly in color but tend to have the same number of melanocytes, which inherit different abilities to make melanin.

When humans are compared, an uninterrupted array of shades of skin color is found. Traits that show such continuous variation are thought to be controlled by several sets of genes (polygenetic inheritance). Thus, several sets of genes control the amount of pigmentation. The observed distribution of human skin color suggests that four or six pairs of genes are involved.

Melanocytes convert tyrosine into melanin by several chemical steps which involve the key enzyme tyrosinase. A functional tyrosinase molecule consists of different amino acids (the building blocks of proteins) and copper. Traces of copper are in the normal human diet and provide the amounts needed for the enzymes.

Tyrosine, the molecule that is converted to melanin, is one of twenty amino acids occurring in biological systems that chain together in various ways to make up different proteins. Eight of these amino acids are essential; that is, they must be present in the diet. The remaining twelve amino acids can be made by chemical modification of the others. Tyrosine is not an essential amino acid. Ample amounts of tyrosine occur in all meats and in most dairy products. If it is not taken into the body in sufficient amounts, however, it will be made from other amino acids. Either way, tyrosine is delivered to the melanocytes and changed into melanin. This product, with its high molecular weight, functions to protect the skin from excessive ultraviolet (UV) radiation.

UV radiation is an invisible part of the sun's radiation having wavelengths from 100 to 400 nanometers. Humans can see the colors of the spectrum from red through violet. Wavelengths of radiation that are slightly longer than red (infrared) cannot be seen but

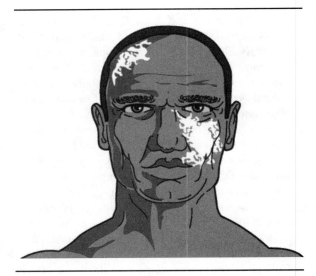

The skin can experience such dysfunctions in pigmentation as the condition known as vitiligo, an autoimmune disease in which the melanocytes that normally produce skin color are absent; the result is light patches on the skin, which are more easily seen on dark-skinned people.

are detected by the body as heat. Wavelengths such as UV that are shorter than violet cannot be seen or felt. Nevertheless, UV radiation penetrates the body. In moderation, UV light is valuable for humans because the body uses its energy to synthesize vitamin D. Vitamin D allows the intestinal absorption of calcium to be used for skeletal growth and for nerve and muscle function.

Ultraviolet radiation poses several risks. A sunburn involves UV radiation damage to epidermal skin cells, which release chemicals that dilate blood vessels, causing redness. Swelling and blistering may occur. When large numbers of cells are destroyed, the skin speeds up production of new cells, which forces the burned cells to peel off. UV radiation also can change the skin's collagen, a protein that holds tissues together in much the same way that concrete is reinforced by steel rods. The changes in the collagen, possibly by causing cross-linkage between fibers, can permanently wrinkle the skin. Finally, many researchers agree that UV light may also inhibit the immune response by damaging Langerhans' cells in the epidermis. When damaged, these large cells lose their ability to alert the other cells of the immune system to infection. The most serious danger is that UV radiation may alter the genetic code within cells, causing cancer.

Melanin protects the cells of the body by blocking and absorbing UV light. People who have more melanin by heredity are not at as high a risk as those who are lighter. (Although this is not to say that dark-skinned people should not protect themselves from the sun.) In all cases, exposure to UV radiation immediately causes the skin to darken by causing oxygen to combine with the melanin that is already present. Exposure also increases the rate of melanin production and speeds its distribution to other cells, producing more darkening.

Melanocytes are found at the bottom of the outer layer of the skin, which is called the epidermis. They are also at the base of the shafts of hairs and in the eye, producing coloration of the iris and in the black membrane of the eye behind the retina. The pigment-producing melanocytes in the skin are found at the base of the epidermis among cube-shaped skin cells that cannot make pigment. About thirty-six of these epidermal cells occur for each melanocyte. Melanocytes have long extensions that reach out to protect the regular skin cells. Furthermore, melanin can also be transferred to epidermal cells. Skin color is also influenced by the distribution and size of the pigment granules in the melanocytes. Very dark skin tends to have single, large granules. Lighter skin tends to have clusters of two to four smaller granules.

On a larger scale, small uneven clusters of pigment are called freckles. These spots of melanin show mostly in lighter-skinned people, are controlled by heredity, and appear with sun exposure to the skin. Because of this uneven distribution of melanin, other cells among the freckles are not protected and can easily be sunburned.

Moles (nevi) are larger, dark spots of melanin that tend to increase as a person ages. Two types occur: The pigment can be deposited into the dermis (intradermal nevi) or can be found between the dermis and the epidermis (junctional nevi). The first type of mole tends to be elevated and have hair growing from it. The second tends to be flat and very dark.

Large amounts of melanin in hair will cause it to be black. Lesser amounts make it brown, and still less causes it to be blond. White or gray hair has no melanin. Yet a separate gene for a reddish, iron-containing pigment can be inherited. If two of these recessive genes are present, then the hair will be red. Depending on the amount of melanin that is also present, such people range from almost purely red hair to a strawberry blond color to a reddish-brown (auburn). Larger amounts of melanin will cover the red pigment completely.

Lack of melanin in the iris of the eye will scatter light and cause the eye to reflect blue. Larger amounts cause the eye color to be darker. The pigment in the iris serves to block radiation that could sunburn the retina. In 1992, investigators at Boston College found that eye sensitivity increases when the amount of melanin is greater.

Melanin breaks down as it moves toward the outer layers of the epidermis, forming a chemical called melanoid in the process. Melanoid can be seen as a yellow color in the thick (calloused) skin of the palms of the hands and the soles of feet.

Carotene is a yellow-to-orange pigment which tends to accumulate in the layer of fat under the skin. This pigment is also responsible for the color of carrots, yellow vegetables, and the yellows in autumn leaves. When taken into the body, carotene is stored in the liver and converted into vitamin A, which is used in vision. Females usually store more carotene than males because of their higher percentages of fat. Asian peoples tend to have combinations of low melanin and higher carotene that produce a yellowish skin hue.

Hemoglobin and oxyhemoglobin are pigments that are found inside red blood cells. Hemoglobin is dark red but looks bluish through the skin. If hemoglobin combines with oxygen, it is called oxyhemoglobin. Oxyhemoglobin is bright red. Skin color from this pigment varies with the amount of blood that is circulated at the surface of the dermis, the relative amounts of hemoglobin and oxyhemoglobin that are present, and the densities of other pigments. Hemoglobin and oxyhemoglobin affect the color of light-skinned people more than of darker people. The skin of lighter people generally looks reddish, with oxygen-poor veins appearing blue.

Rapid change of hair color, from dark pigmented to gray or white, is impossible because of the slow growth rate of hair. Melanin is deposited into the hair shaft at the root. The hairs grow outward at a rate of about 13 millimeters a month. Hence a loss of pigment production would take a long time to show. The myth of rapid change may be based on diseases that cause all the pigmented hair to fall out overnight, leaving only white hairs.

DISORDERS AND DISEASES
Pigmentation can be abnormal and associated with disease. Excess adrenocorticotropic hormone (ACTH)

can increase melanin. ACTH contains several hormones, including MSH. Addison's disease involves the overproduction of ACTH; President John F. Kennedy suffered from this disease. Also, certain injuries such as burns, chemical irritations, or some infections may cause an increase in pigmentation, as can pregnancy. Injuries in which melanocytes are destroyed may result in scar tissue that lacks pigmentation. An excessive intake of carotene can cause light skin to turn orange, a condition called carotenemia.

Skin cancer has been increasing, doubling every decade from the 1960's to the 1990's. There is also evidence that the ozone layer, a thin layer of gas molecules consisting of three oxygen atoms, is being stripped away by chemicals such as refrigerants which are released into the atmosphere. This layer protects life on the planet from the full shower of ultraviolet radiation that comes from the sun. Any changes in the skin, such as a mole that changes in color or begins to grow, should be shown to a doctor. Although moles and other abnormalities in pigmentation are not usually dangerous, some may develop into melanomas.

Researchers have been trying to discover if it is possible to tan safely. Attempts have been made to develop better creams to block UV radiation. Skin cancer is less common among dark-skinned people; it has been reasoned that if melanin could be put into a skin cream, lighter-skinned people could have more of this natural protection. Unfortunately, many sources of melanin are expensive. For example, cuttlefish have an inky defensive spray that contains melanin, but collecting it costs almost three thousand dollars an ounce. In 1986, the Biosource Genetics Corporation used genetic engineering to produce melanin. The gene for melanin was placed into tobacco plants, and the pigment was made for less than one dollar a gram. The company was able to market two skin creams and a lipstick with melanin in some countries.

Presently, the best way to avoid skin cancer is to avoid the sunlight, especially between the hours of 10 A.M. and 3 P.M., when the light is most intense. Additional protection can be found by using a sunscreen lotion with a high sun-protection factor (SPF) of at least 15. SPF 15 permits fifteen times longer exposure before burning (compared to using no sunscreen), and SPF 30 is thought to protect even the fairest skins.

Nevertheless, even with frequent applications of sunscreens, people may be putting themselves at risk of melanoma, the most serious skin cancer. Spe-

cifically, deoxyribonucleic acid (DNA) absorbs and can be directly damaged by the 280 and 320 nanometer range of UV radiation, and it has been assumed that this range, called UV-B, was the only one about which people had to worry. Sunscreens are developed to block UV-B, the "burning rays." Data collected by Richard B. Setlow and his colleagues at Brookhaven National Laboratory in 1993, however, indicated that longer wavelengths, including some visible light and UV-A, can also damage DNA. Setlow suggests that melanin itself absorbs this energy, setting off chemical reactions which produce chemicals that then damage the melanocytes. This process may be the cause of melanoma. He urges people to protect themselves from all sunlight, something that the present sunscreens cannot do. Clearly, the same risks apply to tanning salons. There is no such thing as a safe tan.

Most melanomas are skin cancers. They can also be found inside the eye, as a black spot on the white of the eye, on the iris, or in the center of the field of vision. Treatment of such growths with radiation or surgical removal of the tumor are options. Removal of the entire eye may be necessary. Preventive measures include sunglasses that filter UV light. Sunglasses should block 95 percent of UV-B and 60 percent of UV-A. Most manufacturers label their sunglasses.

In 1991, a controlled study was done in which injections of synthetic MSH were tested. The goal was to help prevent sunburn and skin cancer in high-risk individuals who tan poorly. Those receiving MSH showed significant tanning compared to those who received injections of a placebo. Some mild side effects occurred in the MSH group, including some brief flushing and vague stomach discomfort after the injection.

There are several irregularities of pigmentation. If the tyrosinase enzyme is missing, a person will produce no melanin. This condition is inherited among all races, and such a person is called an albino (Greek for "white"). Actually, the lack of melanin allows hemoglobin to determine the skin color. Albinos have less protection from the sun and, in addition to the risks to the skin, have poor vision because of light reflections off the back of the eye that normally would be absorbed by pigment. With no pigment in the iris, they are also likely to suffer damage to their retinal cells, resulting in blindness.

Especially in lighter-skinned people, a lack of hemoglobin (anemia) will cause paleness. If a person's body circulates more blood into the dermis, the skin will appear more reddish or flushed. This could signal that the body is attempting to cool itself or that a person is embarrassed. If the body is cold or emotionally shocked, it may reduce circulation of blood to the surface of the dermis and the individual will appear pale. Lack of normal sunlight can cause a person to slow the production of melanin. A person who is exercising by swimming in cold water may not circulate blood as quickly as it is needed, and the increase of hemoglobin may turn that person blue, a tone that is noticeable in people with both large and small amounts of melanin.

PERSPECTIVE AND PROSPECTS

Most scientists believe that the first humans probably had their origin in Africa and were darkly pigmented. As people migrated to the higher latitudes, where the radiation from the sun was less direct, having less pigment was adaptive. Less melanin allowed these people to synthesize needed vitamin D where there was less direct sunlight and less UV light. Before individuals began to migrate over long distances, populations were neatly distributed with darker skins near the equator and lighter skins in Northern Europe. Inuits are an interesting exception: They have dark skin and live in a northern latitude. Their diet, however, has always included fish livers with sufficient vitamin D.

The possibility of danger from the sun and other radiation is only a recent discovery. Ultraviolet radiation was discovered in 1801. By 1927, H. J. Muller showed in the laboratory that X rays cause changes in the genetic code of fruit flies that can be inherited. Such changes, called mutations, can be harmful. Further investigations showed that UV light, while not as dangerous as X rays, can also cause mutations. The likelihood of mutation in an organism is proportional to the dose of radiation that is received; spacing out the exposure makes no difference.

Attempts to classify races by description of skin color have given little return. Paul Broca (1824-1880) developed an elaborate table of twenty colors for cross-matching with the eyes and twenty-four colors for cross-matching with the skin. The color of the skin, however, is extremely difficult to judge: The color itself changes with environmental and physiological conditions, the ability of observers varies, and the lighting conditions under which comparisons are made can also make a difference in the results.

To avoid some of these problems, studies have been performed with a device that measures the reflection of various wavelengths by the skin. In 1992, a study

of members of the Jirel population in Nepal showed that the reflections from measurements of upper-arm skin using three different wavelengths varied as if the reflective properties were controlled by only a single set of genes. Evidently, the use of various wavelengths gives little additional information about color differences.

—*Paul R. Boehlke, Ph.D.*

See also Albinos; Dermatology; Grafts and grafting; Plastic surgery; Skin; Skin cancer; Skin disorders; Skin lesion removal; Tattoo removal; Vitamins and minerals.

FOR FURTHER INFORMATION:

Greeley, Alexandra. "Dodging the Rays." *FDA Consumer* 27 (July/August, 1993): 30-33. Discusses the differences in UV radiation types and concludes that all UV is dangerous. Mentions unproven tanning accelerators that have been promoted.

Greener, Mark. "Gene for Red Hair Could Shed Light on Skin Pigmentation." *Dermatology Times* 20, no. 12 (December, 1999): 19. Explains how Jonathan Rees of the University of Newcastle used genetic studies to examine the relationship between UV sensitivity, hair and skin color, and skin phototype.

Guttman, Cheryl. "Pigmentation Disorders Common in Asians." *Dermatology Times* 20, no. 8 (August, 1999): 24. With light, even-coloration of the skin revered as the ideal image of beauty and nobility by Asian patients, these individuals frequently seek treatment for hyperpigmentation problems. Guttman discusses current treatments for hyperpigmentation.

Levine, Norman. *Pigmentation and Pigmentary Disorders*. Boca Raton, Fla.: CRC Press, 1993. Topics discussed include the biochemistry and physiology of melanin, the photobiology of skin pigmentation, the hormonal control of melanogenesis, and congenital and genetic diseases of hyperpigmentation.

Rogers, Spencer L. *The Colors of Mankind*. Springfield, Ill.: Charles C Thomas, 1990. A thorough but accessible review of the various factors that influence human skin color.

PILES. *See* HEMORRHOIDS.

PIMPLES
DISEASE/DISORDER
ANATOMY OR SYSTEM AFFECTED: Skin
SPECIALTIES AND RELATED FIELDS: Dermatology, family practice, pediatrics

DEFINITION: A "pimple" is the term commonly used to denote a papule or pustule. Papules are small, solid elevations in the skin, usually found in the dermis or epidermis. Pustules are papules that have almost reached the surface of the skin and that contain pus, resulting in a white appearance. Both types of pimples are characteristic lesions of acne, the proliferation of papules, pustules, and comedos (hair follicles plugged with matter, often called blackheads and whiteheads). Attempting to remove the pus from pimples can cause open lesions, and possible permanent scarring. Most pimples will resolve themselves with time.

—*Jason Georges and Tracy Irons-Georges*
See also Acne; Dermatology; Puberty and adolescence; Rosacea; Skin; Skin disorders.

FOR FURTHER INFORMATION:

Dvorine, William. *A Dermatologist's Guide to Home Skin Treatment.* New York: Charles Scribner's Sons, 1983.
Flandermeyer, Kenneth L. *Clear Skin.* Boston: Little, Brown, 1979.
Pillsbury, Donald M. *A Manual of Dermatology.* Philadelphia: W. B. Saunders, 1971.
Roenigk, Henry H., ed. *Office Dermatology.* Baltimore: Williams & Wilkins, 1981.

PINWORM

DISEASE/DISORDER

ALSO KNOWN AS: *Enterobius vermicularis*, threadworm, seatworm

ANATOMY OR SYSTEM AFFECTED: Gastrointestinal system, intestines, skin

SPECIALTIES AND RELATED FIELDS: Dermatology, family practice, pediatrics, public health

DEFINITION: A common parasitic nematode that resembles a white thread approximately 0.5 inch in length.

CAUSES AND SYMPTOMS

Infestation with pinworm, a common name for the organism *Enterobius vermicularis*, is characterized by itching around the anus that becomes worse at night, causing sleeplessness, irritability, and general restlessness. There may also be vague gastrointestinal symptoms such as loose stools or nausea. Humans are the only host for the pathogen. Young children are most often affected, and the disease spreads easily to other members of the household.

Adult pinworms live in the large intestine. Females migrate to the anus and deposit eggs outside of the body; this is the cause of the itching. Scratching often causes the eggs to be deposited on food and eaten or transferred directly to the mouth and swallowed. Newly hatched larvae migrate to the large intestine and lay eggs over a four-week period. Pinworm eggs are viable outside of a host for up to two weeks.

Children typically complain of intense itching around the anal area at night. Scratching may cause bleeding in the region. Interrupted sleep may cause irritability during the day. Individual worms are not commonly seen. The most common diagnostic procedure is to apply a piece of pressure-sensitive cellulose tape to the anus and look for eggs under a microscope.

Pinworm infestation must be differentiated from fungal and yeast infections, allergies, and conditions caused by other species of worms. Fungal and yeast infections can be cultured. Allergies may include itching near the anus but usually involve other areas of the body as well. Analyzing their eggs or bodies can identify other species of worms.

TREATMENT AND THERAPY

Pinworm infestation is relatively easy to treat. Drugs requiring a physician's prescription are taken by mouth for three to five days and usually kill the pinworms. Antihistamines can be used to obtain relief from itching.

It is very important to wash one's hands thoroughly with soap and warm water after using the toilet and before meals. Fingernails should be closely trimmed to prevent injury when scratching and to minimize the chance of transferring eggs. All clothing of a patient should be washed after each use. Laundering bedding will kill pinworm eggs.

Although pinworm infestation is annoying, it is otherwise benign. A cure can be obtained readily using appropriate drug therapy. Repeated infestation is common, however, especially among children.

—*L. Fleming Fallon, Jr., M.D., Ph.D., M.P.H.*
See also Gastroenterology; Gastroenterology, pediatric; Gastrointestinal disorders; Gastrointestinal system; Itching; Parasitic diseases; Worms.

FOR FURTHER INFORMATION:

Buchsbaum, Ralph, et al. *Animals Without Backbones.*
3d ed. Chicago: University of Chicago Press, 1987.

Despommier, Dickson D., Robert W. Gwadz, and Peter J. Hotex. *Parasitic Diseases*. 4th ed. New York: Springer-Verlag, 2000.

Donaldson, Raymond Joseph, ed. *Parasites and Western Man*. Baltimore: University Park Press, 1979.

Klein, Aaron E. *The Parasites We Humans Harbor*. New York: Elsevier/Nelson Books, 1981.

Lee, Donald L. *The Physiology of Nematodes*. San Francisco: W. H. Freeman, 1965.

PITYRIASIS ALBA
DISEASE/DISORDER

ANATOMY OR SYSTEM AFFECTED: Skin

SPECIALTIES AND RELATED FIELDS: Dermatology, family practice

DEFINITION: Pityriasis alba is a skin disease that produces round or oval patches which are lighter in color than the surrounding skin. The patches may be flat or slightly elevated, and they may be slightly reddish. They are most often found on the face, neck, upper arms, chest, and back. There is usually little or no itching. The underlying cause of pityriasis alba is unknown. The patches usually disappear without treatment within a few months. Any itching that occurs can be treated with a mild topical steroid.

—*Rose Secrest*

See also Dermatology; Dermatology, pediatric; Rashes; Skin; Skin disorders.

FOR FURTHER INFORMATION:
Lamberg, Lynne. *Skin Disorders*. Philadelphia: Chelsea House, 2001.

Mackie, Rona M. *Clinical Dermatology*. 4th ed. New York: Oxford University Press, 1997.

Rassner, Gernot, and Walter H. Burgdorf. *Atlas of Dermatology*. 3d ed. Philadelphia: Lea & Febiger, 1994.

Sams, W. Mitchell, and Peter J. Lynch, ed. *Principles and Practice of Dermatology*. 2d ed. London: Churchill Livingstone, 1996.

PITYRIASIS ROSEA
DISEASE/DISORDER

ANATOMY OR SYSTEM AFFECTED: Arms, back, chest, hips, legs, skin

SPECIALTIES AND RELATED FIELDS: Dermatology, family practice

DEFINITION: Pityriasis rosea is a viral skin rash that starts as one or more large red spots on the trunk of the body. The spots grow and spread to cover the trunk, upper arms, and upper legs, and the patches become copper-colored with scaly surfaces. Depending on the severity of the itching, a physician may recommend the application of calamine lotion or a steroid cream to the rash or the use of antihistamine tablets. The rash disappears naturally in four to ten weeks.

—*Alvin K. Benson, Ph.D.*

See also Dermatology; Dermatology, pediatric; Itching; Rashes; Skin; Skin disorders; Viral infections.

FOR FURTHER INFORMATION:
Lamberg, Lynne. *Skin Disorders*. Philadelphia: Chelsea House, 2001.

Mackie, Rona M. *Clinical Dermatology*. 4th ed. New York: Oxford University Press, 1997.

Rassner, Gernot, and Walter H. Burgdorf. *Atlas of Dermatology*. 3d ed. Philadelphia: Lea & Febiger, 1994.

Sams, W. Mitchell, and Peter J. Lynch, ed. *Principles and Practice of Dermatology*. 2d ed. London: Churchill Livingstone, 1996.

PKU. *See* PHENYLKETONURIA (PKU)

PLAGUE
DISEASE/DISORDER

ANATOMY OR SYSTEM AFFECTED: Lungs, respiratory system

SPECIALTIES AND RELATED FIELDS: Bacteriology, emergency medicine, environmental health, epidemiology, public health

DEFINITION: An infection transmitted by fleas, which may prove fatal if left untreated.

CAUSES AND SYMPTOMS
Plague is caused by infection with a bacterium called *Yersinia pestis* (formerly *Pasteurella pestis*). *Yersinia pestis* is a gram-negative, bipolar-staining bacillus which predominantly infects rodents, with humans being accidental hosts. The disease is transmitted by the bite of a flea which has become infected after a blood meal from another animal with the bacterium in its bloodstream or by the ingestion of contaminated animal tissues.

There are three cycles that perpetuate plague in animals and humans. Sylvatic or wild plague is maintained in the wild rodent population, such as ground squirrels, rock squirrels, and prairie dogs. Urban rat

Transmission of Plague

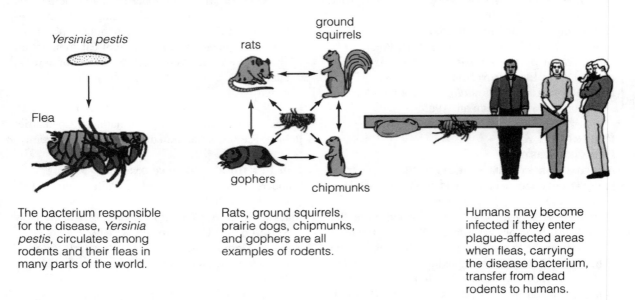

Yersinia pestis

Flea

rats

ground squirrels

gophers

chipmunks

The bacterium responsible for the disease, *Yersinia pestis*, circulates among rodents and their fleas in many parts of the world.

Rats, ground squirrels, prairie dogs, chipmunks, and gophers are all examples of rodents.

Humans may become infected if they enter plague-affected areas when fleas, carrying the disease bacterium, transfer from dead rodents to humans.

A variety of small mammals, particularly rodents, carry the flea that transmits the plague bacterium Yersinia pestis.

plague occurs in developing countries, especially seaports, and is maintained by the infection of urban and domestic rats, which during epidemics may be as high as 10 percent of the rat population. Finally, there is pneumonic plague, a form of the disease limited to humans, which directly transmits the infection via infected aerosol droplets from a person with a lung infection.

The most common plague illness in humans is called bubonic plague. After an incubation period of two to eight days following the bite of an infected flea, there is a sudden onset of fever, chills, weakness, and headache. Within hours, extremely tender oval swellings 1 to 10 centimeters in length appear in one anatomic area of lymph nodes, usually the groin, axilla (armpit), or neck. These buboes presumably result when the bacteria inoculated into the skin by the infected flea migrate to the regional lymph nodes. Many of these patients will have bacteria intermittently present in the bloodstream during the acute stage of the illness.

Less common, but more severe, forms of the illness include septicemic and pneumonic plague. Septicemic plague occurs when the inoculated bacteria proliferate rapidly in the blood, overwhelming the patient before producing a bubo. Pneumonic plague may occur as a secondary pneumonia in bubonic plague, when the lung becomes infected by bacteria carried in the bloodstream, or as a primary pneumonia, through direct inhalation following exposure to a coughing plague patient. Septicemic and pneumonic plague are often fatal, especially if antibiotic therapy is delayed. Rarely, plague can be manifested as a pharyngitis resembling acute tonsillitis or meningitis.

TREATMENT AND THERAPY

A diagnosis of plague is suspected in febrile patients who have been exposed to rodents in areas of the world known to harbor the disease. The causative bacteria are usually identified by microscopic examination and culture of material obtained from aspiration of a bubo. Blood, sputum, throat swabs, or spinal fluid can be processed in a similar manner.

Quarantine, rat control, and insecticides to kill fleas have successfully controlled urban plague in many cities around the globe. Sylvatic plague has been more difficult to control because of the range and diversity of the world rodent reservoirs. A vaccine is available for selected high-risk individuals. Untreated plague has a mortality of more than 50 percent, but this high risk of death can be reduced by the early institution of antibiotic treatment with either streptomycin or tetracycline and the use of modern medical supportive care.

PERSPECTIVE AND PROSPECTS

The first pandemic of plague began in Egypt or Ethiopia in 540 C.E. and continued for sixty years, killing about one hundred million people. The second pandemic, called the Black Death, began in the fourteenth century in central Asia and then spread to Europe, where a quarter of the total population died. The world is currently in the third pandemic, which began in China during the 1890's when infected rats were inadvertently transported on ships to other countries in the Americas, Asia, and Africa.

Currently, about one thousand cases are reported each year to the World Health Organization, with Tanzania and Vietnam leading the list in numbers of cases. The United States reports twenty to twenty-five cases per year, mostly from Arizona and New Mexico. American Indians seem especially susceptible to this disease.

—*H. Bradford Hawley, M.D.*

See also Arthropod-borne diseases; Bacterial infections; Bites and stings; Epidemiology; Pneumonia.

FOR FURTHER INFORMATION:

Altman, Linda Jacobs. *Plagues and Pestilence: A History of Infectious Disease*. Springfield, N.J.: Enslow, 1998. Designed for students in grades six through twelve, this book examines well-known plagues and epidemics in world history, past and present, through the social and historical context of the times.

Biddle, Wayne. *Field Guide to Germs*. New York: Henry Holt, 1995. This comprehensive book is easily accessible to the nonspecialist and includes a discussion of nearly every virus, bacterium, and fungus known to cause human and nonhuman animal disease. The history of the microbe and the treatment of diseases are included.

Cook, G. C., ed. *Manson's Tropical Diseases*. 20th ed. London: W. B. Saunders, 1996. Offers an extensive discussion of plague, including a complete list of rodent reservoirs by country.

Mandell, Gerald L., R. Gordon Douglas, Jr., and John E. Bennett, eds. *Principles and Practice of Infectious Diseases*. 3d ed. New York: Churchill Livingstone, 1990. A standard reference textbook of infectious diseases with a chapter on plague including maps and illustrations.

Woods, Gail L., et al. *Diagnostic Pathology of Infectious Diseases*. Philadelphia: Lea & Febiger, 1993. A pathology reference textbook with a description of host-pathogen interactions and laboratory diagnostic methods.

PLASTIC SURGERY
PROCEDURES

ANATOMY OR SYSTEM AFFECTED: All

SPECIALTIES AND RELATED FIELDS: Dermatology, emergency medicine, general surgery, oncology, physical therapy, psychology

DEFINITION: Plastic surgery uses such procedures as grafting and the implantation of prostheses in order to treat congenital defects and tissue or limb damage resulting from trauma; reconstructive surgery uses the techniques of plastic surgery to repair injured tissues or to reattach severed body parts, while cosmetic surgery employs these same methods to alter body shape or appearance for aesthetic purposes.

KEY TERMS:

congenital: existing at birth; often used in reference to certain mental or physical malformations and diseases, which may be hereditary or caused by some influence during gestation

cosmetic surgery: the application of plastic surgical techniques to alter one's appearance for purely aesthetic reasons

debridement: the excision of contused and devitalized tissue from a wound surface

dermis: the second layer of skin, immediately below the epidermis; it contains blood and lymphatic vessels, nerves, glands, and (usually) hair follicles

epidermis: the outermost thin layer of skin that encompasses structures superficial to the dermis

granuloma: a nodular, inflammatory lesion that is usually small, firm, persistent, and containing proliferated macrophages

plastic surgery: the branch of operative surgery concerning the repair of defects, the replacement of lost tissue, and the treatment of extensive scarring; it accomplishes these ends by direct union of body parts, grafting, or the transfer of tissue from one part of the body to another

reconstructive surgery: the application of plastic surgical techniques to repair damaged tissues

turgor: fullness and firmness; the quality of normal skin in a healthy young person

INDICATIONS AND PROCEDURES

The intent of plastic, reconstructive, and cosmetic surgery is to restore a body part to normal appearance or to enhance or cosmetically alter a body part. The techniques and procedures of all three surgical applications are similar: extremely careful skin preparation, the use of delicate instrumentation and handling techniques, and precise suturing with extremely fine materials to minimize scarring.

Reconstructive surgery. Notable examples of reconstructive surgery involve the reattachment of limbs or extremities that have been traumatically severed. As soon as a part is separated from the body, it loses its blood supply; this leads to ischemia (lack of oxygen) to tissues, which in turn leads to cell death. When an individual cell dies, it cannot be resuscitated and will soon start to decompose. This process can be greatly slowed by lowering the temperature of the severed body part. Packing the part in ice for transport to a hospital is a prudent initial step.

An important consideration in any reconstructive procedure is site preparation. The edges, or margins, of the final wound must be clean and free of contamination. Torn skin is removed through a process called debridement. A sharp scalpel is used gently to cut away tissue that has been crushed or torn. All bacterial contamination must be removed from the site prior to closure to prevent postoperative contamination. Foreign material such as dirt, glass, gunpowder, metals, or chemicals must be completely removed. The mar-

Common Sites for Cosmetic Surgery

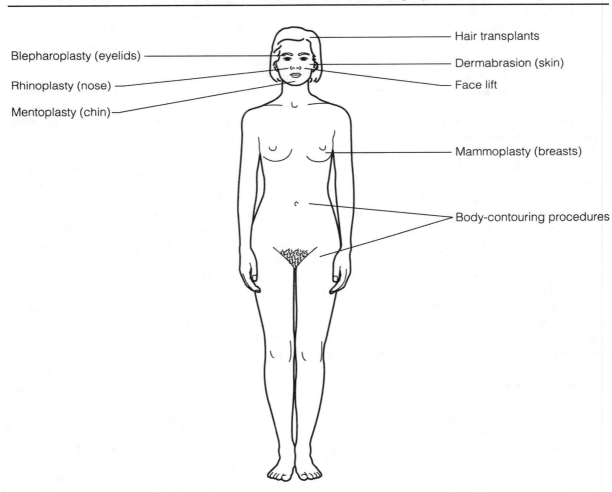

Blepharoplasty (eyelids)

Rhinoplasty (nose)

Mentoplasty (chin)

Hair transplants

Dermabrasion (skin)

Face lift

Mammoplasty (breasts)

Body-contouring procedures

gins of the wound must also be sharply defined. Superficially, this is done for aesthetic reasons. Internally, sharply defined margins will reduce the chances for adhesions to form. Adhesions are bands of scar tissue which bind adjacent structures together and restrict normal movement and function. Therefore, both the body site and the margins of the severed part must be debrided and defined. Reconstruction consists of the painstaking reattachment of nerves, tendons, muscles, and skin, which are held in place primarily by sutures although staples, wires, and other materials are occasionally used. Precise alignment of the skin to be closed is accomplished by joining opposing margins. Postoperative procedures include careful handling of the wound site, adequate nutrition, and rest in order to maximize healing. Abnormalities in the healing process can lead to undesirable scarring from the sites of sutures. Such marks can be avoided with careful attention to correct techniques.

Bones are reconstructed in cases of severe fractures. The pieces are set in their proper positions, and the area is immobilized. Where immobilization is not possible, a surface is provided onto which new bone can grow. These temporary surfaces are made of polymeric materials which will dissolve over time.

Congenital anomalies such as a deformed external ear or missing digit can be corrected using reconstructive techniques. In the case of a missing thumb, a finger can be removed, rotated and attached on the site where the missing thumb should have been. This allows an affected individual to write, hold objects such as eating utensils and generally have a more nearly normal life. Similar procedures can be applied to replace a missing or amputated great or big toe. The presence of the great toe contributes significantly to balance and coordination when walking.

Prosthetic materials are implanted in a growing variety of applications. There are two basic types of materials used in prostheses, which are classified according to their surface characteristics. One is totally smooth and inert; an example is Teflon or silicone. The body usually encloses these materials in a membrane which has the effect of creating a wall or barrier to the surface of the prosthesis. From the body's perspective, the prosthesis has thus been removed. With any prosthesis, the problem most likely to be encountered is infection, which is usually caused by contamination of the operative site or the prosthesis. Infection can also occur at a later, postoperative date because of the migration of bacteria into the cavity

formed by the membrane. This is a potentially serious complication. A smooth prosthesis can also be used to create channels into which tissue can later be inserted. In such an application, the prosthesis may be surgically removed at some time in the future. A second type of prosthesis does not have a smooth surface; rather, it has microscopic fibers similar to those found on a towel. This type of surface prevents membranes from forming, contributing to a longer life for the prosthesis by reducing postoperative infections.

An important procedure in reconstructive surgery is skin grafting. A graft consists of skin that is completely removed from a donor site and transferred to another site on the body. The graft is usually taken from the patient's own body because skin taken from another individual will be rejected by the recipient's immune system. (Nevertheless, fetal pig skin is sometimes used successfully.) Skin grafting is useful for covering open wounds, and it is widely used in serious burn cases. When only a portion of the uppermost layer of the skin is removed, the process is called a split thickness graft. When all the upper layers of the skin are removed, the result is a full thickness graft. Whenever possible, the donor site is selected to match the color and texture characteristics of the recipient site.

A skin flap is sometimes created. This differs from a graft in that the skin of a flap is not completely severed from its original site but simply moved to an adjacent location. Some blood vessels remain to support the flap. This procedure is nearly always successful, but it is limited to immediately adjacent skin.

A wide variety of flaps has been developed. A flap may be stretched and sutured to cover both a wound and the donor site. Flaps may be created from skin that is distant to the site where it is needed and then sutured in place over the donor site. Only after the flap has become established at the new site is it cut free from the donor site. Thus, skin from the abdomen or upper chest may be used to cover the back of a burned hand, or skin from one finger may be used to cover a finger on the other hand. This two-stage flap process requires more time than a skin graft, but it also has a greater probability of success.

Plastic surgery. Plastic surgery consists of a variety of techniques and applications, often dealing with skin. Some common procedures that primarily involve skin are undertaken to remove unwanted wrinkles or folds. Folds in skin are caused by a loss of skin turgor and excessive stretching of the skin beyond which it cannot recover. Common contributors to loss of skin turgor in the abdomen are pregnancy or significant weight loss after years of obesity. Both women and men may undergo a procedure known as abdominoplasty (commonly called a "tummy tuck"). The skin that lies over the abdominal muscles is carefully separated from underlying tissue. Portions of the skin are removed; frequently, some underlying adipose (fat) tissue is also removed or relocated. The remaining skin is sutured to the underlying muscle as well as to adjacent, undisturbed skin. A major problem with this procedure, however, is scar formation because large portions of skin must be removed or relocated. The plastic surgeon must plan the placement of incisions carefully in order to avoid undesirable scars.

Plastic surgery is also used to reduce the prominence of ears, a procedure called otoplasty. In some children, the posterior (back) portion of the external ear develops more than the rest of the ear, pushing the ears outward and making them prominent. By reducing the bulk of cartilage in the posterior ear and suturing the remaining external portion to the base of the ear, the plastic surgeon can create a more normal ear contour. The optimal time to perform this procedure on children is just prior to the time that they enter school, or at about five years of age.

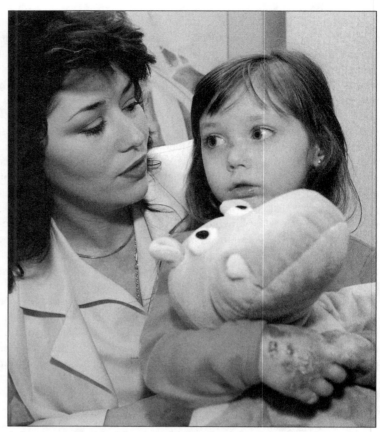

A four-year-old girl with a genetic skin disease waits to undergo a grafting procedure using laboratory-grown skin. (AP/Wide World Photos)

Two other relatively common techniques of plastic surgery are dermabrasion and tattooing. Dermabrasion is the purposeful abrasion of skin using wheels spun at high speeds by compressed air. The effect is similar to that of a plane: Surface defects are removed in thin layers. The technique is widely used to treat scarring caused by severe acne. The edges of an acne scar are abraded, softening the transition from normal skin to the pit of the scar and reducing shadows. As a result, the scar is less noticeable. Dermabrasion is also used to alter the appearance of deep wrinkles and to remove superficially embedded dirt or other debris from a previous injury.

Tattooing is used to blend skin pigmentation or to simulate a structure lost in an injury. Pigment can be injected to alter the color of skin at the graft site. This is most important in areas of sharp contrast, such as the lips; a darker color can be inserted to help camouflage skin taken from a relatively unpigmented donor site. Tattooing is used to color the areolas of nipples in breast reconstructions. It is also used to simulate eyebrows when a healed wound interrupts normal eyebrow contours or continuity. Tattooing is an inexact process due to the difficulty of correctly mixing pigments. Pigmentation varies over the surfaces of single individuals, and it also varies greatly from person to person.

Cosmetic surgery. The most common site for cosmetic surgical procedures is the face. Correction may be desired because of a congenital anomaly that causes unwelcome disfigurement or because of a desire to alter an unwanted aspect of one's body. The cosmetic procedures that have been developed to correct abnormalities of the face include closure of a cleft lip or palate. The correction of a cleft lip is usually done early, ideally in the first three months of life. Closure of a cleft palate (the bone that forms the roof of the mouth) is delayed slightly, until the patient is 12 to 18 months old. These procedures allow affected individuals to acquire normal patterns of speech and language.

Among older individuals, common procedures include blepharoplasty and rhinoplasty. The former refers to the removal of excess skin around the eyelids, while the latter refers to a change, usually a reduction, in the shape of the nose. Both procedures may be included in the more general term of face lift. The effects of aging, excessive solar radiation, and gravity combine to produce fine lines in the face as individuals get older. These fine lines gradually develop into the wrinkles characteristic of older persons. For some, these wrinkles are objectionable. To reduce them—or more correctly to stretch them out—a plastic surgeon removes a section of skin containing the wrinkles or lines and stretches the edges of the remaining epidermis until they are touching. These incisions are placed to coincide with the curved lines that exist in normal skin. Thus, when the edges are sutured together, the resultant scar is minimized. Rhinoplasty often involves the removal of a portion of the bone or cartilage that forms the nose. The bulk of the remaining tissue is also reduced to maintain the desired proportions of the patient's nose. As with any plastic surgical procedure, small sutures are carefully placed to minimize scarring.

A third body area that is commonly subjected to cosmetic procedures is the breast. A woman who is unhappy with the appearance of her breasts may seek to either reduce or augment existing tissue. Breast reductions are accomplished by careful incisions and the judicious removal of both skin and underlying breast tissue. Often the nipples must be repositioned to maintain their proper locations. A flap that includes the nipple is created from each breast. After the desired amount of underlying tissue is removed, the nipples are repositioned, and the skin is recontoured around the remaining breast masses.

Uses and Complications

Reconstructive, plastic, and cosmetic surgeries all have their complications, ranging from severe—such as the rejection of transplanted tissue—to minor but unpleasant—such as noticeable scars. In addition, there is an inherent risk in any procedure that requires the patient to undergo general anesthesia. With

reconstruction, which involves the repair of damaged tissues and structures, the initial injuries sustained by the patient present further obstacles and dangers. The following examples from each type of surgery illustrate the risks involved.

For example, a surgeon who must perform a skin graft can choose between a split or a full thickness graft. A split thickness graft site will heal with relatively normal skin, thus providing opportunities for additional grafting at a later date. It also produces less pronounced scarring. A limitation of this technique, however, is an increased likelihood for the graft to fail. Full thickness grafts are stronger and more likely to be successful, but they lead to more extensive scarring, which is aesthetically undesirable and renders the site unsuitable for later grafts. The surgeon's decision is based on the needs of the patient and the severity of the injury.

The minimization of scarring is a major concern for many patients undergoing plastic surgery. The prevention of noticeable scars involves an understanding of the natural lines of the skin. All areas of the body have lines of significant skin tension and lines of relatively little skin tension. It is along the lines of minimal tension that wrinkles and folds develop over time. These lines are curved and follow body contours. As a rule of thumb, they are generally perpendicular to the fibers of underlying muscle. The plastic surgeon seeks to place incisions along the lines of minimal tension. When scars form after healing, they will blend into the line of minimal tension and become less noticeable. Furthermore, the scar tissue is not likely to become apparent when the underlying muscles or body part is moved. Undesirable scarring is a greater problem in large procedures, such as abdominoplasty, than in procedures confined to a small area, such as rhytidectomy (face lift), because of the difficulty in following lines of minimum tension when making incisions.

One of the most popular cosmetic procedures is breast enlargement. By the mid-1990's, it was estimated that one million women in the United States had undergone breast enlargement, or augmentation. Initially, the most commonly used prosthesis, or implant, was made of silicone. In some patients, silicone leaked out, causing the formation of granulomatous tissue. Such complications led to a voluntary suspension of the production of silicone prostheses by manufacturers and of their usage by surgeons. Different materials, such as polyethylene bags filled with saline solution or solid polyurethane implants, were soon substituted. Saline will not cause tissue damage if it leaks, and few adverse reactions to polyurethane have been reported.

PERSPECTIVE AND PROSPECTS

The origins of plastic, reconstructive, and cosmetic surgery are fundamental to the earliest surgical procedures, which were developed to correct superficial deformities. Without any viable methods of anesthesia, surgical interventions and corrections were limited to the skin. For example, present-day nose reconstructions (rhinoplasty) are essentially similar to procedures developed four thousand years ago. Hindu surgeons developed the technique of moving a piece of skin from the adjacent cheek onto the nose to cover a wound. Similar procedures were developed by Italians using skin that was transferred from the arm or forehead to repair lips and ears as well as noses. Ironically, wars have provided opportunities to advance reconstructive techniques. As field hospitals and surgical facilities became more widely available and wounded soldiers could be stabilized during transport, techniques to repair serious wounds evolved.

Skin grafts have been used since Roman times. Celsus described the possibility of skin grafts in conjunction with eye surgery. References were made to skin grafts in the Middle Ages. The evolution of modern techniques can be traced to the early nineteenth century, when Cesare Baronio conducted systematic grafting experiments with animals. The modern guidelines for grafting were formulated in 1870. Instruments for creating split thickness grafts were developed in the 1930's, and applications of this procedure evolved during World War II.

Plastic, reconstructive, and cosmetic procedures have all become important in contemporary surgical practice. Reconstructive surgery allows the repair of serious injuries and contributes greatly to the rehabilitation of affected individuals. Cosmetic surgery allows individuals to feel better about themselves and their bodies. Both use techniques developed in the broader field of plastic surgery.

There are both positive and negative aspects of plastic surgery. Positively, many individuals who sustain serious and potentially devastating injuries are able to return to relatively normal lives. Burn victims and those having accidents are more likely to return to normal activities and resume their occupations than at any time in the past. Miniaturization and new materials have extended the range of a plastic surgeon's skills. Negatively, there is growing criticism concerning the number of elective procedures undertaken for the repair of cosmetic defects. Charges of abuse have been made. Tattooing is now used to color areas of the head permanently, such as eyebrows and eyelids, thus eliminating the need for some types of cosmetics.

The quest for perfection and physical beauty has prompted some critics to question the correctness of some unnecessary procedures. Although such procedures are not usually covered by insurance policies, their utilization has increased. The continuation of such activities invokes both ethical and personal considerations; there is no clearly defined, logical endpoint. Clearly, while plastic surgical techniques have benefited millions, there are opportunities for abuse. Society must decide if any limitations are to be placed on plastic surgical procedures and what they should be.

In the meantime, advances in materials, instruments, and techniques will benefit plastic, reconstructive, and cosmetic surgery. The advent of magnification and miniaturization and the development of tiny instruments and new suture materials have allowed the reconstruction of many injury sites. Blood vessels and nerves are now routinely reattached. Nine individual sutures are required to join the severed portions of a blood vessel 1 millimeter in diameter. When microsurgical techniques are applied to skin surfaces, they usually result in less noticeable scarring. These techniques have expanded the range of reconstructive and cosmetic techniques available.

—*L. Fleming Fallon, Jr., M.D., Ph.D., M.P.H.*

See also Age spots; Aging; Amputation; Birthmarks; Breast cancer; Breast disorders; Breast surgery; Breasts, female; Burns and scalds; Cancer; Carcinoma; Circumcision, female, and genital mutilation; Circumcision, male; Cleft lip and palate; Cleft lip and palate repair; Cyst removal; Cysts; Dermatology; Dermatology, pediatric; Ear surgery; Face lift and blepharoplasty; Grafts and grafting; Hair loss and baldness; Hair transplantation; Healing; Jaw wiring; Laceration repair; Liposuction; Malignancy and metastasis; Malignant melanoma removal; Mastectomy and lumpectomy; Moles; Obesity; Otoplasty; Otorhinolaryngology; Ptosis; Rhinoplasty and submucous resection; Sex change surgery; Skin; Skin lesion removal; Surgical procedures; Varicose vein removal; Varicose veins; Warts.

FOR FURTHER INFORMATION:

Grazer, F. M., and J. R. Klingbeil. *Body Image: A Surgical Perspective*. St. Louis: Mosby Year Book, 1980. The emphasis in this work is on cosmetic surgery. The authors are skilled plastic surgeons who concentrate primarily on the cosmetic aspects of their profession.

Melmed, E. P. "Polyurethane Implants: A Six-Year Review of 416 Patients." *Plastic and Reconstructive Surgery* 82 (August, 1988): 285-290. This journal article reviews the use of nonsilicone breast implants. Polyurethane is emerging as a preferable alternative to silicone in some but not all applications.

Rutkow, Ira M. *Surgery: An Illustrated History*. St. Louis: Mosby Year Book, 1993. This historical review of surgery includes sections on the evolution and practice of plastic, reconstructive, and cosmetic surgical techniques. This book is useful for individuals who want to know the context from which plastic surgery emerged.

Sabiston, David C., Jr., ed. *Textbook of Surgery: The Biological Basis of Modern Surgical Practice*. 16th ed. Philadelphia: W. B. Saunders, 2001. A standard textbook of surgery containing an extensive discussion of different techniques of plastic, reconstructive, and cosmetic surgery.

PLEURISY

DISEASE/DISORDER

ANATOMY OR SYSTEM AFFECTED: Chest, lungs, respiratory system

SPECIALTIES AND RELATED FIELDS: Pulmonary medicine

DEFINITION: Pleurisy is the inflammation and swelling of the pleurae, the membranes that enclose the lungs and line the chest cavity. It may be one of the complications of tuberculosis, pneumonia, chest injury, viral infection, congestive heart failure, kidney and liver disorders, and lung cancer. The symptoms of pleurisy include chest pain on breathing or coughing, discomfort on moving the affected side, and rapid, shallow breathing. Possible complications include pneumonia, lung compression or collapse, and the restriction of lung expansion. The risk of developing pleurisy increases with obesity, smoking, and the use of immunosuppressive drugs. Treatment consists of addressing the underlying disorder.

—*Jason Georges and Tracy Irons-Georges*
See also Lungs; Pneumonia; Pulmonary diseases;

Pleurisy

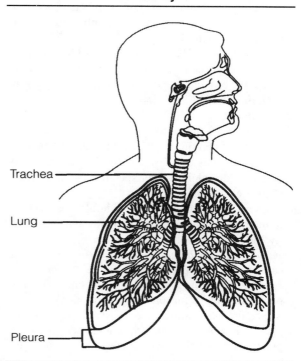

The pleurae are the membranes that encase the lungs; pleurisy is the inflammation of one or both pleurae and may have a variety of causes.

Pulmonary medicine; Pulmonary medicine, pediatric; Respiration.

FOR FURTHER INFORMATION:

Fishman, Alfred, ed. *Update: Pulmonary Diseases and Disorders*. 2d ed. New York: McGraw-Hill, 1992.

Freeman, Neil. *Pleurisy*. Belconnen, Australian Capital Territory: Outlaw! Press, 1989.

James, D. Geraint, and Peter R. Studdy. *A Color Atlas of Respiratory Disease*. 2d ed. St. Louis: Mosby Year Book, 1992.

West, John B. *Pulmonary Pathophysiology: The Essentials*. 4th ed. Baltimore: Williams & Wilkins, 1992.

Widström, Olle. *Pathogenetic Mechanisms in Pleurisy*. Stockholm: Gotab, 1982.

PNEUMONIA

DISEASE/DISORDER

ANATOMY OR SYSTEM AFFECTED: Lungs, respiratory system

SPECIALTIES AND RELATED FIELDS: Emergency medicine, epidemiology, family practice, internal medicine, occupational health, public health, pulmonary medicine

DEFINITION: An inflammation of one of several possible areas of the respiratory system, mainly in the lungs or bronchial passageways, resulting from bacterial or viral infection.

KEY TERMS:

Gram's stain: a laboratory method for tracing the presence of certain bacteria in lung tissue; the procedure involves the observation of different levels of tissue discoloration as specific chemical reactions are induced

pleurisy: a secondary but very painful inflammation of the membranes that line the lungs and chest cavity; often accompanies pneumonia

Pneumocystis pneumonia: a form of pneumonia caused by the single-celled parasite *Pneumocystis carinii*; dangerous primarily to persons with impaired immunity mechanisms, particularly victims of acquired immunodeficiency syndrome (AIDS)

Streptococcus pneumoniae: commonly referred to as pneumococcus; the main bacteria responsible for pneumonia

CAUSES AND SYMPTOMS

Although modern medicine succeeded several generations ago in identifying the key viruses and bacteria responsible for pneumonia and in developing efficient medications for its treatment, a surprisingly high number of deaths from the complications of pneumonia continue to occur. In large part this is the case because pneumonia, which involves infection and inflammation in the respiratory system, occurs not only on its own but also as a complication brought about by other serious illnesses. In aged patients, especially, general deterioration of the body's resistance to bacterial or viral infection can lead in a final stage to death from pneumonia.

Just as the causes of pneumonia can vary, the disease itself may take different forms. Some sources postulate that pneumonia is not a single disease but a group of advanced lung inflammations. Because they are so similar in their symptoms and effects on the body, all members of this family of diseases are labeled as one form or another of pneumonia. Specific forms range from lobar pneumonia (caused by the bacterial invasion of *Streptococcus pneumoniae* into a single lobe of one lung) and bronchopneumonia

(from *Haemophilus influenzae* bacteria colonizing in the bronchi) to viral pneumonia (which may be caused by complications originating from chickenpox or influenza virus). In all cases, symptoms include painful coughing, but other symptoms, such as high fever, reduced sputum production, or discolored (rust-tinged or greenish) sputum, may differ. It follows that the drugs that have been developed to treat pneumonia necessarily vary according to the variety of the disease involved.

Lobar pneumonia and bronchopneumonia are the two main classes of disease. The former occurs when an initial infection attacks only one lobe of one lung. Bronchopneumonia results from an initial inflammation in the bronchi and bronchioles (air passages to

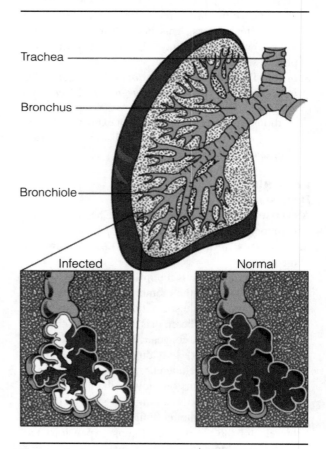

Pneumonia is actually a group of imflammatory diseases that affect the lungs; in lobar pneumonia, only one lobe of the lung is attacked, whereas in bronchopneumonia the bronchi and bronchioles, which lead to both lungs, are affected. The inset shows infection of the alveoli in lobar pneumonia.

the lungs), which then spreads to the internal tissue of one or both lungs. Once the symptoms of pneumonia have become visible, any of the following may occur: fever, chills, shortness of breath, chest pains, or a painful cough that produces yellow-green or brownish sputum. These symptoms occur because of a condition called pleurisy, which is an inflammation of the membrane lining the lungs themselves and the general chest cavity area.

Some assumptions about the causes of pneumonia being limited to bacterial or viral sources have been altered. In particular, clinical observation of patients suffering from AIDS reveals that certain fungi, yeasts, or protozoa can cause pneumonia in these and other cases where immunodeficiency disorders are present.

Although it is apparent that pneumococci can thrive in various parts of the bodies of animals, particularly monkeys and humans, the process that leads to general infection and a concentrated and dangerous attack on the pulmonary system has been the subject of many medical investigations. It is nearly certain that the presence of the common cold virus in the upper respiratory tract can create the conditions needed for the movement of pneumococci from areas of the body where they may be generally present without causing harm (mainly in saliva) into the pulmonary system. Under conditions of normal health, many body mechanisms can stop a potential invasion of the pulmonary system. This process may involve nasal mucus, although it is not itself bactericidal (bacteria-killing), and other mucous membranes in the region of the larynx. Even beyond the larynx and vocal cords, mechanical means associated with the upward sweep of hairlike protrusions called cilia on the inner linings of deeper respiratory membranes tend to protect the bronchial tree.

When normal protective processes are reduced, as when the cold virus is present, pneumococci may reach the lower respiratory zone and the parenchyma of the lung, where they settle and multiply. The metabolic products that accumulate as a result of this reproductive process begin to have injurious effects on the respiratory organs. Such injuries become actual lesions in the internal respiratory tissues. The process of infection that follows involves the deposition of fibrin in the adjacent blood and lymph vessels. This phenomenon actually tends to shield the invading organisms from the effects normally produced by antipneumococcal immune substances carried by the blood. If unchecked by medical treatment, reproduc-

tion of the invading pneumococci can lead to more extensive lesions. If tissue damage occurs, this can cause the formation of edema, a dangerous accumulation of fluids in spaces where fluids are not normally found. At a later stage of the disease, it appears that the pneumococci enter the interstitial and lymphatic tissues. The unchecked advance of pneumonia infection produces a general deterioration of vital breathing processes as excess fluids spread farther into the respiratory system. In weakened or immunocompromised individuals, this process can lead to death.

TREATMENT AND THERAPY
Medical treatment of the two main types of pneumonia is not the same. Lobar pneumonia requires treatment with penicillin. Bronchopneumonia, although also caused by pneumococcus bacteria, must be treated with different antibiotics. Most forms of pneumonia caused by viral infections, including psittacosis and mycoplasmal pneumonia, require one of two specific drugs: tetracycline or erythromycin. When viral pneumonia provides the basic disease to which bacterial infections in the lungs are added, however, antibiotics represent the main general means of treatment.

Since World War II, the progress of medical science in dealing with various types of pneumonia has been marked by the development of antimicrobial drugs that can be used in treating diagnosed cases of pneumonia. One of the earliest such drugs, which eventually turned out to be ineffective, was a derivative of quinine called Optochin. It was used for the first time on mice in 1912. Five years later, when the drug was applied to human patients, it was observed that the pneumococci were able to develop a surprising degree of resistance to these early antimicrobial substances. Thus, just as progress in the field of immunization had to wait for a later generation, so did effective drugs such as penicillin and other antibiotics that have become standard tools in the treatment of forms of pneumonia.

In most cases, advances in drug treatment to cure pneumonia have been strikingly successful. The phenomenon of the nonbacterial, nonviral version of *Pneumocystis carinii* pneumonia arrived very soon after these successes. It posed a particular series of dilemmas for medical science in the 1980's and 1990's. This problem emerged when it became apparent that certain drugs that had been developed to treat pneumonia, in particular the drug combination of trimethoprim-sulfamethoxazole (TMP-SMZ), failed to achieve expected results in a rising number of cases of *Pneumocystis carinii* (*P. carinii*) pneumonia. This particular form of pneumonia turned out to be among the minority strains of the disease caused by single-celled microorganisms called protozoa.

The importance of *P. carinii* in applied medical science soon extended beyond the restricted domain of pneumonia pathology. It had been discovered in 1909 in Brazil and was thought to affect only animals. This research involved local researchers led by the Italian Antonio Carini, whose name was attached to the discovery. It was only much later, in the 1940's and 1950's, that the presence of *P. carinii* could be traced to pneumonia in human infants. This meant that a relatively unusual form of pneumonia belonged to limited number of cases caused not by bacteria or viruses but by fungi, yeasts, or microorganisms, specifically, single-celled protozoa. This form of pneumonia remained a relatively rare occurrence until the number of AIDS cases increased.

What appeared to be a near epidemic frequency of *P. carinii* was in fact a marker or indicator for discovering patients suffering from AIDS. This observation made it possible to immediately test for the presence of AIDS whenever cases of *P. carinii* appeared. Clinical experience during the 1980's revealed that at least 60 percent of all persons suffering from AIDS had contracted or would contract *P. carinii* pneumonia. The presence of *P. carinii* is now assumed to be associated with AIDS unless that diagnosis is excluded by a laboratory test.

It is important to note that relatively rapid advances made by medical researchers in preventing the spread of *P. carinii* and in treating the cases that did occur among infants led to a new appreciation for pneumonia. Applied research dating from 1958 and extending into the 1970's produced surprisingly effective agents to combat *P. carinii* pneumonia. This work led to the early application of drugs to people infected with human immunodeficiency virus (HIV). The concept of multiple drug therapy, patterned on TMP-SMZ, was also successfully applied in the field of cancer treatment.

Another drug, pentamidine, had been used to treat *P. carinii* pneumonia. When TMP-SMZ seemed to provide a superior treatment, pentamidine production was halted. When the potential utility of pentamidine in treating AIDS became apparent, the Centers for Disease Control and the Food and Drug Administration (FDA) had to take special action in 1984 to li-

cense an American supplier. This is how pentamidine quickly became widely available to treat individuals with AIDS. Pentamidine has also been successfully used as an effective treatment for a variety of viral diseases.

A side effect of these AIDS-related developments by the mid-1980's has been to reemphasize the importance of pneumonia. This renewed interest involves both treatments that are most appropriate for different types of pneumonia and research that is still needed to understand fully the role of this family of diseases in modern medicine and society.

PERSPECTIVE AND PROSPECTS

Although modern medicine has not been able to reduce substantially or eliminate totally the number of cases of pneumonia, much has been learned about the disease and its causes. Scientific advances in the campaign to combat the effects of pneumonia in all areas of the world began with the first isolation of *Streptococcus pneumoniae* in France and the United States in 1880. The French discovery of pneumococci is associated with the laboratory of Louis Pasteur. Simultaneously, George Sternberg was completing work in the medical department of the U.S. Army. In the first decade after the isolation of pneumococci, many different researchers contributed to laboratory findings that linked these bacteria to inflammatory infections in the lungs of animals. They extended their research to include the effects on humans.

One of the most important early breakthroughs came in 1884 when the Danish researcher Hans Christian Joachim Gram developed a laboratory method for identifying specific bacteria in tissue specimens. This technique, called Gram's stain, revealed that different chemical reactions occur when samples of lung tissue and secretions from individuals ill with pneumonia and healthy persons are tested. The tissues stain very differently. The next step would lead to research into the phenomenon of phagocytosis, a process within pulmonary tissue that combats inapparent pneumococcus infection in healthy people. This specific discovery became linked with efforts to develop an immunization technology against pneumonia.

Until the 1980's, medical researchers used their knowledge of pneumonia mainly to develop methods of immunization against the disease. They also tried to diversify the drugs used in treating pneumonia. Efforts to produce a vaccine against pneumonia began with experiments by the German researchers George and Felix Klemperer, who tested antiserum in animals in 1891. The Klemperers were able to show that the offspring of adult rabbits which had been immunized were resistant to pneumococcal invasion and infection. Soon thereafter, they carried out the first injections of immune serum into human patients. This research ultimately led to two findings. There was not an actual antitoxin or antibacterial property in the serum. Instead, it promoted phagocytosis, a process of encapsulation around pneumococci that aids in the immunological response of white blood cells in the body. The vaccine stimulates the body to create its own defenses.

In 1911 in South Africa, an experimental pneumonia vaccine program was undertaken. Although the specific program was not successful, the English physician and scientist Frederick Lister extended its theory. Unequivocal success with a pneumonia vaccine did not come until the last year of World War II. In 1945, C. M. MacLeod and several colleagues published research findings proving that pneumococcal infection in humans was preventable through the use of vaccines containing as many as fourteen specific antigens. These were termed capsular polysaccharides. The breakthrough that made those findings possible had been pioneered in 1930 when these antigens were injected into human beings for the first time. Previously, they had been used only in experiments with mice.

Pneumonia vaccines are critically important components of programs to prevent disease among older members of the population. Experts recommend that the elderly receive a pneumonia vaccine each year. The death rate from pneumonia continues to rise, but not as quickly as the percentage of the population that is elderly. Pneumonia is one of the ten leading causes of death in the United States. In 1900, it was the second or third most common killer. Without vaccines, it might easily still be the second or third leading cause of death.

—*Byron D. Cannon, Ph.D.;*
updated by L. Fleming Fallon, Jr.,
M.D., Ph.D., M.P.H.

See also Acquired immunodeficiency syndrome (AIDS); Bacterial infections; Bacteriology; Bronchitis; Common cold; Coughing; Immunization and vaccination; Influenza; Lungs; Microbiology; Pleurisy; Pulmonary diseases; Pulmonary medicine; Pulmonary medicine, pediatric; Respiration; Streptococcal infections; Viral infections.

FOR FURTHER INFORMATION:

Austrian, Robert. *Life with the Pneumococcus.* Philadelphia: University of Pennsylvania Press, 1985. A series of essays on different topics in the history and evolution of medical knowledge regarding the causes of pneumonia and its treatment. Most essays are at a level that can be understood by the layperson.

Hughes, Walter T. *Pneumocystis Carinii Pneumonitis.* 2 vols. Boca Raton, Fla.: CRC Press, 1987. A systematic discussion of various forms of pneumonia caused not by bacteria or viruses, but by a protozoan. Emphasizes the different sectors of the population potentially affected, including infant cancer patients and victims of AIDS.

Karetzky, Monroe, Burke A. Cunha, and Robert D. Brandstetter. *The Pneumonias.* New York: Springer-Verlag, 1993. This multidisciplinary volume addresses the scientific and clinical aspects of pneumonia. Its goal is to enhance the interaction between specialists and generalists in order to ensure more favorable outcomes for patients.

Pennington, James E. *Respiratory Infections: Diagnosis and Management.* 3d ed. Hoboken, N.J.: Raven Press, 1994. This thoroughly updated and revised edition features expanded coverage of HIV-related respiratory tract infections, including a timely discussion of multidrug-resistant tuberculosis. Major sections cover pathogenesis, diagnostic techniques, clinical manifestations, common clinical settings, specific etiologic agents, and therapeutic considerations.

Tierney, Lawrence M., Jr., et al., eds. *Current Medical Diagnosis and Treatment: 2001.* 39th ed. New York: McGraw-Hill, 2000. This book is revised annually and provides complete summaries for the diagnosis and treatment of different varieties of pneumonia. It is an excellent and concise text but is written for professionals.

PODIATRY
SPECIALTY

ANATOMY OR SYSTEM AFFECTED: Bones, feet, nails

SPECIALTIES AND RELATED FIELDS: Dermatology, orthopedics, vascular medicine

DEFINITION: The medical field that involves the diagnosis and treatment of diseases and abnormalities of the feet, ankles, and lower legs.

KEY TERMS:

corticosteroid: a fatlike molecule (or steroid), produced by the adrenal gland or made synthetically, that can be used to treat inflammation

dysfunction: the disordered or impaired function of a body system, organ, or tissue

orthopedics: the surgical or manipulative treatment of any disorder of the skeletal system and the associated motor organs

orthotic device: a podiatric appliance or prosthesis that is used to correct a foot deformity

pharmacology: the aspect of biomedical science that studies therapeutic drugs, their administration, and their bioproperties

SCIENCE AND PROFESSION

The human foot, which is located at the end of the lower leg and connected to the leg by the ankle, is a very complex structure. Feet are designed to optimize both balance and mobility. Each foot is composed of twenty-six bones, ligaments that connect and articulate these bones, blood vessels that provide nutrients and oxygen, sensory nerves, and a very thick covering of tough, strong skin. Heredity and a lack of proper foot care frequently result in painful calluses, corns, bunions, enlarged joints, and ingrown toenails. In addition, a variety of diseases, such as diabetes mellitus and cardiovascular problems, can lead to many other serious foot dysfunctions.

Podiatrists—more correctly called doctors of podiatric medicine—examine, diagnose, and treat dysfunctions of the foot, as well as related problems associated with the ankle and the lower leg. The first record of a process that was associated with podiatric medicine was the creation, in 100 B.C.E., of plasters that were used to treat corns at the Greek city of Smyrna. Although other records of podiatric treatments were found in antiquity and in the Middle Ages, the modern science of podiatry arose from the activities of the fourteenth century barber-surgeons of Europe.

In the United States, the first truly prominent modern podiatrist—then termed a chiropodist—was Isacher Zacharia. Zacharia, foot doctor to President Abraham Lincoln, published the first American podiatry text in 1862. Two other milestones in the history of American podiatry are the founding of the National Association of Chiropodists and the opening of the New York School of Chiropody. Both of these events occurred in 1912.

In 1958, the National Association of Chiropodists was renamed the American Podiatric Medical Association. From the New York School of Chiropody, whose first curriculum required only one year of chiropodic training, arose today's schools of podiatric medicine which require a four-year study period and award to graduates the Doctor of Podiatric Medicine (D.P.M.) degree. This degree derives from a uniform curriculum that all schools follow.

There are presently more than 16,000 licensed podiatrists in the United States. These podiatric practitioners serve patients in American hospitals, in government health programs, and in the armed forces, though most of them are in private, individual practice. Furthermore, modern podiatric medicine is an accepted part of all major health insurance plans, of Medicare, and of Medicaid. To become a licensed D.P.M., it is first necessary to complete the four-year course of postgraduate study at one of the seven American schools of podiatric medicine. These schools are located in California, Florida, Illinois, Iowa, New York, Ohio, and Pennsylvania. The absence of schools of podiatry in many states leads to scarcity of these health care practitioners, particularly in the South and in the Southwestern states.

Admission to all podiatry schools requires the completion of at least three years of a solid bachelor's degree program which must include a year each of biology, inorganic chemistry, and organic chemistry. More than 95 percent of podiatry school entrants have completed a bachelor's degree. In addition, a solid grade-point average and good scores on the Medical College Admissions Test (MCAT) are required for admission.

The first two years of podiatric professional education utilize this background as a springboard that enables laboratory and lecture hall training in anatomy, biochemistry, physiology, pharmacology, diagnostic radiology, and numerous other biomedical sciences. The third and fourth years of training are dedicated to the acquisition of clinical expertise by practicing podiatric medicine in college or community clinics, in hospitals, and in the offices of experienced, well-established podiatrists.

Upon graduation, the new D.P.M. usually completes a hospital residency encompassing three to four years. In the first year, clinical expertise is gained in podiatric orthopedics, biomechanics, and neurology. The first-year podiatry resident engages in supervised primary care, which involves observing, evaluating, and treating many dysfunctions of the feet, ankles, and lower legs. Minor podiatric surgery, such as the correction of a hammertoe, is also carried out during this training period. In the remaining residency years, the resident learns to carry out the more demanding aspects of podiatric surgery of the foot, ankle, and leg. During this time period, the podiatric resident becomes more independent and skilled.

Podiatric practitioners require licenses to practice. In the United States, these licenses are most often gained by passing state board examinations. Satisfactory scores on the separate tests given by the National Board of Podiatric Medical Examiners are also deemed as satisfactory for podiatric licensing by many states. Renewal of podiatry licenses, however, requires that podiatrists undergo extensive continuing education aimed at keeping them at the cutting edge of the field.

Specialization is also possible for podiatrists. Podiatric specialists can be certified by the American Board of Podiatric Surgery, the American Board of Podiatric Medicine, or the American Board of Podiatric Public Health. Each of these podiatric specialty boards requires advanced clinical training, completion of written and oral examinations, and extensive experience in specific aspects of modern podiatric practice. Such board certification indicates that the individuals involved have met much higher standards than those required for licensing alone. Some podiatrists also belong to the American College of Foot and Ankle Surgery of the American Medical Association (AMA).

In modern practice, podiatric surgical procedures designed to prevent or correct podiatric deformities now supplant many of the more conventional methods that originally made up the expertise of most podiatric practitioners. In addition, numerous techniques that cause the improvement of the health and the function of the foot and the ankle, so as to preclude foot deformities, have become key aspects of the modern podiatric profession.

DIAGNOSTIC AND TREATMENT TECHNIQUES

A thorough podiatric examination begins with the complete medical history of the patient, inspection of the patient's gait, and careful examination of both feet, the ankles, and the lower legs. When these procedures point to the diagnosis of a particular podiatric problem, X-ray examination, muscle testing, and neurological consultation may be carried out to search for more subtle problems that the initial examination suggested but did not prove.

Once a clear, complete diagnosis has been obtained, a treatment regimen—including physical ther-apy, various surgical treatments, medications, and the use of podiatric (orthotic) appliances—is prescribed. Often, all aspects of treatment are carried out in the podiatrist's office. Complex podiatric surgery, however, may require the use of a hospital surgical suite or its equivalent.

Among the podiatric problems most often seen are athlete's foot, bunions, calluses, corns, ingrown toenails, hammertoes, heel spurs, traumatic injuries to the ankles or feet, plantar warts, and complaints associated with arthritis, cardiovascular disease, or diabetes mellitus. In many cases—especially those engendered by athletics, diabetes, and cardiovascular problems—the podiatrist refers patients to other health practitioners, such as orthopedists, cardiologists, or endocrinologists. Increasingly, however, podiatrists and other specialists are beginning to work together as teams to solve such health problems.

Bunions are deformities of the big toes and their joints; they may or may not be painful, but they are almost always considered uncosmetic. When a bunion is not painful, it is usually treated by the use of an orthotic device that prevents further damage and pain. In cases where bunion pain is caused by inflammation, oral or injected anti-inflammatory drugs, such as corticosteroids, are often used for the shortest period of time needed to correct the problem. Such short-term treatment is made necessary by the potential health risks caused by this therapy, such as cardiovascular problems. In the most severe cases, surgery is used to remove the bunion. An incision is made near the bunion site, and a surgical burr is used to trim away the region of excess bone that is causing the problem. In cases where manipulative examination and/or X rays show that the bunion problem is in the joint, much more complex surgery is required.

Corns and hammertoes may be considered together, as many corns are caused by hammertoes. Corns are not restricted to occurrence along with hammertoes, however, as they also arise spontaneously on any toe subject to inappropriate biomechanical stress. A corn (or heloma) is a skin protrusion—or thickening—atop or on the side of a toe. Corns can occur wherever a toe has been bent out of shape by a biomechanical problem or by a tight shoe. They can be quite painful. Hammertoe, a contracture of one of the toe joints, produces a toe malformation that makes wearing shoes painful and can lead to corns. Corns may be trimmed periodically or removed surgically. The treatment used by podiatrists depends on the severity of the problem seen. Similarly, hammertoes are corrected surgically. After treatment of these problems, it is important for the patient to wear shoes that fit appropriately, to use corrective orthotic devices that are prescribed, and to follow closely the instructions given by the podiatrist. Failure to do so can counteract the results of the podiatric treatment.

Calluses, like corns, are buildups of tough, thickened skin. Unlike corns, however, they occur most often on the bottoms of the feet. Calluses form to protect the foot from undue stress resulting from uneven weight bearing by the bottom of the foot. Therefore, they will form again after removal wherever the causative mechanical stress recurs. When a callus becomes painful, the appropriate treatment regimen varies greatly from case to case. Often, it is use of an orthotic device to produce evenness of weight bearing by the foot. In other cases, the callus is trimmed. In the most extreme cases, minor surgery is used to correct the anatomical defect in the metatarsal bone that is causing the problem. Again, success in callus treatment is optimized by carefully following the directions of the podiatrist. In the most severe instances, up to three months of diminished physical activity is required to enable complete healing of the trimmed metatarsal bones. Calluses may also occur at the back of the heel, as a result of tight shoes and dermatologic problems. These calluses are usually handled by trimming and subsequent purchase of more appropriate shoes.

Heel spurs, Achilles tendonitis, surgery of the ankles, dermatologic problems of the foot, and diabetic/cardiovascular complications are podiatric problems not discussed here. The interested reader is referred to popular works such as *The Foot Doctor* (1986), by Glen Copeland and Stan Solomon, for preliminary information on these topics. Furthermore, it should be recognized that podiatrists will often repair damaged bones, muscles, and tendons surgically. They can also prescribe medications and treat fractures or sprains by applying casts and braces.

PERSPECTIVE AND PROSPECTS

Many advances in podiatric medicine have occurred in recent years. Most encouraging is the improved ability of podiatrists to handle severe foot problems. This improvement is largely attributable to advances in the field and to more thorough training both in professional school and in postgraduate experiences. The current positive interaction of podiatrists and other health care professionals in the treatment of dermatologic, cardiovascular, and diabetic problems is another great step forward.

It is believed that the job prospects for podiatrists will grow rapidly in the next fifty years, and there will be even greater success in the podiatric treatment of problems that are presently difficult to handle. It is also expected that additional podiatric medical schools will open to meet the need for more D.P.M.'s throughout the United States.

There are two main reasons for the excellent job prospects for podiatrists. First is the increase in the population of senior citizens. Because these individuals have had more wear and tear on their lower legs and feet than younger people, they have foot ailments that require treatment more frequently. Second is the increased interest in jogging and other sports in the general population, which will lead to more injuries that require podiatric intervention.

These factors are also expected to produce advances in the uses of orthotic appliances, generate sophisticated new diagnostic and surgical techniques, and lead to better cooperation between podiatrists and other health care professionals.

—*Sanford S. Singer, Ph.D.*

See also Athlete's foot; Bone disorders; Bones and the skeleton; Bunions; Feet; Flat feet; Foot disorders; Fungal infections; Gout; Hammertoe correction; Hammertoes; Heel spur removal; Lower extremities; Nail removal; Nails; Orthopedic surgery; Orthopedics; Physical examination; Tendon disorders; Tendon repair; Warts.

FOR FURTHER INFORMATION:

Copeland, Glenn, and Stan Solomon. *The Foot Doctor.* Emmaus, Pa.: Rodale Press, 1986. This valuable, chatty book gives useful descriptions of many aspects of podiatric medicine—its surgical and medical techniques and the instruments used. Aspects of numerous useful office and surgical precepts of podiatry are described.

Lorimer, Donald L., ed. *Neale's Common Foot Disorders: Diagnosis and Management.* 5th ed. New York: Churchill Livingstone, 1997. A general clinical guide to foot disorders and diseases and their treatment. Includes a bibliography and an index.

U.S. Department of Labor. Bureau of Labor Statistics. *The Occupational Outlook Handbook.* Lincolnwood, Ill.: VGM Career Horizons, 2000. This broad-based book contains a concise but inclusive description of podiatry, podiatrists, and the working conditions and job outlook of the field.

POISONING

DISEASE/DISORDER

ANATOMY OR SYSTEM AFFECTED: Gastrointestinal system, immune system, muscles, musculoskeletal system, nervous system, respiratory system, stomach

SPECIALTIES AND RELATED FIELDS: Emergency medicine, environmental health, epidemiology, toxicologists

DEFINITION: Exposure to any substance in sufficient quantity to cause adverse health effects, from severe to fatal.

KEY TERMS:

epidemiology: The study of the incidence of diseases or poisonings in affected populations

iatrogenic poisoning: poisoning resulting from medical treatment, which can include overdose, the administration of improper medication by the patient or prescribing physician, and adverse reactions

pharmacology: the science that deals with the chemistry, effects, and therapeutic use of drugs

syrup of ipecac: a plant extract that will induce vomiting when orally administered; the syrup can be used to induce vomiting after ingestion of a poisonous substance

toxicology: the science devoted to the study of poisons

toxidrome: a group of symptoms characteristic of a toxin or group of toxins that act on the same area of the nervous system

CAUSES AND SYMPTOMS

Probably the most accurate statement that can be made about the occurrence of poisoning in the United States is that the numbers vary widely depending on the information source and definition of poisoning. Incidents can be grouped into intentional poisonings, accidental poisonings, occupational and environmental poisonings, social poisonings, and iatrogenic poisonings. There is no single organization that collects and analyzes data from hospitals, physicians' offices, police and court records, and industrial accident and exposure records. One source has reported that as many as eight million people are accidentally or intentionally poisoned each year. It has been stated further that 10 percent of all ambulance calls and 10 to 20 percent of all admissions to medical facilities involve poisonings. A government report which focused on injury-related costs of all kinds cited the number of poisonings classified as injuries in the United States at about 1.7 million in 1985 and ranked poisoning as the fourth most common cause of injury in the country.

Many incidents of poisoning go unreported because a poison control center is not consulted or the effects are not severe enough to require extensive medical treatment. In other cases where exposure to the toxic agent involves constant contact to low but toxic levels of industrial chemicals, such as occupational or environmental exposures, symptoms may be subtle or confused with diseases that are associated with the normal aging process. The degree of illness and/or the number of premature deaths resulting from environmental exposure to naturally occurring or artificial toxic substances—radiation, chemical waste, and other toxins in the air, water, and food supply—is simply not known.

The most consistent and reliable sources of information on accidental poisoning in the United States are the annual statistics compiled by the American Association of Poison Control Centers. While poison control centers receive some calls related to intentional or iatrogenic poisonings, 88 percent of the calls are considered accidental exposures. Combining all the poisoning types together, poison control centers are called concerning about 2.2 million human cases each year. It is important to note, however, that extrapolations from the number of reported poisonings to the number of actual poisonings occurring annually in the United States cannot be made from these data alone.

About 92 percent of exposures occur in the home, almost two-thirds involve children under six, and three-fourths involve ingestion. The great predominance of young children in the accidental poisoning category reflects the inquisitive behavior of that age group. For children under the age of one year, inappropriate administration of medications by the parents is the dominant cause of poisonings. For children over the age of five, exposure to toxic substances often represents the simple misreading of a medication label or the manifestation of family stress or even suicidal intent. These children have increased incidence of depressive symptoms and family problems compared to their nonpoisoned peer group.

Intentional poisoning of children also occurs—usually as a well-planned act of a psychiatrically disturbed parent. Although many of these incidents are clearly homicidal and abusive by design, some have received medical notoriety as cases of Münchausen syndrome by proxy. Münchausen syndrome itself is a psychiatric disorder in which the patient achieves psychological comfort from the attention and treatment received under the pretense of being afflicted with a serious or painful illness. In a variation of this condition, the psychiatric needs of an adult are fulfilled through an induced medical disorder in the child. For example, one parent surreptitiously administered syrup of ipecac to her child, inducing unexplained vomiting and gastrointestinal disorders that required extended hospital care. The phenomenon is rare but well documented in the medical literature and is classified as a form of child abuse.

Intentional poisonings are mostly suicide-related. Various studies have placed the number of attempts per year in the United States at between 200,000 and 4,000,000, indicating the difficulty of collecting accurate statistics. A government report states that 30,000 attempts result in death every year, but at least one source has suggested that the figure is probably 50 percent lower than the actual number that could be at-

tributed to suicide. Although carbon monoxide (as in motor vehicle exhaust) is one of the most common agents used, intentional dosing with large quantities of drugs is also very frequently involved. Of the many thousands of drugs that could be used for overdose incidents, 90 percent of actual cases involve only about twenty products in nine drug groups. Most of these are addictive or abused drugs, including stimulants, antidepressants, tranquilizers, narcotics, sedatives or hypnotics, and antipsychotics. Alcohol alone is seldom lethal but is often consumed along with the more deadly drugs and may make the lethal effects possible.

Social poisoning is related to drug use or abuse, which has significant societal consequences. There are hundreds of thousands of hospital and emergency room admissions each year for overdose treatment as well as for the indirect consequences of recreational drug use, such as violent crime, trauma, and vehicular accidents. Almost 400,000 drug-abuse-related emergency room visits were projected to have occurred in 1990 by the Drug Abuse Warning Network (DAWN), a federal government-sponsored data collection sys-

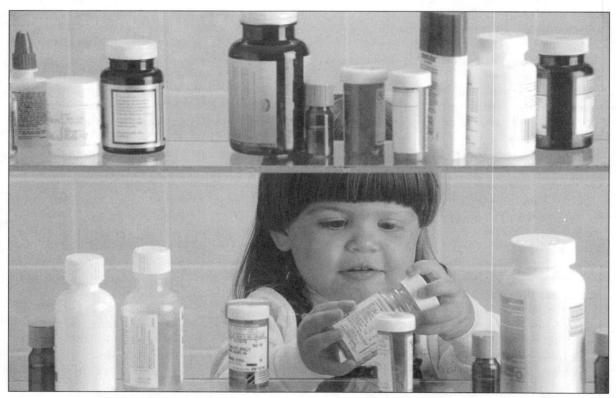

Childproof caps are essential in the prevention of accidental poisoning. (PhotoDisc)

tem. These figures do not include alcohol, however, unless it is mentioned as having been involved in a mixed drug exposure event.

The abuse of alcohol, the most widely available chemical intoxicant legally allowed for recreational use, is a major social problem in the United States. While a majority of the alcohol-consuming public demonstrate a lifelong pattern of little or moderate drinking without the development of addiction-related problems, it has been reported that a small percentage of the population (5 percent to 10 percent) drink one-third or up to one-half of all the consumed alcohol. The causes of alcoholism involve a complex interaction of social, physiological, and genetic risk factors. In the United States, there are approximately 9 million people classified as chronic alcohol abusers, and alcohol is the fourth leading cause of deaths in males between forty and seventy. Alcohol is associated with violence and violent deaths. For example, half of all violent deaths in New York City are associated with acute or chronic alcoholism; these incidents include deaths by homicide, vehicular accidents, falls, fires, drownings, drug abuse, and suicide. Alcohol is the most important single factor in determining the risk of road accidents; half of all drivers involved in fatal automobile accidents in the United States have been drinking.

Similar assertions can be made for tobacco use. Although not closely associated with criminal behavior and vehicular accidents, tobacco use has been connected with increased incidence of cancer, respiratory illnesses, and cardiovascular diseases. In the United States, smoking is responsible for one-quarter of deaths caused by fire and accounts for close to $500 million in other losses. Both smoking and excessive alcohol consumption are becoming increasingly less socially accepted, but the continued wide acceptance of both alcohol and tobacco use obscures their potential to poison.

TREATMENT AND THERAPY

Emergency medical treatment of the poisoned patient is most often based on the relief of symptoms and the provision of life support. If the patient is awake and alert, a medical history is taken and a clinical examination is performed, both of which can help determine substance exposure. The medical staff must never assume that the patient is providing truthful information, especially if clinical impressions conflict with the patient account. If the patient is comatose,

then stabilization and life support take immediate priority over determination of the specific toxic substance involved. The attending physician will want to prevent airway blockage and to maintain respiration and circulation, which may require mechanical aids for breathing assistance. Treatment of cardiac and blood pressure problems can be accomplished with drugs, fluid, or oxygen administration. If the patient is unconscious, the depth of central nervous system depression can be evaluated using a standard test of reactivity to light, sound, pain, and the presence or absence of normal body processes. If the patient is suffering from seizures, drugs that counteract these symptoms can be administered.

Although many hospitals offer in-house toxicology testing in a clinical laboratory, treatment usually must begin before results are available. For this and several other reasons, a comprehensive toxicology testing laboratory is not as useful an asset in the emergency treatment of poisoning as might be believed. It would be impossible for any analytical laboratory to provide timely or cost-effective emergency identification of all potentially toxic substances. Instead, a more efficient strategy concentrates on analyzing those substances for which a specific antidote exists or for which specific medical procedures are required in a critical period of time. A very high percentage of drug overdose cases involve one of a group of six or eight drugs that will vary depending on locality. Pesticide poisoning, for example, is a more prevalent medical problem for rural than urban hospitals. Drug abuse is a problem in all localities, but the frequency and type of drugs abused vary. Regional preferences exist for PCP, cocaine, amphetamines, and opiates. Even prescription drug abuse depends on locality and the patient population.

Common pain relievers found in virtually every home medicine cabinet constitute a large number of both adult and pediatric poisoning incidents. Preparations containing aspirin, as well as nonaspirin analgesics containing acetaminophen (such as Tylenol), are possibly life-threatening when consumed in excess. Acetaminophen poisoning is particularly insidious since death from total and irreversible destruction of the liver will occur unless the antidote, a chemical called Mucomyst, is administered within six hours of ingestion of a lethal dose. Since a specific antidote exists, most hospitals with emergency service will offer around-the-clock testing for acetaminophen levels in the blood. Aspirin, although not as lethal as acetaminophen, can be fatal if a sufficient amount is consumed. Its universal availability and common usage make aspirin a significant poisoning agent encountered in all localities. The symptoms of toxicity are related to aspirin's effects on temperature regulation, rate of breathing, and the body's ability to influence the acidity of the blood. Treatment involves monitoring the patient's vital signs, calculating the severity of the dose taken. Vomiting may be introduced with syrup of ipecac, or charcoal (a very active adsorption agent) may be given orally to limit gastric absorption. Intravenous fluids may also be given to counteract the blood acidity changes.

Prescription drugs that are commonly overused or abused (antiepileptic medication, sedatives and tranquilizers, and antipsychotic or antidepressant drugs) are often routinely assayed in the hospital laboratory as part of the treatment process for patients receiving these medications. The levels in the blood can be monitored to determine the toxicity status of the patient. Usually, supportive care is sufficient for treatment until the drug clears the system. For certain tranquilizers and antidepressants, an antidote called flumazenil can be administered, but it must be used with caution.

Poisoning from an overdose of opiates or morphinelike drugs is a special treatment case. A specific antidote called naloxone can be administered if the patient is treated before irreversible respiratory depression occurs. Recovery is virtually instantaneous and dramatic, with a comatose patient becoming alert within seconds of naloxone administration. For this reason, the routine treatment of comatose patients includes the administration of opiate antidote even when the cause of the unconscious state is unknown.

Although heavy, long-term ethyl alcohol use invariably leads to liver dysfunction and a number of other organ disorders, alcohol is not usually life-threatening unless it is consumed in quantities sufficient to cause a coma. Death most commonly results from respiratory depression and related complications. Other types of alcohols, as well as antifreeze, can be involved in both accidental and intentional poisonings. Methanol or wood alcohol is a common industrial solvent found in materials around the home or work site; consumption can cause blindness and death. Isopropyl alcohol (or rubbing alcohol), although not as toxic as methanol, can also cause severe illness and death when consumed in sufficient quantities. Ethylene glycol, a common ingredient in antifreeze,

is highly toxic and is especially attractive to small children and pets because of its sweet taste. It may also be consumed by alcoholics as an ethanol substitute. When not treated, its consumption can result in kidney failure. It is not the alcohols themselves that are the primary toxins but the degradation products called metabolites that form in the body in an attempt to eliminate the foreign substance. Ironically, the treatment for both methanol and ethylene glycol poisoning is administration of high doses of ethanol, which prevents the formation of toxic metabolites by the liver.

In the United States, lead poisoning is a major medical problem for children living in older, substandard housing; they can become exposed to large amounts of lead from the consumption of lead-based paint. (Even though such paints are no longer used in residential housing, many older buildings remain contaminated.) Another major source of exposure is inhalation of leaded gas fumes and exhaust. Other less common sources of lead poisoning include the consumption of food stored in leaded crystal or pottery or moonshine whiskey distilled in automobile radiators. Intentional gasoline sniffing by adolescents can also be a problem. Lead exposure is extremely hazardous because its effects are both severe and cumulative. Children are especially susceptible to lead poisoning because they absorb and retain more of this substance and have less capacity for excretion than adults.

The nervous system is a major site for lead toxicity, causing both psychological and neurologic impairment. The blood cell production can also be affected, with resulting anemia and decreased oxygen-carrying capacity. Because lead toxicity can result in behavioral and learning disorders that may already afflict children living in substandard conditions, sometimes poisoning cannot be detected by clinical symptoms alone and must be diagnosed through blood testing. Test data indicate that the level of lead associated with nervous system disorders is probably lower than previously believed. In the United States, a major screening effort has been financed by the federal government to detect high lead body deposits in children. The goal is to find affected children and to treat them before permanent damage occurs.

PERSPECTIVE AND PROSPECTS

Poisoning has been a medical problem since the earliest times of human history. A tremendous variety of poisonous substances can be encountered in the natural world alone. It has been estimated that 200,000 plants and animals are known to be toxic to humans, some organisms producing as many as fifty or sixty toxins. The potential of almost any substance to be poisonous was recognized during the Renaissance by Paracelsus, a founder of modern toxicology, who stated, "All substances are poisons. . . . The dose differentiates a poison from a remedy." Many folk remedies and tribal medicine practices were derived from centuries of trial-and-error experiences with toxic plant and animal species in the environment. Historically, the development of the sciences of pharmacology and toxicology is closely related to the study of poisons.

As societies become more urban and technology-based, poisoning problems shift away from natural toxin exposures to those related to drugs and industrial chemicals. For many of these types of poisonings, sustaining the vital life processes until the toxin is cleared from the body is the only method of treatment. Specific antidotes are not available for many drugs or even for many natural poisons. Since a large number of toxins critically affect the nervous system, a diagnostic and treatment system has been developed based on the "toxidrome" concept. If a specific area of the nervous system can be shown to be affected, treatment can begin to counteract those effects even if the identity of the toxin is not known.

The symptoms of acute poisoning or overexposure to a toxic agent are likely to be treated as individual medical problems by physicians in an emergency medicine environment. Meanwhile, social poisons, which often do not create immediate medical emergencies, continue to exact enormous economic and medical costs to society over the long term; these poisoning problems have not been dealt with successfully by social, medical, or governmental agencies. In the case of environmental toxins, little if any well-established information on the long-term toxicity of these substances is available. The science of toxicology, particularly with regard to establishing the risk of exposure of a population to environmental toxins, often becomes a guessing game played by a governmental regulatory agency. Until societal and environmental poisonings can be better evaluated and controlled, they will continue to constitute serious economic and quality-of-life problems.

—*David J. Wells, Jr., Ph.D.*

See also Addiction; Alcoholism; Bites and stings; Domestic violence; Environmental diseases; Environmental health; Food poisoning; Iatrogenic disorders; Intoxication; Lead poisoning; Poisonous plants; Suicide; Toxicology.

FOR FURTHER INFORMATION:

Baselt, Randall C., and Robert H. Cravey. *Disposition of Toxic Drugs and Chemicals in Man.* 5th ed. Chicago: Year Book Medical, 2000. A condensed toxic substances reference book. All toxins are listed alphabetically rather than by class or mechanism of action. The commonly encountered drugs and chemicals are listed with information on toxicokinetics, treatment, analytical techniques, and references for further information.

Ellenhorn, Matthew J., et al. *Ellenhorn's Medical Toxicology: Diagnosis and Treatment of Human Poisoning.* Rev. 2d ed. Baltimore: Williams & Wilkins, 1997. A classic medical reference book on toxic substances. Drugs, industrial chemicals, animal and plant toxins, household products, and pesticides are discussed in depth, with an emphasis on medical symptoms and treatment.

Garriott, James C., ed. *Medicolegal Aspects of Alcohol Determination in Biological Specimens.* Littleton, Mass.: PSG, 1988. Chapters are devoted to discussions of alcoholic beverages and their chemical constituents, the metabolism and disposition of alcohol, methods of analysis, state and federal regulations on drinking and driving in the United States, and the reliability of breath and blood-alcohol testing.

Pesce, John, and Amadeo J. Pesce. *The Lead Paint Primer.* Melrose, Mass.: Star Industries, 1991. An easily understood source of information about lead poisoning. Written for the layperson.

POISONOUS PLANTS
DISEASE/DISORDER

ANATOMY OR SYSTEM AFFECTED: Gastrointestinal system, immune system, skin, stomach

SPECIALTIES AND RELATED FIELDS: Dermatology, environmental health, family practice, gastroenterology, toxicology

DEFINITION: Plants that cause gastrointestinal or dermatological reactions in humans.

Some plants manufacture substances to assist them in survival. These chemicals can cause irritation or allergic reactions in organisms which contact them. Among human beings, the most common reaction is

North American Poisonous Plants

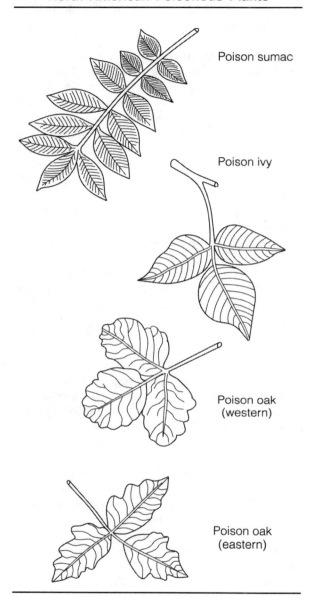

Poison sumac

Poison ivy

Poison oak
(western)

Poison oak
(eastern)

temic reactions when ingested. The reaction of skin to plant toxins is termed dermatitis. These reactions are rarely fatal but have widespread morbidity.

Poison oak, poison ivy, and poison sumac. Poison ivy (*Toxicodendron radicans*) is widely distributed throughout the United States. This is a vine with groups of three shiny green leaves. Poison oak (*Toxicodendron diversilobum*) is a low shrub with leaves that also come in groups of three to a stem; it is found in dry areas. Poison sumac (*Toxicodendron vernix*) is a taller plant with slender leaves arranged in pairs along a stem and a single leaf at the end of the stem. It grows in damp or swampy areas.

Contact with any of these plants leads to a reaction in the skin at the site of contact. An individual's first contact with these plants causes no apparent reaction; sensitization must occur. In the days (usually between five and twenty) following the initial exposure, the immune system causes the entire body to become sensitive to the chemical. If the plant is touched on another occasion, a reaction will occur. The second reaction commonly causes itching (urticaria), redness (erythema), and swelling (edema) at the site of contact. Vesicles filled with a clear fluid may develop. Proper treatment consists of washing the area of contact as soon as possible, then keeping the area dry until the vesicles become crusty and disappear. This process normally requires up to ten days. Physicians sometimes use corticosteroids to manage serious cases of contact dermatitis.

Scratching to relieve urticaria may break the surface of the skin and introduce infection to the affected area. This may prolong the healing time and lead to scarring. The clear, watery fluid found in vesicles does not contain plant material and cannot spread the rash to other parts of one's own body or to other individuals, but a thicker, cloudy material (pus) may be found in vesicles that have become infected by scratching. Pus can transmit the infection, but not the rash, to other individuals.

Sensitivity to poison ivy and poison oak is usually lifelong. Sensitivity to other plants is more individual in nature and is dependent on factors such as the magnitude of the initial exposure, the number of subsequent exposures, and an individual's body chemistry and immune status.

Mushrooms. Although mushrooms appear harmless, they can cause a variety of reactions when ingested. There are five broad types of reactions: gastrointestinal discomfort with nausea, vomiting, and

an allergy. The specifics of an allergic reaction can vary widely and range from no apparent reaction to shock. Allergic reactions to contact with most plants are uncommon and classified on an individual basis. Some plants, however, cause reactions in virtually everyone with whom they come into contact. As a result, they are termed poisonous plants. Many commonly encountered poisonous plants cause reactions in the skin, while some plants can cause adverse sys-

diarrhea; sweating; inebriation or hallucination without sleep; delirium with sleep or coma; and vomiting only when associated with alcohol. Some mushrooms produce reactions only after delays of six hours to three days. These reactions include headaches, extreme thirst, nausea, and vomiting.

The gastrointestinal symptoms associated with mushroom intoxication usually appear within three hours of ingestion. The resulting discomfort is transient. Sweating is caused by the presence of a chemical which is not inactivated by cooking. The symptoms usually subside within two hours.

Psilocybin, a chemical which causes hallucinations, is found in some mushroom species. The effect usually lasts approximately two hours, although the extent of a reaction is determined by the amount ingested, the setting, and the mood and personality of the individual.

Delirium associated with sleep or coma is encountered with ingestion of *Amanita muscaria* and *Amanita pantheria* species. Within approximately thirty minutes of ingestion, an individual becomes drowsy. This may be followed by elation and extreme activity, again followed by a period of drowsiness. This alternating cycle may continue for up to twelve hours. *Coprinus atramentarius* is an edible mushroom but temporally sensitizes the body to alcohol. For approximately three days after ingestion, a chemical contained in the mushroom reacts with alcohol to cause vomiting.

All mushroom species contain some amount of mycotoxins that may or may not be affected by cooking. The best guideline is to avoid eating any mushroom unless it is either purchased in a store or positively identified by an expert.

Other common poisonous plants. Contact with plants called nettles (*Urtica urens* and *Urtica dioica*) can cause intense reactions. The plant is common in well-watered areas throughout North America.

Contact with plants of the carrot (*Umbelliferae*) family such as caraway, dill, parsley, and parsnip can cause a brief sensitivity of the skin to ultraviolet light. Exposure to sunlight or fluorescent light within six to twenty-four hours after contact with the plant may lead to burning of the skin exposed to the chemical—a sunburn. Citrus plants of the rue (*Rutaceae*) family can also cause this skin photosensitivity. It can be prevented by thoroughly washing the skin after contact. Inflammation after exposure can be treated with aspirin.

Inquiries concerning the ingestion of plant materials account for about 10 percent of all calls to poison control centers. The single plant species that is involved in the greatest number of adverse reactions is *Dieffenbachia*. Other house plants, such as philodendron, poinsettia, holly, honeysuckle, jade plant, and yew, may accidentally be ingested by children. Individual reactions to ingested house plants vary; specifics are dependent on the species and amount ingested, the specific plant part ingested, the body size of the individual, and how quickly the plant material is removed from the body. Once in the body, most plants cause vomiting and diarrhea. Other reactions vary and are specific to the plant species involved. *Dieffenbachia* causes immediate burning pain and swelling in the mouth.

Leaves of several plants in the *Solanum* family, such as nightshade, jessamine (jasmine), and the immature fruit of some ground cherries and European bittersweet, contain a chemical that can cause intense gastroenteritis. These plants are especially toxic to small children. If ingested, jimsonweed may cause delirium. Common flowers such as lily of the valley, foxglove, and oleander contain chemical substances that can cause the heart to malfunction.

—*L. Fleming Fallon, Jr., M.D., Ph.D., M.P.H.*

See also Allergies; Coma; Dermatitis; Diarrhea and dysentery; Food poisoning; Gastroenterology; Gastroenterology, pediatric; Gastrointestinal disorders; Gastrointestinal system; Hallucinations; Herbal medicine; Itching; Nausea and vomiting; Poisoning; Rashes; Skin; Skin disorders.

For Further Information:

Ammirati, J. F., J. A. Traquair, and P. A. Horgen. *Poisonous Mushrooms of the Northern United States and Canada*. Minneapolis: University of Minnesota Press, 1985. A comprehensive guide to identification of toxic mushrooms.

Foster, Steven, and Roger A. Caras. *A Field Guide to Venomous Animals and Poisonous Plants: North America, North of Mexico*. Boston: Houghton Mifflin, 1994. Containing excellent information and bright color pictures and written for easy understanding, this book should be in any nature enthusiast's library. Possibly the best plant identification guide around.

Frohne, Dietrich, and H. J. Pfander. *A Colour Atlas of Poisonous Plants: A Handbook for Pharmacists, Doctors, Toxicologists, Biologists, and Veterinar-*

ians. London: Manson, 2000. Colorful illustrations illuminate the text, which covers many different types of toxic plants, focusing on those found in Europe. Includes bibliographical references.

Hardin, J. W., and J. M. Arena. *Human Poisoning from Native and Cultivated Plants*. 2d ed. Durham, N.C.: Duke University Press, 1974. This well-written book, which uses clear language, is intended for parents, camp counselors, and other adults who work with youths.

Lampe, Kenneth F. *Common Poisonous and Injurious Plants*. Washington, D.C.: U.S. Department of Health and Human Services, Public Health Service, Food and Drug Administration, Bureau of Drugs, Division of Poison Control, 1981. This inexpensive bulletin is intended for laypeople. Contains color photographs of the most common poisonous plants found in North America.

Turner, Nancy J., and Adam F. Szczawinski. *Common Poisonous Plants and Mushrooms of North America*. Portland, Oreg.: Timber Press, 1991. This text helps readers identify poisonous mushrooms and plants. Includes an index and a bibliography.

POLIOMYELITIS
DISEASE/DISORDER

ANATOMY OR SYSTEM AFFECTED: Brain, legs, muscles, musculoskeletal system, nerves, nervous system, spine

SPECIALTIES AND RELATED FIELDS: Epidemiology, neurology, pediatrics, public health, virology

DEFINITION: A contagious viral illness capable of causing meningitis and permanent paralysis; in response to a dramatic increase in the frequency of cases in industrialized nations during the twentieth century, a vaccine was developed that has virtually eliminated this disease in Europe and the Western Hemisphere.

KEY TERMS:

endemic disease: a disease that is usually present in a population and does not exhibit marked fluctuations in frequency from year to year

epidemic: a marked increase in the frequency of a disease, relative to the historical experience of the affected population

neurotropic virus: a virus that multiplies in neural tissues

serologic epidemiology: investigation of the history of disease exposure in a population by surveying the incidence of antibodies circulating in the bloodstream

subclinical infection: a disease process characterized by multiplication of the causative organism within the host and production of antibodies by the host without causing apparent illness

CAUSES AND SYMPTOMS

Poliomyelitis, or polio, is a contagious disease affecting humans and some nonhuman primates. It is caused by three closely related strains of a human enterovirus. In its most serious manifestation, it attacks nerve tissue in the spinal cord and brain stem, resulting in paralysis. Polio was one of the most feared diseases in developed countries in the twentieth century. A few medical researchers suspected the connection between the severe neurological symptoms of poliomyelitis and the more typical enteric form of the disease in the first decade of the twentieth century. A complete and accurate picture of the etiology of polio, however, was not demonstrated and accepted until the 1930's, when improved techniques for detecting viruses and antiviral antibodies enabled scientists to trace the disease in all of its phases.

The virus responsible for poliomyelitis is present in large numbers in the intestines of infected individuals. It is excreted in feces, from which it is spread to uninfected individuals through contaminated water, food, hands, and eating utensils and by flies and other filth-loving insects. Once it has been ingested, the poliovirus multiplies in the cells lining the intestine and invades the lymphatic system, producing swelling in the lymph nodes surrounding the intestine and in the neck. The symptoms of the disease at this stage may escape notice altogether, or the infected person may experience fever and a sore throat. These symptoms subside after two or three days as the body's immune system begins producing antibodies to overcome the virus. Most cases never proceed beyond this stage, termed the minor illness of polio.

In a minority of cases, after a period of several days in which a patient is asymptomatic, the minor illness is followed by the onset of neurological symptoms, signaling that the virus has invaded the spinal cord. Symptoms include pain and stiffness in the spine, lethargy, general muscular weakness, and flaccid (that is, not accompanied by spasms) paralysis of muscles, particularly of the legs. Paralysis of the legs occurs because the virus preferentially attacks neurons in the front or anterior horns of the spinal cord,

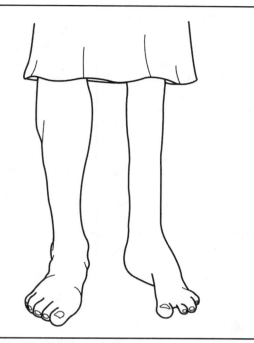

The "wasting" of a limb is typical of advanced poliomyelitis.

including the motor nerves controlling the legs, and often affects one side more than the other. In the most severe cases, viral infection spreads from the spinal cord to the brain stem, attacking neurons serving the diaphragm and esophagus. Without aggressive medical intervention in the form of an artificial breathing apparatus, paralysis of the diaphragm is fatal.

In the absence of brain-stem involvement, a body's normal defenses usually overcome the viral infection. Since the body is unable to replace destroyed neurons, however, acute polio leaves the patient with permanent motor impairment ranging from mild muscular weakness to severe crippling disability. Aided by appropriate physical therapy during the recovery period, patients can usually regain some of the motor function lost during the active disease. As survivors of the polio epidemics of the 1940's and 1950's reached middle age in the 1980's and 1990's, a late phase of the disease called postpolio syndrome was recognized. After decades of apparent normality, muscles affected by the initial paralytic attack experience gradual loss of function without evidence of renewed viral activity.

The proportion of cases resulting in permanent paralysis varies with the age structure of the population affected. Typically, no more than 10 percent of patients who experience a major illness including neurologic symptoms suffer such paralysis. Under premodern conditions, the latter probably accounted for less than 1 percent of the total cases, because subclinical infection, minor illness, and paralytic polio usually occurred in early childhood. Maternal antibodies provided protection for newborns, while a child's own immune system created antibodies following exposure. In this way, lifelong immunity to subsequent infection was acquired. With improving sanitation and an older susceptible population, however, this proportion gradually increased.

During an epidemic, polio is primarily spread by persons with mild and subclinical infections, who may be unaware that they are ill. Infectivity persists for two to three weeks after the onset of the intestinal disease. There is no evidence that lifetime carriers exist. It is virtually impossible to prevent the spread of an asymptomatic, fecally transmitted pathogen among young children in group settings by any behavioral means. Fortunately, vaccines have effectively eliminated polio as an epidemic disease in the developed world and in Latin America.

TREATMENT AND THERAPY

The history of efforts to prevent and treat poliomyelitis illustrates the changing attitudes of the medical community toward disease and the methods by which a once-important pathogen was virtually eliminated. Only time will tell whether the spectacular inroads made by medical science against poliomyelitis are permanent. Persons with compromised immune systems are reminders that vaccines cannot completely protect all individuals. They prevent health professionals from becoming complacent with respect to any infectious disease.

At the end of the nineteenth century, when epidemics of poliomyelitis first began to surface, medical science had made a number of important advances in the understanding and treatment of disease. First and foremost, the role of microorganisms in infectious disease was well established. Although viruses were still poorly defined, the principle that they were transmissible agents was understood. Second, although physicians had few specific remedies at their disposal, they had abandoned most of the drastic, plainly harmful remedies of earlier eras.

As polio became more and more prominent in morbidity statistics and the public imagination, the biomedical community responded on three different fronts. The first was an attempt to prevent transmission by quarantine measures and clinical studies. Scientists attempted to clarify the actual mode of transmission and the natural occurrence of the virus. Second, they attempted to treat paralytic cases in the acute and recovery phases. Lastly, scientists tried to develop a vaccine.

Quarantine measures were never very successful at controlling polio epidemics. Isolating critically ill patients in a sterile environment and restricting travel on the part of their family members, as was done in 1916 in New York, failed to quarantine people with mild infections, who were the main transmitters of the disease. Although the poliovirus can be found in untreated sewage, this is not a major source of infection in the United States. Flies can transmit the virus mechanically and thus may act as vectors, but fly eradication campaigns failed to have any effect on polio occurrence. In the period when it was incorrectly thought that the poliovirus entered through the nose, nasal sprays were touted as offering protection.

In the 1920's, the search for a cure emphasized the use of blood serum from individuals who had recovered from the disease. Theoretically, the idea was a sound one that had been used successfully for other diseases, but it proved ineffective in the case of polio. The gamma globulin used to protect people who have been exposed to hepatitis is a modern refinement of this basic technique. The level of antibodies was not sufficiently high to have a therapeutic effect. More important, by the time that patients developed paralytic symptoms, their bodies were already producing antibodies. Despite disappointing results, serum therapy was used extensively for fifteen years.

In 1920, Philip Drinker of the Harvard School of Public Health introduced the so-called iron lung, a respirator that mimicked the action of lungs by subjecting patients to fluctuations in air pressure. The iron lung gave some hope of survival to patients with paralysis of the diaphragm or lesions in the nervous centers of the brain that govern respiration. Its introduction was accompanied by misgivings that it would only serve to keep alive severely disabled patients who had no hope of survival outside a hospital. Such ethical concerns were justified, but artificial respirators also proved effective in temporarily treating acute cases of respiratory paralysis that subsided with time.

With respect to paralyzed limbs, advances in orthopedics in the early twentieth century allowed for sur-

gical procedures that minimized twisting and deformity and for the design of braces that improved mobility. Observing that deformity could be lessened by bracing and immobilizing limbs at the onset of the paralytic form of the disease, doctors of the 1920's and 1930's had a tendency to encase polio victims, even those with little or no paralysis, in elaborate casts attached to pulley systems. Against this trend, Elizabeth Kenny, an Australian nurse, conducted what amounted to a crusade against immobilization and advocated active physical therapy in acute paralytic poliomyelitis.

In 1921, the future president of the United States, Franklin Delano Roosevelt, was stricken with acute paralytic polio that left him with severe paralysis of both legs. Roosevelt later used his private fortune to establish a center for the rehabilitation of polio victims in Warm Springs, Georgia, where he had spent his convalescence. After he became president in 1933, Roosevelt became a leader in the fight against poliomyelitis. For several years, the principal charitable organization funding polio treatment and research in the United States was the president's Birthday Ball Commission, the immediate forerunner of the National Foundation for Infantile Paralysis (NFIP), better known under the name of its main fund-raising effort, the March of Dimes. Basil O'Conner, a personal friend of Roosevelt, headed both agencies.

Since an attack of polio in any of its forms confers lifelong immunity, researchers from the 1920's onward increasingly concentrated their efforts toward developing a vaccine. Vaccines rely on dead or nonvirulent strains of a pathogenic agent to induce an immune response in a host. To produce a polio vaccine, one must have large quantities of poliovirus, and the only known source of poliovirus prior to 1938 was spinal cord tissue from infected monkeys or humans. In 1935, Maurice Brodie conducted human vaccine trials with a formalin-inactivated virus from monkey spinal cord. At the same time, John Kohler conducted trials with a virus that he claimed had been inactivated by repeated passage through many generations of monkeys. Brodie's vaccine was unsuccessful; Kohler's achieved notoriety as the suspected cause of several cases of paralytic polio.

After World War II, the NFIP concentrated its efforts on funding the development of an effective polio vaccine. Thanks to the work of John Enders and others, a live poliovirus could be produced in tissue culture. Improved serological techniques enabled researchers to assess immunity in chimpanzees without sacrificing the animal. By 1950, a practical vaccination program was beginning to take shape under the direction of Jonas Salk, who headed the development of a formalin-inactivated, injectable vaccine.

In 1954, with the collaboration of the National Institutes of Health and the U.S. Census Bureau, the NFIP conducted a massive nationwide test of this inactivated Salk vaccine, involving 1.8 million children in the first, second, and third grades. In 1955, the number of new cases (or incidence) of polio among inoculated children was two to five times lower than among controls, demonstrating that the vaccine was effective in clinical practice. Thereafter, the inoculation of children against polio became routine, and the incidence per 100,000 people declined dramatically—from 40 in 1952, the last major epidemic year, to 20 in 1955. The number of new cases per 100,000 people was 5 in 1959 and fewer than 1 in 1961 and subsequent years. There have been no domestically acquired cases of paralytic polio in the United States since 1987.

Salk's vaccine conferred only temporary immunity, requiring booster shots to be administered at yearly intervals. This made protection of the population cumbersome in industrialized countries and impractical in developing countries. The NFIP consequently turned its attention toward an effort, under the direction of Albert Sabin, to develop an orally administered attenuated viral preparation. The challenge was to develop a strain of virus that would multiply in the digestive system and stimulate antibody production but that could not attack the human nervous system. This effort was also supported by the World Health Organization (WHO). In 1957, an oral live virus vaccine was tested in Ruanda-Urundi. Between 1958 and 1959, field trials were conducted in fifteen countries, including the United States and the Soviet Union.

The Sabin oral vaccine confers longer-lasting immunity and is easier to administer. It is now routinely used to immunize children and adults against polio throughout the world. WHO has exploited this advantage and undertaken a program to eradicate polio throughout the world. To date, this program has been successful, eliminating polio in Western Europe and the Western Hemisphere. Because of economic and logistic limitations, in the late 1990's it appeared unlikely that the program would reach its goal of worldwide eradication by the year 2000. Sporadic cases of polio still occur. Efforts to eradicate polio in Africa

and tropical Asia are hampered by the existence of a nonhuman primate reservoir for the disease.

PERSPECTIVE AND PROSPECTS

There is evidence that poliomyelitis has afflicted human beings from the beginning of time. There is an Egyptian tomb painting of a priest with a withered leg, and descriptions of individuals with polio-like diseases occur in Greek medical literature. In general, however, polio seems to have been a rare disease; there are no records of epidemics of paralytic polio before the second half of the nineteenth century. The symptoms of paralytic polio are so distinctive and devastating that it is unlikely cases were overlooked.

In the early nineteenth century, a number of physicians published descriptions of cases in which a fever in infants or very young children was followed by paralysis of the lower limbs. At that time, polio was then unknown among older children and adults. As a consequence, the disease came to be known as infantile paralysis. The occurrence was infrequent and sporadic, although Charles Bell, a distinguished English neurologist, recorded an account of an epidemic affecting all the three- to five-year-old children on the isolated island of St. Helena around 1830.

Between 1880 and 1905, several localized outbreaks of epidemic poliomyelitis occurred in rural Scandinavia. In 1894, the United States suffered its first major outbreak, in Rutland County, Vermont. In contrast to earlier experiences, significant numbers of older children and young adults were affected. It was also puzzling to epidemiologists that the outbreaks should have occurred in isolated rural areas rather than in urban centers. Ivar Wickman, a Swedish epidemiologist who tracked the course of the severe Scandinavian epidemic of 1905, obtained evidence for abortive and nonparalytic cases, and postulated that they were important to the epidemiology of the disease. His results were not taken seriously until thirty years later.

In 1916, the northeastern United States suffered one of the most devastating epidemics in the history of poliomyelitis, with more than nine thousand acute cases in New York City alone. Public health authorities, disregarding evidence that acute cases represented less than 10 percent of actual cases, instituted draconian quarantine measures that were largely ineffective. More than 95 percent of those affected in the 1916 epidemic were under nine years of age. By 1931, the date of the next major epidemic in the northeast, the proportion of victims younger than nine had declined to 84 percent; by 1947, it had further declined to 52 percent. Poliomyelitis had somehow been transformed from an uncommon endemic disease affecting only very young children to a sporadic, rural epidemic disease that affected primarily children. Finally, by the end of a century, it had become a widespread epidemic disease affecting all age groups in both rural and urban environments.

In 1905, when Swedish researchers attempted to show the existence of subclinical poliomyelitis infections, there was only one way to demonstrate polio in an unequivocal, scientifically rigorous manner. It involved filtering material from a diseased person to remove bacteria, inoculating the filtrate into the brain of a susceptible monkey, and waiting for paralysis to develop. Cost and logistics precluded large-scale tests. The trials that were conducted often failed because of inadequate sterility. In 1939, Charles Armstrong succeeded in propagating one of the three poliovirus strains in rodents, greatly facilitating research. In 1948, Enders and his colleagues succeeded in growing the poliovirus in tissue culture. In the meantime, reliable techniques for identifying antibodies to specific pathogens had been developed. This development enabled epidemiologists to determine which individuals had the live poliovirus in their bodies and which had developed immunity.

A series of studies conducted in the early 1950's among Alaskan Inuits, urban North Americans, and Egyptian villagers dramatically demonstrated the normal epidemiological pattern of polio occurrence and spread in three very different populations. Among Inuits living in Point Barrow, Alaska, only people over twenty showed antibodies to the virus, as a result of a known and devastating epidemic in 1930. In Miami, the proportion of persons with antibodies rose from 10 percent at age two to nearly 80 percent in adulthood. In Cairo, nearly 100 percent of the population over the age of three proved to have antibodies.

Thus, the following epidemiological picture emerged. Before 1900, sanitary conditions in most of the world approximated those in Cairo, and most people contracted polio before the age of three. The vast majority of infections were subclinical, and paralytic cases occurred only sporadically in infants. As sanitation improved in the United States and Europe, the chances of contracting polio as an infant decreased. Thus, a pool of susceptible individuals of mixed ages arose, and epidemics occurred. Like mumps, measles, and other childhood illnesses, polio is more likely to

cause severe illness in an adult than in a young child. For this reason, paralytic polio became a more serious health problem in Miami than in Cairo. Epidemics occurred first in rural areas in the United States and Scandinavia, where sanitation was relatively good and people were somewhat isolated from major population centers that served as sources of infection.

Defenders of the use of animals in biomedical research often cite the history of the conquest of poliomyelitis to support their point of view. From the earliest days of scientific poliomyelitis research until the discovery of tissue-culturing techniques for viruses in the 1940's, experimental work was dependent on monkeys. For many years, the only way of confirming that the virus was present was to inoculate a monkey with a suspected sample: If the monkey became paralyzed, the test was positive. Cultures were maintained through serial transfer from monkey to monkey, and the earliest vaccines were prepared from monkey spinal cord tissue.

The first successful tissue culture experiments involved fetal intestinal tissue. The experiments depended on having an available source of a characterized viral strain originally isolated from a human but maintained through several generations of transfer through animals. Even after the maintenance and characterization of viral strains and the production of virus for vaccines had moved from animal laboratories to test tubes of cultured cells, the first tests of the safety and efficacy of vaccines were performed with primates. Virtually every step in the conquest of polio involved experimental procedures.

Although the fight against poliomyelitis was spectacularly successful, it would be unwise to be complacent about a disease that is still prevalent in parts of the world and that is selectively virulent under modern urban conditions in developed nations. The percentage of schoolchildren, particularly those living in poorer neighborhoods, who receive routine vaccinations against childhood diseases is decreasing in the United States. Because of the availability of safe drinking water, children are no longer likely to naturally acquire immunity from subclinical infections.

In about 1 in 20 million cases, individuals will develop polio after receiving a vaccine. A naturally acquired case of polio is now exceedingly rare. The number of such cases is less than the number of cases of polio as a result of adverse reactions to the vaccine. For this reason, many parents are not having their children immunized against polio. These well-intentioned people are putting their children at an unnecessary risk of contracting the disease.

Other diseases that were once thought to be virtually extinct, such as measles and tuberculosis, are experiencing a tremendous resurgence because of declining commitment to public and community health and increasing numbers of people with compromised immune systems. There is no guarantee that polio will be excluded from the list of resurgent diseases.

—*Martha Sherwood-Pike, Ph.D.;*
updated by L. Fleming Fallon, Jr.,
M.D., Ph.D., M.P.H.

See also Childhood infectious diseases; Epidemiology; Immunization and vaccination; Meningitis; Paralysis; Viral infections.

FOR FURTHER INFORMATION:

Blume, Stuart, and Ingrid Geesink. "A Brief History of Polio Vaccines." *Science* 288, no. 5471 (June 2, 2000): 1593-1594. In 1988, the World Health Assembly resolved that by the year 2000 paralytic poliomyelitis would be wiped off the face of the Earth. Examines the global eradication campaign in its final stages, with valiant efforts to maintain polio vaccination programs, implement surveillance systems, and eliminate the last remaining reservoirs of poliovirus.

Daniel, Thomas M., and Frederick C. Robbins. *Polio.* Rochester, N.Y.: University of Rochester Press, 1997. This book is written by experts in the field who have experience from the era when polio was a major health problem. It is easily understandable.

Garrett, Laurie. *The Coming Plague: Newly Emerging Diseases in a World out of Balance.* New York: Farrar, Straus & Giroux, 1994. This book contains an excellent discussion of polio and the efforts of the World Health Organization to eradicate it. The author has a style that is easy to read.

Gould, Tony. *A Summer Plague: Polio and Its Survivors.* New Haven, Conn.: Yale University Press, 1995. This is a comprehensive account of the polio epidemic in the West, from the first major outbreak in New York in 1916 to postpolio syndrome. It combines biographical, political, social, and microbiological perspectives and focuses on key individuals, such as President Franklin Delano Roosevelt, Jonas Salk, and Sister Elizabeth Kenny.

Munsat, Theodore L. "Poliomyelitis: New Problems with an Old Disease." *New England Journal of Medicine* 324 (April, 1991): 1206-1207. A review article describing research on the incidence, symptoms, and treatment of postpolio syndrome, with a bibliography citing the most important current studies. The author stresses the importance of recognizing the clinical disease and emphasizes that postpolio syndrome is slow to progress and does not appear to involve new muscular deficits.

POLYP REMOVAL. *See* COLON AND RECTAL POLYP REMOVAL; NASAL POLYP REMOVAL.

PORPHYRIA
DISEASE/DISORDER

ANATOMY OR SYSTEM AFFECTED: Nervous system, skin

SPECIALTIES AND RELATED FIELDS: Genetics, neurology, pediatrics

DEFINITION: One of several rare, genetic disorders caused by the accumulation of substances called porphyrins.

CAUSES AND SYMPTOMS

Porphyria refers to a group of diseases which share a common feature: a defect in the chain of chemical reactions which produce hemoglobin, the protein responsible for the transport of oxygen by the blood. These metabolic errors cause a buildup of porphyrins, resulting in two main types of illness: nervous system attacks and skin lesions.

There are two major groups of porphyrias: erythropoietic and hepatic. In erythropoietic porphyria, the porphyrins are synthesized in the bone marrow; in hepatic porphyrias, they are produced in the liver. Each of these porphyrias has several subtypes. For example, acute intermittent porphyria (AIP) is a hepatic porphyria most common in young adults and adults in early middle age. Its attacks are triggered by alcohol, certain drugs, and hormonal changes (such as those accompanying pregnancy). Some patients experience two to three episodes per year, while others may have as few as three in a lifetime.

Since all forms of porphyria are rare, a physician may not suspect the disease at first. The symptoms of porphyria include abdominal disturbances, nausea, vomiting, reddish urine, and prickling sensations in the hands and feet. The hallmarks that distinguish porphyrias, however, are the skin and nervous system effects. Except for AIP, all the porphyrias cause extreme photosensitivity of the skin because the porphyrins that are deposited in the skin are excited by the ultraviolet aspect of sunlight. This reaction results in skin lesions, which may lead to disfigurement. The neurological disturbances of porphyria range from mild mental confusion to delirium and hysteria. If a porphyria is suspected, urine, stool, and blood tests are done to detect the presence of porphyrins.

TREATMENT AND THERAPY

Avoiding triggering factors is primary in the control of porphyria attacks. Alcohol and drugs, which may cause an attack, should be stopped. Protective clothing should be worn to prevent the irritating effects of sunlight. For certain porphyrias, drugs are available to suppress the formation of porphyrins. In the case of AIP, a simple increase in the consumption of carbohydrates is enough to inhibit the production of porphyrin-forming substances. The treatment of porphyrias is largely aimed at relieving its symptoms.

—*Robert Klose, Ph.D.*

See also Blood and blood disorders; Genetic diseases; Skin disorders.

FOR FURTHER INFORMATION:

Anderson, Karl E. "Diseases of Porphyrins or Metals." In *Cecil Textbook of Medicine*, edited by J. Claude Bennett et al. 20th ed. Vol. 1. Philadelphia: W. B. Saunders, 1996.

Elder, George H. "The Porphyrias." In *Conn's Current Therapy, 1994*, edited by Robert E. Rakel. Philadelphia: W. B. Saunders, 1994.

Lee, G. Richard, et al., eds. *Wintrobe's Clinical Hematology.* 10th ed. Philadelphia: Lea & Febiger, 1999.

Parish, Kathy. "What's Wrong with This Patient?" *RN* 53, no. 7 (July, 1990): 43-45.

POSITRON EMISSION TOMOGRAPHY (PET) SCANNING

PROCEDURE

ANATOMY OR SYSTEM AFFECTED: All

SPECIALTIES AND RELATED FIELDS: Biotechnology, nuclear medicine, radiology

DEFINITION: A noninvasive imaging procedure in which a positron-emitting radiopharmaceutical is administered and a three-dimensional image of an organ, which accumulates the radiopharmaceutical, is obtained by detecting the radiation resulting from positron annihilation.

KEY TERMS:

annihilation: the process whereby an electron and positron combine and their energy is converted into two photons traveling in opposite directions

positrons: a type of radiation, similar to electrons but with a positive charge, emitted by radioactive atoms

tomography: a procedure that yields images of body sections

INDICATIONS AND PROCEDURES

Positron emission tomography (PET) scanning permits the noninvasive determination of biological function, metabolism, and pathology following the administration of short-lived positron-emitting radiopharmaceuticals. Positron-emitting radiopharmaceuticals are drugs that contain a radioactive atom that is transformed to a more stable atom by emitting a positron. A positron is a subatomic particle that has the same mass and charge as an electron, but the charge is positive rather than negative. When an energetic positron is emitted by a radioactive atom, it quickly loses its energy in the surrounding medium and comes to rest. The positron then combines with a free electron in the medium, the two particles are annihilated, and their energy is converted into two 511,000 volt potential (511 keV) photons that travel in exactly opposite directions (180 degrees from each other). The detection of these two photons in coincidence (simultaneously) by placing a ring of small radiation detectors around the patient is the basic principle used in PET scanning. The radiation detectors convert these light photons into electrical signals that are fed to a computer, which reconstructs the distribution of radioactivity in the desired organ and presents the information as an image on a video screen.

USES AND COMPLICATIONS

PET techniques are generally used to measure metabolic rates quantitatively in normal and abnormal tissues. The positron-emitting radionuclides oxygen 15, nitrogen 13, and carbon 11 are well suited for studying tissue metabolism because of their short physical half-lives and their ubiquitous presence in biomolecules. Oxygen 15 gas is useful for studying oxygen metabolism, whereas oxygen 15 water and oxygen 15 carbon monoxide are used to study blood flow and blood volume, respectively, in any organ. Fluorodeoxyglucose (FDG) labeled with fluorine 18 is another positron-emitting radiopharmaceutical which is useful in PET for the quantitative measurement of

PET Scanning Techniques

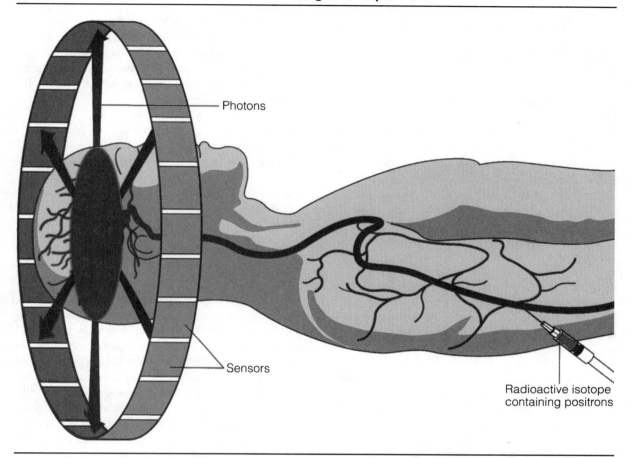

This method of scanning the brain, which can reveal the metabolic and chemical activity of tissue, is used to detect tumors, to evaluate damage resulting from strokes, and to diagnose and assess such conditions as parkinsonism, epilepsy, and certain mental illnesses.

glucose metabolism. Glucose metabolism is high in brain tumors when compared to normal tissue. Hence, PET with fluorodeoxyglucose 18 is widely used in the detection of brain tumors and assessment of the degree of malignancy, since low-grade tumors are less metabolically active than high-grade tumors. Fluorodeoxyglucose 18 PET is also used to identify persistent tumors after surgery.

The radiopharmaceuticals carbon 11 aminoisobutyric acid, rubidium 82 chloride, and gallium 68 citrate are useful for studying the blood-brain barrier permeability. This modality is also being used increasingly in patients with seizure disorders, dementia, and movement disorders. The application of PET in these cases may provide previously unavailable information

about these diseases to help the practicing neurologist. PET imaging is also being used to understand the mechanisms behind normal brain processes. Among the mechanisms studied are language processing, speech, vision, and brain development. Recent improvements in whole body PET scanning technology are useful in clinical oncology. This technique is being employed widely in the qualitative imaging of primary or recurrent tumors, lymph nodes, and distant metastases.

PET is also being used with increasing frequency to measure myocardial perfusion. A number of different perfusion agents which are labeled with rubidium 82, gallium 62, oxygen 15, and nitrogen 13 are being investigated. Some of these agents are being used to measure not only relative perfusion but also the absolute blood flow in selected regions of the myocardium. Carbon 11 palmitate is employed to determine cardiac fatty acid metabolism. These radiopharmaceuticals are generally safe because they involve low doses of radiation with minimal risks.

PERSPECTIVE AND PROSPECTS

The most desirable radionuclides used in PET procedures—carbon 11, nitrogen 13, oxygen 15, and fluorine 18—can be produced only with a cyclotron. Because of their very short physical half-lives, a dedicated cyclotron and fully automated equipment for radionuclide separation is usually necessary. Radionuclides that emit positrons but do not require a nearby cyclotron for their production— such as copper 62, gallium 68, and rubidium 82—are receiving attention because of their reduced cost. Although PET scanning provides valuable diagnostic information that in many cases cannot be obtained using other modalities, the expensive nature of the highly technical equipment necessary may limit the availability of these procedures to specialized medical centers. The changing health care environment and the public demand for cost containment are likely to hinder further advances in this area of diagnostic radiology. Technological advances in PET scanning instrumentation, however, may result in a markedly reduced cost for the procedure in the future.

—*Dandamudi V. Rao, Ph.D.*

See also Brain; Brain disorders; Imaging and radiology; Noninvasive tests; Nuclear medicine; Radiopharmaceuticals.

FOR FURTHER INFORMATION:

Brownell, Gordon. "Clinical Application of PET." In *Physics of Nuclear Medicine: Recent Advances*, edited by Dandamudi V. Rao et al. New York: American Institute of Physics, 1984. A chapter in collection culled from a congress of the AAPM Summer School held at Fairleigh Dickinson University, Madison, N.J., July 24-29, 1983.

Graham, Martin, and Rodney Bigler. "Principles of Positron Emission Tomography." In *Physics of Nuclear Medicine: Recent Advances*, edited by Dandamudi V. Rao et al. New York: American Institute of Physics, 1984. A chapter in collection culled from a congress of the AAPM Summer School held at Fairleigh Dickinson University, Madison, N.J., July 24-29, 1983.

Preboth, Monica. "Use of PET in the Diagnosis of Cancer." *American Family Physician* 61, no. 8 (April 15, 2000): 2548. The Health Technology Advisory Committee has published a report on positron emission tomography for oncologic applications. PET is a three-dimensional imaging technique designed to measure the level of metabolic activity within the cell.

POSTPARTUM DEPRESSION

DISEASE/DISORDER

ANATOMY OR SYSTEM AFFECTED: Endocrine system, psychic-emotional system

SPECIALTIES AND RELATED FIELDS: Gynecology, obstetrics, psychiatry, psychology

DEFINITION: Many women feel emotionally down or even miserable for a few days to the first few weeks after childbirth. Fortunately, most cases are mild and transient.

CAUSES AND SYMPTOMS

Postpartum depression results from several causes. One factor is that the sudden change in body hormones caused by childbirth can affect the mother's mood. There is also a sense of anticlimax after an event that has been anticipated for many months. Many new mothers are very tired, and some are a little apprehensive and lacking confidence about the challenges of motherhood. Another factor is the sudden change that may occur in lifestyle and an associated feeling of shrunken horizons, especially if the mother had been working before the birth. Additionally, environmental, social, and sexual difficulties can predispose some women to develop postpartum depression.

Depressive reactions are fairly common in the first week after childbirth, with approximately 90 percent of women experiencing "fourth-day blues." More severe symptoms of depression, such as insomnia, frequent crying, irrational fears, irritability, guilt, and psychic disturbances, are much less common. On rare occasions, serious depression may set in, and the mother may be unable to care for herself or the baby.

TREATMENT AND THERAPY

It is important for a new mother to avoid becoming too tired. Since the mother needs all the sleep she can get, the baby should be moved to its own bedroom as soon as possible. The loving support of a husband or significant other, relatives, and close friends is extremely helpful. The baby's father should take turns caring for the baby when the baby is unsettled or distressed. During the day, friends or family can help with shopping or looking after the baby while the mother rests. If the depression cannot be shaken off, a physician should be consulted. Antidepressant medication, such as sertraline hydrochloride (Zoloft), is usually effective if administered in the early stages of depression. In severe cases, admission to a psychiatric hospital for treatment may be necessary.

—*Alvin K. Benson, Ph.D.*

See also Depression; Pregnancy and gestation.

FOR FURTHER INFORMATION:

Dalton, Katharina. *Depression After Childbirth: How to Recognize and Treat Postnatal Illness.* 2d ed. New York: Oxford University Press, 1989.

Dix, Carol. *The New Mother Syndrome: Coping with Postpartum Stress and Depression.* Garden City, N.Y.: Doubleday, 1985.

O'Hara, Michael W. *Postpartum Depression: Causes and Consequences.* New York: Springer-Verlag, 1995.

Sebastian, Linda. *Overcoming Postpartum Depression and Anxiety.* Omaha, Nebr.: Addicus Books, 1998.

POST-TRAUMATIC STRESS DISORDER

DISEASE/DISORDER

ALSO KNOWN AS: Shell shock, combat neurosis, battle fatigue

ANATOMY OR SYSTEM AFFECTED: Psychic-emotional system

SPECIALTIES AND RELATED FIELDS: Psychiatry, psychology

DEFINITION: Intense fear, helplessness, or horror, with accompanying reexperiencing, avoidance, and arousal, following a traumatic event.

CAUSES AND SYMPTOMS

Post-traumatic stress disorder (PTSD) sometimes occurs when a person directly experiences intense fear, helplessness, or horror following exposure to a traumatic event (an event outside the range of normal human experiences). The traumatic event involves threatened death, serious injury, or other threat to physical integrity; or, witnessing the death of or threat to another person; or, learning about the death of or threat to a family member or close friend.

PTSD involves reexperiencing, avoidance, and arousal. Reexperiencing includes recurrent and intrusive thoughts, recurrent distressing dreams, feeling as if the event is happening again, intense psychological distress at exposure to any reminders (internal or external) of the event, or intense physical reactivity to any reminders of the event. Persistent avoidance includes anything associated with the event, and a numbing of general responsiveness as indicated by at least three of the following: avoiding thoughts, feelings, or conversations associated with the event; avoiding activities, places, or people that remind one of the event; forgetting an important aspect of the event; experiencing markedly diminished interest or participation in significant activities; feeling detached or estranged from others; having a restricted range of feelings, such as not being able to love; or feeling that the future is foreshortened. Increased arousal includes at least two of the following: difficulty with sleep; irritability or outbursts of anger; difficulty concentrating; hypervigilance; or exaggerated startle response. The reexperiencing, avoidance, and arousal start after the traumatic event, last more than one month, and cause clinically significant distress or impairment in social, occupational, or other important areas of functioning.

Persons with PTSD may describe painful guilt feelings about surviving when others did not, or about what they had to do to survive. Their phobic avoidance of situations or activities that resemble or symbolize the original trauma may interfere with interpersonal relationships and lead to marital conflict, divorce, or job loss.

Likelihood of developing PTSD increases as intensity and physical proximity to the event increase. Recent émigrés from areas of considerable social unrest and civil conflict may have elevated rates of PTSD. Lifetime prevalence rates for PTSD range from 1 percent to 14 percent.

PTSD can occur at any age. Symptoms usually begin within the first three months after the trauma. Duration varies. Complete recovery occurs within three months in approximately half of cases, with many others having persisting symptoms for longer than one year after the trauma.

TREATMENT AND THERAPY

Treatments for PTSD include individual therapy, group therapy, and antianxiety and antidepressant drugs. Combinations of therapies can also be effective. In general, the sooner the victim of PTSD receives treatment, the greater are the chances of complete recovery.

Psychotherapy can help the person come to grips with the traumatic event. Different approaches are used, including exposure (or imaginal) therapy, anxiety management/relaxation training, cognitive therapy, and supportive psychotherapy. Also, hypnosis, journaling (such as thought diaries and grief letters), creative arts, and a critical incident stress debriefing may be used in treating PTSD, either alone or in conjunction with psychotherapy.

Group therapy, in which victims of PTSD can share their experiences and gain support from others, is especially helpful. Groups are typically small (six to eight persons), and are often composed of individuals who have undergone similar experiences. Also, marital and family therapy or parent training may be used in treating PTSD.

In general, the goals of psychotherapy include facilitating victims' emotional engagement with the trauma memory, helping them organize a personal trauma narrative, assisting them in correcting dysfunctional cognitions that often follow trauma, helping them develop increased trust in others, and decreasing their emotional and social isolation. The therapist typically provides empathy, validation, safety, consistency, and sensitivity to cultural and ethnic identity issues.

Antianxiety and antidepressant drugs can relieve the physiological symptoms of PTSD. The major pharmacological agents include benzodiazepines, serotonin receptor partial agonists, tricyclic antidepressants, MAO inhibitors, and selective serotonin reuptake inhibitors. Because of the many biological abnormalities presumed to be associated with PTSD, and because of the overlap between symptoms of PTSD and other comorbid disorders, almost every class of psychotropic agent has been administered to PTSD patients. Whether it includes individual or group therapy, drugs, or some combination of these three, the treatment approach must be tailored to the individual PTSD sufferer and his or her unique situation.

Comorbidity is the rule rather than the exception with PTSD. Depressive disorders, substance use disorders, and other anxiety disorders are the disorders most likely to occur with post-traumatic stress disorder. Treatment must address the comorbid conditions. PTSD can be reliably assessed through semistructured interview and self-report measures. Treatment typically occurs on an outpatient basis, but may also be done on an inpatient basis if the symptoms are severe.

PERSPECTIVE AND PROSPECTS

PTSD was observed in World War I, when some soldiers had intense anxiety reactions to the horrors they were experiencing. At that time, it was called combat neurosis, shell shock, or battle fatigue. It was formally diagnosed as an anxiety-based personality disorder in the 1960's among Vietnam veterans. It is now known that traumatic events may also include violent personal assault, kidnapping, being taken hostage, terrorist attack, torture, natural or manmade disasters, severe automobile accidents, or being diagnosed with a life-threatening illness. For children, sexually traumatic events may include sexual experiences that were developmentally inappropriate, even if no threatened or actual violence occurred. PTSD may be especially severe when the trauma is of human origin (for example, torture).

—*Lillian M. Range, Ph.D.*

See also Accidents; Anxiety; Domestic violence; Psychiatric disorders; Psychiatry; Stress; Stress reduction.

FOR FURTHER INFORMATION:
American Psychiatric Association. *Diagnostic and Statistical Manual of Mental Disorders*. 4th rev. ed. Washington, D.C.: Author, 2000.

Foa, Edna B., Terence M. Keane, and Matthew J. Friedman, eds. *Effective Treatments for PTSD: Practice Guidelines from the Society for Traumatic Stress Studies*. New York: Guilford, 2000.

Horowitz, Mardi J., ed. *Essential Papers on Post-traumatic Stress Disorder*. New York: New York University Press, 1999.

PRECOCIOUS PUBERTY
DISEASE/DISORDER

ALSO KNOWN AS: Sexual precocity, gonadotropin puberty, pubertas praecox

ANATOMY OR SYSTEM AFFECTED: Musculoskeletal system, nervous system, psychic-emotional system, reproductive system

SPECIALTIES AND RELATED FIELDS: Endocrinology, family practice, genetics, neurology, pediatrics

DEFINITION: The early onset of puberty caused by the premature secretion of sex hormones, resulting in the commencement of sexual maturation prior to age eight in girls and age ten in boys.

KEY TERMS:
gonads: ovaries in girls and testes in boys
hormones: chemicals produced by glands such as the

thyroid, pituitary, or adrenals that stimulate bodily changes or growth and that regulate body functions
hypothalamic hamartomas: tumors in the hypothalamic region of the brain, which are usually benign
hypothalamus: the region of the brain that stimulates glands to secrete hormones
idiopathic: having an unidentified cause
puberty: secondary sexual development that involves the maturation of the reproductive system and is typified by significant physical growth

CAUSES AND SYMPTOMS

Secondary sexual development is commonly known as puberty. It is typically characterized by growth of pubic and underarm hair, acne, and rapid physical development until about age eighteen. During puberty, a boy also grows facial hair, his penis and testes enlarge, and he begins to produce sperm. A girl develops breasts and begins to menstruate and ovulate.

Puberty is the result of hormonal changes triggered by the hypothalamus region of the brain. The brain releases luteinizing hormone-releasing hormone (LHRH) in periodic bursts, which causes the pituitary gland to secrete gonadotropin-releasing hormone (GnRH). Gonadotropins stimulate the ovaries in girls and the testes in boys to secrete sex hormones. These hormones—estrogen and progesterone in girls and testosterone in boys—start the sexual maturation process and stimulate rapid physical growth.

Puberty usually begins at about age twelve in boys and age eleven in girls. Approximately one in every ten thousand children begins puberty abnormally early, between infancy and approximately age nine. This condition, known as precocious puberty, affects both sexes but is two to five times more common among girls than boys.

In addition to prematurely developing secondary sexual characteristics, children with precocious puberty are initially tall for their ages. Left untreated, however, they rarely reach their full adult height potential because the same sex hormones that trigger early growth also end it prematurely. Males often grow no taller than 5 feet, 2 inches, and many females remain under 5 feet. Precocious puberty frequently results in adolescent behaviors such as moodiness, irritability, and aggressiveness, as well as the early development of a sex drive. Children with precocious puberty reach sexual maturity at varying rates, and some characteristics may even begin to regress to their normal state.

When an underlying cause for precocious puberty cannot be determined, the condition is known as idiopathic precocious puberty. About 80 percent of cases in females and 40 percent of male cases are idiopathic. Common causes for precocious puberty that can be identified include genetic disorders or tumors in the hypothalamic region of the brain. Such tumors, known as hypothalamic hamartomas, are usually benign. Between 5 and 10 percent of boys with precocious puberty genetically inherit the condition from their fathers or indirectly from their maternal grandfathers. This genetic transmittal of precocious puberty only occurs in about 1 percent of girls with the condition. Less common causes of precocious puberty include other kinds of brain tumors, ovarian tumors or cysts, and adrenal gland disorders such as adrenogenital hyperplasia or congenital adrenal hyperplasia. Precocious puberty can also be caused by hydrocephalus, radiation therapy, nervous system disorders such as neurofibromatosis, and a rare condition called McCune-Albright syndrome.

Children with precocious puberty are often self-conscious about their early physical and sexual development, since they appear older than their ages. Mental development is not affected by the condition, however, so children with precocious puberty are usually not as emotionally mature as they appear.

TREATMENT AND THERAPY

Underlying causes of precocious puberty, if known, are often difficult or impossible to treat. Surgical removal of noncancerous hypothalamic hamartomas and other brain tumors, for example, may not be feasible and rarely halts sexual development. Other causes such as neurofibromatosis are incurable, and treatments for conditions such as adrenal disorders may not stop the effects of precocious puberty.

Therefore, many forms of precocious puberty are treated by changing patients' hormonal balance. The synthetic hormone histrelin acetate, also known by its brand name Supprelin, has been shown to be effective in reducing early sexual changes in both sexes and to slow bone growth. Daily injections of the drug are stopped when the child reaches the appropriate age for the onset of puberty.

Synthetic versions of GnRH or LHRH interrupt the chain of hormonal events that result in sexual maturation. Some research, however, suggests a link between these therapies and bone mineral density loss. Treatments are administered in daily or monthly injections.

Girls with precocious puberty caused by congenital adrenal hyperplasia can be treated by suppressing the hormone known as ACTH with a glucocorticoid. Precocious puberty associated with McCune-Albright syndrome can be treated with testolactone, which blocks the production of estrogens. Some forms of precocious puberty involving the gonadotropins can be treated with the hormone suppressant nafarelin acetate.

Genetic counseling is recommended for families of patients with inherited precocious puberty. Psychological counseling may also benefit patients, since they may not fit in with peers because of the physical ramifications of the condition.

PERSPECTIVE AND PROSPECTS

Previous treatments for precocious puberty included the use of synthetic progesterone, an artificial version of a sex hormone secreted by the ovaries. Synthetic progesterone frequently stops menstruation and reduces breast size in girls, but it has little or no effect on boys. Unfortunately, it fails to stop rapid growth in either sex. Synthetic progesterone can also result in several serious side effects.

Experimental treatments for idiopathic precocious puberty include a combination of spironolactone and testolactone for male patients, as well as another drug called deslorelin or Somagard for either sex.

—*Cheryl Pawlowski, Ph.D.*

See also Endocrine system; Endocrinology; Endocrinology, pediatric; Growth; Hormones; Menstruation; Puberty and adolescence; Sexuality.

FOR FURTHER INFORMATION:

Creatsas, George, et al., eds. *Adolescent Gynecology and Endocrinology: Basic and Clinical Aspects.* New York: New York Academy of Sciences, 1997. Presents fifty-three papers organized in sections on gynecological and endocrine issues from adolescence to adulthood, the endometrium, the menstrual cycle, disorders of the ovarian cycle, pubertal endocrinological disorders, endometriosis, female genital tract malignancies during adolescence, and the reproductive revolution.

Grave, Gilman D., and Gordon B. Cutler, eds. *Sexual Precocity: Etiology, Diagnosis, and Management.* New York: Raven Press, 1993. Proceedings of a conference sponsored by the National Institute of Child Health and Human Development, held October 28-31, 1990, in Airlie, Virginia. Includes bibliographical references and index.

Huffman, Grace Brooke. "Reassessing the Age Limit of Precocious Puberty in Girls." *American Family Physician* 61, no. 6 (March 15, 2000): 1850. Standard textbooks usually define precocious puberty as "development of secondary sexual characteristics" in girls younger than eight years of age. However, puberty seems to be occurring earlier now than in the past.

Walvoord, Emily C., and Ora Hirsch Pescovitz. "Combined Use of Growth Hormone and Gonadotropin-Releasing Hormone Analogues in Precocious Puberty: Theoretic and Practical Considerations." *Pediatrics* 104, no. 4 (October, 1999): 1010-1014. The rationale underlying the use of gonadotropin-releasing hormone analogues to treat patients with central precocious puberty is reviewed. The adult heights attained by these patients often fall short of what would be expected according to their genetic potential.

PREGNANCY AND GESTATION
BIOLOGY

ANATOMY OR SYSTEM AFFECTED: Abdomen, reproductive system, uterus

SPECIALTIES AND RELATED FIELDS: Embryology, gynecology, obstetrics

DEFINITION: The development of unborn young within a woman's uterus and the accompanying physical, biochemical, and developmental changes that occur to both mother and child from conception until birth as genetic material from each parent is joined to create a unique individual.

KEY TERMS:

amniotic sac: the sac that surrounds the fetus in the uterus and is filled with amniotic fluid

blastocyst: the fertilized egg after it has divided several times to form a hollow ball of cells in one of the earliest stages of development

cervix: the constricted lower end of the uterus

chromosomes: rodlike structures inside cells which carry the genetic material

embryo: the unborn child from fertilization through the eighth week of development

endometrium: the lining of the uterus

Fallopian tube: the structure that leads from the internal cavity of the uterus to the ovary

fetus: the unborn child from the eighth week after fertilization until birth

placenta: the organ that connects the mother to the

embryo or fetus through the umbilical cord and is necessary for the child's nourishment

trimester: a division of pregnancy into three equal time periods of about thirteen weeks

PROCESS AND EFFECTS

Pregnancy begins with the fusion of an egg and sperm within a woman's body and continues until childbirth, typically thirty-eight weeks later. This gestational time is divided into three approximately equal periods called trimesters, each associated with specific physical and biochemical hallmarks.

Prior to conception, a mature egg, or ovum, ruptures from a fluid-filled follicle within the ovary and is swept into the Fallopian tube by large fringes on the tube that caress the ovary's surface. The empty follicle is transformed into a structure called the corpus luteum which secretes hormones that help to prepare the woman's body for pregnancy. If the ovum is fertilized within twenty-four hours, pregnancy will occur. If it is not fertilized, the uterine lining will be shed during menstruation.

Sperm ejaculated into a woman's vagina travel through the cervix and uterus and into the Fallopian tubes. Only about two hundred of the original 500 million sperm delivered to the woman may reach the vicinity of the ovum. Enzymes in the sperm heads dissolve through protective outer layers of the egg. When one sperm finally breaks through the plasma membrane, the innermost covering of the ovum, chemical changes on the surface of the ovum prevent additional sperm from entering. The genetic material contained in the sperm and ovum fuse. If the fertilizing sperm carries an X chromosome, the baby will be female; a Y chromosome determines that the baby will be male.

About twelve hours after fusion of the genetic material, the first cell division occurs. Divisions continue at intervals of twelve to fifteen hours, doubling the number of cells each time, and the fertilized ovum is now called a blastocyst. The blastocyst is gently guided through the Fallopian tube to the uterus by the beating of the millions of tiny hairs, called cilia, that line the inner surfaces of the Fallopian tubes. This journey to the uterus takes about three days.

Upon arriving in the uterus, the blastocyst "explores" the endometrium, the uterine lining, for an appropriate site to settle. Prior to this implantation in the endometrium, the blastocyst ruptures from the clear protective sheath that helps to prevent it from settling in the Fallopian tube. By eight days after fertilization, the blastocyst implants securely within the endometrium. At this point, it consists of several hundred cells and is about the size of the head of a pin.

After implantation, chemical signals produced by the blastocyst prevent the mother's immune system from recognizing the blastocyst as a foreign invader and destroying it. Other chemical signals cause the endometrium to thicken and extend blood vessels to the blastocyst for nourishment from the mother. The uterine wall softens and thickens, and the cervical opening is sealed with a mucous plug.

At this point, the cells of the blastocyst divide into two distinct clusters: One part will form the embryo itself, and the other part will join with the woman's tissue to form the placenta, the structure that will provide nourishment from the mother to the growing embryo. These early placental cells produce the hormone human chorionic gonadotropin (hCG). This hormone signals the ovary to cease ovulation and stimulates it to produce the hormone progesterone, which prevents menstruation and causes the endometrium to grow even thicker.

During the second week after fertilization, a cavity surrounding the embryo begins to form. This is destined to become the amniotic sac, which will contain the shock-absorbing amniotic fluid in which the fetus floats during development. At this time, the hormones being produced by the blastocyst and ovaries can be detected by pregnancy tests.

Three weeks after conception, the size of the embryo is about 2 millimeters (0.08 inch). The embryonic cells have divided into germ layers, distinct groupings of cells that are destined to produce specific body parts. The rudimentary brain appears at the end of a long tube. The heart is forming and will be beating within a week. At this point, the mother has missed her menstrual period and may be experiencing symptoms of pregnancy, such as nausea, heartburn, and tender breasts.

During the fifth through seventh weeks of embryonic development, massive physical changes occur. The crown-to-rump length of the embryo increases to around 1.25 centimeters (0.5 inch). The embryo's face, trunk, and limbs grow, and by the end of this period distinct fingers and toes are formed. The backbone is in place, and ribs begin to develop, as do skin, eyes, and all of the organ systems and the circulatory system. At this point, the placenta is connected to the embryo by the umbilical cord, and placental cells pen-

Stages of Fetal Development

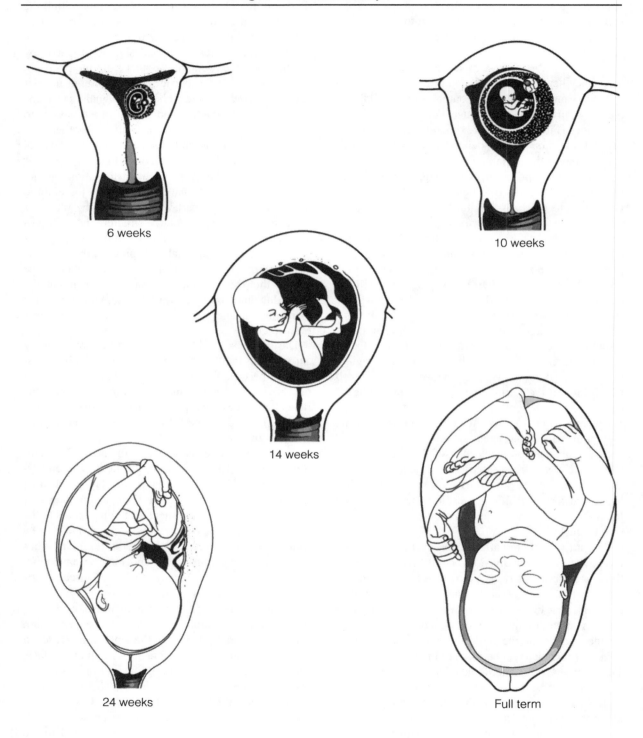

6 weeks

10 weeks

14 weeks

24 weeks

Full term

etrate the blood vessels of the endometrium to provide transit of nutrients from the mother's bloodstream to the embryo. The placenta also filters out some potentially dangerous substances from the mother's bloodstream and aids in disposing of embryonic waste products.

By the eighth week of development, the embryo is about 4 centimeters (1.5 inches) long, weighs about 14 grams (0.5 ounce), and is composed of millions of cells. All organs are formed, and the embryo is officially called a fetus. The woman's uterus has increased in size, and her waistline may begin to enlarge. At this point, hormonal shifts stabilize, which frequently relieves morning sickness and other discomforts of early pregnancy.

Growth and organ system interconnection continues during the third month of fetal life, and the cells of the immune system are formed. During the fourth month, facial features develop and the fetus may begin to respond to sound. Hair on the head and eyebrows coarsen and develop pigment. The distinction between male and female fetuses becomes apparent with a visible vagina or penis. Sixteen to eighteen weeks after fertilization, the mother may feel the first fetal movements. She has gained several pounds, and changes in her body shape are readily visible. Frequently, this second trimester is associated with feelings of joy and minimal discomfort.

The third trimester is largely a period of growth for the fetus. Its weight increases rapidly. The fetus becomes very active within the amniotic fluid and responds to sound from both within and outside the mother. The weight gain may put incredible stress on the mother's body, and pressure on internal organs may cause frequent urination, heartburn, and difficulty breathing and sleeping.

Normal pregnancies vary from thirty-eight to forty-two weeks long. The lungs are the final organs to mature, and by the end of the eighth month all organ systems are established and functional. The fetus continues to gain weight until the end of pregnancy. At this time, the fetus will weigh around 3 kilograms (7 pounds) and have a crown to rump length of approximately 37 centimeters (14.4 inches). The end of pregnancy is heralded by the beginning of uterine contractions, and frequently by the rupture of the amniotic sac and expulsion of its fluid. Labor leads to the birth of a unique individual created from the developmental programs contained in the genetic material inherited from each parent.

COMPLICATIONS AND DISORDERS

Since the developing embryo or fetus is dependent on the placental connection to the mother for nourishment, its health is directly tied to the diet and lifestyle of the mother. Pregnant women must ingest adequate levels of protein, vitamins, and iron to remain healthy and have a healthy baby. Smoking during pregnancy has been linked to cleft palate and eye malformations, and it decreases the amount of oxygen available to the fetus, which causes poor growth. Consumption of alcohol is associated with a host of defects collectively called fetal alcohol syndrome. Whether any level of alcohol consumption is safe during pregnancy is not yet known. The use of drugs such as marijuana and cocaine during pregnancy increases the likelihood of stillbirths and unhealthy babies.

The loss of a fetus before the twentieth week of pregnancy is called a miscarriage. The most common cause of miscarriage during the first trimester is a major genetic defect in which the embryo has missing or extra chromosomes and therefore cannot develop normally. Other common causes are physical abnormalities in the embryo, a malformed uterus in the mother, an "incompetent" cervix that opens as the fetus enlarges, scarring of the uterus, and hormonal deficiencies. Increasing age of the mother, smoking, and alcohol and drug consumption are also correlated with miscarriage. To prevent future miscarriages of a nongenetic cause, hormone therapy, medications, and surgery are options.

Ectopic pregnancies occur when the fertilized egg implants in the wall of the Fallopian tube instead of the uterus. The growing embryo may rupture the tube, endangering the mother's life and necessitating emergency surgery and possible loss of that Fallopian tube. Scarring of the Fallopian tube from an infection can narrow this passage and cause ectopic pregnancy, as can early "hatching" of the blastocyst from its protective covering.

Neural tube defects result from improper closure of the brain and spinal cord in early embryonic development. The outcomes of this defect are anencephaly (absence of a complete brain and part of the skull), a lethal condition, or spina bifida (portions of the spinal cord protruding from the spine), which can vary from mild to severe. These disorders seem to occur in families with a history of neural tube defects in pregnancy. Risk may be increased by vitamin deficiencies. Neural tube defects can be detected prenatally by ultrasound, in which high-frequency sound waves

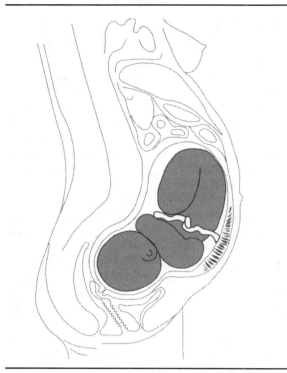

Cross section of a pregnant woman in the third trimester.

are bounced off the contents of the uterus. The echoes are converted to an image, or sonogram, on a screen. Another test for neural tube defects is the alpha fetoprotein test, which measures levels of a fetal protein in the mother's blood; high levels indicate a neural tube defect.

Down syndrome, which results from the presence of one extra chromosome number 21, is the leading cause of mental retardation in the United States and occurs in about 1 in every 800 live births. Many other genetic disorders are caused by missing or extra chromosomes. Some inherited diseases are attributable to errors in small pieces of chromosomes. Examples of these sorts of disorders include cystic fibrosis, hemophilia, Tay-Sachs disease, and sickle-cell disease. Many of these genetic diseases can be detected by prenatal tests.

Amniocentesis is performed between the fifteenth and seventeenth weeks of pregnancy. A needle is inserted through the mother's abdomen, and a sample of the amniotic fluid is removed. Fetal cells present in the fluid are cultured for two to three weeks. The fetal cells are then analyzed for chromosome complement or tested for small genetic changes that can result in

specific genetic diseases. Chorionic villus sampling provides a similar means to examine the genetic material of the fetus. This test is performed as early as the eighth week of pregnancy when a small piece of the chorionic villus, a tissue of embryonic origin which surrounds the early placenta, is removed and genetic analysis is immediately performed. Prenatal diagnosis of a chromosome abnormality or genetic disease allows the parents to terminate the pregnancy or prepare for the birth of an affected child.

Infections acquired by a pregnant woman may be only inconveniences for her, but they may have severe consequences for an unborn child. Rubella, or German measles, can cause fetal death or severe impairment during the first trimester and permanent hearing loss during the second trimester. Vaccination prevents contraction of rubella. Cytomegalovirus (CMV) can cause physical and mental retardation, blindness, and deafness to the fetus if the mother first contracts CMV during pregnancy. Rigorous personal hygiene is the best prevention for CMV infection. Transmission of the sexually transmitted diseases syphilis and gonorrhea to the fetus can be prevented with antibiotic therapy. Human immunodeficiency virus (HIV), which causes acquired immunodeficiency syndrome (AIDS), can be transmitted from mother to fetus through the placenta. Newborns with AIDS have a host of disorders and usually die within one or two years.

Rh factor is a substance on the surface of red blood cells. Individuals with and without this substance are Rh positive and Rh negative, respectively. If a woman is Rh negative and has an Rh-positive fetus, during delivery some of the baby's blood cells will enter the woman, and her body will manufacture antibodies to destroy the foreign cells. If with a subsequent pregnancy the fetus is Rh positive, these antibodies could attack and destroy the fetus. This problem is avoided by bloodtyping of mother and fetus during the first pregnancy and by administering $Rh_0(D)$ immune globulin (human), which destroys the fetal red blood cells entering the mother before her body can produce antibodies. Hence, future pregnancies are not at risk for Rh incompatibility.

A host of medical problems in the mother can develop during pregnancy that could jeopardize both her health and the health of her fetus. Blood pressure problems develop in about 7 percent of pregnant women as a result of the enormous changes in blood volume and pressure. The largest danger is that the fetus will not receive enough oxygen, which may lead to growth problems or sudden death during the final months of pregnancy. Preeclampsia is a cluster of symptoms related to high blood pressure, including edema (swelling caused by water retention) and kidney malfunction. Eclampsia (convulsions and coma) is life-threatening and needs emergency treatment. Bed rest, diet modification, close monitoring by a physician, or hospitalization may be prescribed for mild to severe cases of high blood pressure during pregnancy.

The effect of the hormones induced by pregnancy on the production of insulin, which regulates sugar levels in the body, is not well understood. In some pregnancies, insulin levels are not regulated properly, which results in gestational diabetes. Untreated, this can result in loss of the fetus late in pregnancy, the birth of a baby with high body fat content and an immature pancreas, or maternal convulsions and coma. Proper medical intervention and monitoring can correct or ease the effects of gestational diabetes on both mother and fetus.

Up to half of pregnant women develop anemia, a deficiency in red blood cells, because of a lack of iron or folic acid. The demand for the production of red blood cells in both mother and fetus leads to this disorder, which can cause poor growth in the fetus and increased susceptibility to infection, fatigue, and severe bleeding during childbirth for the mother. Proper diet and dietary supplements can alleviate anemia.

PERSPECTIVE AND PROSPECTS

Until the mid-twentieth century, what was known about fetal development was derived mainly from the study of miscarriages. The development and use of ultrasound techniques in the 1960's allowed a more accurate picture of developmental progression of normal, active fetuses, and such techniques subsequently became indispensable for the detection of some developmental abnormalities.

While physicians had been able to sample the amniotic fluid surrounding a fetus since the late 1800's, it was not until 1970 that they discovered that the fluid contained fetal cells which could be analyzed for chromosomal composition. At this time, amniocentesis became a tool for prenatal genetic analysis and sex determination and a routine test for pregnant women over the age of thirty-five who are at high risk of carrying a fetus with a genetic abnormality. The liberalization of abortion laws in the United

States in the 1960's gave parents of abnormal fetuses the option of pregnancy termination. In the early 1980's, chorionic villus sampling allowed much earlier detection of genetic defects and facilitated decision making for the expectant parents.

In the 1980's, some physicians began performing surgery on fetuses within the mother's uterus to correct problems threatening the life of the fetus, such as kidney disorders. Advanced monitoring and intervention techniques have virtually eliminated maternal deaths during pregnancy and childbirth. Increased knowledge about infectious and toxic agents and about the ill effects of certain lifestyle habits upon a developing fetus has led to better education and prenatal care for both mother and fetus. Because of career and personal considerations, older women frequently wish to begin families. Medical advances have made it not uncommon for women past the age of forty to conceive for the first time and give birth to healthy infants.

Much research has been focused on the initial stages of pregnancy and infertility. Techniques have been developed to circumvent damaged Fallopian tubes. In the procedure called in vitro fertilization, a woman is given hormones to induce ovulation. Several mature eggs are removed from her ovaries and fertilized in a glass dish. The resulting blastocysts are then implanted into the woman's uterus. In some cases in which a woman is unable to carry the fetus herself, a surrogate mother has been used as an "incubator" for the embryo. Unused embryos fertilized in vitro are stored in a deep freeze and may be thawed for future use. Early embryos have been separated into individual cells, which then develop into genetically identical blastocysts, each with the potential to become an infant. These technological advances have raised a host of ethical questions concerning disposal of the embryos and their genetic manipulation.

Human reproductive research is focused on the reversal or circumvention of infertility, the alleviation of maternal and fetal distress, and the prenatal detection and treatment of genetic disease. The knowledge gained about reproduction serves to enhance a sense of awe and wonder at the beauty and complexity of the gestational process.

—*Karen E. Kalumuck, Ph.D.*

See also Abortion; Amniocentesis; Birth defects; Blurred vision; Breast-feeding; Cesarean section; Childbirth; Childbirth complications; Chorionic villus sampling; Conception; Contraception; Ectopic pregnancy; Embryology; Endometriosis; Genetic counseling; Genetic diseases; Genital disorders, female; Gynecology; In vitro fertilization; Infertility in females; Infertility in males; Mastitis; Menstruation; Miscarriage; Multiple births; Postpartum depression; Premature birth; Reproductive system; Sexual differentiation; Sperm banks; Stem cell research; Sterilization; Stillbirth; Tubal ligation; Ultrasonography; Umbilical cord.

FOR FURTHER INFORMATION:

Curtis, Glade B. *Your Pregnancy Week-by-Week*. 4th ed. Tucson, Ariz.: Fisher Books, 2000. In this narrative-style book, each chapter examines one week of pregnancy and includes information on how the baby is growing and developing, changes in the mother, how maternal actions affect the baby, and routine physical exams and special tests.

Eisenberg, Arlene, Heidi E. Murkoff, and Sandee E. Hathaway. *What to Expect When You're Expecting*. New York: Workman, 1996. A standard resource for pregnant women and their families. Offers a wealth of information, sometimes in a question-and-answer format.

Hales, Dianne, and Timothy R. B. Johnson. *Intensive Caring: New Hope for High-Risk Pregnancy*. New York: Crown, 1990. This excellent book defines high-risk pregnancy and who is at risk, supplying helpful information about what can be expected, what can be done to limit problems, and how to deal with potential problems during pregnancy, both physically and psychologically.

Hotchner, Tracie. *Pregnancy and Childbirth*. Rev. ed. New York: Avon Books, 1997. This very readable book addresses a wide range of topics: the physical and psychological changes to mother and fetus; complications; prenatal testing; choosing an obstetrician, midwife, and hospital; labor and delivery; and new baby care.

Morales, Karla, and Charles B. Inlander. *Take This Book to the Obstetrician with You: A Consumer's Guide to Pregnancy and Childbirth*. Rev. ed. Reading, Mass.: Addison-Wesley, 1998. A practical handbook which provides factual information to prospective parents on how to manage the pregnancy and childbirth experience. Contains a wealth of information on prenatal tests, insurance, and alternatives to standard hospital delivery.

Nilsson, Lennart. *A Child Is Born*. Text by Lars Hamberger. Translated by Clare James. New York: Delacorte Press/Seymour Lawrence, 1990. Advanced photographic equipment and fiber optics have enabled Nilsson to capture fantastic color photographs of the developing infant, from conception through birth. Excellent text, which discusses the physical and biochemical changes in fetus and mother, accompanies the spectacular photographs. Includes sections on basic genetics, infertility, and research in human reproduction.

Scher, Jonathan. *Preventing Miscarriage: The Good News*. New York: Harper & Row, 1990. An authoritative book on miscarriage written in an accessible, nontechnical manner by a pioneer in miscarriage research. Includes useful information on how to recognize the first stages of a miscarriage, in-depth discussion as to the causes of miscarriage and how causes are identified, and sections on grieving and the psychological effects of miscarriage on parents.

PREMATURE BIRTH
DISEASE/DISORDER

ANATOMY OR SYSTEM AFFECTED: Reproductive system, uterus

SPECIALTIES AND RELATED FIELDS: Embryology, neonatology, obstetrics, pediatrics, perinatology

DEFINITION: Premature birth is childbirth occurring before the thirty-eighth week of pregnancy; premature infants are those babies born before this time and/or those that are severely underweight.

Babies born later than the thirty-eighth week of pregnancy and before the forty-second are known as term or full-term infants, and birth anywhere during this month is within the window of normal gestation. By definition, babies born before the thirty-eighth week are called preterm or premature infants. (Babies born beyond the forty-second week are post-term infants.) It is common practice to call newborns weighing under 5.5 pounds premature as well. While it is possible to have a newborn who is both full-term and premature (under 5.5 pounds), it is much more important to recognize that both measures, time and weight, are indices of risk. The less of either, the greater the risk.

Every pregnancy carries risk, every birth carries risk, and both carry risk to infant and mother. Preterm and premature infants, however, are at high risk. They have both a lower survival rate and more medical complications with potential lifelong effects than term babies. In the United States, there are 250,000

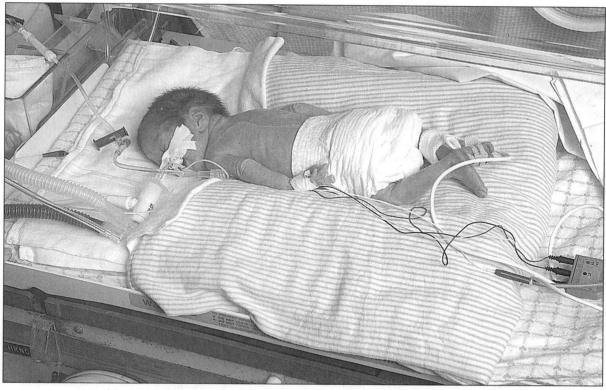

A premature infant in a neonatal intensive care unit. (SIU School of Medicine)

preterm births per year. These infants make up the majority of the 300,000 to 350,000 low-weight births that occur annually.

Developmental prematurity and survivability. Prior to twenty-four weeks of gestation, fetuses are not considered to have developed sufficiently to live outside the womb. Somewhere between twenty-four and twenty-eight weeks of gestation, however, the fetus does become viable, although any baby born between twenty-four and thirty weeks is called very premature. Very premature babies comprise about 1 percent of all live births in the United States (between 35,000 and 39,000 per year). The lengths of these infants range from 11 inches to 18 inches, and weights can range from 1 pound, 5 ounces to almost 4 pounds. At this stage of development, a few ounces more or less make a big difference in the baby's ability to survive. Neonates at 2 pounds have little better than a one in two chance of survival; infants at 3.5 pounds have better than a nine in ten chance.

Babies born between thirty-one and thirty-six weeks of gestation are moderately premature and make up between 4 and 6 percent (150,000 to 200,000) of live births in the United States each year. These babies do well, with a 90 to 98 percent survival rate, and weigh from a little more than 3 to almost 4.5 pounds. Typical lengths range from 16 to 19 inches.

Parents who expect their very premature baby who reaches five to nine weeks of age to resemble a moderately premature baby born at thirty-five weeks will be disappointed. The very premature still appear much less like babies, are significantly lighter, and remain behind developmentally. They are often unready to be bottle-fed or breast-fed or to sleep in an open crib, and they are always less alert and have less behavioral control than the moderately premature. Simply reaching the same number of chronological weeks as moderately premature babies does not negate the substantial differences in their developmental beginnings.

Borderline premature infants are born during weeks thirty-seven or thirty-eight and constitute 16 to 20 percent (600,000 to 700,000) of all live births in the United States. These babies are much like full-term newborns: They have almost the identical survival rate (98 percent) and approach average weights. Nevertheless, they are still at greater risk for respiratory distress syndromes, jaundice, unstable body temperatures, and a variety of problems associated with feeding.

The causes of prematurity and preterm births. Although many conditions result in premature birth, not all causes are known. Some well-known causes include toxemia in the mother (a multistage disease which begins with high blood pressure and rapid fluid retention and may progress to brain hemorrhage, seizure, and coma), placenta previa (when the placenta implants in the lower uterus), placenta abruptio (when a normally positioned placenta detaches from the uterus), premature membrane rupture (when the tissue containing the amniotic fluid tears or leaks before labor begins), incompetent cervix (when the cervix opens mid-pregnancy), and multiple births (twins, triplets, and so on).

Some mothers blame themselves for the premature births of their infants. While it is natural to look for a cause and a target to vent the often-powerful feelings associated with prematurity, it is the rare mother who deliberately causes her baby to be born earlier than necessary. While some factors in the mother—such as high blood pressure, diabetes mellitus, sickle-cell

In the News: The Needs of Premature Infants as They Grow Up

Remarkable advances in neonatal intensive care and technology have improved the survival rate of prematurely born infants. However, the long-term consequences of premature birth are still unclear. The immature brain is at increased risk from bleeding or lack of oxygen. Researchers have found that adolescents who were born prematurely show an increase in thinking and behavioral problems and more than half have abnormal magnetic resonance imaging (MRI) scans. Although early childhood interventions can have compensatory influences on development, they have little influence on structural deficits. Preterm infants are at a greater risk of global cognitive processing deficits. When they become teenagers, they remain at substantial cognitive and educational disadvantage and have a lower global intelligence quotient (IQ), visual short-term memory, and fine and gross motor functioning as compared with peers.

Language problems are compounded by poor-quality speech and grammatical construction. Even allowing for an IQ difference, scores of reading comprehension and mathematics remain lower, with the greatest difficulties in completing nonverbal tasks. Unusual behaviors may be part of a complex of nonverbal learning disabilities such as visual-spatial and visual-motor problems. The gap between prematurely born children and their peers is likely to widen in high school as schoolwork demands increase. In the classroom, underlying learning disabilities are evidently compounded by intrinsic attention and behavior differences which also hinder academic achievement.

Neonatal risk factors have greater effect on neuropsychological outcomes than social risks. Important predictors of cognitive outcomes are the number of days a preterm baby is ventilated, motor skills at age six years, and head circumference at twelve years. Research into therapies to prevent or treat neonatal complications of prematurity rather than early intervention strategies after discharge will probably have the greatest impact on improving the future outcomes of this high-risk population. An important therapeutic innovation is antenatal corticosteroid therapy, which has been associated with improved outcomes in growth and cognitive function at fourteen years of age.

Fortunately, prematurely born adolescents who escape major neurodevelopmental disability experience "catch up" growth and have age-appropriate sexual maturation. While the needs for special education remain high, few children have impairments severe enough to curtail activities of daily living. Researchers indicate good quality of life for the majority of adolescent and young preterm children—even for those with disabilities. Longitudinal studies showed that a large number of premature children who required special education because of cognitive, learning, and behavioral problems had still been able to attend mainstream secondary education and engage in regular work. Some of the small cognitive deficits observed in preadolescent children may disappear during adolescence.

—Paul Moglia, Ph.D.,
and Krishna Bhaskarabhatla, M.D., M.Sc.

disease, and kidney diseases—can contribute to prematurity, these are not volitional conditions and the mother is not at moral fault in any way. She did not will these conditions, and she did not intend for her baby to be born prematurely. In fact, some causes do not involve the mothers at all, but the babies themselves, including congenital defects, intrauterine illnesses, and defective placentas.

The vast majority of women will never deliver prematurely. Those who do, however, run a 25 to 50 percent chance of having a second premature birth. In the rush to understand and find answers to prematurity, it is important not to overinvest in probability statistics and comparative risk factor data which include race (for example, African Americans have a higher prematurity rate than whites), paternity (for example, a few individual males seem to father premature babies even with different mothers without risk factors themselves), the mother's age, and even her mother's exposure to biochemicals (such as diethylstilbestrol, or DES). It is extremely important to realize that many women who are formally classified as high-risk mothers have normal deliveries of full-term babies, and that others, who are healthy and without known risk factors, deliver premature, preterm babies.

The psychological impact. There may be no event with a greater impact on a person's life than becoming a parent, and few events in a parent's life equal the impact of seeing one's tiny, struggling, helpless, and high-risk baby. It is common for parents to have been forewarned of the baby's chances, especially if the infant is very premature. They may, in fact, have begun to prepare themselves psychologically for the death of their baby even as the baby clings to life outside the womb. They may try to protect themselves from bonding to one whose death may be imminent. Parents who expected a bundle of joy can fear that even if their baby lives, he or she will be handicapped, sickly, malformed, and never able to live a life as an independent, functioning, and happy adult.

Parents sometimes confess to not knowing whether they want their baby to live or die, and they feel guilt for not knowing. Their distress, confusion, and contradictory feelings can overwhelm them. Their babies may not look much like the babies they had pictured or prepared for, and they may not feel much like parents. Premature birth can be a crisis rarely equaled in a parent's life.

Some couples react and adapt successfully, while others do not. Nearly all parents of premature infants experience various forms of shock, denial, anger, guilt, and depression. Researchers who study and compare parents who cope better and worse have learned that those parents who accept and express their whole range of emotions (versus only the emotions that they believe they are supposed to have), who seek further information, who accept help in their caring for the babies, and who begin to develop an early relationship with their babies adapt to the crisis well and successfully.

Premature infants were thought, at one time, to be inactive, unaware, and inert. Research and anecdotal observation strongly support the view that these infants are acutely sensitive to their environment, though they usually respond in ways too subtle to be perceived casually. When parents are present, even on the outside of the incubator wall, their babies behave differently, tolerate feedings better, and heal more quickly and completely.

—*Paul Moglia, Ph.D.*

See also Birth defects; Childbirth; Childbirth complications; Multiple births; Postpartum depression; Pregnancy and gestation; Stillbirth.

FOR FURTHER INFORMATION:

Avery, Mary E., and Georgia Litwack. *Born Early.* Boston: Little, Brown, 1983. Presents a case study of a premature birth and the consequent medical challenges. Includes bibliographical references.

Curtis, Glade B. *Your Pregnancy Week-by-Week.* 4th ed. Tucson, Ariz.: Fisher Books, 2000. In this book, Curtis has written a clear, easy to follow guidebook. The tone of the book is informative, chatty, and reassuring. An extensive, excellent glossary adds value. It is especially ideal for very young pregnant women seeking to better understand the changes in their bodies.

Harrison, Helen, and Ann Kositsky. *The Premature Baby Book: A Parents' Guide to Coping and Caring in the First Years.* New York: St. Martin's Press, 1983. This supportive and comprehensive guide helps parents of premature babies deal with the emotional, medical, and practical issues they face. Includes medical information, practical advice, and personal accounts.

Hotchner, Tracie. *Pregnancy and Childbirth.* Rev. ed. New York: Avon Books, 1997. This very readable book addresses a wide range of topics: the physical and psychological changes to mother and fetus; complications; prenatal testing; choosing an obstetrician, midwife, and hospital; labor and delivery; and new baby care.

Hynan, Michael. *The Pain of Premature Parents: A Psychological Guide for Coping.* Lanham, Md.: University Press of America, 1987. This guide is designed to help parents emotionally adjust to having a premature baby. Describes the crises caused by a premature birth, medical complications, and the extended hospitalization of both mothers and babies. The book also details the normal but painful emotional reactions to prematurity, including panic, guilt, anticipatory grief, frustration, depression, and anger.

Pfister, Fred, and Bernard Griesemer. *The Littlest Baby: A Handbook for Parents of Premature Children.* Englewood Cliffs, N.J.: Prentice Hall, 1983. A concise source for information on premature infants, designed for the lay reader. Includes an index.

PREMENSTRUAL SYNDROME (PMS)
DISEASE/DISORDER

ANATOMY OR SYSTEM AFFECTED: Gastrointestinal system, nervous system, reproductive system, skin
SPECIALTIES AND RELATED FIELDS: Gynecology
DEFINITION: PMS (also known as premenstrual tension) is a common condition in some women involving mental tension, irritability, headache, depression, and bloating that begins in the week prior to menstruation and often resolves completely the day after the period starts. Premenstrual syndrome is caused by hormonal fluctuations that induce increased levels of prostaglandin and sodium retention in the bloodstream, resulting in edema in the body tissues. Psychogenic reaction to physical changes in the body plays a large part in initiating behavioral responses. Emotional stress caused by PMS may be severe enough to disrupt a woman's life. Regular, vigorous exercise is known to decrease symptoms.

—*Jason Georges and Tracy Irons-Georges*
See also Gynecology; Hormones; Menstruation; Stress; Stress reduction.

FOR FURTHER INFORMATION:

Dalton, Katharina, and Wendy Holton. *Once a Month: Understanding and Treating PMS.* 6th ed. Alameda, Calif.: Hunter House, 1999.

Golub, Sharon. *Periods: From Menarche to Menopause.* Newbury Park, Calif.: Sage, 1992.

Harrison, Michelle, and Marla Ahlgrimm. *Self-help for Premenstrual Syndrome.* 3d ed. New York: Random House, 1998.

PREVENTIVE MEDICINE
SPECIALTY

ANATOMY OR SYSTEM AFFECTED: All
SPECIALTIES AND RELATED FIELDS: All
DEFINITION: The medical field that seeks to protect, promote, and maintain the health and well-being of individuals and defined populations and to prevent disease, disability, and premature death.
KEY TERMS:

aerospace medicine: the medical specialty concerned with the health of the operating crews and passengers of air and space vehicles, together with support personnel

environmental medicine: the branch of medical science that addresses the impact of chemical and physical stressors and biological hazards on the individual or group in a community

epidemiology: the study of the distribution and dynamics of disease in populations; considers such attributes as gender, age, race, occupation, and social factors and such characteristics of disease as incubation, infectivity, chronicity, and risk factors

incidence: the number of new illnesses or events occurring over a specified period of time among a specific population

occupational medicine: a medical specialty focused on providing all levels of preventive medical services to working men and women in order to preserve, maintain, or restore health and well-being

prevalence: the number of individuals at a particular time who have a disease or a given characteristic

public health: the well-being of humankind, both as a community and as individuals, accomplished by using scientific skills and beliefs that assist in health maintenance and health improvement

risk factors: the situations, circumstances, or conditions that increase the probability of the occurrence of disease or accident

SCIENCE AND PROFESSION

Modern preventive medicine is considered to exist at three levels within the health care community. The initial level, primary prevention, has as its purpose to maintain health by removing the causes of or by protecting the community or individual from agents of disease and injury. These activities are no longer limited to the prevention of infection; they now include improvement in the environment and behavioral changes to reduce risk factors that contribute to chronic disease and injury. An example of primary prevention is immunization programs for children. To reduce the risk of heart attack, one should refrain from smoking, be active, and reduce fat intake—all wise primary prevention actions. Halting the loss of atmospheric ozone, reducing air and water pollution, and developing environmentally friendly technologies form another class of prevention actions.

Secondary prevention seeks to detect and correct adverse health conditions before they become manifest as disease, by reversing, halting, or retarding the disease process. A frequently used secondary prevention technique is health screening. Examples include hypertension (high blood pressure), diabetes, prostate cancer, and glaucoma screening services. In industry, a hearing test is used as a tool to prevent noise-induced hearing loss among the workforce. Once a potential health problem is identified, clinical preventive medicine techniques can be instituted to reverse the condition or prevent further progression.

Tertiary prevention attempts to minimize the adverse effects of disease and disability. Coronary bypass surgery, vocational rehabilitation, and treatment of an incapacitating mental illness are examples.

Specialists in the field of preventive medicine typically focus their efforts within the paradigms of primary and secondary prevention. In epidemiological terms, primary prevention results in a reduction of the incidence of a disease (the new cases occurring over time). Secondary prevention, on the other hand, results in a reduction of the prevalence of a disease (the number of people suffering from a particular illness at a given point in time).

Most physicians provide some degree of preventive medicine services. Pediatricians are practicing preventive medicine when they conduct "well-baby evaluations" and ensure that immunizations are current. Family medicine specialists are providing such services when they perform Pap smears or order mammograms. When the cessation of smoking is discussed and internists prescribe nicotine patch regimens, that too is preventive medicine.

In the United States, approximately one thousand physicians specialize in general preventive medicine. Some use epidemiological methods to design and develop prevention programs that may feature a single intervention or may constitute a strategy which in-

cludes a multitude or matrix of screening technologies and interventions. Other preventive medicine specialists provide services in a clinical setting by ordering a history and physical examination, which may include age- and gender-specific screening tests. The clinical preventive medicine specialist then can counsel the patient on lifestyle alterations recommended to preserve or improve health.

Within the United States, another field of the specialty of preventive medicine is occupational medicine. Practicing in industry or private clinic settings, these specialists are concerned about preventing injury and illness as a result of the physical, biological, and chemical hazards that are present in the workplace. Should workers be injured or made ill as a result of their employment, the occupational medicine physician manages their treatment, rehabilitation, and return to work.

Aerospace medicine physicians limit their practice to those involved in the aeronautical and space transportation fields, including flight crews, support personnel, and passengers. The major task of these physicians is to protect this population group from the adverse environmental conditions of flight, including pressure changes, reduced availability of oxygen, thermal stressors, accelerative forces, and psychosocial factors that might compromise performance.

DIAGNOSTIC AND TREATMENT TECHNIQUES

An example of the application of preventive medicine is a comparison of the leading causes of death in the United States in 1900 with those in 1998. The table on the following page lists the ten leading causes of death in order of greater to lesser numbers for those two years. It only takes a quick glance to realize that there has been a major shift from deaths attributable to infectious disease at the beginning of the twentieth century to deaths attributable to chronic diseases that are often a reflection of individual lifestyle. Preventive medicine has clearly proven itself effective in altering both the cause of death and the age at which death occurs. Accompanying this increased shift to chronic diseases such as cancer and heart disease, moreover, is a significant increase in the life expectancy of the population during the same century. Preventive medicine's focus is now on reducing morbidity and mortality from chronic diseases and accidents, particularly those in which an individual's lifestyle increases the risk for illness and death.

Disease prevention and health promotion are the

Leading Causes of Death in the United States

1900	1998
1. Pneumonia and influenza	1. Heart diseases
2. Tuberculosis	2. Cancer and other malignant tumors
3. Diarrhea, enteritis, and ulceration of the intestine	3. Strokes
4. Heart diseases	4. Chronic obstructive pulmonary diseases
5. Senility (ill-defined or unknown)	5. Accidents
6. Strokes	6. Pneumonia and influenza
7. Nephritis	7. Diabetes mellitus
8. Accidents	8. Suicide
9. Cancer and other malignant tumors	9. Kidney disease
10. Diphtheria	10. Chronic liver disease and cirrhosis

two pillars supporting the discipline of preventive medicine. Beginning in 1987, a consortium was convened to begin to address a preventive medicine strategy to improve the health of Americans. The Institute of Medicine of the National Academy of Sciences worked with the United States Public Health Service and numerous organizations to formulate health objective goals that could be attainable by the beginning of the twenty-first century. Once goals and objectives were established, the next task was to devise methods, technologies, and strategies to achieve the objectives by the year 2000. The resulting report was entitled *Healthy People 2000: National Health Promotion and Disease Prevention Objectives* (1991).

The implementation of what was then known about disease prevention and health promotion was the central challenge. Good health is the result of reducing needless disease, injury, and suffering, resulting in an improved quality of life. A strategy of *Healthy People 2000* was to combine scientific knowledge, professional skills, community support, individual commitment, and the public will to achieve good health. This plan required reducing premature death, preventing disability, preserving the physical environment, and enabling Americans to develop healthy lifestyles. Three broad goals were detailed in *Healthy People 2000*: first, increase the healthy life span for Ameri-

cans; second, reduce health disparity among Americans; and third, achieve access to preventive services for all Americans. A number of examples of the types of programs required to attain these goals were provided.

Tobacco use is the most important single preventable cause of death in the United States, accounting for one of every six deaths, or approximately 390,000 deaths annually. This loss of life is the equivalent of crashing two passenger-filled commercial jumbo jet airliners every day throughout the year. Smoking is a major risk factor for heart and lung disease; cancer of many organs, including the lungs, pancreas, and bladder; and stomach ulcers. Passive or environmental tobacco smoke is a recognized cause of cancer for exposed nonsmokers, and children in smoke-filled homes experience more ear infections. Tobacco use during pregnancy increases the risk of prematurity and low birth weight.

The objectives were to reduce tobacco use by the year 2000 to no more than 15 percent of adults (a 48 percent reduction) and to reduce initiation of smoking to no more than 15 percent by age twenty (a 50 percent reduction).

Among the 120 million people in the United States workforce, it is estimated that 10 million injuries occur annually; one-third are severe, and 10,000 deaths result. The occupations with the highest injury rates include mining, construction, agriculture, and transportation. The prevention of occupational disease and injury requires engineering controls, improved work practices, use of physical protective equipment, and monitoring of the work environment to identify emerging chemical and physical hazards. The objectives to improve occupational safety and health by the year 2000 included reducing work-related deaths to no more than 4 per 100,000 workers (a 33 percent decrease) and reducing work-related injuries to fewer than 6 per 100 workers (a 22 percent decrease).

In the United States, every fifth death is caused by cancer. Nearly one in three Americans will experience a form of this disease. Research has helped to identify many risk factors related to cancer causation, such as tobacco use, low fiber intake, excess fat intake, sunburn, alcohol use, and exposure to chemical carcinogens. Information, education, and early detection have important roles in reducing both the incidence and the prevalence of cancer. Pap smears, prostate examinations, mammography, and oral examinations are secondary prevention procedures that allow for early diagnosis and treatment. Such screening procedures, coupled with education and lifestyle changes, have the potential to reduce cancer rates significantly. To improve cancer prevention and control by the year 2000, the objectives included reversing the cancer death rate to no more than 130 per 100,000 people, increasing breast examinations and mammography at two-year intervals to at least 60 percent of women aged fifty and over (a 140 percent increase), and increasing Pap smears at one- to three-year intervals to at least 85 percent (a 13 percent increase).

Achieving the many objectives of *Healthy People 2000* would require the dedicated commitment of preventive medicine specialists and the broader medical community. Enhanced effectiveness and efficiency of clinical preventive services, screening procedures, immunizations, consultation, and counseling can be achieved only through close relationships between the physician and both the community and the individual. In order to assess whether the goals and objectives for the prevention of disease and health promotion for the year 2000 were realistic, it would be helpful to review a success in the application of preventive medicine. In the decade leading to 1988, there was a 33 percent reduction in the death rate from heart attacks when adjusted for the difference in the age of the population. One might think that this decrease is attributable

to improvements in coronary bypass surgery or to the development of new cardiovascular medications. The true explanation, however, lies with the adoption of more healthful living habits as a result of health education and preventive medicine interventions.

Coronary artery disease and its resultant heart attacks are preventable. A large national clinical trial of preventive medicine procedures known as MRFIT (multiple risk factor intervention trial) not only demonstrated the value of risk factor reduction in preventing disease but also demonstrated that the impact of established disease could be reversed. A subgroup of the MRFIT population made up of those who had established coronary artery disease at the start of the study had 55 percent fewer fatalities than did the control group when both were followed over seven years.

Preventive medicine interventions are not only cost-effective but relatively inexpensive as well. For example, coronary artery bypass surgery or a heart transplant costs many times more than preventive medicine rehabilitation and lifestyle modification programs. The same advantages also accrue for the prevention of strokes. Reducing salt intake, controlling high blood pressure, correcting obesity, performing regular exercise, and quitting smoking reduce the risk factors for stroke. The evidence clearly shows that preventive medicine reduces the death rate for heart attack and stroke and enhances quality of life.

Clinical preventive services have been designed based on the best available scientific evidence to promote the health of the individual while remaining practical and cost-effective. The publication of the *Guide to Clinical Preventive Services* (1989), by the U.S. Preventive Services Task Force, was a major milestone on the road toward reducing premature death and disability. It has been well established that the majority of deaths among Americans under the age of sixty-five are preventable. The guide is the culmination of more than four years of literature review, debate, and synthesis and provides a listing of the clinical preventive services that clinicians should provide their patients. More than one hundred interventions are proposed to prevent sixty different illnesses and medical conditions. The guide is intended to be used by preventive medical specialists and other primary care clinicians. The recommendations are based on a standardized review of current scientific evidence and include a summary of published clinical research regarding the clinical effectiveness of each preventive service.

Although there have been sound clinical reasons for emphasizing prevention in medicine, studies have repeatedly demonstrated that physicians often fail to provide these services. Busy clinicians frequently have inadequate time with the patient to recommend or deliver a range of preventive services. Furthermore, until the publication of this guide, considerable controversy had existed within the medical community as to which services should be offered and how often. In the past, there was skepticism regarding the value of certain preventive interventions and their ability to reduce morbidity or mortality significantly. One result of this review process has been the clear evidence that reducing the incidence and severity of the leading causes of disease and disability is dependent on the personal health practices of individuals.

The periodic health examination was once frequently referred to as an annual examination. The *Guide to Clinical Preventive Services* tailors this examination to the individual needs of the patient and considers factors such as age, gender, and risk. Consequently, a uniform health examination is not recommended. The examination for those between forty and sixty-four years of age is scheduled on a one- to three-year basis, with the more frequent examinations scheduled for those in high-risk groups. Although the examination is not comprehensive, it is focused on identifying the leading causes of illness and disability among people in this age group. During the physical examination, particular attention would be paid to the skin of those individuals at high risk for excessive exposure to sunlight or with a family or personal history of skin cancer. A complete oral cavity examination would be appropriate for individuals abusing tobacco or consuming excessive amounts of alcohol. Counseling would be provided on such items as diet and exercise, substance abuse, sexual practices, and injury prevention. For some women, discussion is recommended regarding estrogen replacement therapy. In discussing patient education and counseling it is wise to remember a comment made by bacteriologist René DuBos: "To ward off disease or recover health, men as a rule find it easier to depend on the healers than to attempt the more difficult task of living wisely."

Approximately 11 million persons in the United States suffer from diabetes mellitus; however, 5 million of them are unaware of their condition. Diabetes is the seventh leading cause of death in the United States, accounting for more than 130,000 deaths per year. In addition, it is the leading cause of kidney failure, blindness, and amputations. The detection of diabetes in asymptomatic persons provides an opportunity to prevent or delay the progress of the disease and its complications.

The *Guide to Clinical Preventive Services* recommends an oral glucose tolerance test for all pregnant women between the twenty-fourth and twenty-eighth weeks of their pregnancy. Routine screening for diabetes in asymptomatic nonpregnant adults, using blood or urine tests, is not recommended. Periodic fasting blood-sugar measurements may be appropriate in persons at high risk for diabetes mellitus, such as the markedly obese, persons with a family history of diabetes, or women with a history of diabetes during pregnancy.

PERSPECTIVE AND PROSPECTS

In the mid-1800's, John Snow provided one of the best examples of preventive medicine by applying what could be called observational epidemiology. During a rather severe cholera epidemic in London, Snow observed an unusual pattern of disease which appeared to be dependent on the particular water supply company providing water to the neighborhood. Recognizing that there was a high incidence of cholera in the Broad Street area, he was able to determine that most of the disease was associated with those families depending on the Broad Street pump for their drinking water. It has been said that he simply removed the handle on the pump and was able to control the epidemic in that area. His discovery occurred before there was a clear understanding of the relationship of bacteria or germs to infectious disease.

Another historic example of the application of preventive medicine was the control of smallpox. In the late eighteenth century, Edward Jenner observed that the milkmaids in the English countryside were not scarred by the scourge of smallpox. On further examination, he determined that these young women had years earlier been infected with cowpox and thus had been spared the more serious smallpox infection. He then advocated intentional infection with the cowpox vaccine. Years later, using this preventive medicine application, the World Health Organization was able to institute a worldwide eradication of smallpox. The last case of smallpox reported in the world was in October, 1977, marking the first time that a major human disease had been eradicated.

Neither the control of cholera in London by Snow nor the eradication of smallpox resulted from medical or surgical treatment of a disease. These results were obtained because of the application of the principles of preventive medicine and public health.

—*Roy L. DeHart, M.D., M.P.H.*

See also Acupressure; Acupuncture; Aging: Extended care; Allied health; Alternative medicine; Aromatherapy; Biofeedback; Cardiac rehabilitation; Cardiology; Centers for Disease Control and Prevention (CDC); Chiropractic; Cholesterol; Chronobiology; Colon therapy; Disease; Electrocardiography (ECG or EKG); Environmental health; Exercise physiology; Family practice; Genetic counseling; Genetics and inheritance; Geriatrics and gerontology; Holistic medicine; Homeopathy; Host-defense mechanisms; Hypercholesterolemia; Immune system; Immunization and vaccination; Immunology; Mammography; Meditation; Melatonin; National Institutes of Health (NIH); Noninvasive tests; Nursing; Nutrition; Occupational health; Osteopathic medicine; Pharmacology; Pharmacy; Physical examination; Physician assistants; Preventive medicine; Psychiatry; Psychiatry, child and adolescent; Psychiatry, geriatric; Qi gong; Screening; Self-medication; Serology; Spine, vertebrae, and disks; Sports medicine; Stress reduction; Tai Chi Chuan; Tropical medicine; Yoga.

FOR FURTHER INFORMATION:

Greenberg, Raymond S., et al. *Medical Epidemiology.* 3d ed. Norwalk, Conn.: Appleton and Lange, 2000. This small study guide will assist the reader in understanding the key concepts of epidemiology. The overview and specific topics create a firm foundation for understanding this important discipline.

Halperin, William, and Edward L. Baker. *Public Health Surveillance.* New York: Van Nostrand Reinhold, 1992. This compact text addresses health surveillance in a wide variety of settings, from the community to the physician's office to the work setting. Provides the medical rationale for establishing and performing health surveillance programs.

Last, John M., and Robert B. Wallace, eds. *Maxcy-Rosenau-Last Public Health and Preventive Medicine.* 13th ed. Norwalk, Conn.: Appleton and Lange, 1992. This textbook enjoys wide use by most preventive medicine training programs in the United States. It provides excellent coverage of all the principles and most of the related topics of preventive medicine. The layperson will find many chapters accessible, although some will require attention and study.

U.S. Department of Health and Human Services. *Healthy People 2000: National Health Promotion and Disease Prevention Objectives.* Washington, D.C.: Government Printing Office, 1991. This book documents the goals, objectives, and strategies for national health promotion and disease prevention. It is an excellent source of data and material related to the United States' health status.

PRION DISEASES
DISEASE/DISORDER

ANATOMY OR SYSTEM AFFECTED: Brain, nervous system

SPECIALTIES AND RELATED FIELDS: Epidemiology, neurology, pathology, and public health

DEFINITION: A variety of fatal neurological illnesses, inherited or transmissible, that are associated with abnormalities in proteins, called prions.

KEY TERMS:

ataxia: the inability to control muscle movements

bovine spongiform encephalopathy (BSE): a prion disease of cattle; also called mad cow disease

Creutzfeldt-Jakob disease (CJD): a human prion disease found worldwide

dementia: the loss of intellectual ability

encephalopathy: any abnormality in the structure or function of the brain

knockout mouse: mouse in which a specific gene has been inactivated or "knocked out"

kuru: a human prion disease formerly found in Papua New Guinea

prion: a protein that can assume an abnormal conformation, aggregate, and disrupt brain function

spongiform: shaped like or resembling a sponge

CAUSES AND SYMPTOMS

Prion diseases are neurological disorders in humans and animals that are associated with abnormalities in proteinaceous molecules called prions. When prions aggregate, they eventually cause spongelike lesions in the brain and disrupt brain function. The resultant illnesses are referred to as spongiform encephalopathies, which can be either inherited or transmissible and are uniformly fatal. Prions are found in all species from yeast to humans, but their normal role is not known. Their evolutionary persistence in so many species implies that they must serve an important purpose, although knockout mice lacking prions do not appear to be deleteriously affected.

Inherited spongiform encephalopathies are primarily attributed to mutations in the prion gene, leading to abnormal prions that adopt an unusual conformation and aggregate over time to cause the brain pathology and neurological symptoms characteristic of the diseases. Transmissible diseases occur when a susceptible animal is inoculated with a fragment or an extract of diseased tissue; inoculation is most effective when insertion is made directly into the brain, although it can occur via intravenous administration and, much less efficiently, oral ingestion. The infectious agent seems to be the abnormal prion itself, which apparently recruits normal prions in the brain to adopt the abnormal conformation, leading to their aggregation and disruption of brain function. This is an unorthodox etiology, in that the infectious agent appears to be devoid of nucleic acid (RNA or DNA); its mode of action is not fully understood, nor is what is understood universally accepted.

These diseases have been described in humans, cattle, sheep, deer, elk, mink, domestic cats, and wild felines, as well as, experimentally, in monkeys, hamsters, and mice. They are usually species-specific. However, the diseases in mink, domestic cats, and wild felines are attributed to consumption of feed derived from diseased ungulates, and a new variant in humans is associated with the consumption of meat from cattle with bovine spongiform encephalopathy (BSE), or mad cow disease.

The most common animal prion disease is scrapie, found in sheep and goats. It is named for the intense itching that causes sheep to rub against hard objects, scraping off the wool. It also causes staggering, tremors, and blindness. It has been known for more than 250 years in Britain and other countries of western Europe. It has been reported in most sheep-raising countries with a few notable exceptions, such as Australia and New Zealand. It first appears at two to five years of age, can last over six months and is eventually fatal. It is generally accepted that it is an infectious disease in which genetics also plays an important role. It has not been shown to be transmissible to humans and poses no risk to human health.

The most famous prion disease in animals is BSE, better known as mad cow disease. First noted in British cattle in 1986, it causes nervousness, aggression, and symptoms similar to scrapie. It appears in adult cattle between two and eight years of age and is fatal. The BSE epidemic, which peaked in 1992, and affected more than 200,000 animals, was apparently caused by feed containing protein from animals with prion disease. A ban on incorporating ruminant-derived protein into cattle feed appeared to be bringing the epidemic to an end in Great Britain as of 2000, although there was a troubling increase in cases in continental Europe.

The best-known prion disease in humans is Creutzfeldt-Jakob disease (CJD), which occurs worldwide at a rate of one per million persons. Its symptoms include dementia and ataxia, leading to death. The disease may be sporadic, inherited, or infectious, or a new variant. The sporadic form, which accounts for 85 percent of the cases, appears in the elderly and has an unknown etiology. The inherited form (15 percent of the cases) is primarily attributed to mutations in the gene for prions, making them more susceptible to aggregation in the brains of affected individuals. The infectious form can be caused by tissue transplants, contaminated surgical instruments, and pharmaceuticals derived from human cadavers. Kuru is an infectious form of the disease, which existed among the Fore people on the island of Papua New Guinea. It was likely spread by ritual cannibalism of deceased relatives, which is no longer practiced. The primary symptoms of kuru were ataxia and tremors, ending in death. A new variant form of CJD was first described in 1996; it differed from the sporadic form by affecting younger individuals and having slightly different symptoms and time course; it has been associated with eating beef from cattle infected with BSE. As of 2000, a cumulative total of eighty such cases had been identified in Great Britain. Because of a long time course and an incompletely known etiology, it is uncertain how many will be affected by this new variant form.

TREATMENT AND THERAPY

No effective treatment for prion diseases existed at the beginning of the twenty-first century. Researchers have speculated that human prion diseases might be treated by preventing the normal prion molecules from adopting the abnormal conformation, aggregating and disrupting brain activity. Another option would be the development of antigene therapy to block the production of normal prions, provided that they truly serve no useful function in humans.

PERSPECTIVE AND PROSPECTS

While the symptoms of scrapie have been noted in sheep and goats for hundreds of years, it was only shown to be transmissible in the 1930's. Creutzfeldt-Jakob disease was first noted in the 1920's, kuru in the 1950's, and BSE or mad cow disease in the mid-1980's. Daniel Carleton Gajdusek began studying kuru in 1955 and won the Nobel Prize in Physiology or Medicine in 1976. Stanley B. Prusiner coined the term "prion" in 1982; he was awarded the Nobel Prize in 1997. In 2000, many scientists were persuaded that prions were the sole cause for transmissible spongiform encephalopathies. Others, in view of unknown aspects in their pathogenesis, suspected that an undetected virus was also involved.

—James L. Robinson, Ph.D.

See also Brain; Brain disorders; Creutzfeldt-Jakob disease and mad cow disease; Food poisoning; Mutation.

FOR FURTHER INFORMATION:

Council for Agricultural Science and Technology. *Transmissible Spongiform Encephalopathies in the United States.* Ames, Iowa: Author, 2000.

Ferry, Georgina. "Mad Brains and the Prion Heresy." *New Scientist* 142, no. 1927 (May 28, 1994): 32-36.

Prusiner, Stanley B. "The Prion Diseases." *Scientific American* 272, no. 1 (January, 1995): 48-57.

_____, ed. *Prion Biology and Diseases.* New York: Cold Spring Harbor Laboratory Press, 1999.

PROCTOLOGY

SPECIALTY

ANATOMY OR SYSTEM AFFECTED: Gastrointestinal system, intestines

SPECIALTIES AND RELATED FIELDS: Gastroenterology, internal medicine, oncology

DEFINITION: The branch of medicine that treats diseases of the colon, rectum, and anus.

KEY TERMS:

anal incontinence: the inability to control defecation

colitis: inflammation of the mucous membranes of the colon

diverticulum: a pouchlike, weakened region of the colon wall which can cause pain and bleeding

endoscope: a lighted, flexible, hollow instrument used for examination and the placement of surgical instruments

fascia: connective tissues such as tendons and ligaments

hemorrhoids: dilated blood vessels in the anus or rectum that are itchy and painful

occult blood: fecal blood, as detected by microscopic or chemical testing

polyp: a tumorlike growth, such as of the colorectal mucous lining

rectal prolapse: the protrusion of the rectum through the anus

SCIENCE AND PROFESSION

The term "proctology" arises from the Greek *proktos,* meaning "anus." In 1961, this field was renamed colon and rectal surgery. The original term, which is still in wide use, will be employed for simplicity. Specialists in proctology are surgeons who are expert in surgery of the colon, rectum, anal canal, and perianal area near the anus. They also carry out surgery of other tissues and organs close to and involved in serious colorectal disease. Moreover, proctologists have special skill in endoscopy of the rectum and colon for the diagnosis and medical treatment of these regions. Proctology involves emergency situations less frequently than many other specialties. Consequently, the hours of these specialists are relatively regular, although no shorter than those of other physicians.

Many conditions encountered by proctologists are clear-cut in diagnosis and treatment. Hence, they often have the satisfaction of providing patients with quick, effective relief of serious pain and discomfort.

Training a proctologist is time-consuming, involving a five-year residency in general surgery, followed by a one- to two-year fellowship in colon and rectal surgery. The specialty is not easily entered because its practitioners are not numerous and there are usually several applicants for each open training position.

The main organ treated in proctology is the large intestine, or colon. This portion of the digestive tract starts at the cecum, a pouch joined to the small intestine. At the far end of the cecum, the colon is subdivided into ascending, transverse, and descending regions. Together, these regions absorb water and minerals from food that has not been digested and absorbed by the stomach or small intestine. The result is feces, which are stored in the colon for elimination from the body. The ascending colon extends upward on the right side of the abdominal cavity and is called the right colon. The transverse colon crosses from right to left in the cavity, and the descending colon (left colon) passes downward along the cavity's left side, ending in the rectum. The short, S-shaped portion of the left colon above the rectum is the sigmoid colon.

The entire colon is made of pouches whose complex series of contractions and expansions moves its contents through quite slowly, enabling optimum water and mineral recovery. The sluggish colon movement enables bacteria to thrive, sometimes causing uncomfortable gas. Normal synchronization of the digestive system leads to absorption of most of this gas, however, as well as the transfer of feces into the rectum for storage and a defecation reflex which releases feces at varied but appropriate intervals. Also synchronized with these digestive processes is the production of both mucus and bicarbonate, which help to propel colon contents through the large intestine and neutralize acid made by bacteria in the colon. These events usually prevent damage to the colorectal system or diseases of its components.

The digestive system does not exhibit frequent dysfunction in early life. Therefore, proctologists for the most part see middle-aged or elderly patients. Furthermore, 60 percent of the problems that they encounter are anorectal, and 40 percent are associated with a diseased colon. Conditions that are often treated by proctologists include, but are not restricted to, anal fissures, cancers, colitis, diverticular disease, hemorrhoids, pilonoidal disease, and polyps.

DIAGNOSTIC AND TREATMENT TECHNIQUES

Thorough colorectal examination starts with a medical history to ensure the clarification of potential problems. Then the proctologist checks the perianal region for abnormalities such as dermatitis, abscesses, hemorrhoids, or lesions that may prove to be tumors. This is followed by digital examination with a lubricated glove, after a warning to patients that this procedure will result in the urge to defecate and cause some discomfort. Tissue irregularity, nodules, or tender areas are sought, and the prostate gland in men and the cervix in women are examined. To ensure complete exploration, a fecal sample is obtained and tested for the presence of occult blood. Other clinical tests of colon, rectum, and related tissues, including biopsy, are also carried out as needed.

Anal fissures may be discovered during this portion of the examination. An anal fissure is a linear tear of the lining of the anal canal, usually originating in the anorectal region. These fissures are common causes of acute anal pain, cutting or burning sensa-

tions beginning at defecation and continuing more mildly for several hours. They are thought to arise from trauma to the anal canal caused by large, dry, hard feces. Other causes of anal fissures include persistent diarrhea, inflammatory bowel disease (IBD), syphilis, leukemia, and anorectal cancer. The treatment of choice is the use of fecal softeners, increased fluid intake, and application of steroids. Surgery is usually carried out only for cases in which treated fissures do not heal.

Pilonoidal disease may also be detected; this is the formation of pits that contain pubic hair that has become trapped under the skin. If an abscess results, the problem is handled by its drainage under local anesthesia. Cleaning out of the pit and the removal of causative hair are also useful. Surgery is required only if the problem becomes chronic.

Anorectal cancers are relatively uncommon. They are treated in an individualized fashion with a varying combination of surgery, chemotherapy, and radiation therapy. Often, they are squamous cell carcinomas. In a smaller number of cases, melanomas, for which the survival rate is less than 5 percent, will occur. Other types of serious anorectal cancers include Paget's disease and basal cell carcinomas. These cancers have better survival rates.

Rectal prolapse, passage of the rectum through the anus, is another common anorectal problem. It is seen either in children under the age of two years or in the very elderly. In childhood, the problem is frequently attributable to anatomic underdevelopment, which cures itself. In adults, rectal prolapse may be partial or complete. Complete rectal prolapse results in the externalization of the entire rectum, bleeding, and excessive mucus discharge.

Rectal prolapse eventually causes anal incontinence, which may become irreversible. For cases in which a patient is feeble, the rectum is first manipulated to return it to a more normal placement. Then, a tightening steel or plastic loop is inserted under the skin at the anal opening to prevent future prolapse. When patients are robust enough for surgery, the rectum is often secured internally by a mesh sling anchored to internal fascia.

The treatment of internal or external hemorrhoids is another major aspect of proctological practice. Internal hemorrhoids are rarely painful because they are covered by insensitive colon mucosa tissue. The external variety, however, are rich in nervous tissue and may be very painful. Internal hemorrhoids are classified into four stages ranging from the relatively innocuous first-degree hemorrhoids, which do not prolapse, to fourth-degree hemorrhoids, which always prolapse.

Treatment for internal hemorrhoids, which depends on the severity of the bleeding and discomfort, ranges from education about proper diet and bowel habits to surgical removal (hemorrhoidectomy). Surgical removal is most often accomplished with a banding technique in which a tight rubber band is placed around the base of the hemorrhoid. Banding normally results in the sloughing off of dead tissue and the creation of a scar that prevents future problems. In cases of severe external hemorrhoids, banding is not used because it is too painful. Instead, more complex surgical excision is required.

Such symptoms as occult blood and lower abdominal pain may signal the need for a colon examination. Barium enemas and colonoscopy are the visualization techniques that are utilized. With a barium enema, a solution of radiopaque barium salt is placed into the colon after fasting and preliminary washing enemas have cleansed the organ. Then the colon containing the radiopaque solution is examined by X-ray techniques. This procedure can reveal diverticula, many colon cancers, large polyps, and other severe colorectal problems.

Colonoscopy, in its various forms, has become a mainstay in the diagnosis of colorectal disease. It is particularly valuable in finding smaller polyps, less developed cancers, and colitis. In addition, because patients who have had colon polyps removed have a one-in-four chance of new polyps forming within the next five years, colonoscopy provides minimally invasive and valuable follow-up. It can also prove useful in the follow-up of cancers and of inflammatory bowel disease.

Furthermore, an endoscope may be used to remove a smaller polyp directly or to determine that a large polyp or extensive carcinoma must be removed by laparoscopy. Colonoscopy is generally safe, and the entire large bowel from rectum to cecum may be examined with little risk to a patient. Moreover, endoscopic surgery greatly reduces hospital stays, recovery time, and the frequency of postsurgical mortality. The most common problems associated with colonoscopy are infrequent colon perforation as a result of diverticula, limited endoscopic access to the colon because of scarring from previous surgery, and flare-ups of ulcerative colitis.

Diverticular disease is quite common after the age of fifty. It is caused by small saclike pouches in the colon, often arising after colon spasms. In mild cases, diverticula can be observed by barium enema in patients exhibiting nonspecific abdominal pain and gas. In many instances, bleeding will occur. In some cases, diverticulitis, widespread diverticular infection and inflammation, can lead to serious colon blockage requiring colostomy, and in those cases where perforation occurs, peritonitis will result. Diverticulitis is most common in the lower left colon, originating in the sigmoid region. It may be painful enough to mimic acute appendicitis.

Polyps, masses arising from the bowel wall, are asymptomatic in many cases but may cause bleeding and pain when they are large. The larger that a polyp becomes, the greater is the risk that it will become cancerous. Polyps are often identified after rectal bleeding and/or cramps and abdominal pain lead to barium enema and colonoscopy. They are then removed completely via colonoscopy or laparoscopy, depending on their size. Thereafter, it is suggested that the entire colon be examined via colonoscope at intervals dependent on symptoms over a five-year period. Polyps tend to recur and may be associated with cancer.

About 70 percent of colorectal cancers occur in the sigmoid colon and rectum. These very common visceral cancers are seen most in people over the age of sixty. The characteristics of these slow-growing tumors—slow growth explains their late appearance—vary with colon site. Treatment is usually surgical removal of the diseased area, and barring spread to noncolon sites, the five-year survival rate is near 90 percent. Considerable variation exists in the size, location, and treatment of this very serious disease.

Major aspects of colitis are Crohn's disease in the colon (most often ileocolitis), ulcerative colitis, and spastic colon. Crohn's disease often appears in early life and is associated with fever, pain, and diarrhea. There is no permanent cure for this baffling disease, which recurs repeatedly. Treatments used include diet manipulation, immunosuppressive drugs, steroids, antibiotics (when colitis is accompanied by bacterial infection), and surgery (when intractable pain and bowel obstruction require it).

Ulcerative colitis is another disease that may appear in early life. It is recurrent, varies in severity from mild to fatal, and in less-severe cases manifests as intermittent attacks of bloody diarrhea. Treatment varies as with Crohn's disease. Particularly dangerous is toxic colitis; very severe cases require immediate surgery.

Spastic colon, or irritable bowel syndrome (IBS), is a much milder form of colitis. It has no known anatomic cause, but emotional factors or other causes of hormone imbalance have been proposed. Periodic abdominal pain, constipation, and/or diarrhea are its usual symptoms. Happily, more than half of colitis complaints are attributable to this relatively mild problem, which is treated by diet modification, observation, and painkillers once the possibility of more serious types of colon disease has been eliminated by physical examination and other methodologies.

PERSPECTIVE AND PROSPECTS

Many advances in proctology have occurred since the 1970's, including the wide use of screening for occult blood in stools, which is easily done and often provides early detection of colorectal cancer.

In addition, sophisticated endoscopic and laparoscopic techniques have been developed. The use of various types of endoscopes has enabled the precise examination of the colon and rectum, allowing the detection of colorectal problems that once would have gone unnoticed even after barium enema and related radiologic techniques were used. Furthermore, endoscopic surgery via colonoscopy and laparoscopy has reduced the severity of surgical intervention and the size of incisions, decreased hospital stays and recovery time, and resulted in higher surgical survival rates and facile follow-up after surgery.

The development of fiber-optic systems to be used with video camera techniques has improved colorectal examinations. Proctologists can review data rather than relying on single-shot views through a colonoscope. Such video records and their ongoing improvement may constitute the most significant innovations in colorectal diagnosis and surgery.

The development of additional clinical tests and drug therapy, including the wide use of steroids and immunosuppressive drugs, has also made some colorectal diseases much more manageable; examples are improved treatment of Crohn's disease and ulcerative colitis. Further advances in drug therapy, laparoscopy, and clinical testing may be major foci of future advances in this field.

—*Sanford S. Singer, Ph.D.*

See also Colitis; Colon and rectal polyp removal; Colon and rectal surgery; Colon cancer; Colonoscopy; Crohn's disease; Cystectomy; Diverticulitis and di-

verticulosis; Endoscopy; Fistula repair; Gastroenterology; Gastrointestinal disorders; Gastrointestinal system; Genital disorders, male; Geriatrics and gerontology; Hemorrhoid banding and removal; Hemorrhoids; Internal medicine; Physical examination; Proctology; Prostate cancer; Prostate gland; Prostate gland removal; Reproductive system; Urology.

FOR FURTHER INFORMATION:

Berkow, Robert, and Andrew J. Fletcher, eds. *The Merck Manual of Diagnosis and Therapy.* 17th ed. Rahway, N.J.: Merck Sharp & Dohme Research Laboratories, 1999. Describes many diseases treated by proctologists, including their characteristics, etiology, diagnosis, and treatment.

Corman, Marvin L. *Colon and Rectal Surgery.* 3d ed. Philadelphia: J. B. Lippincott, 1993. A comprehensive physicians' text that gives timely coverage of proctology and colorectal disorders, such as hemorrhoids; anal fissures; abscesses and fistulas; anal incontinence; rectal prolapse; colon, rectal, and anal cancer; diverticular disease; and colitis. Valuable references and illustrations are included.

Taylor, Anita D. *How to Choose a Medical Specialty.* 4th ed. Philadelphia: W. B. Saunders, 1999. Gives a useful description of many medical specialties, including colon and rectal surgery. Included is information on residency and certification and on the economics of proctology practice, a personal suitability self-examination, and references.

Way, Lawrence W., ed. *Current Surgical Diagnosis and Treatment.* 11th ed. Norwalk, Conn.: Appleton and Lange, 1998. This text is technical but clear to interested readers. The chapters on surgery and other proctological topics are diverse and filled with useful aspects of colon, rectal, and anal biology.

PROGERIA
DISEASE/DISORDER
ALSO KNOWN AS: Hutchinson-Gilford syndrome, Werner's syndrome
ANATOMY OR SYSTEM AFFECTED: All
SPECIALTIES AND RELATED FIELDS: Cardiology, pediatrics, vascular medicine
DEFINITION: Rare disorders characterized by many aspects of premature aging.

CAUSES AND SYMPTOMS

There are two major, unrelated types of progeria: Hutchinson-Gilford syndrome, which begins at about age one, and Werner's syndrome, which develops in late adolescence to young adulthood. Recessive inheritance has been demonstrated for Werner's syndrome, whereas a dominant gene is a suspected source in Hutchinson-Gilford syndrome. Underlying causes have been difficult to determine, although an impaired ability to cope with free radicals appears to play a role in the degenerative course found in each disease.

Hutchinson-Gilford syndrome is characterized by superficial aspects of aging such as deteriorated skin, baldness, repeated nonhealing fractures, and vascular diseases, in addition to short stature and minimal subcutaneous fat. Arteriosclerosis and heart disease lead to a median age of death of thirteen. Werner's syndrome occurs more frequently, with the following symptoms: short stature, thin extremities, a squeaky voice, cataracts, an increased risk of diabetes mellitus, heart disease, tumors, hearing loss, and the loss of bone and teeth. Death usually occurs by the middle forties. Neither disorder is simply accelerated aging. For example, the central nervous system is relatively unaffected in both diseases.

TREATMENT AND THERAPY
No known cures exist for either progeria disease. Suggested treatments include antioxidant supplements (for example, vitamin E), growth hormone therapy, and gene therapy. Therapies have focused on providing a supportive environment and treating the symptoms to make the disorders less painful. Among these treatments are surgery, skin grafting (if skin ulceration occurs), and analgesic drugs.

PERSPECTIVE AND PROSPECTS
Hutchinson-Gilford syndrome was first described by Jonathan Hutchinson in 1886. Hastings Gilford gave the name "progeria" to the disorder in a 1904 article. The first cases of Werner's syndrome were reported in the 1950's.

There are hopes for an eventual genetic solution to progeria diseases. The only definitive prospect for sufferers, however, is premature death.

—*Paul J. Chara, Jr., Ph.D.*
See also Aging; Death and dying; Genetic diseases.

FOR FURTHER INFORMATION:
Bellenir, Karen, ed. *Genetic Disorders Sourcebook: Basic Information About Heritable Diseases and Disorders Such as Down Syndrome, PKU, Hemo-philia, and Von Willebrandt Diseases.* New York: Omnigraphics, 1996.
Gormley, Myra Vanderpool. *Family Diseases: Are You at Risk?* Reprint. Baltimore: Genealogical Publishing, 1998.
Millunsky, Aubrey. *Choices, Not Chances.* Boston: Little, Brown, 1989.

PROSTATE CANCER
DISEASE/DISORDER
ANATOMY OR SYSTEM AFFECTED: Abdomen, lymphatic system, reproductive system
SPECIALTIES AND RELATED FIELDS: Immunology, oncology, proctology, radiology, urology
DEFINITION: Malignancy occurring in the prostate gland, which is the most deadly cancer for men in the United States.

CAUSES AND SYMPTOMS
The normal human prostate gland is a walnut-sized male organ composed of glandular tissue and a thick coat of muscle tissue called the prostatic capsule. Located near the rectum just below the urinary bladder, it secretes an alkaline fluid that makes sperm more

Location of the Prostate Gland

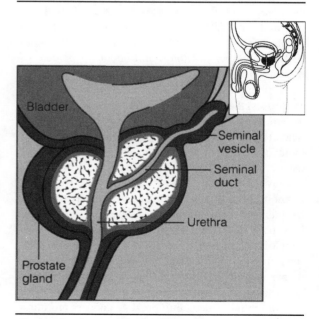

The prostate is one of the major sites where cancer develops in older men; the inset shows the location of the prostate gland in the male reproductive system.

viable after intercourse; substances that cause semen to "clot" temporarily, helping to keep sperm in the female reproductive tract when the penis is withdrawn after intercourse; and fibrolysin, a substance which later breaks down the semen clot and enables the sperm to move on and ensure fertilization where possible.

The urethra, which empties the urinary bladder, passes through the prostate gland. In later life, the prostate gland tends to enlarge. When this occurs, it presses on and constricts the urethra, a disease which is called benign prostatic hyperplasia. The hyperplasia ultimately causes afflicted men to develop difficulty in urination, which may lead to the necessity for surgical removal of the prostate gland.

Much more problematic is prostate cancer. Most often, prostate cancer is detected in asymptomatic men who are found to have lumps within the prostate during a routine rectal examination at a urologist's office. Regrettably, cancers detected in this way are often in a fairly advanced and dangerous stage of growth. Hence, it is advantageous to have routine, yearly urologic examinations after the age of forty, along with clinical testing, so that early detection can prevent the most serious consequences of the disease.

An important adjunct of such testing is the blood test for prostate-specific antigen (PSA). PSA is a glycoprotein produced only by the cells of the prostate, and its levels in the blood correlate well with the presence of malignancy. Normal values are under 4 nanograms per milliliter, and about 25 percent of the men whose blood PSA levels are 4 to 10 nanograms per milliliter will have prostate cancer. In most such cases, the cancer is treatable because the tumors are small and localized inside the prostate capsule. When PSA levels exceed 10 nanograms per milliliter, about 70 percent of test patients are found to have the disease, their cancers are larger, and the prognosis is less favorable.

Another blood test for prostate cancer is the measurement of acid phosphatase levels in the blood. This method is a less sensitive and less reliable indicator of the disease when used alone. Done in conjunction with PSA testing, however, its increased levels are a good indicator of the extent of the spread (metastasis) of prostate cancer. Other useful methods for examining or detecting prostate cancers are ultrasound examinations, needle biopsies guided by ultrasound, and magnetic resonance imaging (MRI). Because of the high cost of these procedures, however, many physicians recommend that they be used only after PSA and rectal examinations are suggestive of serious prostate problems.

Most prostate cancers are graded by a series of designations in a tumor-node-metastasis (TNM) scale, with the main subdivisions T, N, and M indicating increasing severity from T to M. The main subdivisions are themselves divided into twenty-one categories. Small cancers, restricted to the interior of the prostate (from T1 to T2) are most treatable. Those which penetrate the prostate capsule are more problematic (T3 and onward).

TREATMENT AND THERAPY

The handling of localized prostate cancer is controversial and ranges from removal of the entire prostate (radical prostatectomy) to radiation treatment (or both) to surveillance. In radical prostatectomy, the entire prostate, the nearby seminal vesicles, and the vas deferens are removed. This deletes both the prostate—the focus of the cancer—and the nearby male sexual tissues that are most likely to be sites of cancer metastasis. When this procedure is carried out with prostate-confined tumors (categories T1 through T3), cancer recurrence is less than 2 percent. In many cases, radiation therapy, which is viewed as less radical, is carried out on these cancers, and ten-year survival rates approach 70 percent. Surveillance of such cancers is deemed as being unwise by many, but is done by others.

For more severe or metastasized tumors, surgery and radiation treatment are followed by a number of hormone regimens. The latter include androgen deprivation, rationalized by the fact that most prostate tumors are androgen-dependent. The most common hormones used are pituitary antagonists that prevent testicular androgen secretion. Removal of the testes or estrogen administration are other, more radical treatments. The result of castration is unpleasant physically and psychologically. Estrogen therapy has numerous drawbacks, the most common of which is the feminization of appearance. Estrogen treatment must be approached with great care because it can also lead to death by congestive heart failure. Nevertheless, the five- to ten-year survival rate for men found to have nonmetastasized prostate cancer is viewed as good by many physicians, and the survival rates of those with more severe cancers are improving because of the discovery of better therapeutic drugs.

In the News: Managing Prostate Cancer

While the number of cases of prostate cancer in the United States continues to rise, over the past three years prostate cancer deaths have declined, likely as a result of newer diagnostic methods to increase early detection. Prostate specific antigen (PSA) continues to be the principal diagnostic study, with normal PSA below 4 nanograms per milliliter. PSAs above 4 nanograms per milliliter or those which rise more than 0.75 nanogram per milliliter in twelve months should indicate a suspicion of prostate cancer. Newer studies using the percent free PSA or free/total PSA ratio have enhanced the detection of prostate cancer in some men. Using an immunoassay system, PSAs are detected for their total amount in the serum as well as the amount which is not bound to protein (free PSA). A free/total PSA ratio of greater than 25 percent indicates a low probability of prostate cancer, even if that PSA measures greater than 4 but less than 10. If, however, the free to total PSA ratio is less than 25 percent, the risk of prostate cancer rises. This study provides additional helpful information in deciding which patients should undergo prostate biopsy for elevated PSA levels.

The management of localized prostate cancer continues to have the options of expectant therapy, removal of the entire prostate (radical prostatectomy), and radiation therapy. Radical prostatectomy requires removal of the entire prostate and the seminal vesicles. New procedures for prostate cancer surgery, which spare the nerves near the prostate during surgery, have increased the potency rates of men following radical prostatectomy. Lower rates of expected incontinence and erectile dysfunction, and reduced hospital stays have improved the outcomes of radical prostatectomy dramatically. Radiation therapy, an acceptable, but less successful option for treatment of prostate cancer, can be administered by external beam or by the implantation of radioactive seeds in the prostate (brachytherapy) using ultrasound to guide their positioning. Side effects and complications of radiation therapy include bladder, bowel, and erectile function changes.

For prostate cancer that has spread beyond the confines of the prostate or has metastasized, androgen deprivation therapy, which reduces or eliminates circulating testosterone, remains the cornerstone of treatment. This can be provided by surgical removal of the testicles (orchiectomy) or through the use of injectable medications which stimulate the pituitary and decrease circulating testosterone to levels which allow the prostate cancer to recede. This treatment, which is usually effective for three to four years, can reduce prostate cancer growth and improve symptoms of metastatic prostate cancer. Newer combinations of chemotherapy are available for cancers which have stopped responding to androgen deprivation.

—*Culley C. Carson III, M.D.*

PERSPECTIVE AND PROSPECTS

Prostate cancer first became common in the 1960's. In North America, it is the most common cancer detected in men. Moreover, by the 1990's, 150,000 to 200,000 American men per year were found to have the disease and more than 28,000 of them died of it each year. More worrisome is the finding that more than 40 percent of American men fifty years of age or older who were autopsied after death from other causes were found to have prostate cancer as well.

The incidence of the disease varies worldwide and from race to race. For example, the incidence of prostate cancer is very high in North America and Europe but low in the Far East. In the United States, its incidence also varies with race, being highest among African Americans, somewhat lower among Caucasians, and much rarer among Asian Americans. Overall, however, 3 to 4 percent of American men are deemed likely to die of prostate cancer.

—*Sanford S. Singer, Ph.D.*

See also Aging; Cancer; Chemotherapy; Genital disorders, male; Malignancy and metastasis; National Cancer Institute (NCI); Prostate gland; Prostate gland removal; Radiation therapy; Tumor removal; Tumors.

FOR FURTHER INFORMATION:

Bayoumi, Ahmed M., Adalsteinn D. Brown, and Alan M. Garber. "Cost-effectiveness of Androgen Suppression Therapies in Advanced Prostate Cancer." *Journal of the National Cancer Institute* 92, no. 21 (November 1, 2000): 1731-1739. The authors repeated the analysis assuming that the therapies differed in efficacy and basing new efficacy values on the point estimates from the meta-analysis.

Bostwick, David G., Gregory T. MacLennan, and Thayne R. Larson. *Prostate Cancer: What Every Man, and His Family, Needs to Know.* Rev. ed. New York: Villard, 1999. Numerous other books have been written about prostate cancer, but this one—backed by the American Cancer Society's focus on early detection—provides the essential basic information written by a team of internationally recognized experts on the subject.

Del Regato, Juan A., Harlan J. Spjut, and James D. Cox. *Ackerman and Del Regato's Cancer: Diagnosis, Treatment, and Prognosis.* 6th ed. St. Louis: C. V. Mosby, 1985. An in-depth discussion of cancer and tumors, designed for the medical professional. Includes bibliographical references and an index.

"Screening with the Prostate-Specific Antigen Test—Texas, 1997." *The Journal of the American Medical Association* 284, no. 18 (November 8, 2000): 2313-2314. The analysis of the 1999 Behavioral Risk Factor Surveillance System survey relating to prostate-specific antigen testing is discussed. Several screening methods are available for early detection of prostate cancer.

Seppa, Nathan. "Prostate Enzyme Triggers Cancer Drug." *Science News* 158, no. 19 (November 4, 2000): 293. Using a new drug that enlists the aid of an enzyme naturally abundant in the prostate gland, researchers have reversed advanced prostate cancer in mice.

Srikantan, Vasantha, et al. "PCGEM1, a Prostate-Specific Gene, Is Overexpressed in Prostate Cancer." *Proceedings of the National Academy of Sciences of the United States of America* 97, no. 22 (October 24, 2000): 12216-12221. A prostate-specific gene, PCGEM1, was identified by differential display analysis of paired normal and prostate cancer tissues.

PROSTATE GLAND

ANATOMY

ANATOMY OR SYSTEM AFFECTED: Endocrine system, glands, reproductive system

SPECIALTIES AND RELATED FIELDS: Endocrinology, oncology, proctology, urology

DEFINITION: One of several accessory reproductive glands; its main function is to secrete into semen vital additive components that increase the fertilizing potential of sperm.

KEY TERMS:

andrology: study of the physiological functions relating to male reproductive capacity

bulbourethal gland: the bulbous portion of the male urethra adjacent to the posterior prostate zone

gonad: the male or female organ (testis or ovary, respectively) in which the essential gametes are formed for reproduction

hyperplasia: a state of hormonal stimulation causing an increase in the number of cells in a tissue, resulting in an oversized organ

prostoglandular carcinoma: the general pathological nomenclature for cancers located in the prostate gland

vas deferens: the duct that carries the male seminal fluid

STRUCTURE AND FUNCTIONS

The prostate is the largest of several glands that are referred to as the accessory glands of the male reproductive tract; the other accessory glands are the seminal vesicles and the bulbourethral glands. Unlike the latter two, which evolved morphologically in smaller pairs, the prostate evolved as a single gland, approximately 4 centimeters in diameter in adults. It surrounds the urethra, the tubular tract that carries both semen and urine. During the early embryonic stage of life, both urinary organs and accessory sex glands are formed, through the cell division process, out of the same original source of specialized cells in the intermediate mesoderm (called the nephrotome) and the cloaca.

In fact, up to a certain point in the growth of the human embryo, it is not possible to distinguish the pattern that will lead to formation of the male and female gonads. Following what is called the ambisexual stage, the undifferentiated gonad, or reproductive terminus, begins to evolve into a male or female reproductive organ (becoming a testis or ovary, respectively). Then, in the male, the three accessory sex glands begin to form. Their eventual key functions in the reproductive process will not begin, however, until the onset of puberty in the individual's growth cycle. Male puberty, or sexual maturity, is initiated when secretions from the testis and pituitary gland activate secretions from other organs, including the prostate gland. It is at this stage that elevated levels of androgenic steroids in the body cause the prostate to attain its full size and to begin to secrete the fluids that are so essential in the male reproductive function.

The function of all necessary reproductive glands, and of the prostate gland in particular, is to secrete fluids that affect the fertilization potential of the spermatozoa in the seminal fluid as it passes from its source in the testicles through the vas deferens duct. The vas deferens joins the urethra at a point just before the latter is encased by the prostate gland. Thereafter, the urethra serves as a channel for passage of seminal fluid through the penis.

When the adult prostate gland is functioning efficiently, the prostatic secretions that pass into the vas deferens should make up about 30 percent of the volume of the male seminal fluid. Although the process of prostate secretion after puberty is continuous, the composite elements of these secretions may vary. A most notable variation in content occurs between the normal phases of daily life and moments of sexual excitement. A comparison of "resting" prostatic fluids with fluids obtained from ejaculation resulting from sexual stimulation suggests that the latter contains a higher level of certain enzymes (specifically, acid phosphatase) than the former.

All "resting" prostatic fluid is only slightly basic (an approximate pH of 7.2). The pH level may increase (to a pH of 7.7) in men suffering from prostatitis. A listing of the main components of the fluid would include diastase (an enzyme of the amylase group); proteolytic enzymes, especially fibrinolysin; citric acid; acid phosphatase (also an enzyme); cephalin (a chemical group containing amino acids that is found mainly in nervous system tissues); cholesterol; magnesium; zinc; and calcium. In humans, but not necessarily in all mammals, calcium is more highly concentrated in prostatic fluid than in the blood plasma. One may note other differences between humans and other mammals with respect to the glandular origins of separate component elements of seminal fluid. Whereas citric acid originates in the human prostate gland, in other species it flows from the seminal vesicles (as is the case with boars, for example) or in generally equal amounts from each of the accessory sex glands (in rabbits and guinea pigs). In all cases, and specifically in the human prostate, citric acid is synthesized by chemical reactions within the respective glands.

There is general agreement that the fertilizing potential of spermatozoa is enhanced when combinations of these various prostatic fluid constituents join

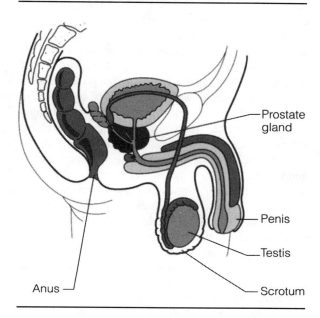

The Prostate Gland

- Prostate gland
- Penis
- Testis
- Scrotum
- Anus

the flow of semen. No evidence has been found, however, of an identifiable "target" effect by any one specific element. One apparent exception to this general assumption has been observed in connection with citric acid. Tests of relative concentration of citric acid in semen suggest an influence on the activity level of testicular hormones, especially androgen. Additionally, and most specifically related to the fertilization potential of male spermatozoa carried in the seminal fluid, citric acid reacts chemically with other component elements in ways that may delay that coagulation of seminal plasma or contribute to its capacity to be absorbed at the appropriate time in the fertilization process.

Research has also tentatively established that the fertilization potential of spermatozoa may depend on levels of zinc contained in secretions from the prostate gland. One chemical effect of zinc is to slow the breakdown of genetically vital chromosomes in individual sperm cells. This function of zinc, however, has not been tied directly to potential fertility levels, since surgical removal of that section of the prostate where zinc is in the highest concentration (the dorsolateral portion of the gland) has not changed reproductive capacities in selected laboratory animals (specifically, in rats). Because prostate surgery involving human patients is almost exclusively connected with attempts to arrest prostate cancer, no research data have been recorded that can be compared with experiments performed on animals.

One area of research that has established irrefutable evidence in connection with fertility levels deals with the effects of certain drugs on the functioning of the accessory sex glands, including the prostate. Tests on morphine and methadone users, for example, have shown a definite reduction in the volume of human seminal ejaculate. Methadone (and, in some cases, morphine) can actually cause a reduction of the weight and volume of the testes, seminal vesicles, and prostate glands of laboratory mice. Specific constituent elements of prostate secretions that appear to be reduced when drugs such as morphine sulfate are administered include prostatic fructose and different forms of glucose that contribute to metabolic activity in the prostate gland itself.

In addition to medically or self-administered drugs, chemicals that enter the body through the food chain (most notably the pesticide DDT) can also affect the functioning of the prostate. In mice, the testosterone metabolic process, which is very much dependent on the prostate, has been shown to be significantly retarded when DDT is administered under close controls. Dieldrin is another pesticide that affects the ability of prostate tissue in mice to absorb testosterone.

DISORDERS AND DISEASES

In general terms, prostate gland diseases tend to fall into two main categories: nonproliferative diseases and proliferative diseases. The latter category is characterized by two forms of dangerous physical change in the tissues of the gland itself: lesions and neoplasms (or tumors).

Diseases of the nonproliferative types, although painful and potentially quite dangerous to the patient's health, may be treated by modern medical means. The first subgroup in this category consists of congenital anomalies. Some of these have slowly developing symptoms and may be discovered only when some other difficulty, such as urinary irregularities or infertility, is the initial cause for the doctor's examination. The most common form of anomaly is the congenital cyst, which occurs as a result of obstructions in the normal flow of secretions through the prostate gland. Secretion blockage is sometimes caused by irregular development of the parenchyma, the functioning tissues of the gland itself. Subsequent

development of a cyst in the prostate itself further impedes the normal flow of secretions within and from the gland.

Congenital cysts usually occur in the prostatic utricle, an oblong protrusion measuring about three millimeters that is palpable when a medical doctor performs a rectal examination. The abnormality is generally discovered in patients in their early twenties. In newborn infants, the fact of recent estrogenic stimulation in utero can have the temporary effect of a utricle that is three times its eventual normal length. If the prostatic utricle does not shorten during childhood and early adulthood, examining doctors will be alerted to the existence of a cyst and the possible need for surgical intervention.

A second form of nonproliferative disease in the prostate involves the formation of tiny calculi, or stones, inside the gland. True prostatic calculi are generally rare, but they may occur when prostatic secretions are altered by one of several possible factors, including infection or some form of metabolic dysfunction. Altered secretions can lead to an abnormal process of chemical deposits inside the organ. These deposits in turn attract mineral concentrations, particularly of calcium salts (the main component of calculi).

Although pathology texts list up to five forms of proliferative tumors that can attack the accessory reproductive glands, the prostate gland itself is mainly vulnerable to two out of the five: prostatic carcinoma and primary prostatic sarcoma. More common and less dangerous proliferative lesions (inflammations, not tumors) affecting the prostate involve many different forms of hyperplasia. Although the causes leading to such lesions in the various tissues that compose the prostate can vary, their effect may be summarized: inflammation leading to the obstruction of normal secretions originating in the prostate and/or to the potentially harmful addition into prostate secretions of "foreign" by-products of the inflammatory process itself.

The most common proliferative lesion of the prostate, nodular prostatic hyperplasia (NPH), leads directly to urological disease, usually in middle-aged and elderly males. Its high incidence is reflected in the widespread need for some form of prostate surgery among men over fifty. The disease derives its name from the fact that it displays multinodular areas of inflammation. This fact makes it very difficult for specialized surgeons to localize areas demanding attention. Doctors are still uncertain of the exact origins of NPH in the tissues in and around the prostate, as well as the complexities of hormonal phenomena associated with the disease. It appears, however, that NPH is a combination of the more simply diagnosed prostatic hyperplasia and a hypertrophy (tissue constriction) of the inner zones of the prostate gland itself.

Although these various forms of lesions affect a high percentage of the adult male population, the greatest pathological menace associated with the prostate gland involves malignant tumors. Prostatic cancers represent the second most common form of cancer occurring among American males. Because of the difficulties associated with diagnosis and the complexities of possible treatments, a quite large percentage of those suffering from prostate cancers die from the disease.

In terms of diagnosis, there is a problem of extended delay in the appearance of symptoms. Approximately 70 percent out of the total recorded cases remain locally latent for years. Yet even the prostatoglandular tumors that have clinical manifestations are often discovered too late for effective medical intervention.

Doctors looking for symptoms of prostate cancer (beyond those that might appear in physical examination via the rectum) pay particular attention to several likely warning signs. These include possible malignant repercussions stemming from prostatic lesions (especially NPH); sacral, low back, or upper pubic pain; excessive urinary retention; and uneven or interrupted urinary flow.

If a physician suspects the presence of cancer in the prostate region, three forms of biopsy may be used. The most accurate (96 percent certain) involves actual surgical opening and removal of sections for laboratory biopsy. This method is the most expensive, however, and is recommended mainly when, for reasons that may not be limited to concerns about cancer, physicians are convinced that a radical prostatectomy should probably follow initial surgical intervention. Of the other two methods of diagnosis, needle injection biopsy and cytologic aspiration biopsy, the former has a slightly higher level of accuracy (82 to 95 percent, as opposed to 73 to 94 percent for needle biopsy). The apparent disadvantage of tissue aspiration compared to needle biopsy, however, is that the former provides a less accurate idea of the tumor grade or its growth pattern. Therefore, physicians

who must decide not only on the malignant or benign nature of prostate tumors but also on the most effective mode of treatment (radiation or surgery) usually prefer to combine both forms of biopsy before proceeding.

An additional complicating factor that makes prostate cancers among the most difficult to treat is similar to what has been observed with NPH. In NPH, which is a proliferative lesion, multinodular development complicates localization of the diseased area for treatment. In the case of prostatoglandular carcinoma, approximately 30 percent of diagnosed patients have diffused, as opposed to focal, growth development patterns. In such cases, radical prostatectomy, despite the fact that it leaves the patient impotent, is usually believed to be the only prognosis for serious consideration.

A second, less common category of prostate cancer is referred to as primary prostatic sarcoma. Although this disease represents only 2 percent of the total prostate cancers, it differs in a very important way from the more common prostatic carcinoma. Sarcoma may occur in male patients of any age and has been diagnosed in infants as young as four months. Another menacing factor is that, if this form of cancer appears in the prostate, it frequently extends directly to other adjacent organs, primarily the bladder, seminal vesicles, or rectum.

PERSPECTIVE AND PROSPECTS

The fact that, by the 1980's, prostate tumors ranked among the most common causes of terminal cancers in American males over fifty would suggest that medical science had amassed considerable data on their occurrence and on possible treatments. Apparently, however, the medical world remained divided, particularly over questions of prognosis.

Doctors called upon by the National Cancer Institute hesitated to reach a consensus about the central question of relative success rates when radiation treatment (as opposed to surgical intervention) is used to attack tumors in the prostate gland. Part of the problem, the institute learned, was that medical data on this subject are not sufficiently random: Prostate cancer diagnoses and recorded treatments tend to reflect cases in a real, but not fully representative, portion of the male population.

Because the average age of diagnosis of patients with prostate cancer is seventy, data gathered on their physical condition do not provide sufficiently random samplings for comparison with the population as a whole. A main reason for apparent dissatisfaction with too focused data is that, because of the typically late discovery of prostate cancer, a central consideration in choosing one of two possible treatments—surgery or radiation treatment—is rendered less vital. Past a certain stage in advanced adulthood, diminished sexual reproductive capacity also diminishes patient sensitivity to the possibility that surgical removal of cancerous growth in the prostate will almost certainly bring about impotence.

For those who are much more likely to be concerned with this eventuality—prostate cancer victims in their forties, fifties, or even sixties—doctors must advise patients that radiation therapy involves a risk of a different and even more weighty nature: Even the most expert therapists cannot know if their treatment is attacking all or just part of the cancerous growth. The risk of fatality from an incompletely eradicated prostate cancer in men of less advanced age has to be weighed against their concern for maintaining a reproductive capacity.

—*Byron D. Cannon, Ph.D.*

See also Aging; Cancer; Colon and rectal surgery; Conception; Endocrinology; Glands; Hormones; Malignancy and metastasis; Oncology; Proctology; Prostate cancer; Prostate gland removal; Puberty and adolescence; Reproductive system.

FOR FURTHER INFORMATION:

Fox, Arnold, and Barry Fox. *The Healthy Prostate: A Doctor's Comprehensive Program for Preventing and Treating Common Problems*. New York: John Wiley & Sons, 1996. This popular work discusses diseases of the prostate gland and offers ways to prevent or control them. Includes a bibliography and an index.
Kolata, Gina. "Prostate Cancer Consensus Hampered by Lack of Data." *Science* 236 (June 26, 1987): 1626-1627. This report of the findings of a 1986 National Cancer Institute conference on prostate cancer indicates that, despite the rather widespread occurrence of prostate cancer, doctors are not fully in agreement concerning the reliability of data that have been gathered on diagnosis and the recommended methods of treatment.
Marieb, Elaine N. *Essentials of Human Anatomy and Physiology*. 6th ed. Redwood City, Calif.: Benjamin/ Cummings, 2000. This introductory anatomy and physiology textbook, easily accessible to those with little science background, is richly illustrated with diagrams and photographs, which help to illuminate body systems and processes. In-depth discussions of prevalent diseases and disorders and of current areas of research make this an all-around useful reference work.
Spring-Mills, Elinor, and E. S. E. Hafez, eds. *Accessory Glands of the Male Reproductive Tract*. Ann Arbor, Mich.: Ann Arbor Science, 1979. Although this book was written by doctors primarily for use by other doctors, the completeness of its treatment, ranging from anatomical descriptions through pathology, offsets its sometimes technical nature.

PROSTATE GLAND REMOVAL
PROCEDURE

ANATOMY OR SYSTEM AFFECTED: Endocrine system, glands

SPECIALTIES AND RELATED FIELDS: General surgery, oncology, proctology, urology

DEFINITION: A surgical procedure to remove all or part of an abnormal prostate gland.

KEY TERMS:

cauterization: a means of sealing blood vessels with heat; used to prevent bleeding
impotence: the inability to achieve an erection
incision: a cut made with a scalpel during a surgical procedure
incontinence: the inability to retain urine
prostate: a gland in males which surrounds the urethra and secretes a fluid into the ejaculate
urethra: the tube that connects the urinary bladder externally

INDICATIONS AND PROCEDURES

The removal of the prostate gland, or prostatectomy, is usually performed when enlargement of the gland blocks or reduces the outflow of urine. Removal may also be indicated in prostate cancer or inflammation of the prostate (prostatitis).

Enlargement of the prostate gland, also known as benign prostatic or nodular prostatic hyperplasia, usually affects men over the age of fifty. Because the prostate gland is situated so that it surrounds the urethra, when it enlarges, it can compress the urethra and reduce the flow of urine. Symptoms usually include gradual reduction in the ability to urinate effectively. Since the flow of urine out the urethra is obstructed by the enlarged gland, the patient experiences difficulty starting urination and a weak stream.

In early stages, the urinary bladder muscle becomes heavier and stronger in order to compensate for the increased resistance in the urethra. Eventually, the bladder is unable to expel all the urine and becomes distended. This urinary retention can cause abdominal swelling and a perceived urgency to urinate. In fact, the bladder may contract frequently and cause a need for frequent urination. This is one sign of bladder muscle failure and the need for medical attention. In some patients, there may be incontinence resulting from the leakage of small volumes of urine.

Prostate cancer is a malignant growth of the prostate gland. Most patients with prostate cancer are in their seventies; this condition also occurs in middle-aged men. The symptoms that develop are similar to benign prostatic hypertrophy. Diagnosis is usually made by a digital rectal examination, ultrasonography, prostate biopsy, and a blood test for prostatic-specific antigens.

The treatment for both benign prostatic hypertrophy and prostatic cancer involves medical management and surgical removal of the gland. In benign prostatic hypertrophy, finasteride (Proscar) can be used to reduce the size of the gland and diminish symptoms. Prostate cancer can sometimes be managed using drugs that block or reduce the production of testosterone. Such agents include flutamide (Eulexin) and leuprolide. If medical management is not effective, surgical removal of the gland is usually indicated.

The most common surgical procedure for the removal of the prostate gland is transurethral prostatectomy, which is performed using an instrument called a resectoscope. The patient is first anesthetized using spinal or general anesthesia. Then the resectoscope is inserted into the urethra at the tip of the penis and directed up toward the prostate gland. The resectoscope allows the surgeon to view the urinary bladder and prostate and insert a cutting instrument or heated wire into the area of the prostate to be removed. As the gland is cut away, it is removed from the urethra by suction. Any bleeding that may occur is stopped by a cauterizing electrode, which seals the vessels. After the prostate gland has been removed, the surgeon withdraws the resectoscope and inserts a catheter into the bladder to drain urine and any remaining blood or tissue.

If the gland is too large to be removed using transurethral prostatectomy, then retropubic prostatectomy is performed. This operation requires that the patient be anesthetized. The surgeon makes a horizontal incision just above the pubic hairline into the abdominal cavity and exposes the urinary bladder and prostate gland. A cut into the capsule that encases the gland is made, and the surgeon begins to remove the prostate gland. To drain excess fluid from the pelvic cavity, the surgeon places a temporary flexible tube near to where the prostate was excised. Bleeding vessels are cauterized, and the abdominal wall is sutured. A urethral catheter is inserted and left in place to aid in draining the bladder of blood and urine.

USES AND COMPLICATIONS

After removal of the urethral catheter, the patient is encouraged to drink large amounts of fluids and to pass urine. Occasionally, the patient may experience frequent and painful urination but should still consume adequate amounts of liquids to help clear the urinary tract of blood and other postoperative debris. A few patients will continue to have incontinence for several weeks.

More severe complications include intra-abdominal bleeding from surgery, infections, and blood clots that obstruct urine outflow from the bladder. Bleeding within the pelvic and abdominal cavities is usually detected and corrected during surgery. If it occurs after prostatectomy, a second operation may be required to find and stop the bleeding. Most infections of the urinary tract can be adequately treated with appropriate antibiotic therapy. Urinary obstruction resulting from a blood clot can be washed out with a catheter in the urethra.

Approximately 10 to 20 percent of men undergoing retropubic prostatectomy experience impotence. This complication is more common in older patients.

For most men, the hospital stay is about two days for transurethral prostatectomy and one week for retropubic surgery. Several weeks after the surgery the patient can resume all activities, including intercourse. Most men are sterile, however, immediately after either procedure because most of the sperm and seminal fluid are expelled backward into the urinary bladder (retrograde ejaculation). The ejaculate is then excreted with the urine during the next urination.

—*Matthew Berria, Ph.D.,*
and Douglas Reinhart, M.D.

See also Aging; Biopsy; Cancer; Colon and rectal surgery; Glands; Incontinence; Malignancy and metastasis; Oncology; Proctology; Prostate cancer; Prostate gland; Radiation therapy; Reproductive system.

FOR FURTHER INFORMATION:

Clayman, Charles B., ed. *The American Medical Association Encyclopedia of Medicine*. New York: Random House, 1994. A concise presentation of numerous medical terms and illnesses. A good general reference.

Stutzman, Ray E., and Patrick C. Walsh. "Suprapubic and Retropubic Prostatectomy." In *Campbell's Urology*, edited by Walsh et al. 6th ed. Philadelphia: W. B. Saunders, 1992. A chapter in a classic urology text, which maintains its encyclopedic approach while following a new organ systems orientation.

Tierney, Lawrence M., Jr., et al., eds. *Current Medical Diagnosis and Treatment: 2001*. 38th ed. New York: McGraw-Hill, 2000. This book is revised annually and provides complete summaries for the diagnosis and treatment of different urologic disorders. It is an excellent and concise text but is written for professionals.

PROTOZOAN DISEASES

DISEASE/DISORDER

ANATOMY OR SYSTEM AFFECTED: Gastrointestinal system

SPECIALTIES AND RELATED FIELDS: Microbiology, public health

DEFINITION: Disease caused by protozoa, a diverse group of free-living, unicellular animals that function as parasites.

Protozoa exist in almost every ecological niche. As parasites, they infect all species of vertebrates and many invertebrates, adapting to nearly all available sites within their hosts' bodies. There are nearly sixty-six thousand known species of protozoa; half of these are represented in the fossil record, and about ten thousand of the living species are known to be parasitic. Unlike many other parasites, however, protozoa replicate within their hosts to produce hundreds of thousands of their kind within several days of infection. Because of their variety, adaptability, and reproductive rates, parasitic protozoa exert a major influence on human existence.

The phylum Protozoa is subdivided into four subphyla, but only the subphylum Sarcomastigophora is of real concern to humans. Within this subphylum are the twelve genera of parasitic protozoa that cause disease to humans and their domestic animals, the most important of which are *Trypanosoma*, *Leishmania*, *Trichomonas*, *Entamoeba*, *Eimeria*, *Toxoplasma*, *Babesia*, *Theileria*, *Giardia*, and *Plasmodium*.

The most startling characteristic of parasitic protozoan diseases in humans is the sheer number of cases that exist. For example, a conservative estimate suggests at least two hundred million persons harbor the protozoa *Entamoeba*, which causes amebic dysentery. Of this number, some fifteen to twenty million suffer severe cases of amebic dysentery. One to two billion humans are estimated to be infected with *Toxoplasma*, the protozoa causing toxoplasmosis. *Trypanosoma* (the agent of sleeping sickness and Chagas' disease) infect fifteen to twenty million people worldwide; *Giardia*, two hundred million; and *Leishmania* (which is responsible for the disease kala-azar), one to two million. The most important of all protozoan diseases, and said to be the greatest killer in history, is malaria. Malaria is caused by the parasite *Plasmodium* and results in the death of two to three million people annually.

Protozoan parasites. Protozoa that infect humans are commonly found in the intestinal tract, various tissues and organs, and the bloodstream. Of the many protozoa that reside in the human gut, only invasive *Entamoeba histolytica* causes serious disease. *E. histolytica* parasites are transmitted by the ingestion of water contaminated with human feces containing *E. histolytica* cysts and can result in the disease amebiasis—or in its severe form, amebic dysentery. If the disease spreads by way of intestinal veins to the liver, the result can be hepatic amebiasis. Though *E. histolytica* can prove highly invasive, mostly it remains in the gut as nonpathogenic infections. Another waterborne intestinal protozoan familiar to campers and vacationers is the flagellate *Giardia lamblia*, which causes giardiasis. Giardiasis results in a mild-to-serious, long-lasting diarrhea. It is usually acquired from the ingestion of water fouled by animal waste. It can also be transmitted by human sources and, if the outbreak occurs in a closed population, frequently results in a rapidly spreading infection.

A number of flagellate parasites infect the human skin, bloodstream, and viscera. The flagellate *Trypanosoma cruzi* is the agent of Chagas' disease, a major cause of debilitation and chronic heart disease among poorly housed populations of Central and South America. *T. cruzi* is transmitted when the liquid feces of an insect (genus *Triatoma*) are scratched into the skin or rubbed in the eye. In Africa, the tsetse fly carries the parasitic agents of the disease trypanosomiasis, also known as African sleeping sickness.

The disease is generated by the flagellate parasites *Trypanosoma brucei gambiense* and *T. brucei rhodesiense*, which infect the bloodstream and can be fatal if the parasites cross the blood-brain barrier. Parasitic flagellates of the genus *Leishmania* are transmitted by blood-sucking midges and sandflies and result in macrophage infection. Cutaneous leishmaniasis is characterized by infected macrophages in the skin, resulting in long-lasting skin lesions. A similar condition, mucocutaneous leishmaniasis, common to the Amazon Basin, begins as skin ulcers and often progresses to the destruction of nasal mucosa, cartilage, and soft facial and pharyngeal tissues. Visceral leishmaniasis, or kala-azar, infects the spleen, liver, bone marrow, and lymph nodes.

Only one species of ciliate protozoa is parasitic in humans: *Balantidium coli*, a free-living, large protozoan covered with rows of cilia. It is found in the large intestine, where it can cause the ulcerative disease balantidiasis.

The group of protozoa known as sporozoans are all parasitic and include many deadly parasites of humans: *Isopora, Sarcocystis, Cryptosporidium,* and *Toxoplasma. Toxoplasma gondii*, the agent of toxoplasmosis, is of great medical concern. It is estimated to infect between 20 and 50 percent of the world's population, and it can penetrate the placenta and subsequently infect the fetus of pregnant women lacking the proper antibodies. The most important sporozoans, however, are the agents of malaria.

Malaria is a disease caused by a group of sporozoans in the genus *Plasmodium* that infect the human liver and red blood cells. Malaria is characterized by periodic chills, fever, and sweats, leading to anemia, enlargement of the spleen, and complications that result in death, especially among infants. The parasites are transmitted to humans by the bite of any of sixty species of infected *Anopheles* mosquitoes. The disease is found in all tropical and temperate regions, but control efforts have eliminated it from North America, Europe, and the northern Asian continent. Despite control efforts and effective medical treatments, malaria is historically the greatest killer of all human infectious diseases, and it remains the single most dangerous threat to humankind from an infectious agent. More than one million children die of malaria in Africa yearly.

—*Randall L. Milstein, Ph.D.*

See also Arthropod-borne diseases; Bites and stings; Diarrhea and dysentery; Epidemiology; Giardiasis; Leishmaniasis; Lice, mites, and ticks; Malaria; Microbiology; Parasitic diseases; Sleeping sickness; Toxoplasmosis; Tropical medicine; Zoonoses.

For Further Information:
Behnke, J. M., ed. *Parasites, Immunity, and Pathology: The Consequences of Parasitic Infection in Mammals.* New York: Taylor & Francis, 1990. Nematode parasites cause widespread mortality in both people and domestic animals and have major economic and clinical implications. This book reviews the latest research in developing better pharmacological control.
Despommier, Dickson D., Robert W. Gwadz, and Peter J. Hotex. *Parasitic Diseases.* 4th ed. New York: Appletree Productions, 2000. Photographs and illustrations illuminate this concise text. Includes bibliographical references and an index.
Gutteridge, W. E., and G. H. Coombs. *Biochemistry of Parasitic Protozoa.* Baltimore: University Park Press, 1977. Discusses such topics as the pathogenic physiology of protozoa and antiprotozoal agents. Includes bibliographical references and an index.
Schaechter, Moselio, Gerald Medoff, and Barry I. Eisenstein. *Mechanisms of Microbial Disease.* 3d ed. Baltimore: Williams & Wilkins, 1999. New edition of a text presenting the material in a pathobiological framework in the context of clinical cases, a format that lends itself to an active form of studying and problem-based learning. New chapters on microbial genetics, viruses, and AIDS.

Pruritus. *See* Itching

Psoriasis
Disease/disorder
Anatomy or system affected: Skin
Specialties and related fields: Dermatology, internal medicine
Definition: A chronic skin disease in which red, scaly patches develop, overlaid with thick, silvery-gray scales, causing physical discomfort as well as damage to self-esteem.
Key terms:
dermatologist: a physician who treats the skin and its structures, functions, and diseases
dermis: the layer of skin directly beneath the epidermis, consisting of dense connective tissue and numerous blood vessels

epidermis: the outermost part of the skin, composed of four or five different layers called strata

methotrexate: a powerful drug, originally developed to treat cancer, that is used to treat patients with severe cases of psoriasis

psoralens: chemicals found in plants that make the skin more sensitive to light

PUVA: a treatment for psoriasis in which the patient is exposed to ultraviolet A (UVA) light after receiving one of the psoralens

stratum corneum: the outermost layer of the epidermis; its cells are normally dead, hard, and constantly removed by normal bathing

ultraviolet light: invisible light composed of waves that are shorter than the ordinary light waves able to be seen by humans

CAUSES AND SYMPTOMS

Psoriasis is a common skin problem which afflicts approximately two of every hundred people, affecting males and females with relatively equal frequency. Although it affects all races, it is most prevalent among northern Europeans (occurring in about 3 percent of this population), less among the Japanese, and least among African Americans and North American Indians (occurring in 0.5 percent of this population). This stubborn, chronic, and as yet incurable disease most commonly appears in one's teens or twenties, although it can appear in early childhood. While 70 percent of those who develop psoriasis do so by the age of twenty, there is another common danger period in the fifties and sixties, with a large number of patients developing their first symptoms at that time.

There are several different types of psoriasis, making diagnosis difficult. By far the most widespread is the plaque-type; because it accounts for 95 percent of all cases, this type is also called common psoriasis. Plaque-type psoriasis gets its name from the appearance of the patches of affected skin. Each patch resembles a plaque or small disk stuck to the body's surface. These dull, wine-colored patches of abnormal skin are often rounded or oval; they may be very irregular in shape when several nearby patches join together. The surface of each thickened patch is rough and scaly, with the scales ranging in color from red to white to the most typical silvery gray. These psoriatic plaques can be small (the size of coins) or become palm-sized and larger. Whatever their final size, they generally begin as a purple or reddened area the size of a pinhead. The original areas expand in size, usually for a few weeks until they reach a stable phase and stop expanding. The average size of a plaque in the stable phase is between 2 and 3 inches. A patch of stable psoriasis may eventually grow pale, less scaly, and disappear completely, or it may begin to enlarge for no apparent reason. Even those plaques that have disappeared may be reactivated and reappear in the same place at some later time.

Certain parts of the body seem most prone to psoriatic lesions; namely, the elbows, the knees, the scalp, and the lower back. The patches may appear elsewhere, including the genitals and the buttocks, but the face, hands, and feet are rarely affected. Severe cases may cover the entire chest or back. In a few cases, psoriasis is symmetrical, appearing in the same area on the left and right sides of the body simultaneously. The patches are, however, more likely to develop in a very random, scattered manner. Almost 50 percent of patients have lesions on their scalps. When these plaques are very large and widespread, they are difficult to treat and very difficult to hide. Although very uncomfortable, scalp psoriasis does not affect the growth of hair or cause baldness. It can cause a temporary thinning of the hair, but the hair grows normally again once the disease is controlled by medication. About one-third of psoriasis patients have affected fingernails and toenails. The diseased nails show pits or pinpoint indentations, loosening, thickening, and a yellowish discoloration. Surprisingly, in some people the condition remains on the nails alone, never developing elsewhere.

In addition to psoriasis of the nails, there are several rare and unusual types of psoriasis that are quite different from the common or plaque type. These include flexural, guttate, pustular, and erythrodermic psoriasis. Flexural psoriasis appears in folds and creases on the body and is often found on people who are particularly overweight and who are in their mid-forties or older. The patches tend to be very moist rather than scaly and are particularly sore and uncomfortable. Guttable psoriasis consists of an enormous number of highly scattered but minute plaques. It is extremely rare and occurs between the ages of eight and sixteen. Although the spots usually clear up in a few weeks, they sometimes recur or change into the large lesions of common psoriasis. Pustular psoriasis is the only form of the disease that never occurs on the palms of the hands and the soles of the feet. It was named for the yellow or white pus-filled spots that form on the skin and eventually drop off.

These spots form when enormous numbers of white blood cells invade the skin even though there is no infection present and, therefore, no need for these infection-killing cells. Erythrodermic psoriasis literally means "red skin." This very rare condition is so named because the entire body is covered by flaming red patches that do not turn scaly. Since the widespread nature of this condition makes internal temperature control very difficult and dehydration inevitable, it can be very dangerous and may require hospitalization.

Common psoriasis, by comparison, is not dangerous or life-threatening. It is usually not painful and does not even cause itching in most patients. It is, however, very annoying because of its unsightly appearance and its tendency to flare up repeatedly. Once the disease has appeared, it stays with the person for life, improving or worsening periodically. After periods of relative quiet, during which the skin may appear quite normal, patients with psoriasis experience new eruptions and scaling for no apparent reason. Plaques continue to form for a given, unpre-

Common Sites for Psoriasis

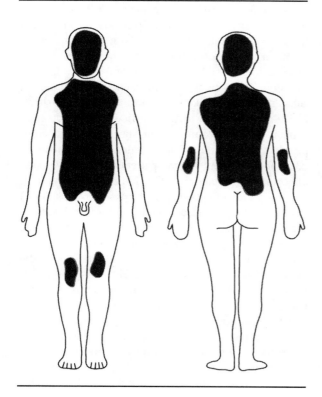

dictable amount of time, until the condition spontaneously quiets down again.

The source of the plaques is a failure in the mechanism by which normal skin renews itself. Ordinarily, the cells at the base of the epidermis reproduce themselves at a slow and steady rate. They then move upward in about twenty-eight days, changing chemically, dying, and detaching from the surface, the stratum corneum. In psoriatic skin, however, there is a huge increase in the number of basal cells in the epidermis, which reproduce so rapidly that they push upward to the surface in only four days, forming thick disks of sticky, abnormal cells. Below the epidermis, the dermis of a patient with psoriasis is also abnormal. Its normally fine blood vessels are wide and extremely twisted, which results in the red appearance of the plaques and causes bleeding to occur easily when the skin is bumped or scratched. An unusually high number of the white blood cells called neutrophils and T lymphocytes are also present. They move up into the epidermis, creating inflammation and swelling within the plaques.

Long before modern dermatology discovered these disturbing facts about the structure and the functioning of psoriatic skin, it was noted that the disease does seem to run in families. If one parent has the problem, there is a one-in-three chance that a child will eventually be afflicted; if both parents have the disease, the risk for their offspring is one in two. With nonidentical twins, there is a 70 percent chance that if one has psoriasis, they both will; with identical twins, the figure can be as high as 90 percent, according to some studies. Investigators suspect that psoriasis is not handed down by a simple pattern, such as with eye color inheritance. It seems more likely that the condition results from a combination of several genetic factors from each parent, much like the manner in which height and intelligence are inherited.

TREATMENT AND THERAPY

More than 90 percent of psoriasis patients can be cleared significantly of their lesions or even made lesion-free by the medicines and methods developed by modern technology. For minor outbreaks, limited to a small area of the body, the first choice for treatment is a corticosteroid cream or ointment applied directly to the plaques. Corticosteroids are hormones, produced by the adrenal glands, that are able to reduce inflammation. Corticosteroids are now produced in the laboratory and combined with other chemicals to reduce inflammation even more effectively by decreasing blood flow to the psoriatic lesions. Dermatologists have a large variety of such preparations ranging from mild to extremely potent. They must find one that is strong enough to suppress the inflammation but not so strong that it causes unwanted side effects.

There are two major undesirable side effects of corticosteroid therapy. Psoriatic skin absorbs all substances more easily than normal skin; the excess hormones enter the bloodstream and can change the output of hormones by the pituitary and adrenal glands, dangerously altering the body's chemical balance. The other danger is to the skin itself, which becomes abnormally thin, easily damaged, and prone to infections. Another drawback to the use of corticosteroids is the tendency for the psoriatic plaques to reappear soon after the creams or ointments are discontinued.

Many patients find relief from a completely different class of medications, those which contain tar. This thick, black, oily liquid is produced from coal. It contains thousands of chemical substances, and biochemists do not know which of those substances actually helps to heal the skin. Tar-containing ointments, creams, gels, shampoos, and bath additives are useful for removing the scales without worrisome side effects. Their major drawback, however, is their tendency to stain clothing, bedding, bathroom tiles, and bathtubs. Some staining can be avoided by covering the treated skin area with bandages, cotton underwear, or a shower cap. In addition to the staining, many patients find the tar odor quite unpleasant; pharmaceutical companies are constantly trying to improve this aspect of these quite effective products.

A third type of preparation is particularly effective for removing very thick scales. These medications contain a compound called salicylic acid. Like the corticosteroids, salicylic acid ointments and gels are most effective when they are in contact with the plaques for a long period of time. After treatment, it is often recommended that patients cover their lesions with plastic gloves, plastic bags (for the feet), or taped-down plastic wrap for four to eight hours.

Patients with psoriasis have noted for years that exposure to the sun is very helpful in clearing their lesions. Daily sunlight exposure is effective for as many as 80 percent of patients. This treatment is relatively accessible for at least part of the year and inexpensive compared to the various medications available. Given the increased risk of skin cancer, it is strongly recommended that patients have repeated but brief sun exposures and avoid sunburn by using creams and lotions. Although sun exposure is helpful to most patients with common psoriasis, it rarely helps and can even worsen the pustulate and erythrodermic types. Since too much exposure to sunlight will damage rather than help any skin, even plaque-type patients are advised to stop their sun exposure once the psoriasis has improved.

For patients in many climates, sunbathing is only possible for a few months of the year. The development of sunlamps for use at home or in a dermatologist's office, hospital, psoriasis care center, or tanning parlor has made this therapy possible all year round. Because of the danger of severe sunburns, sunlamp treatments remain controversial. To reduce their danger, a dermatologist must carefully determine the amount of time of each treatment, the precise distance from the lamp, and the appropriate frequency of treatments for each individual patient to achieve maximal and safe results.

The curative effect of sunlight depends on the presence of the very short wavelength part of the light, called ultraviolet. It is ultraviolet B (UVB) waves that help heal psoriasis, possibly by slowing down the high growth rate of cells in the epidermis. Both natural sunlight and sunlamps contain UVB and, therefore, have the potential to help psoriasis. They also have the potential, however, to burn the skin.

Patients with severe psoriasis may require the use of ultraviolet A (UVA) waves from a special kind of sunlamp. The patient is given a dose of a psoralen, a substance which makes the skin more light-sensitive, and is then exposed to UVA inside a full-body light cabinet. Thirty treatments may be required to completely clear the skin. The psoralen is often given in tablet form, although some patients suffer fewer side effects if it is painted onto the skin or they bathe in it. The early side effects of PUVA (psoralen plus UVA) treatment include nausea, itching, colored blotches on the skin, and occasional worsening of the psoriasis. More worrisome are the possible later side effects: skin cancer and the development of cataracts in the eyes. The danger of developing cataracts also exists from natural sunlight and UVB sunlamps; patients using any light therapy must use excellent sunglasses that block out all rays harmful to the eyes.

For the patient with widespread psoriasis who is not responsive to corticosteroids, tar preparations, or the various light therapies, the drug methotrexate is effective in more than 80 percent of patients. This powerful drug was originally developed to treat various kinds of cancer because it slows down the process of cell multiplication. Thus the psoriatic epidermal cells are prevented from reproducing and forming the scaly plaques. Often methotrexate must be taken for six months or a year, in pill form or by injection, to have a significant impact on an extensive case. Such a dosage poses a risk of numerous and serious side effects, including persistent feelings of sickness, indigestion, and diarrhea. Frequent tests are necessary to monitor the condition of the blood, since methotrexate can interfere with the bone marrow's production of normal blood cells. Most important, periodic liver biopsies, the removal of sample liver cells by means of a special needle, are necessary because methotrexate can cause irreversible damage to this crucial organ. It is very important that a pregnant woman never take methotrexate or that a woman never become pregnant while taking it. The drug's ability to interfere with cell growth can cause many abnormalities in a developing embryo or fetus. Similar fetal abnormalities can be caused by the drugs called retinoids.

For patients with pustular and erythrodermic psoriasis, the retinoids etretinate and acitretin can be very useful, if side effects are carefully monitored. Some dermatologists have been especially successful combining PUVA and etretinate therapies; the improvement in the psoriasis is greater than with either alone, while the lower dosage of each minimizes risk and side effects.

Another medication effective in treating severe psoriasis is cyclosporine. It has brought dramatic improvement to patients with lifelong disabling symptoms. Many people, however, can only tolerate the drug for short periods. Because of its potential to cause high blood pressure and kidney damage, as well as an increased risk of cancer, this medicine is prescribed only with extreme caution.

All the many therapies described can bring partial or total clearing of lesions and even result in the remission of the disease for a period of time. Until the cause of psoriasis is completely understood, however, it is likely that no permanent cure will be developed.

Perspective and Prospects

Descriptions of psoriasis are found in the records of the earliest known civilizations. The term "psora" comes from the ancient Greek language. Psoriasis was considered a form of leprosy in biblical times. Despite this ancient history and extensive modern research, however, the exact cause of psoriasis is still unknown. Unlike many human diseases, psoriasis does not afflict any animals. Therefore, it cannot be studied through controlled laboratory testing.

Early work on psoriasis by dermatologists centered on differential diagnosis. This is the ability to distinguish psoriasis from various rashes caused by fungi, such as ringworm, and from the many forms of eczema or dermatitis caused by allergies. Skin biopsies developed by oncologists can now determine that the condition is not a cancer; the portion of skin removed, when placed under a microscope, will clearly show the dermal and epidermal appearance characteristic of psoriatic skin.

While skin scientists have proven that psoriasis is not contagious, it has been known since the 1930's that many cases develop soon after strep throat and other upper respiratory infections. The bacteria involved are not the cause of the psoriasis, however, but rather a trigger for the development of a condition for which the patient is genetically predisposed. Another trigger, excessive scratching or rubbing of the skin, can precipitate outbreaks in susceptible people; this is named the Koebner phenomenon, for its discoverer. With the help of neurologists and psychologists, it has been proven that the disease is not caused by "nerves." Yet, stress of all kinds is definitely able to make its symptoms worse, and patients must be helped to lower their stress levels if they are to keep the disease under control.

Nutritionists have searched for ways to use diet to help psoriatics, but to no avail. Although no particular foods either help or hinder the course of the disease, most dermatologists now recognize that drinking alcohol can both precipitate and aggravate the disfiguring plaques.

Immunologists have been very involved in the study of psoriasis even though it is not an allergic reaction to any substance in one's environment. In the 1980's, they pursued many possible connections between the streptococci bacteria that cause strep throat, the white blood cells called T lymphocytes that seek to destroy them, and the development of psoriasis. They believe that, in predisposed people, chemicals from the bacteria cause the T lymphocytes to give off substances that trigger the skin's uncontrolled and excessive production of epidermal cells.

Geneticists have been searching diligently for the source of the predisposition to psoriasis. Among the genes children receive from their parents are those that build particular proteins on their white blood cells called HLAs. Out of the hundreds of different HLAs that one can possibly inherit, those who develop psoriasis always seem to possess similar combinations. The identification of the genes responsible for HLAs and the role of those genes in precipitating psoriasis may bring about major improvements in the treatment and possibly a cure for this disease afflicting millions of people throughout the world.

—*Grace D. Matzen*

See also Dermatitis; Dermatology; Eczema; Light therapy; Rashes; Scabies; Skin; Skin disorders; Skin lesion removal.

FOR FURTHER INFORMATION:

Bark, Joseph P. *Skin Secrets*. New York: McGraw-Hill, 1988. This book is written in question-and-answer form and includes all the questions typical patients ask of dermatologists. Solid facts are presented in a lively, interesting style.

Goodman, Thomas. *The Skin Doctor's Skin Doctoring Book*. New York: Sterling, 1984. Provides easily understood explanations of psoriasis and of the various methods and medications used to treat the condition.

Lamberg, Lynne. *Skin Disorders*. Reprint. Philadelphia: Chelsea House, 2001. This brief volume is an introduction to the study of skin problems. Contains very helpful features, including a glossary, a bibliography, and a list of organizations to contact for more information.

Litt, Jerome Z. *Your Skin: From Acne to Zits*. New York: Dembner Books, 1989. Contains a brief but helpful chapter on psoriasis. A useful glossary is included.

Mackie, Rona M. *Clinical Dermatology*. 4th ed. New York: Oxford University Press, 1997. Written for dermatology students but useful to the general public because it offers more precise and detailed information than popular works. Includes color illustrations.

Marks, Ronald. *Psoriasis*. New York: Arco, 1981. An excellent book with clearly worded, detailed information on every aspect of the disease. The author, a dermatologist who has long specialized in the study and treatment of psoriasis, has written a scientifically accurate and very compassionate volume.

Paslin, David. *The Hide Guide: Skin Problems and How to Deal with Them*. Millbrae, Calif.: Celestial Arts, 1981. A clear aid to the recognition, understanding, and treatment of common skin disorders. A highly readable, well-organized, and enjoyable book.

PSYCHIATRIC DISORDERS
DISEASE/DISORDER

ANATOMY OR SYSTEM AFFECTED: Brain, psychic-emotional system

SPECIALTIES AND RELATED FIELDS: Psychiatry

DEFINITION: Clusters of psychological or behavioral symptoms that cause a person to experience serious emotional distress or significant mental impairment; these symptoms must be unusual or unexpected, or the patient must show evidence of more than one behavior that deviates from normal social expectations.

KEY TERMS:

biological model: a way of viewing and understanding psychiatric disorders which emphasizes customary medical practice in identifying and treating a particular disorder from which a person suffers

diagnostic codes: the method used in the *Diagnostic and Statistical Manual of Mental Disorders* (DSM) to record psychiatric diagnoses for statistical and administrative purposes

multiaxial classification: the classification system used in the DSM to account for several factors when making psychiatric diagnoses, including present condition, developmental/personality disorders, physical disorders, life stresses, and overall functioning

neuroscience: the scientific specialization that seeks to understand mental processes, occurrences, and disturbances in terms of underlying mechanisms in the brain and the nervous system

psychodynamic model: a way of viewing and understanding psychiatric disorders which emphasizes the recognition and treatment of underlying psychological and developmental traumas

psychopharmacology: the use of drugs to study effects on brain chemistry; drugs are used to treat mental disorders, study brain chemistry, and promote new disease classifications

psychosocial treatment: a significant specialization in treating people with psychiatric disorders through employing principles of psychology, human behavior, family and group dynamics, and social and occupational learning

somatic treatment: the treatment of people with psychiatric disorders using specialized drugs and electroconvulsive therapy; some major drug groups used are antidepressants, antipsychotics, antimanics, anxiolytics, and psychostimulants

CAUSES AND SYMPTOMS

Physicians who practiced many centuries ago understood that psychiatric disorders such as depression and delirium arose from brain abnormalities. Because the recognition of mental illness came early in its development, medicine has had a profound influence in establishing the biomedical model to define and treat psychiatric disorders. This early medical influence was deepened and broadened by the contribution of neuroscience. Scientists who began studying the brain more intensively, beginning in the late nineteenth century, proved the relationship of brain function to speech, hearing, comprehension, and other important human abilities. Later, the psychodynamic model of understanding the nature of psychiatric disorders began making its contribution, first by promoting the more humane treatment of people with mental illness and then in adding consideration of psychological and social factors when diagnosing patients. Sigmund Freud and other influential psychiatrists broadened the understanding of how emotional pain and trauma experienced during a person's childhood can contribute profoundly to the occurrence and course of mental disorders.

Despite long and exacting efforts to understand mental illness, much remains to be explored. While psychiatrists would prefer to base their diagnoses on knowing the causes and the mechanisms of mental disorders, this knowledge has proved to be elusive. Therefore, most psychiatric diagnoses are based on the psychiatrist recognizing a pattern of symptoms and a typical course of disease. During World War II, psychiatrists learned that their colleagues differed widely in how they recognized and described various mental illnesses. Bureaucratic and professional forces coalesced in a drive to make the diagnosis of psychiatric disorders more systematic. In 1952, the American Psychiatric Association issued a manual which sought to clarify the diagnostic process. Unfortunately, the early manuals proved to be impractical and were largely ignored by psychiatrists. This changed when a more rigorous effort culminated in the publication of the third edition of the *Diagnostic and Statistical Manual of Mental Disorders* (DSM-III) in 1980. This text became widely accepted as the standard reference for psychiatrists to use when diagnosing psychiatric disorders. The manual has been strengthened and revised

several times; a revised fourth edition, known as DSM-IV, was published in 1994. Scientists and clinicians continue their work on the manual to correct flaws, incorporate research findings, and explore new areas. Most psychiatrists have come to agree that standard definitions of psychiatric disorders are needed to clarify their thinking, permit easier communication, improve the ability to predict outcomes, improve treatment planning, and stimulate further research.

When using the DSM-IV, psychiatrists must find that the person presents specific signs and symptoms and has maintained this clinical picture for a sufficient length of time to warrant being diagnosed as having a psychiatric disorder. The DSM-IV assigns a specific code for each psychiatric diagnosis, which facilitates administrative and statistical work. Most are four-digit numbers. The first three indicate a major category of psychiatric disorder, such as affective mood disorder; this is followed by a decimal point, and then another number indicating a more specific illness, such as "Major Depression, Recurrent." A fifth number is added when diagnosing organic mental disorders, schizophrenia, and mood disorders. Additional codes are given when the clinician is unsure of making a specific diagnosis or finds no evidence of a disorder, and V codes are used to indicate significant problems not related to a mental disorder, such as "Marital Problem."

Furthermore, the DSM-IV uses a multiaxial diagnostic system to encourage more complete consideration and recording of important information. Major clinical syndromes are shown on Axis I; Axis II contains information about personality or developmental disorders, personality traits, and disabling defense mechanisms (such as denial); Axis III shows information on any physical disorders that a patient may have that are related to his or her mental condition; Axis IV gives an indication of the amount of psychological and social distress being experienced by a patient; and Axis V contains an assessment of the patient's overall capacity to function.

Several major diagnostic categories of psychiatric disorders are shown in the DSM-IV. These include disorders usually first evident in infancy, childhood, or adolescence; organic mental syndromes and disorders; psychoactive substance abuse disorders; schizophrenia; delusional (paranoid) disorders; psychotic disorders not classified elsewhere; mood disorders; anxiety disorders; somatoform disorders; dissociative disorders; sexual disorders; sleep disorders; factitious disorders; impulse control disorders not classified elsewhere; adjustment disorders; psychological factors affecting physical condition; and personality disorders. This listing demonstrates the breadth of problems that are seen and treated by psychiatrists and other mental health practitioners.

Research shows that, on average, 32 percent of adults in the United States will experience one or more psychiatric disorders during their lives and that 20 percent will have experienced problems related to a diagnosed disorder within the past year. These estimates, based on data collected during an extensive survey conducted in the early 1980's, are somewhat higher than those given previously. The investigator found that the first symptoms of a psychiatric disorder usually begin at a relatively young age; the only exception is cognitive impairment, which increases after the age of seventy.

Researchers learned that people who experience their first symptoms later in life generally have a better chance of recovering, but almost all people who suffer from a psychiatric disorder will experience distressing symptoms for several years. More men than women, the data show, have suffered a psychiatric disorder at some point in life. According to the researchers, the differences in prevalence among the races may be more reflective of survey methods than of ethnic origins. Higher rates of mental illness are found among people who are poor and who fail to complete high school. Where a person lives makes little difference in prevalence rates, unless the person lives in institutional settings such as mental hospitals, nursing homes, and prisons, where rates are high.

Phobias (irrational fears) and alcohol abuse are the most common psychiatric disorders in the United States, according to survey findings, followed by generalized anxiety, major depression, drug abuse, and cognitive impairment (a decrease in a person's ability to perform high-order mental activities such as remembering and learning).

People who suffer from one psychiatric disorder were found by researchers to be at a high risk (60 percent) for having another mental health disorder at some time during their lives. People diagnosed with somatization disorder (in which no medical reason can be found for pain or other physical complaints being experienced), antisocial personality, panic disorder, and schizophrenia are more than 90 percent likely to suffer from another disorder.

TREATMENT AND THERAPY

Making an accurate diagnosis of psychiatric disorders is essential to treating the problem properly, since many can be improved through the application of drug, psychosocial, somatic, and adjunctive therapies. For example, it is said that most people who suffer from major depression can be treated successfully with a course of medication, brief psychotherapy, or a combination of both. The somatic technique of exposing a person each day to a bank of bright lights (light therapy) has been used successfully to treat seasonal affective disorder (depression associated with a specific season, especially winter). Many depressed people and their families have been helped by the adjunctive therapy of participating in a support group.

The use of laboratory tests to clarify psychiatric diagnosis is growing in importance. Only a few disorders can be revealed by laboratory tests, but research is being conducted to validate such testing and to increase its scope and usefulness. Some tests are done routinely to rule out medical problems that may be causing the psychiatric problems the person is experiencing or to ensure that the patient can take needed medication.

Drugs have been used in the United States to treat psychiatric disorders since the early 1950's, and new medications are introduced frequently. The distressing thought disturbances experienced by people suffering from schizophrenia have been treated with antipsychotic drugs. Antipsychotics also are used to treat psychotic symptoms such as the hallucinations and delusions experienced by some people who are suffering from depression or other mood disorders. Nine classes of antipsychotics have been developed. Lithium carbonate is the drug most commonly used to treat people suffering from bipolar disorder, in which patients experience swings in mood from the highs of mania to the lows of depression. Various classes of antidepressants such as tricyclics and monoamine oxidase inhibitors (MAOIs) are used to treat people suffering from depression. Many people experiencing symptoms associated with anxiety disorders have been helped through the use of benzodiazepines and other anxiolytics. Central nervous system stimulants (psychostimulants) are used to treat narcolepsy, a disorder in which people have trouble staying awake. Psychostimulants also are used to treat attention-deficit disorder (ADD) in children, because the stimulants have the paradoxical effect of reducing the behaviors that disrupt classroom work and life at home. The drug decreases excessive physical activity and has been shown to improve the child's attention to adult guidance, increase attention span and memory, and lessen the child's tendency to be distracted from tasks and to act impulsively. The child with ADD also is helped with behavior management techniques and careful control of the child's environment to reduce sources of external stimulation.

Unfortunately, the use of drugs in treating psychiatric disorders is not problem-free. Almost all have side effects that can be serious enough to prevent their use in treatment. Some people must take other prescription drugs that preclude the use of the drug needed to treat the psychiatric disorder. The possibility of overdose by people who have thoughts of taking their lives can limit the use of possibly toxic drugs. Some people are not helped by drug therapy, are reluctant to take drugs, or fail to take drugs properly. For such people, it is fortunate that other forms of treatment can be used.

Many people who suffer from psychiatric illness have been helped by trained psychotherapists, such as psychiatrists, psychologists, social workers, counselors, and members of the clergy. Many forms of psychotherapy are practiced. The aims of psychotherapy can be to help the person deal well with life's stresses and crises, confront and resolve psychological conflict, avoid interpersonal problems, and find more satisfaction and fulfillment in life. Psychotherapy is delivered to individuals, couples, families, and other groups. More emphasis is being placed on conducting psychotherapy only for a limited time, because this approach is preferred by most patients and their insurance companies and because research results support its effectiveness.

Behavioral therapy can be used to help the person to change specific behaviors that cause problems. Behavioral therapy has been used to treat several psychiatric disorders, including alcohol and drug dependence, anxiety, phobia, and eating disorders. Systematic desensitization has been used to help people who have irrational fears. The patient is gradually introduced to the situation that elicits the fearful response and is taught to use relaxation techniques to reduce anxiety and to bring fears under personal control. In behavior modification programs, unwanted behavior is defined, targeted, reduced, and eliminated. At the same time, the person is rewarded for behaving properly.

Electroconvulsive therapy (ECT), formerly called shock therapy, is used generally to treat severely depressed people who fail to respond to less intrusive methods. In ECT, the patient is exposed to an electric current that is passed through electrodes taped to the scalp. The current causes the person to experience a full-blown seizure, usually for less than a minute. This treatment method has been used for many years, and several improvements have been made to make the procedure safer and less damaging to the person's memory. The depressed person usually responds well in fewer than ten ECT sessions.

Treatment of psychiatric disorders is usually delivered in the community where the affected person lives. In the United States, legislation in the 1960's caused federal funds to be used to build and staff community mental health centers. Many health insurance providers will pay part of the fees charged by private therapists, which allows some people to use their services. Alcohol and drug treatment programs generally offer people either short-term residential or outpatient services. Many people are served in institutional settings, such as mental hospitals and nursing homes. Some use services provided by governmental funding.

Many people who have suffered psychiatric disorders recover completely; investigators find a 38 percent remission rate. The researchers were surprised to learn that people are most likely to recover from alcohol and drug abuse, generalized anxiety, and antisocial personality. Complete freedom from distressing symptoms and episodes is less likely for those who suffer from mania, obsessive-compulsive disorder (in which the person performs repetitive rituals such as hand-washing to allay anxiety caused by disturbing thoughts or fears), schizophrenia (a disorder typified by thought disturbances such as hallucinations and delusions, mood changes, communication problems, and unusual behaviors), and phobias.

On the other hand, most people living in the community who suffer mental illness have not been treated. Even in the category most likely to receive treatment, unmarried women who have completed high school, only 27 percent receive treatment. The overall rate of treatment is only 19 percent (14 percent for men and 23 percent for women), a figure that poses a significant problem for those who are concerned with providing adequate mental health care services.

PERSPECTIVE AND PROSPECTS

Early medical documents show that mental illness has always been an area of significant concern. Symptoms of mental illness were described in the Bible, and they were studied and treated in classical times. Interest in understanding mental disorders waned during the medieval period, when it was thought that sufferers were possessed by demons or were being punished by God. Mentally ill people were often maltreated and were sometimes burned as witches. Finally, the foundation was laid in the late sixteenth century for a more complete understanding of psychiatric disorders: In 1586, Timothy Bright, a physician, published the first English-language text on mental illness, entitled *Treatise of Melancholie*.

In late eighteenth century France, Philippe Pinel took over the management of a hospital for insane men and not only advocated more humane treatment of mentally ill people but also took steps to free them from the chains and other punishing devices that they were forced to endure. Pinel instituted the scientific study of mental illness. He tracked the prevalence of mental disorders, conducted studies to learn the natural course of mental illness, and established a treatment model followed by the more progressive psychiatric facilities. Physicians who specialized in the treatment and study of mental illness came to call themselves psychiatrists, and psychiatry became one of the first disciplines in medicine to call itself a specialty.

The brain was studied even more intensely in the nineteenth century. During this era, scientists made important contributions to the understanding of how certain parts in the brain are responsible for specialized functions. They learned that particular brain regions are related to speech and language, movement, sensations, learning, understanding, and emotions. Emil Kraepelin correlated information about the age of onset, natural course, and length of time of particular mental disorders. He used the information that he organized to develop the first classification system of psychiatric disorders. Among the maladies he named were dementia praecox (now called schizophrenia), dementia in the elderly (now called Alzheimer's disease), and manic-depressive illness.

While neuroscientists were making significant contributions to the understanding of the brain, psychiatrist Sigmund Freud was advancing his study of hysteria and its connection with childhood trauma. He used hypnosis and free association to release and resolve underlying traumas and to give the patient lasting freedom from a disabling mental disorder. He also produced theories on psychological function and structure and on psychotherapy.

During the twentieth century, psychiatrists drew on a broad array of disciplines to improve the diagnosis and treatment of psychiatric disorders, including the study of brain chemistry, biology, structure, and functioning. Advances in imaging techniques allowed scientists to study and sometimes diagnose brain dysfunction. Specialized drugs were developed to be used in the treatment of specific mental disorders. Since 1952, the American Psychiatric Association has published a series of diagnostic and statistical manuals designed to bring order to the study, diagnosis, and treatment of psychiatric disorders.

—Russell Williams, M.S.W.;
updated by Nancy A. Piotrowski, Ph.D.

See also Addiction; Alcoholism; Amnesia; Anxiety; Autism; Bipolar disorder; Brain; Delusions; Dementias; Depression; Domestic violence; Eating disorders; Emotions: Biomedical causes and effects; Factitious disorders; Geriatrics and gerontology; Grief and guilt; Hallucinations; Hypochondriasis; Intoxication; Light therapy; Memory loss; Midlife crisis; Neurology; Neurology, pediatric; Neurosis; Neurosurgery; Obsessive-compulsive disorder; Panic attacks; Paranoia; Pharmacology; Phobias; Postpartum depression; Post-traumatic stress disorder; Psychiatry; Psychiatry, child and adolescent; Psychiatry, geriatric; Psychoanalysis; Psychosis; Psychosomatic disorders; Schizophrenia; Sexual dysfunction; Sexuality; Shock therapy; Sibling rivalry; Stress; Stuttering; Suicide.

FOR FURTHER INFORMATION:

Andreasen, Nancy C., and Donald W. Black. *Introductory Textbook of Psychiatry.* 2d ed. Washington, D.C.: American Psychiatric Press, 1995. Designed for use by medical and other students, this book provides basic information on psychiatry, various psychiatric disorders, treatments, and special topics such as suicide, acquired immunodeficiency syndrome (AIDS), and disorders of childhood and adolescence.

Goodwin, Donald W., and Samuel B. Guze. *Psychiatric Diagnosis.* 5th ed. New York: Oxford University Press, 1996. Each chapter in this concise reference is devoted to a separate category of psychiatric disorder. The chapters contain information on prevalence, symptoms, history and nature of the illness, common complications, and treatment methods.

Heston, Leonard L. *Mending Minds: A Guide to the New Psychiatry of Depression, Anxiety, and Other Serious Mental Disorders.* New York: W. H. Freeman, 1992. This text was written expressly for the general reader. The diagnosis, treatment, and typical outcome for several psychiatric disorders are described and illustrated with case histories. Basic information is imparted on how the brain is affected by mental illness, how drug treatment works, and how genetic inheritance relates to mental disorders.

Kaplan, Harold I., and Benjamin J. Sadock, eds. *Kaplan and Sadock's Comprehensive Textbook of Psychiatry VI*. 7th ed. Baltimore: Williams & Wilkins, 2000. A standard text for psychiatry containing an especially helpful section on common signs and symptoms indicating the presence of a psychiatric disorder.

Lickey, Marvin E., and Barbara Gordon. *Medicine and Mental Illness: The Use of Drugs in Psychiatry*. New York: W. H. Freeman, 1991. Assuming no previous knowledge of psychiatry, the authors help the general reader to understand how drugs are used effectively to treat psychiatric disorders. More current findings are included in the discussion of the bases of mental disorders, diagnostic advances, and the use of psychotherapy and drugs in treatment.

Robins, Lee N., and Darrel A. Regier, eds. *Psychiatric Disorders in America: The Epidemiologic Catchment Area Study*. New York: Free Press, 1991. Researchers working for the National Institute of Mental Health collected and analyzed data on twenty thousand people in an effort to define more precisely the prevalence of psychiatric disorders in the United States and the scope of services delivered to people suffering from them.

Psychiatry

Specialty

Anatomy or system affected: All

Specialties and related fields: Critical care, family practice, geriatrics and gerontology, neurology, pharmacology, preventive medicine, public health

Definition: A medical field concerned with the diagnosis, epidemiology, prevention, and treatment of mental and emotional problems.

Key terms:

anxiety disorders: conditions in which physical and emotional uneasiness, apprehension, or fear is the dominant symptom

bipolar disorders: problems marked by mania or mania with depression; historically known as manic-depressive disorders

dementias: disorders characterized by a general deterioration of intellectual and emotional functioning, involving problems with memory, judgment, emotional responses, and personality changes

depressive disorders: problems involving persistent feelings of despair, weight change, sleep problems, thoughts of death, thinking difficulties, diminished interest or pleasure in activities, and agitation or listlessness

personality disorders: pervasive, inflexible patterns of perceiving, thinking, and behaving that cause long-term distress or impairment, beginning in adolescence and persisting into adulthood

psychiatric diagnosis: a clinical labeling process involving the focused study of symptom patterns; physical, emotional, and personality factors; significant relationships; and recent events

psychotic: referring to a disabling mental state characterized by poor reality testing (inaccurate perceptions, confusion, disorientation) and disorganized speech, behavior, and emotional experience

psychotropic drugs: substances primarily affecting behavior, perception, and other psychological functions

schizophrenic disorders: mental disturbances characterized by psychotic features during the active phase and deteriorated functioning in occupational, social, or self-care abilities

Science and Profession

Psychiatrists receive training in biochemistry, community mental health, genetics, neurology, neuropathology, psychopathology, psychopharmacology, and social science. They complete medical school, a four-year residency in psychiatry, and two or more years of specialty residency. Specialty residencies focus on particular treatment methods (such as psychoanalysis) or methods of diagnosis and treatment for particular groups of clients (such as children, adolescents, or elders).

As diagnosticians and treatment providers, psychiatrists must be excellent observers of behavior and be knowledgeable about how nutritional, physical, and situational conditions can be related to mental or emotional problems. An ability to consult with other professionals is also important. Psychiatrists often receive patients from other professionals (general practitioners, psychologists, emergency room staff) and often request diagnostic, legal, case management, and resource advice from other professionals (psychologists, attorneys, social workers). In situations involving abuse, neglect, incompetency, and suicide, such consultation relationships are critical for appropriate referral and treatment.

Given this preparation, psychiatrists are able to diagnose and treat a wide variety of disorders. Some of the most common disorders treated in adult populations include disorders of anxiety (such as phobias, panic attacks, obsessive-compulsive behavior, acute and post-traumatic stress) and mood (e.g. depressive and bipolar problems). Personality, schizophrenic, substance abuse, and dementia-related disorders also are treated frequently by psychiatrists. Such conditions are described in detail in the American Psychiatric Association's *Diagnostic and Statistical Manual of Mental Disorders: DSM-IV-TR* (rev. 4th ed., 2000).

DIAGNOSTIC AND TREATMENT TECHNIQUES

A well-formulated psychiatric diagnosis facilitates treatment planning for mental and emotional disorders. Psychiatric diagnoses, however, are very complex. They are described in a system with five axes of information in order to give a comprehensive picture of how well a person is functioning in everyday life. Axis I pertains to clinical conditions diagnosed in infancy, childhood, or adolescence, as well as other primary mental problems experienced by adults, including cognitive, substance-related, psychotic, anxiety, mood, eating, sleep, impulse control, factitious, somatoform, dissociative, and adjustment disorders. Axis II summarizes problems related to personality and mental retardation. Axis III describes any general medical conditions that are related to a person's mental problems and that may also warrant special attention. Axis IV summarizes psychological, social, and environmental problems that may affect the diagnosis, prognosis, or treatment of a person's mental problems. Axis V is used to give a standardized, overall rating of how well the person has been functioning with his or her disorder.

Once a diagnosis is formulated, a treatment plan is composed. Usually, it involves some combination of medicinal and psychotropic drugs, bibliotherapy, dietary and behavior change recommendations, and psychotherapy for the affected individual or his or her entire family. Treatment compliance is critical, particularly when psychotropic drugs are involved. As such, psychiatric treatment often involves frequent initial contacts and an after-care plan of continued visits with the psychiatrist or a support group able to encourage follow-through on the treatment recommendations.

PERSPECTIVE AND PROSPECTS

The concepts of mental health and illness have been in human cultures since ancient times. As early as 2980 B.C.E., priest-physicians were noted for their treatment of spirit possession involving madness, violence, mutism, and melancholy. In those times, such problems were thought to originate from external, supernatural forces. Later, during the rise of Greco-Roman philosophies in medicine, such states of mind began to be explored more as disturbances of the brain and less as the result of supernatural causes. As such, treatments began to develop greater reliance on methods such as vapors, baths, diets, and emetic and cathartic drugs.

Over time, the field of psychiatry has matured and taken on a major role in medicine. Research into the mind-body relationship has clarified how the mind can influence the healing of medical conditions, as well as how certain medical conditions are rooted in psychological, social, and environmental problems, rather than in a person's biology alone. Additionally, advances in the development of psychotropic drugs have played a major role in the treatment of disabling conditions long thought to be untreatable, such as schizophrenic and bipolar disorders.

In the future, psychiatry is expected to continue developing a broad variety of specialty areas. New techniques for working with children, adolescents, elders, and individuals with particular medical problems or of a particular gender or cultural background are developing rapidly. Finally, understanding the relationship between psychiatric disorders across the life span is likely to increase, as is the need to develop treatments for complex scenarios involving multiple diagnoses.

—*Nancy A. Piotrowski, Ph.D.*

See also Addiction; Aging; Aging: Extended care; Alcoholism; Alzheimer's disease; Amnesia; Anorexia nervosa; Anxiety; Attention-deficit disorder (ADD); Autism; Bipolar disorder; Brain; Brain disorders; Bulimia; Chronic fatigue syndrome; Circumcision, female, and genital mutilation; Delusions; Dementias; Depression; Domestic violence; Eating disorders; Electroencephalography (EEG); Emergency medicine; Emotions: Biomedical causes and effects; Euthanasia; Factitious disorders; Family practice; Fatigue; Geriatrics and gerontology; Grief and guilt; Hallucinations; Hypnosis; Hypochondriasis; Incontinence;

Intoxication; Light therapy; Memory loss; Mental retardation; Midlife crisis; Neurology; Neurology, pediatric; Neurosis; Neurosurgery; Obesity; Obsessive-compulsive disorder; Panic attacks; Paranoia; Pharmacology; Phobias; Postpartum depression; Post-traumatic stress disorder; Psychiatric disorders; Psychiatry, child and adolescent; Psychiatry, geriatric; Psychoanalysis; Psychosis; Psychosomatic disorders; Schizophrenia; Sex change surgery; Sexual dysfunction; Sexuality; Shock therapy; Sleep disorders; Speech disorders; Stress; Stress reduction; Sudden infant death syndrome (SIDS); Suicide; Terminally ill: Extended care.

For Further Information:

American Psychiatric Association. *Diagnostic and Statistical Manual of Mental Disorders: DSM-IV-TR*. Rev. 4th ed. Washington, D.C.: Author, 2000. The bible of the psychiatric community, this is a compendium of descriptions of disorders and diagnostic criteria widely embraced by clinicians. Included is an extensive glossary of technical terms, making this volume easy to understand.

Kass, Frederic I., John M. Oldham, and Herbert Pardes, eds. *The Columbia University College of Physicians and Surgeons Complete Home Guide to Mental Health*. New York: Henry Holt, 1995. This popular work addresses mental health issues within the context of the family. Includes an index.

Mazure, Carolyn, ed. *Does Stress Cause Psychiatric Illness?* Washington, D.C.: American Psychiatric Press, 1995. Twenty contributors discuss recent empirical data relating stress to psychiatric illness and using new models to differentiate types of stress, account for differential responses to stress and the interaction of stressors and psychiatric disorders, and address the neurobiology of stress.

Preston, John, and James Johnson. *Clinical Psychopharmacology Made Ridiculously Simple*. Miami: MedMaster, 1990. Provides a preview of clinical psychopharmacology. Includes general principles, depression, bipolar illness, anxiety disorders, psychotic disorders, miscellaneous disorders, nonresponse and "breakthrough symptoms" algorithms, and case examples. Designed for undergraduates.

Tomb, David. *Psychiatry*. 6th ed. Baltimore: Williams & Wilkins, 1999. Designed for the house officer, this handbook covers the psychological manifestations of general diseases and other aspects of mental illness. Includes bibliographical references and an index.

PSYCHIATRY, CHILD AND ADOLESCENT
SPECIALTY

ANATOMY OR SYSTEM AFFECTED: All

SPECIALTIES AND RELATED FIELDS: Critical care, family practice, neurology, pharmacology, preventive medicine, public health

DEFINITION: The branch of psychiatry concerned with the mental and emotional health and development of infants and teenagers.

KEY TERMS:

development: the process of progressive change that takes place as one matures from birth to death; development can be gradual, as on a continuum, or ordered, as in distinctly different stages

disorder: a persistent or repetitive maladaptive pattern in thinking, behaving, or feeling that necessitates treatment

mental retardation: a condition characterized by a below-average intelligence quotient (IQ) and deficits in adaptive functioning before the age of eighteen years; the degree of retardation ranges from mild to severe

normal: a term of reference that can mean average (as in statistically normal), functional (as in adaptive), or socially appropriate (as in within cultural bounds of acceptability)

SCIENCE AND PROFESSION

Specialists in child and adolescent psychiatry are responsible for the physical and mental health of the individuals whom they treat. They must be acute ob-

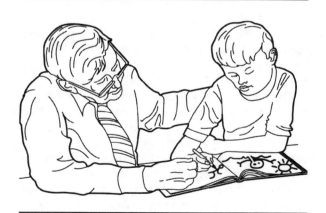

Psychiatrists who treat children may have to use different methods of evaluating the patient's emotional and mental problems, such as asking the child to create drawings that illustrate feelings and states of mind.

servers of individual and family behavior, as well as knowledgeable about how certain nutritional, physical, and situational conditions can manifest themselves as mental or emotional problems. Particularly with infants, this requires keen knowledge of normal and abnormal development, both mental and physical. Additionally, these specialists must be able to consult with a variety of medical and other professionals—from psychologists, who provide behavioral and diagnostic assessments, to social work professionals and lawyers, when child abuse or neglect enters into the clinical picture.

Practitioners in child or adolescent psychiatry receive extensive training. First, they must complete medical school in order to obtain a doctorate in medicine. Next, they must complete a four-year residency in psychiatry and a two-year specialty residency in child psychiatry. Finally, they must go through licensing and certification procedures in order to practice independently.

This training prepares them to diagnose and treat the wide variety of psychiatric disorders experienced by children and adolescents. Anxiety, attention-deficit/hyperactivity, autistic, conduct, learning, mental retardation, mood, oppositional-defiant, pervasive developmental, and substance abuse disorders are some of the most well researched disorders in children. Other problems include asthma, bed-wetting or bed-soiling, child abuse and neglect, conflicts related to sexuality, eating disorders, elective mutism, epilepsy, fire-setting and vandalism, identity disorders, personality disorders, school difficulties, schizoid disorders, sleep-walking, sleep terror, stuttering, and tantrums. Disorders such as these are described in detail in the American Psychiatric Association's *Diagnostic and Statistical Manual of Mental Disorders: DSM-IV-TR* (rev. 4th ed., 2000).

DIAGNOSTIC AND TREATMENT TECHNIQUES

Practitioners of child and adolescent psychiatry are generally introduced to their patients via the parents or an intervening medical professional or agency. In most cases, these specialists diagnose disorders through clinical interviews with the patient, the patient's parents, and sometimes even schoolteachers or other observers of relevant problems. Additionally, diagnoses are sometimes confirmed via a patient's response to drugs (such as Ritalin, antidepressants, or lithium carbonate) or via test results from a psychological or behavioral assessment. Some assessments are based on structured, pencil-and-paper tests that measure intelligence or other personal attributes. Others are based on direct observations of the patient and/or family interactions.

Once a diagnosis is made, practitioners provide therapy to the individual child or adolescent and/or to the entire family. Acute or severe problems might be treated in a hospital setting, while chronic or mild problems might be treated on an outpatient basis. Therapies typically selected include medicinal and psychotropic drugs, dietary recommendations, behavioral therapies and parent training, family therapy, play therapy, and individual psychotherapy. In these situations, a good practitioner will try to involve the child in the process of consent to treatment so as to facilitate trust and gain compliance from the child.

Finally, practitioners in this specialty area perform two other important functions. First, in some cases, no disorder is present, and the psychiatrist provides normative information about child and adolescent growth and development. Second, these professionals must provide protection to suspected victims of abuse or neglect. In such cases, the psychiatrist must report these suspicions to the appropriate authorities, initiate referral to social service agencies, and protect the children or adolescents as necessary.

PERSPECTIVE AND PROSPECTS

Work by Sigmund Freud, the Austrian physician and founder of psychoanalysis, marked the birth of this field of study. By focusing his work on the relationship between childhood experiences and adult functioning, Freud was able to foster interest in child development and welfare. Issues such as family relationships; the emotional, physical, and sexual mistreatment of children; and differences in the way that children and adults perceive and experience the world became highlighted through his work and that of those who followed. Finally, in 1959, child psychiatry became a specialty certified by the American Board of Psychiatry and Neurology, adding credibility and importance to this growing field of practice and research.

Today, child and adolescent psychiatry remains in its infancy compared to other specialties. Relationships between childhood and adult disorders continue to be explored through a variety of epidemiological, genetic, psychiatric, and behavioral studies. Prime topics include connections among attention-deficit/hyperactivity, mood, learning, and a broad spectrum of developmental disorders. Similarly, interest in understanding how trauma, neglect, and family influences relate to childhood mood, learning, and substance abuse disorders is also increasing.

Innovative drug and psychotherapeutic strategies are being explored for the disorders described above. The greatest treatment advances should be expected in the development and application of new drug therapies for childhood and adolescent psychiatric disorders. Further, refinement of behavioral assessment and management strategies for both school and home environments are likely to contribute greatly to this progress. Finally, because this specialty faces growing challenges posed by long-term childhood medical disorders, such as cancer, it is likely that interventions will be improved specifically to meet these needs.

—*Nancy A. Piotrowski, Ph.D.*

See also Addiction; Alcoholism; Amnesia; Anorexia nervosa; Anxiety; Attention-deficit disorder (ADD); Autism; Bipolar disorder; Brain; Brain disorders; Bulimia; Chronic fatigue syndrome; Circumcision, female, and genital mutilation; Dementias; Depression; Domestic violence; Eating disorders; Electroencephalography (EEG); Emergency medicine; Emotions: Biomedical causes and effects; Factitious disorders; Family practice; Fatigue; Grief and guilt; Hallucinations; Hypnosis; Hypochondriasis; Incontinence; Intoxication; Light therapy; Memory loss; Mental retardation; Neurology; Neurology, pediatric; Neurosis; Neurosurgery; Obesity; Obsessive-compulsive disorder; Panic attacks; Paranoia; Pediatrics; Pharmacology; Phobias; Psychiatric disorders; Psychiatry; Psychoanalysis; Psychosis; Psychosomatic disorders; Schizophrenia; Sexuality; Shock therapy; Sleep disorders; Speech disorders; Stress; Stress reduction; Suicide; Terminally ill: Extended care.

FOR FURTHER INFORMATION:

American Psychiatric Association. *Diagnostic and Statistical Manual of Mental Disorders: DSM-IV-TR.* Rev. 4th ed. Washington, D.C.: Author, 2000. Provides comprehensive descriptions of mental disorders, as well as a glossary of technical terms.

Kass, Frederic I., John M. Oldham, and Herbert Pardes, eds. *The Columbia University College of Physicians and Surgeons Complete Home Guide to Mental Health.* New York: Henry Holt, 1995. This popular work addresses mental health issues within the context of the family. Includes an index.

Turecki, Stanley, and Leslie Tonner. *The Difficult Child.* Rev. ed. New York: Bantam Books, 1989. Provides information on childhood behavior problems.

PSYCHIATRY, GERIATRIC
SPECIALTY

ANATOMY OR SYSTEM AFFECTED: All

SPECIALTIES AND RELATED FIELDS: Critical care, family practice, geriatrics and gerontology, neurology, pharmacology, preventive medicine, public health

DEFINITION: A subspecialty of psychiatry which deals with the diagnosis and treatment of psychiatric syndromes experienced by older people.

KEY TERMS:

acute confusion syndrome: a transient condition caused by the action of various biological stressors on vulnerable older persons, who may experience inattention, disorganized thinking, other cognitive impairments, and emotional problems

anxiety: a condition characterized by nervousness or agitation; in older people, it is often caused by the existence of a psychiatric disorder such as depression, a general medical condition such as hypothyroidism, or a side effect of medication

depression: a condition characterized by a persistent mood of sadness, weight loss, greatly decreased interest in life, and sometimes psychotic episodes; biological factors, family history of depression, underlying medical problems, and medication side effects all can contribute to these symptoms

hypochondriasis: a condition in which the patients believe strongly that they are suffering from one or more serious illnesses, even when this belief is unsupported by medical evidence

insomnia: disturbed sleep, which occurs in older people more often than in any other age group; insomnia in older people can be caused by many factors, such as dysfunctional sleep cycles, breathing problems, leg jerking, underlying medical and psychiatric disorders, and the side effects of medication

memory loss syndrome: a condition in which a person gradually but progressively loses capacity in many cognitive areas, but especially in the ability to remember; Alzheimer's disease is considered the most common factor causing serious memory loss in older people

suspiciousness: a range of symptoms from increasing distrust of others to paranoid delusions of conspiracies; changes related to aging are thought to be major factors causing increased suspiciousness in older people

SCIENCE AND PROFESSION

Growing numbers of old and very old people and the increased complexity of diagnosis and treatment of this age group have driven the growth of geriatric psychiatry. Psychiatrists who specialize in working with the geriatric population note that the psychiatric problems experienced by older people often fit poorly in the diagnostic categories set down in the *Diagnostic and Statistical Manual of Mental Disorders: DSM-IV-TR* (rev. 4th ed., 2000). The interplay among declining physical health, decreasing mental functioning, social withdrawal and isolation, and vulnerability to stress makes proper diagnosis and appropriate treatment more difficult. In response to this complexity, practitioners of geriatric psychiatry tend to take a broader approach to diagnosis and to use an interdisciplinary model in developing a treatment plan. The profession of geriatric psychiatry has developed most in Great Britain and Canada but is attracting growing numbers of practitioners in the United States and other Western countries.

DIAGNOSTIC AND TREATMENT TECHNIQUES

Geriatric psychiatrists tend to follow the lead of specialists in geriatric medicine, who have found that taking a syndromal approach to diagnosis appears to work better with older patients. Among the psychiatric syndromes used by geriatric psychiatrists are acute confusion, anxiety, depression, hypochondriasis, insomnia, memory loss, and suspiciousness. Special attention must be given by geriatric psychiatrists to the older person's overall ability to function, general health status, social support system, family history, and preexisting conditions. Geriatric psychiatrists are forced to acknowledge the role played by changes in the brain as it ages and to separate changes that are relatively benign from those that pose real threats to the patient. Hospitalization and significant medical intervention tend to occur more often in the later stages of a person's life, and geriatric psychiatrists are aware that these events can have a great impact on the patient's mental well-being.

When they can, geriatric psychiatrists draw readily upon the help of other health care providers in treating the older person, including the use of specially qualified clinical psychologists, social workers, nurses, occupational therapists, speech pathologists, dietitians, and physical therapists. Improving the understanding of family members and providing them with supportive advice and services can be an important part of the overall treatment plan.

PERSPECTIVE AND PROSPECTS

In the United States, federal funding has expanded for qualified providers, such as clinical psychologists and social workers, to render mental health services to older people, especially those who live in long-term care facilities. Funds have increased for the proper training of those who provide mental health services to older people. Examinations have been established to show evidence of "added qualifications" in geriatric medicine and psychiatry. More textbooks and specialty journals devoted to geriatric mental health are now in circulation. The federal government has sponsored important national conferences on various aspects of geriatric mental health. With the costs of hospital and long-term care continuing to rise, more emphasis has been given to preventive services and day care services.

Furthermore, some hospitals have established specialized geropsychiatric units to improve diagnosis and treatment and to decrease the time that older people spend in the hospital. Services are expected to increase for adult children who care for older parents with mental illnesses. Research efforts have increased concerning the causes and appropriate treatment of psychiatric problems in older people. Older people are becoming healthier as they learn more about how mental health and physical health are affected by the way in which one lives: Older people are advised to stop smoking, eat a better diet, exercise more, and continue to take an active part in family and community life. All these trends are expected to continue in the future.

—*Russell Williams, M.S.W.*

See also Addiction; Aging; Aging: Extended care; Alcoholism; Alzheimer's disease; Amnesia; Anxiety; Bipolar disorder; Brain; Brain disorders; Chronic fatigue syndrome; Delusions; Dementias; Depression; Domestic violence; Electroencephalography (EEG); Emergency medicine; Emotions: Biomedical causes and effects; Euthanasia; Factitious disorders; Family practice; Fatigue; Geriatrics and gerontology; Grief and guilt; Hallucinations; Hypnosis; Hypochondriasis; Incontinence; Intoxication; Light therapy; Memory loss; Mental retardation; Neurology; Neurosis;

Neurosurgery; Obesity; Obsessive-compulsive disorder; Panic attacks; Paranoia; Pharmacology; Phobias; Psychiatric disorders; Psychiatry; Psychoanalysis; Psychosis; Psychosomatic disorders; Schizophrenia; Sexual dysfunction; Sexuality; Shock therapy; Sleep disorders; Speech disorders; Stress; Stress reduction; Suicide; Terminally ill: Extended care.

FOR FURTHER INFORMATION:
Birren, James E., R. Bruce Sloane, and Gene D. Cohen, eds. *Handbook of Mental Health and Aging.* 2d ed. New York: Academic Press, 1992. This is a new edition of a handbook of authoritative reviews and reference sources to the scientific and professional literature on the biological, social, and behavioral aspects of aging. Designed for mental health professionals, researchers, and advanced students.

Busse, Ewald, and Dan G. Blazer, eds. *The American Psychiatric Press Textbook of Geriatric Psychiatry.* 2d ed. Washington, D.C.: American Psychiatric Press, 1996. Revised from the 1989 edition not only to incorporate new scientific knowledge but also to expand the coverage from mental disorders that occur late in life to normal age changes and relevant topics from biomedical and behavioral disciplines.

Whitbourne, Susan Krauss. *Psychopathology in Later Adulthood.* New York: Wiley, 2000. Combining theory, research, and case examples, this book explores both the physical and cognitive changes that occur as adults age. Each chapter focuses on a specific disorder and includes a relevant clinical case study, which is integrated into the substantive content.

PSYCHOANALYSIS
PROCEDURE
ANATOMY OR SYSTEM AFFECTED: Psychic-emotional system

SPECIALTIES AND RELATED FIELDS: Psychiatry

DEFINITION: A psychotherapeutic technique, developed by Sigmund Freud, in which the analyst helps the patient to uncover and resolve unconscious conflicts in order to treat personality disorders and/or deviance.

KEY TERMS:
classical psychoanalysis: the method developed by Freud to help patients achieve insight into why they develop maladaptive ways of relating to others and experience disabling psychological symptoms

dreams: warnings sent from the superego to protect the ego from id impulses

instinctual drives: libido (the seeking of gratification of sexual impulses) and aggression (the seeking of gratification of destructive impulses)

neurosis: a psychic disturbance and defect from childhood that develops into a particular pattern of emotional illness and dysfunctional behavior

Oedipus complex: the experience of having sexual feelings toward the parent of the opposite sex, which is found in young children

psyche: the human mind, which according to Freud is divided into id, ego, and superego; the id contains instincts and repressed feelings, the ego directs everyday behavior, and the superego guides the ego

psychoanalyst: a person, usually a psychiatrist, who has received several years of postgraduate training and supervised practice in using psychoanalysis to diagnose and treat clients

psychosis: a condition occurring when a person's id impulses chronically defeat the control of the ego; schizophrenia and bipolar disorder are two examples of psychoses

transference: the tendency of a person who developed unsatisfying parental relationships to repeat this pattern unconsciously with others; psychoanalytic treatment depends on the development of transference between client and analyst

THE THEORETICAL BASIS OF PSYCHOANALYSIS
Psychoanalysis is a method that is used to understand the workings of the human mind. Adherents to psychoanalysis believe that many forces operate to influence and shape the mind, including some that exist beneath the level of conscious awareness and control. Psychoanalysis permits scientists to observe and collect information about the mind, to develop and test scientific hypotheses about mental processes, and to use the scientific wisdom gained to diagnose and treat mental illnesses. Psychoanalytic theory helps psychiatrists and other mental health practitioners understand more about human emotions and psychological development. Though many psychoanalytic concepts were first developed only in the late nineteenth century, psychoanalysis has made significant and lasting contributions to modern psychiatry and continues to enhance its development.

The precepts of psychoanalysis have been subjected to much scientific scrutiny and criticism. As befits any scientific discipline, psychoanalytic theory has been revised periodically to account for new information, observations, and insights. Psychoanalytic theory also is seen as contributing to other scientific disciplines, such as neurology, the social sciences, and psychology. Psychoanalysis has also broadened understanding in the humanities, the arts, philosophy, ethics, and religion. Psychoanalysis clearly has had a profound and lasting impact upon a broad span of human interests and activities.

Psychoanalytic theory is largely a product of the efforts of Sigmund Freud (1856-1939) to link the physical processes of the human brain with the psychological manifestations of the human mind. While Freud was frustrated in his ultimate goal of demonstrating clearly the relationship between the two, his work informs the same search today. Therefore, an understanding of early and evolving psychoanalytic theory remains important to psychiatry and psychotherapy.

To begin developing an understanding of the complexities of psychoanalysis, one needs to be armed with basic information about psychoanalytic theory. The discussion which follows will touch on instinctual drives, the architecture of the mind, psychological development, mental defense mechanisms, and the psychoanalytic classification of mental illness.

Human behavior is driven from early infancy on by the operation of basic instincts. Freud believed that the primitive and evolving physical needs of humans stimulate instinctual drives. He said instincts possess four essential characteristics: source, impetus, aim, and object. Instincts arise from a particular bodily area, generate varying amounts of energy, aim for gratification, and are directed at particular objects, such as other people. Libido, one of these instincts, drives humans to seek pleasure and provides gratification during all the several stages of human development, beginning with the infant sucking at the mother's breast. Later in his work, Freud expressed his belief that humans possess an aggressive instinct, which appears to be aimed at the destruction of the self and others. His formulation of dual and dueling instincts, as with much of his work, continues to evoke controversy in psychoanalytic circles.

Freud believed that the libido instinct is expressed early in life and continues to be expressed during several stages as a prelude to mature psychosexual development. Infants first experience the oral stage, which centers on feeding. Libido is gratified during the act of nursing, and success experienced at this stage helps the infant develop a sense of trust and self-reliance. Older infants proceed to the anal stage, centering on the retention and expulsion of feces and urine. Successful experience during the anal stage equips children with what they need to develop personal autonomy, independence, guiltless initiative, self-assurance, and willingness to cooperate. Children then move to the phallic stage, finding a new interest in genitalia. Freud's theories about this stage are controversial, and many have been repudiated. He said that the penis holds the interest of both sexes, but girls form an early sense of inadequacy when they see that they do not have one (penis envy). Early sexual feelings are directed, according to Freud, toward the parent of the opposite sex (Oedipus complex). Parents regard these feelings as unacceptable and send signals to the children, who must repress their sexual urges. Boys act out of fear of castration, while girls act out of fear of loss of parental love and of envy of the boy's penis. Children who successfully negotiate this stage are said to have developed a firm basis for sexual identity, uninhibited curiosity, a sense of mastery, and the formation of conscience. Next comes the latency period, from ages five to thirteen, during which previous attainments are integrated and consolidated. Key elements of adaptive behavior develop during this stage. The teenage years are said to be spent in the genital stage, during which the child separates gradually from dependence on parents and begins to attach to new love objects and more mature interests. This stage culminates successfully in a sense of personal identity and acceptance.

Through Freud's study of and work with hysteria, a condition in which emotional conflicts are transformed into bodily maladies, he became convinced that the human mind contains dynamic forces that often oppose one another. For example, a person who experiences significant trauma in early childhood, and the painful emotions that attend it, can mentally oppose or repress memories of the trauma and the traumatic emotions. The repressed memories and emotions remain embedded in the unconscious regions of the mind until they are revived and reexperienced when stimulated by a later event. Thus, the force of emotional material that was repressed but never forgotten can exceed the force used by the conscious mind to hold the memories at bay. The concepts of repression and the needful recognition of repressed material continue to be important principles guiding psychoanalysis.

Freud conceived of the human mind as having three parts: id, ego, and superego. The basic instincts and repressed Oedipal urges of human beings reside in the id. Freud saw the id as a totally undifferentiated mass of energy, constantly seeking gratification without the constraints of reality or morality. In contrast, he saw the ego as being well organized, governed by an accurate perception of the external environment, and honoring certain principles of socially acceptable behavior. The ego seeks to form gratifying relationships with other people. At the same time, the ego must defend itself against the primitive urges of the id. The superego is the last division of the mind to form, which it does through successful resolution of the Oedipus conflict. It forms what is called the conscience and imposes control through guilt. The superego often operates during dreams, Freud said, sending warnings when the ego fails to defend properly against id impulses. Most work of the id and the superego is carried out unconsciously, while much of the ego's work operates at the conscious level.

After Freud had seen his theories confirmed in his clinical and personal experience, he felt comfortable in setting out his thoughts on psychopathology. Among the disorders that he identified were various types of neuroses, phobias, perversions, character disorders, personality disorders, psychoses, hypochondriasis, depressive states, and schizophrenia. He believed that mental illness is caused mainly by intrapsychic conflicts that are poorly managed by the mind or by abnormal mental processes and structures.

INDICATIONS AND PROCEDURES

In relation to medical science and, more specifically, to psychiatry, psychoanalysis is used to diagnose and treat emotional illness.

In diagnosis, psychoanalysts have purposes that differ considerably from those of general psychiatry. The analyst uses diagnosis to determine the patient's potential for analysis, the usefulness of analysis in treating the particular emotional problem experienced by the patient, the patient's level of incapacity, the likelihood that the patient will improve, and the likelihood that the analyst will be able to understand and help the patient. Other mental health specialists typically compare the signs and symptoms demonstrated or described by the patient to those catalogued in one of the editions of the American Psychiatric Association's *Diagnostic and Statistical Manual of Mental Disorders* (DSM) and assign a diagnosis which best fits the patient. The psychoanalytic approach to diag-

nosis, conversely, is based on what the analyst can learn about the patient's inner experiences, especially unconscious conflicts and fantasies.

Psychoanalysis is considered to be the treatment of choice for younger adults suffering from chronic emotional illness not helped by less intensive therapies. People who suffer from hysteria, obsessive-compulsive neuroses, sexual perversions, and certain personality disorders are seen as the best candidates for psychoanalysis. To be considered for psychoanalysis, patients must demonstrate an ability to develop a reasonably good relationship with an analyst and must be willing and able to withstand a long, intensive course of treatment. Psychoanalysis is also expensive, and patients must be able to pay for treatment. Some, but not all, third-party payers will bear part of the cost of psychoanalysis; unfortunately, third-party review of the case compromises analyst-patient confidentiality. Patients who are psychotic or who are alcoholics or drug addicts are considered poor candidates for psychoanalysis. Older adults may have personalities too rigid to tolerate analysis, and others have illness too minor to justify such treatment. Patients who are chronically and deeply depressed may be unsuitable candidates for analysis, as are those who have failed to establish appropriate relationships with both parents. Patients must be deemed able not only to enter analysis but also to tolerate termination of therapy. Patients who need urgent intervention to preserve health and life are not good candidates for analysis; neither are those who have little opportunity to make changes in their lives. Because many factors enter into consideration, analysts give some patients a trial period of analysis before accepting them for treatment.

When a patient enters into psychoanalysis, the patient and analyst must resolve certain practical issues, such as setting up appointment times, payment schedules, and other policy matters. The patient must be willing to spend an hour a day, four or five days a week, for as long as five years to complete analysis.

The analyst and patient must be able to form a therapeutic relationship secure enough to withstand the test of time and the stress of treatment. Early on, the patient and analyst must endure as the patient anxiously defends the ego and resists plunging into deeper emotional material. Eventually, so-called transference neurosis emerges. Patients reexperience and often project onto the analyst infantile desires and conflicts. The process of returning to more primitive emotional states is called regression, and analysts must be skillful in helping the patient to avoid its inherent dangers.

Free association is used to deepen the regression. The analyst instructs the patient to talk freely about issues of current concern and to continue talking about whatever associations come into the patient's awareness, making no effort to censor or restrain the monologue. Despite a patient's apparent willingness to follow the analyst's direction, the patient's resistance to uncovering certain material begins to be demonstrated with silences, pauses, stammers, corrections, slips of the tongue, and so on. The analyst remains alert to these signals of resistance, as the shape of the resistance shows the nature of the neurosis. The analyst gives interpretations of the resistance and related unconscious material; for progress to be made, the interpretation must be accurate, and the patient must accept and make use of it. The patient must work through painful emotional conflicts and find ways to resolve them more satisfactorily. "Working through" consumes much of the time spent in analysis.

The analyst often employs several psychological maneuvers to help patients during analysis. The analyst might offer suggestions, in an effort to induce a mental state which opposes the patient's experiences, expectations, or concept of reality. For example, the analyst may assure the patient that working through repressed emotions will enable the patient to enjoy a more productive life. The analyst may manipulate the patient to facilitate recovery of or to neutralize early unconscious material. The analyst can help the patient by clarifying material that the patient may know only in a semiconscious, disorganized way. The term "countertransference" describes the variety of responses felt by the analyst toward the patient; the analyst must resolve such feelings satisfactorily in order to continue the analytic process.

Dreams are said to be the "royal road to the unconscious," and the analyst will often encourage the patient to recall dreams experienced the preceding night. Dreams not only process waking experiences but often offer clues as to unconscious reactions, wishes, and conflicts as well. The analyst offers interpretations of the dreams in order to bring unconscious material and patterns to the conscious awareness of the patient.

The couch on which the patient reclines during sessions is a trademark of psychoanalysis; it is used rarely in any other form of psychotherapy. The analyst typically is positioned outside the visual range of the patient. This arrangement is considered to be essential in encouraging regression and projection.

As the patient and analyst struggle together to help the patient bring repressed material into awareness, the patient may achieve greater self-understanding and increased ability to find more satisfactory resolutions to emotional conflicts.

The analyst begins to prepare the patient for termination, as the active phase of the analysis comes to a close. Patients must be weaned well from dependence on the analyst and the analytic situation. While the patient may have relived and worked through many primitive wishes and conflicts, the continuing work of resolving conflicts as they arise rests primarily with the patient's ability to work through them independently.

The outcome of psychoanalysis can be difficult to evaluate, but success has been defined as having helped a patient improve adjustment to life, realize a certain amount of contentment, give happiness to others, deal more confidently with inevitable stresses, and maintain mutually satisfying relationships with others. In addition, the patient should experience a reduction in neurotic suffering and inhibitions, have fewer dependency needs, have increased potential for success in all significant areas of life, and function at a more mature level.

PERSPECTIVE AND PROSPECTS

Psychoanalysis was born in the wake of evidence that hysteria can be caused by repressed memories or unconscious wishes. People who suffer from hysteria, now known as conversion disorder, develop physical symptoms such as paralysis or blindness in an otherwise healthy body. Sigmund Freud was influenced by the work of French neurologist Jean-Martin Charcot (1825-1893) and fellow Viennese physician Josef Breuer (1842-1925), both of whom were trying to find effective treatments for hysteria. Charcot relied on the use of hypnosis, while Breuer allowed patients to empty their minds, in an early version of free association. In 1895, Breuer and Freud published accounts of their theories and successful cures of patients suffering from hysteria. Freud also was influenced by the work of others on the hierarchy of the nervous system, philosophical concepts of the unconscious mind, posthypnotic suggestion, and the organization of the brain. He was a prolific author and teacher who fostered the careers of several followers.

Many of those who learned from and were influenced by Freud later developed their own variations or new areas of emphasis within Freudian psychoanalysis. Closer study of the role of the ego in emotional disorders led to the development of ego psychology, which enhanced the understanding of the defense, coping, and adaptive mechanisms of the ego. Others chose to emphasize the role of parents and other significant early childhood caregivers in the subsequent development of emotional health and illness. Still others developed what is known as self-psychology, a variant which emphasizes the importance of a person's cohesive sense of self and emotional well-being; the sense of self is either fostered or hindered by interpersonal relationships formed throughout life. Other variants that draw on the psychoanalytical principle include psychodynamic, insight-oriented, relationship, and supportive psychotherapies. Marital, group, and family therapy also depend heavily on an understanding and application of psychoanalytical theory. Generally speaking, most psychotherapeutic interventions used today are grounded in the psychoanalytic precepts developed by Freud and refined by students of his work.

Classical psychoanalysis is still practiced in the United States, but its use is limited by the relatively few properly trained analysts, the time and expense involved in the treatment process, the lack of widely accepted proof of its superiority as a treatment method, and the demand for brief intervention by patients of psychotherapy and those who pay for it. Modern practitioners of psychoanalysis are concerned by several trends: the ascendence of biological approaches to understanding and treating mental illness, the unwillingness of insurers to pay for psychoanalysis, the growing number of nonphysician analysts, the growing skepticism about its effectiveness, and the establishment of a universal system of psychiatric diagnosis which largely ignores the psychoanalytic perspective.

—*Russell Williams, M.S.W.*

See also Brain; Depression; Emotions, biomedical causes and effects; Hypochondriasis; Neurosis; Obsessive-compulsive disorder; Phobias; Psychiatric disorders; Psychiatry; Psychiatry, child and adolescent; Psychiatry, geriatric; Psychosis; Schizophrenia; Sibling rivalry.

For Further Information:

American Psychiatric Association. Commission on Psychiatric Therapies. *The Psychiatric Therapies.* Washington, D.C.: Author, 1984. Addresses a goal set by the American Psychiatric Association to collect information on psychotherapies in use in the United States. Psychoanalysis is discussed in the section on psychosocial therapies, and psychoanalytic theory is shown elsewhere to be crucial in understanding sexual dysfunction. Another section deals with evaluating psychotherapies.

Clark, Ronald. *Freud, the Man and the Cause.* New York: Random House, 1980. A biography of Sigmund Freud, the founder of psychoanalysis. Presents material uncovered since the publication in the late 1950's of a biography by Freud's protégé Ernest Jones. The reader learns how Freud's own childhood experiences shaped him as he became one of the most influential thinkers of modern times.

Gay, Peter. *Freud: A Life for Our Time.* New York: W. W. Norton, 1988. The author's discussion of Freud's development and revision of his psychoanalytic theories and techniques is particularly valuable for the general reader, who will also appreciate the wealth of detail illuminating significant aspects of Freud's life and the concerns of his time.

Kaplan, Harold I., and Benjamin J. Sadock, eds. *Kaplan and Sadock's Comprehensive Textbook of Psychiatry VI.* 7th ed. Baltimore: Williams & Wilkins, 2000. Contains information on the development of psychoanalysis by Freud, psychoanalytic theory and application, and the development and use of psychoanalytic theory by other pioneers in psychiatry.

Mishne, Judith M. *The Evolution and Application of Clinical Theory: Perspective from Four Psychologies.* New York: Free Press, 1993. The book is intended for use in teaching psychotherapeutic theory and practice. The text introduces four powerful models used for understanding personality: traditional psychoanalysis, ego psychology, self-psychology, and object relations theory.

Psychosis

Disease/disorder

Anatomy or system affected: Psychic-emotional system

Specialties and related fields: Psychiatry

Definition: The most severe mental disorder, in which the individual loses contact with reality and suffers from such symptoms as delusions and hallucinations.

CAUSES AND SYMPTOMS

The individual with a psychosis displays disordered thinking, emotion, and behavior. The individual fails to make sense of his or her surroundings, reacts inaccurately to them, and develops false thoughts or ideas about them. The resulting behavior can be described as peculiar, abnormal, or bizarre. Psychosis runs in families and most often first appears in late adolescence or early adulthood. There are medical and physical causes of some psychoses and some for which the cause is unknown. The treatment of psychoses involves removing or correcting the causes of the psychosis when possible. Psychosis describes a group of symptoms that can be part of several formal psychiatric diagnoses to include schizophrenia. Psychotic symptoms are characterized by delusions, hallucinations, disturbances of movement, and/or speech disturbances.

Delusions are false beliefs that are held despite strong evidence to the contrary. An example of an extreme delusion might be a man who believes that someone has planted a radio transmitter in his brain that sends signals to creatures on Mars. Hallucinations are false perceptions of a sense that, like delusions, are held despite strong evidence to the contrary. Hallucinations can involve any of the five senses. Examples of extreme hallucinations include feeling as if one is covered by ants; seeing green cows walking through the wall; hearing voices that do not exist; and smelling a constant odor when none exists.

Disturbances of movement can occur with psychoses. For example, a woman may become very exaggerated in her movements or, conversely, may become motionless for periods of time. These disturbances of movement are clearly bizarre and unnatural. Finally, speech disturbances are very common in psychoses. A man might speak in a way which is not understandable to others. He may carry on a conversation in which he believes that he is communicating normally but without making sense to others. Alternatively, speech might be clear but the individual shifts from one unrelated idea to another without being aware of doing so. Another psychotic symptom is severe emotional turmoil described as intense shifting moods with accompanying feelings of being confused.

Approximately 2 percent of all people in the world will develop a psychosis sometime during their lifetime. Although psychoses typically first appear in late adolescence or early adulthood, they may begin in middle to late life as well. The symptoms are apparently equally common in males and females. Because there is a strong family pattern to psychoses, some have suggested a genetic predisposition, and such evidence has been found. Environmental factors, however, such as home environment, parenting, and traumatic life events may also play a role in some psychoses.

TREATMENT AND THERAPY

Psychoses are often categorized as organic or functional, which provides a way to communicate the cause of the psychosis and thereby the appropriate treatment. Organic psychoses are attributable to disturbances in the brain. These psychoses can be attributed directly to a problem in the structure, functioning, or chemistry of the brain. Various physical conditions and abnormalities can lead to psychosis, including thyroid disorders, drug reactions, infections, epilepsy, tumors, and circulatory disorders (for example, strokes). The treatment of organic psychoses involves removing or correcting the causes of the psychosis. In the case of a psychosis caused by a disorder of the thyroid gland, the individual might be prescribed medications to correct the thyroid problem or have the gland surgically removed. Certain prescription and illegal drugs can cause a psychosis; these include cocaine, alcohol, heart medications, and pain medications. In these situations, the psychotic symptoms are often eliminated when the medication or drug is discontinued. Organic psychoses may be the result of deteriorating physical conditions, such as Alzheimer's disease. Such a psychosis is typically nonreversible and is treated with tranquilizing medications to decrease the individual's discomfort and disruptive behaviors.

Functional psychoses are those psychoses for which no organic causes can be found. Often the psychotic symptoms are part of a more traditional psychiatric condition such as schizophrenia or depression. The mainstay of the treatment of functional psychoses is medication therapy. As with the organic psychoses in deteriorating physical conditions, tranquilizers are the most appropriate first-line treatment for psychotic symptoms. The goal of therapy is to decrease the frequency and disruption of psychotic thoughts and behaviors.

Individual, group, and family psychotherapy are also a major part of treating individuals with functional psychosis or organic psychosis in deteriorating physical conditions. These therapies help to ensure compliance with the medication therapy, decrease the tendency for relapse, and can even lead to the reduction in the amount of medication required to relieve the individual's symptoms. The goal of psychotherapy is to help the individual maintain optimal functioning.

Occasionally, the patient with a psychosis may require inpatient hospitalization. The experience of hallucinations or delusions can be particularly distressing and can lead to a severe depression. Furthermore, these hallucinations and delusions might be of a homicidal or suicidal nature. While hospitalization is not required in treating individuals with psychosis, when individuals become a danger to themselves or to others, a brief inpatient hospitalization may be required to stabilize the patients and return them to a higher state of functioning. During hospitalization, patients are treated with medication therapy along with individual, group, or family therapy until they can be safely returned to their environments. Occasionally, patients with psychoses have multiple episodes during their lives requiring numerous inpatient hospitalizations.

—Oliver Oyama, Ph.D.

See also Addiction; Alcoholism; Delusions; Dementias; Depression; Domestic violence; Hallucinations; Intoxication; Neurosis; Paranoia; Psychiatric disorders; Psychiatry; Psychiatry, child and adolescent; Psychiatry, geriatric; Schizophrenia; Suicide.

FOR FURTHER INFORMATION:

American Psychiatric Association. *Diagnostic and Statistical Manual of Mental Disorders: DSM-IV-TR.* Rev. 4th ed. Washington, D.C.: Author, 2000. The bible of the psychiatric community, this is a compendium of descriptions of disorders and diagnostic criteria widely embraced by clinicians. Included is an extensive glossary of technical terms, making this volume easy to understand.

Hogarty, Gerard E., Carol M. Anderson, and Douglas J. Reiss. *Schizophrenia and the Family: A Practitioner's Guide to Psychoeducation and Management.* New York: Guilford Press, 1986. Attention is given to techniques for establishing a relationship with the family while the patient is still acutely ill and being seen concurrently on an individual basis by the family clinician.

Torrey, E. Fuller. *Surviving Schizophrenia: A Family Manual.* Rev. ed. New York: Perennial Library, 1988.

PSYCHOSOMATIC DISORDERS

DISEASE/DISORDER

ANATOMY OR SYSTEM AFFECTED: All

SPECIALTIES AND RELATED FIELDS: Psychiatry, psychology

DEFINITION: Physical disorder influenced by psychological stressors, or disorders characterized by symptoms that result from unconscious psychological factors instead of an underlying medical condition.

CAUSES AND SYMPTOMS

In the 1950's, the diagnosis of "psychosomatic disorders" was coined to refer to medical conditions for which there were no clear medical causes, but there was a subtle distinction between psychological processes and physical illness in its definition. The current understanding of medical illness has progressed, however, and health professionals now understand that psychological or sociological factors contribute to most medical illnesses. Thus, the diagnosis of psychosomatic disorders has undergone refinement and more specific diagnostic classification. The two related psychiatric diagnostic classifications are "psychological factors affecting medical condition" and "somatoform disorders."

Psychophysical disorders. The diagnosis of psychological factors affecting medical condition (also occasionally referred to as psychophysiological disorders) describes any physical condition or disorder that is influenced by psychological factors. These psychological factors can range from true psychiatric disorders such as depression to emotional stressors in the person's environment such as the death of a loved one, anger toward a coworker, or the inability to cope with normal life changes. The more common environmental stressors can lead to the initiation or the exacerbation of physical conditions, including headache, ulcer, asthma, arthritis, acne, irritable bowel syndrome, diabetes mellitus, muscular disorders, and essential hypertension. In certain cases, such as headache, the stressor causes the onset of symptoms. In others, such as diabetes, the stressors might cause a worsening of already existing symptoms because of their influence on the person's attitude about the illness and the resultant quality of life, the willingness or the ability of the person to comply with treatment, or the person's capacity to understand the illness and its treatment. For example, in a situation in which a person is faced with the death of a loved one, it would not be unusual to see a corresponding increase in headache frequency or uncontrolled blood sugar levels in the diabetic.

Somatoform disorders. Somatoform disorders are the second diagnostic classification subsumed under the old psychosomatic disorders category. In somatoform disorder, a person displays symptoms that suggest a physical disorder, but no medical evidence exists for such a disorder. In these cases, it is believed that the person possesses psychological stresses, conflicts, or needs that manifest themselves in physical symptoms. The distinction between somatoform and psychophysiological disorders is that in psychophysiological disorders the person has an identified physical illness or disorder that is influenced by psychological stress. In somatoform disorders, there are only physical symptoms and no physical findings or known mechanisms to diagnose any physical illness or disorder.

People with somatoform disorders are presumably unable to tolerate certain forms or intensity of emotional stresses, leading to an expression of their emotional distress through physical symptoms. These disorders typically afflict people in their adolescence or young adult years and cause considerable disruption in life. The symptoms or focus on physical attributes is not intentionally produced or controlled. They are, at the time, outside of the person's capacity to control them. There is no known cause for these disorders, and because they occasionally run in families, some have speculated that environment or genetics may play a role.

An example of a somatoform disorder is conversion disorder. People with conversion disorder display an alteration or loss of physical functioning characterized most often as paralyses, seizures, coordination problems, or visual problems. No physical causes are found for these symptoms. Instead, psychiatric evaluation suggests that the symptoms serve a role in helping the person cope with some type of stress, conflict, or need. A person might become temporarily blind or paralyzed in the right arm as an unconscious way of dealing with an upcoming stressful situation, such as a marriage.

Another somatoform disorder is somatization disorder. People with this disorder complain of at least thirteen unexplained symptoms for which no physical evidence exists. Such people believe that they have acquired a serious physical disorder and often seek out many health care providers to locate a cause for

their symptoms. The disorders are often very disruptive to the person's life and quite costly in terms of medical expenses.

TREATMENT AND THERAPY

Treatment for psychophysiological disorders can include using psychiatric medications to manage intense depression or anxiety; educating the patient about the relationship between stressors and physical illness; challenging maladaptive health care beliefs or any unrealistic assumptions or expectations that the person might possess; teaching physical and emotional relaxation skills; developing and utilizing social support from others in the person's life; and instructing the patient in personal skills to manage better the event or situation causing the stress. These treatments can be very effective with psychophysiological disorders.

Treatment for somatoform disorders involves the use of individual, group, or family therapy to address the stresses, conflicts, or needs that are believed to be at the root of the problem. When patients identify the underlying problems, change their thoughts about these problems, and learn skills to deal more adaptively with them, their physical symptoms typically subside.

PERSPECTIVE AND PROSPECTS

The relationship between the mind and the body has intrigued humankind for centuries. Beliefs about the contribution of the mind in the functioning of the human body have had a mixed history. Scientists and clinicians currently appreciate the influence of psychological and social factors in physical illness and dysfunction, but this has not always been the case. Theories of personality and its influence on health and illness can be found in ancient writings as early as 400 B.C.E. In the late sixteenth and early seventeenth centuries, the view that psychological factors could influence physical illness lost favor as the medical profession began an era of strict scientific study of the body and bodily processes. During this era, an illness or treatment would only be considered legitimate if a scientific explanation could be found for the process. Because of the limits of scientific methodology at the time, many of the traditional beliefs of this mind-body link were abandoned. The mind and body were theoretically separated until the early twentieth century with the introduction of the field of psychobiology and the scientific study of the influence of the mind on the body.

—Oliver Oyama, Ph.D.

See also Anxiety; Depression; Factitious disorders; Hypochondriasis; Midlife crisis; Münchausen syndrome by proxy; Neurosis; Panic attacks; Phobias; Psychiatric disorders; Psychiatry; Psychiatry, child and adolescent; Psychiatry, geriatric; Psychoanalysis; Stress; Stress reduction.

FOR FURTHER INFORMATION:

American Psychiatric Association. *Diagnostic and Statistical Manual of Mental Disorders: DSM-IV-TR*. Rev. 4th ed. Washington, D.C.: Author, 2000. The bible of the psychiatric community, this is a compendium of descriptions of disorders and diagnostic criteria widely embraced by clinicians. Included is an extensive glossary of technical terms, making this volume easy to understand.

Asaad, Ghazi. *Psychosomatic Disorders: Theoretical and Clinical Aspects*. New York: Brunner/Mazel, 1996. A guide to the disorders falling between strict medical or psychiatric diagnosis, presenting definitions, clinical manifestation, course, and prognosis. The text covers somatoform disorders, factitious disorders and malingering, and medical conditions affected by psychological factors.

Gatchel, Robert J., and Edward B. Blanchard, eds. *Psychophysiological Disorders: Research and Clinical Applications*. Washington, D.C.: American Psychological Association, 1993. Leading psychologists and health practitioners explore the epidemiology and etiology, as well as the assessment and treatment, of several prevalent physical disorders and conditions, illustrating the potential for psychological intervention in these traditionally medical areas.

Smith, G. Richard, Jr. *Somatization Disorder in the Medical Setting*. Rockville, Md.: U.S. Department of Health and Human Services, Public Health Service, Alcohol, Drug Abuse, and Mental Health Administration, National Institute of Mental Health, 1990. This manual of somatization disorders is aimed at the family practitioner. Includes bibliographical references.

PTOSIS

DISEASE/DISORDER

ALSO KNOWN AS: Drooping eyelid

ANATOMY OR SYSTEM AFFECTED: Eyes, muscles, nerves

SPECIALTIES AND RELATED FIELDS: Family practice, ophthalmology, optometry, plastic surgery

DEFINITION: Drooping of the upper eyelid, partially or completely covering the eye.

CAUSES AND SYMPTOMS

Ptosis may be congenital or may be associated with other problems, including paralysis of motor and sensory nerve fibers to the eyelids, muscular dystrophy, diabetes, brain tumor, head or eyelid injuries, myasthenia gravis, or a tumor in the upper lobe of a lung. In young children, congenital ptosis is the result of malformation of the levator muscle, which lifts the eyelid, or of a defective nerve supply to the muscle. Congenital ptosis usually does not improve with time. Symptoms include drooping of one or both eyelids, which may vary during different times of the day, as well as associated poor blinking reflexes.

TREATMENT AND THERAPY

Home treatment involves keeping the child's eye moist with artificial teardrops. Medical prescriptions are not necessary for ptosis, but they may be needed for underlying disorders. In most cases, the typical treatment for childhood ptosis is surgery, which involves tightening the levator muscle. The surgeon must be very careful not to raise the eyelid so high that the eye cannot be closed, and also to make it match the other eyelid as closely as possible. In cases involving older children, some ophthalmologists may recommend keeping the affected eyelid raised with a support that is part of a pair of eyeglasses.

PERSPECTIVE AND PROSPECTS

Complications that can arise from ptosis include permanent disfigurement of the face, visual difficulties, and irritation and infection of the eye that is caused by poor blinking reflexes and continual contact between the eyelid and the surface of the eye. If the disorder is not corrected in younger children, it can lead to amblyopia (lazy eye). Since amblyopia persists throughout life if it is not treated early in childhood, ptosis can lead to permanently poor vision. Ophthalmic plastic and reconstructive surgeons who specialize in ptosis and conditions affecting the eyelids, tear system, the bone cavity around the eye, and adjacent facial structures have made significant progress in the successful surgical correction of ptosis.

—Alvin K. Benson, Ph.D.

See also Diabetes mellitus; Eyes; Muscular dystrophy; Optometry; Optometry, pediatric; Plastic surgery; Strabismus; Surgery, pediatric; Visual disorders.

FOR FURTHER INFORMATION:

Anshel, Jeffrey. *Healthy Eyes, Better Vision: Everyday Eye Care for the Whole Family.* Los Angeles: Body Press, 1990.

Converse, J. M. *Reconstructive Plastic Surgery.* 2d ed. Philadelphia: W. B. Saunders, 1977.

Vaughan, Daniel, Taylor Asbury, and Paul Riordan-Eva, eds. *General Ophthalmology.* 15th ed. Norwalk, Conn.: Appleton and Lange, 1999.

PUBERTY AND ADOLESCENCE

BIOLOGY

ANATOMY OR SYSTEM AFFECTED: All

SPECIALTIES AND RELATED FIELDS: Dermatology, endocrinology, family practice, internal medicine, pediatrics, psychology

DEFINITION: Puberty is the onset of the natural biochemical (hormonal) and physical changes that occur in children as they are transformed into sexually mature individuals; adolescence is the period of years during which these transformations take place.

KEY TERMS:

estrogen: the chemical compound produced by the female ovaries that is involved in the regulation of menstrual periods and in the development of female sexual traits

gonadotropins: chemical compounds produced by the pituitary gland of the brain that cause the growth and maturation of the gonads

gonads: the reproductive organs; the ovaries in females and the testes (testicles) in males

hormones: chemical messengers produced in one part of the body that greatly influence activity in another part; examples include the gonadotropins estrogen and testosterone

ovaries: the female reproductive organs, which contain the ova (eggs); the ovaries are almond-shaped and are found in the lower pelvic area

pituitary gland: a small structure located near the base of the brain which produces the gonadotropins

testes: the male reproductive organs and the site of sperm production; also known as the testicles

testosterone: the male sex hormone produced by the testes and responsible for the male sexual traits; a small amount is also produced by the adrenal glands in females and is responsible for the growth of hair during adolescence in both sexes

CAUSES AND SYMPTOMS

The development period known as adolescence encompasses a host of biochemical, physical, and psychological changes in an individual which result in maturation as an adult capable of sexual reproduction. Collectively, the biochemical changes that lead to sexual maturity are called puberty. The process occurs over several years, and its time of onset is difficult to detect because the initial physical changes are quite subtle. For boys and girls in the United States and Western Europe during the last half of the twentieth century, the average age at which the onset of puberty occurred was between eight and thirteen years in girls, and nine and fourteen years in boys.

One of the most dramatic physical changes that occurs in puberty is a tremendous growth spurt. The rate of height increase per year doubles as compared to height gain prior to puberty. On the average, girls gain approximately 3 inches of height during this period, and boys grow by about 8 inches. The bulk of this growth is accounted for by an elongation of the thigh bones, followed by growth in the trunk. During this time, the thighs become wider, and shoulder width also increases. Both sexes accumulate fat during early puberty. Boys frequently appear rather chubby early in adolescence, but they generally lose this excess fat during their growth spurt. Most of this accumulated fat in girls is redistributed on their bodies and results in the typically curved silhouette. The average girl gains approximately 25 pounds during the adolescent period, while boys gain about 40 pounds, most of which is in the form of muscle.

Additional physical changes that occur during adolescence include changes in the facial bones, especially an elongation of the jawbone. Muscle size and strength increase during puberty, with a boy's development in this area extending years past the end of muscle strength increase in the typical girl. Prior to puberty, muscular strength is equivalent in both sexes, but the increase stops at the time of the first menstrual period in girls. Each of the major organs of the body, including the digestive tract, liver, kidneys, and heart, increases in size for both sexes during puberty. The size and activity of various glands adjust to reflect their increasing or decreasing role in the maturing individual.

Both girls and boys experience a characteristic increase in the distribution of hair on their bodies. Axillary (armpit) hair and pubic hair increase in density and coarseness, finally achieving the characteristic adult pattern. Boys also develop facial hair, beginning with a fine fuzz on the upper lip and eventually progressing into a full beard. Sweat glands increase in size as well. Boys undergo an increase in the size of the larynx (voice box), and this change leads to the normal, although psychologically painful, "cracking" of the adolescent male's voice.

Major alterations in the reproductive systems of boys and girls occur during puberty. In girls, the vagina enlarges and undergoes changes in chemical composition and cellular structure, and it begins producing typical adult secretions. Menarche, the first menstrual period, takes place even though ovulation (the maturation and release of an egg by the ovaries) may not occur for many months. The ovaries increase in size, and chemical changes prepare them to ovulate on a monthly basis. Breasts evolve from the preadolescent form to those of adult women. Boys undergo enlargement of the testicles, which are experiencing biochemical changes that prepare them for the continuous process of sperm production.

Because of the complexity of the many physical changes that occur during puberty, and the wide variation in the normal age of onset of this period, physicians have adopted a "sex maturity rating" scale to aid in their assessment of normal adolescent development. For both sexes, a rating of 1 (least mature) to 5 (most mature) is used to rank information collected by the visual observation of secondary sexual characteristics. For girls, breast and pubic hair development are the physical traits assessed. Boys are ranked based on the appearance of their genitals (penis and testicles) and the amount and distribution of their pubic hair.

All these physical changes are the direct result of global biochemical changes occurring in the adolescent's body. Just prior to puberty, a hormone called luteinizing hormone-releasing factor (LHRF) is produced by a portion of the brain called the hypothalamus. The LHRF travels to another structure in the brain, the pituitary gland. Upon receiving this hormonal signal, the pituitary gland produces two additional hormones called gonadotropins. The gonadotropins stimulate the development and enlargement of the ovaries in girls and the testicles in boys. As a result of the stimulation of the gonadotropins, the gonads produce sex hormones; the ovaries produce estrogen, and the testes produce testosterone. Females also produce a small amount of testosterone in the adrenal glands, which are located above the kidneys. These

Physical Changes During Puberty and Adolescence

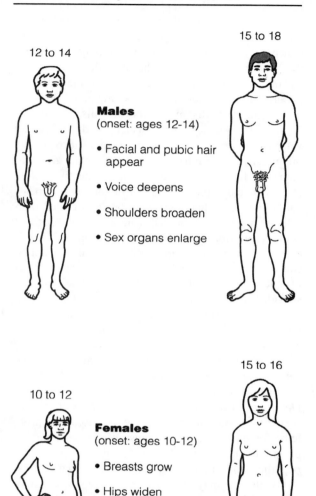

Males
(onset: ages 12-14)

• Facial and pubic hair appear

• Voice deepens

• Shoulders broaden

• Sex organs enlarge

Females
(onset: ages 10-12)

• Breasts grow

• Hips widen

• Pubic hair appears

• Uterus enlarges

• Menstruation begins

sex hormones enter the bloodstream and signal the start of the physical changes associated with puberty.

Examples of the effects of these hormones include the development of axillary hair in both boys and girls, which is initiated and maintained by testosterone. Breast development in girls is triggered by the estrogen produced by the ovaries. Maturation of the larynx in boys is accomplished by the action of testosterone. The other physical changes noted above are the result of sex hormones working alone or in concert with each other and of hormonal action on the genetic information of the individual.

The psychological changes that take place during puberty, although normal, may be dramatic. Thinking and cognitive skills mature during this period, accompanied by a tendency to analyze the rules and values of families, friends, and society. Frequently, this is a period of rebellion against parents and other authority figures. The confusion frequently associated with the rapid changes in adolescents' bodies and minds and their changing perceptions of their role in the world, coupled with the beginnings of adult responsibility, can lead to problems with self-esteem, anxiety, and depression. Critical and unreasonable self-assessment of appearance and abilities may lead to psychological illness. Socialization and self-identity come into prominence in the adolescent's life and can result in additional confusion, feelings of rejection, and experimentation with alcohol and drugs.

Sexual feelings are awakened in the adolescent and can be particularly challenging to understand and channel in an appropriate and responsible manner. Discovery of a sexual orientation contrary to heterosexual interests can create severe psychological problems for the adolescent because of fear of rejection by family and society. The possibilities of pregnancy or fatherhood or the contraction of a sexually transmitted disease may add gravity to early sexual explorations. Many groups argue that adolescents should have access to accurate and nonjudgmental information on contraception and disease prevention.

COMPLICATIONS AND DISORDERS

A number of medical disorders can result from abnormalities in the biochemical processes that mediate puberty. Other, less serious varieties of physical afflictions are natural and temporary side effects of the normal changes that accompany adolescence. Psychological disturbances may be associated with the extensive upheaval in the physical, mental, and social aspects of an adolescent's life, and in most cases they do not reach severe proportions. In some instances, however, professional intervention is indicated.

If the onset of puberty is not evident by age thirteen in girls or age fourteen in boys, or if puberty is initiated but little progression is observed for six to twelve months, detailed medical evaluation of the situation is recommended. Oral histories and a complete physical examination are conducted, and the individual's sex maturity rating is determined. The level of the gonadotropic hormones will first be assessed in order to determine if the delay of puberty is caused by a lack of the gonad-stimulating hormones produced by the brain or if the sex hormone production by the gonads is deficient.

A permanent deficiency in the amount of gonadotropic hormones produced by the pituitary gland prevents the sex organs from maturing and producing the sex hormones estrogen (in girls) and testosterone (in boys). This syndrome is referred to as hypogonadotropic hypogonadism and can be caused by a variety of central nervous system abnormalities. Congenital defects (abnormalities present at birth) in the pituitary gland can inhibit the production of gonadotropins. Likewise, tumors at certain positions in the brain, including the pituitary gland, may block hormone production. Deficiency in another hormone, human growth hormone, results in short stature and delayed puberty. Other conditions, such as genetic abnormalities, chronic disease, pathologies of the thyroid gland or its functions, malnutrition, and excessive exercise, can also be the root cause of delayed puberty.

Delayed puberty can also be caused by failure of the ovaries or testes to mature despite normal levels of gonadotropins produced by the brain. In the vast majority of cases, the root cause of this syndrome, hypogonadotropic hypogonadism, is linked to defects in the normal chromosomal complement of the individual; that is, it is a genetic defect. Usually, it is caused by the presence of abnormal sex chromosomes and is diagnosed by examination of the chromosomes by a procedure called karyotyping.

A third category of delayed puberty is termed "constitutional delay in puberty." At the latest extreme of what is classified as the "average" age of onset of puberty, the individual's stature may be short, menarche may be delayed in girls, and the sex maturity ranking for both sexes would be low. In reality, these individuals are merely slightly beyond the age of onset considered "normal" and will, without medical intervention, proceed through normal puberty and develop into fully mature adults of normal height. Patience and close observation of changes are the best course of action in cases of constitutional delay in puberty.

True cases of "precocious puberty"—that is, puberty with an extremely early onset because of physical or biochemical abnormalities—are extremely rare. In these cases, there is usually a defect in one or more of the glands producing the hormones that initiate puberty. Skilled medical diagnosis is indicated in these cases. Usually, when puberty begins much earlier than expected, no abnormality is present. These individuals are merely "early" according to the accepted range of average age of pubertal onset. Early pubertal onset is considered to be prior to eight and one-half years in girls or nine and one-half years in boys. In these cases, examination by a qualified physician is recommended to check for the rare instance of physical abnormality. Usually, the potential psychological difficulties associated with early puberty greatly outweigh concern for the instances of physical problems.

Acne, pimples and blackheads appearing on the skin of the face and upper back, commonly appears during adolescence. This skin disorder is a by-product of the hormones produced at puberty, which also stimulate the production of oil in the glands of the face and back. Acne may be treated with over-the-counter remedies and frequent washing of the skin, and it usually disappears as the individual approaches adulthood. In some severe cases, however, in which infection and scarring are distinct possibilities, medical intervention is recommended.

Preoccupation with personal appearance, difficulties with self-esteem, and a host of other psychological factors connected with the upheavals experienced during adolescence can lead to eating disorders. Anorexia nervosa is a syndrome characterized by extremely low food intake, preoccupation with losing weight, maintaining a weight that is more than 15 percent below a normal level for age and height, disturbed perception of personal weight (seeing oneself as obese when one is pathologically thin), and (in girls) skipping three or more sequential menstrual periods. This is a serious disorder and is fatal for approximately 5 percent of affected individuals. Death is related to the extremely poor nutritional state of these patients; it may occur from heart failure or kidney failure, among other causes, and is associated with diseases afflicting the entire body. A physician's supervision, psychological counseling, and behavioral modification are very successful in the improvement of patients with this disorder.

Bulimia nervosa is characterized by "binge-purge" cycles of rapid, uncontrolled eating followed by self-induced vomiting, the use of laxatives, and extreme dieting. For a diagnosis of bulimia, these episodes must occur at least twice a week for three months. In contrast to anorectics, bulimics are of normal to slightly above normal weight, so are not as often suspected of having an eating disorder. Binging and purging usually occur in private. Severe medical consequences of the behavior include cardiac arrest, rupture of the esophagus (the tube that runs from the mouth to the stomach), eroding of tooth enamel, and severe dehydration. As with anorexia, medical intervention and psychological counseling are necessary to control and defeat this harmful behavioral pattern.

There are other common physical complaints for some adolescents during this period. "Growing pains" are a very real phenomenon during the rapid growth period of puberty. Sharp pains, especially in the legs, may sometimes awaken the sleeping adolescent. These are best treated with massage or a mild over-the-counter pain reliever. Pain associated with menstrual periods is common in adolescent, as well as adult, females. In most cases, over-the-counter medications provide relief, but in severe cases, or when pain is associated with heavy menstrual flow, a physician's intervention is recommended.

Depression, a feeling of gloom and hopelessness about the present and the future, is a disorder which may afflict the adolescent. Many factors can provoke or heighten depression, including rejection by peers and/or parents, chronic illness, economic turmoil, severe family problems, and stress associated with school. Frequently, the situation quickly resolves itself, but if depression occurs for an extended period (for days or weeks, depending on the teenager), medical intervention and psychological counseling are recommended. Untreated depression can lead to eating and sleeping disorders, a desire to escape problems through the abuse of drugs or alcohol, severe behavioral problems, or psychosomatic disorders such as headaches, chest pains, stomach problems, and fatigue. Anxiety, unfocused fear that sometimes leads to extreme situations including panic attacks, is another psychological disorder sometimes associated with puberty. The most severe outcome of depression and/or anxiety is suicide. Any indication that a teenager is considering suicide, no matter how seemingly inconsequential, must be taken seriously; medical and psychological intervention must be obtained at once.

PERSPECTIVE AND PROSPECTS

Extensive historical evidence dating back as far as the time of Aristotle (384-322 B.C.E.) suggests that the onset of puberty in modern times occurs much earlier than at most other periods of recorded history. Nevertheless, there are many exceptions to this trend. During times of severe stress—for example, in Western Europe during World War II—the age of onset of puberty was several years later than in calmer political times.

Many factors are responsible for the earlier onset of adolescence in Western societies, including improved nutrition and elevated economic status. Improved public health, in terms of immunizations to prevent and treatment to cure childhood diseases, likewise contributes to the improved health of the individual and onset of puberty at an earlier age. Modern society, however, creates stresses that in some cases delay the age of pubertal onset. These factors include poverty, the divorce and remarriage of parents, separation from siblings, and increasing responsibilities assigned to children whose parents are unavailable to the child for much of the day.

In cases of delayed puberty attributable to deficiencies in gonadotropin production or a failure of the gonads to mature despite adequate levels of gonadotropins, medical intervention can compensate for the resulting physical immaturity. Boys can be given increasing doses of testosterone over a period of time, which will lead to the development of the external physical traits characteristic of puberty. Girls initially may be given oral doses of estrogen and then be given a combination of estrogen and another sex hormone, progesterone, as therapy progresses. These hormones lead to normal external pubertal development in most cases.

Some individuals with delayed puberty are deficient in human growth hormone and also experience greatly shortened stature as compared to the normal range of heights for other individuals in their age group. Until the 1980's, human growth hormone was isolated from cadavers, and its cost was prohibitively high for most people. With the revolution in recombinant DNA technology, human growth hormone is synthesized quite cheaply and is available to individuals who need it. Unfortunately, the accessibility of this drug creates the possibility of its abuse by parents who want their normal children to be exceptionally large and strong.

In the latter third of the twentieth century, psychologists and other health professionals began to recognize an increase in the rate of disturbed behavior exhibited by adolescents. These behavioral anomalies included alcohol and drug abuse, promiscuity (with the accompanying risk of infection with sexually transmitted diseases and/or pregnancy), depression, and suicide. Educators, health professionals, and concerned adults recognize these syndromes and address them through counseling, medication when indicated, outreach programs, and peer counseling programs, among other efforts. As the medical and psychological communities gain further understanding of the physical, psychological, and social consequences of puberty, additional interventions will be developed to smooth out this turbulent period of human development.

—*Karen E. Kalumuck, Ph.D.*

See also Abortion; Acne; Anorexia nervosa; Anxiety; Bulimia; Depression; Developmental stages; Eating disorders; Endocrine disorders; Endocrinology, pediatric; Growth; Gynecomastia; Hermaphroditism and pseudohermaphroditism; Hormones; Klinefelter syndrome; Masturbation; Menstruation; Precocious puberty; Pregnancy and gestation; Psychiatry, child and adolescent; Reproductive system; Safety issues for children; Sexuality; Sexually transmitted diseases; Suicide; Tattoo removal; Tattoos and body piercing; Turner syndrome; Wisdom teeth.

FOR FURTHER INFORMATION:

Fox, Stuart I. *Perspectives on Human Biology.* Dubuque, Iowa: Wm. C. Brown, 1991. A textbook designed for the reader with no background in biology. Presents an excellent, well-illustrated discussion of human biology, and contains chapters on human development, including puberty and reproduction.

Greydanus, Donald E., ed. *Caring for Your Adolescent.* New York: Bantam Books, 1991. An excellent resource for those interested in the physical and psychological changes that occur during adolescence. Included are chapters on compassionate parenting as well as specifics on the diseases and challenges commonly encountered during this period.

Kimmel, Douglas C., and Irving B. Weiner. *Adolescence: A Developmental Transition.* 2d ed. New York: John Wiley & Sons, 1995. A text on adolescent psychology that addresses the changes which come with puberty. Includes a bibliography and indexes.

Levine, Melvin D., and Elizabeth R. McAnarney, eds. *Early Adolescent Transitions.* Lexington, Mass.:

Lexington Books, 1988. This book is of interest to everyone from concerned parents to health professionals to adolescents themselves. Explores normal and perturbed pubertal processes and the psychological, social, and health issues that arise from adolescent transitions.

Steinberg, Laurence, and Ann Levine. *You and Your Adolescent.* New York: Harper & Row, 1990. Designed as a parents' guide to children aged ten to twenty, this clearly written book covers the physical aspects of puberty as well as the social, psychological, and health issues confronting adolescents during this period.

Stepp, Laura Sessions. *Our Last Best Shot: Guiding Our Children Through Early Adolescence.* New York: Riverhead Books, 2000. Stepp shows readers the intricacies of teens' lives, schools, friends, and family through case studies of twelve children in Los Angeles; Durham, North Carolina; and Ulysses, Kansas. This book is recommended for teachers, parents, and adults in the community.

PUBLIC HEALTH. *See* ENVIRONMENTAL HEALTH; OCCUPATIONAL HEALTH.

PULMONARY DISEASES
DISEASE/DISORDER

ANATOMY OR SYSTEM AFFECTED: Chest, immune system, lungs, respiratory system

SPECIALTIES AND RELATED FIELDS: Environmental health, epidemiology, immunology, occupational health, oncology, pulmonary medicine, virology

DEFINITION: Diseases of the lungs, which may be serious or fatal; common pulmonary diseases include those caused by infection (bronchitis, pneumonia, tuberculosis), tobacco smoke (emphysema, lung cancer), and allergies (asthma).

KEY TERMS:

alveoli: the many tiny air sacs at the ends of the terminal bronchioles, where oxygen and carbon dioxide are exchanged

asthma: a condition in which spasms of the bronchial smooth muscle cause narrowing and constriction of the airways

bronchi: the branching airways from the single large trachea to the multiple terminal bronchioles

bronchoscopy: a procedure that uses a flexible or rigid fiber-optic telescope to visualize the bronchial tree directly; it also permits samples of tissue to be removed for analysis

cancer: a tumor (or growth) of abnormal, genetically transformed cells that invade and destroy normal tissue; also referred to as a malignancy

emphysema: progressive destruction of the alveolar walls, leading to highly inflated and stiffened lungs

interstitial pulmonary fibrosis (IPF): the scarring and thickening (fibrosis) of the lung tissue, which causes breathing difficulty, chest pain, coughing, and shortness of breath; the lungs become increasingly stiffer until heart failure ensues

pathology: the study of the nature and consequence of disease

pleurisy: the inflammation and swelling of the pleurae, the membranes that enclose the lungs and line the chest cavity; a complication of several pulmonary diseases

pneumonia: an inflammation of the lung tissue in which the alveolar sacs fill with fluid

pulmonary: the Latin word for lung, used to describe both the lung tissue and the bronchial tree

respiration: a process which includes both air conduction (the act of breathing) and gas exchange (oxygen and carbon dioxide transfer between the air and blood)

CAUSES AND SYMPTOMS

Disorders of the pulmonary system are among the most common diseases. Because it acts as an interface between the external and internal environments, the pulmonary system is subject to continual attacks to its health and integrity. A wide variety of disease-causing agents reach the lung with each breath. Infectious organisms (such as bacteria, viruses, and molds), environmental toxins (such as tobacco smoke and air pollutants), and various airborne allergens are the primary causes of lung disease.

The pulmonary system consists of an intricate bronchial tree terminating in very delicate, thin-walled sacs known as alveoli, each of which is surrounded by blood vessels. The entire network is contained within the supporting tissue of the lungs. These individual parts are perfectly suited to carry out efficiently their two life-sustaining functions: air conduction and the gas exchange between oxygen in the air and carbon dioxide (a waste product) in the bloodstream. Disruption of either function renders the person vulnerable to potentially fatal consequences.

All pulmonary diseases can be categorized in two ways: The first is based on the cause, whether a virus, asbestos, or cigarette smoke; the second is based on the result, the specific loss of structure and its function. Infectious diseases are the most common causes of respiratory problems. Infection usually occurs through inhalation, although it can come from another source within the body as well. A vast number of microorganisms are trapped by the hairs, mucus, and immune system cells that line the respiratory tract. Those that are not repelled generally infect the upper tract, namely the nose and throat; but it is the few that reach the bronchi and lungs that cause the most serious illnesses—bronchitis, pneumonia, and tuberculosis. Bronchitis, an inflammation of the bronchial tree, is the result of viruses or bacteria that invade the airways and infect the bronchial cells. In a "counterattack," the body responds by sending large numbers of immune system cells (white blood cells), which destroy the invaders both by direct contact and by releasing chemical substances. The inflamed bronchi begin to leak significant amounts of fluids, producing the most obvious symptom of bronchitis: a frequent cough that yields initially clear white and later yellow or green phlegm. Rarely does bronchitis progress to serious disability; more often it resolves, although recurrence is common.

Unlike bronchitis, pneumonia is extremely serious. It can develop from bronchitis or can occur as a primary infection. Pneumonia is an infection that goes beyond the airways into the alveoli and supporting lung tissue. While the process of the disease is the same as that of bronchitis, fluid accumulates not only in the bronchi but also in the alveolar sacs, which cannot be efficiently cleared by coughing. The normally air-filled sacs, now filled with fluid, cannot perform their vital function of gas exchange. If the fluid continues to accumulate, larger and larger areas of lung become unable to function and the person literally drowns.

In the case of tuberculosis, one specific bacterium (*Mycobacterium tuberculus*) is inhaled, generally from the spray of coughs or sneezes of infected persons. The bacterium settles in the bronchus where it begins to invade and multiply. Unlike the organisms that cause bronchitis and pneumonia, it passes through the airways into the substance of the lung. Again, the body reacts in an attempt to confine the organisms' spread by forming walled-off circular areas (cavities) around the destruction. Up to this point, the person may have been only minimally ill. Deceptively, however, while the cavities are successful at containing the spread, some bacteria within them may not have

been killed and remain dormant for many years. Later, when the person's immune system is weakened by another disease, alcoholism, drug abuse, and so on, the bacteria reawaken and invade the lung, producing massive destruction and the loss of both structure and function. Left untreated, death results.

In ways different from infectious diseases, toxic substances such as tobacco smoke cause severe disability and death either through permanent structural damage (emphysema) or by transforming respiratory cells into abnormal ones (lung cancer). Many toxic chemicals are released when tobacco is burned, and these substances affect the entire lining of the respiratory tract both in the short term and in the long term. In the immediate period, the small hairs that line the upper tract no longer function to filter the air, and large amounts of fluid enter the airways because they are constantly inflamed (producing the familiar smokers' cough). As the irritation continues for years, permanent damage ensues. Emphysema, which is present in nearly all smokers to some degree, is characterized by widespread destruction of the walls of individual alveolar sacs. As adjacent walls break, the alveoli coalesce into very large, balloonlike structures. The supporting lung tissue, which is normally soft and spongy, becomes stiff and hard, making breathing very difficult. Although the lungs become overinflated, the air is stale as it is unable to move in and out with each breath. The picture of a patient with severe emphysema is dramatic: The patient labors forcefully with an open mouth, trying unsuccessfully to draw air in and out. Both air conduction and gas exchange are seriously affected. If lung function falls below a critical minimum, death occurs.

Lung cancer is a major health problem claiming tens of thousands of lives each year in the United States alone, more than any other cancer. The mechanism by which toxic substances transform normal cells into cancer cells is complex but involves damage to the cells' genetic material. Many factors interact to allow cancer cells to grow into tumors, including the failure of the immune system to destroy these abnormal cells. Tumors may form in either the bronchial tree or the substance of the lung itself. In either case, the end result is the same: The tumor destroys normal structure by compression and invasion, replacing large areas of lung. Cancer cells also enter the bloodstream and travel to distant sites in the body, where they can grow into equally destructive tumors.

A pulmonary disease that affects millions of adults

as well as children is asthma. The trachea and bronchial tree of an asthmatic are highly sensitive to a variety of stimuli, as diverse as cold air, dust, exercise, or emotional stress. The bronchial muscles respond to the agent by spasming, producing narrow, constricted airways. Thick secretions are released, which plug the bronchial tree and add to the serious decline in air conduction. An asthma attack may range from mild bronchial contractions to life-threatening closure. Many asthmatic patients have multiple allergies to food, animal dander, plant pollen, dust, and so on, implying that their respiratory systems respond abnormally to otherwise harmless substances. Asthma is usually a lifelong problem, and while most attacks subside, death can occur.

TREATMENT AND THERAPY
The most common symptoms associated with pulmonary disease are coughing, chest pain, and shortness of breath. Because each of these symptoms is present in such a wide variety of pulmonary diseases, it often is necessary to use other tools to determine the specific illness present. The most important of these diagnostic tools is the chest X ray, in which nonspecific symptoms can be correlated with structural and functional abnormalities. A critical advancement in the use of X rays is the computed tomography (CT) scan. Using a computer, a large number of detailed X rays are combined to create a very detailed picture, allowing an ambiguous abnormality on a chest X ray to be visualized with much greater accuracy. If further information is needed in order to determine the exact nature of an abnormality revealed by the chest X ray and the CT scan, a sample of lung tissue must be obtained. The bronchoscope, a flexible or rigid fiber-optic tube, is passed through the mouth into the bronchial tree, allowing direct inspection of the pulmonary system. Performed using anesthesia in the hospital operating room, bronchoscopy can be used to remove a small amount of tissue for biopsy. While the procedure has a higher risk than either the chest X ray or the CT scan, it also has a high yield of information.

Once a specific diagnosis is made, treatment is begun that addresses the particular cause or resulting dysfunction. Infectious agents such as those causing bronchitis, pneumonia, and tuberculosis have the most direct treatment, antibiotics. These drugs, first discovered in the early part of the twentieth century, revolutionized modern medicine. Penicillin, sulfa drugs, erythromycin, and tetracycline are among the

most useful antibiotics for pulmonary infections. The particular microorganisms that are destroyed are specific to each drug, although significant overlap exists. Diseases that once claimed millions of lives can now be successfully cured.

Patients with asthma, lung cancer, and emphysema are not as fortunate. All these conditions are progressive pulmonary diseases: Asthma can remain stable for years but causes significant disability, emphysema slowly worsens, and lung cancer is sometimes curable but is frequently fatal. No cure exists for asthma; treatment is directed at alleviating the symptoms. The drugs that are used fall into three categories: those that reverse the bronchial constriction and open the airways (epinephrine, methylxanthines); those that reduce the inflammation and hence the thick mucus secretions (steroids); and those that attempt to stabilize respiratory cells, decreasing their abnormal response to stimuli (cromolyn sodium). During an asthma attack, epinephrine and similar-acting compounds are administered through inhalation or as injections in order to relieve the spasms that dangerously narrow bronchial airways. Between attacks, patients may use nasal sprays that contain mild doses of epinephrine-like drugs, as well as steroids that reduce the inflammation associated with asthma. Two other commonly used medications are caffeinelike drugs known as methylxanthines, which also serve to open narrowed airways, and comolyn sodium, an interesting substance that appears to stabilize the bronchial cells and prevent their hypersensitive reactions to various allergens. The reality of all these drugs is that, although they reduce the severity of attacks, they do not prevent their occurrence.

Emphysema is more difficult than asthma to treat. The enlarged alveoli and stiffened surrounding lung tissue are permanent structural changes. Progression of the disease can be significantly reduced if, in the early stages, environmental insults, particularly smoking, cease. Patients with emphysema have frequent serious pulmonary infections because the defense mechanisms of the bronchial tree are severely impaired as well. Such repeated infections hasten the decline in respiratory function. Both air conduction and gas exchange are affected. Supplementing oxygen is the mainstay of treatment, both during sudden deterioration and in later stages. Eventually, when the emphysemic's lungs no longer function, mechanical ventilators (artificial respirators) are needed. Need for this technology generally heralds a fatal outcome.

Lung cancer has the most dismal prospects of all the pulmonary diseases. Treatment has met with limited success because it becomes symptomatic relatively late in its course and because it is such an aggressive disease, spreading to other parts of the body. Three main modalities exist in attempting to cure lung cancer: surgical removal of the tumor and surrounding lung tissue, radiation therapy, and chemotherapy. Surgery and radiation are localized treatments, while chemotherapy is systemic, reaching the whole body via the bloodstream. Very often, the latter two are used to alleviate symptoms when attempts at a cure fail. When lung cancer is discovered early, all three procedures may be used. Bronchoscopy allows a sample of the tumor to be analyzed, and based on various other findings, a treatment plan may be instituted that begins with surgically removing the mass. Radiation is then used in very controlled ways to destroy any remaining cancer cells in the surrounding lung tissue. If it is found that cancer cells have already spread to other regions—such as the bone, brain, or liver—then chemotherapy consisting of highly toxic drugs is given directly into the bloodstream in order to reach migrating cancer cells. Unfortunately, because lung cancer (as is true of most malignant diseases) is an extremely destructive disease extending beyond its local site of inception to distant, unrelated organ systems, treatment has been disappointing and fatality rates are high.

A treatment modality that plays a very important role for many pulmonary diseases, and indeed has supported countless lives, is the respirator. This mechanical device, essentially an artificial lung, delivers a preset volume of air rich in oxygen into the lungs through a conducting tube that lies in the trachea, the largest airway, from which the right and left main bronchi divide. Although fraught with ethical issues about unnecessary prolongation of death and suffering, the artificial respirator is clearly indicated when the person will most likely fully recover from a sudden illness. In these cases, mechanical breathing can provide adequate oxygenation to the body as it repairs itself.

Death has long been defined as the cessation of respiration. Artificial respirators have forced a rethinking of that definition, which now requires cessation of brain activity. Many pulmonary diseases in their final stages lead to dependence on these mechanical ventilators. Yet many of these same diseases, and those of other systems that affect the lungs, cause sudden respiratory failure. Cardiopulmonary resuscitation (CPR) is a highly effective emergency procedure that essentially substitutes a rescuer for a machine. By delivering exhaled air into the unconscious person, and simultaneously compressing the chest, the critical functions of breathing and circulation are maintained. CPR is a simple procedure to learn, and one that has saved innumerable victims.

PERSPECTIVE AND PROSPECTS

Pulmonary diseases have caused an extraordinary number of deaths throughout human history. Whereas lung cancer claims the most lives today, infectious diseases, especially pneumonia, claimed many more lives in the thousands of years before the introduction of antibiotics in the early twentieth century. Many potentially fatal illnesses, particularly those that are viral in origin, are transmitted through the respiratory route. Because of the ease with which they can be spread—person to person through coughs and sneezes—epidemics often occur. Rubella, measles, chickenpox, smallpox, mumps, diphtheria, and pertussis (whooping cough) are among such illnesses. Many of these kill by secondary pneumonias that overwhelm the body's defense mechanisms. The well-known rashes that occur in several of these illnesses are simply manifestations of viremia, the passage of viruses through the lungs into the bloodstream. Most of the victims of these diseases were children; indeed, these illnesses were among the principal reasons for the high child mortality rates. While antibiotics are ineffective in treating viral diseases (as opposed to bacterial or fungal diseases), vaccinations have proven very successful, reducing or even eliminating them.

Two epidemic diseases that have killed millions of people throughout recorded history have been the pneumonic plague and influenza. Both have been somewhat controlled because of improved sanitation (in the case of the plague) and improved vaccine programs (as with influenza). General sophistication in caring for the victims of these diseases has minimized mortality in those cases that do occur.

The plague has been feared since ancient times, and at least three major epidemics are known in which large portions of populations were destroyed. The first of these was recorded in Europe and Asia Minor during the sixth century, the second (known as the Black Death) was in the fourteenth century, and the last began in China in 1894, an epidemic which eventually spread to all continents, including North

America, by 1900. The plague is an infectious disease caused by a bacterium that lives in the bodies of rodent fleas. It is transmitted to humans through bites of rat fleas, in particular, and enters the bloodstream. High fever, very enlarged and painful lymph glands, and severe weakness characterize the illness, which occurs a few days after the flea bite. In this stage of the disease, known as the bubonic plague, the fatality rate ranged from 50 to 90 percent, but the disease was not contagious. As the infection spread from the bloodstream to lung tissue, a highly contagious pneumonia resulted that allowed person-to-person transmission through infectious droplets expelled by coughing. This form of the disease, the pneumonic plague, was invariably fatal, with nearly 100 percent mortality within a few days of infection. Approximately one-half of the population of Europe died during the Black Death. Improved sanitation methods that separated the rat population from human habitations have played the most important role in stemming the outbreak of new epidemics. Such problems continue to exist in much of the Third World, however, and plagues occur sporadically there.

While influenza was not recorded well historically, the disastrous epidemic of 1918 proved just as deadly, killing 35 million people worldwide in a few short months. Because of immigration, the disease spread rapidly throughout Europe and North America within a few months. Spread solely by the respiratory route, through inhalation, influenza is caused by a virus. High fever, muscle and joint pain, coughing, chest pain, and weakness are common symptoms. The pneumonia that may develop within a few days of the onset of the illness can rapidly progress to death. Early twentieth century medicine was completely overwhelmed by the number of cases and by the severe pneumonia that followed. Vaccinations with killed virus particles have become routine preventive medicine for those most as risk: the elderly, the sick, and infants. Much of the mortality associated with influenza in the past has been reduced, but definitely not eliminated.

—*Connie Rizzo, M.D.*

See also Addiction; Allergies; Asthma; Bronchiolitis; Bronchitis; Computed tomography (CT) scanning; Coughing; Croup; Cystic fibrosis; Diphtheria; Emphysema; Influenza; Interstitial pulmonary fibrosis (IPF); Lung cancer; Lungs; Multiple chemical sensitivity syndrome; Plague; Pleurisy; Pneumonia; Pulmonary medicine; Pulmonary medicine, pediatric; Respiration; Respiratory distress syndrome; Resuscitation; Smoking; Tuberculosis; Whooping cough.

FOR FURTHER INFORMATION:

Bennett, J. Claude, et al., eds. *Cecil Textbook of Medicine.* 21st ed. Philadelphia: W. B. Saunders, 2000. This superior textbook of internal medicine has an excellent section on respiratory system disease. A perfect place to start for the reader interested in all aspects of a disease. The text is well supplemented with diagrams and photographs.

Fishman, Alfred, ed. *Fishman's Pulmonary Diseases and Disorders.* 3d ed. New York: McGraw-Hill, 1999. A frequently consulted text by health professionals, it is less complex than Fraser and Pare's book but well written and comprehensive. An excellent place to find discussions of current diagnosis and treatment, as well as of research and future directions.

Fraser, Robert G., and J. A. Peter Pare. *Fraser and Pare's Diagnosis of Diseases of the Chest.* 4th ed. Philadelphia: W. B. Saunders, 1999. This bible of pulmonary disease is one of the most extensive textbooks available on the subject. Although used primarily for reference by pulmonary physicians, it is clearly written.

James, D. Geraint, and Peter R. Studdy. *A Color Atlas of Respiratory Disease.* 2d ed. St. Louis: Mosby Year Book, 1992. A wonderfully illustrated text that combines colorful drawings with photographs of X rays, autopsy specimens, and microscopic sections of diseased tissue. Each section is well written, with explanations of both the disease and the findings.

Mulvihill, Mary L. *Human Diseases: A Systemic Approach.* 5th ed. Norwalk, Conn.: Appleton and Lange, 2000. This text, used by nurses and allied health professionals, is a good place to start. Introductory chapters on disease, diagnosis, treatment, the immune system, and cancer provide important background for the chapter on pulmonary disease.

Victor, Lyle, ed. *Clinical Pulmonary Medicine.* Boston: Little, Brown, 1992. A relatively short but concise book that concentrates on signs and symptoms, diagnostic procedures, and treatments. It is easy to understand and interesting to read.

West, John B. *Pulmonary Pathophysiology: The Essentials.* 5th ed. Baltimore: Williams & Wilkins, 1998. Emphasis is placed on understanding the mechanism of disease. After a review of the anatomy and physiology of the respiratory system, diseases are placed in the context of the functional disorder: air conduction or gas exchange. Excellent coverage of the basis of pulmonary disease.

PULMONARY MEDICINE

SPECIALTY

ANATOMY OR SYSTEM AFFECTED: Chest, immune system, lungs, nose, respiratory system, throat

SPECIALTIES AND RELATED FIELDS: Critical care, emergency medicine, environmental health, exercise physiology, immunology, internal medicine, occupational health, otorhinolaryngology

DEFINITION: The field of medicine concerned with all the diseases that may afflict the lungs or in which the lungs may be involved.

KEY TERMS:

acute: referring to a short-term disease process

allergen: a substance that causes an allergic reaction, such as pollen, dust, or animal dander

alveoli: tiny air sacs deep within the lungs

chronic: referring to a long-term disease process

mucus: a fluid excreted by many body membranes as a lubricant

prognosis: the outlook for a patient with a disease condition

SCIENCE AND PROFESSION

Pulmonary medicine is a major specialty requiring years of training in its unique disciplines. The specialist in pulmonary diseases studies the wide variety of pathogens that can infect the human lungs. These include many families of bacteria, viruses, and fungi. Also, the pulmonary specialist learns to treat noninfectious lung diseases, such as asthma, chronic bronchitis, emphysema, and cystic fibrosis, as well as lung diseases that are caused by lifestyle (smoking), the natural environment (pollution, smog, or allergens), and the workplace (toxic chemicals, paints, or airborne dusts). Lung cancer, a major killer in Western societies, is often related to cigarette smoking, although other factors may be involved.

An increasingly visible respiratory problem in modern society is found in premature babies: These infants are often born before their lungs are fully developed. The problem for the caregiver in treating a newborn with respiratory distress is to maintain a steady supply of oxygen for as long as the infant needs it. The services of the pulmonary specialist may be required in the care of these babies.

DIAGNOSTIC AND TREATMENT TECHNIQUES

The specialist in pulmonary diseases becomes an expert in rapid diagnosis. Often, a patient comes into the emergency room or the physician's office in an acute state of discomfort. He or she may require immediate lifesaving measures. The physician must be able to decide quickly what is causing the problem and how to give the patient fast relief. How this is done varies considerably according to the disease.

Some respiratory tract infections progress so rapidly that the patient may require immediate surgical intervention to maintain an airway. Most respiratory infections, however, are considerably more manageable. Many require little more than palliative care.

By far the most common lung infections are attributable to the same organisms that cause the common cold. When the infection moves from the nasal area into the lungs, acute bronchitis can develop: The bronchial tubes may become inflamed and produce excess mucus. The patient coughs to relieve the congestion and may need to take medications and/or breathe in steam in order to break up the mucus deposits. Most common colds are caused by viruses for which there are no drugs that are analogous to the antibiotics taken to treat bacterial infections. Instead, the patient is given medications to relieve symptoms such as fever, hacking cough, and congestion.

Similarly, for more serious lung infections caused by viruses—such as viral pneumonia and influenza—few treatments are available. Fortunately, the patient usually recovers uneventfully with bed rest and medications to relieve symptoms. With certain viral respiratory infections, some new antiviral agents have been developed. For example, ribavirin may be used in children with lower respiratory tract pneumonia, and amantadine or acyclovir may be used to prevent the spread of influenza. During a viral lung infection, it is possible for bacteria to invade as well, a situation which is known as a superinfection. In this case, antibiotics are used to eradicate the bacteria.

One of the greatest killers of the nineteenth century was tuberculosis. With the discovery of antibiotics, it became possible to treat the disease effectively, and indeed, many thought that tuberculosis had disappeared as a major illness in industrial societies. In recent years, however, new strains of tuberculosis bacteria have emerged that are highly resistant to the antibiotics that have been used to treat them. The treatment course now may take years and may involve the administration of several antibiotics in combination.

Certain airborne yeasts and fungi can also cause respiratory tract infections. These diseases include histoplasmosis, aspergillosis, cryptococcosis, and coccidioidomycosis. They are usually not serious, although severe infections can be fatal.

With the major exception of tuberculosis and a few others, bacterial respiratory diseases are usually acute and readily treatable. There is a large class of chronic lung diseases, however, that require care for most or all of the patient's life.

Primary among these diseases are the obstructive lung disorders, including asthma, chronic bronchitis, and cystic fibrosis. The pulmonary specialist uses a wide range of instruments and techniques in the diagnosis and treatment of these patients. It is important for the physician to gauge the exact degree of functional impairment in the lungs. To do so, the physi-

cian uses a battery of pulmonary function tests that give an accurate picture of the patient's status. Among the more familiar functions tests are vital capacity (the maximum volume of air that can be exhaled slowly and completely after a full breath), forced vital capacity (a similar test showing the maximum air volume that can be expelled forcefully), and various other measures of lung volumes and flow rates. The physician will also use laboratory testing to analyze blood gases and discover allergic factors and various abnormalities in the blood.

Asthma is one of the most prevalent obstructive lung diseases. The cause appears to be an inherited allergic tendency. Asthma is most often diagnosed in children, and as many as 90 percent of these patients have allergies that set off the asthma attacks. Nevertheless, many other stimulants and factors can trigger

Anatomy of the Respiratory System

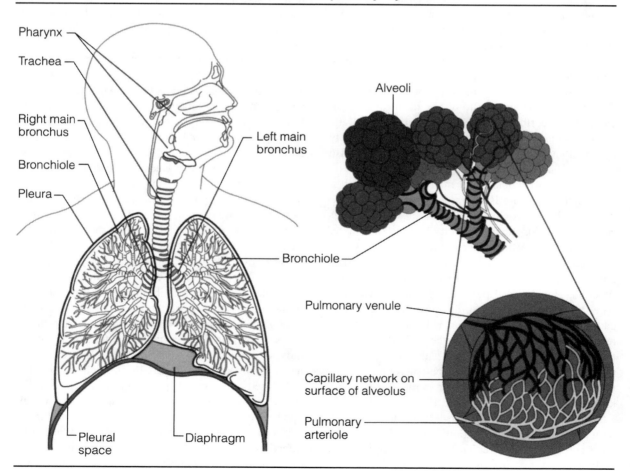

asthma episodes in both allergic and nonallergic patients, including cigarette smoke, airborne chemicals, and exercise.

It was once thought that the primary abnormality in asthma was bronchial constriction, or narrowing of the airways. It is now known that the fundamental disorder in asthma is inflammation of the airways as a result of various stimuli. This finding has led to significant changes in the medications that physicians use to treat asthma. Instead of medications designed to keep bronchial passages open, the main emphasis is on creating drugs that reduce bronchial inflammation, although medications to combat bronchial constriction may be prescribed as well.

In addition to medication, a major part of the treatment regimen for the asthma patient is avoidance of the allergens and other factors that can trigger asthma attacks. When possible, the physician will recommend immunization of the asthma patient against diseases that could be harmful such as influenza.

Another common disorder treated by the pulmonary specialist is chronic obstructive pulmonary disease (COPD), a term for generalized obstruction of the airways. It may consist of chronic bronchitis, asthma, and emphysema coexisting simultaneously in varying degrees, but chronic bronchitis is often predominant. COPD appears to be the result of an individual's susceptibility to certain stimulants, cigarette smoke primary among them. Smoking is definitely the main cause of chronic bronchitis, but it can also be caused and aggravated by pollution, dusts, toxic fumes in the workplace, and many other stimulants.

Cigarette smoking is also the major cause of emphysema. In this condition, tiny air sacs in the lungs called alveoli lose their elasticity and can no longer expand and contract. At the same time, the smaller breathing passages narrow. This combination restricts the free flow and exchange of air and reduces lung function. Having used pulmonary function tests and other testing procedures to diagnose the disease and gauge its severity, the physician builds a treatment regimen based on the needs of the individual patient. For patients with emphysema, cigarette smoking is strictly taboo, and, like asthma patients, they are advised to avoid any allergens or stimulants that are known to affect them.

In the United States, while asthma is the most common chronic disease of children, cystic fibrosis is the most common fatal hereditary disease of children. A child with cystic fibrosis has inherited the disease from both parents, carriers who experience no symptoms. In these children, heavy, thick mucus deposits build up in the lungs. Ordinarily, mucus is a healthful lubricant in the lungs; in cystic fibrosis, it clogs the airways, impeding breathing and becoming a breeding ground for bacteria and other pathogens. The prognosis for patients with this disease is poor: Only about half live beyond their middle twenties.

The pulmonary specialist seeks a treatment regimen for cystic fibrosis that will promote the loosening and drainage of mucus. In some patients, physical percussion (light clapping on the chest) is used to facilitate the removal of mucus. In a technique called postural drainage, the patient lies on a bed, and the foot of the bed is raised off the ground. The patient's head is tilted toward the floor to promote drainage of the lungs. Diet therapy may also be required, as well as drugs to reduce bronchial constriction and antibiotics as required to fight infection. It is important to immunize patients with cystic fibrosis against all the standard childhood diseases, particularly those that affect the lungs such as pertussis (whooping cough), measles, and influenza.

Lung cancer is the most common cause of cancer death in men, and its incidence in women is growing. The primary cause is cigarette smoking. The outlook for patients is variable: If untreated, patients with bronchogenic carcinoma succumb within nine months. Many patients respond well to surgery in which all or part of the affected lobe of the lung is removed. These patients often survive at least five years after surgery, although 6 to 12 percent may develop cancer in the other lobe. Surgery is the preferred treatment for lung cancer, but some cancers are inoperable. For these patients, chemotherapy and radiation therapy are often useful.

PERSPECTIVE AND PROSPECTS

Until the discovery of antibiotics, infectious diseases of the lungs were among the major killers of humankind. Diphtheria epidemics were common, and tuberculosis was rampant throughout the world. Today, most children in the industrialized world are vaccinated against diphtheria early in life. Tuberculosis has resurfaced as a major problem, however, because strains resistant to ordinary antibiotics have developed. For these patients, a long, tedious, multiantibacterial regimen is the only way to eradicate the infection. At least two antibiotics are recommended, often three, and the course of therapy may take years.

Pneumonia has become a major infection in hospitals, where outbreaks among patients are common. Hospital infection control teams are active in reducing the incidence of outbreaks, and extensive immunization programs are in operation in many hospitals to vaccinate against pneumococcal pneumonia. Most other bacterial lung diseases respond to antibiotic therapy.

A major area of research today is in antiviral medications. So far, most of the viruses that cause lung diseases are beyond the reach of antibiotics. Nevertheless, inroads have been made with amantadine, ribavirin, and some others.

The treatment of asthma continues to improve. The main course of therapy for many patients is corticosteroids to reduce bronchial inflammation. Oral corticosteroids often have undesirable side effects, however, particularly when taken over a long time. Fortunately, these patients can usually take the steroid in inhalable form, which greatly reduces the incidence of side effects and delivers medication directly to the affected areas in the lungs. Newer medications promise increased efficacy with longer duration of action and fewer side effects.

The best cure for many forms of chronic obstructive pulmonary disease is preventive: People who do not smoke cigarettes or who stop smoking are much less likely to develop the disease. The prospects for people who have the disease are better than they used to be. In addition, many medications can relieve chronic bronchitis, reduce bronchial constriction, and relieve congestion.

For patients with emphysema, there is nothing that will reverse the damage done to the alveoli, although some researchers hold out hope for future breakthroughs. Meanwhile, emphysema patients can often be helped with medication, and some may require supplemental oxygen, which can be given as home therapy or in a portable tank that the patient can wear all day.

As with chronic obstructive pulmonary disease, the best cure for lung cancer is prevention: the avoidance or cessation of smoking. Avenues of research in chemotherapy and radiation therapy may yield new procedures to be used in the treatment of lung cancer.

—*C. Richard Falcon*

See also Asthma; Bronchiolitis; Bronchitis; Catheterization; Chest; Choking; Coughing; Critical care; Critical care, pediatric; Croup; Cystic fibrosis; Diphtheria; Edema; Emergency medicine; Emphysema; Endoscopy; Environmental health; Exercise physiology; Fluids and electrolytes; Forensic pathology; Fungal infections; Gene therapy; Geriatrics and gerontology; Internal medicine; Interstitial pulmonary fibrosis (IPF); Lung cancer; Lung surgery; Lungs; Multiple chemical sensitivity syndrome; Occupational health; Oxygen therapy; Paramedics; Pediatrics; Physical examination; Pleurisy; Pneumonia; Pulmonary diseases; Pulmonary medicine, pediatric; Respiration; Respiratory distress syndrome; Smoking; Systems and organs; Terminally ill: Extended care; Thoracic surgery; Tracheostomy; Tuberculosis; Tumors; Whooping cough.

FOR FURTHER INFORMATION:

Larson, David E., ed. *Mayo Clinic Family Health Book.* 2d ed. New York: William Morrow, 1996. Perhaps the best general medical text for the layperson, this book covers the entire medical field. While the information is derived from a wide variety of highly technical sources, the articles are written to be easily understood by a general audience.

Wagman, Richard J., ed. *The New Complete Medical and Health Encyclopedia.* 4 vols. Chicago: J. G. Ferguson, 2000. The chapters on upper respiratory diseases in this work are thorough and clear, with good illustrations.

PULMONARY MEDICINE, PEDIATRIC
SPECIALTY

ANATOMY OR SYSTEM AFFECTED: Chest, immune system, lungs, nose, respiratory system, throat

SPECIALTIES AND RELATED FIELDS: Critical care, emergency medicine, environmental health, exercise physiology, immunology, internal medicine, neonatology, occupational health, otorhinolaryngology, pediatrics

DEFINITION: The diagnosis and treatment of disorders of the respiratory tract in infants and children.

KEY TERMS:

asthma: a reversible disorder of the lungs, experienced as wheezing and mucus blockage of the bronchi

biopsy: the removal of a small piece of tissue (such as respiratory tissue) for laboratory study

bronchoscopy: the visual examination of the respiratory system using a flexible tube composed of optic fibers

SCIENCE AND PROFESSION

The pediatric pulmonary specialist is a pediatrician who has received extra training in the diagnosis and

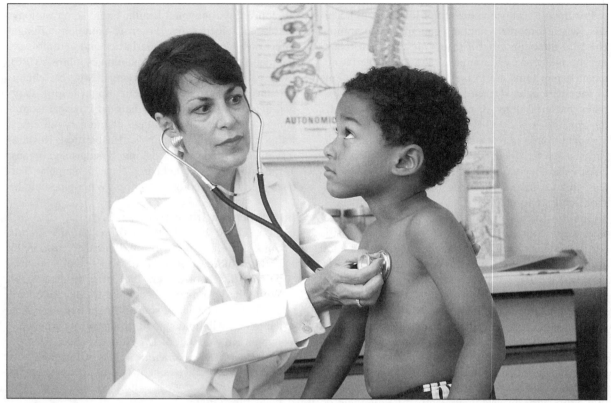

Pediatric pulmonary specialists use stethoscopes to evaluate the health of the respiratory system. (Digital Stock)

treatment of respiratory diseases. The full course of training requires a medical degree followed by three years of pediatric residency plus an additional three years of intensified study of children's respiratory diseases. The six years of postdoctoral training are almost always conducted at a large teaching hospital.

The respiratory system has several responsibilities. Most important for life, it allows the body to take in oxygen and to eliminate carbon dioxide. It also cleans and humidifies the air that is breathed. The system contains major sensory components, particularly hearing and smell. The respiratory system is divided into two parts, the upper and lower tracts. The upper respiratory tract includes the nose, ears, paranasal sinuses, throat, and larynx. The remainder of the respiratory system, the lower respiratory tract, is within the chest and includes the trachea, lungs, and pleura (the lining between the lungs and the rib cage).

Disorders of the respiratory system are extremely common in childhood. In the first year of life, at least half of illness-related visits to the doctor are for respi-

ratory ailments, especially ear infections and upper-respiratory infections.

A child's respiratory system is subject to a wide variety of disorders. Infections include ear infections, sinusitis, throat infections, croup, bronchitis, and pneumonia. Asthma, or reactive airway disease, is a common chronic inflammatory disease of the respiratory system that affects 5 to 10 percent of all children. The pediatric death rate from asthma rose steadily in the late twentieth century. By the 1990's, this ominous trend had slowed, as a result of new medications and an emphasis on patient education.

Cystic fibrosis, although much less common than asthma, is a serious inherited respiratory disorder that involves the abnormal production of mucus by the respiratory system and pancreas. Children with cystic fibrosis have a shorter-than-usual life span, although by the 1990's many of them were able to survive to young adulthood.

Pulmonary specialists often work in pediatric critical care, the provision of medical care to seriously ill or injured children. These children require careful monitoring of vital functions and management of fluids and medications. They frequently need respiratory support, such as oxygen or a ventilator. Critical care is provided in an intensive care unit.

The survival of severely premature infants has led to an increase in chronic lung disorders caused by prolonged ventilator and oxygen therapy in the intensive care nursery. Pediatric pulmonary specialists are responsible for the long-term care of these patients, along with neonatologists, specialists in newborn care.

The majority of a pediatric pulmonary specialist's time is spent in the clinic, examining and treating children with respiratory ailments. Patient education is important in this specialty, particularly for families of children with chronic respiratory diseases such as asthma. Because pulmonary specialists hospitalize more patients than many other pediatric specialists, a substantial amount of their time is spent in the hospital. The care of critically ill children, in particular, is extremely time-consuming.

The two most severe adult respiratory diseases, lung or laryngeal cancer and chronic pulmonary disease resulting from smoking, virtually never occur in children. Nevertheless, the behaviors and habits that lead to these diseases may begin in childhood. Pediatric pulmonary specialists are active advocates of child and parent education regarding the risks of these behaviors.

DIAGNOSTIC AND TREATMENT TECHNIQUES

A careful medical history and a thorough physical examination of the entire body, not simply of the respiratory system, are the pulmonary specialist's most important tools. The physician augments this information with a variety of laboratory tests, radiographic studies, and special pulmonary procedures.

Pulmonary function tests involve the measurement of various volumes of air in the lungs during the cycle of inhaling and exhaling and a determination of the speed with which the patient can exhale. It helps to diagnose whether the patient suffers from restriction of lung movement or obstruction of air movement in and out of the lungs. It is most useful in evaluating chronic pulmonary disorders but is not practical for young children because of the amount of patient cooperation it requires.

Bronchoscopy is performed by using a flexible, small-diameter tube of optic fibers with an external light source in order to inspect the larynx, trachea, and larger bronchi visually. Biopsies of tissue, in-

cluding lung tissue, can be obtained, as can samples of mucus for laboratory testing. Bronchoscopy is helpful in pediatric pulmonary medicine for finding and retrieving objects and particles of food that have been breathed into the lower respiratory tract. This procedure is also helpful in bronchoalveolar lavage, which is the rinsing out of a segment of chronically infected or obstructed lung tissue to remove pus, mucus, and other inflammatory products.

Respiratory infections generally respond to antibiotics and, in some cases, to antiviral agents. Asthma is treated with oral and inhaled medications that counteract the swelling and congestion of the bronchi, preferably before an attack of wheezing even begins. Cystic fibrosis requires aggressive treatment to keep mucus from obstructing the lungs, as well as occasional courses of intravenous antibiotics.

PERSPECTIVE AND PROSPECTS

Pediatrics, as a medical specialty, developed in the late nineteenth century. The pediatric subspecialties, including pulmonary medicine, generally became organized in the mid-twentieth century. Major advances in the 1990's, such as the discovery of the gene responsible for the molecular defect of cystic fibrosis, promise a bright future for pediatric pulmonary medicine.

—*Thomas C. Jefferson, M.D.*

See also Asthma; Bronchiolitis; Bronchitis; Catheterization; Chest; Choking; Coughing; Critical care, pediatric; Croup; Cystic fibrosis; Diphtheria; Emergency medicine, pediatric; Environmental health; Exercise physiology; Fluids and electrolytes; Fungal infections; Gene therapy; Internal medicine; Lung surgery; Lungs; Multiple chemical sensitivity syndrome; Oxygen therapy; Paramedics; Pediatrics; Physical examination; Pleurisy; Pneumonia; Pulmonary diseases; Pulmonary medicine; Respiration; Respiratory distress syndrome; Systems and organs; Thoracic surgery; Tracheostomy; Whooping cough.

FOR FURTHER INFORMATION:

Johnson, Kevin B., and Frank A. Oski. *Oski's Essential Pediatrics*. Rev. ed. Philadelphia: Lippincott-Raven, 1997. This is a clinical text on the essential elements of pediatrics, for medical students preparing for clerkships. Problem-based perspective, featuring 176 contributors.

Kercsmar, Carolyn M. "The Respiratory System." In *Nelson Essentials of Pediatrics*, edited by Richard

E. Behrman and Robert M. Kliegman. 3d ed. Philadelphia: W. B. Saunders, 1998. A chapter in a great text for medical students rotating through pediatrics. It has thorough explanations of diseases and treatments.

PYLORIC STENOSIS
DISEASE/DISORDER

ANATOMY OR SYSTEM AFFECTED: Gastrointestinal system, stomach

SPECIALTIES AND RELATED FIELDS: Gastroenterology, general surgery, pediatrics

DEFINITION: An obstruction of the stomach in infancy caused by muscular hypertrophy of the gastric outlet.

CAUSES AND SYMPTOMS

The exact cause of pyloric stenosis is unknown. The condition is usually characterized by nonbilious projectile vomiting beginning at three weeks of age, although it may occur as early as the first week of life or as late as five months of age. The vomiting is progressive and leads to poor growth and dehydration. Initially, the vomit resembles the fluid that the infant ingested, but it may become brownish in later stages of the disease.

TREATMENT AND THERAPY

Pyloric stenosis is diagnosed through palpation of a small, firm mass, similar to the size and shape of an olive, in the mid-upper abdomen. This mass is not palpable in all infants with pyloric stenosis. In these cases, imaging procedures such as an upper gastrointestinal (GI) series or ultrasound of the upper abdomen can confirm the diagnosis.

The initial treatment of pyloric stenosis involves correction of dehydration with intravenous fluids. The surgical treatment is called a pyloromyotomy. After the infant is anesthetized, an incision is made in the right-upper abdomen, through which the pyloric mass is removed. The pyloric muscle is split down to the mucosa, or lining of the stomach. Postoperative vomiting is common and is probably caused by slow emptying of fluids from the stomach. The vomiting usually resolves, however, such that the infant may resume feeding within twenty-four hours after surgery, with advancement to regular feeding within two days. This operation is usually curative, with low mortality and recurrence rates.

PERSPECTIVE AND PROSPECTS

Pyloric stenosis was first described in 1788. Harald Hirschsprung coined the term "congenital hypertrophic pyloric stenosis" in 1888. At that time, approximately one-fourth of infants affected by pyloric stenosis died without treatment, while more than half of the infants with this condition died after surgery. A significant advance in the treatment of pyloric stenosis came in 1912 when Conrad Ramstedt reported performing a pyloromyotomy. The procedure that he described remains the standard treatment.

—*David A. Gremse, M.D.*

See also Birth defects; Dehydration; Failure to thrive; Gastroenterology; Gastroenterology, pediatric; Gastrointestinal disorders; Gastrointestinal system; Nausea and vomiting; Neonatology; Pediatrics; Surgery, pediatric.

FOR FURTHER INFORMATION:

Christian, Janet L., and Janet L. Greger. *Nutrition for Living*. 4th ed. Redwood City, Calif.: Benjamin/Cummings, 1994.

Cockburn, Forrester, et al. *Children's Medicine and Surgery*. New York: Oxford University Press, 1996.

Garrow, J. S., and W. P. T. James, eds. *Human Nutrition and Dietetics*. 10th ed. New York: Churchill Livingstone, 2000.

Keet, Albertus D. *The Pyloric Sphincteric Cylinder in Health and Disease*. New York: Springer-Verlag, 1993.

QI GONG

PROCEDURE

ANATOMY OR SYSTEM AFFECTED: All

SPECIALTIES AND RELATED FIELDS: Alternative medicine, preventive medicine

DEFINITION: A Chinese meditative exercise that improves cardiovascular circulation, restores deep breathing, and relieves stress, qi gong is both a martial art and an ancient form of healing. The many forms of this exercise center on the concept of C'hi, the vital energy force that circulates freely in the body of a healthy person. Unbalanced C'hi can cause disease, and stress alters the balance and distribution of C'hi in the body. One form of qi gong involves practitioners sitting calmly and visualizing their own C'hi, directing it to specific parts of the body. The motion form of qi gong is a series of graceful, flowing movements practiced by individuals while they meditate on the movement of C'hi through their bodies. It is believed that qi gong initiates a relaxation response heralded by a decrease in blood pressure and heart rate. Qi gong may be prescribed as part of a stress reduction program or as therapy for patients with Alzheimer's disease. Some people believe that Chinese qi gong masters are able to radiate C'hi from their fingertips and thereby heal people; however, there is no scientific evidence to support this phenomenon.

—*Karen E. Kalumuck, Ph.D.*

See also Alternative medicine; Alzheimer's disease; Anxiety; Disease; Exercise physiology; Healing; Stress; Stress reduction; Tai Chi Chuan.

FOR FURTHER INFORMATION:

Jacobs, Jennifer, ed. *The Encyclopedia of Alternative Medicine: A Complete Family Guide to Complementary Therapies*. Rev. ed. Boston: Journey Edition, 1997.

Pelletier, Kenneth R. *Holistic Medicine*. New York: Delacorte Press, 1979.

Salmon, J. Warren, ed. *Alternative Medicines*. New York: Tavistock, 1984.

QUADRIPLEGIA

DISEASE/DISORDER

ANATOMY OR SYSTEM AFFECTED: Legs, muscles, musculoskeletal system, neck, nerves, nervous system, spine

SPECIALTIES AND RELATED FIELDS: Neurology, physical therapy

DEFINITION: Quadriplegia is partial or complete paralysis of both the arms and the legs caused by spinal cord damage in the neck; this damage may be the result of an accident, a spinal cord tumor, or a birth defect. If the spinal cord is seriously damaged or severed, total paralysis below the neck will result, while lesser damage may cause only partial paralysis. If the damage is minimal, there is a chance of recovery. With physical therapy, some cases of quadriplegia can be overcome, but the prognosis depends on the severity of the damage.

—*Jason Georges and Tracy Irons-Georges*

See also Birth defects; Head and neck disorders; Nervous system; Neurology; Neurology, pediatric; Paralysis; Paraplegia; Physical rehabilitation; Spinal cord disorders; Spine, vertebrae, and disks; Tumor removal; Tumors.

FOR FURTHER INFORMATION:

Carey, Joseph, ed. *Brain Facts: A Primer on the Brain and Nervous System*. Washington, D.C.: Society for Neuroscience, 1990.

Jenkins, David B. *Hollinshead's Functional Anatomy of the Limbs and Back*. Rev. 7th ed. Philadelphia: W. B. Saunders, 1998.

Kandel, Eric R., James H. Schwartz, and Thomas M. Jessell, eds. *Principles of Neural Science*. 2d ed. New York: Elsevier, 1991.

QUINSY

DISEASE/DISORDER

ANATOMY OR SYSTEM AFFECTED: Ears, throat

SPECIALTIES AND RELATED FIELDS: Family practice, otorhinolaryngology

DEFINITION: Quinsy is acute inflammation of the tonsils that may arise from streptococcal or staphylococcal tonsillitis. Peritonsillar abscesses typically occur several days after the onset of acute tonsillitis. As the symptoms of tonsillitis begin to resolve, increasing pain develops in one side of the throat or ear. Symptoms of quinsy also include a high temperature, headache, drooling, and impaired speech. Inflammation creates a partial obstruction to swallowing. Historically, this condition was treated with quinsy-wort (*Asperula cynanchia*). Today, antibiotics are used to clear the infection in its early stages. Otherwise, the abscesses need to be surgically drained. Normally, the tonsils are also removed, with the adenoids, to prevent recurrence.

—*John Alan Ross, Ph.D.*

See also Abscesses; Antibiotics; Bacterial infections; Otorhinolaryngology; Respiration; Sore throat; Strep throat; Tonsillitis; Tonsillectomy and adenoid removal.

FOR FURTHER INFORMATION:
Finegold, Sydney M., and William J. Martin. *Bailey and Scott's Diagnostic Microbiology.* 6th ed. St. Louis: C. V. Mosby, 1998.

Gest, Howard. *The World of Microbes.* Menlo Park, Calif.: Benjamin/Cummings, 1987.

Joklik, Wolfgang K., and Hilda P. Willett, eds. *Zinsser: Microbiology.* 20th ed. East Norwalk, Conn.: Appleton and Lange, 1992.

Rabies

Disease/Disorder

Anatomy or system affected: Brain, muscles, musculoskeletal system, nervous system, psychic-emotional system

Specialties and related fields: Epidemiology, neurology, public health, virology

Definition: A virus that attacks the nerve cells and is most often transmitted by the bite of a rabid animal; control of the disease is accomplished through vaccination of pets and immediate immunization of humans if exposed to the disease; once symptoms occur in humans, the disease is nearly always fatal.

Key terms:

anticoagulant: a chemical which blocks the clotting of blood; some stimulate internal bleeding when ingested by vampire bats and can be used as a method of extermination

epidemiology: the study of the maintenance and spread of disease in a population

fixed virus: a virus which has been repeatedly cultured in the laboratory so that it has lost its natural variation and is more predictable in experiments

passage: one of the culture steps in the production of a fixed virus

replication: the reproduction of a virus; many copies are made within a host cell, then released to infect other host cells

reservoir: the host species in which a parasite is maintained in a given area and from which it may infect other species, initiating an epidemic

street virus: a virus derived directly from a natural source; a fixed virus is produced from a street virus by several passages through an artificial culture system

sylvatic rabies: rabies in wild animal populations (as opposed to rabies in domestic animals and pets)

Causes and Symptoms

Rabies is caused by a bullet-shaped virus that attacks warm-blooded animals, especially mammals. The virus can enter many types of mammal cells and cause them to produce and bud off new viruses, but it is particularly adept at attacking nerve cells and glandular cells. This combination enhances the virus's chance of being transmitted to another host.

The following sequence of events occurs in an untreated human being after being bitten by a rabid animal. The bite introduces large amounts of saliva, which contains abundant rabies virus because of the virus' efficient growth in salivary glands. The virus enters muscle cells in the vicinity of the bite and replicates there. The new viruses then enter the nerve cells that carry signals from the brain and spinal cord to the muscle cells. They move along these nerve cells to the spinal cord, eventually making their way to the brain. The viruses replicate at certain sites as they ascend the nerve and spinal cord. In the brain, they replicate especially well in the centers that control emotions. Once established in the brain and spinal cord, the virus replicates move out of these organs along the nerves to most organs of the body. The salivary glands are favored targets in this migration.

As a result of its extensive migrations, the virus is present in many tissues of the body, but the critical ones for the pathology and transmission of the disease are the brain and salivary glands, where the virus reproduces especially well. To understand this relationship between transmission and pathology, consider the dog or other animal that bit the human being described above. A sequence of events similar to that described for the human being has occurred in the animal. The viruses attacking the emotional centers of the animal's brain initiated the characteristic aggressive state in which it wandered aimlessly, attacking anything it encountered. Viruses attacking the brain also stimulated the production and release of copious amounts of saliva, giving rise to another familiar symptom of rabies: frothing at the mouth. The viruses reproducing in the salivary glands, and the excessive salivation, assured that an abundance of virus would be chewed into the wound.

The time sequence and pathology of a human victim include an incubation period that may range from ten days to a year; in most victims, however, it is between two and eight weeks. During this time, the virus is replicating in cells at the site of the bite and moving to the central nervous system. As the nervous system begins to be involved, generalized symptoms begin. These include fever, headaches, and nausea and last about a week. Neurologic symptoms then develop, including hyperactivity, seizures, and hallucinations. The throat sometimes becomes so sore and prone to spasms that the patient has trouble swallowing and fears choking while drinking. Another common name for rabies, hydrophobia (literally, fear of water), is based on this aspect of the disease. Paralysis and coma occur about a week after the onset of the neurologic symptoms, and death follows a few days later. Once the symptoms begin in a human being, the disease is nearly always fatal.

In dogs, a similar sequence of events occurs, though the timing is somewhat different and dogs occasionally recover. The aggressive stage described above is called the furious stage in animals, and the gradual development of paralysis is called the paralytic, or dumb, stage. Both phases may occur in dogs or the furious stage may be bypassed, but death commonly occurs shortly after symptoms begin.

Rabies in wildlife is called sylvatic rabies, and the species of wildlife involved differ according to geographic area. Some species act as the virus' reservoir and as the source of rabies epidemics in humans or their pets. In arctic regions of North America and Eurasia, arctic foxes and wolves are the most important hosts of sylvatic rabies. Red and gray foxes and skunks play important roles in spreading the disease in various parts of eastern Canada and the United States, as do raccoons. Some investigators believe that weasels and their relatives are important carriers in maintaining the virus in nature in many areas, although they are not particularly important in the direct transfer of the virus to humans. Bats are common sources of rabies throughout the United States, but especially in the southern part of the country. They play a major role in rabies epidemiology in Mexico and Central and South America, where the disease often occurs in vampire bats.

Other mammals, both wild and domestic, are attacked by the virus, but they are not important in transmitting rabies between species or in acting as reservoirs. Examples of these species are grazing and browsing animals such as cattle and deer, which seldom bite other animals and so are not likely to pass the virus to other creatures. Many of these animals die from rabies, however, and the economic and ecologic impact of these deaths may be great.

These animals are attacked by the virus in the same manner as are humans and dogs, and they show similar symptoms. Rabid wild animals do not always suffer a furious stage. Raccoons, for example, often skip the furious stage and go directly into the dumb stage. Early in this stage they may lose their fear of humans and appear to be friendly. If left alone, they seldom attack, but humans who approach these "friendly" raccoons may be bitten and exposed to rabies. Many bat species also do not go through the furious stage; a bat suffering from dumb rabies is easily caught and may bite if handled, exposing the handler to rabies. Unlike humans, bats, skunks, raccoons, and other wildlife often survive the symptoms of rabies.

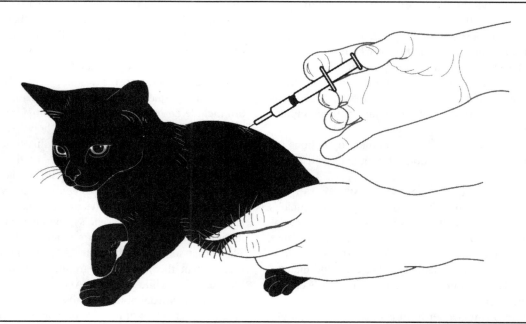

Rabies is a deadly disease that can be transmitted between humans and other mammals; inoculation of household pets against rabies is important to minimize risk to both pets and their human companions.

In addition to the disease it causes in humans and their pets, the rabies virus has had other negative impacts on human society. Rabies transmitted to cattle by vampire bats has had a devastating economic effect on the cattle industry in all of Latin America. Rabies in red foxes has occasionally had a detrimental effect on Canada's fur industry. Wildlife populations in many parts of the world may be periodically decimated by rabies epidemics, sometimes reducing the population of a species of recreational importance to humans or one critical to the ecological stability of a region.

TREATMENT AND THERAPY

Active immunization by vaccination can be used after exposure to rabies because of the relatively long latency period of the virus. If a person has been bitten by a rabid animal, symptoms usually do not appear for two or more weeks. Prompt vaccination after the bite induces the production of antibodies that attack the virus and neutralize it before it reaches the central nervous system. Two other precautions are often taken. The wound is cleaned and treated with antiviral agents, and passive immunity is often produced by injecting antirabies antiserum into the victim.

The rabies inoculations of early immunization series were numerous, extremely painful, and not always successful. Since the early twentieth century, it has been possible to determine whether the attacking animal was rabid and thus whether this painful treatment was necessary. The animal was sacrificed, and its brain was sectioned and stained. Treated in this way, a rabid animal's brain cells often display Negri bodies, named for the scientist who first described them. They are the sites of production of new virus in the brain cell, and their presence indicates the need for vaccination of the victim. Even though the immunization sequence that was first developed was painful, the certain death that followed the onset of symptoms made immunization imperative if there was any possibility of rabies exposure.

Improved immunization sequences and rabies tests have been developed. Refined and nearly infallible, these immunization sequences require only three inoculations and are no more painful than most shots. Tests using antibodies are more rapid and reliable at detecting the presence of the rabies virus than the test for Negri bodies.

Pre-exposure immunization, in contrast to the postexposure immunization described above, is used to protect persons who might be exposed to rabies in their normal activities and to protect pets from contracting rabies. Since the overwhelming majority of human cases of rabies come from dog bites, pet vaccination is the most important part of the successful rabies control programs of developed countries. Laws requiring the immunization of pets against rabies and leash laws (which require that pets be controlled and not allowed to wander freely) have been very effective in reducing human rabies in these countries.

Because wildlife may harbor rabies, attempts have been made to control or eliminate the disease by killing (culling) or immunizing wildlife. Neither approach has been particularly successful, and the first is accompanied by troublesome side effects. The purpose of culling members of host species is to reduce the host population below the point that will sustain the rabies virus' population. This method is based on the idea that each infected host must, on the average, infect at least one other susceptible host before it dies in order for the parasite to persist in the population. The lower the host population, the lower the chance of one host meeting another and thus the lower the probability of an infected host infecting other members of the population. Yet many of the methods of culling (trapping and poisoning, for example) are not species-specific, and members of other species are killed, sometimes in large numbers. Culling has also been ineffective in many cases. It is most successful in small, isolated areas with a low probability of reinvasion.

Instead of reducing the population size of the host, the goal of immunization is to reduce the number of members that are susceptible to rabies by increasing the number that are immune. Oral immunization by scattering bait containing a rabies vaccine has shown promise in the reduction of fox rabies. Whether this method would work with raccoons and whether it is worth the expense of application have been debated.

An argument against immunization of wildlife to control human rabies is based on the success of the control programs in effect and can be stated as follows. Immunization and regulation of pets, preexposure immunization for humans regularly exposed to rabies, and effective postexposure treatment have already minimized the incidence of human rabies in developed nations. Therefore, wildlife immunization is not necessary for the control of human rabies. In developing nations, where human rabies is still a serious disease, all the potential solutions strain the available resources, but the most cost-effective solution would be the one in use in developed countries. There is general agreement, however, that wildlife immunization might be an effective way to increase the population size of a wildlife species that is normally susceptible to rabies, if desirable.

In order to control vampire bats in Latin America, where rabies carried by vampire bats burdens the cattle industry, culling has been attempted repeatedly, often unsuccessfully, and with serious side effects. For example, other bat species, some of which are important to insect control and the pollination of fruit trees, have been regular victims of indiscriminate attempts at vampire bat control by culling.

A more effective, and less ecologically disruptive, method for the control of vampire bats employs anticoagulants. These chemicals stimulate bleeding in the digestive tract of vampire bats that swallow them, resulting in death. The anticoagulant can be applied directly to the backs of the vampire bats and will spread through the bat population when the bats groom one another at the roosting colony. Alternatively, anticoagulant can be injected into a cow's rumen, the enlarged first chamber of its four-part stomach. The anticoagulant is then absorbed into the animal's blood and spread to vampire bats when they feed on the cattle.

In test areas, each method has reduced the number of vampire bat bites in cattle by 90 percent, but each has drawbacks. Direct application to these bats requires extensive netting or trapping, special equipment, and workers skilled in vampire bat identification. The rumen injection technique requires expensive equipment for, and workers experienced in, handling large numbers of cattle. In developing countries, either combination can be difficult to finance.

Education is another important aspect of rabies control. While dogs are the most common source of human rabies, humans occasionally contract the disease after being bitten by a wild animal. In addition, there are potential avenues of transfer other than bites. These include skinning rabid animals, being licked by a rabid animal on broken skin, and breathing air infested with the rabies virus. All these alternative transmission mechanisms are exceptionally infrequent, but there are documented cases of aerial transmission to humans. For example, two men who were not bitten died of rabies contracted while exploring a bat cave in Texas. To be transmitted in this way, the rabies virus must be highly concentrated in the air.

These concentrations probably occur only in caves occupied by a large number of bats, and many of them must be carrying the rabies virus.

While educating spelunkers and hunters to these dangers would have a minimal effect on the incidence of rabies, as these transmission mechanisms are so infrequent, such educating could be of the utmost importance to an individual who is spared a rabies infection by the knowledge. Educating people, especially children, to leave animals acting in an unnatural fashion alone would have a somewhat greater effect on rabies incidence. Most wild animals that can be caught or approached closely are sick and may be suffering from dumb or paralytic rabies. They should be avoided and reported to the appropriate authorities, as should any dog or cat that behaves unnaturally. Educating the public about the importance of pet vaccination and pet control is the most important role of education in the regulation of rabies.

PERSPECTIVE AND PROSPECTS

Rabies in humans and its association with attacks by mad dogs have been known for more than two thousand years. Despite the fact that rabies has never caused epidemics accompanied by mass mortality as have smallpox and bubonic plague, its frightful symptoms and ability to turn a loving family pet into a vicious animal have given the disease a terrifying and mysterious aura. As a result, cures and preventions have been sought throughout history.

In the late 1800's, Louis Pasteur and his associates performed a series of experiments in which the rabies virus was isolated from a dog and injected into rabbit brains. Pasteur called this virus a "street" virus because it was isolated directly from dogs in the street. The virus replicated in the rabbit brain and could be transferred into another rabbit's brain where it again replicated. Growth of the virus in one of the rabbit brains was called a "passage." A sequence of such passages resulted in a virus which had a more predictable and shorter incubation period. This virus was called a "fixed" virus because of its fixed incubation period. After a hundred such passages, the virus had lost much of its ability to infect dogs.

Pasteur then developed an immunization sequence which protected dogs from the street virus. He air-dried rabbit spinal cord tissue infected with the fixed virus for varying amounts of time and developed a series of virus solutions, ranging from those that could not infect rabbits through those that could occasionally establish weak infections to those that were maximally infective. He then injected dogs daily for ten days, beginning with the noninfective preparation the first day and increasing the infectivity with each day's injection until, on the tenth day, he was injecting highly infective virus. Dogs so treated were resistant to experimentally injected street virus.

Pasteur was still refining his immunization system when a boy who had been attacked by a rabid dog was brought to him. Knowing that the latency period of the virus might allow time for the development of immunity before the symptoms appeared, and aware of the almost certain fatal result if nothing was done, Pasteur treated the boy with the sequence that he had used on the dogs. The boy lived, with no apparent side effects, and Pasteur's treatment became the standard for rabies. The modern treatment sequence is a refinement of Pasteur's. While the immunization sequence for rabies was not the first to be used successfully—smallpox immunization nearly a century earlier holds that distinction—the possibility of immunization after exposure to diseases with long incubation periods was established by Pasteur's work.

Considerable work has been done on the epidemiology of rabies. Mathematical and computer models have been developed that attempt to predict the characteristics of the disease spread under different conditions, and thus suggest means of controlling and preventing rabies epidemics. Arguments over the effectiveness of wildlife vaccination are partially based on such models. The usefulness of these models is not restricted to rabies epidemiology, but contributes to an understanding of epidemiology in general. Thus research on rabies continues to enhance the control and prevention of that terrifying disease and to add to the general knowledge base of medicine as well.

—*Carl W. Hoagstrom, Ph.D.*

See also Bites and stings; Coma; Immunization and vaccination; Paralysis; Seizures; Viral infections; Zoonoses.

FOR FURTHER INFORMATION:

Bacon, Philip J., ed. *Population Dynamics of Rabies in Wildlife.* New York: Academic Press, 1985. Deals primarily with models of rabies epidemiology, but also contains good discussions of the virus and disease. Each chapter was written by an active investigator. Illustrations, an index, and references are provided.

Baer, George M., ed. *The Natural History of Rabies.* 2d ed. Boca Raton, Fla.: CRC Press, 1991. Probably the most thorough coverage of all aspects of rabies available. Each chapter was written by an active investigator in the field. Includes illustrations, an index, and extensive reference lists.

Biddle, Wayne. *Field Guide to Germs.* New York: Henry Holt, 1995. This comprehensive book is easily accessible to the nonspecialist and includes a discussion of nearly every virus, bacterium, and fungus known to cause human and nonhuman animal disease. The history of the microbe and the treatment of diseases are included.

Bruggemann, Edward P. "Rabies in the Mid-Atlantic States: Should Raccoons Be Vaccinated?" *BioScience* 42 (October, 1992): 694-699. Argues that vaccination of wild raccoons to control human rabies is expensive, probably would not be effective, and is certainly unnecessary. Contains illustrations and an extensive reference list, including several references to articles arguing in favor of vaccinating wild raccoons.

Campbell, James B., and K. M. Charlton, eds. *Rabies.* Boston: Kluwer Academic, 1988. An excellent source covering most aspects of rabies. The first chapter provides an especially interesting history of the disease. Each chapter is written by an active investigator.

Constantine, Denny G. "Health Precautions for Bat Researchers." In *Ecological and Behavioral Methods for the Study of Bats,* edited by Thomas H. Kunz. Washington, D.C.: Smithsonian Institution Press, 1988. Pages 504 through 515 deal with rabies in general but especially in bats. An appendix gives some sources for an array of protective products and services. An index and an extensive reference list are provided.

Finley, Don. *Mad Dogs: The New Rabies Plague.* College Station: Texas A&M University Press, 1998. Finley, a newspaper medical reporter, describes the canine rabies outbreak that began in Texas in 1988 and the epidemic of raccoon rabies that swept the East Coast from Florida to New York.

Kaplan, Colin, G. S. Turner, and D. A. Warrell. *Rabies: The Facts.* 2d ed. New York: Oxford University Press, 1986. An excellent summary of rabies, the virus and the disease, written for the layperson. Contains illustrations, an index, and a bibliography.

Levy, Richard L. "A Cautionary Tale: Bitten by a Dog in Kathmandu." *Patient Care* 31, no. 9 (May 15,

1997): 212-214. This article tells of a young woman who died in Massachusetts after being bitten by a dog in Nepal and failing to find treatment in Thailand and Australia.

Pace, Brian, and Richard M. Glass. "Rabies." *Journal of the American Medical Association* 284, no. 8 (August 30, 2000): 1052. The symptoms and treatments for rabies are discussed. Anti-rabies treatment should begin as soon as possible, ideally within twenty-four to forty-eight hours after exposure to rabies.

RADIATION SICKNESS
DISEASE/DISORDER

ANATOMY OR SYSTEM AFFECTED: Gastrointestinal system, hair, skin, stomach

SPECIALTIES AND RELATED FIELDS: Critical care, emergency medicine, occupational health, oncology, public health, radiology

DEFINITION: An acute illness that occurs when an individual is exposed to a sudden, large dose of nuclear radiation or X rays.

Typical symptoms of radiation sickness are nausea, diarrhea, skin burns, internal bleeding, and severe anemia. The production of blood corpuscles in the bone marrow is inhibited, and the ability of the body to fight infection is reduced.

The severity of radiation sickness depends on the dose, which is commonly measured in units called rads (an acronym for radiation absorbed dose). For humans, a whole-body dose greater than 600 rads is usually fatal. At 450 rads, there is a 50 percent survival rate. Below 50 rads, no symptoms of radiation sickness are observable, although the risk of cancer is somewhat higher than normal. Radiation therapy for cancer patients typically prescribes doses of about 5,000 rads. Such large doses are not fatal for two reasons: First, only a small region of the body (the actual cancer site) is irradiated; and second, the therapy is given over a period of several weeks, so that the body has time to recover between treatments.

Once radiation damage occurs, however, little can be done to repair it directly. Treatment focuses on helping the body's natural processes of recovery. Vomiting and diarrhea can be controlled with drugs, while bacterial infections and wounds are treated with antibiotics. In extreme cases, bone marrow transplants can be performed to reestablish the formation of new blood cells. Donor cells are not likely to be rejected because the body's immune system has been inactivated temporarily by the radiation.

—Hans G. Graetzer, Ph.D.

See also Bone marrow transplantation; Burns and scalds; Environmental diseases; Occupational health; Radiation therapy.

FOR FURTHER INFORMATION:

Frigerio, Norman. *Your Body and Radiation.* Washington, D.C.: U.S. Atomic Energy Commission, 1967. This very concise guide offers details on the physiological effects of radiation. Includes bibliographical references, a glossary, and an index.

Hall, Eric J. *Radiation and Life.* 2d ed. New York: Pergamon Press, 1984. Covers the physiological effects of radiation and outlines safety measures. Also covers radiation in the medical setting, such as radiology and nuclear medicine. Includes an index.

Prasad, Kedar N. *Handbook of Radiobiology.* Rev. 2d ed. Boca Raton, Fla.: CRC Press, 1995. This handbook presents the most current information on the effects of ionizing radiation on mammalian cells, with emphasis on human tissues. The dose-effect relationship is emphasized in a quantitative manner.

RADIATION THERAPY
PROCEDURE

ANATOMY OR SYSTEM AFFECTED: All

SPECIALTIES AND RELATED FIELDS: Nuclear medicine, oncology, radiology

DEFINITION: The use of X rays or radioactivity in the treatment of cancer patients, frequently in combination with surgery and chemotherapy.

KEY TERMS:

computed tomography (CT) scanning: from the Greek word *tomos,* meaning "section"; the process of using X rays to obtain a computer picture of an interior cross-section from a patient's body

gamma rays: penetrating radiation that comes from a radioactive source, such as cobalt 60

internal radiation: therapy in which a small radioactive source is implanted close to the cancer site, such as on the cervix or inside the chest cavity

magnetic resonance imaging (MRI): a diagnostic technique using large magnets (not X rays) to outline the shape and size of a tumor

metastasis: the spread of cancer cells from one part of the body to another

oncologist: a physician who specializes in the treatment of cancer *radiation dose:* the amount of radiation absorbed, depending on the intensity of the source and the time of exposure; measured in units of rads or grays

tumor: an abnormal mass of tissue which may be malignant (growing larger) or benign (not spreading)

X rays: penetrating radiation produced by means of a high-voltage machine; useful for both diagnosis and therapy of cancerous tissue

INDICATIONS AND PROCEDURES

When a person is diagnosed with cancer, three main methods of treatment may be used: surgery, radiation, and chemotherapy (drugs). Surgery and radiation are most useful if the cancer is a localized tumor whose shape and size can be determined. Radiation is the treatment of choice if the tumor is at an inoperable location, such as inside the brain, liver, or spine. In some cases, radiation is used following surgery in order to prevent recurrence of a malignant growth.

The amount of energy absorbed in radiation therapy can be expressed quantitatively in a unit called a gray. It was named after a British radiobiologist, Louis Harold Gray, who studied the biological effect of various ionizing radiations. One gray corresponds to the absorption of a fixed amount of radiation energy. Before 1984, radiation doses were commonly measured in rads, which was an acronym for radiation absorbed dose. The conversion factor is "100 rads = 1 gray." Since most references continue to use the more familiar rad, it will be adopted here. For converting to grays, each rad value is divided by one hundred.

In order to develop a feel for typical dose levels in radiation therapy, it is helpful to remember two numbers for comparison: First, the maximum safe dose established by the Nuclear Regulatory Commission (NRC) for radiation exposure in the workplace is 5 rads per year; second, a lethal dose for 50 percent of humans, called LD-50, is about 450 rads. LD-50 means that, statistically, 50 percent would die and 50 percent would recover from such a massive dose.

The numbers given above must be interpreted with care. For example, a dental X ray gives a dose of about 2 rads. Four such X rays give a total exposure of 8 rads, exceeding the NRC yearly maximum of 5 rads. Only a small part of the body, however, perhaps 1 percent, is irradiated during a dental X ray. Therefore, the radiation dose averaged over the whole body is only 1 percent of 8 rads.

A patient with malignant cancer might be given twenty radiation treatments of 250 rads each, for a to-

tal dose of 5,000 rads. Even though this far exceeds the LD-50 of 450 rads, it is not lethal because it is spread out over time. The patient may develop symptoms of radiation sickness—skin reddening, nausea, loss of hair, and blood changes—but the body has time to heal partially between irradiations. The healing process can be compared to recovery from a serious burn injury, in which the skin and flesh repair themselves but permanent scars may be left behind. The present trend in radiology is to subdivide the total dose into more and smaller increments, reducing patient discomfort.

One of the most common elements used for cancer therapy is called cobalt 60, which is created by irradiating ordinary cobalt in a research reactor. Because the radioactive form of cobalt emits gamma rays with a penetrating power that is equivalent to a 2 million-volt X-ray machine, it is useful for the treatment of deep internal cancers. The radioactive source must be kept in a thick lead shield. When a patient is to be treated, the source is positioned near the cancer site, and a small port is opened briefly to irradiate it. Sometimes, the cobalt source is moved around the patient so that the gamma rays enter the body from different angles, thus reducing the damage to healthy tissue lying above the cancer site. The irradiation procedure is done by remote control so that the radiologist and other medical personnel will not be exposed.

Radioactive gold is another useful source for radiation therapy and one that is especially suitable for internal placement in the body, such as in the treatment of uterine or ovarian cancer. The half-life of radioactive gold is less than three days, so it can be left in the body to provide continuous treatment for a short time. The gamma rays from gold are of much lower energy than those from cobalt, so they penetrate only a few centimeters of tissue around the source. This limits damage to healthy cells farther from the irradiation site.

X rays are seldom used today for cancer therapy because radioactive sources are much more convenient. A large number of radiopharmaceuticals, with various half-lives and energies, are available for different applications. Beams of electrons, protons, and other particles coming directly from nuclear accelerators also have been used to irradiate tumors, with some excellent results. The personnel and equipment costs to operate an accelerator, however, are too great for most hospitals. Also, patients may find the experience of being bombarded by the output beam from a large and noisy accelerator to be too traumatic.

The various types of radiation, including X rays, gamma rays, and particle beams, all produce damage in living tissue by the process of ionization. The radiation strikes individual atoms and breaks the bonds that hold molecules together. The breakup of normal molecules produces positive and negative ions, which act as toxic chemicals. The internal structure of cells is disrupted so that they can no longer replicate themselves. Fortunately, cancer cells tend to be more sensitive to radiation damage than normal cells.

Radioactive needles, grains, and other sealed-source designs may be used when there is a suitable body cavity or opening. Such internal sources are common for treating cancer of the prostate, vagina, uterus, rectum, throat, and larynx. One problem with implanted sources is the radiation dose received by the physician during the surgery. Sometimes, it is possible to use "afterloading," in which a hollow tube or shell is positioned in the patient and radioactive material is loaded into it at a later time.

Breast cancer is the leading cause of death for American women in their thirties and forties. In the United States, about 180,000 new cases are diagnosed per year, and 15 percent of these patients will die within five years. Early detection and treatment are the keys to improving the chances for survival. A radical mastectomy (breast removal) can be an emotionally traumatic experience. If the cancer is not too advanced, however, radiation therapy is an alternative. In some cases, daily treatment with a cobalt source can be done on an outpatient basis, with only minor disruptions of schedule and no long-term disfigurement.

During treatment for any type of cancer, the radiologist needs to determine whether the radiation therapy is shrinking the tumor. Therefore, computed tomography (CT) scanning or magnetic resonance imaging (MRI) will be used during and after treatment to monitor the size of the tumor. The radiation dose then can be adjusted to take into account the individual characteristics of various patients.

The goal of radiation therapy is to deliver a dose of several thousand rads to a cancer site while minimizing the damage to surrounding tissue and nearby organs. The shape of a malignant cancer may be a simple round lump, or it can be a complex group of nodules with tentacles extending through the flesh. For effective treatment, it is essential to determine the location and shape of the tumor as precisely as possible. An ordinary X-ray photograph is not very useful for diagnosing a tumor. The problem is a lack of contrast between tumor and surrounding tissue, because there is very little difference in their densities. An X ray of the head, for example, provides an excellent outline of the skull, but it cannot distinguish between tumor and brain material on the inside. In the 1970's, a major advance in X-ray technology called CT scanning was developed in England, which is sometimes also called a computed axial tomography (CAT) scan. CT scanning replaces the film of conventional X rays with pictures on a computer screen.

A narrow X-ray beam with the diameter of a pencil scans across the region of interest, while an electronic detector measures the transmitted intensity and sends the data to the computer. A tumor is slightly denser than surrounding tissue, so a small decrease of intensity is recorded by the detector. The X-ray beam and detector system are rotated by a small angle, and another scan is recorded. Altogether, 180 scans may be used to record one "slice" of the body. The region where beams of decreased intensity from all the scans intersect defines the location of a tumor in that slice. Next, the X-ray beam and detector are moved along the body a small distance, and another 180 scans are made to obtain a second slice. Several more slices will be recorded. Eventually, the computer assembles all the information into a three-dimensional picture of the region of interest.

The sharpness and contrast obtained with CT scans are remarkable improvements over X-ray film. A radiologist can view the computer display of a tumor from various angles and with different enlargements. The computer screen can be photographed to provide a permanent record. The two scientists who developed the CT scan, Allan Cormack and Godfrey Hounsfield, shared the Nobel Prize in Physiology or Medicine in 1979.

An entirely different method to determine the location and outline of an internal tumor is called MRI. Instead of using X rays, MRI utilizes the magnetic properties of hydrogen nuclei, which can be aligned by a very strong magnet.

The patient lies on a couch in a magnetic field produced by coils around his or her body. Radio waves are used to reverse the direction of alignment of the hydrogen. The concentration of hydrogen atoms in a tumor differs slightly from that in the surrounding tissue, so the output signal will differ correspondingly.

Several methods are used to identify the precise location in the body where the magnetic reversals occur. A computer is used to convert the information into a pictorial display on a screen. Since bones contain virtually no hydrogen, the MRI picture shows them as shadows while emphasizing the structure of soft organs, tumors, and tissue.

Both MRI and CT scanning are complex diagnostic procedures. In order to diagnose and treat a cancer, radiologists, medical physicists, physicians, and computer specialists must work together as a team. New techniques for obtaining and displaying information are under continuing development.

USES AND COMPLICATIONS

The way in which radiation therapy is used depends on many factors, such as tumor location, the age and overall health of the patient, and the extent and stage of the cancer. Consider a young woman who has symptoms of back pain and loss of feeling in her legs. Use of MRI clearly shows a tumor growing inside her spinal column. For cancer in this location, treatment using radiation therapy, rather than surgery or chemotherapy, is indicated.

A treatment plan is devised that will minimize the radiation dose to the patient's lungs, heart, and liver; the direction of entry for the beam of radiation must avoid passing through these sensitive organs. Furthermore, the radiologist has to make sure that the proper dose will be received at various depths below the skin. A plastic dummy to simulate the patient, called a phantom, can be irradiated with detectors placed inside it to measure the dose. Scattering of radiation and shielding effects by bones can be very complex and must be determined by computer calculations supplemented by careful measurements.

The radiation pattern can be shaped with filters and baffles so that it will conform to the shape of the tumor as closely as possible. A useful computer display for planning the therapy, called the "beam's-eye view," shows the tumor and its surroundings as if the observer's eye were at the source of radiation.

Two final considerations in treatment planning for this patient are how the total radiation dose is to be subdivided and what the time interval between exposures should be. The radiologist must make a decision based on a judgment of the patient's stamina, as well as of the urgency of treatment.

Consider another patient, a man who has developed a cancerous tumor of the tongue. Surgery is un-

desirable because his speaking ability would be impaired. Instead of an external radiation beam, the radiologist will probably recommend that radioactive needles be inserted directly into the affected region. Five to ten needles containing radioactive radium or cesium deliver the appropriate dose directly to the cancer site. The needles are left in place for several days and then removed. An alternative to needles in this case is the use of very small grains of radioactive material that can be implanted into the tumor. Sources with a short half-life, such as radioactive gold or radon, lose almost all their activity within two weeks, so the grains do not have to be removed.

The overall effectiveness of radiation therapy can be summarized approximately by the "half-half-half" rule. About half of all cancers are treated with radiation. Half of those patients are given a large enough dose to attempt a cure. (For the others, radiation is used simply for pain relief.) Finally, about half of these patients are actually cured by radiation. Out of about 800,000 new cases of cancer reported annually in the United States, about 100,000 patients are cured with radiation therapy. The success rate is encouraging, but clearly there is much room left for improvement.

The survival rate after radiation treatment varies greatly depending on the site of cancer in the body. For example, patients with localized cancer of the prostate, larynx, or uterus have five-year survival rates that range from 80 to 90 percent. At the other end of the scale, stomach or lung cancers that have spread show only about a 10 percent survival rate. Radiation therapy for ten different kinds of cancer—breast, cervix, larynx, prostate, uterus, bladder, testicle, tongue, and mouth cancers and Hodgkin's disease—results in cure rates that are equal to or greater than those with surgery while preserving the organ function.

Many people are apprehensive about the hazards of radiation, with good reason. In the 1920's, some workers who were hired to apply radium paint to watch dials (to make them glow in the dark) developed cancer when they ingested radioactive material. At Hiroshima and Nagasaki, many people developed radiation sickness and died from the aftereffects of the atomic bombs dropped on those cities. For medical applications of radiation, regulatory agencies which are responsive to the general public must evaluate potential benefits and risks. Sometimes, sensationalized articles are published that present frightening scenarios of highly unlikely hazards. The perception of risk from low-level radioactive waste, for example, far exceeds the actual hazard. The advantages of radiation therapy would be lost if permits for hazardous waste storage were denied. The responsible use of any technology should balance concerns for safety with the benefits of that technology.

Ensuring the health and safety of medical personnel who administer radiation therapy to patients requires proper training. All workers must wear radiation monitors, which are checked daily. Radiation areas have to be posted with warning signs. The nuclear medicine department at a hospital must keep an accurate inventory of radioactive materials. The shipment and disposal of radiopharmaceuticals are strictly regulated. Periodic on-site visits by Nuclear Regulatory Commission inspectors also are part of the licensing procedure. Careless overexposure of personnel must be avoided if the benefits of radiation therapy are to find continued acceptance by the medical profession and the general public.

PERSPECTIVE AND PROSPECTS

Radiation therapy most commonly makes use of X rays or radioactivity. It is interesting to note that both types of radiation were discovered only a year apart in the 1890's. Wilhelm Röntgen, a German physicist, discovered X rays in 1895. He received the Nobel Prize for his work in 1901, the first year in which the award was given. He used high voltage to accelerate an electron beam; when the electrons hit a metal target, they released a new kind of penetrating radiation. Röntgen made a now-famous X-ray photograph of his wife's hand which clearly showed the bones inside the flesh. The medical profession adopted X rays with great enthusiasm, primarily for the diagnosis of broken bones, swallowed objects, and bullet or shrapnel fragments.

Radioactivity was first observed in 1896 by Henri Becquerel, in Paris. By chance, Becquerel had placed a uranium rock next to unused photographic film that was still wrapped in its container. He was amazed to find that radiation from the uranium had penetrated the wrapping and had exposed the film inside. His discovery and follow-up experiments earned for him the Nobel Prize in 1905.

Marie Curie, a graduate student under Becquerel, became famous for isolating a new radioactive element from uranium ore, which she named radium. It emits radiation at a rate that is a million times greater than an equivalent weight of uranium. In her doctoral thesis in 1904, Curie described an experiment in which she placed a small capsule containing radium on her husband's arm. It produced a sore that took more than a month to heal. The hazards of handling radioactivity and the possibility of using it to destroy cancer cells were recognized quite early.

The element radium is very rare on earth. In fact, the world's total supply is less than 1 kilogram. Only after the invention of nuclear particle accelerators and neutron sources in the 1930's was it possible to create artificial radioactive elements in substantial amounts.

Radiation therapy has since become a treatment of choice in oncology. Such treatment will likely remain necessary for some time to come: It is not reasonable to expect a cure for cancer soon because there are too many different types. Much has been accomplished, however, in the area of prevention. The strong correlation between lung cancer and smoking has received wide publicity, so many people have stopped, at least in the United States. Research with animals has linked cancer to certain food additives and industrial pollutants, leading to legal restrictions on their use. In addition to surgery, radiation, and chemotherapy, other treatment methods are under investigation. For example, one procedure involves blocking the blood supply from reaching a tumor so that the malignant cells die from lack of nutrients. Other researchers hope to use genetic engineering, trying to stimulate the body's immune system to produce specific antibodies that will fight against the cancer cells.

—Hans G. Graetzer, Ph.D.

See also Cancer; Chemotherapy; Computed tomography (CT) scanning; Hair loss and baldness; Magnetic resonance imaging (MRI); Malignancy and metastasis; Oncology; Nuclear medicine; Nuclear radiology; Radiopharmaceuticals, use of.

FOR FURTHER INFORMATION:

Cameron, John R., James G. Skofronick, and Roderick M. Grant. *Medical Physics: Physics of the Body.* Madison, Wis.: Medical Physics, 1992. A textbook for college students who are preparing for a career in the health professions. Pertinent chapters deal with X rays, radiation therapy, nuclear medicine (radioactivity), and radiation safety. Offers clear explanations and well-chosen photographs.

Hall, Eric J. *Radiation and Life.* 2d ed. New York: Pergamon Press, 1984. An excellent introduction to X rays and radioactivity for nonspecialists. One chapter gives a good overview of radiation in medicine, with applications for both diagnosis and therapy. Other topics include industrial uses of radioactivity and a discussion of radiation risks versus benefits.

Hendee, William R., and Geoffrey S, Ibbott. *Radiation Therapy Physics*. 2d ed. St. Louis: C. V. Mosby, 1996. A fairly technical book for radiology students. Shows how doses are calculated from various sources of radiation, such as radioactive cobalt, radium, cesium, and particle beams.

Laws, Priscilla W., and the Public Citizen Health Research Group. *The X-Ray Information Book*. New York: Farrar, Straus, & Giroux, 1983. This book is billed as a consumers' guide to avoiding unnecessary medical and dental X rays. The author gives a balanced, factual presentation about the benefits and risks of diagnostic X-ray procedures.

Saha, Gopal B. *Physics and Radiobiology of Nuclear Medicine*. New York: Springer, 2000. A textbook and study guide for medical residents preparing to take the American Board of Radiology examination, especially those specializing in nuclear radiology. Reviews the fundamental physics of radiology, the instrumentation, radiobiology, dosimetry, and safety regulations.

Smith, F. A. *A Primer in Applied Radiation Physics*. River Edge, N.J.: World Scientific, 2000. This volume, intended for students of radiology, includes bibliographical references and an index.

Sochurek, Howard. *Medicine's New Vision*. Easton, Pa.: Mack, 1988. Contains many excellent computer-generated pictures taken with ultrasound, X-ray tomography, and MRI. One extensive chapter is devoted to radiation therapy. The author relates actual case histories of cancer patients in order to personalize the applications of this high-technology apparatus.

RADIOLOGY. *See* IMAGING AND RADIOLOGY; NUCLEAR RADIOLOGY.

RADIONUCLEOTIDE SCANNING. *See* NUCLEAR MEDICINE; RADIOPHARMACEUTICALS.

RADIOPHARMACEUTICALS
PROCEDURE

ANATOMY OR SYSTEM AFFECTED: All

SPECIALTIES AND RELATED FIELDS: Endocrinology, internal medicine, oncology, radiology

DEFINITION: Imaging techniques involving radioactive chemical agents that are designed to localize in specific organs and emit radiation, which can be detected outside the body with a camera in order to provide visual images of the organ.

KEY TERMS:

becquerel: the international unit of radioactivity, defined as a radioactive sample which is decaying at the rate of one disintegration per second

electron volt: a unit of energy defined as the energy acquired by an electron traveling through a potential difference of 1 volt

gamma camera: a type of radiation detection instrument that detects gamma rays external to the body and makes an image of the radionuclide distribution in body organs; also known as a scintillation camera

gamma ray: a type of electromagnetic radiation that has the same physical properties as X rays but is emitted by unstable nuclei in their decay process; gamma rays are capable of penetrating soft tissue, thereby allowing their detection outside the body to produce images of organs

half-life: the time required for one-half of the nuclei in a radioactive sample to decay

radioimmunotherapy: a cancer therapy using radionuclides; the radionuclides attach themselves to antibodies that tend to target cancer cells in the body, thus eradicating the cancer cells through selective irradiation

radionuclide: an unstable atomic nucleus which, in the process of decay, emits radiation; also referred to as a radioisotope

THE FUNDAMENTALS OF RADIOACTIVITY

All matter consists of atoms, which contain a central nucleus and tiny particles called electrons that revolve around the nucleus. Electrons carry a small negative charge, while the nucleus is made up of particles called neutrons, which have no charge, and protons, which carry a positive charge. Atoms are generally neutral, with the number of protons in the nucleus equaling the number of electrons. Most objects are made up of atoms in which the neutron and proton numbers in their nuclei are arranged in such a way that they are stable. If the proton number or the neutron number in the nucleus is altered, the atom may become unstable. Such unstable atoms are termed radioactive and tend to reach a stable state by emitting radiation. This process is referred to as radioactive decay, and the elemental atoms that emit radiation are called radioisotopes or radionuclides. All stable elements can be made into radioactive elements by either adding or removing neutrons or protons, a process known as the artificial production of radioactivity. The few naturally occurring radioisotopes, such as radon 222 and uranium 235, are not used in nuclear medicine.

Radioactivity was first discovered by the French scientist Antoine-Henri Becquerel in 1896, when he observed that a photographic plate sitting next to a uranium sample had darkened. Appropriately, the international unit of radioactivity was chosen to be the becquerel. Radioactivity is a property of unstable atomic nuclei, and the rate of decay cannot be affected by normal physical and chemical processes such as heat, pressure, or the presence of magnetic or electric fields. The nuclei in a radioactive sample do not decay spontaneously or all at once. Rather, they decay randomly at a rate that is characteristic of the given radioisotope. While it is impossible to tell when a particular nucleus will decay or disintegrate, the fraction of nuclei in a sample that will decay in a given time can be determined. The decay rate of a radioactive sample is usually expressed in terms of its half-life, the time required for one-half of the original sample nuclei to decay. Half-life is a characteristic property of a particular radionuclide. The half-lives of radioactive isotopes vary from a small fraction of a second to millions of years. For example, carbon 14 has a half-life of 5,730 years, while the half-life of iodine 123 is 13 hours. Naturally occurring uranium 238 decays with a half-life of 4.5 billion years, which is the approximate age of the earth itself. Hence, at present there remains only half of the original uranium 238 that was formed when the earth was born.

Radionuclides emit three types of radiation: alpha particles, beta particles, and gamma rays. Alpha particles are positively charged ions containing two protons and two neutrons. Beta particles are either positively (positron) or negatively (electron) charged and have the same mass as an electron. In contrast, gamma rays are electromagnetic waves that have no mass or charge and are sometimes called photons. Because alpha particles are relatively massive, they can be totally absorbed by a sheet of paper. Beta particles can penetrate up to about a centimeter or so into an object, depending on their energy. On the other hand, gamma rays of moderate energy can easily penetrate through the body, as with X rays. When radionuclides

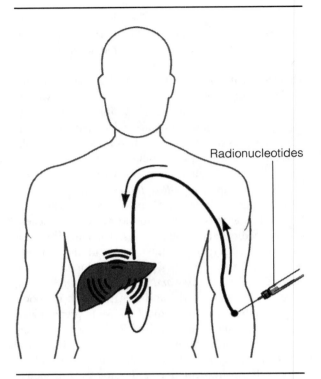

One use of radiopharmaceuticals is to deliver radioactivity to a target organ, such as the liver, that may otherwise be inaccessible to radiation treatment.

that emit gamma rays are administered to patients, the gamma rays exit the body and are captured by a scintillation camera, which produces an image. The desirable energy of the gamma rays for external detection and imaging with gamma cameras is generally in the range of 100 kilo-electron volts to 300 kilo-electron volts. The half-life of the radionuclide emitting the gamma rays should be long enough to allow its uptake by the organ of interest, and subsequent imaging with a gamma camera, and short enough so as not to irradiate the patient long after the image is obtained. Half-lives between three hours and three days are considered optimal for diagnostic purposes. When radionuclides are used for therapy, the half-life is generally required to be in the range of several days, and the preferred form of radiation consists of beta particles because they tend to deposit their energy near the disintegration site.

USES AND COMPLICATIONS

If the physician is interested in imaging a particular organ, drugs that take the radionuclide preferentially to that organ are necessary. This is achieved by chemically attaching the radionuclide to a pharmaceutical carrier. Once the radiopharmaceutical is localized in the organ, the gamma rays that it emits are detected by a gamma camera, which electronically displays an image that is representative of the radionuclide distribution. Such images are of substantial diagnostic value. Similarly, radionuclides attached to drugs that selectively target cancer cells can potentially deliver lethal doses of radiation to the cancer cells, a process called radioimmunotherapy. Hence, radiopharmaceuticals play an important role in medicine, providing new and promising avenues for diagnosis and therapy.

Radiopharmaceuticals are generally administered intravenously to patients. Blood flow to the organ of interest determines the fraction of the administered radioactivity that will be delivered. The ability of the organ to accumulate the circulating radiopharmaceutical is also an important determinant of the pathological condition of the organ. Such considerations are usually taken into account in developing appropriate pharmaceuticals.

Although many radionuclides are available, the most preferred one is called technetium 99m, an excited (metastable) state of technetium 99. This radionuclide is readily available, has a convenient half-life of six hours, and has very desirable radiation properties. Accordingly, many pharmaceuticals are labeled with this radionuclide for diagnostic nuclear medicine purposes. A few other radionuclides, such as thallium 201, iodine 123, gallium 67, and indium 111, can be used when technetium 99m compounds are not available.

The most widely used radiopharmaceutical for brain imaging is technetium 99m pertechnetate. The primary advantage of this chemical is that it is inexpensive and can be easily prepared. Other radiopharmaceuticals used for brain studies are technetium 99m diethylenetriamine-pentacetic acid (DTPA) and technetium 99m glucoheptonate. Brain imaging usually consists of a dynamic study immediately after bolus intravenous injection of the compound in which rapid sequential images are obtained as the radiopharmaceutical enters the brain. This is followed by a static image one hour later. When a brain lesion is suspected, a delayed static image is sometimes necessary three to four hours after an injection. These imaging techniques are valuable in detecting neoplastic tissue, inflammatory processes, infarction, Alzheimer's disease, and stroke. Another class of radiopharmaceuticals

has also been developed to study brain function. These compounds, such as carbon 11 N-methylpiperone, use very short-lived radionuclides that need on-site radionuclide production facilities and require a sophisticated imaging system called a positron emission tomography (PET) scanning unit. Imaging of cerebrospinal fluid is performed using DTPA labeled with indium 111 after an intrathecal administration. Radiopharmaceuticals for such administrations are tested carefully for their safety.

Lung imaging using radiopharmaceuticals is usually performed to study either pulmonary perfusion or ventilation. For perfusion studies, the radiopharmaceutical of choice is microaggregated albumin (MAA) labeled with technetium 99m. Ventilation studies are performed using the radioactive inert gas xenon 133. The patient breathes while the images are obtained with a gamma camera. These lung studies are used extensively to detect several conditions, including pulmonary embolism, asthma, bronchitis, tumors, inflammatory disease, congestive heart failure, and deep-vein thrombus.

Bone imaging with radiopharmaceuticals often provides earlier diagnosis and better detection of lesions than other radiographic procedures. Furthermore, the extent of metastatic disease may be determined using radionuclide imaging techniques. Other applications of bone imaging include determination of the viability of bone, detection of infections in prosthetic joints, necrosis, and infarction, and evaluation of fractures and bone pain. Bone-seeking compounds are usually similar to calcium or phosphates in their chemical behavior. Hence, diphosphonate labeled with technetium 99m and its analogs are the compounds of choice for this purpose.

Radionuclide imaging techniques play an important role in evaluating the function of the heart. Coronary artery perfusion is studied using thallium 201 chloride. The patient is asked to exercise on a treadmill, and the radionuclide is injected at peak stress. The patient continues to exercise for an additional minute, and redistribution of the thallium 201 within the myocardium occurs immediately after cessation of the exercise. Gamma camera images are obtained soon thereafter. Abnormal thallium distribution is the basis for the detection and diagnosis of stress-induced ischemia and permanent myocardial damage. Acute myocardial infarction can be detected using pyrophosphate labeled with technetium 99m within twenty-four to seventy-two hours after the onset of symptoms.

Other radiopharmaceuticals using technetium 99m as a label are also under development. In order to evaluate ventricular function, the radiochemical is administered intravenously and images are obtained during the first pass of the radionuclide through the heart, lungs, and great vessels. An alternate technique for this purpose is to obtain images of the cardiac blood pool after the radiopharmaceutical has achieved equilibrium in the intravascular space. Such noninvasive studies are invaluable in the diagnosis of heart problems and in the management of patients with heart disease.

Evaluation of thyroid function using radioisotope techniques marked the beginning of the field of nuclear medicine. The element iodine is actively transported into the thyroid gland, where it is retained. Therefore, the readily available radioiodines iodine 131 and iodine 123 have been used for this purpose. Technetium 99m pertechnetate is sometimes used because of its low cost and favorable radiation characteristics. Thyroid uptake tests usually involve administration of a small dose of sodium iodide 131 in either liquid or capsule form and measurement of the radioiodine in the thyroid eighteen to twenty-four hours later. Significantly higher uptake compared to the normal value is a reflection of an overactive gland (hyperthyroidism). Conversely, a lower uptake indicates an underactive gland (hypothyroidism). Thyroid imaging is performed using either sodium iodide 123 or technetium 99m pertechnetate to detect cancer. Effective treatment of benign and malignant cancers, as well as hyperthyroidism, is accomplished by administering larger doses of iodine 131. Although the strong uptake of radioactive iodine by the thyroid gland is useful in nuclear medicine, uptake of iodine 131 in the thyroids of people living in nuclear-fallout zones, such as the one around the Chernobyl nuclear reactor, is a major concern. The risk from such exposure can be reduced by saturating the thyroid with nonradioactive iodine using orally administered doses of Lugol's iodine solution.

Radiopharmaceutical studies of kidneys are sometimes necessary to evaluate structural and functional abnormalities. Renal imaging is indicated to assess renal blood flow and the differential and quantitative functioning of natural or transplanted kidneys. Among the radiopharmaceuticals used for these studies are technetium-labeled glucoheptonate, 2,3-dimercaptosuccinic acid (DMSA), and DTPA. Iodine 123 hippurate is also employed for glomerular filtration studies.

Nuclear medicine techniques to image the liver and spleen are also available. Alcohol-related liver diseases can be readily diagnosed using liver images obtained after injection of technetium-labeled sulfur colloid. Primary liver cancers and metastases can also be detected, and the physiological functioning of transplanted livers can be assessed. Spleen imaging with technetium 99m sulfur colloid has been useful in detecting hepatomas, cysts, infarctions, and neoplasms. Gastrointestinal hemorrhaging and associated bleeding are identified by removing a small portion of the patient's red blood cells, labeling them with technetium 99m, and injecting the labeled cells back into the patient. Similarly, white blood cells labeled with indium 111 are used to image abscesses and inflammation. Radionuclide procedures also provide a method to assess digestive disorders and esophageal transit noninvasively. A variety of tumors can be diagnosed when gallium 67 citrate is used for imaging. This radionuclide is also used in studying patients with acquired immunodeficiency syndrome (AIDS).

Radiopharmaceuticals are also playing an important role in treating many functional disorders and cancers. As pointed out above, hyperthyroidism and thyroid carcinoma are best treated with iodine 131. Malignant pheochromocytomas and other neuroendocrine lesions can be treated with metaiodine 131 benzylguanidine. Gold 198 colloid has been used to assist in the therapy of peritoneal metastases and recurrent malignant ascites. Phosphorus 32 colloids are employed in treating malignant pericardial effusion associated with breast and lung carcinomas. Intraarterial injection of phosphorus 32 colloid to treat inflammatory arthritis of bone joints is also common. The uncontrolled proliferation of bone marrow cells is checked by administering phosphorus 32 orthophosphate. Patients with advanced bone metastases and intractable bone pain are also often treated with single or multiple doses of phosphorus 32 orthophosphate. Other radionuclides that are useful for this purpose are strontium 89, rhenium 186, and yttrium 90.

The implementation of monoclonal antibodies labeled with suitable radionuclides to treat cancer has received considerable attention. This approach involves selecting an antibody that is directed against a tumor-specific antigen and labeling the antibody with an energetic beta particle-emitting radionuclide. If the tumor selectively concentrates these labeled antibodies, then it can be lethally irradiated without seriously affecting the normal tissues and organs. Thus far, however, clinical trials using this approach have met with limited success because of insufficient tumor uptake and bone marrow toxicity. Nevertheless, labeled antibodies are becoming useful in diagnosing a variety of primary and metastatic tumors.

PERSPECTIVE AND PROSPECTS

Although radioactivity was discovered in the late nineteenth century, application of radionuclides as biological tracers did not begin until 1924, when Georg von Hevesy used a bismuth radionuclide to study circulation in rabbits. In that same year, bismuth 214 was used in humans to measure the blood circulation time after injecting the radionuclide in one arm and then following the arrival of radioactivity in the other arm. They found that it takes eighteen seconds in normal patients, and longer in patients with heart disease. The discovery of artificial radioactivity by Frédéric Joliot and Irène Joliot-Curie in 1934 led to the wider use of radionuclides as tracers. When Enrico Fermi artificially produced several radionuclides, Hevesy used phosphorus 32 to study phosphorus metabolism in rats. Such artificial production of radionuclides became possible after the pioneering work of Ernest Lawrence, who invented the cyclotron in 1929. Cyclotrons are still widely employed to produce a variety of radionuclides for medical use. The most commonly used one in nuclear medicine imaging is technetium 99m; this radionuclide is generated in the decay of another radionuclide called molybdenum 99, which was first produced by a cyclotron in 1938.

Radiopharmaceuticals and nuclear medicine took a major leap forward when technetium 99m, the radionuclide of choice for imaging, became readily available. Concurrent development of the scintillation camera by Hal Anger in 1958 advanced the field of nuclear medicine imaging. Radiolabeled compounds are also used extensively in biomedical research to trace biologically important molecules. The radioimmunoassay is another area in which labeled compounds are used to diagnose diseases; here, an antigen-antibody interaction is utilized. These procedures require only a trace amount of radioactivity, along with a blood sample of the patient.

Radiopharmaceutical imaging techniques have become important for the diagnosis and treatment of many diseases, and they will continue to play a major role in improving the quality of health care. Improvements in imaging instrumentation technology and the availability of computer technology to process the images are likely to further the accuracy of nuclear medicine images. Future developments in biotechnology should also assist in designing new pharmaceuticals that are more target-specific, thus further reducing the risks and enhancing both the diagnostic quality of the images and the therapeutic efficacy of radiolabeled compounds.

—*Dandamudi V. Rao, Ph.D.*

See also Angiography; Catheterization; Imaging and radiology; Invasive tests; Magnetic resonance imaging (MRI); Nuclear medicine; Nuclear radiology; Positron emission tomography (PET) scanning; Radiation therapy.

FOR FURTHER INFORMATION:

Harbert, John C. *Nuclear Medicine Therapy.* New York: Thieme Medical, 1987. An excellent source of practical information that nuclear medicine physicians need to plan and conduct therapy in which radiopharmaceuticals are administered. Most of this book deals with clinical applications. Each chapter treats historical background and the clinical complications that may result from radionuclide therapies.

Mettler, Fred A., and Milton J. Guiberteau. *Essentials of Nuclear Medicine Imaging.* 4th ed. Philadelphia: W. B. Saunders, 1998. An introductory text in nuclear medicine imaging. The authors cover concepts and medical examinations in an easy-to-understand way. Numerous medical diagnostic procedures involving radiopharmaceuticals are described and their usefulness illustrated.

Sorenson, James A., and Michael E. Phelps. *Physics in Nuclear Medicine.* 2d ed. New York: Grune & Stratton, 1987. This excellent book covers the necessary physical principles in detail for an understanding of radionuclide properties and the nuclear medicine instrumentation techniques for imaging. The authors have considerable experience in this field.

RASHES

DISEASE/DISORDER

ANATOMY OR SYSTEM AFFECTED: Skin

SPECIALTIES AND RELATED FIELDS: Dermatology

DEFINITION: General eruptions of the skin that are often associated with communicable diseases and that are most often temporary; most are some shade of red.

KEY TERMS:

erythematous: red
pruritic: itchy
systemic: affecting the whole body
wheal: a flat, firm, and raised area of the skin

CAUSES AND SYMPTOMS

Rashes may have many different causes: infection, inflammation, irritation, an allergic reaction, and systemic disease. Rashes usually vary in color from pale pink to red. They take many different forms: flat, raised, puffy, scaly, blistery, or crusted. They may be pruritic. Rashes may involve a small portion of the skin or cover much of the body. They may come in characteristic shapes, such as a bull's eye, or may appear irregular. A rash may be accompanied by other signs and symptoms that help the health care provider determine the cause of the rash, or a rash may form part of a constellation of signs and symptoms diagnostic of another disease or disorder.

Infectious rashes may be caused by bacteria, viruses, or fungi. For example, impetigo is caused by either staphylococcal or streptococcal bacteria, cold sores are caused by a herpesvirus, and athlete's foot is caused by a fungus. Some infectious rashes are highly contagious to other children or to family members and others.

Rashes associated with inflammation include allergic responses to drugs, certain foods, stings, and poison ivy. Allergic rashes are typically red and itchy. They may be flat or may arise as wheals. Many allergic rashes are merely annoying, but some can be part of a life-threatening condition called anaphylaxis. Symptoms of anaphylaxis include blockage of the airways, a rash, and cardiac problems. Children can go into anaphylactic shock after eating a food to which they are highly allergic (such as shellfish, peanuts, or strawberries) or after being stung by a bee.

A common, but not usually serious, rash in infants is heat rash, or miliaria rubra. It is also called "prickly heat." This rash is most common in hot and humid environments and on areas of the body covered by tight clothing.

Many of the so-called childhood diseases are characterized by fever and rash: measles, rubella (German measles), chickenpox, and fifth disease. The rash as-

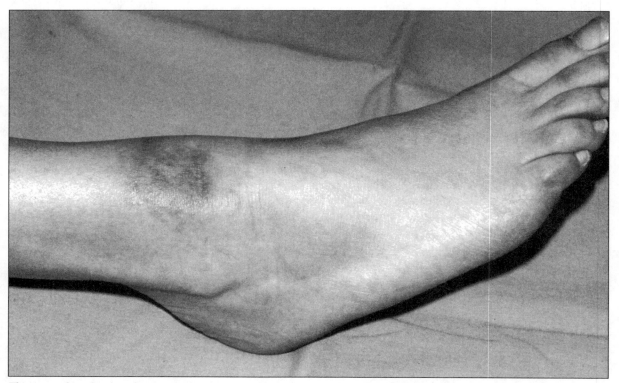

This insect bite developed into a rash, which can result from an allergic reaction or from excessive scratching of the site. (SIU School of Medicine)

Common Rash-Producing Infections

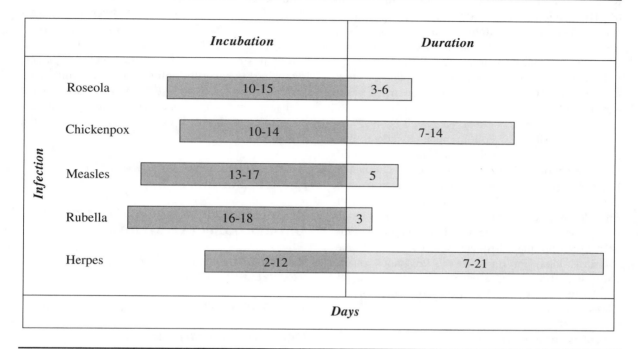

Infection	Incubation	Duration
Roseola	10-15	3-6
Chickenpox	10-14	7-14
Measles	13-17	5
Rubella	16-18	3
Herpes	2-12	7-21

Days

sociated with each of these has distinctive features that help in the diagnosis of the disease. For example, the child with fifth disease has bright red cheeks, the so-called "slapped cheek" phenomenon, and a fine lacy rash on the trunk and extremities. The rash of rubella begins on the face and spreads rapidly to the trunk, arms, and legs. All these childhood diseases are related to systemic viral infections. Scarlet fever, on the other hand, is a streptococcal infection accompanied by a rash. Again, the characteristics of the rash help in making the diagnosis: It has a fine sandpaper-like feeling when touched.

TREATMENT AND THERAPY

The treatment of rashes depends on the cause. A common rule of thumb is that if a rash is wet, the treatment is to dry it, and vice versa. For example, an oozing rash such as that caused by poison ivy may be relieved by a drying paste that relieves itching, while a dry rash may be best treated with an ointment or by an oatmeal bath.

Some rashes will resolve on their own, and the main job of parents and health care providers is to relieve a child's unpleasant symptoms, such as itching, that go along with the rash. Patients with rashes that itch need to receive medications to relieve itching, such as antihistamines, so that they will not complicate their condition by scratching the affected skin. Most antihistamines, however, cause the side effect of sleepiness. Soothing oatmeal baths or moisturizing lotions can relieve itching without causing sleepiness.

Treatments for rashes can be either topical or systemic. Topical treatments are put directly on the skin. For example, athlete's foot is treated with topical ointment or powder containing an agent that will kill the fungus that causes the condition. Impetigo, on the other hand, is usually treated with systemic antibiotics to kill the causative bacteria.

A mainstay of dermatological treatment is steroid medications. Topical steroids such as hydrocortisone cream or ointment are applied directly to the skin and may be covered with a dressing. In some cases, as in a serious case of poison ivy, steroids may be given orally or by injection. Steroids have potential serious adverse effects, so most health care providers use them sparingly. They should almost never be used on the face or eyelids unless so prescribed by a physician.

PERSPECTIVE AND PROSPECTS

Rashes are an extremely common problem in childhood and adolescence. Parents can often diagnose rashes themselves and treat them with appropriate over-the-counter products. Rashes that are associated with other symptoms, whose origin is unclear, or that fail to clear up in a reasonable amount of time, should be evaluated and treated by a qualified health care provider.

—*Rebecca Lovell Scott, Ph.D.*

See also Allergies; Autoimmune disorders; Bacterial infections; Bites and stings; Chickenpox; Childhood infectious diseases; Cradle cap; Dermatitis; Dermatology; Dermatology, pediatric; Diaper rash; Diphtheria; Eczema; Epidermolysis bullosa; Fever; Fifth disease; Fungal infections; Hand-foot-and-mouth disease; Herpes; Hives; Itching; Lupus erythematosus; Measles; Multiple chemical sensitivity syndrome; Pityriasis alba; Pityriasis rosea; Poisonous plants; Psoriasis; Ringworm; Roseola; Rubella; Scabies; Scarlet fever; Scurvy; Skin; Skin disorders; Sunburn; Thrush; Viral infections.

FOR FURTHER INFORMATION:

Berkow, Robert, ed. *The Merck Manual of Medical Information, Home Edition.* New York: Pocket, 2000. A best-selling medical reference book is now available in a new home edition. Easy to understand and full of up-to-date information, this volume contains over fifteen hundred pages on diseases, causes, treatments, and drugs. Includes over three hundred drawings.

Clayman, Charles B., ed. *The American Medical Association Family Medical Guide.* New York: Random House, 1994. An excellent reference for the beginner. The scientific accuracy of the text is not compromised by its accessibility.

Goldsmith, Lowell A., Gerald S. Lazarus, and Michael D. Tharp. *Adult and Pediatric Dermatology: A Color Guide to Diagnosis and Treatment.* Philadelphia: F. A. Davis, 1997. A well-written, richly illustrated, user-friendly book with an appealing layout. The authors have admirably succeeded in producing a valuable resource of knowledge for any dermatologist.

Schmitt, Barton D. *Your Child's Health: The Parents' Guide to Symptoms, Emergencies, Common Illnesses, Behavior, and School Problems.* Rev. ed. New York: Bantam Books, 1991. Offers parents complete and authoritative advice from one of the nation's leading pediatricians in a step-by-step, quick-reference format.

Spock, Benjamin, and Steven J. Parker. *Dr. Spock's Baby and Child Care.* 7th ed. Rev. ed. New York: Pocket Books, 1998. For more than a half a century, this book has been a virtual bible for parents seeking trustworthy information on child care. Informative, easy to use, and responsive to the changes in society, this revised and updated seventh edition makes a classic work more essential than ever.

RECONSTRUCTIVE SURGERY. *See* PLASTIC SURGERY.

RECTAL POLYP REMOVAL. *See* COLON AND RECTAL POLYP REMOVAL.

RECTAL SURGERY. *See* COLON AND RECTAL SURGERY.

REFERRED PAIN. *See* PAIN.

REFLEXES, PRIMITIVE
DEVELOPMENT

ALSO KNOWN AS: Newborn reflexes

ANATOMY OR SYSTEM AFFECTED: All

SPECIALTIES AND RELATED FIELDS: Family practice, pediatrics, perinatology

DEFINITION: Involuntary patterns of behavior that can be elicited in the newborn infant.

KEY TERMS:

in utero: a Latin phrase meaning "in the uterus"; refers to the period of fetal development

subcortical centers of the brain: the parts of the brain that control and regulate basic physiological functions, including breathing, body temperature, sleeping, and waking; these parts are contrasted with the cortex, where voluntary control of behavior originates

PHYSICAL AND PSYCHOLOGICAL FACTORS

Primitive reflexes range from very simple reactions such as the blinking and startle reflexes to more complex patterns of behavior such as the stepping and crawling reflexes. Primitive reflexes appear to be important for orienting the infant to its environment and for protecting it against potential threats to its safety. The reflexes are automatically elicited when an appropriate stimulus is present, such as liquid in the

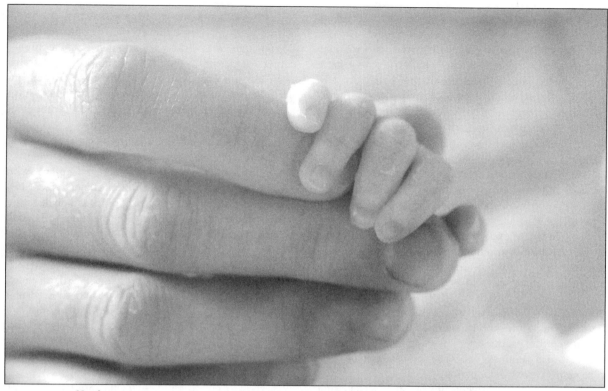

Newborns possess a grasping reflex that allows them to hold tightly to objects. (PhotoDisc)

mouth or pressure on the bottom of the feet, and they take the same form on every occasion.

Several primitive reflexes exist for the head and face. Blinking is elicited when an object approaches the eye. This reflex functions to protect the eye from harm. The head-turning reflex is seen when an infant is placed face down on a soft surface such as a mattress. The infant will turn its head to one side to allow breathing to continue. Similarly, the defensive reaction reflex is seen when a cloth is placed over an infant's face. The infant will turn its head and make swiping movements with its arms in an attempt to clear away the obstruction. Rooting and sucking are two important reflexes of the face that assist in feeding. The rooting reflex is elicited when an object gently touches an infant's cheek; the infant will turn its mouth in the direction of the touch. Sucking is elicited whenever a nipple-sized object is placed in an infant's mouth.

The reflexes of the arms include the Moro reflex and the tonic neck reflex. The Moro reflex is seen when an infant's head is dropped slightly. The infant's legs and its arms, with hands extended, will spread wide, then come together in an embracing movement as the hands clench. This sequence of behaviors appears to be a defense against falling, as the reflexive response could allow the infant to grasp on to something. The Moro reflex is seen in other primates as well. The tonic neck reflex is seen when an infant, lying on its back, has its head turned to one side. The infant's arm on the same side will extend, and the other arm will move up to the back of its head, to assume a "fencing position." This reflex is also called the fencer's reflex.

The primitive reflex of the hand is the palmar or grasping reflex. If an object touches an infant's palm, then the hand will clench into a fist. If the object is small enough for the infant to get a grip on it, then the infant's grip will be strong enough to support its own weight. A newborn infant grasping an adult's fingers with both hands can be pulled to a sitting or standing position.

The swimmer's reflex is seen when an infant is lying on its stomach. If the infant is gently tapped along its side above the waist, then it will turn its torso in the direction of the touch. Another primitive reflex of the torso is the crawling reflex. If an infant is lying on its stomach and pressure is applied against the soles of its feet, then it will move its arms and legs in a crawling movement. This reflex may be a precursor for later voluntary crawling behavior.

Two reflexes of the legs also appear to prefigure later-developing motor behavior. If an infant is held upright under the arms and its feet are allowed to touch a surface, then the infant will demonstrate the standing reflex by straightening its legs and supporting some of its body weight. If the infant is then tilted forward and moved forward slightly, then it will make high stepping movements characteristic of the stepping reflex.

The plantar reflex is similar to the palmar reflex. If an infant's foot is stimulated with an object touching the sole just below the toes, then the toes will curl around the object as if to grasp it. The Babinski reflex is another reflex of the foot; if the outside edge of an infant's foot is gently stroked, then the toes will fan out. The Babinski reflex, unlike many of the other primitive reflexes, does not have an obvious function; the lack of a Babinski response, however, may indicate neurological dysfunction.

Some of the primitive reflexes, such as sucking and grasping, have been detected in utero. Most of the reflexes disappear within a few months after birth, although some primitive reflexes, such as blinking, persist throughout life. Still other reflexes, such as the crawling and walking reflexes and the defensive reaction, are later replaced by behaviors that are voluntarily controlled.

DISORDERS AND EFFECTS

Because the absence of primitive reflexes can indicate neurological damage, most infants are tested for some of the reflexes soon after birth. Reflexes of the face, hands, and feet are components of neurological examinations such as the Brazelton Neonatal Behavioral Assessment Scale.

Despite the fact that the primitive reflexes are involuntary, infants show variability in their reflexive responses. There are individual differences among infants, such that some infants may show stronger or weaker primitive reflexes than others. Within individual infants, there is variation in the strength with which the reflexes may be elicited on different occasions. The age of the infant, its state of arousal, and the interval since its last feeding are all factors that can affect an infant's reflexive responses.

PERSPECTIVE AND PROSPECTS

Traditionally, it was believed that primitive reflexes disappeared with brain development, as the higher centers of the brain took over some motor functions from the subcortical centers of the brain. Recent investigations of the stepping reflex, however, have shown that other factors can affect the development of the reflexes.

Esther Thelen and Linda B. Smith, in their book *A Dynamic Systems Approach to the Development of Cognition and Action* (1994), report that infants who no longer show the stepping reflex under typical circumstances do demonstrate stepping if their legs are submerged in water. Similarly, the stepping reflex can be suppressed in very young infants by adding weights to their legs. Another study by Philip Zelazo, as described in an article found in *Developmental Psychobiology: The Significance of Infancy* (1976), provided infants with daily stepping practice and showed that under those conditions, the stepping reflex did not disappear. These findings suggest that experience, growth, and weight gain, as well as brain development, influence the developmental course of the primitive reflexes.

—*Virginia Slaughter, Ph.D.*

See also Breast-feeding; Cognitive development; Developmental stages; Motor neuron diseases; Motor skill development; Neonatology.

FOR FURTHER INFORMATION:

Brazelton, T. Berry, and J. Kevin Nugent. *Neonatal Behavioral Assessment Scale*. 3d ed. Clinics in Developmental Medicine 137. London: MacKeith Press, 1995. This widely used test of infant development includes items that assess primitive reflexes.

Field, Tiffany. *Infancy*. Cambridge, Mass.: Harvard University Press, 1991. The chapter "Motor Development and Learning" gives an overview of the primitive reflexes in the context of motor development and learning.

Stanley, Jenna. "Reflex Action." *Parents* 73, no. 5 (May, 1998): 24-25. Babies are born with more than seventy built-in responses that can help parents assess their development. Some of the most fascinating include the stepping reflex, moro reflex, galant response, and placing reflex.

Thelen, Esther, and Linda B. Smith. *A Dynamic Systems Approach to the Development of Cognition and Action*. Cambridge, Mass.: MIT Press, 1994. The chapter "Lessons from Learning to Walk" describes a series of studies on the stepping reflex and the implications of the results for the study of motor development in general.

RENAL FAILURE
DISEASE/DISORDER

ANATOMY OR SYSTEM AFFECTED: Kidneys, urinary system

SPECIALTIES AND RELATED FIELDS: Internal medicine, nephrology

DEFINITION: Renal failure is the inability of the kidneys to process waste products out of the blood and excrete them through the urine. Acute cases feature a sudden onset and a short, severe course which is often curable; they can be caused by conditions in the kidney or in another area of the body that causes the kidneys to stop functioning, leading to a buildup of waste products in the blood and tissues. Untreated acute renal failure can lead to chronic kidney failure or death. In chronic cases, onset is gradual and symptoms may not be noticed until only half a single kidney is functioning; these cases may be linked to other chronic and long-term abnormalities and diseases, as well as to drug overdoses. Treatment of acute symptoms involves medication, rest, and strict dietary control.

—Jason Georges and Tracy Irons-Georges
See also Cystitis; Glomerulonephritis; Kidney disorders; Kidneys; Nephritis; Nephrology; Nephrology, pediatric; Urethritis; Urinary disorders.

FOR FURTHER INFORMATION:

Brenner, Barry M., and Floyd C. Rector, Jr., eds. *Brenner and Rector's The Kidney*. 2 vols. 6th ed. Philadelphia: W. B. Saunders, 1999.

Cameron, Stewart. *Kidney Disease: The Facts*. 2d ed. New York: Oxford University Press, 1986.

Catto, Graeme R. D., and David A. Power. Nephrology in Clinical Practice. London: Edward Arnold, 1988.

Dische, Frederick E. *Concise Renal Pathology*. 2d ed. Oxford, England: Oxford University Press, 1995.

Legrain, Marcel, and Jean-Michel Suc Legrain et al. *Nephrology*. Translated by M. Cavaille-Coll. New York: Masson, 1987.

REPRODUCTIVE SYSTEM
ANATOMY

ANATOMY OR SYSTEM AFFECTED: Abdomen, genitals, uterus

SPECIALTIES AND RELATED FIELDS: Embryology, genetics, gynecology, obstetrics, proctology, urology

DEFINITION: The organs of the female (the vagina, uterus, Fallopian tubes, ovaries, and mammary glands) and the male (the penis, testes, vas deferens, and prostate gland) that are necessary for the production of offspring.

KEY TERMS:

bladder: the pouch in the abdominal cavity that collects urine until it can be eliminated from the body; while not a part of the reproductive system, it is located adjacent to the reproductive organs and is an important landmark

fertilization: the process in which the sperm head penetrates the ovum, resulting in the formation of an embryo

gametes: the reproductive cells in either sex (the sperm and the ova)

hormone: a chemical signal that is carried in the blood from its site of production to the area where it has an effect

menstrual cycle: the cycle of ovum development, hormone production, and menstruation in female primates; in humans, the average duration is about twenty-nine days

ovulation: the release of an ovum from its follicle in the ovary

ovum: the female gamete; a large round cell that carries the female's chromosomes

sperm: the male gamete; the mature sperm has an oval head that contains the male's chromosomes and a long tail that allows it to swim in fluid

STRUCTURE AND FUNCTIONS

The reproductive system in each sex includes the organs that produce the gametes, called the gonads, and those that transport the gametes. In addition, the female mammary glands (breasts) are also considered reproductive organs since they produce milk to nourish the newborn, a critical step in survival of the species.

The male gonads are the testes, which are located within the scrotum, a pouch of skin and muscle that is suspended from the body wall. In the adult, each egg-shaped testis measures about 2.5 centimeters by 4.0 centimeters. Internally, the testes contain seminiferous tubules, hollow tubes in which the sperm develop. Besides the sperm cells, the seminiferous tubules also contain Sertoli cells, large cells in which the developing sperm are embedded. The Sertoli cells produce hormones, pass nutrients to the sperm, protect them from blood-borne toxins, and control their development. In spaces between adjacent seminiferous tubules are the interstitial cells of Leydig, which produce testosterone and other hormones.

Lying near each testis within the scrotum is the epididymis. Sperm undergo several stages of development within the testis, then move into the epididymis where they proceed through further steps in maturation, including the development of the swimming ability that is necessary for fertilization of an ovum.

The narrow end of the epididymis is continuous with the long (45-centimeter) tubule called the vas deferens. The vas deferens leads upward from the epididymis and passes through a narrow ring of tissue, the inguinal canal, to enter the abdominal cavity. Within the abdominal cavity, the vas deferens loops over the top of the bladder, then turns downward to enter the prostate gland below the bladder. Near the end of the vas deferens, an enlarged area called the ampulla serves as a storage site for mature sperm.

Within the prostate gland, the vas deferens becomes a short segment of tubule known as the ejaculatory duct. The two ejaculatory ducts (one on each side) empty into the urethra, the tube that extends downward from the bladder. In the male, the urethra carries either sperm or urine, but not both at the same time: A valvelike structure below the bladder prohibits urine outflow when sperm are moving through the system. The urethra passes through the penis to open to the outside at the tip of the penis.

Besides the urethra, the penis contains three columns of erectile tissue, spongy material with a large blood supply. During sexual excitement, the blood flow into the erectile tissue increases while the outflow decreases; the accumulation of blood within the erectile tissue causes the penis to increase in both length and diameter, a process known as erection. Erection allows the penis to become stiff enough to be inserted into the female's vagina during intercourse. On the outside of the penis, the enlarged area at the tip, the glans penis, is well supplied with touch receptors that play a role in sexual excitement.

During intercourse, stimulation of the touch receptors on the penis results in ejaculation, the expulsion of sperm from the male's body. During ejaculation, sperm move out of the vasa deferentia, through the ejaculatory ducts, and then through the urethra. This sperm movement is caused not by the swimming of

The Male Reproductive System

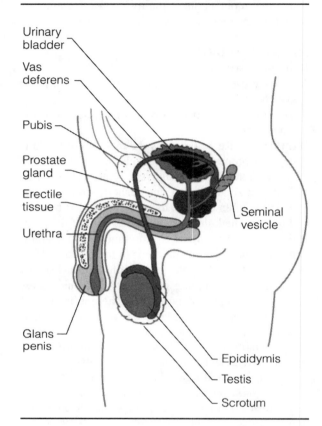

the sperm but by the contractions of involuntary muscles in the walls of the tubules. As sperm pass through the tubules, they are mixed with fluid secreted by three glands: the prostate, located immediately below the bladder; the seminal vesicles, which open into the vas deferens above the prostate; and the bulbourethral or Cowper's gland, which lies below the prostate and opens into the urethra. The fluid secreted by these glands contains chemicals and nutrients that will ensure the survival of the sperm within the female tract.

The female's vagina serves as the repository for sperm released during ejaculation and as the outlet for the fetus during childbirth. The outer opening of the vagina is located behind the urethra, which carries only urine and does not have a reproductive role in the female. Bartholin's and Skene's glands are located near the urethral and vaginal openings; these glands supply moisture and mucus to the female external genitals. The vaginal and urethral openings are located between folds of tissue, the labia majora and the labia minora. At the front junction of these folds is the clitoris, a small round structure containing many touch receptors; stimulation of the clitoris during intercourse is important in promoting sexual gratification in the female. The area that includes the labia, the vaginal and urethral openings, and the clitoris is known as the vulva.

Internally, the vagina consists of a recess with elastic walls and a large blood supply, but little sense of feeling since there are only sparse touch receptors. The vagina slants upward and slightly backward from its outer opening. Near its upper end is the cervix, the lowest portion of the uterus. The cervix consists of strong connective tissue and contains glands that secrete mucus. The cervix has a narrow passageway, the cervical canal, that opens into the main part of the uterus.

The uterus is about 7.5 centimeters long and 5.0 centimeters wide in the nonpregnant woman. The wall of the uterus is composed primarily of involuntary muscle controlled by nerves and hormones. The inner part of the uterus is hollow and is lined with a spongy layer of cells, the endometrium; the endometrium has a large blood supply and contains glands that secrete nutrients for the embryo during pregnancy. The endometrium undergoes growth during the menstrual cycle and is shed as the menstrual discharge if the woman does not become pregnant.

At either side of the upper end of the uterus are the oviducts, or Fallopian tubes, hollow tubes that open into the cavity of the uterus. The oviducts lead upward and sideways away from the uterus toward the ovaries, with their funnel-shaped ends adjacent, but not attached, to the ovaries.

The ovaries are the female gonads; they produce ova, the female gametes. Each 3-centimeter-long ovary contains thousands of follicles, spherical structures that each contain one ovum. Hormonal signals cause growth of some of the follicles during the menstrual cycle, and, as they grow, the ova within them mature. The follicles are also sites of production of the hormones estrogen and progesterone. In the middle of the menstrual cycle, one follicle will ovulate, releasing its ovum, which will enter the oviduct to be transported toward the uterus.

During intercourse, after sperm are deposited in the vagina, the sperm will swim in the fluids of the female tract, passing upward through the cervical canal, the uterus, and the oviducts. If an ovum is present in one of the oviducts, it may be fertilized by a sperm. The fertilized ovum will then move downward to the uterus, where it will attach to the endometrium and develop into an embryo. At birth, uterine muscle contractions will cause stretching of the cervical canal and movement of the fetus through the cervix and vagina.

Milk production (lactation) in the woman's breasts after childbirth will allow for the nourishment of the newborn. Milk is produced in glands within the breast; ducts carry the milk to openings in the nipple. In between the milk-producing glands are wedges of fat; it is the fat tissue that determines the size of the breast in the nonpregnant woman. Breast size is not related to milk-producing ability.

The Female Reproductive System

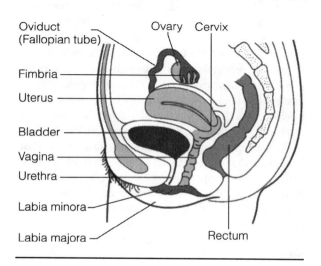

Oviduct (Fallopian tube)
Ovary
Cervix
Fimbria
Uterus
Bladder
Vagina
Urethra
Labia minora
Labia majora
Rectum

DISORDERS AND DISEASES

Abnormalities may exist in either the male or the female reproductive tract as a result of deviations during embryonic development, injury, or disease. Anatomical abnormalities in the reproductive system often can be corrected surgically.

In hypospadias, a problem during embryonic development of the male reproductive organs causes the urethral opening to be on the underside of the penis rather than at its tip. Hypospadias can occur independently or can be a sign of more serious problems. Urethral stricture or stenosis refers to a narrowing of the urethra; this can occur anywhere along its length, from the tip of the penis back to the prostate gland. Urethral stenosis causes difficulty in urination; it may be present from birth or result from later damage or infection. Cryptorchidism is the presence of one or both testes in the abdominal cavity instead of in the scrotum. In the male embryo, the testes begin development in the body cavity near the kidneys and then migrate into the scrotum during the last month or two before birth. In some male infants born with undescended testes, the testes will spontaneously move into the scrotum shortly after birth. If not, then the cryptorchidism must be corrected surgically, usually within the first year of life, in order to prevent later infertility and other complications.

In females, problems during embryonic development can also lead to malformed reproductive organs. The vagina may be present but may not have an outer opening, or conversely, the outer opening may lead to an abnormally shallow vagina. The uterus may be divided into two separate halves (bicornuate uterus), and the vagina may also show such a division. It is also possible for a normal uterus to have an abnormal placement in the abdomen: It may be tilted backward or bent forward at an atypical angle. Surprisingly, variations in the anatomy of the uterus often have little effect on fertility.

Malfunctions in embryonic development of the reproductive organs can lead to hermaphroditism, a rare condition in which an individual has a mixture of male and female reproductive organs. A hermaphrodite may be either a genetic male or a genetic female. Hormone treatment and surgery can usually assure a fulfilling sex life in adulthood for such individuals.

In inguinal hernia, the wall of the inguinal canal between the scrotum and abdominal cavity becomes weakened and stretched. A loop of the intestine may then become lodged in the canal, or the testis and epididymis may move upward to block the canal. The symptoms of inguinal hernia include pain during movement, especially during the lifting of heavy objects, and the presence of a soft lump in the herniated area.

A varicocele is a group of enlarged blood vessels within the scrotum. Varicoceles are thought to arise because of impaired blood flow from the testis. Normally, the blood flowing through the scrotum maintains the temperature of the testes a few degrees below that of the rest of the body. When the blood flow out of the scrotum is reduced in the presence of a varicocele, the temperature in the testes tends to increase. This increased temperature can cause infertility, since sperm production requires a local temperature that is lower than the normal body temperature. Increased scrotal temperature can be the cause of infertility in other situations as well: the wearing of tight clothing, prolonged soaking in hot water, or during episodes of fever. Infertility in these situations is usually temporary and self-correcting.

In women, stretching of the pelvic area during childbirth sometimes leads to uterine prolapse, a condition in which the uterus sags into the vagina. Other causes of prolapse are developmental abnormalities, lifting heavy objects, and loss of muscle and tissue strength with aging. A prolapsed uterus is associated with pain during intercourse and may cause difficulty in urination. Temporary relief from a uterine prolapse can be achieved with the use of a pessary, a device worn in the vagina to support the uterus. Surgery to restore the supporting tissues in the pelvis may be necessary for long-term relief, but in some cases the uterus cannot be returned to its proper position and so must be removed, a process called hysterectomy.

In endometriosis, patches of endometrial tissue from the uterine lining attach to and grow on other organs in the pelvic cavity, affecting the shape and function of these organs. It is thought that the endometrium escapes into the pelvis through the oviducts during menstruation. The abnormally placed endometrial tissue can cause pain and infertility. Endometriosis can be treated with hormone therapy or with surgery to remove the endometrial patches. In more severe cases and when the woman does not wish to bear children in the future, the removal of the uterus may be required to control the invasion of other organs by the endometrial patches. The ovaries may also be removed in order to eliminate the source of hormones that produce the growth of the endometrium.

In polycystic ovary syndrome, one or both ovaries contain cysts that are formed from follicles that have failed to ovulate. Women with polycystic ovaries either do not menstruate or have irregular patterns of bleeding. Because ovulation does not occur, they are infertile. Another symptom of polycystic ovary syndrome is growth of hair in a male pattern on the face, neck, and chest; the hair growth is caused by certain hormones that are produced in abnormal amounts by the ovaries. Therapy usually involves hormone treatment in an attempt to establish ovulation and to prevent the deleterious effects of abnormal hormone levels on the body.

Both benign (nonspreading) and cancerous tumors may appear in the reproductive organs. Potential sites of tumor growth are the testes and prostate gland in the male and the ovaries, uterus, and breasts in the female. Only rarely do tumors cause pain, but they may be detected during routine self-examination of the testes or breasts or during a doctor's examination. Treatment usually begins with surgery to remove the tumor, and X-ray therapy or chemotherapy prevents further tumor growth. Hormone treatment can also be useful in controlling the growth of some reproductive tumors. The exact factors that cause tumors to form are not well understood, but a family history of such problems, abnormal hormone levels and exposure to radiation, pollutants, and toxins have all been implicated.

Prostate tumors should not be confused with nodular prostatic hyperplasia, an increase in the size of the prostate gland that occurs in about 75 percent of men over sixty years old. The enlargement appears to be caused by dihydrotestosterone (DHT), a hormone related to testosterone; the prostate gland itself is one site of conversion of testosterone into DHT. Prostate enlargement is associated with difficulty during urination and ejaculation. It has traditionally been managed with surgery to remove the gland or to reduce its size. More recently, a drug that prevents the production of DHT has been made available to treat prostatic enlargement.

PERSPECTIVE AND PROSPECTS

Rituals involving alteration of the reproductive organs have been performed since ancient times. Castration (removal of the testes) has been carried out for various reasons. In early times, men who were guards of noble women were castrated to control their sexual activity. During the Renaissance, castration of boys was performed to produce singers who would retain their clear, high-pitched voices, since it is testosterone that causes the deepening of the voice at puberty. More recently, castration has been espoused as a "treatment" for habitual rapists: Some judges sentence convicted sex offenders to castration, despite the fact that many authorities believe that rape is a manifestation of violent tendencies, rather than the result of excessive sexual desire.

In the United States and elsewhere, it is common for boys to undergo circumcision, or the removal of the foreskin, a flap of tissue that covers the glans of the penis. Parents have their sons circumcised in order to conform to religious and cultural practices. In the United States, the procedure is usually performed shortly after the boy's birth, but in other cultures circumcision may occur during puberty rituals. One rationalization for performing circumcision is that removal of the foreskin helps to prevent the buildup of smegma, a thick secretion produced by glands located under the base of the foreskin. In fact, some studies have shown that circumcised boys are less likely to have urinary tract infections. There are no apparent effects of circumcision on sexual functioning. Researchers debate the advisability of circumcision, however, and the medical establishment has not established a definitive recommendation.

It is less well known that circumcision of women is practiced in some cultures. Indigenous groups who perform female circumcision are are found in the Pacific Islands, Asia, the Mideast, and Africa, and the practice has been carried to the United States by immigrants. The term "female circumcision" refers to three procedures that may be carried out singly or together. In simple circumcision, the flap of tissue covering the clitoris is removed. The entire visible part of the clitoris is removed in clitoridectomy. Infibulation is the sewing together of the labia to cover the vaginal opening, leaving only a small hole for the discharge of urine and menstrual fluid. A woman who has been infibulated cannot have intercourse or give birth; the tissue must be cut open to allow either of these events, after which the area may be sewn closed again.

Female circumcision may take place shortly after a girl's birth or at puberty, and it is performed for a variety of reasons. Infibulation is a means of enforcing female abstinence from sexual activity. A wish to control women's sexual desire is also given as a reason for performing simple circumcision and clitoridectomy. Also involved are the society's views of what the ideal female organs should look like. From a medical standpoint, female circumcision is of concern because of pain and discomfort caused by the development of scar tissue in the vulva area. It is not known how many women die from infection or bleeding following these procedures, which are usually performed by other women under less-than-sanitary conditions.

—*Marcia Watson-Whitmyre, Ph.D.*

See also Abortion; Amenorrhea; Amniocentesis; Anorexia nervosa; Breast-feeding; Breasts, female; Candidiasis; Catheterization; Cervical, ovarian, and uterine cancers; Cervical procedures; Cesarean section; Childbirth; Childbirth complications; Chlamydia; Circumcision, female, and genital mutilation; Circumcision, male; Conception; Contraception; Culdocentesis; Cyst removal; Cysts; Dysmenorrhea; Ectopic pregnancy; Electrocauterization; Endocrine disorders; Endocrinology; Endometrial biopsy; Endometriosis; Episiotomy; Estrogen replacement therapy; Fistula repair; Genital disorders, female; Genital disorders, male; Glands; Gonorrhea; Gynecology; Herpes; Hormone replacement therapy; Hormones; Hydrocelectomy; Hypospadias repair and urethroplasty; Hysterectomy; In vitro fertilization; Infertility in females; Infertility in males; Laparoscopy; Masturbation; Menopause; Menorrhagia; Menstruation; Miscarriage; Multiple births; Myomectomy; Obstetrics; Orchitis; Ovarian cysts; Pelvic inflammatory disease (PID); Penile implant surgery; Pregnancy and gestation; Premature birth; Premenstrual syndrome (PMS); Prostate cancer; Prostate gland; Prostate gland removal; Puberty and adolescence; Sex change surgery; Sexual differentiation; Sexual dysfunction; Sexuality; Sexually transmitted diseases; Sterilization; Stillbirth; Syphilis; Systems and organs; Testicles, undescended; Testicular surgery; Testicular torsion; Tubal ligation; Ultrasonography; Vasectomy; Warts.

FOR FURTHER INFORMATION:

Gilbaugh, James H. *A Doctor's Guide to Men's Private Parts.* New York: Crown, 1989. As the title implies, the author of the book is a physician who specializes in urology. The text covers all aspects of the male reproductive system in a straightforward manner and using nontechnical terms.

Jones, Richard E. *Human Reproductive Behavior.* San Diego, Calif.: Academic Press, 1991. This book was designed as a textbook for college courses in human reproduction. Noteworthy for its completeness, which makes it a valuable reference.

Marieb, Elaine N. *Essentials of Human Anatomy and Physiology.* 6th ed. Redwood City, Calif.: Benjamin/Cummings, 2000. This introductory anatomy and physiology textbook, easily accessible to those with little science background, is richly illustrated with diagrams and photographs, which help to illuminate body systems and processes.

Quilligan, Edward J., and Frederick P. Zuspan, eds. *Current Therapy in Obstetrics and Gynecology.* 5th ed. Philadelphia: W. B. Saunders, 1999. Intended as a reference for physicians and other medical personnel, this book offers the most complete and up-to-date information on the diagnosis and treatment of disorders of the female reproductive system.

Yen, Samuel S. C., and Robert B. Jaffe. *Reproductive Endocrinology: Physiology, Pathophysiology, and Clinical Management.* 4th ed. Philadelphia: W. B. Saunders, 1999. The role of hormones in normal reproductive function is discussed as the basis for understanding the various abnormalities of hormone secretion that can disrupt reproduction. Those who are interested in reading about research in reproduction will find the citations to original research papers helpful.

RESEARCH VS. ANIMAL RIGHTS. *See* ANIMAL RIGHTS VS. RESEARCH.

RESPIRATION
BIOLOGY

ANATOMY OR SYSTEM AFFECTED: Chest, lungs, muscles, musculoskeletal system, nose, respiratory system, throat

SPECIALTIES AND RELATED FIELDS: Biochemistry, exercise physiology, otorhinolaryngology, pulmonary medicine, vascular medicine

DEFINITION: A basic physiological process in which an organism takes in oxygen (which is utilized as a source of energy) and produces carbon dioxide (which is excreted as a waste product).

KEY TERMS:

capillaries: the smallest and most numerous blood vessels in the cardiovascular system; these vessels connect the arteries to the veins and are where all exchange of oxygen and nutrients occurs

diffusion: the process in which substances move from an area of high concentration to an area of low concentration; if given enough time, the concentration of the substance will be the same everywhere

hemoglobin: a special molecule, found only in red blood cells, that binds oxygen very efficiently in the lung and releases it to the tissues

partial pressure of a gas in a gas: the measure of the contribution of one gas of a mixture of gases to the total pressure pushing on the walls containing it; it is the pressure that would be exerted if all the other gases were removed from the container, leaving only the gas of interest

partial pressure of a gas in a liquid: the measure of how much of a gas dissolves into a liquid when the liquid is in contact with a gas mixture; if the gas and liquid are in contact long enough, the liquid is said to have the same partial pressure as the gas mixture; the absolute measure of the amount of gas in a liquid is the partial pressure multiplied by the ability of the gas to dissolve in liquid (solubility)

plasma: the fluid of blood in which the blood cells (white and red) are suspended

pressure: the measure of how much a gas or a liquid pushes on the walls of its container

THE MECHANICS OF RESPIRATION

The primary function of respiration is performed by the lungs and their associated tissues. Air must be breathed in through the mouth and nose through the larynx (voice box) into the main airway, the trachea (windpipe). Inside the chest, the trachea branches into the two main airways called bronchi, which in turn successively branch many times into small bronchi called bronchioles. These airways end in very small sacs called alveoli. These alveoli have a very thin membrane separating the air space from the blood in the capillaries. Oxygen (O_2) diffuses through the alveolar membrane across the capillary membrane and into the blood to be taken to all the tissues of the body. Tissues excrete carbon dioxide (CO_2) into the blood that is carried back to the lungs. Carbon dioxide diffuses from the blood into the alveoli and is carried back through the airways and out of the lungs with the exhaled air. The mouth and nose humidify dry air to ensure that the linings of the lower airways do not dry out. The main airway divides to supply the left and right lungs. These large airways are cylindrical. Their circular shape is maintained by C-shaped cartilage in the walls. The stiff walls prevent collapse of the airways and the loss of gases through the walls of these "conducting" airways. The airways branch repeatedly into smaller airways. As the airways become smaller, they have less cartilage, until, in the very smallest airways, the cartilage is absent. These thin airways, which are called respiratory bronchioles, have alveoli budding from their walls. Gases may diffuse through the walls of these airways. These bronchioles become alveolar ducts and then erupt into lobular sacs of alveoli. There are about 300 million alveoli in an individual's lungs, which provide about 70 square meters of extremely thin membrane through which most gas exchange occurs.

The lungs are elastic in nature and have a tendency to collapse. They do not because they adhere to the inside surface of the chest wall in much the same way that a moist suction cup adheres to a smooth surface. The two surfaces may slide against each other without separating. The chest wall has a tendency to expand because the rib cage and the muscles between the ribs (the intercostal muscles) tend to pull the chest out and up. The balance of these forces (elastic recoil and chest wall expansion) keeps the lungs slightly expanded at all times. Like balloons, the alveolar sacs have a tendency to collapse. The lungs produce a substance called surfactant that keeps the small air sacs from collapsing.

Air gets into and out of the lungs in the following way. The lungs expand, drawing air into them. The lungs adhere to the diaphragm in the same way that they adhere to the chest wall. When the muscles of the diaphragm contract, the lungs are pulled down. At the same time, the intercostal muscles contract slightly, making the chest wall rise up and out. These actions cause the lungs to expand. This expansion causes the pressure inside the lungs to decrease, sucking in air. When the intercostal muscles and diaphragm relax, the elasticity of the lungs causes them to deflate again to their resting state. This passive recoil of the lungs causes the pressure inside them to increase and pushes air out of the lungs.

The amount of air breathed in each breath is called the tidal volume. Each breath contains about 500 milliliters of air. Normally, a human being breathes in and out about twelve times in one minute. This results in about 6,000 milliliters of air being breathed each minute. Not all air that enters the mouth reaches the area of the lung where gases are exchanged. About 150 milliliters of each breath stay in the larger airways. Therefore, 4,200 milliliters of air reach the alveolar space each minute. Since the chest wall and the chemical surfactant tend to keep the lungs partially inflated even after the breath is normally exhaled, additional air can be blown from the lungs, if one exhales consciously and forcefully. The volume of air blown out in this manner, which is called the expiratory reserve volume, is normally about 1,000 milliliters. Additional air can also be drawn into the lungs after a normal inspiration. This volume, the inspiratory reserve volume, is normally about 3,000 milliliters. The sum of the tidal, inspiratory reserve, and expiratory reserve volumes, which is called the vital capacity of the lungs, is about 4,500 milliliters. If these reserves are called into play, tidal volume can be increased tenfold. The breathing rate can also be increased at least twofold. Therefore, total alveolar ventilation can be as great as 120,000 milliliters per minute.

The oxygen that is drawn into the lungs diffuses into the blood, and carbon dioxide diffuses out of the blood into the alveolar spaces to be exhaled. Fresh air exerts a pressure (barometric pressure) of 760 millimeters of mercury (mmHg). Oxygen is 21 percent of air; therefore, it has a partial pressure of about 160 mmHg. It mixes with air in the lungs which has lost oxygen to the blood. This results in a reduction in the partial pressure to about 100 mmHg by the time the breathed air reaches the alveoli. Blood pumped by the right ventricle of the heart into the lungs to be oxygenated has only 40 mmHg of oxygen. Oxygen diffuses from an area of high concentration in the alveoli to the blood, which has a low concentration. This diffusion process is rapid enough that the partial pressure in the blood becomes equal to that of the alveoli before it courses one-half the distance through the lung capillary. Although the partial pressure is 100 mmHg, the amount of oxygen carried in blood fluids (plasma) is low. Therefore, without red blood cells containing hemoglobin, blood cannot carry much oxygen to the tissues.

Hemoglobin is a very efficient carrier of oxygen. Each molecule of hemoglobin can carry four molecules of oxygen. In the same way that a disposable diaper absorbs water, hemoglobin absorbs oxygen from the plasma, allowing more oxygen to diffuse into the blood from the alveoli. As hemoglobin absorbs oxygen, it turns from a bluish purple to red. Between partial pressures of 20 and 100 mmHg, hemoglobin can absorb a large amount of oxygen. Hemoglobin does have a maximum capacity for oxygen that is reached at about 100 mmHg. Hemoglobin is called saturated at this point, and it can hold no more even if the partial pressure of oxygen increases. Hemoglobin is filled to half capacity by the time the plasma partial pressure reaches 30 mmHg. When the partial pressure increases from 20 to 100 mmHg, the increase in the amount carried by the plasma is 2.1 milliliters of oxygen per liter of blood. With the same change in partial pressure, hemoglobin increases the amount of oxygen carried by approximately 150 milliliters per liter of blood. Blood can carry more than seventy times the amount that plasma alone can carry at this range of partial pressure. If the partial pressure does increase beyond 100 mmHg, little more oxygen is added to the blood. Oxygen is added to plasma in the dissolved form at a rate of 0.03 milliliters of oxygen per liter of plasma for each mmHg change in the partial pressure.

Oxygen is carried to the tissues by the blood, where it is efficiently removed from hemoglobin. The partial pressure in the tissues is between 20 and 60 mmHg, depending upon the particular tissue and the rate at which the tissue uses oxygen. Inside the tissues, the partial pressure can be as low as 1 mmHg, providing a large difference to stimulate diffusion into the tissues. Oxygen is quickly absorbed by the tissue. Just as rapidly, carbon dioxide diffuses out of the cells and into the blood. There are also special ways in which the blood carries carbon dioxide to increase its capacity.

Carbon dioxide dissolves in plasma in much the same way that oxygen does, but supplemental mechanisms are required to carry the large amounts of carbon dioxide produced by the body. Carbon dioxide is also absorbed by red blood cells. It diffuses into the red blood cells, where it is changed in chemical form. Stimulated by an enzyme, carbonic anhydrase, carbon dioxide is combined with water and converted to a new chemical (the bicarbonate ion). The bicarbonate ion can attach to hemoglobin in this form. This, in effect, keeps the concentration of carbon dioxide in the plasma low, allowing more to diffuse. In the normal range of operation (40 to 50 mmHg), blood can absorb about 470 milliliters of carbon dioxide per liter of blood. With this large capacity, the partial pressure need change only a few mmHg to carry all the carbon dioxide that is produced by the tissues.

The anatomy of the lungs and the functioning of the respiratory system are well suited to meet most of the challenges that life presents. Exercise is a good example of how the respiratory system can handle a challenge. At rest, a fit young man breathes 6,000 milliliters of air per minute and uses about 250 milliliters of oxygen per minute to supply his body's needs. When exercising to his maximal capacity, the same individual may use as many as 4,000 milliliters of oxygen per minute. To supply this increased demand, the respiratory system must utilize all the reserve volumes discussed above and increase the breathing rate nearly threefold, to a total of 120,000 milliliters of air per minute. The brain senses the movement of the arms and the legs. It also senses the greatly increased amount of carbon dioxide produced by the exercising muscles. In turn, the brain sends signals to the chest and diaphragm to breathe much deeper and faster.

Another example of the large reserve capacity of the human lungs is the ability to hold the breath. Since only a small amount of oxygen from each breath is used, a person can take a deep breath and hold it easily for nearly one minute. Some pearl divers can take a deep breath and swim under water for four minutes or longer. The urge to breathe that one experiences while holding one's breath is produced when the brain senses the buildup of carbon dioxide and the decrease of oxygen in the blood.

The brain also uses its ability to sense the oxygen in the blood to adjust to unusual environments. At high altitudes, there is less oxygen in the air. With less oxygen in the air, less gets into the blood. The brain senses this condition and signals the respiratory system to breathe more air. Therefore, when one travels into the mountains, one will breathe slightly deeper and faster. One is not aware of the increased breathing until fairly high altitudes are reached (above 10,000 feet). If one begins to exercise, however, performing even mild exercise such as brisk walking, one will be very aware of breathing heavily. This situation is greatly intensified if the person has diseased lungs. With some severe lung diseases, even people living at low altitudes (sea level) have shortness of breath, and some need to breathe air supplemented with extra oxygen.

DISORDERS AND DISEASES

The major type of lung disease, which is called obstructive disease, has three subclasses. The first is general obstruction, a disease in which material is abnormally present in an airway. The second is disease in which the large airways are narrowed. The third is disease in which the small airways and alveoli are diseased.

The case of general airway obstruction is simple. The simplest form is one in which a foreign body such as food or part of a child's toy is lodged in a large airway, such as the trachea or a main bronchus. The Heimlich maneuver (standing behind the affected individual, clasping the hands in a fist just below the rib cage, and thrusting up and in with the fist) is very effective in dislodging food caught in the trachea or larynx. An object that is small enough (such as a peanut), however, can get farther into the lung, in which case special instruments or surgery are necessary to remove the object. Tumors can also grow into the opening of an airway and obstruct it. Severe cases of tonsillitis are examples of this type of obstruction. Surgery is sometimes necessary to remove such a tumor if it limits airflow.

Large-airway narrowing is another type of related airway obstructive disease. Asthma and bronchitis are examples of this type of disease. The walls of the tra-

chea and larger bronchi become thickened and thus make the passageway for air smaller. In addition, the specialized muscle (smooth muscle) surrounding the large airways has a tendency to contract, making the opening in the airway even smaller. These conditions result in difficulty of breathing, particularly when inhaling. Relatively rapid airway narrowing caused by smooth muscle contraction is called an asthma attack. Irritants such as air pollution, tobacco smoke, and pollen can start an asthma attack. Exercise, particularly in cold weather, can also stimulate an attack in some asthmatics. Asthma attacks can last for hours and sometimes days. There are some drugs, frequently taken in an inhaled form, that help relieve the symptoms by relaxing the smooth muscle. Many cases of asthma, however, are resistant to these drugs. Some asthmatics have benefited from drugs that help decrease the frequency and severity of attacks. Asthma usually begins in childhood and has a tendency to run in families.

Chronic obstructive pulmonary disease is the term that characterizes obstructive disease of the smallest airways and alveoli. Emphysema and chronic bronchitis belong to this class of lung disease. Emphysema consists of enlargement of the smallest bronchioles and the alveolar sacs. The walls of the alveoli disappear, and with them the capillaries. Therefore, the area previously used to exchange oxygen and carbon dioxide is lost. Since the air sacs are enlarged, the oxygen must travel farther to diffuse into the blood. Emphysema can be indicated by chest X rays and pulmonary function tests but cannot be definitely identified until after death. Emphysema is frequently associated with chronic bronchitis. Chronic bronchitis is characterized by enlargement of the mucous glands and by excessive mucus (sputum) production in the bronchial tree. The enlargement of the mucus glands alone can increase the resistance to airflow. Bronchitis is considered chronic when mucus is produced for three months of the year for at least two years. The sputum can be very thick and may form into plugs to completely block off areas of the lung from airflow. Chronic obstructive pulmonary disease is generally a combination of both emphysema and chronic bronchitis of varying degrees. Persistent cough with expectoration is a normal symptom of this lung disease. With the destruction of airways and alveoli, some of the elastic recoil of the lungs is lost. As a result, exhalation is very laborious. Excess air is left in the lungs at the end of the exhalation, causing the chests of sufferers to be enlarged. Chronic obstructive disease is commonly found in long-term smokers.

Restrictive lung disease is another major classification of lung diseases. The main general feature of this class is primary changes in respiratory system tissues that restrict the movement of the lungs and thus respiration. Cystic fibrosis is the primary example of this disease. Cystic fibrosis appears to be caused by a malfunction of the immune system that produces a thick scarlike substance in the walls of the alveoli. The walls of the alveoli become thick and very stiff (fibrous). In some cases, the scar tissue grows across the small airway opening and closes off the airway. These closed air pockets are called cysts. The stiffness of the airways increases the elastic recoil of the lungs, making it very difficult to inhale.

PERSPECTIVE AND PROSPECTS

Hippocrates (c. 460-c. 370 B.C.E.) recognized the breathing of air as an important function. He believed, however, that the function of breathing was to cool the generator of heat, the heart. Aristotle (384-322 B.C.E.) believed that air was breathed into the arteries, which carried it in the gaseous form to the rest of the body. Galen (129-c. 199 C.E.) transformed medicine from a hypothetical (philosophical) science into an experimental science by performing the first experiments on animals. He found that the arteries did not contain air, and he deduced that a quality of air (oxygen had not yet been discovered), not air itself, was important to life. In the seventeenth century, William Harvey discovered that blood circulated from arteries to veins in both the lung and the rest of the body, and oxygen was identified at the end of the eighteenth century by Joseph Priestly. Claude Bernard described the union of oxygen and hemoglobin at the end of the nineteenth century.

Many major technological advances have been made. Machines have been developed to assist and in some cases completely take over the function of respiration. Respirators can assist patients who have difficulty breathing on their own. Victims of poliomyelitis whose muscles for respiration are no longer functional and paralyzed patients have been greatly helped by respirators. Respirators maintain breathing during surgery when the patient receives general anesthesia. They also assist premature babies whose lungs are not fully developed. Scientists can now make the chemical surfactant that helps keep the lungs open. Premature babies frequently do not make enough sur-

factant; therefore, administration of synthetic surfactant can be lifesaving. Some machines can completely assume the function of the lung. These machines, called extracorporeal membrane oxygenators, can do the job of both the heart and the lungs. They are used in heart transplantation operations. They are also used to function in the place of severely damaged lungs of newborns until those lungs can repair themselves.

Knowledge of the functioning of the respiratory system has allowed humans to function in unusual environments. Humans are able to travel to high altitudes (for example, the top of Mount Everest) with the assistance of supplemental oxygen. Travel into outer space, where there is no oxygen, is now possible because an atmosphere can be created that is suitable for long-term living in space. Experimental work is being performed with the breathing of special liquids instead of air. Success with liquid breathing may allow humans to exist in different environments, such as the deep sea, and may also have therapeutic value.

—*J. Timothy O'Neill, Ph.D.*

See also Asthma; Blood and blood disorders; Bronchitis; Choking; Circulation; Cystic fibrosis; Emergency medicine; Emphysema; Exercise physiology; Lung cancer; Lung surgery; Lungs; Otorhinolaryngology; Pulmonary diseases; Pulmonary medicine; Pulmonary medicine, pediatric; Resuscitation; Tonsillitis; Tracheostomy; Tumors.

FOR FURTHER INFORMATION:

Asimov, Isaac. *The Human Body: Its Structure and Operation.* Rev. ed. New York: Penguin Books, 1992. This text provides an understandable overview of the body's organ functions, including those relating to respiration.

"Fresh Breathing Strategy for ARDS." *Nursing* 29, no. 10 (October, 1999): CC14. A recent study shows that the traditional uses of mechanical ventilation to treat acute respiratory distress syndrome (ARDS) can actually increase levels of cytokine, an inflammatory mediator that contributes to ARDS.

Kittredge, Mary. *The Respiratory System.* Edited by Dale C. Garell. New York: Chelsea House, 1989. This text explains respiration in animals with and without lungs. Covers the historical development of respiratory knowledge and addresses many pathologies of the lung.

Parker, Steve. *The Lungs and Breathing.* Rev. ed. London: Franklin Watts, 1989. An excellent text on the anatomy of the lung and its elementary functions.

The presentation of function is simple and understandable, and the excellent pictures and drawings are a very strong asset.

Ware, Lorraine B., and Michael A. Matthay. "The Acute Respiratory Distress Syndrome." *The New England Journal of Medicine* 342, no. 18 (May 4, 2000): 1334-1349. Acute respiratory distress syndrome is a common, devastating clinical syndrome that affects both medical and surgical patients. Ware and Matthay provide an overview of the definitions, clinical features, and epidemiology of this syndrome.

West, John B. *Pulmonary Pathophysiology: The Essentials.* 5th ed. Baltimore: Williams & Wilkins, 1998. This is an advanced discussion of lung diseases and their diagnoses. Also discusses function testing: normal and abnormal values. A simply written book about a very difficult subject.

RESPIRATORY DISEASES. *See* EMPHYSEMA; LUNG CANCER; LUNGS; PNEUMONIA; PULMONARY DISEASES; RESPIRATION; RESPIRATORY DISTRESS SYNDROME.

RESPIRATORY DISTRESS SYNDROME
DISEASE/DISORDER

ANATOMY OR SYSTEM AFFECTED: Heart, lungs

SPECIALTIES AND RELATED FIELDS: Neonatology, pediatrics, pulmonary medicine

DEFINITION: A deficiency of surfactant in the neonatal lungs, causing generalized alveolar collapse leading to respiratory failure.

KEY TERMS:

air bronchograms: a term used in radiology to describe the presence of air in the terminal bronchi that does not reach the alveoli because they are collapsed

alveoli: the small air sacs in the lungs where gas exchange occurs

endotracheal intubation: the placement of a plastic tube in the trachea to deliver a combination of oxygen and air under pressure to the lungs

mechanical ventilation: the delivery by mechanical means of air and oxygen to the lungs under fine control of pressure and inspiratory/expiratory times by electronic and mechanical equipment

prematurity: the status of being born before thirty-seven weeks of gestation or less than 259 days after conception

respiratory failure: the inability of the lungs to perform adequate gas exchange, resulting in insufficient oxygen absorption and carbon dioxide elimination to sustain life

reticulogranular pattern: a term used in radiology to describe a lack of air in the alveoli

surfactant: a mixture of phospholipid and protein substances produced by cells lining the alveoli that reduces surface tension and prevents their collapse

CAUSES AND SYMPTOMS

Respiratory distress syndrome (RDS) is a condition observed mainly in premature infants and children born to diabetic patients. It is also known as premature lungs, pulmonary immaturity, hyaline membrane disease, and surfactant deficiency syndrome. In 1959, researchers discovered that surfactant deficiency is the cause of RDS in premature infants; this discovery has been the basis for treatment since that time.

The main symptom is a rapid respiratory rate involving the use of accessory muscles to increase the amount of air taken into the lungs. The forceful closure of the vocal cords while contracting the abdominal muscles and diaphragm causes a particular grunting sound. The premature rib cage is very flexible, and affected infants must use extra effort to maintain expanded lungs.

A diagnosis of RDS is made on clinical basis including a history of premature delivery and the symptoms listed above. A chest X ray is also useful; in RDS, a reticulogranular pattern and air bronchograms are observed together with a whited-out appearance in the lung fields. Respiratory function is determined by measuring the amount of oxygen and carbon dioxide in the arterial blood. The samples are obtained using a catheter inserted in an arterial vessel and analyzed in a blood gas machine. In newborns, the catheter is usually placed in one of the umbilical arteries, but samples from radial, posterior tibial, or dorsal pedis arteries are acceptable for analysis. Respiratory failure is defined as the inability of the lungs to perform adequate gas exchange, resulting in insufficient oxygen absorption and carbon dioxide elimination to sustain life.

TREATMENT AND THERAPY

Initially, the treatment for RDS was nonspecific. Physicians used various methods to maintain open airways and waited until the infant's lungs matured on their own. The treatment of RDS was one of the main areas of research that helped in the development of the subspecialty of neonatology.

At present, the pregnant patient who is in imminent danger of delivering a child prematurely, between twenty-four and thirty-four weeks of gestation, is given antenatal steroids. The use of prenatal steroids has been associated with accelerated maturity of the lungs in infants born prematurely. Once a premature infant is born, endotracheal intubation, mechanical ventilation, and natural or artificial surfactants are used in order to maintain open airways and to prevent the development of atelectasis, the defective expansion of the alveoli.

Mechanical ventilation became a standard of care across the United States in teaching institutions. It has helped decrease mortality rates for premature infants and has evolved into a fine art assisted by advanced technology. Mechanical ventilation uses a variety of techniques to maximize lung expansion and to minimize the damage to lung tissues caused by high concentration of oxygen and pressures. Pressure, volume, and high-frequency ventilators are among the current equipment available to neonatologists for use with infants suffering from RDS.

In 1980, a report was published concerning the use of bovine surfactant mixed with saline solution administered endotracheally in infants with RDS. This treatment offered significant improvement in the outcome of this disease. Natural surfactants have been extracted from the lung tissues of calves and pigs, and surfactant has even been harvested from amniotic fluid in humans. The main difference between natural and artificial surfactants is the presence of surfactant-associated proteins. Surfactant-associated proteins function as dispersing agents for the lipid components that line the internal surface of the alveoli, thus preventing the collapse of these air sacs. Artificial surfactants are pure chemicals mixed in the laboratory without surfactant-associated proteins; other chemical substances are used as dispersing agents.

At least seven different types of surfactant have been tested in humans in clinical trials; controversy still exists regarding the proper timing of surfactant replacement, either as prophylaxis or as a rescue treatment. In addition, concern remains about the possible increased incidence of two major complications, pulmonary hemorrhage and intraventricular hemorrhage, in premature infants with RDS following the use of surfactant treatment.

Overall, the use of surfactants and mechanical ven-tilation have decreased mortality and complications in premature infants, but the number of patients with long-term complications, such as chronic lung disease with oxygen dependency, has increased considerably.

PERSPECTIVE AND PROSPECTS

In 1960, the son of John Fitzgerald Kennedy, then president-elect of the United States, died of respiratory distress syndrome. Since then, significant advances in the understanding and treatment of this condition have been made, but the elimination of this disease will be achieved only when premature births are prevented. Until then, RDS will continue to exist in nurseries everywhere.

—*Fortunato Perez-Benavides, M.D.*

See also Critical care; Critical care, pediatric; Lungs; Multiple births; Premature birth; Pulmonary diseases; Pulmonary medicine; Pulmonary medicine, pediatric; Respiration.

FOR FURTHER INFORMATION:

Gerstmann, D. R., S. D. Minton, and R. S. Stoddard et al. "The Provo Multicenter Early High-Frequency Oscillatory Ventilation Trial: Improved Pulmonary and Clinical Outcome in Respiratory Distress Syndrome." *Pediatrics* 98 (December, 1996): 1044-1057. A study was conducted to compare the hospital course and clinical outcome of preterm infants with respiratory distress syndrome treated with surfactant and managed with high-frequency oscillatory ventilation or conventional mechanical ventilation as their primary mode of ventilator support.

Turner, Joan, Gwendolyn J. McDonald, and Nanci L. Larter, eds. *Handbook of Adult and Pediatric Respiratory Home Care*. St. Louis: C. V. Mosby, 1994. Text for home care nurses on the etiology, assessment, treatment, and nursing care of physical and psychosocial problems often encountered in the home care of adults and children with chronic lung disease. Features thirty U.S. contributors.

RESUSCITATION

PROCEDURE

ANATOMY OR SYSTEM AFFECTED: Chest, circulatory system, heart, lungs, respiratory system, brain

SPECIALTIES AND RELATED FIELDS: Critical care, emergency medicine

DEFINITION: The physical act of reviving a person in cardiac or respiratory arrest, which involves such techniques as artificial respiration, chest compressions, and defibrillation.

KEY TERMS:

advanced life support (ALS): a variety of life support procedures, including the administration of drugs and electrical defibrillation

arrhythmia: an abnormal heart rhythm, either in speed or force; arrhythmias do not always lead to a heart attack

basic life support (BLS): a variety of life support procedures, including rescue breathing and chest compressions, often given to a heart attack victim by the first person responding to patient; public training in such procedures is available from the Red Cross and the American Heart Association

cardiopulmonary resuscitation (CPR): a method of producing some breathing and circulation of blood to a patient in cardiac arrest using chest compressions and artificial ventilation

defibrillation: the application of electrical energy through the chest in order to correct abnormal heart function and restore a normal heart rhythm

electrocardiogram (EKG) monitor: a machine which records the electrical activity of the heart onto a monitor and paper strip, which is then used by medically trained personnel to determine further treatment

THE PHYSIOLOGY OF RESPIRATION AND CIRCULATION

Every cell in the human body needs a constant and steady supply of oxygen. The delivery of oxygen is only possible through a continuous movement of oxygen-rich blood, with the heart and lungs working efficiently together. In order to survive, the body must have a functioning heart and lungs, or an outside force that makes both organs function artificially. Two major life-threatening conditions include respiratory arrest (cessation of breathing) and cardiac arrest (cessation of heartbeat). Death is certain unless something is done to put oxygen into the blood and circulate it throughout the body. Cardiopulmonary resuscitation (CPR) is the artificial action of putting oxygen into the lungs and making the heart pump blood throughout the body. By understanding the anatomy and physiology of the heart and lungs, and their entire systems, it is easier to see how CPR can help a person who is not breathing and whose heart is not pumping blood.

The respiratory system. This system has many parts, from the nose down to the smallest sacs of the lungs. After air is taken in through the nose or mouth, it moves further down into the throat (pharynx), past the larynx (voice box) and the trachea (windpipe). Next, the inhaled air goes through specialized tubes called bronchi, one connected to each lung. From this larger tube, the air passage narrows into smaller tubes called bronchioles. The bronchioles become smaller and end at the air sacs, called alveoli. Alveoli are actually millions of tiny air sacs that allow oxygen to move into the bloodstream and carbon dioxide to be removed from the blood and exhaled. The alveoli are hollow and surrounded by a very thin, specialized membrane that is only one or two cells thick. This transfer of needed oxygen, along with the removal of the carbon dioxide waste products, happens through the small capillaries surrounding the alveoli. In the blood, oxygen attaches to the hemoglobin found in red blood cells, and, in return, carbon dioxide crosses back into the lungs in order to be exhaled.

It is this carbon dioxide buildup in the blood that stimulates how deep and how often one breathes. An area of the brain called the medulla is considered the body's respiratory center because it is responsible for sending electrical signals to the chest muscles that control breathing. A check-and-balance system monitors the amount of carbon dioxide in the bloodstream. When the level increases, the rate and depth of respirations also increase so that the excess amount can be exhaled.

The brain sends messages via the nerves to the muscles of the ribs. In addition to smaller muscles between each rib, the neck and shoulder muscles must also help during breathing. The diaphragm, a large, sheetlike muscle that separates the chest from the abdominal organs, also plays a major role in inspiration and expiration. The diaphragm extends from front to back by attaching to the lower part of the ribs. During inhalation, the muscles raise the ribs up and forward while the diaphragm moves downward toward the abdominal cavity, thus making room for the lungs to expand. As a result, the pressure inside the lungs becomes less than that of the surrounding air. It is this difference in air pressure, not an actual sucking in of air, that causes air to move into the lungs. The act of exhaling occurs when these muscles relax, causing the ribs to move back down and the diaphragm to rise. The size of the chest cavity decreases, the elastic nature of the lungs causes them to become smaller, and air moves out of the lungs.

The circulatory system. Life cannot be sustained simply by air moving in and out of the lungs. Once the oxygen moves from the tiny air sacs in the lungs and across into the bloodstream, it must be moved to every cell in the body. This transportation is only possible because of the circulation of blood within the many vessels. At the center of this circulatory system, the heart acts as the pump, pushing blood out through the large arteries and the smaller arterioles and capillaries. After reaching the capillaries, the oxygen is delivered to the cells, and waste products such as carbon dioxide are picked up. The capillaries branch into larger venules and then into even larger veins. The major veins, from all areas of the body, return blood to the heart that is no longer rich in oxygen. Instead, it contains carbon dioxide that needs to be removed. It is this lack of oxygen that makes the blood in veins appear blue, whereas the oxygen-rich blood found in arteries is more red in color.

The heart is responsible for sending out oxygen-carrying blood to all body tissues and moving carbon dioxide-rich blood to the lungs so that it can be exhaled. The right side of the heart is responsible for receiving blood that no longer has enough oxygen, called deoxygenated blood. The blood is next pumped through the bottom half of the heart (right ventricle) into a specialized artery called the pulmonary artery and then into each lung. Although the term "arteries" is usually reserved for vessels carrying blood with high levels of oxygen, there is one exception: The pulmonary artery does not carry oxygen-rich blood. The blood then flows into smaller capillaries surrounding the alveoli in the lungs, where it exchanges carbon dioxide for oxygen. On the return trip to the left side of the heart, after leaving the lungs, the oxygenated blood moves through the pulmonary veins. Blood then travels from the left upper portion of the heart (left atrium), to the left ventricle that is the major muscle of the heart responsible for pumping blood to all the cells of the body.

In summary, the right side of the heart carries deoxygenated blood from the body to the lungs. The left side of the heart receives the oxygenated blood from the lungs and pumps it throughout the body. The huge network of connections in the circulatory system, from the heart all the way out to the tip of the toe and returning to the heart, makes up a closed system that must not have any large leaks which occur during bleeding.

INDICATIONS AND PROCEDURES

Whether the heart is functioning is not a matter of yes or no, black or white. There are many gray areas which represent a heart that is beating but not working in a manner that will support life. One of these gray areas includes many types of abnormal beats, known as arrhythmias, or abnormal rhythms. If the heart is beating too fast (tachycardia) or extremely slowly (bradycardia), then it cannot supply body tissues with needed oxygenated blood. A constant and even pressure of blood flow must also be maintained.

The amount of pressure inside the circulatory system varies. Blood pressure is measured as diastolic pressure over systolic pressure. In a blood pressure reading of 120/70, the top number, 120, indicates the amount of pressure on the walls of the vessels when the heart is beating (contracting). The bottom number, 70, reflects the amount of pressure on the vessel walls between beats when the heart is at rest. In cases when both numbers are extremely low or high, the system is not working properly and urgent measures must be taken to identify and fix the problem.

When either the circulatory or the respiratory system is not able to perform properly, the entire body suffers quickly. Without oxygenated blood, brain damage begins within four to six minutes. While sitting, the human heart pumps sixty to one hundred times each minute, moving about 5.5 liters of blood throughout the body every minute. The average 150-pound man has a total of about 6.75 liters of blood that must be kept constantly moving. The heart acts like a pump because it is a special muscle with its own electrical system. Much the same way as a light switch turns on a light bulb, the heart pumps because an electrical message at the top of the heart, in the sinoatrial (S-A) node, makes the entire heart muscle contract. This natural pacemaker keeps the heart beating when all things are in proper working order. If the heart stops beating correctly or the lungs do not work, however, the person will die unless resuscitation is started.

Resuscitation means making the heart pump blood and getting oxygen into and out of the lungs. In an example of the most severe case, a person is found not breathing and without a pulse. Cardiopulmonary resuscitation (CPR) courses teach that the first step is to open the airway and be sure that nothing is blocking the flow of air in and out of the lungs. If a blockage is found, it must be removed immediately. If the person is not breathing, the rescuer must breathe for him or her. Artificial respiration, or mouth-to-mouth ventilation, in which one individual breaths air into another's mouth, will force oxygen-containing air into the lungs so that it can be picked up in the bloodstream and transported to body cells. Pinching the patient's nose and blowing into the mouth forces air into the lungs in much the same way as taking a deep breath. Yet this artificial breathing alone is not enough. The oxygen put into the lungs must be moved around the body, which can only be done through circulating blood.

In order to move the blood through the circulatory system, something must be done to make the heart pump. This can be accomplished through chest compressions. Since the heart lies between the breastbone (sternum) and the spine, it is surrounded by hard, bony structures. By pressing in the correct position, with sufficient pressure and depth, the heart muscle can be squeezed. This squeezing action will result in blood being forced out of the heart and onto its path around the body. The oxygen blown into the lungs will be picked up by the passing blood and moved out to necessary areas of the body.

Even with the use of proper techniques, however, cardiopulmonary resuscitation should only be a temporary measure for a person who has no pulse and who is not breathing. CPR is only a momentary first-aid measure. Yet this procedure is a vital one: Until further medical assistance can be given, it is extremely important that oxygen circulate in the patient's body.

CPR is usually done by the first responder who finds the victim. This form of resuscitation is known as basic life support (BLS). The administration of BLS is the step just before advanced life support (ALS), which offers additional treatment measures given by medically trained personnel. ALS is given by emergency medical technicians (EMTs), paramedics responding in ambulances, or other health care professionals. While continuing CPR, the medical team will start advanced care before or during the drive to a hospital emergency department.

In order to provide the proper treatment, paramedics must determine the electrical activity of the heart. The heart's rhythm is recorded on an electrocardiograph (ECG or EKG) machine, which helps the med-

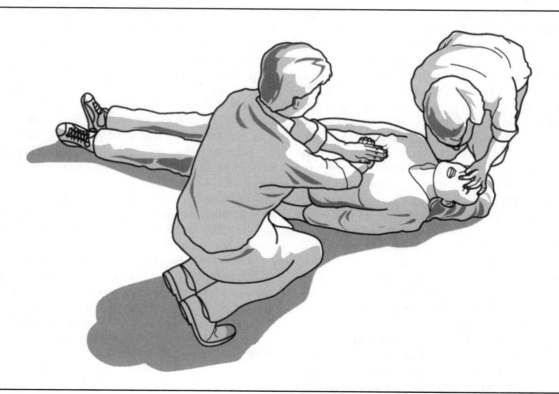

One of the most common methods of resuscitation that can be performed by nonmedical rescuers is cardiopulmonary resuscitation (CPR), which consists of a combination of artificial respiration and manual chest compressions.

ical team find the cause of the problem. The portable ECG machine, which is commonly called a cardiac monitor, displays the electrical activity in the heart. When the electrical impulses are not producing a rhythmic beating pattern, various treatment procedures may follow, depending on how the heart is pumping or if it is working at all. It is possible to correct a heart that has an irregular beat caused by abnormal electrical activity. A total lack of electrical activity in the heart is called asystole and is recorded on the monitor as a flat line. The ALS team can attempt to adjust the abnormal electrical signal but usually cannot mechanically restart a heart that has no electrical impulses. Other heart problems produce other types of tracings on the monitor. In one type of arrhythmia called ventricular fibrillation, the heart has a rapid, chaotic electrical activity that does not allow the heart to beat; the patient will stop breathing and will have no pulse. In this case, CPR is needed to reduce brain damage caused by decreased oxygen to cells, while paramedics and other health care professionals begin advanced life support in an attempt to reverse the dying process.

Many different protocols exist on how ALS treatment should progress, and the following is merely one example. The medics may use an electrical machine known as a defibrillator to deliver electrical shocks through the chest and toward the heart in the hope of correcting the rhythm. Three electrical shocks, given at increasing strengths, are followed by continued CPR. A needle and special catheter are placed in a vein to allow for the starting of an intravenous (IV) drip in which medications can travel to the heart through the veins. A high concentration of oxygen is delivered through a tube inserted through the mouth or nose and passed into the upper part of the lung so that artificial ventilation can aid in the movement of concentrated oxygen. Next, adrenaline (also known as epinephrine) is given through the IV; this drug will increase the blood flow to the heart and brain by narrowing other vessels and will also increase the heart rate and blood pressure. After this drug is given, another electrical shock is administered. The next drug given is lidocaine, which helps to calm a heart that is beating too fast or erratically. Another electrical shock is given, followed by a third drug called bretylium tosylate. This drugs works through interactions with the nervous system to increase the flow of blood from the heart. If the irregular rhythm has still not been corrected, then sodium bicarbonate will be given to reduce the acids produced in the body because of the lack of oxygen. Another electrical shock is given, followed by a repeat dose of either bretylium tosylate or lidocaine. This entire scenario is repeated until the heart is beating in a manner which will sustain life. Other drugs that are used for specific heart problems include atropine, procainamide, verapamil, dopamine, and adenosine. All these drugs target specific problems during a cardiac episode.

When the heart slows or weakens to the point that it is barely beating, life can be artificially maintained in a few cases by using a cardiac pacing unit to create an artificial heartbeat electrically, a procedure called cardiac pacing. This artificial heartbeat may be sufficient until a permanent pacemaker can be implanted.

PERSPECTIVE AND PROSPECTS

Over the years, huge advances have been made in resuscitation measures. More lives have been saved by the training of medical personnel to administer advanced life support before a patient reaches the hospital. Lifesaving drugs and defibrillation have greatly decreased the death rate for heart attack victims and cardiac patients. With the continued training of emergency medical technicians, the survival rate can improve as a result of earlier and more aggressive medical treatment.

Medical treatment could be avoided entirely, however, if more preventive health measures were implemented. With continued research identifying risk factors, the public can be educated about how to prevent conditions that lead to heart attacks. Among the known risk factors are cigarette smoking, hypertension (high blood pressure), high cholesterol and triglycerides, lack of exercise, excess weight and improper nutrition, stress, and diabetes mellitus. Three risk factors cannot be changed: predisposing heredity, gender (men are more likely to have heart attacks), and increasing age.

With further research, the first group of risk factors may be addressed in society through extensive education, but heart attack rates cannot be curbed unless people change their lifestyles. An understanding of heredity, gender, and age risk factors can only bring changes in these rates through further research into their relationship to heart attacks.

Until people are willing to change their lifestyles, early recognition of the warning signs of a heart attack may be the easiest method of increasing survival rates. These warning signals include a squeezing tightness in the chest, sweating, nausea, weakness, and shortness of breath. Too often, people deny that they could be suffering a heart attack, with many believing that the pain is heartburn or indigestion. If medical attention is sought immediately, however, severe damage can often be reduced or stopped. Special drugs such as streptokinase or tissue plasminogen activator (TPA) can dissolve clots that interfere with blood flow, while surgical techniques such as coronary artery bypass surgery (CABG) or angioplasty (PTCA) can open clogged arteries. Heart transplants offer a solution for patients with extensive heart damage. Research continues to decrease the rejection rates for heart transplants. Medications are being developed to decrease the buildup of plaque in arteries. The fields of genetics and gene therapy hold many keys to the prevention and treatment of heart disease.

It is important to note that all medically trained personnel, from the EMT to the emergency medicine physician, must perform life support measures. Unless patients have given appropriate "do not resuscitate" orders, they will receive some form of the above-mentioned procedures. A living will is a legal document that stops CPR or advanced life support from being given. Future resuscitation measures will be influenced by ethical questions regarding when to sustain life.

In February, 2000, more than five hundred experts from around the world met to update guidelines on how to provide CPR and emergency heart care. The goal of the meeting was to improve resuscitation rates from cardiac arrest, and to reduce the devastating complications of brain damage in survivors of cardiac arrest. Recommendations were made according to the results of the most recent human and laboratory research. A variety of changes were made for both BLS and ALS. Updated resuscitation care guidelines were also made for children and newborns.

Bystander CPR (initiation of CPR by the first person to find a cardiac arrest victim) was reaffirmed as a vital component in the chain of survival between BLS and ALS. However, it was recognized that very few people were willing to perform mouth-to-mouth rescue breathing, a vital component of success for CPR. Therefore, it was acknowledged that it was better to at least open the victim's airway by extending the neck and doing chest compressions alone versus doing nothing at all. The layperson will no longer be taught to check for a pulse before initiating CPR. Checking for a pulse was removed from the recom-

mendations because it was demonstrated that laypersons could not be taught to reliably check for a pulse. Instead, they will be taught to look and examine for "signs of circulation," which include breathing, coughing, or chest movements, before starting CPR. Another recommendation for BLS was to train nonmedical professionals such as police, firemen, security officers, and others exposed to large populations in the use of the automated external defibrillator (AED). The AED has two pads that, when applied to the chest of the cardiac victim, analyzes the electrical heart activity. The AED then administers the electrical shock (defibrillation) necessary to restart a heart if the cause of cardiac arrest was ventricular fibrillation, the most common arrhythmia of cardiac arrest. Bystander CPR and early defibrillation by the AED have been shown to do more to reduce morbidity and mortality from cardiac arrest than all current therapies for cardiac arrest combined.

Vasopressin and amiodarone were added to the list of medications to be used during ALS. Vasopressin was recommended as an alternative to adrenaline for increasing blood circulation during CPR. Amiodarone was suggested as an alternative to lidocaine, the current medication used for reducing heart arrythmias during cardiac arrest and resuscitation. Greater emphasis was placed on methods to reduce brain damage in patients resuscitated from cardiac arrest. Passive cooling of the brain (hypothermia) was promoted as the most effective postresuscitative method for reducing irreversible brain damage in survivors of cardiac arrest. Finally, the importance of respecting the wishes of those who do not want to be resuscitated—Do Not Resuscitate (DNR) or living wills—was reaffirmed.

—Maxine M. Urton, Ph.D.;
updated by Laurence Katz, M.D.

See also Arrhythmias; Bypass surgery; Circulation; Critical care; Critical care, pediatric; Electrocardiography (ECG or EKG); Emergency medicine; Ethics; Heart; Heart attack; Lungs; Malpractice; Pacemaker implantation; Paramedics; Pulmonary medicine; Pulmonary medicine, pediatric; Respiration; Thrombolytic therapy and TPA; Tracheostomy.

FOR FURTHER INFORMATION:

Bledsoe, Bryan E., Robert S. Porter, and Bruce R. Shade. *Brady Paramedic Emergency Care.* 3d ed. Upper Saddle River, N.J.: Brady Prentice Hall Education, Career & Technology, 1997. A book used to train emergency medical technicians at the paramedic level. Some of the text is technical, but the anatomy and physiology of the body are covered in an understandable format. Extensive drawings and photographs explain the anatomy of the heart and lungs, CPR, and defibrillation.

Circulation 102, no. 8 (August 22, 2000): I1-I357. This journal provides a detailed description of all the new CPR guidelines made by the panel of experts at the International Consensus conference in February, 2000. The journal can be accessed on the web at http://circ.ahajournals.org/content/vol102/suppl_1

Crosby, Lynn A., and David G. Lewallen, eds. *Emergency Care and Transportation of the Sick and Injured.* 6th rev. ed. Rosemont, Ill.: American Academy of Orthopaedic Surgeons, 1997. This book is often used in the training of emergency medical technicians, yet its chapters are easily understood by nonmedical lay readers. The information given goes a step beyond basic first aid.

Handal, Kathleen A. *The American Red Cross First Aid and Safety Handbook.* Boston: Little, Brown, 1992. A comprehensive, fully illustrated guide outlining basic first aid and emergency care procedures to be given by the first responder until medical assistance arrives.

Heartsaver Manual: A Student Handbook for Cardiopulmonary Resuscitation and First Aid for Choking. Dallas: American Heart Association, 1987. This handbook is used when teaching the CPR courses offered by the American Heart Association. Offers easy-to-understand descriptions of anatomy and physiology, and lists health risk factors. Intended to be read during formal classes. The American Heart Association is revising the manual based on the 2000 guidelines.

Henry, Mark C., and Edward R. Stapleton. *EMT: Prehospital Care.* Philadelphia: W. B. Saunders, 1992. This comprehensive training manual begins with a thorough explanation of prehospital emergency care and includes well-organized chapters depicting a wide range of medical emergencies. Photographs and drawings of specific procedures, including defibrillation, are provided.

Hodgetts, Tim, and Nick Castle. *Resuscitation Rules.* London: BMJ Books, 1999. This book provides a discussion of practical issues and pitfalls in the management of critically ill people, in order to prevent cardiorespiratory arrest. The content is based on the various 1998 guidelines from the European Resuscitation Council.

Safar, Peter, and Nicholas G. Bircher. *Cardiopulmonary Cerebral Resuscitation.* 3d ed. Philadelphia: W. B. Saunders, 1988. Written by the father of CPR, Dr. Peter Safar. He provides detailed information on the past, current, and future practices of resuscitation medicine. The book emphasizes the brain as the target organ for a successful resuscitation.

Thygerson, Alton L. *First Aid and Emergency Care Workbook.* Boston: Jones and Bartlett, 1987. Concise information packed into a workbook format, produced in cooperation with the National Safety Council. Charts, drawings, photographs, and tables outline common emergency care and cover a wide range of topics for the general public. Designed to be used as a textbook in a first aid course.

RETINAL DISORDERS. *See* VISUAL DISORDERS.

REYE'S SYNDROME
DISEASE/DISORDER

ANATOMY OR SYSTEM AFFECTED: Brain, circulatory system, heart, kidneys, liver, nervous system, urinary system

SPECIALTIES AND RELATED FIELDS: Emergency medicine, internal medicine, neurology, pediatrics

DEFINITION: A somewhat rare, noncontagious disease of the liver and central nervous system that strikes individuals under the age of eighteen.

CAUSES AND SYMPTOMS
The exact cause of Reye's syndrome has not been determined, but the majority of patients develop the disease while recovering from a mild viral illness, such as chickenpox, influenza, or a minor respiratory illness. It is theorized that the virus combines with another unknown substance(s) in the body to produce a damaging poison.

The first symptom of the disease is a sudden onset of vomiting, then high fever, headache, and drowsiness. As the disease progresses, alternating states of excitation and confused sleepiness may occur, as well as convulsions and a loss of consciousness. In the final stages of the disease, damage occurs to the liver, kidneys, and brain. The brain cells swell and pressure builds in the skull, followed by a coma, permanent brain damage, and, in some cases, death.

TREATMENT AND THERAPY

There is no known cure for Reye's syndrome. Early recognition and specialized care may be lifesaving. Treatment consists of helping the victim survive the first few days of the illness through intake of fluids, glucose, and other nutrients. If the patient survives the first three or four days, the symptoms usually subside and recovery follows. Medication, such as mannitol, or surgery will reduce the pressure within the skull if it reaches dangerous levels. Although it has not been proven that aspirin causes or promotes Reye's syndrome, based on a variety of medical studies, it is recommended that aspirin not be given to children with viral infections, especially chickenpox and influenza. With few exceptions, acetaminophen or ibuprofen are safe alternatives.

PERSPECTIVE AND PROSPECTS

Reye's syndrome was first described by an Australian pathologist, R. D. K. Reye, in 1963. In the early 1980's, approximately 50 percent of the cases were fatal, but improved diagnosis and treatment of the disease had reduced that number to about 10 percent by the 1990's.

—*Alvin K. Benson, Ph.D.*

See also Chickenpox; Influenza; Pediatrics; Viral infections.

FOR FURTHER INFORMATION:

Crocker, John F. S., ed. *Reye's Syndrome II.* New York: Grune and Stratton, 1979.

Hoekelman, Robert, ed. *The New American Encyclopedia of Children's Health.* New York: New American Library/Dutton, 1991.

Pollack, J. D., ed. *Reye's Syndrome.* New York: Grune and Stratton, 1975.

Taubman, Bruce. *Your Child's Symptoms.* New York: Simon & Schuster, 1992.

RH FACTOR

BIOLOGY

ANATOMY OR SYSTEM AFFECTED: Blood, immune system

SPECIALTIES AND RELATED FIELDS: Embryology, genetics, hematology, neonatology, obstetrics, serology

DEFINITION: Also called the Rhesus factor; an important chemical sometimes found on the surface of red blood cells in humans, the presence or absence of which can complicate pregnancy and blood transfusions.

KEY TERMS:

agglutination: a clumping of blood cells caused by antibodies joining with antigens on the cell surfaces

antibody: a protein made by B lymphocytes that is found in blood; a specific antibody binds with a specific antigen

antigen: a substance that is capable of causing an immune response if it is foreign to the body that it enters; antigens may be free or located on cell surfaces

antisera: the fluid portion of blood that contains specific antibodies

blood type: a blood classification group based on the presence or absence of certain antigens on red blood cells

serum: the fluid part of blood without red blood cells and clotting factors

transfusion: the injection of whole blood or its parts into the bloodstream

STRUCTURE AND FUNCTIONS

Blood replacement in emergency or surgery can be critical: Blood loss exceeding 40 percent can lead to a condition called shock in which the heart cannot pump efficiently, resulting in death. In the search for human blood replacements, scientists have found that animal blood is not compatible. More important, they have discovered that even the blood from different humans does not always mix. Sometimes the red blood cells will agglutinate; that is, they will settle out of the plasma in clumps. Consequently, these red blood cells will be destroyed by the body, and jaundice and death may follow. To prevent this reaction, human blood must be classified into types and cross-matched. The two most important general groupings are the ABO and Rh types.

Human blood is classified into types according to the antigens that might be present on the red blood cells as a result of heredity. Antigens are usually large, complex molecules made of protein alone, protein with attached carbohydrates, or lipids with attached fatty acids and alcohol. They may be free molecules, as in the case of toxins released by invading bacteria, or they may be located on a cell's surface and serve to label or mark the cell. The markers attached to cell surfaces identify the cell as "self" or "foreign." Such antigens are the basis of blood types.

Karl Landsteiner was able to show that there were four major blood types on the basis of two antigens which might be present or missing. He called the markers A and B. People with both markers on their cells are called type AB, people with one of the two are type A or type B, and those without either marker were called C (later changed to O). Landsteiner's system of classifying blood according to the presence of the A and B antigens is now termed the ABO system. Landsteiner demonstrated the chemistry of the antigens and the antibodies by mixing blood from himself and coworkers in his laboratory and observing that some combinations agglutinated.

The next major breakthrough came with Philip Levine and Rufus Stetson's study of the blood of a woman whose fetus had died six weeks before birth. The mother's immune system had produced antibodies against the Rh factors on the blood cells of her developing child. She was Rh negative while her child was positive, having inherited an Rh-positive gene from the father. The positive blood of the child caused the mother's immune system to react. The importance of the discovery was twofold. It not only explained why some babies suffered from an immune reaction in their mothers but also showed that blood transfusions could be typed as ABO compatible and still fail if the Rh factor was not considered.

The term "Rh factor" came about because of a misunderstanding. Working independently and believing that they had found the same factor first in their laboratory animals, Landsteiner and Alexander Wiener claimed discovery and named the Rh antigen after the rhesus monkey. They injected the monkey blood into rabbits, and the rabbits developed antibodies against the foreign factor. Hypothesizing that closely related primates might share the factor, the rabbit antibodies in a serum were then mixed with samples of human blood. Further work verified that there was indeed a new important human factor, but it differed from the one in monkeys. By this time, however, it was too late to change the misleading name. To clear up the confusion, the factor in humans kept the name of Rh factor, while the monkey antigen was labeled the LW factor.

Even if it is inappropriately named, the Rh factor is an important discovery. People with the marker on their blood cells are Rh positive, while people without it are Rh negative. Rh-negative people can give blood to people who are positive if all other antigens such as those found in the ABO types are compatible.

If the reverse is attempted, however, the Rh-negative person will develop antibodies against the Rh marker. Clumping of the red blood cells will occur, and illness and death are likely.

Discovery of the presence of these markers was the key to understanding both the blood types and what happens in immune responses. When a foreign protein or antigen enters the body, antibodies are produced by the immune system and released into the blood and lymph. These antibodies are specific in the sense that a particular antibody will only combine with a particular antigen. (If a particular antigen is present on a person's own blood cells, the individual would not normally produce and carry antibodies for this molecule. Otherwise, the antibodies would attack a person's own blood cells.) The antibodies fasten the cells together in what is called agglutination. Agglutinated cells are destroyed by white blood cells.

Combining the ABO and Rh systems, a person could be A+, A−, AB+, AB−, B+, B−, O+, or O−. Because an AB+ individual has A, B, and Rh antigens and no antibodies against them, this person can receive blood from all others. An O− individual has no antigens and is a universal donor, assuming that the O− person has no other important antigen differences from other, more rare types. The importance of the ABO and Rh systems is shown by the standard practice of hospitals in typing and sorting by these systems.

Unlike the ABO types, Rh-negative blood does not normally contain antibodies for positive blood unless the person has been previously exposed (sensitized) to positive blood. The A and B antibodies are developed early in people because A and B antigens are common in the environment. They are found not only on red blood cells but also in milk, colostrum, saliva, and other body fluids. Should a transfusion of Rh-positive blood be given to an Rh-negative person, the negative blood produces the antibody, which will have a violent reaction with the next similar transfusion.

The Rh factor is inherited, as are all blood types. A person inherits one gene involving the factor from each parent. If the person inherits two genes (DD) for the factor, it will be present on the red blood cells. If a person inherits one gene for the factor and one that does not produce it (Dd), the individual will still be Rh positive. If a person inherits two recessive genes (dd), that person will be Rh negative. Consequently, the gene for production of the Rh factor is called dominant; the other gene is recessive.

The original Rh factor can also be called the D factor. Additional investigation has shown that the entire Rh factor is not a single factor caused by one pair of genes; at least three pairs of genes may be involved. Antisera have been found not only for the most reactive D antigen but also for four other factors. The situation can be explained by imagining Rh to be determined by a combination of three genes, which are probably closely linked on the same chromosome. Ronald Fisher labeled the genes C, c, D, d, E, and e. An Rh gene complex could then be any of these combinations: CDE, CDe, CdE, Cde, cdE, cDe, cde, or cDE. An individual would have two of these complexes, one from each parent. The number of different Rh types then reaches sixty-four.

To illustrate, a person with CDe/cdE would test Rh positive using standard anti-D sera because of the D gene. So would people with any combination of C, c, E, e with a least one D. Nevertheless, the other nearby genes can cause agglutination problems. Each of them, except d, produces an antigen on the red blood cells. The antigens cause antisera to form in human blood that recognizes them as foreign. One can also choose to think of the situation as having eight different alleles for Rh. Then a single symbol can stand for each combination: $r = cde$, $r' = Cde$, $r'' = CdE$, $r^y = cdE$, $R^0 = cDe$, $R^1 = CDe$, $R^2 = cDE$, and $R^z = CDE$. Any r is an Rh-negative combination in the classic sense, and any R is Rh positive. Additional discoveries of new Rh antisera have caused some investigators to hypothesize about the possibility of more than thirty antigens: some which are variant forms of the above and some which require more genes.

R^1r (or CDe/cde) is the most common Rh blood gene combination, at about 32 percent of the population in Great Britain. The R^1R^1 (or CDe/CDe) combination follows at 17 percent, rr (or cde/cde) at 15 percent, R^1R^2 (or CDe/cDE) at 14 percent, R^2r (or cDE/cde) at 13 percent, and R^2R^2 (or cDE/cDE) at 3 percent. All the other combinations total about 6 percent.

Rh has turned out to be quite complex. Nevertheless, the system can be understood and applied at a very basic and useful level of Rh positive or Rh negative which involves consideration of the very reactive D antigen on the blood cells. In that case, the Rh symbol is often labeled Rh_0.

DISORDERS AND DISEASES

The discovery of the ABO system allowed transfusions to proceed with some confidence of success

Rh Incompatibility

First pregnancy

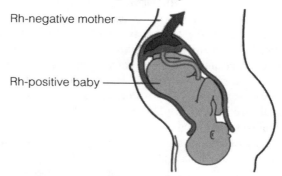

During childbirth, the baby's blood enters the mother's circulation, causing antibodies to form against Rh-positive blood.

Second pregnancy

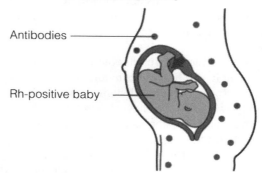

If a second baby is Rh positive, these antibodies may cross the placenta and destroy the baby's red blood cells.

during World War I. Still, some transfusions produced problems, and some minor independent blood-type systems (MNS, P) were discovered. Clearly, people were members of more than one blood-type system. The additional discovery of the highly reactive Rh factor or D antigen was critical for safe transfusions.

Another immediate application of the discovery was in the area of childbirth. Rh incompatibility explained why some babies either died at birth or were born in serious trouble. The attack of the mother's antibodies on the fetal blood cells can lead to various forms of hemolytic disease of newborns, or erythroblastosis fetalis. Incompatibility between mother and child is also one of the causes of spontaneous miscarriage early in pregnancy. Knowing the existence of the Rh factor has saved countless infants.

Recall that the Rh factor is inherited. If an Rh-negative woman (dd) marries an Rh-positive man (DD or Dd), the child may be Rh positive. During pregnancy, there is no direct blood flow from mother to child because red blood cells cannot cross the placenta. At some time during the pregnancy or at birth, however, blood will probably mix, and the mother will then be sensitized. She then will form antibodies against the Rh factor. Many of these antibodies are of the IgG type and are smaller than A or B antibodies (IgM). The small IgG antibodies can cross the placenta into the blood of the fetus. Nevertheless, the first Rh-positive child usually escapes harm by being born. A second positive child will be in great danger, however, because the mother's preformed antibodies will cross the placenta and attack the red blood cells of the fetus. Blood cells are likely to be broken open, releasing hemoglobin. The fetus will become anemic and jaundiced and may suffer brain damage or be stillborn.

The occurrence of erythroblastosis fetalis can be prevented if an Rh-negative mother is given an injection of Rhesus gamma globulin (RhoGAM) within seventy-two hours of the delivery of her first Rh-positive child. This approach was developed by C. A. Clark, P. M. Sheppard, and others working at Liverpool University. The gamma globulin destroys the fetal blood cells in the mother and prevents the production of antibodies that would affect the next positive child. Miscarriages or abortions of Rh-positive pregnancies count as an exposure to the antigen and can cause the mother's immune system to react. Therefore, these events also require the injection to protect future children. Also, any Rh-negative woman accidentally given a transfusion of positive blood would be in danger herself, as would the fetuses in any of her future pregnancies.

Amniocentesis, a sampling of fluid from the sac around the developing fetus, can reveal such difficulties as Rh incompatibility. An Rh-negative woman can also be given a series of blood tests (Rh titers) during her pregnancy. If the tests show that the antibodies are increasing in number, intrauterine transfusion of negative blood may be attempted. Moreover, if the child is nearing full term, delivery may be induced to prevent the blood of the fetus from being completely destroyed. If the child is born with signs of circulatory problems, a blood transfusion can help.

Anthony Smith notes that the ABO type has an effect on trouble with Rh during pregnancy. If the mother is Rh negative, the child is positive, and their ABO types are also incompatible, then the Rh reaction is diminished. The reason may be that the mother already has antibodies against incompatible ABO types. When the red blood cells leak into the mother's circulatory system, they are immediately destroyed by already existing maternal ABO antibodies before any antibodies against Rh factor can be formed.

Some interesting associations with Rh have been discovered but are not understood. Typhoid, mumps, mononucleosis, and viral meningitis are more common in Rh-negative people. Viral diseases tend to be more common in the nonantigenic types of both the ABO and Rh systems (O and Rh negative).

Perspective and Prospects

Few successful blood transfusions took place before 1900. In that year, Karl Landsteiner discovered that there were different types of blood. Some would mix, while others would clump. He and his coworkers identified four major human blood groups: A, B, AB, and O. Even so, eight years passed before the first transfusion using Landsteiner's ABO types was attempted. Transfusions now were more likely to succeed. People could be typed by the antigens on their blood cells, and donors could be matched with the patient. Yet sometimes the transfusions still did not work as predicted. In 1930, Landsteiner won the Nobel Prize in Physiology or Medicine for his discovery of ABO blood types.

Landsteiner and Philip Levine discovered the MNS types in 1927; these are not important in transfusions but are of great help in cases of doubtful paternity. Levine, beginning his own work, had agreed with Landsteiner not to study new blood groups; Landsteiner had reserved that project for himself. Nevertheless, in 1939 Levine and Rufus E. Stetson published a report showing that the blood of a mother with a stillborn child was able to react hemolytically with 80 out of 104 ABO compatible donors. They correctly concluded that the mother's blood lacked an antigen which many others had: an unknown marker that was independent of the known ABO, MNS, and P blood groups. Levine and Stetson had correctly analyzed the problem but did not name their new antigen. Clearly, they had discovered what would be called the Rh factor.

Less than a year later, Landsteiner and Alexander Wiener immunized rabbits and guinea pigs with the blood of the monkey *Macacus rhesus*. They found that the resulting rabbit serum agglutinated not only the rhesus monkey blood but also about 85 percent of blood samples from people in New York City. They called these people Rh positive and the remaining 15 percent Rh negative. Wiener and H. R. Peters attempted to show that the Rh antibody in the rabbits was the same as that found in the serum of people who had suffered incompatible transfusion reactions not explained by ABO blood typing.

A bitter exchange between Levine and Wiener occurred about who had discovered the Rh factor. This was resolved when it was shown that the antigen on the rhesus monkey cells was not the same as the human Rh factor. Unfortunately, the name Rh was too well established to be changed by this time. To avoid further confusion, Levine suggested that the factor in the monkeys be called the LW factor after Landsteiner and Wiener. Despite this controversy, R. R. Race and Ruth Sanger called the discovery of the Rh factor the most important event in blood group science since the discovery of the ABO system forty years before.

Soon different investigators were able to derive sera with different antibodies for the Rh factor. Clearly, the Rh factor was not simply a single antigen. By 1943, Ronald Fisher studied the different antisera that had been developed and proposed that eight different Rh gene complexes were involved.

The existence of the Rh factor is useful in other ways. In addition to transfusions, another application of blood typing (including the presence or absence of the Rh factor) is in criminology. Blood left at the scene of a crime can be powerful evidence against a suspect. London's Blood Research Unit reports that the most common type of blood for a person in England is O, MNS, P1, CDe/cde, Lu^b Lu^b, kk, Le^u Le^u, Fy^a Fy^b, Jk^a Jk^b. Even this most common type occurs only once in every 270 cases. Furthermore, blood types can eliminate individuals as possible fathers in paternity suits. For example, if both parents are Rh negative, the child cannot be Rh positive. A more complete typing of the blood would allow further strong evidence. Yet it must be remembered that such typing does not prove paternity: Even if a man could be the father, he still might not be.

Blood typing also allows anthropologists to develop theories about the relationships among various human groups and how people may have migrated. The breakdown between being Rh positive or negative varies among the races. The Basques, a group of people near the Bay of Biscay between Spain and France, are only 64 percent positive. About 85 percent of the Caucasian population in general is Rh positive. Races other than Caucasian generally are nearly 100 percent Rh positive. According to Sir Peter Medawar, however, the advantages of being one type or another are obscure. Why there are so many different blood types remains an interesting question.

The discoveries of the ABO types and the Rh factor stand as fundamental achievements in medical science. Even though many other types continue to be uncovered, ABO and Rh determinations remain the most basic steps in matching blood for many purposes, especially for safe transfusions.

—Paul R. Boehlke, Ph.D.

See also Amniocentesis; Blood and blood disorders; Blood banks; Blood testing; Embryology; Genetic counseling; Genetics and inheritance; Hematology; Hematology, pediatric; Hemolytic disease of the newborn; Neonatology; Obstetrics; Perinatology; Pregnancy and gestation; Transfusion.

For Further Information:

Bibel, Debra Jan. *Milestones in Immunology: A Historical Exploration.* Madison, Wis.: Science Tech, 1988. Offers the reader selections from the original papers of important scientists. The commentary is valuable in understanding the importance of the work. Both Landsteiner and Levine are included.

Jandl, James H. *Blood: Textbook of Hematology.* 2d ed. Boston: Little, Brown, 1996. Discusses the field of hematology and diseases of the blood. Includes a bibliography and an index.

Page, Jake. *Blood: The River of Life.* Washington, D.C.: U.S. News Books, 1981. A beautifully illustrated book on blood, with good biographies of the scientists involved in new discoveries. Contains a useful glossary and a section on blood types.

Smith, Anthony. *The Body.* New York: Viking Press, 1986. Provides a good chapter on blood groups. Smith's popular style and love for odds and ends are engaging. His error that Rh-positive parents cannot conceive an Rh-negative child does not detract much from an exciting physiology book.

Starr, Douglas P. *Blood: An Epic History of Medicine and Commerce.* New York: Quill, 2000. This work credits Dr. Louis K. Diamond with first describing the problem of blood group incompatibility between mother and unborn child commonly known as the Rh factor and then solving it in 1946 through whole-body blood transfusions.

RHEUMATIC FEVER

DISEASE/DISORDER

ANATOMY OR SYSTEM AFFECTED: Heart

SPECIALTIES AND RELATED FIELDS: Cardiology, family practice, immunology, pediatrics

DEFINITION: An inflammatory disease of the heart that may follow a streptococcal throat infection.

KEY TERMS:

B hemolytic streptococci: streptococcal bacteria that secrete an enzyme capable of dissolving red blood cells

pharyngitis: inflammation of the pharynx (throat), which is sometimes associated with streptococcal infection

polyarthritis: pain and inflammation in multiple joints

rheumatic heart disease: damage to heart muscle or valves as a result of rheumatic fever

rheumatic nodules: accumulations of white cells in soft tissue or over bony areas in patients with rheumatic fever

CAUSES AND SYMPTOMS

Rheumatic fever is an inflammatory disease affecting the heart that may follow infection by the bacterium *Streptococcus pyogenes*. The streptococci constitute a large number of gram-positive cocci, some of which are pathogens. They were originally classified in the 1930's by Rebecca Lancefield into groups based on characteristics of carbohydrates and proteins in their cell walls. *S. pyogenes* is the sole species of streptococci in group A. Group A streptococci cause a wide array of illnesses, most notably pharyngitis (causing strep throat) and impetigo. The most serious complication associated with infection by specific strains of *S. pyogenes* is rheumatic fever.

Rheumatic fever may develop one to five weeks after recovery from a streptococcal infection, often strep throat. The onset is sudden, with the child exhibiting severe polyarthritis, fever, and abdominal pain. There may be chest pain and heart palpitations. Transient circular lesions may develop on the skin. While there is no specific diagnostic test for rheumatic fever, the combination of clinical symptoms may suggest its onset, particularly if there was a recent sore throat.

The production of serum antibodies against strep-tococcal antigens is also indicative of rheumatic fever. Rheumatic nodules may be noted on joints and tendons along the spine and even on the head. Sydenham's chorea, the exhibition of irregular body movements, may also appear during the course of the illness. In severe cases, the patient may become incapacitated.

Most of the time, the symptoms subside with bed rest. Mild cases generally last three or four weeks, while more severe cases may last several months. A single bout with rheumatic fever may be followed by recurrent episodes with additional infections by B hemolytic streptococci.

Rheumatic fever is an autoimmune phenomenon. Certain proteins in specific strains of group A strep-tococci contain segments that cross-react with heart tissue, including that found in muscle and valves. As the body responds to the streptococcal infection, the immune response may also involve cardiac tissue, resulting in inflammation and possible damage. Since the immune reaction occurs over a period of days to weeks, the onset of rheumatic fever may be considerably removed from the actual infection.

TREATMENT AND THERAPY

Because rheumatic fever represents an autoimmune reaction to an earlier streptococcal infection, antibiotic treatment is of limited value. Penicillin or similar antibiotics may be administered for their prophylactic value, preventing further streptococcal infection and recurrence of the illness during the recovery period.

Bed rest and restriction of activities is recommended during the course of the illness. The child should receive large amounts of fluids. Steroids or other anti-inflammatory compounds may also be administered in response to severe polyarthritis or valvular inflammation. The duration of such inflammation is generally no more than two weeks.

Repeated infections with streptococci may trigger additional episodes of rheumatic fever, so antibiotics may be administered on a regular basis. While not all streptococcal infections trigger rheumatic fever, any previous cardiac episode is likely to be repeated after an additional streptococcal infection, often resulting in greater damage. For this reason, prophylactic antibiotic treatment may be long term.

If rheumatic heart disease has resulted in permanent damage to heart tissue, additional therapies may be necessary. Often, such damage may not be apparent for years. Thickening or scarring of the heart valves, particularly the mitral and aortic valves, may necessitate valve replacement at some point in the future.

PERSPECTIVE AND PROSPECTS

Thomas Sydenham, called the "English Hippocrates," in 1685 provided the first description of what was probably rheumatic fever. He also described what has become known as Sydenham's chorea, now known to be symptomatic of rheumatic fever. In 1797, London doctor Matthew Baillie noted the damage to heart valves among patients suffering from the illness. The association of rheumatic fever with bacterial infection, however, was not established until well into the twentieth century.

In part this delay resulted from the inability to isolate an organism either from the diseased heart or from blood of patients with rheumatic fever. In 1928, Homer Swift, a New York physician, suggested that rheumatic fever was an allergic response following streptococcal infections. A few years later, the role of serologic group A, B hemolytic streptococci as the actual agent associated with the disease was established by Alvin Coburn.

A decline in the incidence of rheumatic fever in the United States began in the first decades of the twentieth century. The reason is unclear in this period before antibiotics; this decrease may have been attributable in part to the presence of less-virulent strains of the bacteria. With the introduction of penicillin in the 1940's as an effective treatment for streptococcal infections, the incidence of acute rheumatic fever continued its decline.

A resurgence of the disease was first noted in the 1980's. The reasons remain unclear. Since different strains of streptococci differ in their ability to induce rheumatic fever, it is suspected that the increase may have resulted from the introduction of new bacterial strains into the population. The disease has also been seen to cluster in families, suggesting that a genetic predisposition may exist in the general population which contributes to the rise in numbers of cases. Fortunately, the streptococci have not yet established the widespread resistance to antibiotics seen among other bacteria, and rheumatic fever as a sequela to streptococcal pharyngitis may be prevented with proper treatment.

—*Richard Adler, Ph.D.*

See also Antibiotics; Arrhythmias; Bacterial infections; Cardiology; Cardiology, pediatric; Childhood infectious diseases; Endocarditis; Fever; Heart; Heart disease; Heart failure; Heart transplantation; Sore throat; Strep throat; Streptococcal infections.

FOR FURTHER INFORMATION:

English, Peter C. *Rheumatic Fever in America and Britain: A Biological, Epidemiological, and Medical History.* New Brunswick, N.J.: Rutgers University Press, 1999. In this volume, English, a primary care pediatrician and medical historian, provides a detailed and comprehensive history of rheumatic fever during the nineteenth century and the first half of the twentieth century in the United States and Great Britain.

Kiple, Kenneth, ed. *The Cambridge World History of Human Disease.* New York: Cambridge University Press, 1993. In addition to being an encyclopedia describing human diseases, this book provides an epidemiological history of disease and discusses possible origins and treatments.

Murray, Patrick, et al. *Medical Microbiology.* 3d ed. St. Louis: C. V. Mosby, 1998. A comprehensive textbook providing the medically important information that students need to know—in a format of concise presentations supplemented by numerous tables, color illustrations, and summary boxes.

Steeg, Carl N., Christine A. Walsh, and Julie S. Glickstein. "Rheumatic Fever: No Cause for Complacence." *Patient Care* 34, no. 14 (July 30, 2000): 40-61. Resurgences of rheumatic fever during the past two decades emphasize that primary care physicians cannot afford to relax their vigilance. The latest thinking on diagnosis, treatment, and prevention is discussed.

RHEUMATOID ARTHRITIS
DISEASE/DISORDER

ANATOMY OR SYSTEM AFFECTED: Hands, hips, joints, knees, legs, muscles, musculoskeletal system

SPECIALTIES AND RELATED FIELDS: Internal medicine, rheumatology

DEFINITION: Rheumatoid arthritis is a disease involving the muscles and the membrane linings of the joints and cartilage. Its onset can be slow or sudden, and it involves redness, pain, warmth, and tenderness in the affected joints. Other symptoms include stiffness in the mornings, a low-grade fever, and sometimes nodules under the skin. Chronic rheumatoid arthritis can cause painful swelling and sometimes crippling deformities of the hands. The disease can affect persons of any age; however, it commonly begins between the ages of thirty and fifty. The cause of the disease is unknown, but both immunologic and infectious factors are implicated.

—*Jason Georges and Tracy Irons-Georges*
See also Arthritis; Arthritis, juvenile rheumatoid; Massage; Muscle sprains, spasms, and disorders; Muscles; Osteoarthritis; Rheumatology.

FOR FURTHER INFORMATION:

Dong, Collin, and Jane Banks. *New Hope for the Arthritic.* New York: Ballantine Books, 1990.

Eades, Mary Dan. *Arthritis: Reducing Your Risk.* New York: Bantam Books, 1992.

Fries, James F. *Arthritis: A Take-Care-of-Yourself Guide to Understanding Your Arthritis.* 5th ed. Reading, Mass.: Addison-Wesley, 1999.

Shlotzhauer, Tammi L., and James L. McGuire. *Living with Rheumatoid Arthritis.* Baltimore: The Johns Hopkins University Press, 1993.

RHEUMATOLOGY

SPECIALTY

ANATOMY OR SYSTEM AFFECTED: Bones, hands, hips, immune system, joints, knees, legs, musculoskeletal system

SPECIALTIES AND RELATED FIELDS: Geriatrics and gerontology, immunology, orthopedics, pharmacology

DEFINITION: The field of medicine concerned with the diagnosis and treatment of joint inflammation and bone or joint destruction and with the surgical repair of damaged joints.

KEY TERMS:

acute: referring to a disease process of sudden onset

arthritis: joint inflammation

capillary exudate: a group of substances secreted by the capillaries as part of the inflammatory process

chronic: referring to a lingering disease process

joint: the conjunction of two or more bones

SCIENCE AND PROFESSION

Rheumatology is concerned with the major diseases of bones and joints: arthritis, osteoarthritis, other arthritic disorders such as gouty arthritis, and ankylosing spondylitis, among a host of others.

The onset of rheumatoid arthritis is usually in middle age. It strikes three times as many women as men. To understand the disease, it is necessary to understand the body's skeletal system—the bones and bone structures, as well as the tissues between and around bones and joints.

There are 206 bones in the human body. Some function as support mechanisms that hold the body erect and support the weight, such as the spine and the bones of the hips and legs. Some bones form defensive "cages" that protect body organs, such as the skull and the ribs. Some bones are involved in movement, specifically the bones in the spine, shoulders, arms, hands, hips, legs, and feet.

Bones are composed of three main sections. The tough membranous tissue that covers the bone, the periosteum, contains the blood vessels that nourish bone cells and the nerve fibers that sense pain and pressure. The outer layer of the bone itself is called compact bone; it forms the hard exterior. Inside is a spongy inner structure called cancellous (chambered) bone. Cancellous bone contains the marrow that manufactures blood cells, and it also stores fat cells.

When bones meet, the structure formed is called a joint, or articulation. Some joints are fixed, such as the ribs and the bones of the skull; they are called fibrous joints because a tough, fibrous adhesive material connects them, prohibiting movement and maintaining the integrity of the protective cage.

Some joints are capable of motion. Moving joints are of two types: synovial joints and cartilaginous joints. An example of the latter is the spine, where each vertebra is connected to its neighbor by a spinal disk made of cartilage. Cartilaginous joints are capable of movement, but they have nowhere near the mobility of the synovial joints, so-called because they are filled with synovial fluid, a liquid resembling the white of an egg.

There are six kinds of synovial joints: ball-and-socket, ellipsoidal, hinge, pivot, saddle, and gliding joints. Ball-and-socket joints are found in the shoulders and hips. In these joints, a long bone—the femur in the leg and the humerus in the arm—end with a ball-shaped structure that fits neatly into a round, concave socket. Ball-and-socket joints are capable of the widest range of movement. Ellipsoidal joints are modifications of the ball-and-socket structures, where the bones are not round but oval. They are found in the wrists and ankles. The elbows and knees are hinge joints, which permit only bending and extending motions, up and down or side to side, as with a common door hinge. In pivot joints, one bone contains a small cup or arch that accepts a point of another bone, permitting it to rotate on its axis. The two

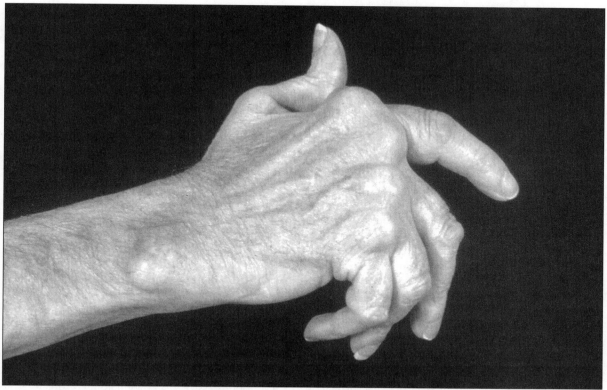

The hand of an elderly patient showing severe rheumatoid arthritis. Rheumatologists diagnose and treat such joint inflammation. (SIU School of Medicine)

bones at the top of the spine, which govern the range of motion of the head, are examples. A saddle joint consists of two bones, shaped rather like saddles; they fit snugly into each other and allow a wide range of movement. The joint connecting the thumb to the rest of the hand is the only saddle joint in the human body. The bones of gliding joints are almost flat; their surfaces slide over one another, permitting limited motion forward and back or from side to side. Some of the wrist bones are gliding joints.

The synovial joints are the most intricate and mobile of all the joints, and they are also the most prone to disease. The synovial joint capsule is a complex structure that encloses the moving bones and other tissues. It consists of the capsular ligament, which forms the joint capsule; the joint cavity, an open space between bones that allows free mobility; and the synovial membrane, a thin, smooth tissue that secretes synovial fluid. The synovial fluid fills the joint cavity and lubricates bone surfaces. Bones do not actually rub against each other; they are too rough and would become abraded. They are separated by a cov-

ering of smooth, white tissue called articular cartilage that permits smooth movement and absorbs impact. Just outside the joint capsule are bursae, small pouches that store synovial fluid.

In rheumatoid arthritis, the first signs of disease are pain and inflammation in the synovial joint capsule. This initial manifestation may be attributable to a number of factors, such as bacterial infection or injury. The reasons that an acute episode of pain and inflammation in the synovial joints progresses to chronic rheumatoid arthritis are unknown. It is suspected that genetic factors may be involved; the disease often runs in families. Blood components called rheumatoid factors are present in the majority of rheumatoid arthritis patients. The role of these factors in the development of disease, however, is unclear because rheumatoid factors are also found in people who do not develop rheumatoid arthritis.

In some patients, rheumatoid arthritis is relatively benign, with pain and inflammation that can be controlled by medication and other support techniques. In other patients, the disease progresses to devastating bone deformities and complete loss of mobility in the affected joints. How this degeneration occurs is related to a disruption in the body's normal reaction to infection or injury. Pain and inflammation are protective mechanisms with which the body attempts to compensate for a disease or disorder. The following sequence of events is what normally occurs when a synovial joint is damaged by infection, physical injury, or a toxic substance.

Tissue injury—from trauma or infection—causes the release of chemical mediators from surrounding cells. These chemicals include prostaglandins, leukotrienes, histamine, serotonin, and bradykinin. Collectively, they cause the local blood vessels to enlarge (vasodilate), increasing blood flow to the affected area and causing redness and heat.

Ordinarily, the capillaries, the tiny blood vessels that supply nutrients to the cells, have openings in their walls so small that only tiny bits of matter can get through. During inflammation, they become more permeable; that is, the openings in the capillary walls enlarge so that the capillaries can deliver larger substances to the affected area. This group of substances forms the capillary exudate, and it flows copiously into the affected area, causing swelling. The exudate consists of lymphocytes, which produce antibodies to fight infection; neutrophils; and macrophages, specialized white blood cells that facilitate the removal of tissue debris, dead cells, and other material. These white blood cells can also release other substances, such as superoxide, an agent used by white blood cells to kill bacteria but which can also damage healthy tissue. Another is interleukin-1, an agent that promotes healing and stimulates lymphocytes to produce antibodies. The spread of inflammation is prevented by a third agent released by the white blood cells, fibrinogen, which effectively closes off the area of inflammation.

In normal situations, the agent causing the inflammation is neutralized, the capillaries return to their normal size, certain white blood cells remove the protective shield, and the healing process begins. In rheumatoid arthritis, the orderly process that begins with pain and inflammation and ends with healing is disrupted by various events. Instead of neutralizing the trauma, the anti-inflammatory phase can set off a chain of events that makes the condition progressively worse.

Why this disruption occurs is not yet known, but four major theories have been suggested. The first is the theory of genetic predisposition to the disease, a factor which may or may not relate to the other three. The second theory is that rheumatoid arthritis is an immune-complex disease. Ordinarily, when the body fights an infectious microorganism that has invaded the body, lymphocytes produce antibodies that combine with the antigens characteristic of the microorganism. This antigen/antibody combination is the immune complex, and it is removed by other white blood cells. In this theory, the process is altered. Instead of being removed by white blood cells, the immune complex lodges in the synovial membrane and causes continuing inflammation. Capillaries continue to release exudate, whose constituents cause cell proliferation, thickening of the synovial membrane, and destruction of articular cartilage and bone tissue.

The autoimmune theory is similar, but in this case the causative agent is not a foreign substance but something natural within the body. For example, if a specific protein released by a gland finds its way into a joint, it may be regarded as a foreign, infective agent. Thus it will set off an immune response and cause inflammation, initiating the same process described above.

The fourth theory links rheumatoid arthritis to viral or bacterial infection. It has been noted that fever, malaise, and enlarged lymph nodes—common symptoms of infection—are often seen in patients with rheumatoid arthritis. Furthermore, rheumatoid arthritis sometimes occurs simultaneously with bacterial pneumonia, tuberculosis, hepatitis, and sexually transmitted diseases, as well as with diseases caused by viruses, such as mumps and measles.

The progress of rheumatoid arthritis is variable. In some patients, it is characterized by occasional flare-ups (episodes of acute pain and inflammation) and periods of remission (times when the patient is relatively comfortable). In others, the disease causes progressive, insidious destruction of the joint and may involve other organs of the body. Articular cartilage may be destroyed, and the joint may become immobilized, an extremely painful condition. The bones in the joint may fuse together, becoming one solid mass. The bones may also become dislocated. In about 30 to 35 percent of patients, rheumatoid nodules develop. These hard, solid lumps usually occur at the elbows but may also be found at the knees, ankles, and feet. In advanced cases, nodules may be discovered in the heart muscle, the lungs, and other organs where they could impair organ function.

The diagnosis of rheumatoid arthritis has been codified by the American Rheumatism Foundation. This organization lists seven symptoms and suggests that the presence of any four should confirm the diagnosis of rheumatoid arthritis (although patients with two or more of the symptoms should not be excluded). The seven symptoms are morning stiffness lasting an hour or more; arthritis in three or more joints; arthritis in hands, fingers, or wrists; arthritis occurring symmetrically (for example, in both hands, elbows, or knees); rheumatoid nodules; the presence of rheumatoid factor; and X-ray evidence of bone deterioration.

Diagnostic and Treatment Techniques

Once a patient is suspected of having rheumatoid arthritis, the physician may wish to conduct further laboratory tests to assess the severity of the disease and, from that analysis, develop a treatment regimen. In addition to testing for rheumatoid factor, the physician will check the patient's erythrocyte (red blood cell) sedimentation rate (ESR). This test helps to determine the presence of inflammatory activity. Another blood test looks for C-reactive protein (CRP). CRP also indicates inflammatory activity; levels rise during an acute attack and fall during a period of remission. Synovial fluid is analyzed to discover changes that occur during inflammation. For example, during inflammatory episodes, the color of the fluid becomes significantly darker, turning yellow or green. Ordinarily quite clear and viscous, it becomes cloudy and thinner in consistency. Many more tests are available to the physician to help him or her evaluate the severity of the disease, including an analysis of the various substances involved in the immune process.

There is no cure for rheumatoid arthritis, but most patients can be helped with the therapies available. In spite of treatment, however, 5 to 10 percent will eventually be disabled by bone deterioration and destruction.

Treatment depends on the severity of the condition. The regimen can simply involve rest and immobilization of the affected joint, or it may include any of a wide range of medications, from aspirin to potent, often-toxic compounds. In advanced cases, joint deformity may be so severe as to require surgery and/or prosthetic implants.

The goals of therapy are to relieve pain, reduce inflammation, and maintain the function of the joint. Ideally, the physician would also like to halt the progress of the disease. Some medications in use today promise to slow or stop the progress of the disease, but nothing is available to cure it.

For the relief of pain, the physician has a large number of medications available, many of which will also reduce inflammation. These include a group of drugs called nonsteroidal anti-inflammatory drugs (NSAIDs). NSAIDs as a class include the salicylates, such as aspirin, ibuprofen, acetaminophen, and at least twenty other drugs currently in use in the United States.

Far and away the largest number of patients with rheumatoid arthritis are being treated with NSAIDs. Many of the NSAIDs are perfectly safe when used in lower doses. At the high doses often required to control the pain of rheumatoid arthritis, however, they can cause significant adverse reactions. A significant percentage of patients given some NSAIDs develop side effects severe enough to warrant stopping the drug. Many develop gastrointestinal (GI) problems ranging from stomachaches to bleeding ulcers, which can be fatal.

One of the ways in which NSAIDs work is to reduce the production of prostaglandins, substances released in the capillary exudate that are partially responsible for the inflammatory process. At the inflamed synovial joint, this attribute of NSAIDs is a desirable one. In the stomach, however, NSAIDs can cause problems. One of the prostaglandins helps to protect the stomach lining from damage by the organ's highly acid contents. NSAIDs can remove this protection, allowing stomach acids to attack the lining, causing irritation and inflammation. Therefore, some physicians prescribe an NSAID with a prostaglandin analog, such as misoprostol, in the hope of avoiding or reducing GI distress. Misoprostol has problems of its own, however, such as causing severe diarrhea in some patients.

For the patient with severe rheumatoid arthritis—defined as painful, debilitating illness that does not respond to NSAIDs and is progressing to deformity—the available medications are both more potent and more toxic. A group of agents called disease-modifying drugs promise to reduce the degenerative processes in rheumatoid arthritis. These drugs include gold compounds, D-penicillamine, drugs used to treat malaria, and sulfasalazine. They appear to alter the course of rheumatoid arthritis, but they do not relieve pain or inflammation, so they must be given with NSAIDs. They all have a high potential for toxicity and must be used carefully, with constant monitoring, to avoid serious side effects.

In some cases, physicians find it necessary to prescribe corticosteroids to patients with rheumatoid arthritis. These drugs present a problem, because rheumatoid arthritis is a lifelong condition, and toxicity and physical changes often occur with long-term steroid therapy. Sometimes corticosteroids are given as short-term therapy to achieve a rapid reduction of inflammation. In this case, there is a danger of a severe rebound reaction when the drug is stopped. A corticosteroid may be administered as an injection into the joint, which is an effective short-term procedure to bring fast relief of pain and inflammation in an acute situation.

Immunosuppressive therapy is sometimes prescribed for patients with rheumatoid arthritis. Immunosuppressive agents have the potential to be highly toxic, and their use is reserved for patients who have not responded to other treatment.

Exercise and physical therapy are useful to the patient with rheumatoid arthritis. During acute inflammation, passive exercise within pain limits, with the limb manipulated by another person or the patient, will help keep the joint mobile and prevent muscle tightening. After the inflammation has subsided, active exercise is recommended to maintain muscle mass and mobility, but the activity should never be strenuous or fatiguing.

Flexion contracture, a condition in which the muscles that move the joint become stiff and shortened, may respond to exercise. If the contracture has become established, however, then more intensive exercise, splinting, or orthopedic treatment may be necessary.

Orthopedic surgery to correct fused or dislocated joints can be performed on any joint in the body, and in some cases, a fused or badly deteriorated joint can be replaced with an implant of metal and/or plastic (arthroplasty). The two most successful implant procedures are total replacement of the hip or knee. When a hip is replaced, the surgeon reveals the joint where the ball of the femur nests in the socket of the acetabulum, a cavity in the hipbone. The ball of the femur is replaced by a metal or plastic ball attached to a shaft that is anchored inside the femur. The socket is replaced as well, usually with a plastic cup that is anchored into the hipbone. The implant can give the patient instant relief from pain and restore mobility. The length of time that the hip replacement

will last varies, but many patients receive years of relief from a single operation. A similar procedure is used to replace the hinge joint of the knee, and, although knee replacement is not as successful as hip replacement, it has helped many patients.

PERSPECTIVE AND PROSPECTS

Rheumatoid arthritis afflicts about 1 percent of all populations and approximately 2.5 million people in the United States. While the disease is not life-threatening, it is one of the most significant crippling disorders in the world. Most patients can be treated successfully by medication, exercise, and other support measures. The disease is progressive in most patients. After ten years, 80 percent of patients will have some degree of deformity, ranging from minor destruction of bone and cartilage to complete fusion of the joint.

Some patients medicate themselves with over-the-counter painkillers and rarely, if ever, see a physician. It is to be expected that, in these patients, the disease is mild, with acute episodes occurring only sporadically. The majority of patients with moderate-to-severe rheumatoid arthritis are seen by physicians.

Currently, there is no perfect therapy for rheumatoid arthritis, in the sense that there is no one agent or family of agents that promises to be safe and effective in all patients. The danger of significant adverse reactions exists with most drugs that are effective, particularly in those patients who require high doses to control the pain and inflammation of the most severe forms of the disease.

Pharmaceutical science continues to search for new medications that will relieve pain and inflammation without damaging side effects. New drugs that will stop the progress of the disease safely and effectively are also sought. There is also the hope that rheumatoid arthritis will be curable or preventable one day.

Orthopedic surgeons continue to improve the techniques for alleviating the effects of bone and joint destruction that occur in some patients. New prosthetic appliances are designed and produced constantly in an effort to widen the range of joint replacement procedures.

—*C. Richard Falcon*

See also Aging; Aging: Extended care; Arthritis; Arthritis, juvenile rheumatoid; Arthroplasty; Arthroscopy; Autoimmune disorders; Bone disorders; Bones and the skeleton; Bursitis; Geriatrics and gerontology; Gout; Hydrotherapy; Inflammation; Lyme disease; Orthopedic surgery; Orthopedics; Orthopedics, pediatric; Osteoarthritis; Physical examination; Rheumatic fever; Rheumatoid arthritis; Spondylitis; Sports medicine.

FOR FURTHER INFORMATION:

Cook, Allan R., ed. *Arthritis Sourcebook: Basic Consumer Health Information About Specific Forms of Arthritis and Related Disorders.* Detroit: Omnigraphics, 1999. This volume includes information about medical, surgical, and alternative treatment options and offers strategies for coping with pain, fatigue, and stress.

Eades, Mary Dan. *Arthritis: Reducing Your Risk.* New York: Bantam Books, 1992. This book, from a series entitled If It Runs in Your Family, deals with the possibility that genetic factors are involved in the development of rheumatoid arthritis. Suggests that a person who is genetically predisposed to the disease can take certain steps to minimize its effects.

Kiple, Kenneth F., ed. *The Cambridge World History of Human Disease.* New York: Cambridge University Press, 1993. It seems that rheumatoid arthritis has afflicted humans from the beginning of recorded history. This volume is useful for learning about the history and progression of rheumatoid arthritis and other diseases around the world.

Larson, David E., ed. *Mayo Clinic Family Health Book.* 2d ed. New York: William Morrow, 1996. Compiled with the aid of physicians from the renowned Mayo Clinic, this is an excellent medical text for the lay reader. The section on rheumatoid arthritis and other bone diseases is concise and thorough.

Maddison, P. J. *Oxford Textbook of Rheumatology.* New York: Oxford University Press, 1998. Presents information on rheumatology, diseases of the joints and connective tissues, and arthritis. Includes bibliographical references and an index.

Shlotzhauer, Tammi L., and James L. McGuire. *Living with Rheumatoid Arthritis.* Baltimore: The Johns Hopkins University Press, 1993. An illustrated text for the lay reader. Covers the causes and progression of rheumatoid arthritis, as well as contemporary treatment modalities.

RHINITIS. *See* ALLERGIES; COMMON COLD; HAY FEVER.

RHINOPLASTY AND SUBMUCOUS RESECTION
PROCEDURES
ANATOMY OR SYSTEM AFFECTED: Nose
SPECIALTIES AND RELATED FIELDS: General surgery; otorhinolaryngology; Plastic surgery
DEFINITION: Surgical procedures that correct cosmetic and health problems related to the nose.
KEY TERMS:
cartilage: white, fibrous connective tissue attached to the articular surfaces of bones
inspired air: air that is breathed in
pharynx: the part of the respiratory-digestive passage that extends from the nasal cavity to the larynx (voice box)

INDICATIONS AND PROCEDURES

The nose, in addition to being an important organ for breathing and smelling, is cosmetically significant because of its prominence on the face. Hence, surgery to improve the nose may be of utilitarian origin or for cosmetic reasons to enhance facial appearance. In modern society, the latter type of nasal surgery is the most common. Nasal surgery, however, usually involves both. Before examining rhinoplasty and submucous resection, it is useful briefly to denote the function of the nose, its anatomy, and its interconnections with the body's respiratory and olfactory systems.

Air breathed in enters the nose through the nostrils, which are separated by a wall of cartilage and bone called the nasal septum. In most cases, the septum produces two nostrils of similar size. In some cases, however, injury or heredity causes the septum to become thickened on one side or to exhibit ridges or bumps. In minor cases of such deviated septum, the irregularity may make one nostril smaller than the other and can affect breathing and sinus drainage adversely during colds. In very severe cases, it can obstruct and irritate the nose enough so that relatively permanent nasal tissue swelling requires chronic, uncomfortable breathing through the mouth.

In most individuals, inspired air passes into two nasal passages which lead into the upper part of the throat. They allow the air to pass through the pharynx and trachea (windpipe) to reach the lungs. Each nasal passage is lined with a soft, moist mucous membrane which is covered with fine cilia (hairs) that catch dust and other particles and keep them from reaching the lungs. The nose and the nasal passages also raise the temperature of inspired air before it enters the lungs.

Furthermore, the nose plays a large part in the sense of taste, as shown by the inability of people with severe colds to taste food.

Submucous resection is performed when the nasal septum is so distorted that it causes discomfort to the patient, especially chronic nasal pain, the need for continuous and uncomfortable mouth breathing, or repeated and prolonged colds. In these cases, the septum is reshaped in order to cure the problem, allowing the patient to breathe normally again through the nose. Septum resection may be accomplished with fine scissors, a scalpel, and/or bone rasps.

Cosmetic nose alterations are collectively referred to as rhinoplasty. The most common procedures correct prominent bumps, bulbousness, drooping tip, and overly large or small size. Perusal of any text on cosmetic surgery of the nose provides picturesque terms that graphically identify the surgical problems encountered in rhinoplasty, such as "saddle nose," "short nose," "pig nose," and "hook nose." Rhinoplasty is also used to repair damage caused by accidents and cancer. Furthermore, it is an essential part of repairing a deviated nasal septum, which can greatly impair the breathing of afflicted individuals if left untreated.

Most often, nasal surgery is performed by use of intranasal incisions. The nasal skin is temporarily freed and pulled back from underlying bone and cartilage. Then, this hard framework is altered by partial removal, rearrangement, augmentation with synthetic materials, or bone and cartilage grafts from various parts of the patient's body. The site in the nose and the shape of the grafts used depend on the procedure to be carried out. Once all necessary procedures have been completed on cartilage and bone, the skin is redraped over them. In some cases, especially where nose size is to be reduced, portions of the soft tissues of the nose are removed.

After nasal surgery—whether rhinoplasty, submucous resection, or some combination of techniques is used—the nostrils are packed with sterile gauze to prevent bleeding and to support the nasal mucosa during its initial healing, as incisions are usually sutured only minimally and with resorbable suture materials. The packing is often removed after several days. A nasal splint is also used in many cases. It provides external support and aid in maintaining nasal recontouring. The splint also protects the altered nose from damage during the several weeks usually required for most swelling to subside. After the removal of the splint, it takes at least several months for

normal feeling and final nose shape to be attained as postsurgical swelling subsides entirely.

USES AND COMPLICATIONS

Nasal surgery can be done under local or general anesthesia in a hospital or in a surgeon's office. Hospitalization and general anesthesia are most often used, although frequently they are not needed. Most reconstructive surgeons prefer these operative conditions for the patient's sake and because they allow easier physical manipulation of the patient.

Most procedures attempted are quite safe and uncomplicated. Occasional problems include excessive bleeding, internal scarring of nasal mucosa, recurring airway obstruction, and unexpected contour irregularities. Infections after nasal surgery are rare except in cases where cartilaginous nasal implants are used. The incidence of infection may increase, however, as surgeons add forehead and chin alteration to rhinoplasty to optimize the overall cosmetic results.

Overall, nasal surgery is straightforward and has few real risks. Patients should be aware, however, that the procedure can fail to yield a chosen cosmetic improvement and that airway obstruction can be generated by the process or can recur after repair.

PERSPECTIVE AND PROSPECTS

Among the exciting advances being made in rhinoplasty and submucous resection are the replacement of deficient nostril parts and septa with cartilage from other body parts or with synthetic materials. It is projected by some doctors that implants obtained from other individuals will eventually be used to repair function and appearance in individuals whose noses are irreversibly damaged by accidents and cancer.

Another aspect of importance to cosmetic nasal surgery is the growing realization that the chin, forehead, and other parts of the face are important to the appearance of the nose. This has led some surgeons performing nose recontouring to expend much effort toward examining these features and designing complementary surgical procedures to achieve optimum results.

—*Sanford S. Singer, Ph.D.*

See also Nasal polyp removal; Nasopharyngeal disorders; Otorhinolaryngology; Plastic surgery.

FOR FURTHER INFORMATION:
Berkow, Robert, and Andrew J. Fletcher, eds. *The Merck Manual of Diagnosis and Therapy.* 17th ed.

Rahway, N.J.: Merck Sharp & Dohme Research Laboratories, 1999. Describes many diseases treated by proctologists, including their characteristics, etiology, diagnosis, and treatment. Designed for physicians, the material is also useful to less specialized readers.

Gruber, Ronald P., and George C. Peck. *Rhinoplasty: State of the Art.* St. Louis: Mosby Year Book, 1993. This text discusses the methods used in the practice of rhinoplasty. Includes bibliographical references and an index.

Professional Guide to Diseases. 7th ed. Springhouse, Pa.: Springhouse, 2001. A comprehensive yet concise medical reference covering more than six hundred disorders, this book includes information about the latest AIDS treatments, new parameters for defining diabetes, current information on cancers, updates on Alzheimer's disease, and more.

RICKETS
DISEASE/DISORDER

ANATOMY OR SYSTEM AFFECTED: Bones, musculoskeletal system, teeth

SPECIALTIES AND RELATED FIELDS: Nutrition, orthopedics, osteopathic medicine, pediatrics

DEFINITION: A disorder involving the softening and weakening of a child's bones, primarily caused by lack of vitamin D and/or lack of calcium or phosphate.

CAUSES AND SYMPTOMS
Rickets is a relatively rare bone disease that most frequently afflicts children. It is the result of insufficient or inefficient absorption of vitamin D in the body, which causes a progressive softening and weakening of the bone. Certain physical conditions can reduce digestion or absorption of fats and may also diminish vitamin D absorption by the intestines. The loss of calcium and phosphate from the bone eventually causes destruction of the supportive bone matrix. In adult deficiency, demineralization (osteomalacia) may occur in the spine, pelvis, and lower extremities causing osteoporosis (an adult disorder causing brittle bones).

Symptoms of rickets may include pain or tenderness of the long bones and pelvis, skeletal deformities such as bowlegs, bumps in the rib cage (rachitic rosary), spinal and pelvic deformities (including kyphosis or scoliosis), pigeon breast, an asymmetrical or odd-shaped skull, increased tendency toward frac-

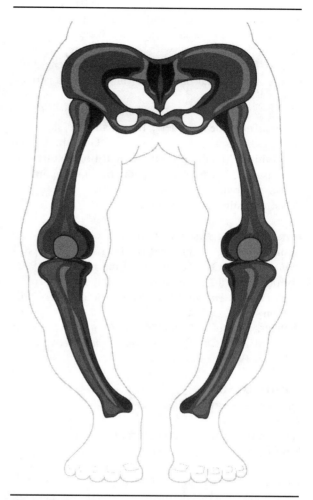

Bowed legs is a sign of a skeletal deformation that is a classic effect of rickets.

tures, dental deformities and cavities, night fevers, muscle cramps, impaired growth, decreased muscle tone and growth, and general weakness and restlessness.

Hereditary rickets is a sex-linked vitamin D-resistant disorder that occurs when the kidney is unable to retain phosphate. Rickets may also occur in children with liver or biliary disorders, when vitamin D and fats are inadequately absorbed.

TREATMENT AND THERAPY
Uncomplicated infantile rickets can be cured with a daily replacement of deficient calcium, phosphorous, and vitamin D. Clinical testing reveals improvement after one week. Dietary sources of vitamin D include

fish, liver, and processed milk. In addition, moderate exposure to sunlight is therapeutic. Skeletal deformities can be corrected with good posture or body braces. If rickets is not corrected in children, short stature and skeletal deformities may become permanent.

—*John Alan Ross, Ph.D.*

See also Bone disorders; Bones and the skeleton; Bowlegs; Fracture and dislocation; Growth; Lower extremities; Malabsorption; Malnutrition; Nutrition; Orthopedics; Orthopedics, pediatric; Osteoporosis; Scoliosis; Spinal cord disorders; Spine, vertebrae, and disks; Vitamins and minerals.

For Further Information:

Bentley, George, and Robert B. Greer, eds. *Orthopaedics*. 4th ed. Oxford, England: Linacre House, 1993.

Tortora, Gerard J., and Sandra R. Grabowski. *Principles of Anatomy and Physiology*. 9th ed. New York: John Wiley & Sons, 2000.

Wenger, Dennis R., and Mercer Rang. *The Art and Practice of Children's Orthopaedics*. New York: Raven Press, 1993.

Ringworm
Disease/disorder

Also known as: Tinea

Anatomy or system affected: Skin

Specialties and related fields: Dermatology, family practice

Definition: A group of fungal diseases caused by several species of dermatophytes and characterized by itching, scaling, and sometimes painful lesions.

Causes and Symptoms

Ringworm is a skin disease characterized by itching and redness. Despite its name, it is caused by a fungal infection, not a worm. The skin in areas affected with ringworm often contains round lesions that are colored red, have scaly borders, and contain normal-appearing skin in their centers. Alternatively, the lesions can simply be scaly, red patches with no clearly defined shape. Typically, these lesions are relatively small, approximately 1 inch in their largest dimension. Complications of ringworm include spread to the scalp, hair, or nails of the fingers or toes.

The lesions of ringworm are caused by species of fungi that are members of the genus *Trichophyton*. The most common pathogen is *Trichophyton rubrum*. Ringworm appears on exposed areas of the body, often on the face and arms. Cats are the most common means of transmitting the *Trichophyton* pathogen from one person to another.

Examination of scrapings from skin lesions is used to diagnose ringworm. Species of *Trichophyton* can be tentatively identified by their microscopic structure. Culturing material from a skin lesion provides a definitive diagnosis.

Treatment and Therapy

The treatment of ringworm involves both the patient and any carriers. The patient can be treated effectively with any of several creams applied to the skin that are available without a prescription. Their use should be continued for one to two weeks after the skin lesions have cleared. Other drugs are available but require a physician's prescription. They are used for more extensive lesions or when fingernails or toenails are involved. Body ringworm usually responds within four weeks of treatment. The carrier should be identified and treated. Avoiding contact with infected household pets or clothing that has been worn by an infected person can prevent ringworm.

Perspective and Prospects

Tinea species cause infections in other parts of the body: tinea capitis on the scalp, tinea pedis on the feet, and tinea cruris in the groin region. Ringworm must be differentiated from several other diseases that also cause round skin lesions: psoriasis, syphilis, pityriasis rosea, and lupus erythematosus. The lesions of psoriasis usually appear on the elbow, knees, and scalp. Syphilis lesions usually appear on the mucous membranes of the genitals or on the palms of the hands or soles of the feet. Although pityriasis rosea often begins with a single round lesion, many more usually follow. The classic skin lesion of lupus erythematosus is butterfly-shaped and covers the nose and cheeks. The presence of a cat or other domestic pet is often an important element in establishing a diagnosis of ringworm.

—*L. Fleming Fallon, Jr., M.D., Ph.D., M.P.H.*

See also Athlete's foot; Dermatology; Dermatology, pediatric; Fungal infections; Itching; Lupus erythematosus; Pityriasis rosea; Psoriasis; Rashes; Skin; Skin disorders; Syphilis.

For Further Information:

Burns, Tony. *Lecture Notes on Dermatology*. 7th ed. London: Blackwell Science, 1997.

Goldsmith, Lowell A., Gerald S. Lazarus, and Michael D. Tharp. *Adult and Pediatric Dermatology: A Color Guide to Diagnosis and Treatment.* Philadelphia: F. A. Davis, 1997.

Lamberg, Lynne. *Skin Disorders.* Philadelphia: Chelsea House, 2001.

Mackie, Rona M. *Clinical Dermatology.* 4th ed. New York: Oxford University Press, 1997.

Rassner, Gernot, and Walter H. Burgdorf. *Atlas of Dermatology.* 3d ed. Philadelphia: Lea & Febiger, 1994.

RNA. *See* DNA AND RNA.

ROOT CANAL TREATMENT
PROCEDURE

ANATOMY OR SYSTEM AFFECTED: Gums, mouth, teeth

SPECIALTIES AND RELATED FIELDS: Dentistry

DEFINITION: The removal of irreparably damaged tooth pulp and its replacement with inert materials.

INDICATIONS AND PROCEDURES

At the center of every tooth is soft pulp tissue. Among its main components are blood vessels that nourish teeth, sensory nerves, and supportive connective tissue. Tooth fractures or deep dental caries (cavities) irreparably damage this pulp. When this happens, root canal treatment is rendered. All dentists can carry out this procedure, but specialists who limit their practice to such efforts—endodontists—are the most skilled.

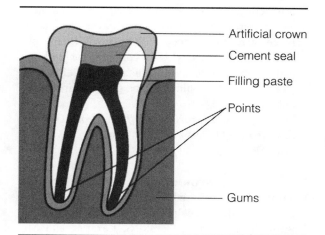

Artificial crown

Cement seal

Filling paste

Points

Gums

Root canal treatment may become necessary when the dental pulp is damaged; the pulp is removed and replaced with artificial material, and a crown is fitted.

The symptoms that often require root canal treatment are steady throbbing pain and sensitivity to pressure on or tapping of the tooth. Because pulp disease is associated with bacterial infection, gum abscesses may occur in extreme cases.

Root canal therapy is carried out when upon examination the pulp is found to be irreversibly damaged. The tooth is opened by drilling an access channel. Then, the pulp is removed from the center and from the tooth root portions—the root canals—that it also fills. Next, the pulp chamber and root canals are cleaned and reshaped by drilling and with specialized endodontic files. Lastly, the canals are filled with inert materials such as gutta-percha (a rubberlike substance), and a temporary filling is put in place. At a later time, when it is clear that the procedure has been successful, a permanent filling or an artificial crown is substituted.

USES AND COMPLICATIONS

Root canal therapy prolongs the life of teeth by creating a tooth which retains much of its strength over time. Without pulp, however, the blood supply and support of the tooth are reduced. Hence, teeth that have undergone root canal treatment are likely to become brittle and susceptible to fracture.

The success of root canal therapy is greater than 90 percent. Nevertheless, it can produce later complications, including fine, virtually undetectable canal fractures that may allow the entry of bacteria; imperfectly filled canals can have the same result. In such cases, repeated root canal therapy may be needed or the tooth may require extraction. These problems, although relatively uncommon, occur because of the nature of this delicate surgery. For example, it is not possible to view the surgical site directly. Rather, the site is approximated by X-ray pictures taken at each treatment stage.

PERSPECTIVE AND PROSPECTS

Root canal treatment has improved markedly in recent years, and further advances are expected, such as better surgical tools and filling materials and an enhanced ability to evaluate the success of the procedure. In addition, efforts to preserve and/or regenerate damaged tooth pulp are ongoing.

—*Sanford S. Singer, Ph.D.*

See also Dental diseases; Dentistry; Endodontic disease; Periodontal surgery; Teeth; Tooth extraction; Toothache.

FOR FURTHER INFORMATION:

Anderson, Pauline C., and Martha R. Burkard. *The Dental Assistant*. 6th ed. Albany, N.Y.: Delmar, 1995.

Cranin, A. Norman. *A Modern Family Guide to Dental Health*. New York: Stein & Day, 1971.

Klatell, Jack, Andrew Kaplan, and Gray Williams, Jr., eds. *The Mount Sinai Medical Center Family Guide to Dental Health*. New York: Macmillan, 1991.

Smith, Rebecca W. *The Columbia University School of Dental and Oral Surgery's Guide to Family Dental Care*. New York: W. W. Norton, 1997.

ROSACEA

ALSO KNOWN AS: Acne rosacea, adult acne, rhinophyma

DISEASE/DISORDER

ANATOMY OR SYSTEM AFFECTED: Nose, skin

SPECIALTIES AND RELATED FIELDS: Dermatology

DEFINITION: A chronic inflammation and redness of the face that usually affects people between the ages of thirty and fifty; it is more common in women but is more severe in men.

CAUSES AND SYMPTOMS

Guy de Chauliac, a French surgeon, first described rosacea medically in the fourteenth century, attributing the condition to the excessive consumption of alcoholic drinks. It is now known that, although alcohol may exacerbate the condition, rosacea can develop in individuals who have never consumed alcohol. While the actual cause is unknown, rosacea is more common in fair-skinned people who flush easily. The most common triggers for this flushing are hot drinks, alcohol, spicy foods, stress, sunlight, and extreme heat or cold. There is no cure for rosacea, but it can be treated with oral and topical antibiotics and avoidance of triggers.

Untreated, rosacea may progress from facial redness to slight swelling, pimples, pustules, and prominent facial pores on the nose, mid-forehead, and chin. In some patients, particularly in men, the oil glands enlarge, causing a bulbous, enlarged red nose and puffy cheeks. Thick bumps can develop on the lower half of the nose and nearby cheeks. This stage is known as rhinophyma, a condition made famous by actor W. C. Fields with his red, bulbous nose. Rhinophyma can be extremely disfiguring, and its mistaken association with alcoholism can cause embarrassment and affect self-esteem.

TREATMENT AND THERAPY

Rosacea and rhinophyma cannot be cured, but the symptoms can be lessened or even eliminated. Rhinophyma is usually treated with surgery. The excess tissue that has developed can be removed with a scalpel or a laser, or through electrosurgery.

—Lisa M. Sardinia, Ph.D.

See also Acne; Dermatology; Rashes; Skin; Skin disorders.

FOR FURTHER INFORMATION:

Dvorine, William. *A Dermatologist's Guide to Home Skin Treatment*. New York: Charles Scribner's Sons, 1983.

Pillsbury, Donald M. *A Manual of Dermatology*. Philadelphia: W. B. Saunders, 1971.

Roenigk, Henry H., ed. *Office Dermatology*. Baltimore: Williams & Wilkins, 1981.

Sauer, Gordon C. *Sauer's Manual of Skin Diseases*. 8th ed. Philadelphia: J. B. Lippincott, 2000.

ROSEOLA

DISEASE/DISORDER

ANATOMY OR SYSTEM AFFECTED: Skin

SPECIALTIES AND RELATED FIELDS: Pediatrics, virology

DEFINITION: Roseola is a common and contagious childhood disease characterized by high fever and skin rash. It affects infants and children ages one to three. Symptoms include fever, irritability, drowsiness, and a flat, reddish skin rash after three to four days of fever. The cause is unknown, although it is believed to be caused by a virus with an incubation period of five to fifteen days. The occurrence of roseola seems to be seasonal with exposure to public places. It is common for children and infants to recover spontaneously after one week; children should never be given aspirin to reduce fever.

—Jason Georges and Tracy Irons-Georges

See also Childhood infectious diseases; Fever; Pediatrics; Rashes.

FOR FURTHER INFORMATION:

Behrman, Richard E., ed. *Nelson Textbook of Pediatrics*. 16th ed. Philadelphia: W. B. Saunders, 2000.

Goldsmith, Lowell A., Gerald S. Lazarus, and Michael D. Tharp. *Adult and Pediatric Dermatology: A Color Guide to Diagnosis and Treatment*. Philadelphia: F. A. Davis, 1997.

Korting, G. W. *Diseases of the Skin in Children and Adolescents*. Philadelphia: W. B. Saunders, 1970.

ROUNDWORM
DISEASE/DISORDER
ANATOMY OR SYSTEM AFFECTED: Abdomen, gastrointestinal system, intestines, respiratory system, stomach

SPECIALTIES AND RELATED FIELDS: Gastroenterology, internal medicine, nutrition, pediatrics, public health

DEFINITION: Roundworms, or nematodes, are one of two main types of worms (helminths)—the other is flatworms. Some roundworms are intestinal parasites in humans which thrive in the gastrointestinal tract. Roundworm eggs enter the human body through contaminated water and food or from dirty hands. The larvae hatch in the small intestine, make their way into the bloodstream, and become lodged in the lungs. Upon returning to the small intestine, they develop into adults and lay eggs which are excreted in the feces. Roundworms are found in all ages but are more common in children. Symptoms include irritability, restlessness at night, poor appetite, frequent fatigue, weight loss, abdominal discomfort, diarrhea, and sometimes coughing and wheezing. If the infestation is untreated in children, malnutrition may occur. Round-

Roundworm

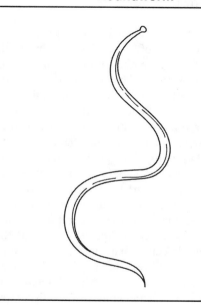

worms are treated with medication and improved hygiene.

—*Jason Georges and Tracy Irons-Georges*
See also Elephantiasis; Parasitic diseases; Trichinosis; Worms.

FOR FURTHER INFORMATION:
Buchsbaum, Ralph, et al. *Animals Without Backbones*. 3d ed. Chicago: University of Chicago Press, 1987.
Despommier, Dickson D., Robert W. Gwadz, and Peter J. Hotex. *Parasitic Diseases*. 4th ed. New York: Springer-Verlag, 2000.
Donaldson, Raymond Joseph, ed. *Parasites and Western Man*. Baltimore: University Park Press, 1979.
Klein, Aaron E. *The Parasites We Humans Harbor*. New York: Elsevier/Nelson Books, 1981.
Lee, Donald L. *The Physiology of Nematodes*. San Francisco: W. H. Freeman, 1965.

RUBELLA
DISEASE\DISORDER
ALSO KNOWN AS: German measles

ANATOMY OR SYSTEM AFFECTED: Joints, lymphatic system, nervous system, skin

SPECIALTIES AND RELATED FIELDS: Family practice, pediatrics

DEFINITION: An acute, contagious childhood disease caused by a virus and characterized by a rash.

KEY TERMS:
arthralgia: pain in a joint or joints
arthritis: inflammation of a joint or joints
congenital: present at birth; having to do with a fetus carried by a pregnant woman

CAUSES AND SYMPTOMS
Rubella can be either acquired, infecting both children and adults, or congenital, infecting a fetus before birth. Acquired rubella is typically a mild disease with few complications. The incubation period is usually sixteen to eighteen days, but it can last fourteen to twenty-one days. For children, the first symptom is typically a rash that is small, red, and spotty. It starts on the face and behind the ears and spreads downward in the next one or two days. This rash is much milder than the rash of measles. In adults, the rash is preceded by symptoms that include a low-grade fever, headache, loss of appetite, mildly red eyes, a stuffy nose, a sore throat, coughing, and lymph node enlargement in the neck. Typically, this enlargement occurs behind the ears and in the back of the neck.

Complications of rubella are more common in adults, particularly in young women. The most common complications are arthralgia and arthritis. These joint manifestations can occur in any time from when the rash subsides to several weeks later. Rarer complications include effects on the blood, the heart, and the nervous system.

Congenital rubella is associated with multiple birth defects in the infant. The most common manifestations of congenital rubella affect three areas: growth, the blood, and the central nervous system. The effects on growth include prematurity and intrauterine growth retardation. The effects on the blood include thrombocytopenia (a decrease in platelets), anemia, and an enlarged liver and spleen. The effects on the central nervous system include microcephaly (a small head), deafness, eye damage (including cataracts and retinal damage), mental retardation, and behavioral disorders. Whether these effects of congenital rubella are manifested depends on the timing of the infection during pregnancy and the severity of the infection. Some newborns may appear normal at delivery and develop manifestations during their first five years of life.

The diagnosis of acquired rubella primarily hangs on the clinical symptoms, such as a rash and lymph node enlargement in the back of the neck. The diagnosis of congenital rubella may be confused with other congenital or perinatal infections, such as syphilis, toxoplasmosis, herpes simplex, and cytomegalovirus (CMV). These congenital infections can all lead to intrauterine growth retardation, deafness, mental retardation, and thrombocytopenia.

TREATMENT AND THERAPY

Infants with congenital rubella must be viewed as having a continually involving disease, since there is no present method to stop or decrease the replication of the rubella virus in the infected newborn. No antiviral medications or antibody preparations have been found to be of therapeutic benefit in children with congenital rubella. Thus, therapy is supportive and requires a multidisciplinary approach. Hearing disabilities require testing, which involves special equipment for infants. If hearing loss is found, support for the child's language and communication development must take place; specially designed educational programs are available. A full eye examination should be performed by an ophthalmologist.

Acquired rubella infection is fairly benign, and its management usually involves allowing the virus to run its course. Since the greatest damage done by rubella virus is to a developing fetus, the management of rubella should focus on prevention of infection in women of childbearing age. Because acquired rubella infection is commonly asymptomatic or subclinical, the only adequate way to prevent this disease and its effects on the fetus is immunization.

A vaccine is available and has been shown to produce an excellent immune response in its presently used form. Two doses of rubella vaccine are recommended, given as the combined vaccine known as measles, mumps, rubella (MMR). The first dose is given to a child at twelve to fifteen months of age. The second dose should be given prior to the child's entry into school. The vaccine should also be given to adult women who have not received the vaccine previously.

Although it is not recommended that the vaccine be given to pregnant women because of the theoretical risk of inducing congenital rubella, no infants whose mothers were vaccinated during pregnancy have shown congenital defects. Rubella vaccine should not be given after the administration of antibody preparations. The vaccine also should not be given in immunosuppressed patients unless recommended by a doctor. The side effects of the vaccine, occurring in about 10 percent of children, include fever, a rash, and lymph node enlargement. Adult women are prone to developing arthralgia after receiving the rubella vaccine. Other, very rare complications of the vaccine have also occurred.

PERSPECTIVE AND PROSPECTS

Since the introduction of the rubella vaccine in the United States in 1969, the rates of rubella disease and the associated congenital rubella syndrome have decreased dramatically. Before mass vaccination was practiced in the United States, rubella was typically a childhood disease among children aged five to fourteen. The occasional outbreaks of rubella that occur today are found in groups of the population that do not receive vaccines, such as certain religious communities and poor, typically urban African American or Latino communities. Rubella continues to be a health problem in developing countries around the world.

—*Peter D. Reuman, M.D., M.P.H.*

See also Birth defects; Cataracts; Childhood infectious diseases; Eyes; Fever; Hearing loss; Immunization and vaccination; Measles; Mental retardation; Mumps; Rashes; Viral infections; Visual disorders.

FOR FURTHER INFORMATION:

Bellenir, Karen, and Peter D. Dresser, eds. *Health Reference Series: Contagious and Noncontagious Infectious Diseases Sourcebook*. Detroit: Omnigraphics, 1997. A handy reference source on infectious diseases. Includes bibliographical references and an index.

Berkow, Robert, and Andrew J. Fletcher, eds. *The Merck Manual of Diagnosis and Therapy*. 17th ed. Rahway, N.J.: Merck, Sharpe & Dohme Research Laboratories, 1999. Describes many diseases treated by proctologists, including their characteristics, etiology, diagnosis, and treatment. Designed for physicians, the material is also useful to less specialized readers.

Clayman, Charles B., ed. *The American Medical Association Family Medical Guide*. New York: Random House, 1994. An excellent reference for the beginner. The scientific accuracy of the text is not compromised by its accessibility.

Rakel, Robert E., ed. *Conn's Current Therapy 2000: Latest Approved Methods of Treatment for the Practicing Physician*. Philadelphia: W. B. Saunders, 2000. Concise reference for recent advances in therapy. Includes information on treatment of conditions frequently encountered in practice. Presented by international authorities, with new section on travel medicine.

Shaw, Michael, ed. *Everything You Need to Know About Diseases*. Springhouse, Pa.: Springhouse, 1996. This well-illustrated consumer reference, compiled by more than one hundred doctors and medical experts, describes five hundred illnesses and conditions, their causes, symptoms, diagnosis, treatment, and prevention.

Safety issues for children

Procedures

Anatomy or system affected: All

Specialties and related fields: Critical care, emergency medicine, family practice, pediatrics, sports medicine

Definition: Measures taken to prevent accidents among children.

The Importance of Safety Measures

Each year in the United States, approximately 1 million children receive medical care as a result of unintentional injury. Of these, forty thousand to fifty thousand suffer permanent damage and four thousand die. The first years of a child's life are the most dangerous: Unintentional injuries are the primary cause of death in children up to the age of five.

Foresight, common sense, and vigilance are required to prevent injuries to children, particularly those under the age of two, who do not communicate verbally. Between the ages of two and four, although a child has a sense of cause and effect (a boy who kicks a ball knows that it may roll into the street), the child is unable to consider outside effects (a car could hit him if he runs into the street after the ball).

Basic information in case an emergency occurs should be accessible in all homes with children. The phone number of the family physician, the nearest hospital and emergency service, and the local poison control center should be posted adjacent to the phone. When caregivers are employed, they should be given transportation fare, copies of children's medical cards, the doctor's phone number, and the phone number where the parents can be reached. For optimum communication, parents should travel with a cellular phone. The number of a relative to contact in the event of an emergency occurring to the parents should be included as well.

Safety in the Home

All parents should develop a childproofing plan before a newborn arrives and modify it when the baby begins to crawl and walk. Hazards change with age. The Consumer Product Safety Commission urges families to do a room-by-room check of their house. The best way to do this is to put oneself in the place of the child, getting down on one's hands and knees and imagining what would be interesting or constitute an obstacle.

Equipment. Surprisingly, almost as many children are injured or die from using objects designed for their use as from automobile accidents. In the United States, accidents related to playing with toys send 120,000 children to the emergency room annually. Most standards for baby equipment went into effect in the early 1970's, so extra caution must be exercised with equipment manufactured prior to that date.

Baby walkers, which are involved in more than twenty-eight thousand injuries annually, are not approved by the American Academy of Pediatrics. Tipping is the most common cause of injury; it can be prevented by using a walker with at least six wheels and a base wider than the seat height. Walkers can also fall down stairs.

Falls from high chairs sent another seven thousand infants to the hospital. High chairs should have a safety strap and a wide base to prevent tipping. Cantilevered high chairs that hook to a table are more unstable. They should lock to the table and be attached only if the table is strong enough to support them.

Despite standards to ensure safe cribs, up to 30 million potentially dangerous cribs are in use in the United States, and approximately fifty babies suffocate or strangle in cribs annually. Cribs more than twenty-five years old are the most hazardous because the slats are too wide. Moreover, they may have lead-based paint. Even newer cribs with decorative cutouts can trap a baby's head. In addition, corner posts can catch clothing, resulting in strangulation.

The first safety measure is to ensure that crib slats are spaced no more than $2\frac{3}{8}$ inches apart and that corner posts extend no more than $\frac{1}{16}$ of an inch above the railing. Cribs should never be placed next to a wall lamp, electrical outlet, window, radiator, or vent. To prevent the possibility of suffocation, puffy gear such as large stuffed animals, adult pillows, or comforters should not be used in cribs until a child reaches one year of age. Securely fastened bumpers, however, may be used until the baby is able to stand (and thus able to climb on them to exit the crib).

Bunk beds pose a similar threat as cribs. To safeguard these beds, wooden bars should be added to ensure that any spaces, such as those between the guardrail and the bed frame or cutouts in the headboard and footboard, do not exceed 3 inches.

Portable playpens may have faulty latches that can cause the enclosure to collapse, trapping a child's head in the top rails. Latches on a playpen should click audibly, signifying that they are securely locked. Also, the side of a mesh playpen should never be left lowered, as an infant can be trapped in the slack mesh.

The Consumer Product Safety Commission's hot line, (800) 638-2772, provides information about specific models of child's equipment that are hazardous and repair information from manufacturers.

Windows. Children aged five and younger are most likely to fall from windows because they are mobile but do not comprehend the danger of an open window. In the United States, about fifteen thousand children aged ten and younger are injured annually from window falls, with three-quarters of the accidents happening in the spring and summer. Surprisingly, the majority of falls occur when children play on furniture adjacent to an open window and topple out as a result of losing their balance, rather than because they leaned against the window.

The following safeguard measures are recommended, and in some U.S. cities required, for any household with young children. All windows from the second floor up must have window guards. Each guard should have a quick-release mechanism for swift exit in case of a fire. Screens do not support a child's weight, so windows should be opened at the top rather than the bottom; if they are opened on the bottom, they should not be wide enough to allow a child to fit through them. Above all, furniture should not be placed under a window. Drapery and blind cords should be secured so that a child is unable to play with them.

Electrical outlets. The most important safety procedure is to cover unused electrical outlets with a safety plug. In wet areas, such as the kitchen or the bathroom, a ground-fault circuit interrupter can be installed in outlets to prevent electrocution if an appliance comes in contact with the water. Tempting electrical appliances such as hair dryers should be unplugged and stored out of reach of a child when not in use.

Household furniture. If toddlers are in the house, any standing object such as bookcases, dressers, desks, or a television stand may tip onto a child, who may be tempted to climb on it or any open drawers. To diminish the hazard of household furniture, angle braces

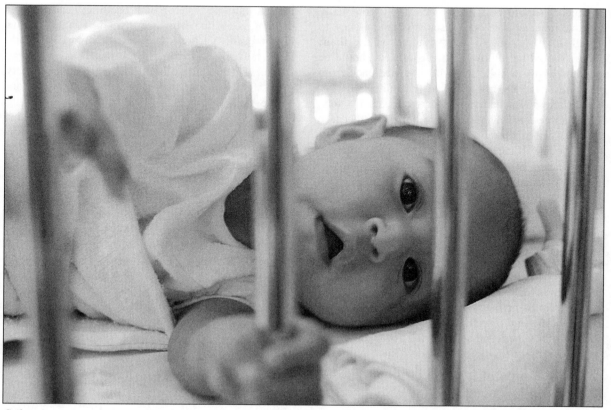

Cribs can pose serious health threats to babies; the government issues guidelines regarding dimensions and spacing between slats. (PhotoDisc)

Number of Injuries Among U.S. Children and Teenagers in 1993

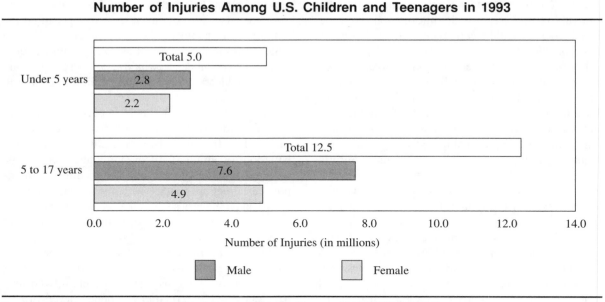

Source: Statistical Abstract of the United States 1997. Washington, D.C.: GPO, 1997.

or anchors should be used to secure any potentially unstable item, such as bookcases or china hutches, to a wall. Heavy furniture must rest flat on the floor; gliders should be removed. Television sets should be mounted above a child's reach or set far back from the edge on a very low piece of furniture.

Furniture poses many unsuspected threats to safety. For example, bean bag chairs are hazardous because a toddler can unzip the chair, inhale the foam pellets, and suffocate. If such a chair must be in the house, it should have a permanent seam or sealed zipper. Automatic locks on furniture that is big enough to climb into, such as certain types of chests, should be replaced with safety locks.

A recliner is another unsuspected hazard, as openings of 5 inches or more between the footrest and the seat can trap a child's head. Hammocks are dangerous as well if they do not have spreader bars at each end to hold the netting apart to prevent entrapment of a child's limbs or head.

Tablecloths and place mats should not be used, as a child can grab them and spill hot food or heavy items. Drawers within a child's grasp should have automatic safety latches to prevent spilling sharp items such as knives.

Rugs on slippery areas, such as linoleum tile or the bathroom floor, should be stabilized with nonskid backing. Any edge that could cut a child, such as on a table, should be covered with padding; heat-resistant padding is available for hearths. Glass tables should not be used. All breakable items should be kept on high shelves.

Stairs. If young children are in the home, safety gates should be installed at both the top and bottom of the stairs. Stair gates should have a straight top edge and be filled with a rigid mesh screen containing slats less than 4.25 inches apart. According to the Consumer Product Safety Commission, accordion gates made before February, 1985, are unacceptable, as the openings are wide enough to trap a child's head. The V-shaped openings at the gate's top edge should be no more than 1.5 inches wide. All gates should be at least 32 inches high.

Hardware-mounted gates securely attached to a solid structure, such as a stair post or wall, should be used at the top of the stairs rather than an expanding-pressure gate, which can be dislodged by the weight of a toddler. Gates should be removed as soon as a child attempts to climb over them.

OUTDOOR SAFETY MEASURES

Summer is a magic time for many children, but most parents are unaware that hospital emergency room staffs call May through August "the trauma season." Long daylight hours, no school, and more outdoor activities add up to increased opportunity for accidents.

Prevention consists of three facets: supervision, education (of both parent and child), and safeguarding.

Playgrounds. Shockingly, more than 200,000 injuries occur annually on playgrounds to children fourteen years old or younger in the United States. While most parents assume that a playground is safe simply because it is designed for children, in truth, there are no mandatory safety standards for this equipment. More than half of playground injuries result from a fall onto a hard surface, including asphalt, concrete, and even grass and dirt. A significantly higher risk for serious injury is associated with a fall of more than 4 feet for preschoolers or more than 8 feet for school-age children. One problem is that most parents are unaware that playground equipment is specifically designed for one of two age groups: two to five years old or five to twelve years old. To address this issue, equipment made after 1994 is supposed to be marked with a sign indicating its intended age group.

To optimize safety on playgrounds, children should use a playground covered with pea gravel, sand, chips, rubber, or a soft synthetic surface. This protective surface should extend at least 6 feet around slides and twice the height of the swings in front and back to create a safety fall zone. Playgrounds should be checked for sharp edges, loose joints, and protruding hardware, such as unclosed "S" hooks. Swings that are not at least 2 feet apart and 2.5 feet lower than the swing support should be avoided. Platforms and ramps are usable only if they have guardrails. Above all, a toddler should play on equipment lower than 4 feet high, while a school-age child should be restricted to structures 8 feet high or lower.

Drowning. Drowning is known as the "silent death" since young children do not scream or splash while drowning. Each year in the United States, one thousand children aged fourteen and younger drown, while four thousand more are treated for near-drowning injuries. Of these, 20 percent end up with permanent neurological damage. More than three hundred children aged four and under drown in residential pools annually. Accidents in children five and older tend to occur in lakes or the ocean as well as in pools and to occur as a result of "horsing around."

The American Red Cross and the National Safe Kids Campaign issued guidelines to optimize safety near water. The most important rule is that a pool should be enclosed with a four-sided fence at least 5 feet high that is filled with vertical bars 3.5 inches apart or less. The gate should be self-locking and self-closing, with the latch out of reach of children.

Parents and caregivers should know cardiopulmonary resuscitation (CPR), and the CPR instructions should be posted near the pool. Basic life-saving equipment, including a pole, rope, and flotation device, should be next to the pool. Many parents also keep a phone near the pool. In addition, children who cannot swim should wear an approved flotation device that has a collar to keep the head upright and the face out of the water.

Children should never have access to the pool while unsupervised, which includes exiting the back door while a parent is on the phone. Once discovered, the pool is a fascinating place. Caregivers should be mindful of this, as drowning happens in a matter of minutes. Toys and floats that attract young children should be kept away from the pool when not in use, and furniture that enables climbing over a pool fence should be moved to a different location. A toddler should be taught repeatedly not to go near the pool without a parent. Many parents install a motion-sensing device that sounds an alarm if something has fallen into the water.

Hot tubs are dangerous for young children; children under the age of four years should not be allowed in them. Most parents are unaware that hot tubs and spas manufactured prior to 1987 have strong suction that could injure a child; children should be cautioned to keep their head above water and their hair tied up and to sit away from a drain. The water temperature should not exceed 104 degrees Fahrenheit.

Animals and insects. Children, especially babies, are more likely to be bitten by pets than are adults. Animals should never be left alone with infants. Any animal bite that breaks the skin, no matter how minor, necessitates a visit to the pediatrician.

Shrubbery should be trimmed, since it is a breeding ground for disease-carrying rodents and ticks. In areas with a high frequency of Lyme disease, such as New Jersey and Connecticut, children should be checked and bathed daily, especially if they have been outdoors or around animals. The health department and certain medical centers test ticks for Lyme disease. The tick must be alive and in a plastic container. Ticks removed within twenty-four hours usually do not transmit disease. To prevent infection, the tick should be removed gently with tweezers. The area around the bite should be squeezed, so that pus is pushed outward, and then sterilized.

MEDICAL EMERGENCIES

Burns. The kitchen is considered the most dangerous room in the home for children by experts. A burn may occur when a hot pan or liquid falls on a child or when a child presses hands against an oven door or pulls a pan off the stove. The insulation on oven doors may wear out and cause second-degree and third-degree burns, even when the oven is at a relatively low temperature.

To prevent such injuries, the following precautions should be instituted. Above all, the child should be placed at a safe remove from the potential source of burns. Counter space should be well-organized and spacious, so that a hot pan placed there is far enough from the edge to prevent it from falling off. Pots should be placed on the back burners, with their handles turned toward the rear, so a child cannot reach them. In addition, stove knobs may be removed or covered when the stove is not in use if they are especially accessible or tempting to a child.

The oven door, and the window in particular, should be checked to ensure that it is not hot enough to cause even a slight burn. The manufacturer or a repair company should be called immediately if it is too hot. Several working fire extinguishers should be readily available, and smoke detectors should be installed outside sleeping areas and tested regularly.

To prevent scald burns from hot water, the temperature on hot water heaters should be set to a maximum of 120 degrees Fahrenheit. In addition, a parent should always test the water before putting a child in the bathtub.

If a child is burned, the immediate goal is to prevent heat from penetrating deeper into the skin. Clothing, which retains heat, must be removed from the burned area immediately. If fabric is stuck to the skin, it should not be pulled away, as this can tear the skin, but cut away as best as possible. A physician should remove the remainder.

Cold water should be applied to the burn at once until the pain subsides and the skin is no longer hot to the touch, usually at least five minutes. Nothing else should be applied to the area, including ice cubes, which may cause frostbite, and butter, grease, or ointment, which may impel the heat deeper into the skin.

If the burn is not oozing, a sterile gauze dressing should be applied, taking care not to break blisters or remove any skin. Medical attention should be sought immediately if the burn is on a child six months or younger or if the burn affects a child's eyes, face, mouth, hands, feet, or genitals. In addition, blisters, oozing, severe pain, dizziness, breathing problems are all reasons to seek medical attention.

Choking. Choking is the most common cause of accidental death in children under age one. Choking is life-threatening if a child swallows an object that blocks the flow of air to the lungs. The child will be unable to talk, and his or her face will turn blue. A child who is coughing should not be interrupted, as this strong natural reflex may dislodge the object.

Parents must be familiar with the emergency medical procedures for choking; approved first-aid courses are sponsored by the American Heart Association and the American Red Cross. The Heimlich maneuver is not recommended for infants; rather, they are to be turned face down on the forearm or lap and administered rapid blows between the shoulder blades. If this fails, the infant is turned on the back and four rapid chest thrusts over the breastbone are given with only two fingers. If all else fails, mouth-to-mouth or mouth-to-nose respiration should be performed.

Items that can be swallowed should be kept away from babies, including marbles, coins, safety pins, and small refrigerator magnets. Particular caution must be exercised with toys. Hazards include rattles less than 1⅝ inches across, eyes or ribbons that come off stuffed animals, balloons, and small parts of toys that break off. Toys labeled for ages three and under must meet federal guidelines requiring they have no small parts. Young children can choke on certain foods. Those foods to be avoided include peanuts, candy, whole grapes, or any hard, smooth food that must be chewed with a grinding motion.

Drawstrings in clothing pose a hazard, as they can strangle a child if the drawstring is caught on a slide, school bus door, or handrail. Drawstrings should not be worn at the neck. If they are at the waist of a garment, then knots should be untied, as they may catch on objects. A child should not use playgrounds while wearing clothing with drawstrings. In 1994, the Consumer Product Safety Commission asked clothing manufacturers to remove drawstrings from the hoods of children's garments; hand-knit or second-hand clothing still poses a risk.

Poisoning. Ironically, although most parents are aware of the poisonous hazard posed by cleaning products, they do not consider the toxicity of household plants. For example, ivy, geraniums, and philodendrons are poisonous if ingested. In addition, many plants in the yard are toxic. A poison control center can provide names of hazardous plants in a particular region.

A poison control center should be called immediately if a child ingests a toxic substance. The number of the regional center is listed on the inside cover of the telephone book and should be posted next to the phone. The parent should report what was ingested, how much, and, if it is a plant, the common and botanical name. Syrup of ipecac to induce vomiting should be readily available, but it should not be administered until instructions are received from the poison control center, since in some cases vomiting causes more harm. If a child gets poison in the eyes or on the skin, the area should be flushed immediately with lukewarm water for a period of fifteen minutes as the poison control center is being called.

To prevent the ingestion of poisons, safety locks should be installed on low-level cabinets containing cleaning products and on the medicine chest. Over-the-counter and prescription medicines, soaps, cosmetics, and shampoos are all potentially toxic if ingested by a child. Many people are unaware that vitamins consumed in a sufficient quantity can cause an overdose reaction. Shampoo and soap in the tub should be kept out of a child's reach. Many parents opt to keep medicines and vitamins, as well as sharp items such as razors, in a separate, high, and locked place.

Many automobile and building products are poisonous as well as flammable; they should be kept in locked metal cabinets away from children. In addition, lawn products, such as fertilizer and weed killer, should be kept in a locked area away from toddlers.

Lead poisoning. Lead poisoning constituted one of the most underrated afflictions of children until education efforts raised awareness. In the late 1990's, about 1 million children in the United States had elevated blood lead levels. Any building constructed before 1978, the year that lead paint was banned, probably has lead in the paint. This puts a child at risk, especially if the paint is chipped or sanded or renovations are being done. Lead is also found in pipes, which were made entirely of lead in the United States until the 1950's; lead was used to fuse copper pipes until 1986.

Safety measures include determining if lead paint exists in the home or soil. The local department of health may be contacted for further information. Repainting a home built prior to 1977 is recommended. Even if an area has been covered with nonleaded paint, precautions should be taken when children are not in the house. Chipped and peeling paint should be removed with a wet cloth. If extensive peeling has occurred, the area should be sanded and painted over. Guidelines for the removal of lead paint are available from the National Association of Homebuilders.

Tap water should be run for ninety seconds before using it, as water that as been standing in the pipes has a higher concentration of lead. Cold water should be used for drinking and cooking, as it is less likely to leach lead. High-phosphate detergents are recommended for cleaning.

All infants should be tested for lead, no matter how safe the home is. The Centers for Disease Control and Prevention (CDC) and the American Academy of Pediatrics (AAP) recommend that babies be tested at ages one and two, the ages when they are most likely to put objects that may be covered with lead dust into their mouths. Risk factors for lead exposure in children include living in cities; being poor, African American, or Hispanic; or living in areas where houses were built prior to 1950. Parents should remain alert to any possible exposure, if even their children are not considered at risk.

—Lee Williams

See also Accidents; Allergies; Bites and stings; Bleeding; Burns and scalds; Choking; Concussion; Critical care; Critical care, pediatric; Electrical shock; Emergency medicine; Emergency medicine, pediatric; Food poisoning; Fracture and dislocation; Frostbite; Hives; Lead poisoning; Lice, mites, and ticks; Poisoning; Poisonous plants; Snakebites; Sunburn; Zoonoses.

FOR FURTHER INFORMATION:

American Academy of Pediatrics. *Baby Alive*. Elk Grove Village, Ill.: Author, 1994. Describes procedures for dealing with a medical emergency.

_____. *Choking Prevention and First Aid for Infants and Children*. Elk Grove Village, Ill.: Author, 1994. Describes procedures for dealing with choking and other first aid issues.

_____. *Playground Safety*. Elk Grove Village, Ill.: Author, 1994. This brochure reviews the safety hazards of playgrounds and offers prevention measures.

Bentz, Ric, and Christine Allison. *Street Smarts for Kids: What Parents Must Know to Keep Their Children Safe*. New York: Fawcett Books, 1999. Detective Bentz of the Kenosha, Wisconsin, Police Department and Allison, a children's writer, have compiled an outstanding tool for parents and care-takers concerning child safety. They cover topics such as pedophiles, child abductors, and cyberspace safety threats and identify certain characteristics in children that might make them vulnerable to strangers.

Shelov, Steven P., et al., eds. *Caring for Your Baby and Young Child: Birth to Age Five.* Rev. ed. New York: Bantam Books, 1998. Offers a comprehensive discussion of the accidents that commonly occur with young children, accident-prevention techniques for the home and outdoors, and emergency measures to enact if an accident does take place.

SAFETY ISSUES FOR THE ELDERLY
PROCEDURES

ANATOMY OR SYSTEM AFFECTED: All

SPECIALTIES AND RELATED FIELDS: Critical care, emergency medicine, family practice, geriatrics and gerontology

DEFINITION: Measures taken to prevent accidents among the elderly.

THE IMPORTANCE OF SAFETY MEASURES

The age-related changes that elderly people experience often alter what constitutes a risk to their safety. The family home environment can be dangerous for an elderly person, not because the aspects of the house have changed, but because of the change in the physical abilities of the elderly person. Elderly people with intact cognitive abilities may choose to take the risk of staying in their familiar home environments with full knowledge of the increased risk. The dilemma for others, especially health providers, is defining what constitutes an acceptable level of risk for the elderly.

Unintentional injuries (accidents) are the sixth leading cause of death in people over sixty-five years of age. The death rate is 51 per 100,000 people for those sixty-five to seventy-four years of age, rises to 104 per 100,000 for those aged seventy-five to eighty-four, and reaches a high of 256 per 100,000 for those who are eighty-five years of age or older. In the over-eighty-five age group, accidental injury is the fifth leading cause of death. Injuries cost the United States between 75 billion and 100 billion dollars each year. Accidents are usually viewed as random events over which individuals have little or no control. Many other types of injuries are preventable, and safety enhancement may decrease the number of serious outcomes.

FALLS

Falls account for a considerable number of deaths and injuries among elderly people. They are the second leading cause of death related to unintentional injury, after motor vehicle deaths. Falls are not an uncommon event for elderly people; approximately 30 percent of noninstitutionalized elders report a fall each year. One-half of the people who report falls experience multiple falls. Although falls are a common occurrence, they are not always dangerous: Only 11 percent result in a serious injury, and an estimated 1 percent result in hip fractures. The number of hip fractures yearly in the United States (200,000) is substantial and serious. They lead to death in 12 percent to 20 percent of cases and account for 2 percent of the mortality rate in the United States. More than 40 percent of deaths from falls occur in the home. Stairs account for a large proportion of falls, many occurring because the elderly individual misses the last step. Falling injuries account for 40 percent of nursing home admissions; however, more than 20 percent of all fatal falls occur in the nursing home setting.

Falls among the elderly may be caused by a variety of factors: physical frailty, pathological states, psychological stress, drug interactions, and multiple environmental hazards. The risks of falling increase with increasing age, the number of chronic diseases present, the number and type of medications being taken, cognitive impairment, and physical disability. The risk of falling is often associated more with the intake of some types of drugs (antidepressants, sedatives, or vasodilators) than with medical conditions. Most doctors provide elderly patients with information concerning the effects of drugs that they may be taking, including the risk of a drop in blood pressure related to these medications. Instruction concerning how to decrease the effects of orthostatic hypotension, such as dangling feet before getting out of bed and rising slowly from a sitting or reclining position, is important in the prevention of falls.

Falls may cause bruises, abrasions, pain, swelling, or fractures. Changes in cognitive function related to pressure from edema or blood clots within the brain may also be evidenced. Psychological damage resulting from falls is more subtle. An older person who sustains little or no injury in a fall may delay or avoid discussing it in order to avoid embarrassment or risk of being viewed as less competent. Falls may also prompt changes in behavior, such as decreased thoroughness in housekeeping tasks or discussion of fears of living alone. Changes in grooming, dress, and personal appearance may also be observed. Increased fear of venturing out into the neighborhood may lead to a decreased ability to meet the daily requirements of shopping and food preparation.

Falls are better prevented than treated. Because quality of life is as important as length of life, limiting activity in the hope that falls will not occur is the least acceptable method of prevention. A more realistic approach is to modify the environment. Although cost may be a limiting factor, many alterations can be implemented that are both acceptable to the older person and minimal in expense. Many environmental modifications are relatively easy to perform.

Many falls occur in the bathroom. Non-slip bath mats and adhesive-backed, non-skid strips in the bathtub or shower are important safety measures. Grab bars may be placed at critical locations near the bathtub and toilet to lend support. Railings may be installed on stairways for support. A piece of fabric, a knob, or some other marker can be attached to the rail to indicate the level of the top and bottom steps.

The need for light increases with age. The environment can be lighted at a safe level by increasing either the number of lights or the intensity of the light bulbs. Adequate illumination that does not cause shadows, which may cause problems with perception, is extremely important in high-hazard areas, such as stairways and stair landings. Night lights or lighted switches enable those who get up at night to orient themselves more easily within the environment and minimize the risk for falling. The removal of obstructions and obstacles can also help increase the safety of the home. Among the objects that may cause elderly people to trip are extension cords and long phone cords, low furniture, carpet edges, and throw rugs. These can easily be removed from high-traffic areas or taped down to minimize the risk of causing injury.

TRAFFIC INJURIES

In modern societies, an important rite of passage for adolescents is to receive a driver's license. Driving an automobile is viewed as the first step toward adult life because it

fosters independence. On the other hand, driving a car also calls for a sense of responsibility to others who share the roads. Many roads are crowded, and traffic moves at a rapid and sometimes confusing rate. Drivers must be physically and mentally alert to handle the hazards of the roads. Elderly people with impaired physical capabilities must make a choice between continuing to drive, and therefore maintaining their independence, or taking measures to increase safety for themselves and others on the road.

Traffic injuries in the elderly population are divided into two categories: pedestrian injuries and vehicle-related injuries. Elderly people are more at

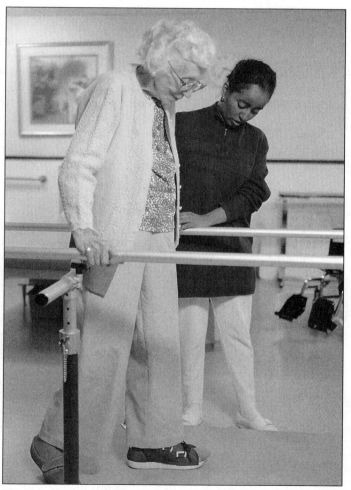

The elderly may experience problems with mobility that can pose a threat to safety. Falls are much more serious with advanced age because bones and tissues do not heal as quickly or completely as in youth. (PhotoDisc)

risk for injury at street intersections than anywhere else, both as pedestrians and as drivers or passengers in an automobile. As pedestrians, many elderly people are at risk because of an inability to cross the street in the time allotted between changes in the traffic lights. Factors that may influence pedestrian injuries are curb height, driver error, and physical and cognitive impairment of the elderly pedestrian.

A major problem for older drivers is the multivehicle accident, and the risk for injury in these crashes increases dramatically with age. The majority of such accidents take place in daylight, on good roads, and with no alcohol involvement. Elderly people experience a higher mortality rate with less severe injuries in vehicle crashes; the risk of death is three times greater for a seventy-year-old person than for a twenty-year-old person. The major factor that influences the high susceptibility of involvement in traffic injuries may be the decreased skill of the elderly person in operating an automobile. This change in skill level may be caused by age-related changes, such as decreased visual acuity or a slower neurological response time.

Citations for traffic violations, such as failure to yield right-of-way and failure to obey traffic signs, increase after the age of sixty. Although older adults have lower accident rates and fewer traffic violation citations than those under twenty-five years of age, elderly people have an increased risk of fatality in traffic accidents. One group of elders at increased risk for vehicle-related injury are those who are experiencing the early signs and symptoms of dementia. The American Association for Retired Persons (AARP) operates special classes in driver education to help older adults cope with age-related changes that affect their driving abilities.

SAFETY CONSIDERATIONS

Safety is a major concern when assessing living conditions. Many older adults live in unsafe housing. Relatively minor nuisances—such as excessive clutter, loose flooring or floor coverings, poor lighting, and unstable stairs—can pose safety risks for the older adult. Financial constraints may prompt older adults to settle for living in less desirable areas. Other safety concerns are related to the older adult's physical or mental functioning. People who have trouble walking or climbing stairs are prime examples of those at risk as the result of impaired physical functioning. People who are forgetful or who wander off and get lost pose a significant risk to themselves and others as the result of impaired mental function.

It may be necessary to observe the elderly actually moving about in their environment to locate any potential problems. If the elderly person uses an assistive device, such as a cane, walker, or wheelchair, the environment may require further modifications. Ramps may need to be installed, or living arrangements may need to be changed to accommodate these ramps.

Most elderly people prefer to stay in their own homes in familiar communities for as long as possible. As people get older, they often fear that they may have to leave home for health reasons. Such fears are realistic because acute and chronic health problems associated with aging often dictate at least temporary changes in environment, leading the elderly to reside in places they do not prefer. Their desire to stay at home challenges the health care system to study their special needs and devise solutions that will accommodate them in the most acceptable way.

Elderly individuals who live alone are well advised to learn how to summon emergency help and to make home adaptations to compensate for decreased mobility and dexterity. Cognitive impairments often present a more serious threat to safety than physical impairment. People who know they are having problems are likely to call for help and remain safely in the home until help arrives. However, individuals with impaired judgment may present a hazard to themselves, as well as to their neighbors, through such behavior as forgetting to turn off the stove. In isolated instances, a choice may be made to preserve such a person's autonomy at the risk of serious injury; however, few would agree that the impaired older person has a right to put others at risk of serious injury.

Medication usage is another important factor to consider when evaluating whether or not an older person can safely remain at home alone. Sometimes the deciding factor in whether a cognitively impaired individual can remain at home alone is the nature of the medication regimen. Some individuals must have regular medication to maintain health. There are various systems to help forgetful people take their medicines. Preparing and labeling medications for each day is one strategy for simplifying medication administration. Medication calendars, which show each type of pill with its time of administration and which have a space for marking when the pill is taken, are useful to individuals with early memory impairment. Functionally impaired individuals who want to stay at home but require assistance or supervision with activities of daily living are often helped by paraprofessional personnel.

—*Jane Cross Norman, Ph.D., R.N.*

See also Accidents; Aging; Aging: Extended care; Alzheimer's disease; Balance disorders; Critical care; Death and dying; Dementias; Emergency medicine; Fracture and dislocation; Geriatrics and gerontology; Hip fracture repair; Hip replacement; Hospice; Memory loss; Nursing; Osteoporosis; Psychiatry, geriatric.

For Further Information:

Gill, T. M., C. S. Williams, J. T. Robison, and M. E. Tinetti. "A Population-Based Study of Environmental Hazards in the Homes of Older Persons." *American Journal of Public Health* 89, no. 4 (1999): 553-556. An environmental assessment was completed in the homes of one thousand persons seventy-two years and older. Weighted prevalence rates were calculated for each of the potential hazards and subsequently compared among subgroups of participants.

Howland, J., et al. "Covariates of Fear of Falling and Associated Activity Curtailment." *Gerontologist* 38, no. 5 (1998): 549-555. With a sample survey of elderly adults residing in six housing developments in Massachusetts, the authors used logic regression to identify covariates of fear of falling among all subjects and identify covariates of activity curtailment among the subset of subjects who were afraid of falling.

Lachman, M. E., et al. "Fear of Falling and Activity Restriction: The Survey of Activities and Fear of Falling in the Elderly (SAFE)." *Journals of Gerontology Series B—Psychological Sciences and Social Sciences* 53B, no. 1 (1998): 43-50. A new instrument was developed to assess the role of fear of falling in activity restriction. The instrument assesses fear of falling during performance of eleven activities, and it gathers information about participation in these activities as well as the extent to which fear is a source of activity restriction.

Lachs, Mark S. "Caring for Mom and Dad: Can Your Parent Live Alone?" *Prevention* 50, no. 10 (October, 1998): 155-157. Information on how to develop a care plan for an aging parent who is having problems with activities of daily living is offered.

Lisak, Janet M., and Marlene Morgan. *The Safe Home Checkout: A Professional Guide to Safe Independent Living.* 2d ed. Chicago: Geriatric Environments for Living and Learning, 1997. Covers safety measures for older buildings, accident prevention, and self-help devices for the disabled. Includes bibliographical references.

Raiche, Michel, Rejean Hebert, Francois Prince, and Helene Corriveau. "Screening Older Adults at Risk of Falling with the Tinetti Balance Scale." *The Lancet* 356, no. 9234 (September 16, 2000): 1001. Although many balance characteristics are associated with an individual's risk of falling, a standardized and valid screening instrument to identify people at risk of falling is still unavailable.

SALMONELLA INFECTION
DISEASE/DISORDER

ANATOMY OR SYSTEM AFFECTED: Blood, gastrointestinal system

SPECIALTIES AND RELATED FIELDS: Bacteriology, family practice, gastroenterology, pediatrics, public health

DEFINITION: A broad spectrum of clinical diseases caused by many types of salmonella bacteria.

KEY TERMS:

asymptomatic: without symptoms

bacteremia: the presence of bacteria in the blood, which is usually associated with chills and fever

gastroenteritis: infection of the gastrointestinal tract, usually accompanied by nausea, vomiting, diarrhea, and abdominal pains

typhoid fever: a particular disease syndrome most often associated with infection by *Salmonella typhi* but occasionally caused by other types of salmonella bacteria

CAUSES AND SYMPTOMS

Salmonella are a group of bacteria that cause enteric or typhoid fever. All types can cause gastrointestinal infections, blood infections, and various local infections. All types of salmonella can be carried in the gastrointestinal tract without symptoms after recovery from infection.

The clinical disease caused by salmonella depends on the type of bacteria, the amount of organisms ingested, and the age and immune status of the person infected. Infection with salmonella can take place with the ingestion of one or 100 million organisms. Increasing in the dosage of bacteria decreases the incubation period and increases the severity of the resulting disease. After ingestion, the bacteria adhere to and invade the gastrointestinal tract. In the wall of the intestinal tract, salmonella survive and multiply in immune cells and then enter the bloodstream, where they proceed to any area of the body. Young infants and people with immune deficiencies and hemolytic anemia are at increased risk for severe and complicated infections.

Typhoid fever or enteric fever is very rare in the United States, causing less than five hundred cases per year; it is primarily seen in people coming from developing countries. Classically, this disease is caused by *Salmonella typhi* bacteria, but it can also be caused by other types of salmonella. Symptoms during the first week of illness include progressively increasing fever with associated headache, muscle aches, abdominal pains, and lethargy. In the second week, the heart rate decreases, the liver and spleen enlarge, small red bumps form on the trunk, and the patient enters into a stupor. During the third to fourth week, intestinal hemorrhage and perforation are common. The fever begins to remit in the fifth to sixth week of illness. Diarrhea usually starts in the first week and resolves within six weeks. Without treatment, death can occur from gastrointestinal hemorrhage and perforation. Infants tend to have much more severe disease than older children.

Salmonellosis caused by nontyphoid salmonella is more common in United States, causing about fifty thousand cases per year. The major reservoir of nontyphoid salmonella is the gastrointestinal tract of many animals, including mammals, reptiles, birds, and insects. Farm animals and pet reptiles commonly carry salmonella. Some antibiotic resistance is caused by the use of antibiotics in animal feeds. Salmonella can be isolated from 50 percent of chicken, 16 percent of pork, 5 percent of beef, and 40 percent of frozen eggs in retail stores. Contaminated eggs and milk

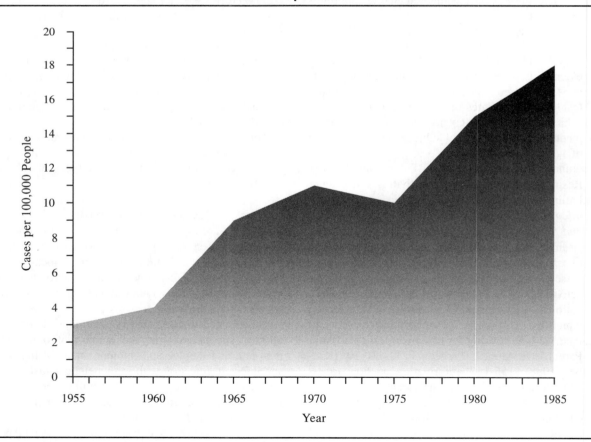

Cases of Salmonellosis Reported in the United States

Source: Professional Guide to Diseases, 4th ed., 1992.

products are common sources of human infection.

Gastroenteritis is the most common disease caused by nontyphoid salmonella. The incubation period for this disease is about one day, with a range from six hours to three days. Symptoms include nausea, vomiting, and abdominal pain. Diarrhea typically contains blood and white cells. Usually, symptoms disappear in less than a week in healthy children, but in young infants and in children with immune deficiencies, symptoms may persist for several weeks.

Bacteremia can occur in 1 to 5 percent of patients with salmonella gastroenteritis. Bacteremia is generally associated with fever, chills, and toxicity in the older child but may be asymptomatic in the infant. Children with an increased risk of bacteremia include those with acquired immunodeficiency syndrome (AIDS) or other immune deficiencies and hemolytic anemias such as sickle-cell anemia.

Bacteremia can lead to infection of almost any organ. Children with sickle-cell anemia are more prone to bone infections and meningitis. Salmonella may localize to areas of the body that have received trauma or that contain damaged tissue or a foreign body. Meningitis, inflammation of the covering of the spine and brain, is primarily seen as a complication of bacteremia in infants. Meningitis has a 50 percent death rate, and residual developmental and hearing defects are commonly found in survivors. Patients who have persistent bacteremia should be evaluated for heart infection.

The diagnosis of a salmonella infection is best made by culturing stool and blood samples. With enteric fever, it is important to culture multiple sites multiple times. Antibiotic susceptibility testing must be performed routinely to guide therapy. Other bacterial causes of gastroenteritis can be confused with salmonella infection.

TREATMENT AND THERAPY

Treatment for gastroenteritis usually does not require antibiotics. Antibiotics do not speed the resolution of disease but instead lead to prolonged excretion of salmonella. Therapy is primarily focused on the correction of fluid and salt abnormalities and on general supportive care. If the patient has indications of sepsis, shock, or chills, however, then antibiotics should be administered. Infants under three months of age and children with immune deficiencies should also be treated with antibiotics. Ampicillin is usually used as the initial treatment in uncomplicated cases, and

third-generation cephalosporin antibiotics are used in severe and complicated cases. About 20 percent of nontyphoid salmonella in the United States is resistant to ampicillin as well as to other antibiotics. Antibiotic treatment should last ten days to two weeks in children with bacteremia and four to six weeks in children with bone infection or meningitis. Local infections may require surgical drainage.

Typhoid fever is treated for a minimum of two weeks. It is important to perform susceptibility testing for the possibility of resistance so that proper antibiotic therapy can be chosen. Chronic carriers of *Salmonella typhi* should be treated with antibiotics. If eradication is unsuccessful, surgical assessment of the biliary tract should be sought.

Prevention of the spread of salmonella requires a number of public health procedures. Hand washing is critical to the prevention of transmission. Persons who are carriers of salmonella should be excluded from food preparation and from child care settings. Hospitalized infants and children should be isolated. Proper sewage disposal, water purification, and chlorination are essential public health measures. In developing countries, the promotion of prolonged breast-feeding also reduces the infection rate.

Several vaccines are available for the prevention of *Salmonella typhi* infection. The efficacy of each vaccine is similar and in the range of 50 to 75 percent over two to three years. Heat-phenol inactivated vaccine has the most side effects when compared with the live, oral vaccine and the capsular polysaccharide vaccine. The live, attenuated, oral vaccine should not be administered to immunocompromised persons. The use of typhoid vaccines in children is limited to those traveling to areas where the disease is endemic.

PERSPECTIVE AND PROSPECTS

Salmonella was identified as the cause of typhoid fever in 1880 and was first cultured in 1884. Since 1920, improvements in sanitation, water supplies, and sewage disposal have resulted in a marked decrease of typhoid fever in the United States. In 1920, 36,000 cases were reported; after 1965, the number of cases per year has rarely exceeded 500. Since then, the number of cases has remained fairly constant because of the importation of disease by tourists, immigrants, and migrant laborers. About 62 percent of *Salmonella typhi* infections are acquired through foreign travel. Direct person-to-person transmission is rare except in the homosexual population.

Recent research is focused on public health. Measures to decrease food contamination such as improved cleanliness, decreased use of antibiotics in animal feeds, and food irradiation are being evaluated and used to decrease transmission to humans. Research into alternate vaccines with fewer side effects and improved immune response is also being performed.

Nontyphoid salmonella causes 500,000 infections per year in the United States. One-third are in children less than five years of age, and 40 percent are in adults over thirty years of age.

—Peter D. Reuman, M.D., M.P.H.

See also Antibiotics; Bacterial infections; Diarrhea and dysentery; Food poisoning; Gastroenterology; Gastroenterology, pediatric; Gastrointestinal disorders; Gastrointestinal system; Immunization and vaccination; Meningitis; Poisoning; Zoonoses.

FOR FURTHER INFORMATION:

Bellenir, Karen, and Peter D. Dresser, eds. *Health Reference Series: Contagious and Noncontagious Infectious Diseases Sourcebook.* Detroit: Omnigraphics, 1997. A handy reference source on infectious diseases. Includes bibliographical references and an index.

Berkow, Robert, and Andrew J. Fletcher, eds. *The Merck Manual of Diagnosis and Therapy.* 17th ed. Rahway, N.J.: Merck, Sharpe & Dohme Research Laboratories, 1999. Describes many diseases treated by proctologists, including their characteristics, etiology, diagnosis, and treatment. Designed for physicians, the material is also useful to less specialized readers.

Clayman, Charles B., ed. *The American Medical Association Family Medical Guide.* New York: Random House, 1994. An excellent reference for the beginner. The scientific accuracy of the text is not compromised by its accessibility.

Rakel, Robert E., ed. *Conn's Current Therapy 2000: Latest Approved Methods of Treatment for the Practicing Physician.* Philadelphia: W. B. Saunders, 2000. Concise reference for recent advances in therapy. Includes information on treatment of conditions frequently encountered in practice.

Shaw, Michael, ed. *Everything You Need to Know About Diseases.* Springhouse, Pa.: Springhouse, 1996. This well-illustrated consumer reference, compiled by more than one hundred doctors and medical experts, describes five hundred illnesses

and conditions, their causes, symptoms, diagnosis, treatment, and prevention.

SARCOMA

DISEASE/DISORDER

ANATOMY OR SYSTEM AFFECTED: Bones, immune system, musculoskeletal system

SPECIALTIES AND RELATED FIELDS: Cytology, immunology, oncology, radiology

DEFINITION: Sarcomas are malignant tumors originating in the connective tissue, which includes bone and muscle. They are differentiated from carcinomas, malignant tumors that are composed mainly of cells similar to those of the skin and mucous membranes. Sarcomas are less common than carcinomas. Another form of sarcoma, called reticulum cell sarcoma, originates as a malignant tumor in the lymph glands. Sarcoma tumors are commonly treated with radiation therapy and anticancer drugs.

—Jason Georges and Tracy Irons-Georges

See also Bone cancer; Bone disorders; Bone grafting; Bones and the skeleton; Cancer; Chemotherapy; Kaposi's sarcoma; Muscle sprains, spasms, and disorders; Muscles; Oncology; Orthopedic surgery; Orthopedics; Orthopedics, pediatric; Radiation therapy.

FOR FURTHER INFORMATION:

Cady, Blake, ed. *Cancer Manual.* 7th ed. Boston: American Cancer Society, 1986.

Dollinger, Malin, Ernest H. Rosenbaum, and Greg Cable et al. *Everyone's Guide to Cancer Therapy.* 3d ed. Kansas City, Mo.: Andrews and McMeel, 1997.

Dorfman, Howard D., and Bogdan Czerniak. *Bone Tumors.* St. Louis: Mosby, 1998.

Editors of Time-Life Books. *Fighting Cancer.* Alexandria, Va.: Time-Life Books, 1981.

Murphy, G., L. Morris, and D. Lange. *Informed Decisions: The Complete Book of Cancer Diagnosis, Treatment, and Recovery.* New York: Viking Press, 1997.

SARCOPENIA

DISEASE/DISORDER

ANATOMY OR SYSTEM AFFECTED: Bones, immune system, musculoskeletal system

SPECIALTIES AND RELATED FIELDS: Cytology, immunology, oncology, radiology

DEFINITION: Reduction in muscle mass with aging, which is associated with weakness, decreased physiological functioning, and decreased physical activity; it can result in functional impairment, disability, loss of independence, and increased risk of fall-related fractures.

CAUSES AND SYMPTOMS

Sarcopenia, when translated from its Greek roots, means "flesh" (*sarx*) "loss" (*penia*). Thus, the syndrome for the loss of muscle mass (also known as lean body mass or fat-free mass) that often accompanies aging is called sarcopenia. This is differentiated from the general terms "wasting," which refers to the unintentional loss of weight attributable to a loss of both fat and muscle mass from insufficient caloric intake, and "cachexia," which refers to the loss of muscle mass without weight loss as a result of an overactive metabolism. Therefore, the term "sarcopenia" is often used to describe muscle wasting in old age.

Since skeletal muscle stores great quantities of protein for the body, tracking protein synthesis can verify subsequent muscle mass loss. A reduction in muscle mass occurs when muscle protein content is reduced. The protein content is determined by assessing the balance between protein synthesis and protein breakdown. With aging, protein synthesis slows, thereby resulting in decreased muscle synthesis. This can be aggravated by poor nutritional status, low caloric intake, and low protein intake.

The combination of inadequate dietary intake combined with decreased strength from declining muscle mass results in a progressive decline in physical activity and accelerates muscle atrophy, or shrinkage, as a result of disuse. This condition adversely affects functional mobility, as evidenced by slower walking speeds, shorter walking strides, and a decrease in the amount of work a muscle can tolerate.

Nutritional surveys have reported that individuals over age sixty-five consume an average of 1,400 Calories (kilocalories) a day, or less than 25 Calories per kilogram of body weight (1 kilogram = 2.2 pounds; 1 pound = 3,500 Calories). This average daily caloric intake of 1,400 Calories is approximately 500 Calories less than that which is recommended for optimal health for individuals over fifty years of age. Thus, based upon the average energy allowance recommendations, older adults should be consuming 5 Calories more for every kilogram of their body weight if they are to meet or exceed the current U.S. recommended daily allowances (RDAs) for caloric intake and optimal health. Lower caloric

intakes imply lower nutritional status: less fat, carbohydrate, and/or protein consumption, potentially leading to nutritional deficiencies in important vitamins and minerals.

The current nutritional guidelines also suggest that adults in the United States only need 0.8 gram of protein per kilogram of body weight daily; however, some researchers contend that this value is based primarily on the needs of young adults, not older adults. Based on data which showed that many adults over the age of sixty consume less than 0.8 gram per body weight daily, researchers from the Noll Research Laboratory at Pennsylvania State University suggested that older adults should consume between 1.0 and 1.25 grams of high-quality protein per kilogram of body weight daily. This would potentially help to prevent the compensatory loss in muscle mass resulting from long-term deficits in dietary protein intake.

The negative age-related changes in body composition are reflected in decreased muscle, bone density, and water content of the body, with a corresponding increase in body fat. Muscle tissue plays an important role in the regulation of metabolic rate (the burning of calories). It is generally agreed that muscle mass is maintained up to about age forty; however, the gender issue as to who loses muscle mass faster is not resolved. Some reports state that men begin to lose muscle mass between forty and sixty years of age, with women not experiencing similar declines until after age sixty; other reports declare the opposite or find no difference between the genders. Regardless of gender, however, by eighty years of age, the cumulative muscle mass loss is estimated to average 30 percent, with a corresponding decline in muscle strength. Ultrasound estimates of muscle mass loss suggest that older subjects lose between 0.5 and 0.7 percent of muscle annually. Muscle tissue is more metabolically active than fat tissue, meaning that muscle burns more calories than fat. Beginning in the third decade of life, metabolic rate, or the rate at which calories are burned by the body, decreases 2 to 3 percent per decade. Taken together, the loss in muscle tissue and the decrease in metabolic rate results in a gradual percent body fat increase from the second through the eighth decades of life, resulting in a net percent body fat gain of 20 percent for men and 10 percent for women. Hence, as muscle tissue atrophies, the unused "leftover" space is replaced by fat tissue, which is not used to perform muscular work.

Cross-sectional studies comparing athletes to sedentary controls, as well as studies with nonathletes, suggest that large muscle mass is predictive of higher bone mass. Thus, age-related sarcopenia and osteopenia (loss of bone) may be related. Research suggests that age-related changes in the dynamics of muscular contractions might contribute to bone remodeling imbalances, resulting in bone loss. The loss of motor units, activation, and synchronization of these units not only impairs bone integrity but also contributes to the loss of strength that accompanies muscle mass loss. Muscle strength is the ability to generate a maximal force by a muscle group. This strength is determined not only by total muscle mass but also by the individual muscle fibers. When muscle mass atrophies with aging, there is a decrease in fiber size, fiber number, and selective shrinking of type II, or fast-twitch, muscle fibers. Fast-twitch fibers are responsible for anaerobic, power-type strength activities. In addition, the loss of muscle mass may contribute to the reduction in aerobic capacity as the total amount of mitochondria, the powerhouses of cells, is reduced when muscle mass is lost.

TREATMENT AND THERAPY

Research is inconclusive as to whether age-related skeletal muscle wasting is preventable. It appears to be an inevitable part of aging. It may be, however, that the rate of skeletal muscle loss can be slowed down with progressive resistance (strength) training. This type of exercise has been shown to increase muscle size and strength even in the oldest of old. If strength training is to be used as a potential preventive measure, research suggests that high-intensity training (50 to 70 percent of one's maximal strength) with low repetitions should be implemented no later than fifty years of age; after age sixty, strength training is considered to be therapeutic, compensating for the age-related muscle mass wasting.

This is not to say, however, that after age sixty strength training should not be done. The situation is quite the contrary. While sarcopenia may not be preventable after age fifty, it has been proven that the frail elderly as well as community-dwelling healthy elderly can increase muscle mass by as much as 17 percent and maximal strength by as much as 110 percent with an aggressive strength training program. Contrary to the "moderate" exercise guidelines used for improving aerobic fitness, low-level resistance training only yields modest increases in strength and muscle mass. In addition to the use of exercise for

maintaining and improving muscle mass and strength, the judicious use of hormone replacement therapy (estrogen, testosterone, growth hormone) may also assist in maintaining muscle protein synthesis, thereby preventing and/or reducing muscle wasting.

PERSPECTIVE AND PROSPECTS

The extent of sarcopenia in the aged population suggests that less than 25 percent of persons under seventy years of age are afflicted with this syndrome, whereas more than 50 percent of those aged eighty or more are likely to be affected. Beginning in the seventh decade of life, approximately 25 percent of people report difficulty in walking and carrying heavy packages. Those older than seventy years of age report decreased ability to carry out common daily activities such as going down stairs or performing housework, and some even have difficulty using the toilet without assistance. These self-reported difficulties in functional ability occur regardless of gender, ethnicity, income, or other health behaviors.

—*Bonita L. Marks, Ph.D.*

See also Aging; Balance problems; Estrogen replacement therapy; Exercise physiology; Malnutrition; Nutrition; Weight loss and gain.

FOR FURTHER INFORMATION:

Dutta, Chhanda. "Significance of Sarcopenia in the Elderly." *Journal of Nutrition* 127, no. 5 supplement (May, 1997): 992S-993S. Sarcopenia in the elderly leads to gait and balance problems and increased risk for fall and can also lead to an increased risk for chronic diseases, such as diabetes and osteoporosis.

Evans, William J. "Reversing Sarcopenia: How Weight Training Can Build Strength and Vitality." *Geriatrics* 51, no. 5 (May, 1996): 46-47, 51-53. Sarcopenia, the loss of skeletal muscle mass with age, has consequences ranging from decreased bone density to poor glucose tolerance. Sarcopenia can be reversed and patient function can be improved with weight training.

_____. "What Is Sarcopenia?" *The Journals of Gerontology, Series A* 50A (November, 1995): 5-8. Sarcopenia is the age-related loss in skeletal muscle. The preservation of muscle mass and prevention of sarcopenia can help prevent the decrease in metabolic rate in the elderly.

Nair, K. Streekumaran. "Muscle Protein Turnover: Methodological Issues and the Effect of Aging."

The Journals of Gerontology, Series A 50A (November, 1995): 107-112. Theoretical and practical problems related to the methodologies used to measure protein turnover in humans are noted. Intervention studies such as exercise-training, nutritional supplements, and hormone replacement will make it possible to find out if changes in protein synthesis are reversible.

Roubenoff, Ronenn. "The Pathophysiology of Wasting in the Elderly." *Journal of Nutrition.* 129, 1S (January, 1999): 256S-259S. Aging is associated with changes in body composition, energy, and protein metabolism that are due both to the direct effects of aging and to the effects of age-related diseases. The authors differentiate these changes into three categories: wasting, cachexia, and sarcopenia.

_____. "Sarcopenia and Its Implications for the Elderly." *European Journal of Clinical Nutrition* 54 (June, 2000): S40-S47. Sarcopenia is the loss of muscle mass and strength with age. Sarcopenia is a part of normal aging and occurs even in master athletes, although it is clearly accelerated by physical inactivity.

Rowe, John W., and Robert L. Kahn. *Successful Aging.* New York: Pantheon Books, 1998. Based on a MacArthur Foundation study, this book explains how diet, exercise, pursuit of mental challenges, and social involvement positively or negatively affect aging.

Sexell, Jon. "Human Aging, Muscle Mass, and Fiber Type Composition." *The Journals of Gerontology, Series A* 50A (November, 1995): 11-16. Invasive and noninvasive techniques were used to estimate the muscle structure and fiber type composition to assess the age-related loss of muscle mass and to determine the mechanisms behind aging atrophy.

Shepard, Roy J. *Aging, Physical Activity, and Health.* Champaign, Ill.: Human Kinetics, 1997. Covers demographics and current theories of aging, physical activity, and health in older people.

Tseng, Brian S., Daniel R. Marsh, Marc T. Hamilton, and Frank W. Booth. "Strength and Aerobic Training Attenuate Muscle Wasting and Improve Resistance to the Development of Disability with Aging." *The Journals of Gerontology, Series A* 50A (November, 1995): 11-16. Aging-associated muscle wasting is defined as a progressive neuromuscular syndrome that will lower the quality of life in the elderly by decreasing the ability to lift loads and decreasing endurance.

SCABIES

DISEASE/DISORDER

ANATOMY OR SYSTEM AFFECTED: Skin

SPECIALTIES AND RELATED FIELDS: Dermatology, family practice

DEFINITION: Skin infestation by mites, causing a rash and severe itching.

CAUSES AND SYMPTOMS

The human scabies mite *Sarcoptes scabiei*, a small arachnid, approximately 0.4 millimeter long, produces intense pruritus (itching) and a red rash. Though scabies is most commonly noted on the fingers and hands, almost any skin surface can be affected. After fertilization, the female mite burrows into the upper layer of the host's skin and deposits several eggs. Upon hatching, the young migrate to the surface, where they mature; this life cycle lasts three to four weeks. In most cases, an affected human host will have an average of eleven adult females. The elderly and immuno-compromised patients are susceptible to a more severe, widespread variant called Norwegian scabies. In cases of Norwegian scabies, a human host may carry more than two million adult females.

A patient with scabies generally complains of severe itching, and the skin may be inflamed from scratching. Examination with a magnifying lens reveals characteristic burrows several millimeters in length, especially in the spaces between the fingers. A skin scraping aids in the diagnosis, producing a specimen for microscopic viewing which reveals the adult mite, eggs, or feces.

TREATMENT AND THERAPY

The treatment of scabies is straightforward. Clothing and bed linen should be washed in hot water. Shoes or other articles that cannot be washed may be sealed in a plastic bag for a week; this kills the mites, which need a human host to survive for more than a few days. Patients are treated with a 5 percent preparation of permethrin applied from head to foot (sparing the mouth and eyes) and left on overnight. An alternative treatment is lindane, which is less commonly used because of the risk of nerve toxicity in children. With either treatment, the medication is rinsed off in the morning shower. Rapid diagnosis and treatment decrease the chance of the mites spreading to other individuals.

—*Louis B. Jacques, M.D.*

See also Dermatology; Itching; Lice, mites, and ticks; Parasitic diseases; Rashes; Skin; Skin disorders.

FOR FURTHER INFORMATION:

Chosidow, Oliver. "Scabies and Pediculosis." *The Lancet* 355, no. 9206 (March 4, 2000): 819-826.

Gach, J. E., and A. Heagerty. "Crusted Scabies Looking Like Psoriasis." *The Lancet* 356, no. 9230 (August 19, 2000): 650.

Haag, M. L., S. J. Brozena, and N. A. Fenske. "Attack of the Scabies: What to Do When an Outbreak Occurs." *Geriatrics* 48 (October, 1993): 45-46, 51-53.

Levy, Sandra. "The Scourge of Scabies: Some Ways to Treat It." *Drug Topics* 144, no. 22 (November 20, 2000): 56.

Stewart, Kay B. "Combating Infection: Stopping the Itch of Scabies and Lice." *Nursing* 30, no. 7 (July, 2000): 30-31.

SCALDS. *See* BURNS AND SCALDS.

SCARLET FEVER
DISEASE/DISORDER

ANATOMY OR SYSTEM AFFECTED: Immune system, skin

SPECIALTIES AND RELATED FIELDS: Bacteriology, family practice, internal medicine, pediatrics

DEFINITION: An acute, contagious childhood disease caused by bacterial infection.

CAUSES AND SYMPTOMS

The bacteria *Streptococcus pyogenes* that cause scarlet fever (which is also known as scarlatina) produce erythrogenic toxins A, B, and C. Historically, scarlet fever has been associated with toxin A-producing streptococcal strains, but by the late twentieth century there was a prevalence of toxins B and C. Nevertheless, a resurgence of toxin A-producing streptococci has also been observed.

The bacteria are spread by inhalation of air that has been contaminated by the coughing or sneezing of an infected person. After exposure, the incubation period is between two and four days. The disease is characterized by a sore throat, fever, and rash; it may follow throat infections and, occasionally, wound infection and septicemia (blood poisoning). The face is flushed, resembling sunburn with goosebumps, with a pale area around the mouth. The mucous membranes of the mouth, throat, and tongue become strawberry red. The irritation usually appears first on the upper chest but quickly spreads to the neck, abdomen, legs, and arms.

TREATMENT AND THERAPY

Penicillin and erythromycin (given to people who are allergic to penicillin) have reduced the complications of scarlet fever to a minimum. In mild cases, recovery takes two to three days. To decrease its contagious effect, isolation for the patient for the first twenty-four hours is recommended. A few days after the body temperature returns to normal, peeling off of the skin takes place at the site of the rash, especially on the hands and feet. The rare complications that might arise include ear infections, rheumatic fever, and kidney inflammation (nephritis). A child with scarlet fever should rest and be given plenty of fluids and antipyretics (fever-reducing agents), such as acetaminophen, to reduce discomfort.

PERSPECTIVE AND PROSPECTS

Scarlet fever was first clearly distinguished from measles and other rash-producing diseases in 1860. Fifty years later, Russian scientists associated its cause to streptococcus, a hemolytic microorganism (one that destroys red blood cells). In 1924, George and Gladys Dick isolated the rash-causing substance in the medium used to grow hemolytic streptococci. They applied it to susceptible individuals in an attempt to establish immunity in them, but the technique was not successful. The loss of human life as a result of scarlet fever continued until the development of antibiotics in the 1940's. For an unknown reason, the incidence of the disease had declined drastically by the end of the twentieth century.

—*Soraya Ghayourmanesh, Ph.D.*

See also Antibiotics; Bacterial infections; Childhood infectious diseases; Fever; Pediatrics; Rashes; Septicemia; Streptococcal infections.

FOR FURTHER INFORMATION:

Clayman, Charles B., ed. *The American Medical Association Encyclopedia of Medicine*. New York: Random House, 1994. A concise presentation of numerous medical terms and illnesses. A good general reference.

McGraw-Hill Encyclopedia of Science and Technology. 7th ed. Vol. 16. New York: McGraw-Hill, 1994. This complete reference for the nonspecialist offers thousands of articles written by world-renowned scientists and engineers. It includes many new and revised articles and extensive cross-references and bibliographies and is fully illustrated.

Professional Guide to Diseases. 7th ed. Springhouse,

Pa.: Springhouse, 2001. This book covers more than six hundred disorders, organized by body system. Each disease entry is complete in itself, defining the disease and describing signs and symptoms, causes and complications, and relevant diagnostic tests.

SCHISTOSOMIASIS
DISEASE/DISORDER
ANATOMY OR SYSTEM AFFECTED: Bladder, liver

SPECIALTIES AND RELATED FIELDS: Internal medicine, public health, urology

DEFINITION: Schistosomiasis is a chronic illness caused by parasitic worms that live in the blood vessels around the liver and bladder. It is one of the leading causes of ill health, lethargy, and premature death in tropical countries. People are infected with the parasite by swimming or wading in contaminated water. The infectious larvae enter the

Cycle of Schistosomiasis Infection

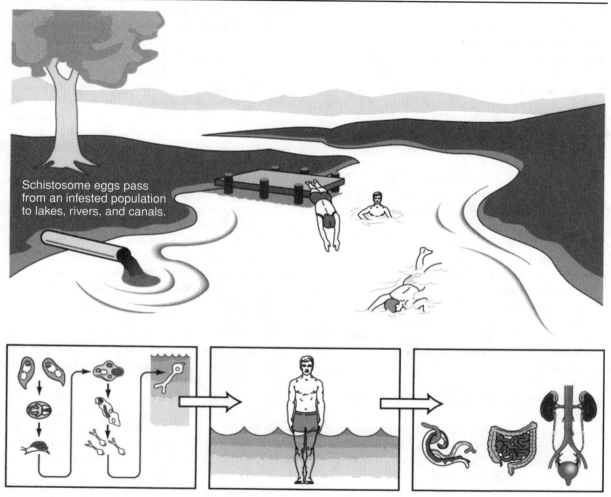

Schistosome eggs pass from an infested population to lakes, rivers, and canals.

Eggs hatch into larvae, enter and live in freshwater snails; larvae later leave snail hosts as cercariae.

Cercariae burrow through the skin of swimmer, find their way to the bloodstream, and mature into adult worms.

Adult worms (male and female) settle in the veins of the bladder and intestines; the females produce eggs that go through the walls of the bladder or intestine and are passed in the urine or feces.

bloodstream and make their way to the veins around the bladder. As adults, schistosome worms can grow to two centimeters in length, live for thirty years, and produce three thousand eggs daily. Schistosomiasis produces few symptoms until the infection is heavy, at which point the victim may pass blood in the urine, have diarrhea, and experience weakness, malaise, and abdominal pain. Untreated, schistosomiasis leads to either kidney or liver failure and eventually to death.

—Jason Georges and Tracy Irons-Georges
See also Parasitic diseases; Tropical medicine; Worms.

FOR FURTHER INFORMATION:

Buchsbaum, Ralph, et al. *Animals Without Backbones.* 3d ed. Chicago: University of Chicago Press, 1987.

Despommier, Dickson D., Robert W. Gwadz, and Peter J. Hotex. *Parasitic Diseases.* 4th ed. New York: Springer-Verlag, 2000.

Donaldson, Raymond Joseph, ed. *Parasites and Western Man.* Baltimore: University Park Press, 1979.

Klein, Aaron E. *The Parasites We Humans Harbor.* New York: Elsevier/Nelson Books, 1981.

Smyth, James D. *The Physiology of Trematodes.* San Francisco: W. H. Freeman, 1966.

SCHIZOPHRENIA

DISEASE/DISORDER

ANATOMY OR SYSTEM AFFECTED: Brain, psychic-emotional system

SPECIALTIES AND RELATED FIELDS: Psychiatry

DEFINITION: A disease of the brain characterized by withdrawal from the world, delusions, hallucinations, and other disorders in thinking.

KEY TERMS:

delusions: a false view of what is real

genetic cause: something that is handed down through the genes

hallucinations: a false or distorted perception of objects or events

hereditary: something that is passed down from generation to generation through the genes

CAUSES AND SYMPTOMS

Schizophrenia is a disease of the brain. Eugen Bleuler (1857-1939), a Swiss psychiatrist, first named the disease in a 1908 paper that he wrote entitled "Dementia Praecox: Or, The Group of Schizophrenias." In 1911, he published a book with the same title describing the disease in more detail. Bleuler served as the head of an eight hundred-bed mental hospital in Switzerland and treated the worst and most chronic cases. Beginning in 1896, he embarked on a project to understand the inner world of the mentally ill. He developed work therapy programs for his patients, and he visited them and talked to them almost every day. Bleuler insisted that the hospital staff show the same kind of dedication and support for his clients that he did.

Bleuler's discoveries challenged the traditional view of the causes and treatment of the disease. The traditional view, based on the work of the great German psychiatrist Emil Kraepelin (1856-1926), held that dementia, as it was called, always got worse and that the patient's mind continued to degenerate until death. Kraepelin suggested that the disease, which he called dementia praecox, was hereditary and was the result of a poisonous substance that destroyed brain cells. Bleuler's investigation of living victims led him to reject this view. Instead, he argued, continuing deterioration does not always take place because the disease can stop or go into remission at any time. The disease does not always follow a downhill course. Bleuler's views promised more hope for patients suffering from schizophrenia, which means "to split the mind."

The symptoms of schizophrenia are more well known than the cause. Diagnosis is based on a characteristic set of symptoms that must last for at least several months. The "psychotic symptoms" include a break with reality, hallucinations, delusions, or evidence of thought disorder. These are referred to as positive symptoms. "Negative" symptoms can also be displayed; they include withdrawal from society, the inability to show emotion or to feel pleasure or pain, total apathy, and the lack of a facial expression. The patient simply sits and stares blankly at the world, no matter what is happening.

Schizophrenia can take many forms. Among the most frequent are those that display acute symptoms under the following labels. Melancholia includes depression and hypochondriacal delusions, with the patient claiming to be extremely physically ill but having no appropriate symptoms. Mania is characterized by withdrawal and a mood of complete disinterest in the affairs of life. Schizophrenia can also be catatonic, in which patients become immobile and seem fixed in one rigid position for long periods of time. Delusional states accompanied by hallucinations frequently involve hearing voices, which often scream and shout abusive and derogatory language at the patient or make outrageous demands. The delusions are often visual and involve frightening monsters or aliens sent to do harm to the afflicted person.

The above symptoms can often be accompanied by disconnected speech patterns, broken sentences, and excessive body movement and purposeless activity. Victims of the disease also suffer through states of extreme anger and hostility. Cursing and outbursts of uncontrolled rage can result from relatively insignificant causes, such as being looked at "in the wrong way." Many times, anniversaries of important life experiences, such as the death of a parent or the birthday of a parent or of the patient, can set off positive and negative symptoms. Hallucinations and mania can also follow traumatic events such as childbirth or combat experiences during war.

The paranoid form of schizophrenia is the only one that usually develops later in life, usually between the ages of thirty and thirty-five. It is a chronic form, meaning that patients suffering from it usually become worse. Paranoid schizophrenia is characterized by a feeling of suspiciousness of everyone and everything, hallucinations, and delusions of persecution or grandiosity. This form becomes so bad that many victims, perhaps one out of three, eventually commit suicide simply to escape their tormentors. Others turn on their alleged tormentors and kill them, or at least someone who seems to be responsible for their terrible condition.

Other chronic forms of the disease include hebephrenic schizophrenia. In this case, patients suffer disorders of thinking and frequent episodes of incoherent uttering of incomprehensible sounds or words. The victims move quickly from periods of great excitement to equally exhausting periods of desperate depression. They frequently have absurd, bizarre delusions such as sex changes, identification with and as godlike creatures, or experiences of being born again and again. Those suffering from "simple" schizophrenia exhibit constant feelings of dissatisfaction with everything in their lives or a complete feeling of indifference to anything that happens. They are usually isolated and estranged from their families or any other human beings. Patients with these symptoms tend to live as recluses with barely any interest in society, in work, or even in eating or in talking to anyone else.

The various types of schizophrenia start at different times in different people. Generally, however, except for the paranoid form, the disease develops during late adolescence. Men show signs of schizophrenia earlier than women, usually by age eighteen or nineteen. It is unusual for signs of the disorder to appear in males after age twenty. In women, symptoms may not appear until the early twenties and sometimes are not evident until age thirty. Sometimes, there are signs in childhood. People who later develop schizophrenia tended to be withdrawn and isolated as children and were often made fun of by others. Not all withdrawn children develop the disease, however, and there is no way to predict who will get it and who will not.

Schizophrenia is a genetic disease. Individuals with the disease are very likely to have relatives—mothers, fathers, brothers, sisters, cousins, grandmothers, or grandfathers—with the disorder. Surveys indicate that 1 percent of all people have the disease. A person with one parent who has the disease is ten times more likely to develop schizophrenia than a member of the general public. Thirty-nine percent of people who have both parents afflicted with the disease also develop schizophrenia.

Other factors are involved in the disease in addition to heredity. E. Fuller Torrey, a leading researcher into the causes of schizophrenia, discovered important information about the origins of the disease in studies that he made of the brains of identical twins. Magnetic resonance imaging (MRI) of their brains showed that individuals diagnosed with the illness had slightly smaller brains than those without the disease. The difference in size was most apparent in the temporal lobe, the area that controls emotions and memory. Apparently, something goes wrong in the development of the temporal lobe of the fetus during the fourth to sixth month of pregnancy. Torrey speculated that this abnormality might result from a viral infection. The antibodies that normally protect the brain seem to get mixed up and attack the brain itself. Why or how this happens is not known. One possibility is that a nutritional deficiency in the mother might cause the temporal lobes to grow in an abnormal manner.

As to why the disease develops later in life rather than at birth, investigators provide the following information. First, the brain develops more slowly than other organs and does not stop developing until late adolescence. Many genetic diseases remain dormant until later in life, such as Huntington's chorea and multiple sclerosis.

Schizophrenia operates by disrupting the way in which brain cells communicate with each other. The neurotransmitters that carry signals from one brain cell to another might be abnormal. Malfunction in one of the transmitters, dopamine, seems to be a source of the problem. This seems likely because the major medicines that are successful in the treatment of schizophrenia limit the production or carrying power of dopamine. Another likely suspect is serotonin, a transmitter whose presence or absence has important influences on behavior.

TREATMENT AND THERAPY

Since the 1950's, many medications have been developed that are very effective in treating the symptoms of schizophrenia. Psychotherapy can also be effective and beneficial to many patients. Drugs can be used to treat both positive and negative symptoms. Some such as Haldol, Mellaril, Prolixin, Navane, Stelazine, and Thorazine are used to treat positive symptoms. Clozapine and Risperidone can be used for both positive and negative symptoms. These medications work by blocking the production of excess dopamine, which may cause the positive symptoms, or by stimulating the production of the neurotransmitter, which reduces negative symptoms. Clozapine blocks both dopamine and serotonin, which apparently makes it more effective than any of the other drugs.

The chief problem resulting from the use of such drugs are the terrible side effects that they can produce. The most dreaded side effect, from the point of view of the patient, is tardive dyskinesia (TD). This problem emerges only after many years of use. TD is characterized by involuntary movement of muscles, frequent lip-smacking, facial grimaces, and constant rocking back and forth of the arms and the body. It is completely uncontrollable.

Dystonias are another side effect. Symptoms include the abrupt stiffening of muscles, such as the sudden contraction of muscles in the arms, neck, and face. Most of these effects can be controlled or reversed with antihistamines. Some patients receiving medication are afflicted with effects similar to those movements associated with Parkinson's disease. They suffer from the slowing of movements in their arms and legs, tremors, muscle spasms. Their faces seem frozen into a sad, masklike expression. These effects can be treated with medication. Another problem is akathisia, a feeling developed by many patients that they cannot sit still. Their jumpiness can be treated with Valium or Xanax. Some of these side effects are so severe or embarrassing that patients cite them as the major reason that they do not take their medicine.

Many patients report great value in family or reha-bilitation therapy. These therapies are not intended to cure the disease or to "fix" the family. Instead, they are aimed at helping families learn how to live with mentally ill family members. Family support is important for victims of schizophrenia because they usually are unable to live on their own. Therapy can also help family members understand and deal with their frustration and the constant pain that results from knowing that a family member is very ill and probably will not improve much. Rehabilitation therapy is an attempt to teach patients the social skills that they need to survive in society.

The results of treatment are not always positive, even with medication and therapy. Ten percent of people with schizophrenia commit suicide rather than trying to continue living with the terrible consequences of the disease.

PERSPECTIVE AND PROSPECTS

Hopes for improving the treatment of schizophrenia rest mainly on the continuing development of new drugs. Several studies suggest that psychotherapy directed at improving social skills and reducing stress helps many people with the disease improve the quality of their lives. It is known that stress-related emotions lead to increases in delusions, hallucinations, social withdrawal, and apathy. Therapists can help patients find ways of dealing with stress and living in communities. They encourage their patients to deal with feelings of hostility, rage, and distrust of other people. Family therapy can teach all members of a family how to live with a mentally ill family member. Such therapy, along with medication, can produce marvelous results.

One study of ninety-seven victims of schizophrenia who lived with their families, received individual therapy, and took their medications showed far fewer recurrences of acute symptoms than did a group that did not get such help. Among those fifty-four individuals who received therapy but lived alone or with nonfamily members, schizophrenia symptoms reappeared or worsened over the same three-year period of the study. People living alone usually had more severe symptoms to start out with and found it difficult to find housing, food, or clothing, even with therapy. The demands of life and therapy apparently were too much for them. The major problem with this kind of treatment, which seems to work for people in families, is that it is expensive.

—*Leslie V. Tischauser, Ph.D.*

See also Anxiety; Depression; Hallucinations; Hypochondriasis; Manic-depressive disorder; Paranoia; Psychiatric disorders; Psychiatry; Psychiatry, child and adolescent; Psychoanalysis; Psychosis; Suicide.

FOR FURTHER INFORMATION:

Gorman, Jack M. *The New Psychiatry: The Essential Guide to State-of-the-Art Therapy, Medication, and Emotional Health.* New York: St. Martin's Press, 1996. A well-written, easy-to-understand book by a doctor and researcher that provides the latest information concerning the development of new medications, treatments, and therapies. Valuable information on the new antipsychotic drugs, how they work, and what their possible side effects are.

Gottesman, Irving I. *Schizophrenia Genesis: The Origins of Madness.* New York: W. H. Freeman, 1991. The author, a leading researcher into the genetic causes of schizophrenia, describes recent discoveries on the origins of the disease. He also evaluates different treatments and the many kinds of counseling and therapeutic techniques.

Johnstone, Eve C., et al. *Schizophrenia: Concepts and Clinical Management.* New York: Cambridge University Press, 1999. Written in conjunction with colleagues from Edinburgh, Eve Johnstone's book is a useful summary of current knowledge. The suggestion that psychosis can be thought of as occurring along three dimensions—positive, negative, and disorganized—with distinct pathological mechanisms, is well argued but probably still falls short of being an accepted theory.

Marsh, Diane T. *Families and Mental Illness: New Directions on Professional Practice.* New York: Praeger, 1992. A good book on the role of families in the care and treatment of the mentally ill. Written for professionals but very useful for anyone who must learn to deal with schizophrenia.

Sheehan, Susan. *Is There No Place on Earth for Me?* Boston: Houghton Mifflin, 1982. A book that provides an accurate, compassionate view of the course of chronic schizophrenia, including the many difficulties faced by victims of the disease. Describes the ineffective care available for many patients in public facilities.

Torrey, E. Fuller. *Surviving Schizophrenia: A Manual for Families, Consumers, and Providers.* 3d ed. New York: Harper & Row, 1995. Perhaps the best single book on the topic, by a leading medical researcher and advocate of more humane care for the mentally ill. Describes the latest research into the origins of the illness and provides useful information and evaluations of the newest drugs and best forms of treatment.

Woolis, Rebecca. *When Someone You Love Has a Mental Illness: A Handbook for Family, Friends, and Caregivers.* New York: Jeremy P. Tarcher/Perigree Books, 1992. A brief, practical guide that gives useful tips on handling the anger, hostility, and bizarre behavior exhibited by people with the disease. Also describes how to help patients to live at home and what to do if suicide is threatened.

SCIATICA
DISEASE/DISORDER

ANATOMY OR SYSTEM AFFECTED: Back, hips, legs, nerves, nervous system, spine

SPECIALTIES AND RELATED FIELDS: Family practice, internal medicine, neurology

DEFINITION: Painful inflammation of one of the sciatic nerves.

CAUSES AND SYMPTOMS

The two sciatic nerves are the largest nerves in the body. One runs from the spine down the left leg, the other down the right leg; they supply the tissues of the thigh, lower leg, and foot. The roots of the sciatic nerves are in the lower spinal column. It is here that difficulty is most likely to occur. Inflammation of these nerves is most often caused by a pinching of one or more spinal nerve roots between the vertebrae of the lower back.

Sciatica is characterized by shooting pain down the sciatic nerve and extending into the hip, the thigh, and the back portion of the leg. The pain may occur in all these points at once or skip about from point to point. Sciatica often begins with a long period of intermittent, mild low back pain. Suddenly, however, the slightest movement, such as lifting a weight or merely bending over, may bring about intense sciatic pain.

A mild case of sciatica can be brought on by vitamin deficiencies or by arthritic inflammation in the lower spine. Prolonged constipation can build pressure on the nerve and cause sciatic pain. Occasionally, a tumor may develop near the nerve and press on it. Sometimes, a herniated, or slipped, disk at the level where the nerve roots emerge in the low back may protrude and press on the nerve, thereby causing sciatica.

TREATMENT AND THERAPY

If the sciatic nerve is being compromised, surgery may be indicated. More than 50 percent of patients with sciatica, however, recover on their own in six weeks. In the acute stage, rest is essential. Heat may give temporary relief from pain. The type of medication used depends on the cause of the sciatica. Ultimately, a therapeutic exercise program to develop stabilizing strength and endurance in the trunk muscles is essential for functional recovery.

—Genevieve Slomski, Ph.D.

See also Nervous system; Neuralgia, neuritis, and neuropathy; Neurology; Slipped disk; Vitamins and minerals.

FOR FURTHER INFORMATION:

Brown, Mark D., and Bjorn L. Rydevik, eds. *Causes and Cure of Low Back Pain and Sciatica.* Philadelphia: W. B. Saunders, 1991. Discusses the etiology and treatment of low back pain and sciatica. Includes bibliographical references.

Fishman, Loren, and Carol Ardman. *Back Talk: How to Diagnose and Cure Low Back Pain and Sciatica.* New York: Norton, 1997. Discusses the mechanisms of backache and offers some treatment options. Includes bibliographical references and an index.

Gillette, Robert D. "A Practical Approach to the Patient with Back Pain." *American Family Physician* 53, no. 2 (February 1, 1996): 670-678. When treatment is based on a specific diagnosis, when patients are followed proactively to recovery, and when psychosocial factors receive appropriate attention, then the management of back pain will probably be effective.

Hooper, Paul D. *Preventing Low Back Pain.* Baltimore: Williams & Wilkins, 1992. Discusses such topics as the prevention of backache and its treatment, including chiropractic. Includes bibliographical references and an index.

SCOLIOSIS

DISEASE/DISORDER

ANATOMY OR SYSTEM AFFECTED: Back, bones, musculoskeletal system, spine

SPECIALTIES AND RELATED FIELDS: Orthopedics, physical therapy

DEFINITION: Abnormal curvature of the spine, often progressive, which can result in severe deformity and associated medical problems.

KEY TERMS:

adolescent scoliosis: curvature of the spine that is diagnosed in the early stages of puberty

Cobb angle: the commonly used measure of the degree of spinal curvature; the angle created by perpendiculars to the top of the first and bottom of the last vertebrae in a curve

idiopathic: referring to a medical condition with no known cause

skeletal or bone age: a measurement of age based on a comparison by an X ray of the bone structure in the left hand with the standards of the Gruelich and Pyle Atlas

spine: the combined spinal cord and the spinal column, a structure central to erect posture and the complex nervous communications system of the body

*vertebra (*pl. *vertebrae):* the individual bones that are stacked upon one another to form the vertebral column, or spine

CAUSES AND SYMPTOMS

Of all the structures making up the human body, the spine is second only to the closely associated brain in its centrality to human characteristics. Two distinct aspects of human life are deeply involved in the proper functioning of the spine. First, the spinal column protects the spinal cord, which carries out critical message-carrying functions in the body. Second, the spinal column also holds the body erect, a distinctly primate feature. An abnormal curvature of the skeletal structure of the spinal (or vertebral) column is known as scoliosis.

The usual term for the spine, the backbone, is completely misleading. If one really had a backbone, one would be unable to bend, nod, or stretch. The normal spine consists of approximately thirty-three separate bones whose very name, vertebrae, is derived from the Latin verb "to turn." Furthermore, it is essential to know that the normal spine takes the form of four separate curves. Each of these curves is associated with a distinct set of vertebrae. At the very top of the spine are the cervical vertebrae. In the chest area are found the thoracic vertebrae, which support the body when one leans backward and which are the sites of attachment of the twelve pairs of ribs. The largest of the vertebrae, which support the upper body weight, are called lumbar from the Latin for "loin." At the very base of the spine are two sets of small vertebrae called the sacrum and coccyx.

Although these curves are a vital part of a healthy spine, they are not always obvious because one usually sees people from the front or rear, so that the spine appears straight. If one looks at a person with good posture from the side, however, the gently S-shaped curve of the spine is clearly visible. Deformities involving abnormal spinal curvature toward the front or back are well known, but they are not called scoliosis. The side-to-side curvature of scoliosis is referred to as a lateral curve.

As important as the bones are, the vertebral spine is a much more complicated structure. Along its entire length is a surrounding complex of ligaments and muscles making it possible for the body to bend and straighten again. Within the vertebral column are rubbery cylinders of cartilage called disks. These disks absorb shocks, relieving the body from the countless pressures of movement. With this array of closely balanced mechanisms and associated forces, it is no wonder that the curvature of the spine is a complex subject for diagnosis and treatment.

Scoliosis can result from a number of different causes. While a birth defect, an accident, poliomyelitis, or muscular dystrophy can all result in lateral curvature, the cause is unknown in the majority of cases. Some authorities believe that 80 percent of all scoliosis has no known cause. The technical term for this important class of malady is "idiopathic scoliosis." Within this general subdivision, three separate forms are recognized, based on the age of the patient at the onset of the curvature.

The adolescent form of scoliosis, which is usually recognized between ten and thirteen years of age, is by far the most common form. A brief look, however, at infantile (birth to three years) and juvenile (four to ten years) scoliosis will help to illustrate the difficulty faced by researchers in this area and the enormous problems yet to be solved. (All these age groupings refer to the age at which the deformity is first noted, not the age at which the curvature began.)

When the scoliosis is recognized in the youngest range, it is more common in males, with one study giving a 3:2 ratio. By contrast, in the far more common adolescent condition one finds a striking shift to females, who are three times more likely to be affected. While it is often observed that infantile idiopathic scoliosis corrects itself (that is, it spontaneously resolves), this natural remission is rarely observed when the diagnosis is made later. More fascinating but puzzling is the noted absence of the infantile con-

Scoliosis

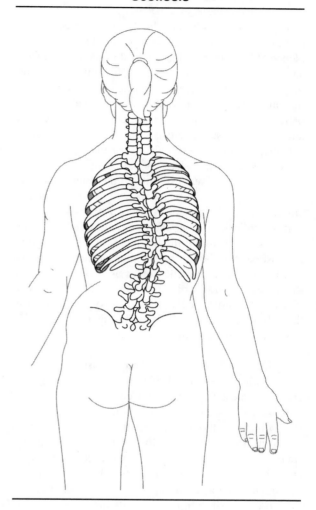

ditions in the United States and Canada, while its occurrence is well documented in Great Britain and France. J. I. P. James, who studied scoliosis extensively at the University of Edinburgh for many years, reported this form to be as common in Europe as the adolescent variety is worldwide. At a subtler level of research, one finds that 90 percent of the curves in infants are formed to the left, whereas 90 percent of those in adolescent girls lie to the right.

It is small wonder that James's collaborator, Ruth Wynne-Davies, calls the cause of infantile scoliosis "multifactorial" and states, "The exact cause in each individual is likely to be different." Wynne-Davies has made important studies of the influence of heredity in producing scoliosis. She, like many others, sees infantile idiopathic scoliosis in a different class from the adolescent variety.

The juvenile condition is likely to be related closely to adolescent scoliosis. As before, there is marked evidence of hereditary influence. In this age range, males and females share equally in the likelihood of being diagnosed. The chance of significant progression of the curvature is so variable that close watching of the patient is the single point of common agreement among specialists. There is concern among parents, patients, and practitioners alike over the excessive use of X rays for diagnosis.

Some research suggests intriguing clues about the cause of scoliosis from unexpected sources. For example, studies at the University of Rochester suggest that in scoliosis patients there may be significant differences in the side of the brain that processes sound. In most people, the left hemisphere of the brain hears and understands phonetic sound as in language, but those people with scoliosis seem much more likely to use both sides or the right side of the brain for these functions. It may be possible that a simple listening test can determine who is at risk for spinal curvature.

A dozen different types of curves associated with scoliosis have been identified, but four major classes are of greatest frequency and concern. In the chest area, one finds the most common of all curve patterns, the right thoracic curve. It is possible for this condition to progress rapidly. Early treatment is essential. As the curve develops, the ribs on the right side shift and create a deformity which not only is unattractive but also can squeeze the heart and lungs; this so-called rib hump can result in serious cardiopulmonary difficulties.

A similar, but gentler, curve is the thoracolumbar curve. It begins in the same region of the thoracic vertebrae and ends further down the back, in the lumbar region. The twist may be either right or left and is generally less deforming in its appearance. A lumbar curve is found far down in that region of the back, producing a twist in the hips. In pregnant women and other adults, this twist often causes severe back pain.

The three curves described thus far are single, or C-shaped, curves. The double major curve is an S-shaped curve and is the most common of that type. Curvature begins in the thoracic or chest area and is complimented by a second curve in the opposite direction found in the lumbar region. To some extent, the two curves offset each other and the scoliosis is less deforming. The double major curve can progress and become the source of a rib hump.

These and the other less common curves demand an accurate description beyond their location. John Cobb searched for such an important tool and developed the widely used Cobb angle measurement. His suggestion was to relate the top of the first and the bottom of the last vertebrae of a curve by determining the angle formed by the intersection of lines perpendicular to them. It is not difficult, using an X ray of the spine, to draw lines above and below the vertebrae, construct the required perpendiculars, and measure the angle of their intersection. This technique allows physicians to communicate accurately and have a useful measure with which to note the progression, remission, or stabilization of the patient's scoliosis. In addition to degree of curvature, the complex structure of the spine shows rotation in scoliosis. The rotation causes the pedicles or indentations of the vertebrae to shift closer to the midline drawn on the X ray. The relative shift is described as a rotation of +1, +2, and so on.

TREATMENT AND THERAPY

Scoliosis can result from many different causes, each of which demands treatment, as well as the idiopathic variety under discussion. Since there is no known cause, prevention is impossible, and since there are enormous difficulties in predicting the course of the disease, the most that can be achieved is satisfactory correction.

A diagnostic examination for scoliosis demands specific attention to accurate family history. Particularly important is information concerning the first recognition and previous treatment of the condition. Then a detailed evaluation of the nature and extent of the curvature must be made. The examining physician should make certain that the patient is standing straight with the knees unflexed. A simple plumbline is used to examine the patient's back to determine any curvature in the spine. Then the forward bending test is conducted. This observation is considered one of the most reliable diagnostic tools. Various forms of curvature, including scoliosis, can be seen by the trained observer. When viewed, at eye level from both front and back, one side of the thoracic or lumbar regions is higher. An accurate measurement of the degree of difference can be made with a level. The use of X-ray photographs also forms a vital part of the diagnostic data.

Even with the best diagnostic skill, training, and experience, the decision concerning the treatment of scoliosis is hardly straightforward. One important consideration is the patient's bone age. Because people grow and mature at such different rates, chronological age may not correspond well to the degree of maturity of that person's skeleton. Many clues are used to determine the bone age, including the degree of fusion observed in the individual vertebra or the bony pelvic girdle. A catalog of X rays of hands is available and provides a useful measure of the bone age. The central concern is that curvature is more likely to progress if the growth and development of the patient's skeleton is still incomplete.

The treatment of scoliosis varies from none at all to extensive surgical procedures. In general, treatment is undertaken for the prevention of further curvature or for the correction of the curvature already present. Some treatments, such as exercise, are of benefit to the patient in general but are seen as having no prospect of arresting or correcting the spinal curvature. Research has also suggested that copper in the diet may play a key role in scoliosis treatment. These studies were carried out with chickens, which show scoliosis very similar to that found in humans, but much remains to be learned about these and similar studies on rabbits, salmon, and quail before much confidence can be placed in the applicability of the data to human treatment or prevention.

Of all the methods proposed, the use of braces and casts is certainly the oldest and the most common. The many modifications of design and material used in braces over the centuries have had the central purpose of forcing the spine to become straight. The evolution of the brace has reached the point of an active or kinetic apparatus called the Milwaukee brace, developed by Walter Blount and Albert Schmidt. It is a carefully designed assembly of a molded plastic pelvic girdle, three metal bars which keep the wearer erect and allow a neck ring to be attached. The neck ring and its associated axillary sling keep the torso balanced and prevent listing to the right or left.

In order for the Milwaukee brace (or any modified versions of it) to be effective, it must be worn day and night and until the growth period of the patient has been completed. It is also imperative that exercise be carried out on a daily basis. There are many advantages of the modern brace over older systems. For example, it can be removed for showering and swimming, and much greater activity is allowed. The one serious drawback is that a patient must not expect correction of the scoliosis. The value of the brace is that it can, with good use and exercise, maintain the already present curvature and prevent further progression.

Only in certain cases will braces be of benefit to the patient. With curves of 40 or 50 degrees, pain that does not respond to treatment, or the failure of the brace to stop the curve's progression, surgery is the most reasonable approach. Surgery can offer some degree of correction, but it is important to recognize that only a partial correction is possible. Even with the safest techniques, pressure must be applied to the spine, creating a serious risk of damage to the spinal cord. Most authorities estimate reasonable correction to be about 60 percent.

Once it is agreed that surgery is the proper route of treatment, a wide range of methods are available. The most common, and generally considered the safest, method is the Harrington rod technique. The incision is from the back (as opposed to front or side entries), and metal hooks are inserted at the highest and lowest points in the curve. These hooks hold metal rods used to straighten the spine and then to hold it in place. Small chips of bone are then taken from the hip or ribs and inserted between especially prepared vertebrae. In a period of six to eight months, solid bone will grow and fuse the vertebrae, giving a solid bone mass of a single elongated vertebra. After the surgery, the patient is usually placed in a brace or cast for four to six months.

The success of the Harrington rod technique has inspired several modifications, such as using two rods to achieve more balance and greater correction. With a patient who has unusually soft bones, a system of wires is used to hold the rods in place. This method is considered superior because the normal hooks might break off. Several variants of the wire technique are also available. Some surgeons thread the wires through the neural canal, and others drill small holes to avoid coming near to the spinal cord.

Another technique which is growing in popularity avoids the use of a Harrington rod. Many small wires are attached through the neural canal and twisted around two thin rods, one on either side of the curvature. This Luque method provides greater stability, and usually there is no need to wear a cast after surgery. These advantages must be balanced, however, against a significantly greater risk of paralysis and a smaller amount of room for new bone growth in fusion.

Another modern technique which is showing some success involves placing small electrodes near the spine and transmitting tiny electrical impulses to nerve endings periodically during sleep. This electronic bracing, or electrosurface stimulation, appears to stop scoliosis curves from progressing in about 80 percent of the cases studied. The application of these devices has about the same limitations as conventional braces—that is, curves of greater than 40 degrees, curves treated after the end of bone growth, and certain types of lumbar curves will fail to benefit from this treatment.

PERSPECTIVE AND PROSPECTS

One finds the beginning of serious study of the spine in the writings of Hippocrates (c. 460-c. 370 B.C.E.). He described the curves of both the normal and the abnormal spine. He may not have been as clear in his description of scoliosis as in those of the clubfoot or epilepsy, but he was well aware of the difficulty of its treatment and recognized its possible relationship to pulmonary disease. Another celebrated physician of antiquity, Galen, first suggested the medical term for this deformity, scoliosis, in the late years of the second century. Among the complications faced by early medical science were the inadequate methods and equipment available for making subtle diagnoses. Thus it was not until the sixteenth century that Ambrose Pare carefully described the various types of spinal curves. He also noted for the first time that scoliosis is largely a condition of children.

Over the centuries, many men and women added to the array of methods and instruments as well as the store of knowledge and thoughtful speculation about scoliosis. Many possible causes were presented on the basis of observation and research. Many approaches to the treatment of these deformities were described and tested. Yet, in spite of all this research, scientists are just beginning to appreciate the complexity of the problem of scoliosis.

—K. Thomas Finley, Ph.D.

See also Birth defects; Bone disorders; Bones and the skeleton; Muscular dystrophy; Orthopedic surgery; Orthopedics; Orthopedics, pediatric; Pediatrics; Poliomyelitis; Puberty and adolescence; Spinal cord disorders; Spine, vertebrae, and disks.

FOR FURTHER INFORMATION:

Eisenpreis, Bettijane. *Coping with Scoliosis*. New York: Rosen, 1998. Designed for students in grades seven to ten, this clearly written and well-organized book looks at the patterns of spinal curvature, treatment options, and emotional effects of this condition.

Griesse, Rosalie. *The Crooked Shall Be Made Straight*. Atlanta: John Knox Press, 1979. While this book does not pretend to offer specific medical information concerning scoliosis, it contains valuable insights for those facing the painful task of fighting this crippling malady. A truly inspiring story.

Neuwirth, Michael, with Kevin Osborn. *The Scoliosis Handbook: A Consultation with a Specialist*. New York: Henry Holt, 1996. This popular work educates the general reader about scoliosis. Includes a bibliography and an index.

Sachs, Elizabeth-Ann. *Just Like Always*. New York: Atheneum, 1981. A beautifully written story of two young ladies who share so much more than their hospitalization for surgery. Dated technical information is nevertheless skillfully woven into this essential book for anyone suffering from scoliosis.

Schommer, Nancy. *Stopping Scoliosis: The Complete Guide to Diagnosis and Treatment*. New York: Doubleday, 1987. One of the best books written for the layperson that is devoted to the discussion of a medical problem. Includes many references to other information, specialists, and organizations concerned with the study and treatment of scoliosis.

SCREENING

PROCEDURE

ANATOMY OR SYSTEM AFFECTED: All

SPECIALTIES AND RELATED FIELDS: Genetics, oncology, preventive medicine, public health

DEFINITION: A strategy used by physicians and public health professionals to diagnose disease or the potential for disease at an early stage, when it may be treatable or preventable; screening may be a mandatory procedure for a specific population or a voluntary activity requested by individuals.

KEY TERMS:

efficacy: the extent to which a drug or procedure works as expected under ideal conditions, such as in the laboratory; efficacy must be proven before a drug or procedure may be applied in a clinical environment

nulliparity: having never given birth to a viable infant

primary medical care: medical care provided by a generalist physician or health care provider, who assumes responsibility for a patient's total health care needs and manages subspecialty referrals and medical care provided by subspecialists

reliability: the concept that repeated tests will produce the same result

sensitivity: the ability of a screening technique to identify correctly people who have a disease

specificity: the ability of a screening technique to identify correctly people who do not have a disease

validity: a preliminary indication of a screening technique's capability to identify persons with preclinical disease as test-positive and those without preclinical disease as test-negative

INDICATIONS AND PROCEDURES

Screening is an activity that is intended to identify a condition or a disease before symptoms develop in a person, at which time the condition becomes apparent to a clinician or has a negative impact on the individual or society. From a clinical perspective, screening and early detection are intended to prevent disease in or provide early treatment for an asymptomatic, apparently healthy person. Detection and treatment of high cholesterol and abnormal lipids, for example, will prevent heart attacks, strokes, and other cardiovascular problems. Early detection of a cancer may mean the difference between survival and death. Screening is distinguished from testing persons who have developed symptoms of a disease or condition. Screening programs for infectious diseases also serve the public's health by identifying infected persons and directing them to appropriate health care, thereby limiting disease transmission.

Screening techniques vary in the sophistication of the technology used and the cost to the consumer. They may be quick, simple, and inexpensive, such as a total blood lipid profile obtained from a booth in a shopping mall (about five minutes, from the finger prick for a blood sample to a printed profile, and usually available at no cost) or time-intensive, technologically advanced, and costly, as in the case of a mammogram for the detection of breast masses indicative of breast cancer (two to three hours from the time of the appointment to the completion of the procedure, with potential adverse effects from radiation and at a high cost to the patient). In the United States, the costs associated with screening for the presence of a disease are often not reimbursable from standard, commercial health insurance policies; however, insurers are increasingly encouraging periodic screening for individuals associated with defined populations and reimbursing providers for much of the costs associated with the procedures involved. Health maintenance organizations (HMOs) routinely offer patients comprehensive periodic screenings to afford diagnosis and treatment at a stage when the disease or condition is relatively easy and inexpensive to treat. The appropriateness of screening for a disease or condition rests primarily upon the disease or condition in question and the screening technique chosen.

The natural process of the disease studied is an important determinant for whether and when a screening procedure may be practical. There is a time lag associated with every condition, from initial exposure to the onset of infection or development of a cancer or other disorder and the point at which early diagnosis is possible. Screening is ineffective if it occurs during this time interval, called the biologic onset of disease. For some diseases, biologic onset occurs immediately or within days upon the initial interaction with the causal agent. There is an eight- to thirteen-day period between exposure to the measles virus and onset of fever. For other conditions, early diagnosis becomes possible after a more prolonged period as in the case of tuberculosis, in which the onset of infection occurs about four to twelve weeks after exposure. In the case of infection from the human immunodeficiency virus (HIV), which causes acquired immunodeficiency syndrome (AIDS), early diagnosis as a result of screening is not possible until about three to six months following the initial exposure. It is during this second period in the natural history of HIV that changes within the infected body become apparent and subsequently measurable with the screening tools available. The individual usually remains free of specific symptoms during this period; however, antigens to the virus become apparent and indicate that the individual is indeed infected.

Screening protocols can be organized as unlinked, anonymous, or confidential. Unlinked screening occurs when a blood, fluid, or tissue specimen is examined without the possibility of identifying its source. In anonymous screening, samples are identified by a code that is known only to the person tested, and the results of the test are made known to the person tested. Confidential screening occurs when a health care provider orders a test and receives the test results.

Participation in screening programs may be voluntary, routine, or mandatory. The nature of the condition examined, its significance for the public's health, and the situation in which a potentially infected person is identified all pose guidelines for the means of structuring participation in a screening program. Mandatory screening occurs when the individual has no choice but to undergo the screening procedure. For example, a government may require all military recruits to be screened for a variety of infectious diseases to prevent epidemics from occurring within the military. In the United States, some federal and state statutes call for screening newly incarcerated prisoners, the mentally ill, and other institutionalized groups to avoid transmission of infection among the larger group. Some states require that all marriage certificate applicants undergo screening for syphilis to protect potential unborn children from the consequences of congenital infection.

From the individual's perspective, there is little to differentiate mandatory screening from routine screening. The difference lies in whether enabling legislation exists requiring an individual to undergo the screening procedure. Blood banks routinely screen donated blood for hepatitis B and antigens to HIV. Many hospitals routinely screen surgery patients for the presence of HIV antigens to protect health care workers. Commercial life insurance applicants are almost always required to undergo a physical examination and to provide samples of blood, urine, and even feces for screening tests. The rationale for routine screening is sometimes disputed. For example, health care professionals are expected to maintain vigilance regarding virus transmission by avoiding direct contact with blood and body fluids of all patients in accord with universal precautions, which were developed by the Centers for Disease Control and Prevention (CDC). Presumably, knowledge of a patient's infection status should not justify altering the way in which a health care provider encounters the patient, nor should it justify altering patient care. Hospitals and surgeons reason that alternative methods may be employed for some surgical procedures that may potentially reduce the chances of the physician receiving an injury from a needle or a bone fragment while suturing a wound or manipulating organs within the body. Routine screening for

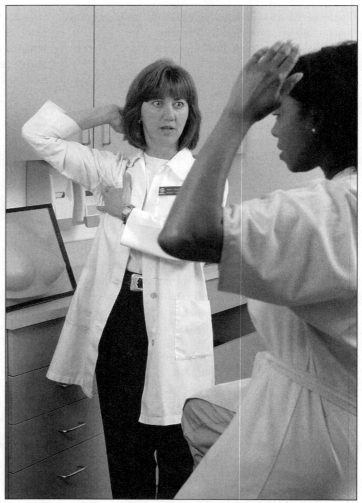

A doctor shows a woman how to perform a breast self-examination. Combined with periodic mammograms, such screening procedures can catch many cases of breast cancer. (PhotoDisc)

blood-borne diseases is also recommended by some hospitals and law enforcement agencies for employees who come into contact with blood or body fluids through needle pricks or human bites.

Mandatory screening is most effective and scientifically useful in cases where testing is anonymous or unlinked (such as blood banks or research protocols for the purpose of surveying the epidemiology of an infection). Routine screening may be justified when implemented within a defined group of people who, by nature of their living or working situations, are at greater risk for infection than the general public (soldiers, prisoners, the institutionalized, hemophiliacs, health care workers, law enforcement officers) or who fall into a high-risk group for other disorders such as cancer. Routine hospital screening for preoperative patients is considered justified by the CDC only when the institution can document a high prevalence of HIV within the population likely to access its services. Mandatory and routine screening for most conditions, however, are usually too costly and inefficient to justify.

Voluntary screening occurs when individuals avail themselves of a screening procedure for no other reason than personal knowledge of infection or disease status. In some cases, when a condition may be engendered through lifestyle choices rather than by airborne transmission or casual contact, and may be more predominant in specific subpopulations or minority groups, mandatory screening is probably counterproductive. HIV is an example of an infection for which screening individuals on a voluntary basis is expected to yield more positive results than a mandatory program. Transmission of the AIDS virus only occurs through intimate contact, not casual contact. Although a required mass screening program may appease public anxiety about widespread infection, it may also have the unintended result of causing infected individuals to be secretive about their disease status. Pulmonary tuberculosis, on the other hand, is an example of a disease that is highly transmissible through casual contact and for which well-structured screening programs for specific populations are likely to benefit the public's health. Although the epidemiology of tuberculosis is such that the antibiotic-resistant strain, the cause of the disease's resurgence in the 1990's, is most prevalent among intravenous drug users and their sexual partners, the benefits of restraining infection through screening far outweigh the potential dangers of a mass-screening program.

Screening should never occur without a full disclosure by the health care professional regarding the concomitant risks and benefits and without the individual's consent. The concept of informed consent is a hallmark of the scientific and medical code of ethics in the United States. The recognition that informed consent is a crucial part of any medical study or screening program grew out of several striking and severe abuses of medical power that occurred during the twentieth century.

The ideal screening tool is one that is noninvasive, quick, inexpensive, and always accurate. Although these characteristics may appear simple to evaluate, the scientific and medical communities apply rigorous criteria to screening techniques to assess the extent to which they conform to the ideal. A screening technique should be valid; that is, it should appropriately do what it intends to do by categorizing persons accurately who have a preclinical disease as test-positive and those who do not have a preclinical disease as test-negative. Validity consists of two components: sensitivity and specificity. Sensitivity is defined as the ability of a test to identify correctly those who have the disease, while specificity is the ability to identify those who do not. Sensitivity and specificity are complements of each other; therefore, a single test cannot be both highly sensitive and highly specific. The best screening tests sacrifice a small degree of sensitivity to gain specificity, and vice versa. In some cases, these thresholds are arbitrarily set. For example, if in a hypertensive screening program the threshold for positivity for diastolic blood pressure, indicating hypertension, were set low, most people who actually have the disease would be identified. Many people who are not hypertensive, however, those whose diastolic blood pressures are greater than the threshold, would be falsely diagnosed with hypertension. False-positive and false-negative results can have significant consequences when they lead to subsequent treatment for the incorrectly diagnosed condition or lack of treatment for the undiagnosed condition.

A screening technique must be reliable to be considered useful. A highly reliable, or precise, screening technique is one that provides consistent results when the technique is performed more than once on the same individual under the same conditions. The reliability of a technique can be increased by minimizing the variability of interpreting its results and by defining and quantifying its end points.

Finally, a screening technique must be beneficial; it must do more good than harm. It must provide adequate results (both reliable and valid) by identifying presymptomatic individuals at a cost that is less than what would be spent on potential morbidity and mortality from the disease or condition if it went undetected. Expenses incurred by both the individual and the society should be considered when estimating the economy and benefits of a screening tool. Individual expense would include specific medical costs, transportation costs, and the less tangible costs of submitting to potentially unpleasant medical care. Societal costs would include such issues as a measure of resources used to benefit one individual and the loss of productivity for a period of time. Rigorous scientific evidence has not yet been developed to determine the effectiveness of some screening techniques that society has come to accept as beneficial. Rather, as in the case of screening for cervical cancer, the evidence for its benefit lies mainly in the comparison of trends of deaths from cervical cancer among countries that have well-organized screening and those that do not.

USES AND COMPLICATIONS

Examples of screening techniques that take these principles into consideration are those that are used to detect infection with HIV and cancer.

The epidemiology of HIV dramatically shifted during its history in the United States; by the early 1990's, it had come to reflect patterns of infection that were consistent with international patterns. Among the heterosexual population, the prevalence of HIV disease was increasing at a greater rate than among such groups as hemophiliacs, homosexuals, and intravenous drug abusers. There was a high prevalence of HIV disease among persons aged twenty to twenty-nine years, many of whom were likely to have become infected during their adolescent years. Although scientists are working hard to develop a vaccine to cure or an immunization to prevent infection with HIV, medicine is capable only of prolonging survival with HIV disease and perhaps enhancing the quality of life of those who suffer from it. Early detection of infection through screening is important for the initiation of pharmaceutical therapy.

There are two primary serologic screening tools used to detect indirectly the presence of HIV in humans. These tools, the enzyme-linked immunosorbent assay (ELISA) and the Western blot, identify antibodies to the virus rather than the virus itself. Just as the body's immune system develops antibodies to infectious diseases from viral agents such as influenza, mumps, and measles, the body likewise generates antibodies to HIV when it is exposed to this virus. Direct identification in host tissues by virus isolation is the most specific means of diagnosing HIV infection, but it lacks sufficient sensitivity for practical use. HIV suppresses the body's immune system from responding to opportunistic infections caused by bacteria and viruses, ultimately progressing to the series of opportunistic infections that are used as markers to make a clinical diagnosis of AIDS.

There is a standard method for testing an individual's blood for the presence of antibodies to HIV. A sample of blood is initially exposed to the ELISA. If the test result is negative, no additional testing is performed and the individual is considered free of the disease. If the test result is positive, then the ELISA is repeated on the same sample. If the second ELISA is positive, then the Western blot is used to confirm the results of the ELISA. A confirmatory test is important because of the Western blot's high specificity, that is, its probability of correctly identifying people who are not infected with the virus. When screening for HIV in the general population, where there is a low probability that individuals are truly infected with the virus, the ELISA's high sensitivity will cause it to return a small percentage of false-positive results. Therefore, basing infection status upon the ELISA alone will risk incorrectly diagnosing HIV disease when the virus is absent, consequently exposing an individual to the psychological, social, legal, and medical issues that accompany such a diagnosis. The Western blot, on the other hand, is highly specific for antigens to HIV; that is, there is an extremely small probability that a Western blot will return a false-positive result on a blood sample that has been subjected to the ELISA on two occasions. Individuals whose blood samples receive two positive results from ELISA tests fall into a group other than the large, general population described above. Instead, they may be characterized as more likely to be infected with the virus.

When screening for outcomes as severe as HIV disease, a confirmatory test is included in the screening protocol for the general population. In the case of HIV screening, blood samples are first exposed to a highly sensitive test, the ELISA, to rule out exposure. Samples for which exposure is not ruled out and remains possible are then exposed to a highly specific test, the Western blot, to check the results of the previous test, thereby ruling in exposure. All patients with an indeterminate Western blot test result after ELISA-positive results must have repeat testing after three months.

Cancer of the breast, which is responsible for approximately 32 percent of the total cancer incidence among American women, is another condition for which screening is available and is considered efficacious. In 1988, there were about 105 cases of breast cancer per 100,000 women, accounting for 18 percent of all female cancer deaths that year. Breast cancer is the leading cause of cancer death for women aged fifteen to fifty-four, and it is estimated that one in nine women in the United States will develop breast cancer during their lifetime. The set of factors that place a woman at an increased risk for breast cancer is well studied, but such characteristics as family history of breast cancer, nulliparity or late age at first full-term pregnancy, history of breast-feeding, earlier age at menarche (onset of menstruation), and use of oral contraceptives account for only 21 percent of the breast cancer risk in women aged thirty to fifty-four and 29 percent of the risk in women aged fifty-five to eighty-four.

While women at increased risk for breast cancer should be vigilant regarding the onset of breast masses indicative of carcinoma of the breast, established risk factors do not explain about 70 percent of breast cancer cases. Several screening techniques are available with which to identify carcinoma of the breast at an early stage, before the onset of advanced malignancy. These are breast self-examination (BSE), clinical breast examination (CBE), and mammography.

BSE, the least invasive of breast cancer screening techniques, is the practice of examining one's own breasts on a monthly basis to detect any noticeable changes in breast size, shape, and mass. BSE has been widely promoted by the American Cancer Society and the National Cancer Institute; however, the U.S. Preventive Services Task Force and the World Health Organization suggest that the data regarding the effectiveness of BSE in reducing breast cancer mortality are equivocal. Furthermore, some researchers suggest that BSE may not be efficacious because of the risk of unwarranted reassurance associated with false-negative results and the potential adverse effects from medical investigation of false-positive findings. To practice BSE, a woman should first undress to the waist in a well-lit room and sit or stand in front of a mirror. She should first examine the general appearance of her breasts and then methodically palpate each breast to detect lumps or thickening of the skin. The American Cancer Society recommends that women older than twenty years of age self-examine their breasts monthly.

In CBE, a physician or health professional visually examines and methodically palpates a patient's breasts to detect irregularities. The American Cancer Society recommends that women aged twenty to forty receive a CBE every three years and that women older than forty receive a CBE annually. The U.S. Preventive Services Task Force does not recommend CBE for women younger than forty, but it too suggests that women older than forty receive an annual CBE. In order to rule out the presence of an abnormality, health professionals must be even more thorough in a screening examination than when a patient comes to the health care provider for evaluation of a lump.

Breast mammography is a radiological technique that relies upon soft-tissue X rays to illustrate breast structure. Early cancers may be more easily detectable with mammography than with BSE or CBE. The mammogram may also confirm a physician's clinical diagnosis by ruling out disease. The technique is useful by identifying nonpalpable cancer or early cancer that may be present in the breast in question or in the opposite breast and that is likely to remain unnoticed by the physician or patient. Mammography can also be helpful by differentiating benign lesions from malignant ones.

As a screening tool, mammography is effective because of its capability to detect cancer in the asymptomatic or minimally symptomatic woman. A study that is frequently used to justify the effectiveness of mammography was conducted by the Health Insurance Plan of Greater New York under contract with the National Cancer Institute of the U.S. Public Health Service, in which 33 percent of the cancers went undetected with CBE but were detected with mammography. Women are recommended by the American Cancer Society to receive their first mammogram between the ages of thirty-five and forty. They should receive mammograms every year or two from age forty to forty-nine and annually thereafter. The U.S. Preventive Services Task Force recommends a mammogram every one to two years for women aged fifty to seventy-five, with mammograms earlier than age forty for women at high risk for breast cancer.

PERSPECTIVE AND PROSPECTS

Screening before disease is clinically apparent or to identify risk for infection has enhanced the quality of the public's health by controlling disease. Unfortunately, apparent success in controlling infectious disease through screening and early treatment has led to decreased vigilance in the case of some infectious diseases. Partly as a result of decreased funding for surveillance, gonorrhea, syphilis, and tuberculosis all increased in incidence in the last quarter of the twentieth century, sometimes in antibiotic-resistant forms. For example, during the first half of the twentieth century, the ability to detect and to treat syphilis received the benefit of federal public health expenditures in the United States, leading to a dramatic reduction in its incidence. Achieving success in its effort to reduce the consequences of this major sexually transmitted disease (STD), the government and clinicians then focused on a program to control gonorrhea in the 1970's. Again, medical and scientific progress allowed a reduction in infection and the serious sequelae associated with gonorrhea. By the early 1980's, however, other STDs such as chlamydia, herpes, and infection with the human papillomavirus became major threats. HIV became an important concern by the middle of the 1980's. During the second half of the 1980's, while attention was diverted to these diseases, the incidence of infectious syphilis increased to the highest level in forty years. Gonorrhea increased in epidemic proportions in a form that was resistant to recognized treatment.

Clinicians and public health authorities value the role of detection, prevention, and treatment for infectious diseases and other disorders at the primary care level, when the condition is asymptomatic. To this end, authorities recommend that primary care providers complete sexual and drug histories on all adolescent and adult patients and assess their risk categories for other diseases such as hypertension and cancer. The history is a screening technique that enables providers to identify patients at risk for specific disorders. The value of the history lies in its ideal clinical attributes: It is sensitive, nonintrusive, inexpensive, and quick. Providers should conduct laboratory screening tests on individuals suspected of being at risk for a serious medical condition and, regardless of test outcome, encourage behavior modification to prevent it.

Prenatal and postnatal screening have significantly reduced childhood morbidity and mortality by enabling clinical interventions during pregnancy or immediately following birth. Based on screening of the parents, the health care provider may assess an infant's risk for intrauterine problems or for health problems during infancy and childhood. For example, certain babies born to Rh-negative mothers and Rh-positive fathers may be at risk for a life-threatening anemia. Screening women during a first pregnancy identifies those who should receive an immunization to prevent problems in future infants. For those who do not receive this immunization, screening tests during pregnancy indicate which babies need therapy before they are born. Current medical treatments allow an affected baby to receive blood transfusions even in the womb.

Another example is that of sickle-cell anemia, an inherited disorder of the red blood cells. If both parents carry genes for sickle-cell anemia (even if they do not have the disease themselves), their infants are at risk for development of the disease. Screening of the parents allows genetic counseling to take place prior to or during pregnancy. Screening of the infants identifies those at risk for serious medical problems associated with sickle-cell disease.

Screening for the sickle-cell trait is an example of an existing test for a genetic disease. As the Human Genome Project progresses, scientists will have a better understanding of the causes of many diseases that have a genetic component, resulting in more accurate diagnosis and more effective treatments for them. Medical researchers will be able to develop screening tests for a multitude of genetic disorders. In the late 1990's, for example, scientists identified the genes associated with susceptibility to sarcomas and other tumors before age forty-five, predisposition to breast and ovarian cancer, tumors of the retina, Wilm's tumor, and familial colon cancer. In leukemias, genetic analysis allows classification of the disease. Lymphomas are under study.

Complex ethical and practical issues arise with this increased ability to screen for genetic disorders. In the first place, not every person with a genetic predisposition to a given disorder will develop that disorder. Understanding of the other, nongenetic, factors that allow one person with a given gene or set of genes to remain healthy throughout life and those factors that cause another person with the same genes to fall ill is still limited. Questions arise about how to treat people with a genetic predisposition to a disorder. Some worry that people with certain gene patterns will be unable to obtain health or life insurance. Others worry about the mental health of a person shown by genetic screening to be at risk for a serious disease. Genetic manipulation for the treatment or prevention of disease is yet another controversial issue that society as a whole must address.

—*John G. Ryan, Dr.P.H.;*
updated by Rebecca Lovell Scott, Ph.D.
See also Acquired immunodeficiency syndrome (AIDS); Apgar score; Biostatistics; Blood testing; Breast cancer; Cancer; Childhood infectious diseases; Colon and rectal polyp removal; Colon cancer; Colonoscopy; Down syndrome; Genetic counseling; Genetic diseases; Genetics and inheritance; Gonorrhea; Hepatitis; Human Genome Project; Human immunodeficiency virus (HIV); Immunization and vaccination; Laboratory tests; Mammography; Noninvasive tests;

Phenylketonuria (PKU); Physical examination; Pregnancy and gestation; Preventive medicine; Rh factor; Scoliosis; Sexually transmitted diseases; Sickle-cell anemia; Spina bifida; Syphilis; Tuberculosis.

FOR FURTHER INFORMATION:

Bennett, Rebecca, and Charles A. Erin. *HIV and AIDS: Testing, Screening, and Confidentiality.* New York: Oxford University Press, 1999. This book sets out the different points of view that have been gathered by the University of Manchester under the direction of John Harris.

Dawson, Deborah A. *Breast Cancer Risk Factors and Screening: United States, 1987.* Hyattsville, Md.: U.S. Department of Health and Human Services, Public Health Center, Centers for Disease Control, and National Center for Health Statistics, 1990. Dawson consistently contributes to an understanding of health in the United States by thoroughly examining data from the National Health Interview Survey (NHIS).

McBride, David. *From TB to AIDS: Epidemics Among Urban Blacks Since 1900.* Albany: State University of New York Press, 1991. Infectious diseases capitalize on social situations that facilitate their transmission: poverty and immune systems compromised by other infectious diseases or drugs.

Miller, Anthony B., ed. *Screening for Cancer.* Orlando, Fla.: Academic Press, 1985. This book focuses on the principles of screening and of its evaluation, the available tests for specific types of cancer, and the issues associated with specific cancer sites (such as the breast).

SCURVY
DISEASE/DISORDER

ANATOMY OR SYSTEM AFFECTED: Blood, gums, skin

SPECIALTIES AND RELATED FIELDS: Internal medicine

DEFINITION: Scurvy is a disease caused by a prolonged inadequate intake of vitamin C, also known as ascorbic acid. The average person needs 75 milligrams of vitamin C per day. In infants and children, it is characterized by tender and swollen legs, bleeding under the skin, anemia, tender ribs, bleeding gums, and fever. In adults, the symptoms include bleeding gums, loss of teeth, rough skin, weakness, hallucinations, and an increased susceptibility to infection. Treatment includes large daily doses of vitamin C for several months beyond the disappearance of symptoms.

—Jason Georges and Tracy Irons-Georges
See also Malnutrition; Nutrition; Vitamins and minerals.

FOR FURTHER INFORMATION:

Garrow, J. S., and W. P. T. James, eds. *Human Nutrition and Dietetics.* 10th ed. New York: Churchill Livingstone, 2000.

Kreutler, Patricia A., and Dorice M. Czajka-Narins. *Nutrition in Perspective.* 2d ed. Englewood Cliffs, N.J.: Prentice Hall, 1987.

Whitney, Eleanor Noss, and Sharon Rady Rolfes. *Understanding Nutrition.* 8th ed. St. Paul, Minn.: West, 1999.

Winick, Myron, Brian L. G. Morgan, Jaime Rozovski, and Robin Marks-Kaufman, eds. *The Columbia Encyclopedia of Nutrition.* New York: G. P. Putnam's Sons, 1988.

SEIZURES
DISEASE/DISORDER

ANATOMY OR SYSTEM AFFECTED: Brain, head, muscles, musculoskeletal system, nerves, nervous system

SPECIALTIES AND RELATED FIELDS: Neurology, pediatrics

DEFINITION: Asynchronous, paroxysmal discharges of neurons in the brain that result in body movements, unusual sensations, altered perceptions, and/or hallucinations that interfere with normal function and behavior.

KEY TERMS:

aura: the initial event signaling the beginning of a seizure

clonic: referring to the alternate contraction and relaxation of muscles

convulsion: an involuntary contraction of the body musculature, tonic or clonic, that can be of either cerebral or spinal origin

epilepsy: a chronic brain disorder of various causes, characterized by recurrent seizures resulting from the excessive discharge of cerebral neurons

seizure: an unsynchronized, paroxysmal discharge of neurons in the brain that results in body movements, unusual sensations, altered perceptions, hallucinations, or various mixtures of such symptoms; also called an ictus

tonic: characterized by tension or contraction, especially muscular tension

CAUSES AND SYMPTOMS

Seizures can be divided into two fundamental groups—partial and generalized. In partial seizures, the abnormal discharge of neurons usually arises in a portion of one hemisphere and may spread to other parts of the brain during a seizure. Generalized seizures, however, have no evidence of localized onset; the clinical manifestations and abnormal electrical discharge give no indication of the locus of onset of the abnormality, if such a locus exists.

Partial seizures are divided into three groups: simple partial seizures, complex partial seizures, and partial seizures secondarily generalized. Simple partial seizures are associated with the preservation of consciousness and unilateral hemispheric involvement. The area of seizure may spread until the entire side is involved. This type of seizure, with motor, sensory, or autonomic signs was originally called Jacksonian epilepsy. Complex partial seizures are associated with alteration or loss of consciousness and bilateral hemispheric involvement. A partial seizure secondarily generalized is a generalized tonic-clonic seizure that proceeds directly from either a simple partial seizure or a complex partial seizure. The distinction between simple partial seizures and complex partial seizures is clarified by the observation that neurologic problems that are confined to one hemisphere, such as a unilateral cerebral stroke, generally spare consciousness, whereas bilateral cerebral (or brain stem) involvement causes alteration of consciousness.

If there is no evidence of localized onset, then the attack is a generalized seizure. Generalized seizures are more heterogeneous than partial seizures. The generalized seizures include generalized tonic-clonic (grand mal), absence (petit mal), atonic, myoclonic, clonic, and tonic seizures.

Tonic-clonic seizure is a common seizure pattern with sudden loss of consciousness, tonic contraction of muscles, loss of postural control, and a cry caused by contraction of respiratory muscles forcing exhalation. This is followed by a generalized contraction of the muscles of the four extremities. After two to five minutes of unconsciousness and the cessation of clonic contractions, the individual gradually regains consciousness. Fecal and urinary incontinence, as well as biting of the tongue, may occur. The individual does not remember the event and may not be completely functional for several days.

The absence seizure usually begins in childhood or early adolescence, and in many cases individuals out-grow the condition. Although unresponsiveness is the rule, motionlessness occurs in less than 10 percent of absence attacks; in fact, phenomena such as mild clonic motion and increased or decreased postural tone may accompany such attacks. Absence seizures are generally brief, usually lasting less than ten seconds and very rarely longer than forty-five seconds. The attacks are not associated with auras, hallucinations, or other symptoms characteristic of partial seizures, generalized tonic-clonic seizures, or infantile spasms. Individuals exhibiting these seizures are normal except for the seizures, but the seizures may occur as frequently as one hundred times a day.

Atonic seizures are characterized by a sudden loss of muscle tone. Myoclonic seizures are sudden and brief contractions of a single group of muscles or of the entire body. The patients fall but do not lose consciousness. Clonic and tonic seizures are characterized by alternation of contraction and relaxation and by contraction, respectively.

Infantile spasms are generalized seizures occurring in the first year of life. These are synchronous contractions of the muscles of the neck, trunk, and arms. About 90 percent of infants experiencing these attacks are mentally deficient.

Seizures may be further subdivided into epileptic (those involving recurrent seizures) and nonepileptic. The term "nonepileptic seizure," however, is somewhat problematic. For example, a seizure caused by hypoglycemia (low blood sugar) may not be considered an epileptic attack by some because it is a transient event easily corrected by metabolic manipulation. Of the organic nonepileptic seizures, the most common are of cardiovascular origin; others are caused by transient cerebral ischemia, movement disorders, toxic or metabolic problems, sleep disorders, and even headaches. Nonepileptic attacks may also be of nonorganic or psychiatric origin, such as with hysteria and schizophrenia, in which case they are called psychogenic seizures or pseudoseizures.

Attempts to find a cause for the sudden abnormal discharge of cerebral neurons has not been possible in all types of seizure activity. In some cases, a brain tumor, scar tissue remaining from trauma to the brain, or a progressive neurological disease may be responsible. In the great majority of cases, however, no pathologic basis for the seizures is evident, either during life or at autopsy. The latter type of seizure has been classified as "idiopathic." In certain circumstances, for example, fever, infection, or hyperglycemia, the response may include seizure. In many instances, these events are isolated and do not recur, and for this reason they are not categorized as epilepsy.

The cause of a seizure is related to the age of onset of the first attack. When seizures begin in the neonatal and infant period, the most likely causes are perinatal anoxia (a deficiency of oxygen), congenital brain defects, meningitis, birth injuries, or other metabolic problems, such as hypoglycemia or hypercalcemia (excessive calcium). Less common causes of seizures in young children include toxins such as lead poisoning, as well as rare degenerative diseases. In older children or adults, although metabolic or degenerative processes must be considered, other causes become more probable.

Head trauma accounts for the origin of many partial epileptic seizures in young adults, whereas brain tumors and vascular diseases are the major cause of such seizures in later life. Brain tumor is not a common cause of epilepsy in children, since 60 to 70 percent of brain tumors in children are located in the posterior fossa. Arteriosclerotic cerebrovascular disease is the most common cause of seizures in patients over the age of fifty. In about 4 percent of patients with brain infarction and 10 percent of those with intracerebral hemorrhage, seizures accompany the stroke; an additional 3 percent of patients who experience a stroke have recurrent seizures in later life, presumably generated by the cerebral scar.

Most idiopathic seizure activity appears to have its origin in an inherited propensity to cerebral dysrhythmia. Although there is a high incidence of electroencephalographic (EEG) abnormalities in close relatives of persons with recurrent seizures, not all family members have clinical seizures. In general, genetic factors are particularly important when recurrent seizures begin in childhood and decrease in importance with age.

In most studies of early seizures predicting future epilepsy, the conditions that are associated with high risk include a depressed skull fracture, an acute intracerebral hematoma, post-traumatic amnesia lasting more than twenty-four hours, and the presence of tears in the dura mater of the brain or focal neurologic signs.

Generalized tonic-clonic seizures sometimes develop during the course of chronic intoxication with alcohol or barbiturates, almost always in association with withdrawal or reduction of the drugs. How long a period of chronic drug intoxication or abuse must last to produce seizures upon withdrawal is uncertain, but such patients often give a history of many years (sometimes decades) of drug dependence. Usually, the patients experience one or more seizures or short bursts of two to six seizures over a period of hours. An episode of alcohol withdrawal rarely precipitates more than a single burst of convulsions, while convulsions may recur for several days after barbiturate withdrawal. Studies have shown that among those who have had withdrawal seizures without other evidence of neurological damage, seizures almost always occurred during the seven-hour to forty-eight-hour period following cessation of drinking. With alcohol withdrawal seizures, tremor, anorexia, and insomnia follow the seizure in perhaps 20 to 30 percent of cases. Delirium tremens is a less frequent event.

TREATMENT AND THERAPY

Prior to treatment, it is necessary for the physician to conduct a thorough investigation of the patient to identify any remedial cause of the seizures. This investigation would include metabolic diseases, endocrine system disturbances, cerebral tumors, abscess of the brain, or meningitis.

Persons who have recurrent convulsions controlled by medications can participate in sports and lead a relatively normal life; most countries will permit a person to drive an automobile if he or she has experienced no seizures for six months to one year. If seizures are uncontrolled, however, then automobile driving, swimming, the operation of unguarded machinery, and ladder climbing are not advised.

Drug therapy varies with the type of seizure presented. In the case of recurrent seizures, it generally consists of at least two to four years of daily medication. Careful neurologic examinations every four to six months, monitoring of seizure frequency correlated with drug blood level, and serial EEG's about once a year are also required. If there is a change in seizure frequency despite adequate drug blood levels, if there are focal neurologic signs or signs of increased intracranial pressure, or if evidence of focal changes on EEG's develop, further evaluation, including a computed tomography (CT) scan, is necessary. A small brain tumor may not be apparent even on a CT scan at the time of the initial evaluation, particularly in a patient with adult-onset epilepsy or in an older child or adolescent with partial seizures without a documented specific cause.

Absence seizures present less urgency. The patient rarely seeks medical advice until repeated episodes have occurred. Early treatment and prevention or reduction of repeated seizures can be beneficial. The drugs of choice for absence epilepsy are ethosuximide or valproate sodium. Medication is generally discontinued after two to four seizure-free years, depending on the presence or absence of generalized tonic-clonic seizures and the results of the EEGs. After the medication is discontinued, and after follow-up for fifteen to twenty-three years, there is about a 12 percent incidence of recurrence.

If the seizure process is strong enough to require more than one drug, multiple drug administration needs to be maintained. The aim of the treatment is to achieve the best possible seizure control with the least amount of side effects. This goal may necessitate a compromise in patients with resistant seizures; such patients may prefer having an occasional seizure to being continuously sedated or unsteady. This is particularly true with patients who experience partial seizures that are not excessively disruptive.

The side effects of drugs may cause impairment of liver function in susceptible individuals. Thus, periodic monitoring of the patient's complete blood count and platelet count is necessary, as are liver function tests. This monitoring is done more frequently at the onset of therapy or after an upward adjustment of dosage.

The selection of specific drugs to be used for the prevention and control of seizures depends on the type of seizure. The most commonly used drugs include phenytoin, carbamazepine, phenobarbital, primidone, ethosuximide, methsuximide, clonazepam, valproate sodium, and trimethadione.

The pharmacokinetics and side effects of these drugs in infants and children differ somewhat from those observed in older children and adults. Absorption, plasma-protein binding, and metabolism are subject to age-specific variations. Younger children usually require a higher dose per kilogram to maintain a therapeutic blood level than do adults. Some of the classic signs of toxicity to the medications that are seen in adults may not be obvious in children.

If the seizures are related to a lesion in the brain, neurosurgical treatment is indicated. Surgery is the obvious form of treatment for demonstrable structural lesions such as cysts lying in accessible areas of the cerebral hemispheres. In a more restricted sense, surgical therapy is considered in patients without a mass

lesion when the seizures are unresponsive to drug treatment and the patient has a consistent, electrophysiologically demonstrable focus emanating from, for example, a scar. Specific surgical treatments vary from case to case.

Up to 80 percent of properly selected patients have been found to benefit to some extent from surgical removal of the focal lesion. In some cases of intractable seizures associated with behavior disorders and hemiplegia of childhood, removal of a damaged cerebral hemisphere has been found to control the intractable seizures and improve the behavior disorder without causing further neurological deficit.

Perspective and Prospects

In the twentieth century, major developments were made in diagnosis and therapy. In 1929, Hans Berger recorded the first human electroencephalogram. Descriptions of EEG patterns and their correlation with clinical absences, partial seizures, and generalized tonic-clonic seizures led to important developments in classification and treatment. Special EEG recordings with activation techniques, depth recordings, and long-term recordings for patients with intractable seizures became available to aid in the diagnosis and medical management of patients and in the selection of candidates for possible neurosurgical treatment.

Prolonged EEG recording by telemetry (the transmission of data electronically to a distant location) and ambulatory monitoring became helpful in making a diagnosis in patients who have brief spells of uncertain type. Electrical activity at the time of the attack can be documented. Videotaping with split-screen EEG recording and patient observation allows excellent correlation between the clinical and EEG manifestations, which aids in the classification and determination of appropriate therapy in difficult clinical problems. In those patients with intractable epilepsy, prolonged recording can document the frequency of seizures and correlation with anticonvulsive drug blood levels.

Radiological advances and CT scans in the 1970's, and later positron emission tomography (PET) scans, improved diagnostic skill in delineating potentially remediable lesions in patients with seizures.

During the twentieth century, many other medications became available for patients with seizures. The use of the operating microscope and technical advances in microsurgical techniques refined surgical treatments and improved the outlook for patients with structural lesions such as brain tumors, vascular malformations, and scars.

—*Genevieve Slomski, Ph.D.*

See also Addiction; Alcoholism; Arteriosclerosis; Bites and stings; Brain; Brain disorders; Eclampsia; Electroencephalography (EEG); Epilepsy; Head and neck disorders; Headaches; Hypoglycemia; Ischemia; Lead poisoning; Neuralgia, neuritis, and neuropathy; Neurology; Neurology, pediatric; Rabies; Schizophrenia; Sleep disorders; Snakebites; Strokes and TIAs; Tetanus; Tumors.

FOR FURTHER INFORMATION:

Levy, Rene H., Richard H. Mattson, and Brian S. Meldrum, eds. *Antiepileptic Drugs.* 4th ed. New York: Raven Press, 1995. This useful work offers a quantitative analysis and interpretation of the drugs most often used in the treatment of recurrent seizures.

Millichap, J. Gordon. *Febrile Convulsions.* New York: Macmillan, 1967. This work discusses febrile seizures, which are usually associated with upper-respiratory tract infection, pharyngitis, or otitis media. The author states that fever may be the triggering factor in the developing brain, since febrile seizures rarely occur in older age groups.

Rowan, A. James, and John R. Gates, eds. *Non-Epileptic Seizures.* 2d ed. Boston: Butterworth-Heinemann, 2000. This book draws together a multidisciplinary perspective on the most current state of knowledge of paroxysmal events that suggest a diagnosis of epilepsy but that are not of epileptic origin.

Solomon, Gail, et al. *Clinical Management of Seizures.* 2d ed. Philadelphia: W. B. Saunders, 1983. Offers comprehensive treatment of seizures. After a brief historical perspective, the authors discuss the physiology, chemistry, and pharmacology of seizures; their classification; epidemiology and predisposing factors; treatment; and special management problems. Contains numerous charts, graphs, and illustrations.

SELF-MEDICATION

TREATMENT

ALSO KNOWN AS: Self-treatment, medications management

ANATOMY OR SYSTEM AFFECTED: All

SPECIALTIES AND RELATED FIELDS: All

DEFINITION: Self-administration of drugs without the direction or supervision of a physician.

KEY TERMS:

compliance: taking drugs as directed by a physician; completing therapeutic activities in proper fashion, as directed by a health care provider

drug interactions: the chemical effects of taking drugs in combination, where the effects will reduce, magnify, or alter the desired effects of the drug

illicit drugs: drugs that are illegal to possess, have addiction potential, and lack approved medical uses

over-the-counter drugs: pharmaceutical products, vitamins, herbal remedies, and other medicines that can be purchased by anyone, without a doctor's prescription

palliative care: care that decreases the suffering associated with health conditions by reducing the severity of symptoms, but does not provide a cure

prescription drugs: medicines that can only be obtained with the prescription of a doctor

INDICATIONS AND PROCEDURES

Every day, millions of people take medicinal drugs. Usually this is because they are experiencing symptoms, want to experience a particular feeling, or want to prevent a problem from developing and have information leading them to believe that the drug is the answer. For some, this occurs under the direction of a physician through the use of prescription medications. For others, this occurs through self-medication as a form of treatment. Most popularly, there are those who, through advertisements or personal experience, have learned that certain over-the-counter medications or popular legal drugs (such as cigarettes or alcohol) can be used to alleviate symptoms, provide palliative care, or cause certain symptoms or feelings. Others, via self-knowledge or guidance from alternative medicine specialists, will use teas, herbal remedies, and vitamins to achieve these same goals. Similarly, others may use illicit drugs to self-medicate in order to adjust their mood, physical feelings, or other abilities. For these individuals, it may be that they have didactic knowledge about drug properties or have learned about drug effects through their experience with drugs. Relatedly, even those receiving prescribed drugs may abuse those drugs by using them in ways unapproved by their doctor. This may be due to judgments that they need more of less of the drug or need to mix it with something else to get the desired effect(s). Together, access to drugs, knowledge of dosages and drug effects, and having a culture that encourages use of medicinal remedies and drugs all contribute to self-medication.

USES AND COMPLICATIONS

Drug interactions are one of the biggest dangers of self-medication. When individuals mix different medicines, legal, or illegal drugs, there is a risk that they may cause themselves harm. Some drug interactions can cause medicinal drugs to be less effective for treating the condition needing attention. Others can lead to substantial discomfort or more serious conditions such as seizures or death. Similar problems can come from mixing certain medicinal substances and herbal remedies with each other or with certain foods. As such, anyone using self-medication as a treatment strategy should learn as much as possible about the drug(s) they are taking.

Another problem of self-medication as a style of treatment is that unsupervised medical problems can often worsen without proper care. Using alcohol, cigarettes, or marijuana to alleviate conditions such as anxiety or depression may provide relief in the short term, but in the long term such use may worsen the mood problems and lead to substance abuse or dependence. Similarly, taking an antacid or laxative can be helpful for minor gastrointestinal problems, but prolonged use of such drugs can result in dangerous physical conditions not getting much-needed medical attention. Therefore, the limits of self-medication as a strategy must be known.

PERSPECTIVE AND PROSPECTS

More than 30 percent of individuals living in the United States use an over-the-counter drug in any two-day period. It is estimated that 54 percent of three-year-olds receive over-the-counter drugs in any thirty-day period. Elderly adults use 25 percent of all over-the-counter drugs. Research also shows that 70 to 95 percent of all illnesses are managed without physician assistance. Additionally, over-the-counter drugs, herbal remedies, legal drugs, and illicit drugs constitute multibillion-dollar industries. Given these trends, self-medication as a treatment strategy is likely to continue. Increases can be expected as well because it is becoming easier to gain knowledge about how to use drugs safely. Further, the practice of self-medication has the potential to decrease health care costs substantially by reducing the need of health care services, conserving valuable physician time.

The presence of self-medication as a positive force, however, must be balanced against problems such as a lack of compliance with medication regimens and the use of illicit and legal drugs to manage untreated mental and physical illnesses. When people do not take medicines as directed or fail to get proper medical treatment, problems can worsen. Work in the health care field therefore will need to address the longer-term problems that can develop as a result of these types of practices. Such investments may require increased time from service providers for purposes such as assessment and diagnosis, so as to uncover the hidden illnesses causing individuals to look for medicinal help in the first place. Additionally, barriers to treatment will have to be brought down so as to allow individuals who need medical and other health care to get the help they deserve.

—*Nancy A. Piotrowski, Ph.D.*

See also Addiction; Alcoholism; Alternative medicine; Antioxidants; Herbal medicine; Internet medicine; Pain management; Pharmacology; Pharmacy; Smoking; Supplements; Vitamins and minerals; Weight loss medications.

FOR FURTHER INFORMATION:

Chamberlain, Logan. *What the Labels Won't Tell You: A Consumer's Guide to Herbal Supplements*. Loveland, Colo.: Interweave Press, 1998.

Gorman, Jack M. *The Essential Guide to Psychiatric Drugs*. 3d ed. New York: St. Martin's Press, 1997.

Graedon, Joe, and Teresa Graedon. *The People's Guide to Deadly Drug Interactions: How to Protect Yourself from Life-Threatening Drug/Drug, Drug/Food, Drug/Vitamin Combinations*. New York: St. Martin's Press, 1995.

Hazelden Foundation. *The Dual Disorders Recovery Book*. Center City, Minn.: Author, 1993.

Rapp, Robert P., and Aimee R. Gelhot, eds. *The Pill Book Guide to Over-the-Counter Medications: The Illustrated Guide to the Most Commonly Used Non-Prescription Medications*. New York: Bantam, 1998.

Vandeputte, Charles. *Alcohol, Medications, and Older Adults: A Guide for Families and Other Caregivers*. St. Paul, Minn.: Johnson Institute, 1991.

Weil, Andrew, and Steven Petrow. *Common Illnesses: Ask Dr. Weil*. New York: Ivy Books, 1997.

Woolis, Rebecca. *When Someone You Love Has a Mental Illness: A Handbook for Family, Friends, and Caregivers*. New York: Tarcher/Putnam, 1992.

SENILITY. *See* **DEMENTIAS.**

SENSE ORGANS
ANATOMY
ANATOMY OR SYSTEM AFFECTED: Ears, eyes, gastrointestinal system, mouth, nerves, nervous system, nose, skin

SPECIALTIES AND RELATED FIELDS: Audiology, dentistry, dermatology, neurology, ophthalmology, optometry, otorhinolaryngology

DEFINITION: Specialized structures anatomically suited to a particular sense—the eyes for vision, the nose for smell (olfaction), the taste buds for taste, the ears for hearing and balance, and the skin for such cutaneous sensations as warmth, cold, light touch, deep pressure, and pain.

KEY TERMS:

chemoreception: sensitivity to chemical stimuli

cochlear: referring to the parts of the ear concerned with hearing

cutaneous: occurring within the skin

photoreception: sensitivity to light

retina: the light-sensitive part of the eye

stimulus: anything capable of producing a response

vestibular: referring to the parts of the ear concerned with balance

STRUCTURE AND FUNCTIONS

The sense organs of the body include the cutaneous sense organs, the organs of chemical reception, the organs of vision or sight, and the organs of hearing and balance. The skin is the major organ of sensation for touch, pressure, cold, warmth, and pain; the nasal epithelium and taste buds are the major organs of chemoreception; the eyes are the major organs of vision or sight; and the ears are the major organs of both hearing and balance.

There are five types of cutaneous receptors within the skin, each with a different type of sensory nerve ending and each with a different spatial pattern of distribution. Free (naked) nerve endings are sensitive to pain and are widely distributed over the body's skin surface, especially at the base of each hair. Overstimulation of any type of nerve ending also results in a sensation of pain, but these nerve endings are so exposed that any stimulation at all is felt as an overstimulation. All the remaining cutaneous receptors are encapsulated in one of several types of end organs. Of these, the end bulbs of Krause are sensitive to cold; they are most numerous around the conjunctiva

of the eye and along the glans of the penis and the glans of the clitoris.

The Pacinian corpuscles each contain a single central nerve fiber, enclosed in many concentric layers of semitransparent tissue resembling the bulb of an onion. These structures, which are about 2 to 4 millimeters in diameter, are sensitive to deep pressure and are distributed throughout the skin, principally within the dermal papillae. They are most numerous on the palm of the hand, the sole of the foot, and on the insides of many joints such as the front of the elbow or the back of the knee. The tactile (Meissner's) corpuscles each consist of an oval, bulblike swelling in which the nerve endings run around in spiral patterns at right angles to the long axis. Meissner's corpuscles are sensitive to light touch and are most numerous along the fingertips (and the hand in general), the tongue and lips, parts of the eye, and the skin of the mammary nipple or papilla. The corpuscles of Ruffini are enclosed in connective tissue sheaths perpendicular to the nerve which serves them. The axons of this nerve branch repeatedly within the corpuscle and these branches intertwine, each ending in a tiny knob. Corpuscles of Ruffini are sensitive to warmth and are very numerous over the fingertips, the forearm, and the skin of the face. The evidence to associate particular nerve endings with particular sensations (such as the Meissner's corpuscles with light touch) comes largely from patterns of spatial distribution: The areas of the body most sensitive to touch are also those with the highest densities of Meissner's corpuscles.

Neuromuscular spindles occur in most voluntary muscles and are sensitive to the state of contraction or relaxation of the muscle fibers. The spindle consists of a muscle fiber or small bundle of such fibers, around which are wrapped several turns of infrequently branching sensory nerve endings. The tendons of many muscles also frequently contain neurotendinous spindles, encapsulated structures in which a bundle of tendon fibers receive branched nerve endings. These nerve endings branch slightly just before reaching the tendon fibers, but then lose their sheaths and branch profusely within the tendon. These neurotendinous spindles act as stretch receptors, sensitive to the state of stretching of the tendon.

Chemoreceptors of the body include those tissues sensitive to certain chemicals. The carotid body, a swelling within the carotid artery of the neck, contains tissue sensitive to the carbon dioxide or acid

The Five Senses

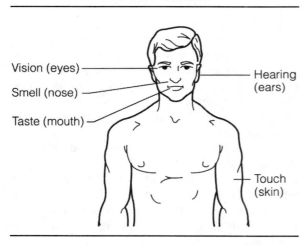

Vision (eyes)

Smell (nose)

Taste (mouth)

Hearing (ears)

Touch (skin)

content of the blood; it stimulates the breathing reflex when the carbon dioxide level is too high. The taste buds of the tongue are sensitive to the taste of a variety of chemical substances present in moderate concentrations. Each taste bud contains gustatory cells along with nonsensitive supporting (sustentacular) cells. Experimental evidence points to four basic types of taste sensations: sweet (like sugar), bitter (like quinine), sour (like vinegar or citric acid), and salty (like sodium chloride). Sensitivity to each of these four basic tastes has its own characteristic pattern of distribution over the tongue and palate.

The nasal epithelium is responsible for olfaction or smell, which is a sensitivity to chemical substances in much smaller concentrations. Most of the nasal epithelium is associated with the nose and the nasal passages, but a small part of this epithelium has become attached instead to the roof of the mouth, where it forms the vomeronasal (Jacobsohn's) organ, which "smells" the contents of the mouth (mostly food). The nasal epithelium is structurally unusual in that the cell bodies of the sensory cells originate within the epithelium and their nerve endings (axons) migrate inwardly to the brain, through the cribriform plate, forming the first cranial nerve or olfactory nerve. All other sensory nerves in the body grow outward from the central nervous system, and their cell bodies are located where their growth began.

Attempts have been made to classify smells according to a scheme similar to the bitter-sweet-sour-salty system used for tastes, but there are many more basic smells than there are tastes—lists vary from seven to twenty to more than ninety—and there is no general agreement on any of these schemes.

The eyes are the body's principal visual receptors. (Some evidence also exists of the brain's own ability to sense daily changes in the level of light intensity, especially in the pineal body.) The primary parts of the eye include the eyelids, cornea, lens, ciliary body, iris diaphragm, pupil, aqueous humor, vitreous humor, retina, choroid coat, scleroid coat, and optic nerve. The eyelids protect the front of the eye and prevent injury to the eye by closing. The cornea is the transparent covering of the front of the eye, the lens is the transparent, almost spherical body that focuses rays of incoming light onto the retina, and the ciliary body is a largely connective tissue structure (also containing some muscle tissue) that supports the lens. The colored part of the ciliary body is the iris diaphragm; muscle fibers within the iris diaphragm adjust the size of the pupil for different brightness levels of light. The opening in the middle of the iris diaphragm is called the pupil. The aqueous humor is the watery fluid in front of the lens, while the vitreous humor is the thick, jellylike fluid behind the lens.

The light-sensitive portion of the eye is the retina. It is almost spherical in shape and consists of two layers: a sensory layer on the inside (closer to the front) and a pigment layer surrounding and behind the sensory layer. Within the sensory layer are contained both the rods, which are sensitive to finer details, and the cones, which are sensitive to colors. The eye's most sensitive area is called the area centralis; it is centered upon a depression called the fovea. The choroid coat is the connective tissue layer immediately surrounding the retina, which is continuous with the pia mater that surrounds the brain. The scleroid coat is the stronger connective tissue layer that surrounds the choroid coat; it is continuous with the dura mater surrounding the brain. The optic nerve fibers originate from the sensory layer of the retina, where they converge toward a spot called the blind spot, marking the place where the nerve fibers turn inward toward the brain. A majority of the optic nerve fibers cross over to the opposite side of the brain via the optic chiasma, but a small proportion of the fibers remains on the same side without crossing over. Experiments on the physiology of vision have led researchers to conclude that there are three separate types of color receptors (cones) in the retina, sensitive principally to red, green, and blue regions of the spectrum. All other color sensations can be simulated experimentally in people with normal vision by a suitable combination of red, green, and blue stimuli.

The ears are special sense organs devoted to the two distinct functions of hearing and balance. The ear may be divided anatomically into outer, middle, and inner portions or functionally into a cochlear portion for hearing and a vestibular portion for balance. The outer (external) ear consists of a flap called the pinna (or external ear flap) and a tubelike cavity called the external acoustic meatus. Within the external ear, sound impulses exist as waves of compressed or decompressed (rarefied) air, forming a series of longitudinal waves that vibrate in the same direction in which they are transmitted. The tympanic membrane (eardrum) is a vibrating membrane which marks the boundary between the outer and middle ears.

The middle ear consists of a cavity containing three tiny bones, the auditory ossicles. Within the middle ear, the vibrations of the tympanic membrane set up a series of vibrations within these tiny bones. The three auditory ossicles are called the malleus (hammer), incus (anvil), and stapes (stirrup). The malleus gets its name from its hammerlike shape, which includes a long handle (the manubrium) extending across the tympanic membrane. The incus, the second of the auditory ossicles, rests against the malleus at one end and the stapes at the other. The stapes is shaped like a stirrup, in which the foot is placed when riding a horse. The flat base of the stapes is called the footplate, in analogy to the corresponding part of a stirrup; this footplate rests against the fenestra ovalis of the inner ear. The opening in the stapes is penetrated by an artery called the stapedial artery. The cavity of the middle ear connects to the pharynx by means of a tube, the pharyngotympanic or Eustachian tube.

The inner ear is entirely housed within the petrosal bone. It can be divided into cochlear (hearing) and vestibular (balance) portions. The cochlear portion of the inner ear begins with two windows, the fenestra ovalis (oval window) and fenestra rotundum (round window), communicating between the middle ear and the inner ear. Behind the fenestra ovalis lies a vestibule, filled with a fluid called perilymph and extending into a long scala vestibuli. Behind the fenestra rotundum lies another long tube, the scala tympani, also filled with perilymph and running parallel to the scala vestibuli. Between these two tubes lies a third, the scala media or cochlear duct, filled with a different fluid called endolymph. Together, the

three are prolonged into a spiral coil called the cochlea (Latin for "snail"), which has a bit more than three complete turns. At the end of this coil, the scala media ends, and the scala vestibuli and scala tympani join with one another by means of an intervening loop called the helicotrema. The basilar membrane separates the scala tympani and the cochlear duct. The spiral organ (organ of Corti) runs within the cochlear duct along the basilar membrane, not far beneath a tectorial membrane that is suspended within the cochlear duct.

The outer ear receives vibrations that travel through the air and transmits these vibrations to the tympanic membrane. In the middle ear, the vibrations of the tympanic membrane are transmitted through the malleus, incus, and stapes to the oval window. These vibrations are transmitted through the perilymph of the inner ear (vestibular portion), where they cause vibrations of the basilar membrane. The vibrating basilar membrane causes vibrations within the endolymph and also in the tectorial membrane, but the tectorial membrane is less flexible than the basilar membrane, creating regions of greater and lesser pressure within the endolymph. The hair cells of the spiral organ are sensitive to these pressure differences and send out nerve impulses to the brain, where they are interpreted as sounds.

The vestibular portion of the inner ear includes two interconnected chambers called the sacculus and the utriculus, both filled with endolymph. The sacculus has a downward extension called the lagena, and it also connects into the scala media of the cochlear portion of the ear. From the utriculus emerge three semicircular ducts, approximately at right angles to one another, all filled with endolymph: an anterior vertical duct, a posterior vertical duct, and a horizontal duct. Each semicircular duct runs through a bony semicircular canal, filled with perilymph. Each duct has a bulblike swelling, the ampulla, at one end. Each ampulla has a patch, or macula, of sensory structures called neuromasts, which are sensitive to movements in fluids such as endolymph. Other maculae, or patches of neuromasts, are located in the sacculus, the utriculus, and the lagena.

The vestibular portion of the inner ear is sensitive to movements and especially to acceleration. Normally, this acceleration is caused by gravity, but nonlinear movements (such as the swerving of a fast-moving vehicle around a curve) may also result in accelerations that cause fluid movements within the semicircular canals. These movements are perceived by the sensitive hair cells (neuromasts) within each ampulla. Spinning around or other sudden acceleration causes temporary dizziness (vertigo) and a consequent loss of balance.

DISORDERS AND DISEASES

Several types of medical specialists deal with problems of the various sense organs: Ophthalmologists deal with diseases of the eye; otorhinolaryngologists deal with diseases of the ears (oto), nose (rhino), and throat (larynx); and neurologists deal with all the senses. All these specialists first conduct diagnostic tests in order to detect any sensory malfunction and to determine the probable cause; they then provide whatever treatment may be available for each condition.

The ability to distinguish tastes diminishes gradually with age in older persons as the number of gustatory cells declines, but complete loss of taste is rare. Persons with diminished taste are at greater risk for accidental poisoning. Except for the decline of taste among the elderly, other defects of smell or taste are rare and are usually indicative of more serious neurological problems such as brain damage or nerve damage. The inability to smell is a rare condition known as anosmia. Loss of cutaneous sensations, even over a small portion of the body, is usually indicative of nerve damage.

Disorders of the eye range from easily correctable visual problems to total blindness. Impaired function of one or more of the three types of color receptors results in one of the several types of color blindness. The most common type, red-green color blindness, is inherited as a sex-linked recessive trait and is thus more common in men than in women. Blindness may result from various defects or injuries: A defective lens or cornea may limit vision to large objects, and a defective retina may limit perception to light and darkness only. Total blindness results if the optic nerve is damaged or missing. More common visual defects include myopia (nearsightedness), hyperopia (farsightedness), and astigmatism (differences in vision along different axes), all of which can be corrected with glasses or contact lenses or by surgical procedures. A failure of the mechanism that drains fluid from the interior of the eyeball may result in a buildup of ocular pressure, a condition known as glaucoma. In times past, when treatment for glaucoma was not readily available, most cases resulted in permanent blindness.

Glaucoma can now be treated, however, either surgically or with drugs. Several changes occur to the lens of the eye in older individuals. As the lens becomes more rigid with advancing age, reading and other near-vision tasks become more difficult, a condition known as presbyopia. Also frequent among older people are cataracts, tiny opaque grains that cloud up the lens and reduce the ability to see clearly. Untreated cataracts may eventually result in blindness, but various forms of treatment are available to prevent this from occurring.

Diseases of the ear should always be treated as serious. Tinnitus, or ringing in the ears, can result from damage to the hair cells of the organ of Corti. Damage to the auditory nerve can result in deafness. Upper-respiratory infections can travel up the Eustachian tube and cause a common childhood infection of the middle ear known as otitis media. Infections of the vestibular portion of the inner ear can result in recurrent or permanent dizziness (vertigo) because the inflamed cells transmit impulses that the body wrongly interprets as resulting from accelerations in unusual directions. Some plant poisons (or the drugs derived from them, such as ipecac) can also impair the function of the inner ear and result in sensations of dizziness, often followed by nausea and by the vomiting of the plant containing the poison. This reaction may have evolved as an adaptive response to possible poisons; the same reaction also results in vomiting in other situations that cause unusual accelerations in the vestibular portion of the inner ear, as in the case of seasickness or other motion sickness.

PERSPECTIVE AND PROSPECTS

The many biblical references to deafness and blindness show that ancient civilizations were concerned about the proper functioning of the sense organs. The Greek philosopher Aristotle, also considered the greatest biologist of antiquity, enumerated five senses: touch, hearing, taste, smell, and sight. Detailed anatomical descriptions of the sense organs were made during the Renaissance by Bartolommeo Eustachio (or Eustachius) (1520-1574), after whom the Eustachian tube is named; by Giulio Casserio (1552?-1616); and by Andreas Vesalius (1514-1564), whose superbly illustrated texts set new standards for art as well as science. Further discoveries were made by such anatomists as Alfonso Corti (1822-1876), who first described the detailed internal structure of the inner ear. The detailed cellular structure of the retina was first elucidated by the Nobel Prize-winning anatomist and histologist Santiago Ramón y Cajal (1852-1934). Other anatomists who expanded the understanding of the microscopic anatomy of sensory structures include Abraham Vater (1684-1751), Filippo Pacini (1812-1883), Georg Meissner (1829-1905), and Jan Evangelista Purkinje (1787-1869).

—Eli C. Minkoff, Ph.D.

See also Aromatherapy; Astigmatism; Audiology; Cataract surgery; Cataracts; Dermatology; Ear surgery; Ears; Eye surgery; Eyes; Hearing loss; Microscopy, slitlamp; Myopia; Nasal polyp removal; Nasopharyngeal disorders; Nervous system; Numbness and tingling; Ophthalmology; Optometry; Otorhinolaryngology; Skin; Skin disorders; Smell; Systems and organs; Taste; Touch; Visual disorders.

For Further Information:

Agur, Anne M. R., and Ming J. Lee. *Grant's Atlas of Anatomy.* 10th ed. Baltimore: Williams & Wilkins, 1999. This text contains many excellent, detailed illustrations.

Crouch, James E. *Functional Human Anatomy.* 4th ed. Philadelphia: Lea & Febiger, 1985. A very readable book with good explanations. A good reference work for the general reader.

Davson, Hugh, ed. *The Eye.* 4 vols. 3d ed. Orlando, Fla.: Academic Press, 1984. A very thorough compendium of the anatomy, physiology, and optics of the eye.

Gray, Henry. *Gray's Anatomy.* Edited by Peter L. Williams et al. 38th ed. New York: Churchill Livingstone, 1999. A great classic with the most thorough descriptions. The excellent color illustrations offer realistic detail in most cases and well-selected highlights in a few cases.

Rosse, Cornelius, and Penelope Gaddum-Rosse. *Hollinshead's Textbook of Anatomy.* 5th ed. Philadelphia: Lippincott-Raven, 1997. A very thorough, modern, detailed reference with good descriptions and illustrations.

Wertenbaker, Lael T. *The Eye: Window to the World.* Washington, D.C.: U.S. News Books, 1981. Easy to read and understand, with good illustrations. Written for a popular audience.

Wolf, K. P. *Eyewise: Eye Disorders and Their Treatment.* Philadelphia: Harper & Row, 1982. Written by a practicing ophthalmologist, this book is a well-written description of various treatments for eye disorders, especially radial keratotomy.

Separation anxiety

Development

Anatomy or system affected: Psychic-emotional system

Specialties and related fields: Psychiatry, psychology

Definition: Distress shown at the departure of a caregiver. It is common from ten to eighteen months of age; some children show distress throughout the preschool years.

Physical and Psychological Factors

Infants are often wary or even fearful when someone other than the usual caregiver tries to pick them up. This may be partly attributable to anticipation of separation. In the second year of life, negative reactions to strangers are compounded by toddlers' concerns about separation from the caregiver.

Self-initiated separations and those that are brief, in familiar settings, and explained by the departing caregiver are less likely to elicit distress. Factors that do not seem to be related to separation distress are gender, birth order, and experience within the normal range for a given culture and economic class. Usually, separation anxiety subsides by about three years of age.

Disorders and Effects

Researchers used to think that the intensity of separation distress was an index of the strength of the attachment bond. However, the child's reaction during reunion with the caregiver is a better indicator of the security of attachment.

Child psychiatrists have described an uncommon disorder (with a prevalence of 4 percent) called separation anxiety disorder. This disorder may develop in early childhood after a life stress such as the death of a relative or a change in school or neighborhood. Children with this disorder show excessive anxiety about separation from the caregiver or home. Separation anxiety disorder is long lasting and causes significant disruption to functioning, such as school avoidance, excessive worry about losing caregivers, and fear of being left alone.

A relationship may exist between very strong and long-lasting separation anxiety as an infant and separation anxiety disorder in later life, but infant distress about separation is very common, almost universal, and is usually relatively short-lived. Thus, there is usually little reason to be concerned about separation anxiety in infancy.

—George A. Morgan, Ph.D.,
and Robert J. Harmon, M.D.

See also Anxiety; Bonding; Developmental stages; Emotions: Biomedical causes and effects; Phobias; Psychiatry, child and adolescent.

FOR FURTHER INFORMATION:

Caplan, Theresa. *The First Twelve Months of Life: Your Baby's Growth Month by Month.* New York: Bantam, 1995.

Craig, Grace J., and Marguerite D. Kermis. *Children Today.* Englewood Cliffs, N.J.: Prentice Hall, 1994.

Leach, Penelope. *Your Growing Child: From Babyhood Through Adolescence.* New York: Alfred A. Knopf, 1991.

SEPTICEMIA
DISEASE/DISORDER

ANATOMY OR SYSTEM AFFECTED: Blood, circulatory system

SPECIALTIES AND RELATED FIELDS: Hematology, internal medicine, serology

DEFINITION: Serious, systemic infection of the blood with pathogens that have spread from an infection in a part of the body, characteristically causing fever, chills, prostration, pain, headache, nausea, and/or diarrhea.

KEY TERMS:

antibacterial therapy: treatment for patients with septicemia, best initiated with a combination of antibiotics when the infecting organism is unknown; when cultures define the causative microbe(s) or other data point to a specific organism, therapy can be tailored to the most appropriate, most specific, least toxic, and least expensive single antibiotic

bacteremia: also known as blood poisoning or septicemia; the rapid multiplication of bacteria and the presence of their toxins in the blood, a serious, life-threatening condition

bacteria: microorganisms with a wide variety of biochemical, often pathogenic, properties

septic shock: a dangerous condition in which there is tissue damage and a dramatic drop in blood pressure as a result of septicemia

shock treatment: the immediate treatment of septic shock, including the use of antibiotics and surgery and rapid fluid replacement by infusion

CAUSES AND SYMPTOMS

The rapid multiplication of bacteria and the presence of their toxins in the blood is a condition commonly known as blood poisoning, septicemia, or bacteremia. It is always a serious condition and represents a medical emergency that requires the prompt institution of therapy. A person in whom septicemia develops suddenly becomes seriously ill, with a high fever, chills, rapid breathing, headache, and often clouding of consciousness. Skin rashes or jaundice may occur, and sometimes the hands are unusually warm. In many cases, especially when large amounts of toxins are produced by the circulating bacteria, the person passes into a state of septic shock, which is life-threatening.

Bacteria in the bloodstream can produce two different types of complications: microbiologic and inflammatory. The microbiologic complications result from the local and systemic proliferation and seeding of the bacterial causative organism, which causes direct tissue or organ damage. The inflammatory complications are produced locally and can result in tissue or organ destruction independent of the toxic factors produced by the causative organism. Bacteremia triggers intravascular activation of the same inflammatory systems that are protective within tissues. These systems, which combine with stress-generated endocrine responses, produce a sequence of metabolic events, the end stage of which is the systemic vascular collapse traditionally called septic shock.

Shock symptoms vary with the extent and site of major tissue damage. They are similar to those for septicemia, with additional symptoms including cold hands and feet, often with blue-purple coloration caused by poor blood flow; a weak, rapid pulse; and markedly reduced blood pressure. There may be vomiting and diarrhea, and a poor output of urine may indicate that damage to the kidneys is occurring and that there is risk of renal failure. Heart failure and abnormal bleeding may also occur.

Septic shock is a dangerous condition in which there is tissue damage and a dramatic drop in blood pressure as a result of septicemia. Septic shock is usually preceded by signs of severe infection, often of the genitourinary or gastrointestinal systems. Fever, tachycardia, increased respiration, and confusion or coma may occur during shock. The classic septic shock syndrome results primarily from the sequence of events triggered by bacteremia, during which the bacterial toxins activate compounds that impair the functioning of surrounding cells in several ways. In many cases, the bacterial toxins are the main cause of trouble because they can cause damage to cells and tissues throughout the body and promote clotting of blood in the smallest blood vessels, seriously interfering with circulation. Consequently, damage occurs especially to tissues in the kidneys, heart, and lungs. The bacterial toxins may cause leakage of fluid from blood vessels and a reduction of the ability of the vessels to constrict, leading to a severe drop in blood pressure. Therefore, septic shock is a systematic vascular collapse, in which the systolic blood pressure of the patient is less than 90 millimeters of mercury. In septic shock, the low blood pressure has become unresponsive to adequate volume replacement. Morbidity and mortality associated with septic shock are high: About two-thirds of patients die.

Septicemia and septic shock can precipitate multiple organ failure. As the patient becomes hypermetabolic and febrile with progressive failure of one or more organs, the mortality rate can be as high as 90 percent. Septicemia is most common in people hospitalized with major disorders such as diabetes mellitus, cancer, or cirrhosis and who have a focus of infection somewhere in the body (often the intestines or urinary tract). Progression to septic shock is especially likely for people who have immunodeficiency disorders or are taking immunosuppressant drugs for cancer or an inappropriate antibiotic treatment. Newborn infants are also particularly at risk if septicemia develops.

TREATMENT AND THERAPY

A presumptive diagnosis of septicemia is often made on the basis of historical, physical, and laboratory data even in the absence of proof. The setting in which the episode is occurring should be evaluated promptly. Crucial to appropriate initial decision making are the background history, which may help to define the type of host-defense defect present, and prior blood culture data, which might predict the infecting organism. The physical examination should be quick and thorough, searching for the septic source as well as signs that might indicate progression to shock.

A diagnosis can be confirmed and the infective bacteria identified by growing a culture of the organisms from a blood sample. Several laboratory tests are often helpful in the evaluation of a potentially septic patient. In general, patients with fever should be considered septic until proved otherwise, and ther-

apy should always be initiated for high-risk febrile patients in advance of a microbiologic confirmation of septicemia.

Common microorganisms which enter the bloodstream when the body's defenses break down include staphylococci from boils, abscesses, and wounds; streptococci from the tonsils, throat, or cuts; and pneumococci from the lungs. Other invaders of the bloodstream include the gonococci, the typhoid bacilli in typhoid fever, and *Escherichia coli* in bowel infections. All these bacteria may be detected by taking a blood culture.

Antibacterial therapy should be started as soon as septicemia is suspected. It is normally started by intravenous infusion of antibiotic drugs and glucose and/or saline solution. The focal site of infection is sought immediately and may be surgically removed. Surgical debridement (removal) and drainage of septic foci are especially important, and all severe localized infections should be widely debrided and drained. If the infection is recognized and treated promptly, there is usually a full recovery.

Broad antibacterial coverage is required in patients with severe septicemia. It is best to initiate therapy with a combination of antibiotics when the infecting organism is unknown. When cultures define the causative microbe(s) or other data point to a specific organism, therapy can then be tailored to the most appropriate, most specific, least toxic, and least expensive single antibiotic. Penicillin is usually used to combat staphylococcic, streptococcic, pneumococcic, and gonococcic infections; chloramphenicol and ampicillin are used against typhoid and paratyphoid infections; and neomycin is used against *E. coli* infections. Extreme care must be taken with the administration of chloramphenicol and neomycin because of their toxic side effects.

Antibiotics limit the microbiological complications of bacteremia, but other metabolic events, whether initiated by or independent of bacterial proliferation, may still produce substantial morbidity and mortality. Therefore, therapy in addition to antibiotics is recommended to counter this metabolic sequence.

Septic shock requires immediate treatment, including the use of antibiotics and surgery, rapid fluid replacement by infusion, and the maintenance of urine flow to prevent the effects of renal failure. Other measures must also be taken to raise the blood pressure and to promote a better supply of important nutrients to tissues, such as through intravenous infusion and oxygen therapy. The use of anti-inflammatory drugs is under active investigation.

PERSPECTIVE AND PROSPECTS

Most febrile patients lacking other signs of severe septicemia will usually do well. Such patients usually respond quickly to fluid administration, antibacterial therapy, and drainage of the primary focus of infection. The presence of septic shock, however, dramatically increases morbidity and mortality. Even when the inciting infection is localized, shock is associated with at least 50 percent mortality. Full-blown septic shock has greater than 70 percent mortality. A favorable outcome in a patient in severe shock depends on the skill of management in the intensive care unit. Early diagnosis and therapy of severely septic patients will greatly decrease the morbidity and mortality of these individuals. The best means of preventing bacteremia is the proper care of burns and wounds and prompt application of antiseptic tinctures or preparations to ordinary cuts and tears.

Infections most commonly occur in the hospital setting, where many infected patients become bacteremic. About 5 percent of all hospital patients either are admitted with or develop an infection during hospitalization. This means that the number of patients at risk of developing septic shock is large. The clinician must be familiar with the manifestations and differential diagnosis of the patient who appears to suffer from septic shock and must have in mind rapid, comprehensive diagnostic and therapeutic plans of action. It is important to develop the concept of a preshock phase of septic shock predicated on identifying a subgroup of infected patients more likely than others to develop shock. In such patients, fluids should be administered and broad antibiotic coverage started early. Treatment before shock develops undoubtedly prevents some of the morbidity and mortality associated with septicemia.

—*Maria Pacheco, Ph.D.*

See also Antibiotics; Bacterial infections; Bacteriology; Infection; Poisoning; Shock; Staphylococcal infections; Streptococcal infections; Toxemia; Toxicology.

FOR FURTHER INFORMATION:

Anderson, Kenneth N., ed. *Mosby's Medical, Nursing, and Allied Health Dictionary*. Rev. 5th ed. St. Louis: C. V. Mosby, 1998. Offers a basic presentation of medical terms and concepts.

Bennett, J. Claude, et al., eds. *Cecil Textbook of Medicine*. 21st ed. Philadelphia: W. B. Saunders, 2000. An excellent, concise presentation of the topic. It is recommended that the reader have a good biology/science background.

Clayman, Charles B., ed. *American Medical Association Encyclopedia of Medicine*. New York: Random House, 1994. Offers a good presentation of basic medical concepts in an easy-to-understand way.

Landau, Sidney I., ed. *International Dictionary of Medicine and Biology*. New York: John Wiley & Sons, 1986. An accessible and concise presentation of various medical terms and subjects.

Miller, Benjamin Frank, and Claire B. Keane. *Encyclopedia and Dictionary of Medicine, Nursing, and Allied Health*. 6th ed. Philadelphia: W. B. Saunders, 1997. Gives the reader a good nontechnical presentation of medical terminology.

Strand, Calvin L., and Jonas A. Shulman. *Bloodstream Infections: Laboratory Detection and Clinical Considerations*. Chicago: American Society of Clinical Pathologists, 1988. A technical monograph reviewing the concepts and factors important in the selection and development of optimal blood culture systems for the detection of septicemia.

SEROLOGY

SPECIALTY

ANATOMY OR SYSTEM AFFECTED: Blood, immune system

SPECIALTIES AND RELATED FIELDS: Bacteriology, cytology, hematology, immunology, microbiology, oncology, pathology, preventive medicine, public health, virology

DEFINITION: The study of serum, the liquid portion of blood, the testing of which is used in blood typing, vaccination, diagnosis, and therapy.

KEY TERMS:

antibody: a protein substance produced by lymphocytes in response to an antigen in order to combat bacterial, viral, chemical or other invasive agents in the body

antigen: a chemical substance often on a bacterial or viral surface, containing antigenic determinants that initiate the body's immune response

antigenic determinant: a molecule on the surface of a cell or microorganism that is specific for evoking an immune response

bacteria: single-celled microorganisms that exist throughout the environment

host: the body of the person or animal infected

immunoglobulin: antibody; the globulin fraction of serum protein

microorganism: any bacterium, virus, or other minute organism. Some microorganisms are harmless in the body and in fact many are involved in essential body processes. Some are harmful and cause disease

pathogen: any disease-causing microorganism, such as bacteria, viruses, yeasts, fungi, and spirochetes

seronegative: the test result seen when blood does not contain the specific antibody or antigen being sought and the particular antigen-antibody reaction is not present

seropositive: the test result seen when blood contains the specific antibody or antigen being sought and the particular antigen-antibody reaction is present

SCIENCE AND PROFESSION

The term "serology" comes from the Latin *sero* (serum, a blood liquid) and *ology* (the study of). Many serologic testing procedures have been developed to determine the amount of specific antibodies the individual has circulating in his or her bloodstream. These tests can help the physician diagnose disease conditions and develop appropriate treatment regimens. In order to understand serological testing in relation to blood typing and immunity—two major uses of serology—it is necessary to understand the structure and nature of blood cells and the workings of the human immune system.

The surface of red blood cells contains antigenic determinants that define the individual's blood group. There are more than twenty blood grouping systems; the most common, the ABO system, identifies individuals as being in A, B, AB, or O groups, depending on the antigenic determinant present on their red blood cells. The red blood cells of people in the A group are covered with A antigen, in the B group with B antigen, and in the AB group with both antigens. Red blood cells in the O group have neither A nor B antigens. The antigenic determinant causes the body to produce antibodies against other blood types. For example, if an individual's red blood cells are coated with A antigen, the body will produce antibodies against B antigen. Therefore, if a person with A blood is given B blood cells, these cells will be regarded as foreign, and the body's anti-B antibodies will dissolve them, leading to a severe, life-threatening hemolytic reaction.

All the blood groups in the ABO system are also classified as either negative or positive for Rh factor, another antigen found on the red blood cells, and so named because a similar antigen was first found in rhesus monkeys. About 85 percent of the population is Rh positive; that is, these individuals have Rh antigens on their red blood cells. If an Rh-negative person is given Rh-positive blood, he or she may tolerate the first transfusion, but a severe, even fatal, reaction can occur if a second is given. Furthermore, if an Rh-negative woman becomes pregnant with an Rh-positive baby, she may be exposed to Rh-positive red blood cells and may develop anti-Rh antibodies. This reaction may be of no significance for the first baby, but if a subsequent baby is also Rh-positive, the mother's antibodies will attack and dissolve the red blood cells of the fetus and may cause intrauterine anemia, heart failure, or miscarriage.

As on the red blood cells, there are antigenic determinants on the surfaces of invading microorganisms that trigger the body's immune process: When a virus, bacterium, or other infective agent enters the body, the immune system recognizes the invader as foreign. Once the organism is recognized as an enemy, the body begins to respond with the host-defense mechanism, an intricate process that not only destroys the offending pathogen but also protects against future infection by it.

Two factors determine whether an organism is antigenic and thus will trigger the immune response: First, there must be antigenic determinants present on the organism's surface that the body identifies as foreign, or nonself. Second, the organism must be large enough to carry antigenic determinants on its surface. Antigenic determinants are large molecules; the more there are on the organism's surface, the greater the antigenicity.

Antigens induce the production of certain white blood cells called lymphocytes. There are two basic types of lymphocytes involved in the immune process. One is the T cell, which originates in the bone marrow and travels to the thymus gland, where it becomes specialized for its immune function. The other lymphocyte is the B cell, which originates in the bone marrow and develops fully in the lymph system. T cells and B cells each develop into cells specialized for specific tasks in the immune process.

About 70 percent of T cells become helper-inducer cells, which have various functions. They promote the production of B cells, support B-cell activity, and increase the production of macrophages (cells that destroy foreign substances and dead cells). They also become "memory cells" capable of recognizing a pathogen to which the body has been exposed. If the particular pathogen reenters the body, the memory cells trigger the immune system to synthesize antibodies against it. T cells also become "killer" T cells that attack pathogens directly.

B cells produce the antibodies that are detected in seropositive blood tests. Antibodies, also called immunoglobulins, are rings, chains, or Y-shaped proteins that are carried in blood plasma. There are five groups of immunoglobulins involved in the immune system: IgG, IgA, IgM, IgD, and IgE. IgG makes up about 80 percent of all immunoglobulins and is found in tissue fluid and plasma. Its major function is to combat bacteria and viruses and to neutralize poisonous substances. IgA (13 percent) is found in the secretions of seromucous glands in the nose, gastrointestinal tract, eyes, and lungs. It also combats bacteria and viruses. IgM (6 percent) is found in blood plasma. It reacts with antigens during the first exposure to the disease organism. IgD (less than 1 percent) is found on the surface of most B cells. Its activities are not fully understood, but it is thought to be involved in the production of antibodies. IgE (less than 1 percent) is bound to mast cells found in connective tissue. It promotes allergic reactions.

Antibodies work in two ways—by direct attack on an antigen and by activating a protein complex called a complement. In direct attack, there are four ways in which antibodies destroy antigens: agglutination, which causes antigens to clump together; precipitation, which causes antigens to form insoluble substances; neutralization, which prevents antigens from producing toxic substances; and lysis, which causes the cell walls of antigens to rupture.

The activation of a complement causes three main activities: chemotaxis, which attracts macrophages and other white blood cells to the area, where they can eliminate the pathogens that are present; opsonization, which alters the structure of the antigen cell wall, making it easier for macrophages to engulf and destroy it; and inflammation, a process that helps to prevent the spread of pathogens.

Like T cells, some B cells become memory cells that help prevent reinfection by recognizing and destroying a pathogen that they have previously encountered.

DIAGNOSTIC AND TREATMENT TECHNIQUES

The major use for seronegative-seropositive testing is in blood typing. The patient's blood type is recorded as part of his or her medical history and is required for a blood transfusion to ensure that the patient receives blood from a compatible donor. Blood typing is an activity conducted in, or readily available to, virtually every medical facility. A major example is the Coomb's test, which detects antibodies on red blood cells in the bloodstream and establishes whether the patient has sensitized cells. This information is helpful in cross-matching donor and patient blood and in the diagnosis of hemolytic anemia.

Another important aspect of serologic testing is to determine the immune status of an individual—that is, whether a person or a local population is immune to a specific disease or is susceptible and therefore should be vaccinated. Such tests are geared to the identification of antibodies that protect against certain diseases. These antibodies are created by exposure to the disease-causing microorganism as a result of infection by the organism itself; vaccination, in which a modified form of the microorganism is used to trigger the body's immune response; or immunity that is acquired by a newborn baby from a mother, an immune state that lasts only a few months. A test that comes back seronegative or with very low antibody levels indicates that the patient is not immune to a given disease. A test that comes back seropositive indicates that the patient has circulating antibodies characteristic of a specific disease and that, if the amount of antibodies is high enough, the patient is immune to the disease.

A good example of immune status determination is the testing for hepatitis B surface antigen among health care workers. Hepatitis B is a blood-borne disease that can be transmitted when infected blood or other body fluids enter the bloodstream of another person. Transmission often occurs among health care workers because they are often exposed to the blood and body fluids of patients during operating procedures, dental procedures, or even when the nurse or other health care worker draws blood and is inadvertently stuck with the needle. Tests show that health care workers are seropositive for hepatitis B surface antigen at rates far above the general population. For example, 25 percent of surgeons and dentists become seropositive after five to ten years in practice. These tests prove that some health care workers are at high risk for contracting hepatitis B from their patients.

Therefore, routine vaccination is recommended for those health care workers who are likely to be exposed to the blood and body fluids of patients carrying the hepatitis B virus.

Seronegative-seropositive testing can also reveal whether a person who has been vaccinated against a certain disease has achieved immunity (has "seroconverted" and developed antibodies in response to the antigen), whether the individual has not achieved immunity, or whether the individual has achieved immunity and then lost it.

No vaccine is 100 percent effective, but the better ones induce an immune response in 90 to 98 percent of individuals. For example, measles vaccine is about 95 percent effective. This means that most of the children who have received it are immune to measles, but 5 percent or so remain susceptible.

A few vaccines produce lifelong immunity. With most, however, the amount of antibody diminishes after time, and the vaccination must be repeated to maintain immunity. In other words, the patient is given a "booster" shot. In the late 1980's, many children who had received measles vaccine and who had seroconverted were found to be seronegative: They had lost their immunity to measles. This finding suggested that the measles vaccine conveyed an immunity that could diminish with time. Therefore, medical authorities and public health organizations revised their recommendations for mass vaccination against measles. Instead of only one vaccination of the infant at twelve to fifteen months of age, the protocol now recommends repeating the vaccination at a later date.

Serologic tests are used in virtually all branches of medicine. One group of seronegative-seropositive tests is used to detect fetal abnormalities. Another group, autoantibody tests, detects such diseases as autoimmune hepatitis, thyroiditis, and lupus erythematosus. One example is testing for rheumatoid factor, an antibody that appears in the blood of adult patients with rheumatoid arthritis. Its presence will help the physician make a diagnosis and determine a course of treatment for a patient with joint inflammation. Similarly, specific antibodies will indicate specific disease conditions. A patient with lupus erythematosus has antinuclear antibody (ANA). Rheumatic fever diagnosis requires evidence of the bacteria *Streptococcus pyogenes*. Syphilis patients have antibodies to the spirochete *Treponema pallidum*. Patients with mononucleosis are seropositive for heterophile antibodies.

Viral, bacterial, and fungal tests detect antibodies or antigens developed in response to infection. These include the antistreptolysin-O test for streptococcal antibodies, the febrile agglutination test to detect diseases caused by salmonella, and the latex particle agglutination (LPA) tests for antigens of other bacteria. Also in this group are the hepatitis-B surface and core antigen tests, which are used to screen blood donors as well as to identify persons who have been exposed to hepatitis B. Fungal serology tests are used to detect various fungal infections. The fluorescent treponemal antibody absorption test is used to diagnose syphilis.

Serologic tests called general humoral tests are used to detect and diagnose various bodily dysfunctions. Another group called the general cellular tests includes the lymphocyte transformation test to determine whether transplant donors and recipients are compatible. In this group, the terminal deoxynucleotidyl transferase test is used to diagnose leukemias and lymphomas, as well as to monitor the progress of treatment. In cancer therapy, the carcinoembryonic antigen test (CEA) is used to gauge the response of certain cancers to treatment or to detect the recurrence of certain cancers.

A major new field for serology is emerging with monoclonal antibody research. In this science, antibodies can be manufactured in the laboratory. Instead of injecting a patient with modified antigen and inducing the body to create antibodies to it (as in vaccination) physicians can provide the patient with the antibodies themselves. Because these antibodies are absolutely identical to their parent protein or cell and to one another, they are not subject to the variables present in antibodies produced by other methods. They have properties that make them ideal for treating certain diseases.

Once the analysis of tissue identifies a specific antigen, it may be possible to program monoclonal antibodies to search out and destroy them. It is also possible to link the antibodies to chemotherapeutic agents. Thus, monoclonal antibodies not only can target specific antigens but also can bring medication to the specific tissues where it is required. In cancer therapy, these qualities promise to improve the efficiency of treatment greatly. With monoclonal antibodies, cancer-destroying drugs can be brought directly to the cancer cell and can destroy it without harming other body tissues, thus reducing the severity of side effects from chemotherapy.

PERSPECTIVE AND PROSPECTS

The science of serology and serological testing for antibodies and antigens in the body have become mainstays of modern medical diagnosis and treatment for a wide range of diseases. Virtually every individual in the industrialized world and most members of the Third World urban populations undergo serologic testing as part of their regular medical routine.

Serological testing is part of every hospital workup, almost every routine medical examination, every blood transfusion, all transplant procedures, many diagnostic procedures, and many treatment regimens. It is the basis for most epidemiological studies that enumerate the extent of susceptibility to individual diseases in various populations and hence directs the development of immunization programs. It is an integral part of vaccine production and is critical in the development of new vaccines. With the development of monoclonal antibody research, serology enters a new era where the possibilities of improved serologic testing and therapeutic modalities seem almost unlimited.

So far, serological testing and therapy have been based on the manipulation and modification of living organisms. It is theoretically possible to develop vaccines and therapeutic agents that are completely synthetic in structure. This science promises greater specificity and efficacy, both for vaccines and for disease treatment.

—C. Richard Falcon

See also Anemia; Blood and blood disorders; Blood testing; Cholesterol; Cytology; Cytopathology; Dialysis; Fluids and electrolytes; Forensic pathology; Hematology; Hematology, pediatric; Hemophilia; Hodgkin's disease; Host-defense mechanisms; Hypercholesterolemia; Hyperlipidemia; Hypoglycemia; Immune system; Immunology; Immunopathology; Jaundice; Laboratory tests; Leukemia; Malaria; Pathology; Rh factor; Septicemia; Sickle-cell anemia; Thalassemia; Toxemia; Transfusion.

FOR FURTHER INFORMATION:

Bryant, Neville J. *An Introduction to Immunohematology.* 3d ed. Philadelphia: W. B. Saunders, 1994. This book was written as a background text for laboratory personnel and students. Somewhat technical, but the writing is clear and the author covers the subject well.

Chase, Allan. *Magic Shots.* New York: William Morrow, 1982. An excellent history of immunization that covers ancient medical practice and describes the work of such early pioneers as Edward Jenner and Louis Pasteur. Details the major discoveries that have taken place in the twentieth century, such as the development of the polio vaccine and the eradication of smallpox.

Griffith, H. W. *Complete Guide to Medical Tests.* Tucson, Ariz.: Fisher Books, 1988. A complete compendium of all tests used in hospitals and other medical facilities. All current seronegative-seropositive tests are described and categorized according to their diagnostic and therapeutic uses.

Larson, David E., ed. *Mayo Clinic Family Health Book.* 2d ed. New York: William Morrow, 1996. A superior medical reference for the general reader.

Widmann, Frances K. *An Introduction to Clinical Immunology and Serology.* Philadelphia: F. A. Davis, 1998. Discusses immunology, immunopathology, and serologic testing methods. Includes bibliographical references and an index.

SEX CHANGE SURGERY

PROCEDURE

ANATOMY OR SYSTEM AFFECTED: Breasts, endocrine system, genitals, glands, reproductive system, uterus

SPECIALTIES AND RELATED FIELDS: Endocrinology, general surgery, gynecology, plastic surgery, psychiatry, psychology, urology

DEFINITION: A set of procedures designed to convert the secondary sexual characteristics of an anatomic male to a female or an anatomic female to a male.

KEY TERMS:

labia: the folds of tissue along the external portion of a woman's vagina and urethra

testosterone: the male sex hormone that gives rise to male fertility and secondary sexual characteristics, such as body hair and musculature

transsexuals: individuals who genuinely believe that they exist in a body of the wrong sex, despite the fact that they are anatomically normal

urethra: the tube through which urine is conducted from the bladder to the outside of the body

INDICATIONS AND PROCEDURES

Sex change surgery is performed to allow an individual's gender identity to conform to his or her anatomic sex. In some cases, an individual is born with ambiguous genitalia and this condition is not corrected shortly after birth to conform to chromosomal sexual identity. Anatomical changes at puberty may

The Steps Involved in Sex Change Surgery

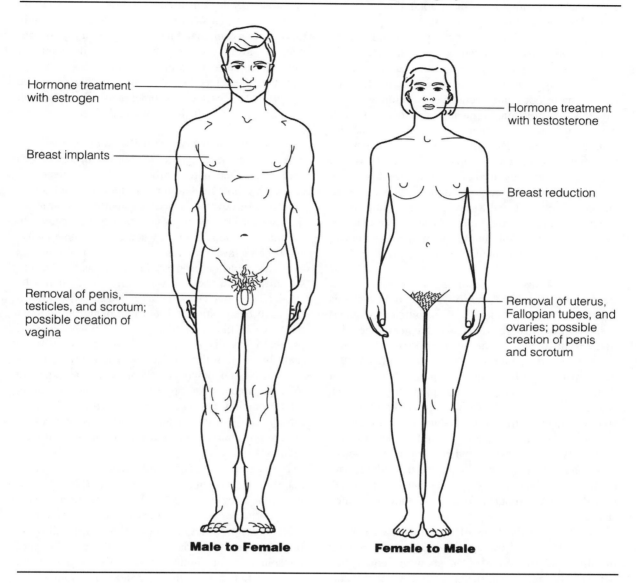

Hormone treatment with estrogen

Breast implants

Removal of penis, testicles, and scrotum; possible creation of vagina

Male to Female

Hormone treatment with testosterone

Breast reduction

Removal of uterus, Fallopian tubes, and ovaries; possible creation of penis and scrotum

Female to Male

conflict with such an individual's gender identity, and thus surgery may be used to correct the discrepancy. More commonly, this surgery is performed on adult individuals who are absolutely certain that they are trapped within the body of the wrong sex, which causes them severe distress. Extensive psychological tests are performed on individuals seeking to embark on the irreversible change of their anatomic sex.

In male-to-female surgery, the penis, testicles, and scrotum are removed and may be replaced by a va-

gina and labia. Prior to surgery, the patient has taken estrogen supplements. In the surgery itself, the surgeon dissects out each testicle through an incision at the base of the penis and ties off the spermatic cords. The skin and urethra are separated from the penis, and a tunnel for the vagina is created from skin at the base of the urethra. A scalpel is used to remove the base of the penis. The lower abdominal and penile skin is sutured to the pubic bone, and some of this skin is used to create a vagina. A lubricated glass mold is inserted into the vagina to prevent shrinkage, and labia are formed from the scrotal skin.

During female-to-male surgery, breasts and hormone-secreting reproductive organs are removed and replaced with male secondary sexual characteristics. Prior to surgery, the patient undertakes a program of body-building exercises and testosterone supplements that promote body and facial hair development and suppress menstruation. Surgical procedures begin with the removal of excess breast tissue, in a procedure similar to breast reduction, and with a hysterectomy to remove the uterus, Fallopian tubes, and ovaries, with their female sex hormones. At a later date, a penis may be constructed from abdominal wall tissue and/or a skin graft and a scrotum containing plastic "testicles" formed from labia. An inflatable cylinder in the penis and a fluid pump within the scrotum can be used to simulate erection.

USES AND COMPLICATIONS

Because of the critical and irreversible nature of this type of surgery, the American Psychological Association has developed guidelines for diagnosing genuine transsexualism and for defining who should be considered for sex change surgery in the United States. Transsexuals must feel an inappropriateness about their anatomic sex, have attempted to obtain sex change surgery persistently for at least two years in spite of rejection for the procedure, have no genetic defects or psychiatric disorders, and be past the age of puberty. In earlier cases, when such rigorous selection criteria were not in effect, some individuals who obtained sex change surgery experienced such social, sexual, and psychological trauma that they committed suicide.

Potential complications of male-to-female surgery include infection of incisions, closure of the urethral opening, and formation of an abnormal connection between the vagina and rectum, all of which are correctable. Long-term effects include dryness and potential shrinkage of the artificial vagina, unless the mold is worn the majority of the time, and an inability to achieve orgasm except through mental stimulation. Individuals may opt for breast augmentation surgery and must take female hormones for at least one year, perhaps for life, to maintain fat deposits on breasts and hips. Additional cosmetic surgery may be undertaken to achieve feminization of features.

Female-to-male surgery carries serious potential side effects from the hysterectomy, including pain, infection, and debilitation. Most individuals do not undertake penile construction and instead use a dildo or prosthetic penis. Constructed penises are usually unsatisfactory in that they are significantly shorter than the average erect penis and are incapable of transmitting sexual sensation. In some cases, pumps have become defective and required further corrective surgery. Male hormone supplements must be taken for the remainder of the individual's life.

PERSPECTIVE AND PROSPECTS

For centuries, rare individuals born with ambiguous genitalia, called hermaphrodites, were subjected to severe psychological trauma as they reached adulthood and/or developed a sexual anatomy contrary to the gender identity in which they were reared. In the mid-twentieth century, when chromosome analysis became available, those born with ambiguous genitalia could be properly identified as to chromosomal sex, and their outward ambiguities could be surgically corrected soon after birth. Transsexuals too have been ostracized and humiliated throughout the ages; in the latter half of the twentieth century, psychologists diagnosed these individuals as genuinely being born the wrong sex. The cause of transsexualism is unknown, and theories such as exposure to large amounts of opposite-sex hormones during fetal gestation have been proven wrong. Research into the cause of this disorder is progressing and may lead to prevention or early treatment of affected individuals.

Individuals who undergo sex change operations do not experience normal physical sensations in their new genitalia. They are also sterile and therefore unable to reproduce or become pregnant. Research into neurobiology may lead to future procedures allowing physical sensations, as well as to the possibility of transplanting functioning reproductive organs. Even in the current state of the procedure, individuals who are properly psychologically and physically prepared find peace and fulfillment in—for them—a normal gender role.

—*Karen E Kalumuck, Ph.D.*

See also Breast surgery; Breasts, female; Estrogen replacement therapy; Genetics and inheritance; Grafts and grafting; Hermaphroditism and pseudohermaphroditism; Hormone replacement therapy; Hormones; Hysterectomy; Penile implant surgery; Plastic surgery; Psychiatry; Reproductive system; Sexual differentiation; Sexual dysfunction; Sexuality.

FOR FURTHER INFORMATION:

Gorman, Christine. "A Boy Without a Penis." *Time* 149, no. 12 (March 24, 1997): 83. A boy who was one of a set of infant twin sons born in 1963 had his penis damaged beyond repair by a circumcision that went awry. After seeking expert advice, his parents decided to raise the boy as an anatomically correct female.

Simpson, Joe Leigh. *Disorders of Sexual Differentiation*. New York: Academic Press, 1976. Although this book is a bit dated, its detailed descriptions of disorders is still useful and largely accurate. The last chapter deals with diagnosis.

Youngson, Robert M. *The Surgery Book: An Illustrated Guide to Seventy-three of the Most Common Operations*. New York: St. Martin's Press, 1993. The author presents descriptions of surgical procedures. Topics range from cosmetic surgery to heart and lung transplants. The first four chapters cover hospital routines, preoperative testing, transfusions and transplants, and the operating room.

SEXUAL DIFFERENTIATION
BIOLOGY

ANATOMY OR SYSTEM AFFECTED: Endocrine system, genitals, glands, reproductive system, uterus

SPECIALTIES AND RELATED FIELDS: Embryology, endocrinology, genetics, gynecology, urology

DEFINITION: The process by which an embryo becomes male or female under the influence of genetic and hormonal factors.

KEY TERMS:

differentiation: the process of gradual remodeling of tissues in the embryo or fetus; in this context, the process of formation of the male or female reproductive organs

external genitalia: in the male, the penis and scrotum; in the female, the clitoris, the vaginal opening, and the folds (labia) around it

gender identity: the mental view of oneself as male or female

gonad: the internal organ in either sex that produces the reproductive cells (ova and sperm); the ovary in the female and the testis in the male

hormone: a chemical that is produced by a gland in the body and secreted into the blood; hormones act as coordinating signals

hormone receptor: a molecule contained in or on a cell that allows it to respond to a hormone; if re-

ceptors are not present, the hormone will have no effect

Müllerian ducts: the pair of tubes in the early embryo that will develop into the internal female organs (uterus, oviducts, and upper vagina)

urethra: the tube that drains the bladder; in the male, the urethra passes through the penis and carries sperm during ejaculation, while in the female, the urethra opens in front of the vagina but does not have a reproductive function

Wolffian ducts: the pair of tubes in the early embryo that will develop into the internal male organs (the epididymis, the vas deferens, the seminal vesicles)

X and Y chromosomes: the chromosomes that determine genetic sex; males carry an XY pair, and females carry an XX pair

THE FUNDAMENTALS OF SEXUAL DIFFERENTIATION

The chromosomal sex of each individual is determined at the time of conception, when the ovum from the mother is fertilized by a single sperm from the father. All ova (eggs) produced by a female contain one chromosome, denoted X. Sperm from the male can carry either an X or a Y chromosome. The Y chromosome is smaller than the X and contains fewer genetic codes. Men normally produce equal numbers of X- and Y-bearing sperm. The type of chromosome carried by the one sperm that fertilizes the ovum will determine the sex of the embryo. A Y-bearing sperm joining with the ovum will result in an embryo with one X and one Y; this embryo will develop as a male. If the ovum is fertilized with an X-bearing sperm, the embryo will have two X's and will develop as a female.

Although the genetic sex is determined at conception, male and female embryos initially look alike, both internally and externally. For the first seven weeks of development, each human embryo has the anatomical potential to develop in either a male or a female direction: This period is referred to as the sexually indifferent stage. Internally, the gonads, which lie in the kidney region, cannot yet be identified as ovaries or testes. The other internal reproductive organs are represented in every embryo by two pairs of ducts: the Müllerian ducts, which will later develop in the female but will be lost in the male; and the Wolffian ducts, which will later develop in the male but will regress in the female. Externally, male and female embryos possess the same rudimentary genital organs, which will later be remodeled to become either male or female genitalia.

The first organ to differentiate in the embryo is the gonad. Starting at about seven weeks of development in a male embryo, the cells within the gonad are reorganized to form a testis. This reorganization is brought about by the presence of the Y chromosome, which contains the codes for the production of a substance called testis-determining factor (TDF). The chemical nature of TDF has not yet been determined, but its existence is clear from experimental evidence. TDF acts on the gonad to cause it to become a testis. In the absence of a Y chromosome and TDF in a female embryo, the gonad develops into an ovary at about twelve weeks of development. If an individual has only one X chromosome (a condition known as Turner syndrome), the gonads will develop into ovaries, but these ovaries will not contain ova and so the person will be infertile.

The development of the other reproductive organs is not directly determined by the X and Y chromosomes, but rather by hormones secreted by the gonads. In the male, the fetal testes begin to produce testosterone by the tenth week of development, and this testosterone acts on the Wolffian duct system to cause it to develop into the epididymis, vas deferens, and seminal vesicles. The Müllerian duct system in the male regresses under the influence of another hormone from the testes, called Müllerian-inhibiting hormone (MIH). In the female, MIH is not produced, and the Müllerian ducts develop into the oviducts, uterus, and upper part of the vagina. The Wolffian ducts in the female regress in the absence of testosterone. Normal female development does not, at this stage, require any hormone produced by the ovaries, but instead occurs spontaneously in the absence of testicular hormones. Thus, the presence or absence of the Y chromosome determines which type of gonad develops, and the presence or absence of gonadal hormones determines which type of internal reproductive organs develop.

Similarly, the development of the external genitalia is hormonally directed. In the male, testosterone is converted by the action of the enzyme 5-alpha-reductase to 5-alpha-dihydrotestosterone (DHT). DHT acts on the undifferentiated external genital tissue, causing it to take on a male appearance: A pea-shaped structure (the genital tubercle) at the front of the crotch area grows to become the penis; a slitlike opening (the urethral groove) is enclosed within the penis to become the urethra when two folds behind the genital tubercle fuse together; and two swellings on the sides of the urethral groove become enlarged as the scrotum. In the female, it is the absence of DHT that causes development in the female direction: The genital tubercle remains as the relatively small clitoris; the folds do not fuse, allowing the urethral groove to remain as an open area where the vagina and urethral openings are located; and the swellings that become the scrotum in the male remain separated as the labia in the female.

Hormones also cause sexual differentiation of the brain, but the mechanism is not fully understood in humans. The most obvious result of brain differentiation is the difference in adult hormone production patterns. In the adult male, hormone production is relatively constant from day to day, and this results in constant production of sperm in the testes. In the female, hormone production changes in a monthly cycle that is associated with ovum maturation and ovulation. The difference in the pattern of hormone release in adult males and females appears to be attributable to hormonal programming of the fetal brain. Animal studies indicate that the development of the male pattern results from exposure of the fetal brain to testosterone or one of its derivatives. The female pattern of development is prevalent when testosterone is absent. In humans, testosterone also affects brain differentiation, but the effect appears to be less permanent than in animals.

It is not known for sure if there is any direct influence of the chromosomes or prenatal hormones on male and female behavior. Most researchers agree that human behavior is heavily influenced by social and cultural factors, so the importance of prenatal programming is difficult to assess. Indeed, it appears that gender identity, the internal view of oneself as male or female, is so heavily influenced by learning that a child with a disorder of sexual differentiation can be successfully reared in the gender that is opposite to that of the chromosomes. For example, a child born with female-appearing genitalia, but with XY chromosomes and internal testes, can be reared as a girl and will firmly adhere to this identity even if some masculinization occurs at the time of puberty.

DISORDERS AND DISEASES

Disorders of sexual differentiation result from errors in the signaling systems that normally direct male and female anatomical development. There are several different classes of these disorders, some of which result in a mixture of male and female reproductive organs. These disorders are rare, with the number of documented cases numbering only in the hundreds for most types.

True hermaphrodites are defined as individuals who possess both ovarian and testicular gonadal tissue. There may be one ovary and one testis, two gonads in which ovarian and testicular tissue are combined (ovotestes), or an ovotestis on one side and a normal ovary or testis on the other. True hermaphroditism can result from several distinct genetic anomalies. Some hermaphrodites have been shown to be chimeras: individuals that develop from the fusion of two separate embryos at an early stage. These individuals possess two distinct cell populations, one with an XX pair of chromosomes and one with XY. It is thought that expression of both of these chromosome pairs leads to the mixture of ovarian and testicular tissue seen in true hermaphrodites. A similar condition is mosaicism, in which the mixture of XX and XY cells is caused by errors of chromosome replication in a single early embryo. Other true hermaphrodites are neither chimeras nor mosaics; they appear to have a normal pair of XX or XY chromosomes, but on closer examination, one of the chromosomes is found to have a defect. For example, a Y chromosome may be missing a tiny piece, or an X chromosome may contain a portion of a Y.

There is much variation in the anatomical features of true hermaphrodites. One basic guideline is that the effects of the presence of testicular tissue are local. Thus, a true hermaphrodite with a testis on the left side and an ovary on the right will have Wolffian duct-derived (male) organs on the left side, but Müllerian duct-derived (female) organs on the right. The external appearance depends on the relative levels of estrogen and testosterone, but might include a typical male penis along with enlarged breasts. There are documented cases of ovulation and even pregnancy in true hermaphrodites. Successful sperm production appears to be less frequent than ovulation, and sperm production and ovulation are not seen in the same individual.

Pseudohermaphrodites are individuals whose external reproductive organs do not match their gonadal sex. Male pseudohermaphrodites have testes but external organs that appear to be female; female pseudohermaphrodites have ovaries and varying degrees of external male development.

Female pseudohermaphroditism has only one basic cause: the exposure of an XX fetus to masculinizing hormones. These hormones might come from the fetus itself, as in certain disorders involving the adrenal gland, or synthetic hormones given to a pregnant woman may have a masculinizing effect on a female fetus. The extent of masculinization depends on the timing of the hormone exposure, with earlier exposure leading to more extensive malelike appearance of the external genitalia, including fusion of the urethral folds and enlargement of the clitoris. The internal organs are normal female.

Male pseudohermaphroditism arises from a wide variety of causes. There may be failure of testosterone production, or the reproductive organs may lack testosterone receptors, causing them to fail to respond to the hormone. Because of the hormonal abnormalities, the Wolffian duct organs may fail to develop, and the external genitalia will appear female to some extent. If MIH production is normal, internal female organs will not be present. The appearance at puberty is variable, depending on the exact hormonal deficiency. Some individuals undergo the typical male responses of increased muscle mass, deepening of the voice, and growth of beard and chest hair; others do not. Most male pseudohermaphrodites are infertile because of the hormonal problems.

Treatment of disorders of sexual development depends on the exact symptoms and their cause, but the prevailing overall philosophy is to attempt to produce an individual who will be able to function sexually as an adult, even if that means sacrificing fertility and rearing the child in the sex opposite to that of the chromosomes. Early diagnosis is a key, since most authorities agree that gender identity is irrevocably set by the age of eighteen to twenty-four months. After that time, few physicians would be willing to try to alter the individual's gender identity from that which has already been established.

For true hermaphrodites, the choice of sex for rearing usually depends on the predominant appearance of the external genitalia. If the genital tubercle has remained small, like a clitoris, the decision is usually for a female sex assignment; if the tubercle appears more penislike, the individual can be reared as a male. Usually, the gonadal tissue that does not correspond to the sex of rearing will be removed, to prevent the production of hormones that would interfere with the desired appearance. Appropriate hormone treatment and surgery can enhance the body form of the chosen sex. For example, testosterone treatment will cause beard growth, and estrogen treatment will cause breast development.

In the case of female pseudohermaphrodites, most can successfully be reared as girls. Surgical alteration of the external genitalia and hormone treatment to correct the original problem may be necessary. Assuming early diagnosis and treatment, most female pseudohermaphrodites will be fertile as adults.

Similarly, hormonal treatment of male pseudohermaphrodites who do not produce testosterone can allow these individuals to be reared as boys, even if they are not fertile later. There is no treatment, however, that will allow a male pseudohermaphrodite who is unresponsive to testosterone to develop a male appearance; these individuals are usually reared as girls, with female pubertal development induced by estrogen treatment.

A fascinating form of male pseudohermaphroditism is seen in the *guevedoces* (meaning "penis at twelve") of the Dominican Republic. In this island nation, the extensive intermarriage of related individuals has produced a population in which a certain genetic defect is seen in relatively high numbers. This genetic defect results in absence of the 5-alpha-reductase enzyme necessary to convert testosterone to DHT. Affected individuals are born with external genitalia that appear more female than male. The internal reproductive organs, which are stimulated by testosterone rather than by DHT, are normal for a male, although the testes may remain in the body cavity instead of descending into a scrotum. Female internal organs are absent, since MIH production is normal. Traditionally, these individuals were reared as girls until the time of puberty, when growth of the penis occurred under the influence of increasing levels of testosterone. (Although the penis would enlarge, the opening of the urethra would remain misplaced for a male, being on the bottom of or behind the penis, a condition known as hypospadias.) At this time, these individuals would make a transition to a male gender identity and sex role. Although initially reared as female, the *guevedoces* were typically heterosexual as adult males, participating in sexual activity with females. Physicians and psychologists have been puzzled by the fact that the *guevedoces* could switch their gender identity at such an advanced age, in the face of evidence suggesting that this should be impossible. This traditional switch of sex role at puberty is no longer seen, since most

guevedoces are now diagnosed at birth and reared as males from the start.

PERSPECTIVE AND PROSPECTS

Anatomical descriptions of people with disorders of sexual development are found in writings beginning in the pre-Christian era. The word "hermaphrodite" itself derives from the Greek myth about Hermaphroditos, the son of Hermes and Aphrodite, whose body was permanently merged with that of a nymph in a loving embrace. The myth probably arose from a desire to explain the existence of hermaphrodites.

Although the existence of hermaphrodites was known long ago, there was no understanding of the mechanism of sexual differentiation until modern times. During the nineteenth century, embryological studies firmly established the concept that the early human embryo is sexually indifferent anatomically. In the twentieth century, genetic and hormonal studies revealed the controlling factors in male and female development.

It was in the 1920's that the X and Y chromosomes were first discovered and recognized to be important in sex determination. Since the 1960's, researchers have had the ability to pinpoint the exact chromosome sites associated with many disorders of sexual differentiation. Ongoing efforts deal with the identification of the TDF coded by the Y chromosome and the mechanism by which TDF causes testicular development.

The nature of the hormonal control of sexual differentiation was determined by experiments such as those performed on rabbit embryos by A. Jost in the 1940's and 1950's. Jost systematically removed or transplanted embryonic testes and ovaries, and treated the embryos with estrogen and testosterone, in order to demonstrate the importance of hormones from the testis on the development of the internal and external reproductive organs.

Jost's conclusions for rabbits were confirmed in humans by studying individuals with disorders of sexual differentiation caused by genetic factors. Additional confirmation came from observations of the offspring of pregnant women treated with synthetic hormones as a possible preventive for miscarriage. Such treatment was later found to be ineffective in preventing miscarriage, but worse, the treated women often gave birth to masculinized female fetuses. It is now recognized that synthetic hormones in oral birth control pills can also masculinize female fetuses.

Discovery of the causes of true hermaphroditism and pseudohermaphroditism have allowed physicians to make important distinctions between these disorders, with a clear physical cause and manifestation, and the psychological disorders of sexuality that were previously confused with them. For example, up to the middle of the twentieth century, the term "hermaphrodite" was used to refer not only to people with a mixture of male and female reproductive organs but also to those with a psychological confusion of gender identity. The latter individuals are now called transsexuals; they identify themselves as the gender opposite to that of their reproductive organs (such as a male "trapped" in a female body, or vice versa). Transsexuals possess a complete set of normal reproductive organs and have no known chromosomal or hormonal abnormality. Another condition is transvestitism, which refers to the wearing of clothing of the opposite sex. Most transvestites are male heterosexuals who engage in this behavior to achieve sexual arousal; like transsexuals, transvestites have normal anatomy, chromosomes, and hormones. Finally, homosexual orientation is now considered to be a personality trait, rather than a disorder. Homosexual individuals are sexually and romantically attracted to individuals of the same sex; their reproductive organs, chromosomes, and hormone levels are the same as those of heterosexuals.

—*Marcia Watson-Whitmyre, Ph.D.*

See also Embryology; Genetic diseases; Genetics and inheritance; Hermaphroditism and pseudohermaphroditism; Reproductive system; Sex change surgery; Sexual dysfunction; Sexuality.

For Further Information:

Barbin, Herculine. *Herculine Barbin: Being the Recently Discovered Memoirs of a Nineteenth-Century French Hermaphrodite.* Translated by Richard McDougall. New York: Pantheon Books, 1980. This translation from the French tells the true story, in his own words, of a male pseudohermaphrodite who was reared as a girl but underwent masculinizing changes at the time of puberty.

Carlisle, David Brez. *Human Sex Change and Sex Reversal: Transvestism and Transsexualism.* Lewiston, N.Y.: E. Mellen Press, 1998. This helpful resource discusses aspects of transvestism and transsexualism. Includes bibliographical references and an index.

Khan, Aman U., and Joseph Cataio. *Men and Women in Biological Perspective.* New York: Praeger, 1984. This book will be useful for the reader who, after learning that male and female embryos are indistinguishable at first, asks if there are indeed any differences between males and females.

Money, John. *Sex Errors of the Body and Related Syndromes: A Guide to Counseling Children, Adolescents, and Their Families.* 2d ed. Baltimore: Brookes, 1994. Written by one of the leaders in the treatment of sexual disorders, this book is remarkable for its easy-to-read straightforward approach.

Simpson, Joe Leigh, and Mitchell S. Golbus. *Genetics in Obstetrics and Gynecology.* 2d ed. Philadelphia: W. B. Saunders, 1992. Chapter 11 deals with the genetic basis of disorders of sexual differentiation and provides a detailed, technical account of the results of various genetic defects.

Wilson, Jean D., and Daniel W. Foster, eds. *Williams Textbook of Endocrinology.* 9th ed. Philadelphia: W. B. Saunders, 1998. Chapter 11, "Disorders of Sexual Differentiation," begins with a description of normal sexual differentiation and then covers all the known disorders, including appearance, chromosomes, hormone levels, fertility, and treatment.

Sexual dysfunction
Disease/disorder

Anatomy or system affected: Genitals, psychic-emotional system, reproductive system

Specialties and related fields: Endocrinology, gynecology, psychiatry, psychology, urology

Definition: Impotence is the persistent inability of a man to achieve and maintain an erection adequate for vaginal penetration and the successful completion of sexual intercourse; frigidity is the disinterest in sex, usually applying to women, because of inadequate or unpleasurable sensation during intercourse.

Key terms:

corpora cavernosa: two passageways in the penis containing spongy reservoirs of tissue and blood vessels

etiology: the science of causes or origins, especially of diseases

neuropathy: malfunction of the nerves

organic disease: a disease caused or accompanied by an alteration in the structure of the tissues or organs

psychogenic: psychologic in origin

Causes and Symptoms

It is evident from the term "performance anxiety" that sexual anxiety is more easily recognized when it involves performance (that is, erections and orgasms) than when it involves subjective arousal. The most extreme example of this way of thinking is the familiar notion that women do not experience performance anxiety because it is only men who have to perform. When researchers searched for a corresponding term that refers not to performance but to subjectively felt arousal, they devised the oxymoronic-sounding term "pleasure anxiety." Performance anxiety refers to the fear of not being able to perform, while pleasure anxiety refers to the fear of feeling pleasure. Sex therapists have traditionally been much more concerned with the fear of not being able to perform.

To explain this blind spot in the field, it is clear that, historically, lack of desire has been considered a female disorder, whereas lack of performance has been considered a male disorder. From the male-identified point of view, the failure to perform is relatively understandable; it is often treated with humor, sympathy, or indulgence. Traditionally, however, the same indulgence has not been extended toward a woman when she cannot fulfill the role expected of her.

If there are any doubts that "frigidity" is a more accusatory term than "impotence," "impotence" as a diagnostic term retains its currency, whereas "frigidity" has largely been dropped. Researchers William H. Masters and Virginia E. Johnson were the first authorities to drop the term, and as a result of their influence it is rarely used in the field of sex therapy and research. It is still used, however, in the psychoanalytic literature.

The category of "inhibited sexual desire" in the American Psychiatric Association's *Diagnostic and Statistical Manual of Mental Disorders* (3d ed., 1980, DSM-III) indicated the difficulty in finding a nonjudgmental means of referring to the lack of erotic arousal: The term "inhibition" implies that the conditions for desire are present but that desire is being withheld. One of the implied accusations in the term "frigidity" is that the woman who does not experience erotic arousal is a cold, unfeeling, or withholding person. The work group on psychosexual disorders for the revision of the DSM-III published in 1987 recognized this difficulty and recommended that "inhibited sexual desire" be renamed "hypoactive sexual desire disorder," arguing that this more awkward term is necessary because it reflects greater neutrality in terms of etiology.

One researcher points out that between the years of 1974 and 1976 roughly 32 percent of couples seeking help received a diagnosis of low sexual desire. In the years 1977 and 1978, this figure increased to 46 percent of couples. In 1981-1982, the incidence of low-desire cases was 55 percent. The sex ratio of identified patients within couples also changed over these years. From 1974 to 1976, the female was the identified patient about 70 percent of the time. In 1977 and 1978, this figure had declined to only 60 percent. In 1982 and 1983, in a noteworthy change, 55 percent of all low-desire cases involved male low desire. Thus low sexual desire, or "frigidity," is clearly a problem affecting both men and women.

Most of the knowledge of the causes of low sexual desire is based on clinical experience, rather than on more empirical and objective research. It has become clear that there is no single cause for low sexual desire. Rather, many cases involve several causal factors working simultaneously.

Virtually every standard work on sexual dysfunction lists religious orthodoxy as a major cause of sexual dysfunction. Some patients suffer from low sexual desire because they essentially lack the capacity for play (the obsessive-compulsive personality). Specific sexual phobias or aversions also may cause low sexual desire. Low-desire men almost uniformly have some degree of aversion to the vagina and female genitals. Women who have been sexually molested as children, or raped as adults, often have specific aversion reactions.

Some patients fear that if they allow themselves to feel any sexual desire at all, they will lose all control over themselves and begin acting out sexually in ways that would have disastrous consequences. Fear of pregnancy is often a "masked" cause of low sexual desire among women. Depression, hormonal issues, the side effects of medication, relationship problems, lack of attraction to one's partner, fear of closeness, and an inability to fuse feelings of love and sexual desire are among the many causes of low sexual desire in both men and women.

With regard to impotence, although the exact number is not known, it has been estimated that there are approximately ten million men in the United States suffering from impotence. In the past, it was thought that psychogenic causes accounted for 90 percent of impotence, with only 10 percent attributable to medical or postsurgical diseases, so-called physical or organic impotence. As medical knowledge increased, in the early 1990's it was estimated that medical or organic causes accounted for 50 to 70 percent of all patients suffering from impotence.

Until the 1980's, it was difficult to determine whether any given patient was impotent as a result of psychogenic causes or physical, organic ones. The availability of blood tests to measure hormone levels and of penile tumescence sleep laboratory testing now allows for accurate determination of the true cause of impotence in patients. Yet even when it is attributable to organic causes, impotence has significant psychological implications for the male-female relationship.

Impotence can be defined as the persistent inability to attain and maintain a rigid penis adequate for vaginal penetration and successful completion of intercourse. There are two types of impotence: primary and secondary. Primary impotence is the term used to describe the male who has never been able to achieve an erection adequate for sexual intercourse. This is a relatively rare condition. Except in very unusual circumstances that might have involved a surgical procedure on the penis during childhood, primary impotence is not caused by any physical defect but instead has a psychologic basis. Men with primary impotence are most often found to have had a severely repressive childhood with strong religious or mother-figure relationships. These patients generally exhibit considerable conflict in their relationships with women and have hostile or fearful attitudes toward females.

The majority of men with impotence have secondary impotence; that is, at one time in their lives they were capable of full erections and intercourse but have subsequently lost that ability. In the 1980's, other medical terms for impotence came into common use, such as "erectile dysfunction." As in the case of "frigidity," the word "impotence" has had negative connotations.

Diabetes mellitus is a rather common organic medical problem accounting for impotence in many men. It has been estimated that 50 percent of men who have had diabetes for twenty years become impotent. It is thought that diabetes results in impotence by causing neuropathy or malfunction of the nerves, as well as narrowing of the blood vessels. Arteriosclerosis, or hardening of the arteries, causes a narrowing of the blood vessels. Many patients who have arteriosclerosis involving the aorta or smaller blood vessels that supply blood to the penis will experience impotence.

Chronic kidney failure, cirrhosis (chronic liver disease), neurological diseases such as Parkinson's disease and multiple sclerosis, malfunction of the spinal cord (such as spina bifida or spinal cord injury), and low levels of testosterone are also frequent organic causes of impotence. Masters and Johnson have stated that alcoholism is the second most common cause of impotence. Pelvic fractures and trauma, radiation therapy, radical pelvic surgery (including removal of the prostate, bladder, or rectum), and aortic aneurysm repair can cause nerve and blood vessel injuries that can result in impotence and/or problems with ejaculation. Penile cancer, Peyronie's disease (curvature of the penis as a result of scar tissue formation), and priapism (prolonged erection of the penis) are also causes of organic impotence. It has been reported that prescription drugs may account for 25 percent of patients with impotence. By far the most common group of drugs resulting in impotence are those taken for treatment of hypertension, or high blood pressure.

Treatment and Therapy

There are several difficulties inherent in devising a treatment program for low sexual desire. While most of the behavioral exercises devised by Masters and Johnson may enhance arousal and orgasm, they often fail in increasing sexual desire or motivation, since they were not designed to deal specifically with low sexual desire. A second problem is that many cases of low sexual desire not only are quite complex but are diverse in apparent etiology and maintenance factors as well. Each case of low desire must be examined on its own terms, and treatment must be tailored to the specific needs of the individual.

Behavior therapy and social learning theory contributed most of the effective techniques that constituted sex therapy in the 1980's. Other therapeutic approaches, however, have been used as adjunct techniques or proposed alternatives. One broad-spectrum approach attempts to integrate interventions from many theoretical orientations into a comprehensive treatment program, while remaining sensitive to the need to fine-tune the program to the individual.

The first step in this broad-spectrum approach is experiential/sensory awareness. Many patients with low sexual desire are unable to verbalize their feelings and are often unaware of their responses to situations involving sexual stimulation. The goal of this phase of therapy is to help patients recognize, using bodily cues, when they are experiencing feelings of anxiety, pleasure, anger, or disgust.

The second stage is the insight phase of therapy, in which patients, with the help of the therapist, attempt to learn and understand what is causing and maintaining their low desire. Frequently, patients with low sexual desire have misconceptions and self-defeating attitudes about the cause of the problem. Patients are helped to reformulate attitudes about the cause of the problem in a way that is conducive to therapeutic change.

The third stage, the cognitive phase of therapy, is designed to alter irrational thoughts that inhibit sexual desire. Patients are helped to identify self-statements that interfere with sexual desire. They are helped to accept the general assumption that their emotional reactions can be directly influenced by their expectations, labels, and self-statements. Patients are taught that unrealistic or irrational beliefs may be the main cause of their emotional reactions and that they can change these unrealistic attitudes. With change, patients can reevaluate specific situations more realistically and can reduce negative emotional reactions that cause low desire.

The final element of this treatment program consists of behavioral interventions. Behavioral assignments are used throughout the therapy process and include basic sex therapy as well as other sexual and nonsexual behavior procedures. Behavioral interventions are used to help patients change nonsexual behaviors that may be helping to cause or maintain the sexual difficulty. Assertiveness training, communication training, and skill training in negotiation are examples of such behavioral interventions.

The treatment of psychogenic impotence includes supportive psychotherapy and behavior-oriented tasks. If, during the course of evaluation, symptoms of depression such as loss of libido and appetite or sleep

In the News: New Treatments for Erectile Dysfunction

The treatment of men with sexual dysfunction, particularly erectile dysfunction (ED), has undergone a revolution in the past few years. The introduction of sildenafil (Viagra) has allowed as many as 80 percent of men suffering the disorder to be treated with minimally invasive oral medication that is safe and effective. Recent studies have demonstrated the safety and effectiveness of sildenafil in men with erectile dysfunction caused by diabetes, spinal cord injury, vascular disease, cardiac disease including ischemic heart disease and congestive heart failure, nerve-sparing radical prostatectomy, and erectile dysfunction associated with depression. The major contraindication to sildenafil continues to be the use of nitroglycerin or long-acting nitrates in any form. These nitrate medications in combination with sildenafil produce significant blood pressure drops and are dangerous, especially to patients with compromised cardiac status.

Newer medications for ED are being investigated and will be available soon. These include additional drugs similar to sildenafil, which are classified as phosphodiesterase V (PDE V) inhibitors. These drugs facilitate erectile function by stimulating the relaxation of smooth muscle tissue in the erectile bodies of the penis. This relaxation allows rapid blood flow into the penis and facilitates erectile function in men with erectile dysfunction. Additional drugs, including cialis and vardenafil, will be available soon. Other agents, including apomorphine (Uprima), will stimulate central nervous system functions, providing improved erectile function. Uprima, which has been approved by the FDA Advisory Panel, is the first agent to act on the central nervous system to improve erectile dysfunction.

Recent studies have documented the success and support of the outcome measurements of penile implants for the treatment of erectile dysfunction. Inflatable penile prostheses, which encompass two cylinders placed in the erectile bodies of the penis, a small pump placed in the scrotum allowing the two cylinders to inflate and produce an erection of normal size, sensation, and function, have been available since the mid-1970's. Recent studies have demonstrated mechanical reliability of more than 90 percent at five years, with patient satisfaction of greater than 90 percent at five and ten years. In patients with sexual partners and functioning penile prostheses, more than 70 percent use their prostheses twice monthly ten years after surgery. These prosthetic devices continue to be useful in patients who cannot use medical treatment for erectile dysfunction.

—*Culley C. Carson III, M.D.*

difficulties are present without a physical basis, the patient is often treated with an antidepressant medication. As mental depression lessens, sexual interest and potency will often return. Depression is the most common mental disorder detected when impotent patients undergo psychological studies.

There are certain causes of organic impotence that may be reversible with appropriate therapy. The alcoholic patient, for example, may regain his potency if his drinking problem can be resolved. The heavy cigarette smoker may similarly experience improvement in his general health and regain erections following cessation of smoking. Patients with newly discovered diabetes mellitus and high blood sugars may regain their erections following control of their diabetes with insulin, diet, or oral medications. This improvement will not be seen, however, in those individuals with long-standing diabetes who lose their erections.

Treatment programs for organic impotence are geared toward the problems of each individual and are often age-dependent. From 1980 to 1990, there were major advances not only in the diagnosis but also in the treatment of erectile insufficiency; moreover, many of those major treatment advances were nonsurgical. As a result of these nonsurgical advances and their positive rate of success, men often are encouraged to begin their treatment program with the most conservative technique possible. It has been estimated that approximately 90 percent of patients with erectile insufficiency are adequately treated with one of the following (conservative) medical programs: oral medication, self-injection, and vacuum tumescence devices.

Often the first step to medical management of erectile dysfunction is oral medication. Generally, these medications cause smooth muscle relaxation, thereby enhancing the blood flow into the penis. The drug Viagra (sildenafil), introduced in 1998, allows sufficient blood flow for an erection over a four- to five-hour period. Viagra boasted a success rate of almost 80 percent and was immediately in great demand. Concerns arose, however, about its misuse to enhance sexual performance instead of to treat impotence. Medications to increase sexual desire are also being investigated by various pharmaceutical companies in conjunction with the Food and Drug Administration (FDA). These medications became available for experimental use in the early 1990's.

Penile injection with drugs is a treatment for male impotence that was popularized in 1982 by Dr. Ronald Virag of Paris, France. Penile injection with vasoactive compounds to effect an erection, however, had not yet been approved by the FDA in the United States by the early 1990's. Thus patients were required to sign a legal release of liability if this method of treatment was chosen.

In 1990, there were approximately 80,000 males using self-injection therapy (for the treatment of erectile impotence) in the United States. This method of treatment has gained much international acceptance and continues to be the focus of much clinical and laboratory research. This technique is relatively painless and quick, producing results in ten to twenty minutes. Treatment is initiated by administering a test dose of the medication. During this initial stage of treatment, the medication dosage level is adjusted. The patient is then taught the injection technique, given instructions on how to care for the medication and equipment, and given an assessment of erectile response. This method is considered simple, safe, and highly successful (with a success rate of approximately 75 to 80 percent). The major complications are priapism and penile scarring, which occurs in 1 to 2 percent of cases.

Another nonsurgical option available is vacuum tumescence therapy. This device enables the patient to attain penile enlargement and rigidity by inducing blood flow into the penile shaft. Once the blood flow is induced by the creation of a vacuum, it is trapped by the use of an occlusive device applied at the base of the penis. Although it produces a successful erection in approximately 75 percent of cases, the vacuum tumescence device and the accompanying obstructing rubber occlusive device prevent the ejaculate from being expelled in most cases.

Many men with erectile dysfunction are best treated by surgical reconstruction. This group represents approximately 10 percent of the entire impotent population. Penile revascularization is one option. The patients who are best treated with penile revascularization are typically men under fifty years of age. Generally, these men are nonsmoking, healthy individuals whose potency problems are caused by a single lesion or injury. The purpose of penile revascularization is to channel more blood into the corpora cavernosal and thereby increase the corpora cavernosa pressure. Pressure can be increased by a variety of methods, including bypass artery-to-artery, bypass artery-to-vein, or closure of specific leaking areas in the corpora cavernosa.

Although available since the mid-1930's, penile prosthetics made their greatest strides after the introduction of synthetic materials (plastics) in the 1950's. Since then, major changes in design, function, and surgical technique have evolved. The prosthetics available by the 1990's were of three basic varieties: simple rods, flexible rods, and hydraulic devices (one-piece, two-piece, and multicomponent). Once implanted, prosthetics give the patient a return to "normal erectile dynamics." Although the tumescence-detumescence cycle is a result of the patient's prosthesis, sensation, satisfaction, and often even ejaculation remain as they were prior to surgery.

PERSPECTIVE AND PROSPECTS

Anthropologists have found that impotence (erectile dysfunction) and frigidity (inhibited or low sexual desire) have been observed in both primitive and highly developed societies. During most of human history, it was taken for granted that women attain sexual gratification in the same manner as men. Little attention was paid to the failures.

One of the most significant social changes affecting attitudes toward these sexual dysfunctions has been the altered status of women in contemporary society. During the Victorian era, whether they worked or not, women were legally the wards of men and had virtually no civil rights. Many of the Victorian attitudes toward sex—fears, prejudices, taboos, and superstitions— remained powerful influences into the late twentieth century.

Researchers, however, have learned that they cannot understand the problem of impotence in women by comparing it with impotence in men, since the dynamics as well as the treatments for each disorder differ greatly. With the women's movement and the Masters and Johnson research into human sexuality, the archaic terms "impotence" and "frigidity" were called into question. More gender-neutral terms were used, and, particularly in the case of erectile insufficiency, organic as opposed to psychogenic etiologies were acknowledged. By the 1990's, erectile insufficiency had become a disorder more often treated by urologists than by psychiatrists.

With this changing attitude toward these sexual dysfunctions among the medical community as well as the public at large, more research was devoted to treating the problems effectively and to reassuring the patients. Age-old stereotypes came under attack, such as the notion that performance anxiety affects only

men and that "frigidity" or low sexual desire is a disorder that affects only women. As more organic etiologies for both erectile dysfunction and low sexual desire are acknowledged, patients feel increasingly comfortable seeking medical attention, and the stigma of sexual dysfunction being purely psychological is slowly beginning to vanish.

—Genevieve Slomski, Ph.D.

See also Alcoholism; Anxiety; Arteriosclerosis; Cirrhosis; Diabetes mellitus; Genital disorders, female; Genital disorders, male; Hormones; Hypertension; Menopause; Multiple sclerosis; Parkinson's disease; Prostate cancer; Psychiatry; Psychiatry, geriatric; Psychosomatic disorders; Renal failure; Sexuality; Spina bifida; Stress; Urinary disorders.

FOR FURTHER INFORMATION:

Kaplan, Helen Singer. *The Sexual Desire Disorders: Dysfunctional Regulation of Sexual Motivation.* New York: Brunner/Mazel, 1995. This book provides current thinking on disorders of sexual desire and directions for contemporary treatment.

Leiblum, Sandra R., and Raymond C. Rosen, eds. *Sexual Desire Disorders.* New York: Guilford Press, 1988. A groundbreaking collection of papers on disorders of sexual desire. One of the questions raised in the volume is "Are there unknown genetic or constitutional factors that can account for low sexual desire?"

Miller, Karl E. "Treatment of Antidepressant-associated Sexual Dysfunction." *American Family Physician* 61, no. 12 (June 15, 2000): 3728. Many classes of antidepressants, including the selective serotonin reuptake inhibitors (SSRIs), can impair sexual function. Michelson and associates evaluated the effectiveness of buspirone and amantadine in the treatment of sexual dysfunction associated with fluoxetine use.

Phillips, Nancy A. "Female Sexual Dysfunction: Evaluation and Treatment." *American Family Physician* 62, no. 1 (July 1, 2000): 127-136. Sexual dysfunction includes desire, arousal, orgasmic, and sex pain disorders. Basic treatment strategies, which may be successfully provided by primary care physicians for most sexual dysfunctions, are discussed.

SEXUALITY

BIOLOGY

ANATOMY OR SYSTEM AFFECTED: Genitals, psychic-emotional system, reproductive system

SPECIALTIES AND RELATED FIELDS: Family practice, genetics, gynecology, internal medicine, obstetrics, pediatrics, psychiatry, psychology

DEFINITION: A complex, multidimensional, umbrella term referring to the identification of male and female gender, qualities associated with each gender, capacities for erotic stimulation, behaviors causing erotic stimulation, the biology of reproduction, and fundamental elements of individual personality and personal identity that relate to these; it has procreational, recreational, and relational dimensions.

KEY TERMS:

bisexuality: the capacity to be sexually attracted to and aroused by both genders; the term further implies a significant and consistent capacity for such arousal and does not refer to occasional attraction to or activity with both sexes

celibacy: originally meaning unmarried, it also refers to the willful or circumstantial refraining from sexual intercourse, and by implication, erotic behavior; though sometimes misconstrued as asexual, celibates are no less sexual than noncelibates

erogenous zones: bodily areas that are especially sensitive to touch, leading to sexual arousal; although a dozen or so such zones are common (for example, the clitoral glans and labia, penile glans and shaft, breasts, buttocks, inner thighs), these zones can differ from person to person

erotic: referring to sensory perceptions that are sensual (gratifying or pleasurable) and sexual; the context in which they occur will determine whether the perceptions become erotic (for example, breast and testicle examinations are typically not erotic, while caressing these same body parts in romantic settings typically is)

gender: strictly speaking, the behavioral and social aspects of being one sex versus the other; the term is more loosely used to refer to the biological and physical aspects of being male or female as well

gender identity: a person's inner sense and feeling of maleness and/or femaleness; it implies that one clearly identifies with one gender more than the other, although some people identify with both genders equally or near equally

gender role: behaviors and self-presentations that are associated with being male or female and that one uses to identify or recognize others as male or female; the term also implies societal and/or cultural expectations of males and females

heterosexual: being principally attracted to and aroused by opposite-gender persons; a synonymous term, "straight," refers to persons of either gender who are primarily heterosexual

homophobia: obsessive fear of and anxiety about homosexuals and their social and sexual activities; while several causes of homophobia are known, the most common is a homophobic's private, often unconscious fear and doubt about his or her own sexuality and sense of sexual adequacy

homosexual: being principally attracted to and aroused by persons of one's own gender; two synonymous terms are "gay," which can refer to all homosexuals or to homosexual males exclusively, and "lesbian," which only refers to homosexual females

HISTORICAL OVERVIEW

Sexuality is usually manifested and experienced as orientation toward and attraction to people of the same gender, opposite gender, or both. Sexual orientation is also referred to as "sexual preference." The term "preference," however, can imply that sexual attraction and orientation are chosen and voluntary, that one can will oneself to find someone else sexually appealing. In fact, most research suggests the opposite: People find themselves attracted to an individual or gender without having thought about it or having consciously willed it. The attraction and orientation are not chosen. People can wish not to be attracted in the ways that they are, and they may choose not to act on these feelings, but the attraction felt and experienced is outside voluntary control.

A female athlete may wish not to have the sexual feelings she does for her teammates. A male chemistry major may want himself not to find a female classmate as distracting as she is. A female attorney who is happily married may want the sexual feelings that she experiences for her male client to cease. A celibate priest may desire the sexual feelings that he has toward some male and female members of his congregation to go away. As much as these individuals may want to will such feelings away, success in this endeavor is unlikely. Each, instead, must choose how to cope with the feelings, from acting on them directly, to carrying on in spite of them, to pretending that the feelings are not there.

The historical evidence suggests that the prevailing belief in most societies was that people had either a homosexual or a heterosexual orientation; regardless of what made people attracted to their own or to the opposite sex, sexual orientation was "either-or." In the twentieth century, most social scientists and sex researchers came to think about sexual orientation as lying on a continuum marked by degrees of likelihood of finding one's own or the opposite sex attractive. In 1948, Alfred C. Kinsey and his associates published their landmark work, *Sexual Behavior in the Human Male*, in which they used a continuum of sexual orientation to quantify a range of attraction, from those who found only members of the opposite sex attractive (whom they defined as "heterosexual") to those who found only members of the same sex attractive (whom they defined as "homosexual"). Between the two extremes were the majority of people, who find both sexes attractive and arousing in varying degrees.

In determining sexual orientation, researchers once focused on the gender of sex partners, which was also the criterion on which laypeople generally focused. If a male usually had female partners, they would consider him heterosexual; if a female usually had female partners, they would consider her homosexual. Yet sexual orientation, how one is attracted by and toward others, is more accurately considered to be primarily the subjective experience of how one feels inside, not the overt behavior that one demonstrates outside.

Research has shown that, in any given individual, there can be a large discrepancy between the sex of one's actual partners and the sex to which one is more attracted and drawn. Social and cultural circumstances often affect, even determine, whether one will behave the way one feels. People who are primarily attracted to opposite-sex persons may be influenced to have, and even pursue, same-sex partners by particular religious beliefs, certain restricted environments (such as prison), or the sense that this behavior is or is not permissible. Orientation is better understood in the mind and feelings of persons themselves: which sex attracts, how often, and how much. Personal histories that include facts such as procreating children, marriage, homosexual activities, and bisexual experimentation cannot be used to identify sexual orientation.

Although many studies followed their early work, most experts believe that Kinsey and his colleagues produced the most valid observations about sexuality and sexual orientation. Conducting research in this field is difficult. Different studies use different survey tools, and not all are equally reliable. In addition, many people will not candidly or honestly discuss their sexual attitudes, attractions, or behaviors. Nevertheless, the best estimates which rely and build on the Kinsey group's earlier work suggest that about 10 percent of the population in Western countries is primarily gay or lesbian and that an additional 10 percent of the population is primarily bisexual. (There is less research available on non-Western nations, and much of what is available is methodologically less reliable.) In the United States, 20 to 30 million people are likely to be homosexual or bisexual. Far more important than the numbers, however, is the reality that gay, lesbian, and bisexual orientations are neither unusual nor peculiar. This remains true even though heterosexuality is the more common pattern of most people, most of the time—a finding true for all societies ever studied. Yet a minority pattern of attraction cannot, simply on the basis of numbers, be considered abnormal.

Expert and lay opinions about how sexual orientation develops differ, often considerably. Yet expert, if not lay, opinions do converge on when it develops: at about age four or five, which is a year to two earlier than when experts believe an individual's personal traits and characteristics emerge intact as an identifiable personality. Because erotic behavior and erogenous stimuli do not usually become an important part of one's personal world until puberty begins (the developmental marker used to interpret when childhood ends and adolescence begins), many do not learn what their orientation is until late adolescence or even well into adulthood. People who eventually come to have nearly exclusive heterosexual fantasies, attractions, and sexual affiliations often have had earlier, adolescent homosexual experiences. Likewise, people who eventually come to discover that their orientation is strongly homosexual have often married, borne children, and had long periods of gratifying heterosexual dating experiences.

Most people eventually come to identify their orientation, at least implicitly, in terms of direction and strength. Direction refers to the direction of sexual orientation, toward one's own or one's opposite sex. Strength refers to the degree of exclusivity associated with the direction of one's orientation: only attracted by the same or opposite sex, sometimes attracted by each, always attracted to each.

Bidirectional orientation is the least researched and least understood of sexual orientations. As with homosexual and heterosexual behavior, bisexual encounters, even if gratifying, do not in themselves mean that someone is bisexually oriented, and therefore bisexual. All sexual orientation is internal, not behavioral.

Some people, while learning about their sexual selves and their accompanying orientation, engage in experimental bisexual behavior. Some, with limited access to the sex toward which they are more predominantly or exclusively oriented, become sexually active with the sex toward which they are not oriented but which is more available. Some are sexually active with both sexes for money. Some are sexually stimulated and aroused regardless of sex. (William H. Masters and Virginia E. Johnson, perhaps the leading sex researchers and sex educators of all time, label this group "ambisexual.") Some indicate that they have a definite orientation toward sexual activity with both genders. Among this last group, there are those who report having long-term, one-sex relationships that followed long-term, other-sex relationships, and there are others who report having concurrent sexual relationships with partners of both sexes.

Although descriptions of active bisexuality are readily available in the research, the sheer variety of patterns substantially challenges research-based understandings of how sexual orientation originates and develops. What is known is that people with bisexual orientations are neither poorer nor better psychologically adjusted than heterosexuals or homosexuals, and that bisexuality, while poorly understood, reflects a comfortable and fulfilling sexual lifestyle and identity for a significant percentage of the general population.

THEORIES OF SEXUAL ORIENTATION

No other area of sexuality has generated more interest, theory, or research than orientation and how it originates. No one theory stands alone as proven, and not-yet-explained data shake the foundations of even the most useful theories. Nevertheless, scientific inquiry has disproven many earlier theories. The most promising theories fall into several categories, some of which can overlap to a degree: genetic, hormonal, psychodynamic, parental, familial, behavioral, societal, and cultural.

The first significant study of genetic causality for sexual orientation was published in 1952. The research compared one group of male identical twins with one group of male fraternal twins. In both groups, one twin was known to be homosexually oriented. Reasonably assuming that both twins of a pair would be

exposed to essentially the same environments, the study counted how many second twins, whose sexual orientations were unknown at the start of the study, were also gay. If the rate of homosexuality for twins was higher among the group of identical twins than in the group of fraternal twins, it would evidence that genetic makeup, which is virtually the same between identical twins, would be the main cause of sexual orientation.

Twelve percent of fraternal twins who were homosexual had a homosexual twin. Because male fraternal twins are genetically as similar and dissimilar as any pair of brothers, and the rate of homosexuality among the fraternal set was close to the rates that the Kinsey group found in the general population, the results were initially considered a breakthrough. The study also showed, however, that the twin of every known homosexual in the identical set was also homosexual. One hundred percent concordance rates are rare in studies of identical twins (even studies which might compare heights or weights between identical twins would not achieve 100 percent concordance) and are almost nonexistent in all other social groups on any variable ever studied. This particular study and its unique finding needed replication to be believed. Two later studies, published in 1968 and 1976, had quite different results, and the view that sexual orientation was principally a product of genetic conditions and variability was abandoned, though most researchers still believe genetics provides contributory influence.

Investigation into the role hormonal factors play in sexual orientation divides between research on animals and research on humans. Studies clearly show that altering prenatal hormone exposure leads to male or female homosexual behavior in at least several animal species. Among humans, a number of studies have had findings that link prenatal exposure to specific sexual orientation outcomes. For example, females who were exposed to male hormones (androgens), especially testosterone, were more likely to develop lesbian orientations; males with Kleinfelter's syndrome, a chromosomal abnormality marked by a deficiency in androgens, are known to develop gay orientations at a greater frequency than the population average.

Other research on humans has shown that there are different hormone levels between adult homosexuals and heterosexuals. Some studies have found lower testosterone in homosexual males; some have found higher levels of estrogens (though present in both sexes, they are usually considered female hormones) in homosexual males; and other studies have found both. At least one study found higher blood testosterone in homosexual females than heterosexual females.

While this evidence seems illuminating on the surface, it is far from conclusive. First, although many studies show different hormone levels between straight and homosexual persons, several studies have also found hormone levels to be the same in both groups. Second, administering sex hormones to adults does not affect their orientation in any way. Third, prenatal overexposure or underexposure to sex hormones is relatively rare. It would not account for the differences in orientation that are observed in the general adult population, nor is it beyond reason to view cases of abnormal hormonal prenatal environments as extraordinary and unrepresentative of how sexual orientation usually develops. Fourth, while animal studies often describe processes in particular species that are readily analogous to processes in humans, this does not seem to be the case with human sexuality in general or human sexual orientation in particular.

What seems clear is that there is no one-to-one link between sex hormones and sexual orientation. Prenatal hormones, which are known to influence brain development in many ways, may play an indirect role in predisposing individuals toward adapting certain adult sexual behavioral patterns of greater or lesser bisexuality.

Psychodynamic explanations focus on the nature of parent-child relationships and how parents encourage or discourage the growth of their children. Several studies showed homosexual males to have been reared in homes where mothers were dominant and overprotective and fathers were weak, passive, or emotionally uninvolved, a family constellation seen with less statistical frequency among heterosexual males. Other studies, however, showed strained, distant relationships between homosexual men and their fathers but could not find evidence of maternal dominance and overprotectiveness. One study even described the fathers of homosexual males as underprotective, generous, good, and dominant, while the mothers were not found to be overly protective or bossy. Another study simply found no differences in family constellation and dynamics between psychologically well-adjusted heterosexual and homosexual males and females. Given the varied results, the research outcomes from psychodynamic, parental, and familial studies lack cohesive evidence that homosexuality or any orienta-

tion results from poor parent-child relationships or dysfunctional family environments.

Behavioral, societal, and cultural theories assume that orientation is primarily learned as people become culturally assimilated and psychologically conditioned (rewarded and punished) for specific sexual feelings, thoughts, and behaviors. Therefore, in an environment where homoerotic feelings were accepted and valued, people would be more likely to develop homosexual, and perhaps bisexual, orientations. In an environment where homophobic attitudes were considered the norm, homoerotic feelings would more likely be abandoned. While these theories have utility in explaining certain sociological phenomena such as atypical gender role behavior (for example, tomboys) and observed shifts toward lesbianism among some female rape victims, they seem to have less utility in explaining how orientation develops in the majority of the population.

PERSPECTIVE AND PROSPECTS

Although answers to the question of how orientation develops are complex, researchers Alan P. Bell, Martin S. Weinberg, and S. K. Hammersmith published the two-volume work *Sexual Preference: Its Development in Men and Women* (1981) in an attempt to reveal the causal chain of sexual orientation development in more than 1,300 adult homosexual, heterosexual, and bisexual men and women. They based their findings on both lengthy face-to-face interviews with every person in their study and a sophisticated and reliable statistical technique called "path analysis." Their research represents the most extensive collection of data on a large number of people in existence, and most experts are taking at least some of their findings to be conclusive. These results show that sexual orientation is strongly established in most people by late adolescence and that sexual feelings rarely undergo directional changes in adulthood. Atypical gender role behavior in childhood, such as boys preferring to play with dolls and not having an interest in more competitive activities, was found to be more likely than not to proceed homosexual orientations in adolescence and adulthood. Adult homosexuals and bisexuals had, on average, the same amount of heterosexual experience as heterosexual adolescents, though their heterosexual experiences were less rewarding and enjoyable than either their own homosexual experiences or the heterosexual experiences of heterosexuals. The study found that girls choosing their fathers as role models does not cause lesbianism (as several theories had maintained) and that the parental combinations of a domineering, powerful mother and a weak, inadequate father does not cause homosexuality in males (as was once believed).

Although their study was methodologically well planned and statistically sound, Bell, Weinberg, and Hammersmith could not find solid support for any of the prevailing theories about the causality of orientation. Some theories explain some of the observed data, and some theories seem to enhance understanding of the origins of sexual orientation in some elements of the population, but no theory or combination of theories explains all the data.

If this research has moved medical science along to some degree, it also serves to remind everyone, professional and nonprofessional alike, that the very complexity of human experience and how humans develop their identity warrants caution if it is ever to be accurately understood. The evidence is not complete. It is known that some aspects of the theories of the origins of sexual orientation are true and that others are false.

Learning one's own sexual orientation is a complex process requiring self-observation, self-reflection, and self-recollection. People discover what they like, who they like, what is the content and orientation of their sexual fantasies, and which sex feels closer to their sexual identity as persons (rather than the gender role that they feel a societal obligation to play). It is their own experiences of what is, and is not, sexually gratifying that teaches people how they are oriented.

—*Paul Moglia, Ph.D.*

See also Hormones; Masturbation; Precocious puberty; Psychiatry; Psychiatry, child and adolescent; Psychiatry, geriatric; Psychoanalysis; Puberty and adolescence; Reproductive system; Sex change surgery; Sexual differentiation; Sexual dysfunction; Sexually transmitted diseases.

FOR FURTHER INFORMATION:

Altman, Dennis. *The Homosexualization of America.* New York: St. Martin's Press, 1982. A thoughtful, well-researched, and well-written analysis of the cultural and social changes that the gay minority community has brought about in the majority, heterosexual community in the United States.

Bayer, Ronald. *Homosexuality and American Psychiatry: The Politics of Diagnosis.* New York: Basic Books, 1981. While most laypeople imagine that psychiatric diagnoses are empirically, clinically, and objectively derived, this is a fascinating account of the mental health field's susceptibility to political pressure and social stereotyping, and a reminder that psychiatry is first a human and then a scientific discipline.

Berzon, Betty. *Permanent Partners: Building Gay and Lesbian Relationships That Last.* New York: E. P. Dutton, 1988. A practical, realistic guide for same-sex partners in primary relationships. Berzon addresses the main conflict and confusing areas of relationships typically experienced by gay and lesbian couples.

Brown, Gabrielle. *The New Celibacy.* New York: McGraw-Hill, 1980. A secular and nonsectarian discussion and validation of abstinence.

Byer, Curtis O., and Louis W. Shainberg. *Dimensions of Human Sexuality.* 5th ed. Dubuque, Iowa: Wm. C. Brown, 1999. An excellent, thorough, well-organized textbook on all areas of sexuality, with highlighted topics of special interest.

Fairchild, Betty, and Nancy Hayward. *Now That You Know: What Every Parent Should Know About Homosexuality.* Updated ed. New York: Harcourt Brace Jovanovich, 1989. An excellent, sensitively written guide for parents of homosexually oriented persons. It is intended to answer questions, allay fears, and improve communication between the generations.

Gardner-Loulan, JoAnn. *Lesbian Passion: Loving Ourselves and Each Other.* San Francisco: Spinsters/Aunt Lute, 1987. A classic work by a national authority on the societal, interpersonal, and personal issues that particularly affect homosexual women, whether single or in primary relationships, and that undermine their sexuality and self-esteem.

Masters, William H., Virginia E. Johnson, and Robert C. Kolodny. *Human Sexuality.* 5th ed. New York: HarperCollins College, 1995. A well-organized, highly readable textbook covering biological, psychological, social, cultural, ethical, and religious perspectives on human sexuality.

Silverstein, Charles. *Man to Man: Gay Couples in America.* New York: William Morrow, 1981. Silverstein is the founding editor of the *Journal of Homosexuality*, a professional psychology journal. In this book, he provides detailed accounts of primary relationships among gay men, along with insightful commentary on the intimacy, psychology, and sociology of homosexuality.

SEXUALLY TRANSMITTED DISEASES
DISEASE/DISORDER

ANATOMY OR SYSTEM AFFECTED: Genitals, reproductive system

SPECIALTIES AND RELATED FIELDS: Epidemiology, gynecology, internal medicine, public health, urology, virology

DEFINITION: Diseases acquired through sexual contact or passed from a pregnant woman to her fetus, including diseases such as syphilis, gonorrhea, chlamydia, genital herpes, genital warts, viral hepatitis, and acquired immunodeficiency syndrome (AIDS).

KEY TERMS:

antibody: a protein found in the blood and produced by the immune system in response to contact of the body with a foreign substance

asymptomatic: an infection without any symptoms

bacteria: microscopic single-celled organisms that multiply by means of simple division; bacteria are found everywhere, and most are beneficial—only a few species cause disease

immunity: the capacity to resist a disease caused by an infectious agent

infertility: the inability to produce offspring by a person in the childbearing years who has been having sex without contraception for twelve months

inflammation: a response of the body to tissue damage caused by injury or infection and characterized by redness, pain, heat, and swelling

latent: lying hidden or undeveloped within a person; unrevealed

pelvic inflammatory disease (PID): an extensive bacterial infection of the pelvic organs, such as the uterus, cervix, Fallopian tubes, and ovaries

protozoan: a single-celled organism that is more closely related to animals than are bacteria; only a few drugs are available that will kill protozoa without harming their animal hosts

virus: a noncellular particle of protein and nucleic acid; viruses, which can reproduce only inside cells, usually cause damage to their hosts by killing the cells they enter

CAUSES AND SYMPTOMS

Sexually transmitted diseases, or STDs (formerly called venereal diseases), have plagued humankind for centuries. The most prevalent, serious STDs are syphilis, gonorrhea, nongonococcal urethritis, trichomoniasis, genital herpes, genital warts, viral hepatitis, and AIDS. Others, troublesome but not as serious, in-clude lice, scabies, and vaginal yeast infections. They are passed on from one person to another mostly by sexual contact, although some of these diseases may be acquired indirectly through contaminated objects or blood. In addition, nearly all these diseases can be passed on from an infected mother to her fetus, which may cause birth defects, severe and damaging infections, or even death. A person can acquire several STDs at the same time, and since recovery from an STD does not confer immunity, a person can get them again and again. Many of these diseases are asymptomatic, which allows them to spread and cause serious complications before a victim is aware of being infected. Finally, some STDs are treatable and some are not.

Syphilis is caused by *Treponema pallidum*. This bacterium normally infects the penis in males and the vagina or cervix in females, but it can also enter through a cut on the mouth or other parts of the skin. Once inside, the bacteria grow at the site of entry, then spread throughout the body through the lymph and blood vessels. The symptoms of syphilis are caused by the efforts of the immune response of the patient to fight off the infection. The disease occurs in three stages: primary, secondary, and tertiary. In primary syphilis, a flat, firm, painless, red sore called a chancre appears at the site of entry two to ten weeks

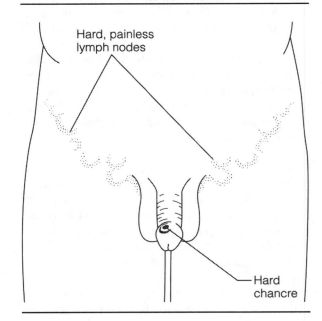

Symptoms of Syphilis

Hard, painless
lymph nodes

Hard
chancre

after infection. Secondary syphilis is characterized by a red rash that appears two to ten weeks after the disappearance of the primary lesion. The rash will disappear in a few weeks. Without treatment, 40 percent of patients will progress to the tertiary stage within three to ten years. Tertiary syphilis is characterized by the formation of severe lesions called gummas on the skin, bones, or internal organs. Gummas on the spinal cord, brain, or heart can lead to seizures, insanity, or death. Almost all pregnant women with untreated primary or secondary syphilis will transmit the bacteria through the placenta to the developing baby, who will develop congenital syphilis. Many babies with congenital syphilis are spontaneously aborted or stillborn. Many others are born with characteristic birth defects, secondary or tertiary syphilis, or neurological damage, and may die shortly after birth.

Gonorrhea is caused by the *Neisseria gonorrhoeae* bacterium (also known as gonococcus). The bacterium infects the urethra in males and the cervix, vagina, or urethra in females. Most infected males get urethritis (inflammation of the urethra) along with symptoms of a pus-containing discharge from the penis and painful urination. Untreated, 1 percent of these men will develop complications of urethral blockage, epididymitis (inflammation of the epididymis, a sac through which sperm passes as it leaves the testicles), prostatitis (inflammation of the prostate, a gland that secretes fluid for semen), and infertility. Between 20 and 80 percent of women infected with gonococcus are asymptomatic or show only mild symptoms. Symptoms include burning or high frequency of urination, vaginal discharge, fever, and abdominal pain. In 20 to 30 percent of untreated women, gonococcus will spread to the Fallopian tubes and cause pelvic inflammatory disease (PID), which can lead to infertility. Infected mothers can transmit the bacteria to their babies as they pass through the birth canal, causing ophthalmia neonatorum, a type of conjunctivitis (inflammation of the eye) that can cause blindness if untreated.

Most cases of nongonococcal urethritis (NGU) are caused by *Chlamydia trachomatis* types *d* through *k*. This bacterium infects the urethra in males and the cervix or urethra in females. The symptoms of chlamydia infection are often mild and go unnoticed. Males experience mild urethritis with a watery discharge, frequent urination, and painful urination. Females are either asymptomatic or experience mild

cervicitis (inflammation of the cervix) or urethritis. Complications include epididymitis in males and PID and infertility in females. Infants born to mothers with cervicitis can develop eye (inclusion conjunctivitis) or lung (infant pneumonia) infections.

Trichomoniasis is caused by the protozoan *Trichomonas vaginalis*. In both sexes, the disease is often mild or asymptomatic. In males, the organism infects the prostate, seminal vesicles, and urethra. About 10 percent of infected males show signs of mild urethritis, with a thin, white urethral discharge. Secondary bacterial infection can lead to more severe urethritis and inflammation of the prostate and seminal vesicles. In females, the organism can infect the vulva, vagina, and cervix. Females may suffer from severe vaginitis, which includes a tender, red, and itchy genital area, and a profuse, frothy, foul-smelling, greenish-yellow discharge. Newborns may acquire the infection from an infected mother during delivery.

Most genital herpes infections are caused by herpes simplex virus type 2, but some are caused by herpes simplex virus type 1. The virus infects the penis in males and the cervix, vulva, vagina, or perineum in females. Two to seven days after infection, painful blisters appear in the genital area that ulcerate, crust over, and disappear in a few weeks. Herpesviruses are unique in that they can remain latent in the nerves and cause a recurrent infection at any time in the future. Fever, stress, sunlight, or local trauma may trigger the virus to come out of hiding and cause a recurrent infection. The virus can be transmitted from an infected mother to her baby either congenitally, through the placenta, or neonatally, as it passes through the birth canal. In congenital or neonatal herpes, the virus can infect all parts of the body, the death rate is high, and survivors commonly have long-term neurological damage and recurrent infections.

Viral hepatitis is also an STD. At least three variants of the virus—hepatitis A virus (HAV), HBV, and HCV—are known to be transmitted sexually. HBV is the form most commonly transmitted sexually. Vaccines are available to immunize persons at risk for HAV and for HBV.

Genital warts are caused by human papillomaviruses (HPVs). In males, the warts appear on the penis, anus, and perineum. They are found on the vagina, cervix, perineum, and anus in females. The warts themselves may be removed, but the infection remains for the life of the patient. HPV infection seems to increase a woman's risk for cervical cancer.

AIDS is caused by the human immunodeficiency virus (HIV). This virus is acquired through sexual contact as well as through intravenous drug use and blood transfusions. HIV infects and inactivates the T helper cell that is needed by the immune system to respond to and fight off infections. Without T helper cells, the immune system eventually becomes nonfunctional, and the affected person becomes susceptible to every type of infection possible. Two-thirds of all AIDS patients get pneumonia caused by *Pneumocystis carinii*. Other common diseases associated with AIDS patients are tuberculosis and other mycobacterial infections, viral infections such as those caused by cytomegalovirus and herpesviruses, fungal infections, cancers such as Kaposi's sarcoma, and neurological disorders. HIV can also be transmitted from an infected mother to her baby through the placenta. Virtually every person infected with HIV will eventually die of AIDS, usually within six years.

TREATMENT AND THERAPY

Sexually transmitted diseases can be diagnosed in several ways. One way is by observing the symptoms and case history of the patient. Characteristic sores or symptoms can lead a doctor to suspect a particular disease, and a sample of a scraping from a lesion or an unusual discharge can be examined under a microscope to identify the infecting organism. The syphilis, gonorrhea, chlamydia, and trichomoniasis organisms all have unique shapes that a doctor can recognize. For those STDs with mild symptoms or no symptoms, a doctor can try to grow the organism in the laboratory from samples taken from appropriate sites on the body. All organisms that cause STDs can be grown in the laboratory, and since these organisms are not normally present in humans, isolation of the organism from the body is a sign that the body has been infected by that organism. Finally, there are many blood tests that have been developed to test whether a person has specific antibodies in his or her blood that bind to one of these organisms. The presence of antibodies to an organism implies that one has been or is currently infected with that organism. In many cases, doctors will use several of these methods to confirm a diagnosis of an STD.

Specific treatment recommendations for each sexually transmitted disease are subject to periodic revision. Current recommendations are reviewed by the Centers for Disease Control and are published in the *Morbidity and Mortality Weekly Report* every three

or four years. It is important for physicians to review these recommendations in order to prescribe the best method for treating STDs. All the bacterial and the protozoal STDs can be treated and cured with antibiotics. It is important to seek early diagnosis and treatment of these diseases for three reasons: First, to prevent the disease from spreading; second, to prevent the various complications associated with the diseases; and third, to prevent the infection of infants by pregnant mothers. There is no cure for STDs caused by viruses; there are only drugs that slow the progress of the infection.

Syphilis is commonly treated with penicillin, or with erythromycin, tetracycline, or cephaloridine in patients who are allergic to penicillin. In most patients receiving appropriate therapy during primary or secondary syphilis, the active disease is totally and permanently arrested. Treatment during the latent stage stops the development of symptoms of the tertiary stage. There is no successful treatment for patients in tertiary syphilis. Treatment of gonorrhea includes penicillin, ampicillin, tetracycline, or spectinomycin. In the mid-1970's, an antibiotic-resistant strain of gonococcus appeared called penicillinase-producing *Neisseria gonorrhoeae* (PPNG), which is resistant to killing by penicillin. Cases of PPNG are treated with cephalosporins. Tetracycline or erythromycin is used to treat NGU caused by chlamydia, and trichomoniasis is treated with metronidazole.

Genital herpes is treated with antiviral agents such as acyclovir. Topical application of acyclovir is helpful in reducing the duration of primary, but not recurrent, infections. The use of oral acyclovir to suppress recurrent infections may cause more severe and more frequent infections once the therapy has stopped. Neonatal herpes is treated with acyclovir or vidarabine, which can reduce the severity of the infection but cannot reverse any herpes-related neurological damage or prevent recurrent infections. Genital warts can be removed by chemicals, freezing, electrocautery, or laser therapy. Antiviral drugs are useful in treating some STDs: acyclovir for genital herpes, zidovudine for AIDS, and interferon for hepatitis virus. They slow the progress of the disease in some persons, but they do not cure it.

As with any disease, prevention is the most desirable means of controlling STDs. With the exception of viral hepatitis, there are no vaccines for STDs; although much research is being done and many potential vaccines have been developed and tested, none is yet satisfactory for general and routine use. There-fore, behaviors resulting in disease avoidance are the only means of preventing most STDs. The only 100 percent effective way to prevent venereal disease is abstinence. Abstinence means to refrain voluntarily from engaging in sexual activity. Since many of these diseases can be spread through sexual activity other than intercourse, abstinence must include all sexual activity. Choosing to exercise one's sexuality within the confines of a monogamous relationship for life can also help prevent sexually transmitted disease. The use of a condom or any other barrier method is only somewhat helpful in the prevention of STDs. Prevention of transmission of STDs from infected mothers to their babies involves early diagnosis and treatment of the mothers before birth and preventive medication of the babies after birth. In the past, oph-thalmia neonatorum was the cause of blindness for half of the children admitted to schools for the blind. Therefore, the government made it mandatory to treat all newborns' eyes with silver nitrate, tetracycline, or erythromycin, to prevent this disease. The instillation of silver nitrate in babies' eyes does not prevent chla-mydia eye infections, so babies born to mothers with chlamydia need additional antibiotic treatment. Pre-vention of neonatal herpes may involve delivery by cesarean section to avoid infection of the child as it passes through the birth canal. Preventing the spread of AIDS includes screening blood supplies, organ do-nors, and semen donors, and avoiding contact with infected body fluids through sexual contact, blood transfusions, or intravenous drug use.

Control of STDs in a population is complex, since it is both a medical and a social problem. First, it is important that persons who contract a sexually trans-mitted disease receive early diagnosis and adequate treatment that will prevent further spread of the dis-ease, serious complications, and infection of infants. This is difficult because many STDs are asymptom-atic; therefore, people do not know they have the dis-ease and have no reason to seek treatment. Many per-sons contract STDs from asymptomatic carriers. In addition, social stigma or embarrassment reduces the motivation of a victim to seek prompt medical care. Adequate treatment of STD victims is difficult if they do not want to return for subsequent treatment or will not take all their medication. Finally, people often contract several STDs at the same time, so detection of one STD should routinely instigate testing for other STDs.

Not only does the person with an STD need to be treated, but all the sexual contacts of that person need to be contacted, tested, and treated as well. Public health officials interview victims of STDs to deter-mine the names and addresses of contacts and then try to find and treat the contacts. This is difficult if a victim does not remember who those contacts are, if he or she does not want to discuss his or her sexual activity, or if the contacts do not want to be bothered by the health department. In addition, many private physicians do not report cases of STDs to the public health department; therefore, in many cases, the sources of STDs are never interviewed.

A reduction in promiscuity would aid in the con-trol of STDs. Effective education to change sexual behavior must be predicated upon the motivation and cognitive development of the student. One-third of all cases involve teenagers and young adults; sexual ac-tivity in this age group is on the rise, and members of this group are more likely to have multiple sex part-ners. Prostitution for money or drugs also increases the incidence of STDs. Other control measures in-clude development of vaccines for these diseases, mandatory reporting of all STDs, and education of the population regarding the dangers and risks in-volved in acquiring these diseases.

PERSPECTIVE AND PROSPECTS

Syphilis was first recognized at the end of the fif-teenth century in Europe, where it rapidly reached epidemic proportions and was called the "great pox." Gonorrhea was described and given its present name by the Greek physician Galen in 150 C.E. From the fifteenth century to the eighteenth century, there was much confusion as to the nature of syphilis and gonorrhea, and many persons thought they were dif-ferent stages of the same disease. In 1767, an English physician named John Hunter inoculated himself with a urethral discharge from a patient with gonor-rhea in order to determine once and for all whether they were one disease or two. Unfortunately, that pa-tient also had syphilis, so when Hunter developed symptoms of both gonorrhea and syphilis he con-cluded they were a single disease. It was not until 1838 that it was clearly proved that they were two separate diseases. Traditionally, 95 percent of all cases of sexually transmitted disease were either syphilis or gonorrhea. Since the late 1900's, how-ever, there has been a dramatic increase in the inci-dence of several other sexually transmitted diseases, such as genital herpes, NGU, AIDS, genital warts, and trichomoniasis.

The rise in incidence of STDs is of epidemic proportions. Worldwide in the 1990's, about 250 million new cases of STDs occurred annually. In the United States, about 12 million new cases, including 3 million in teenagers, occurred annually. By 1997, chlamydia had become the most frequently diagnosed STD in the United States, estimated at more than 4 million annually. Other STDs with high incidence included gonorrhea (1.3 million new cases annually) and genital herpes (0.5 million annually). Because there is no cure for genital herpes, it may be present in 20 percent of Americans. In 1997, about 1 million Americans were HIV-positive; only a portion of these had AIDS. That year, the U.S. government announced that the incidence of new cases of AIDS, about 56,000 annually, had begun to decline. A decline in the numbers of persons dying from AIDS was also announced. It is estimated that there are 3 to 5 million new cases of NGU per year. One in five couples in the United States is infertile, and much of that infertility is caused by the complications associated with STDs, with chlamydial infection being the primary preventable cause of sterility in women. In the United States, it is estimated that 25 percent of all women are infected with trichomoniasis and more than 20 million people are infected with herpes simplex virus type 2.

Despite the fact that most STDs can be controlled, the incidence of many of the diseases is still quite high; thus, STDs obviously present a social as well as a medical problem. An increase in education concerning the signs and risks of these diseases, a reduction in promiscuity, and development of vaccines would help in controlling these destructive and fast-spreading diseases.

—Vicki J. Isola, Ph.D.;
updated by Armand M. Karow, Ph.D.

See also Acquired immunodeficiency syndrome (AIDS); Antibiotics; Bacterical infections; Candidiasis; Chlamydia; Contraception; Epidemiology; Genital disorders, female; Genital disorders, male; Gonorrhea; Gynecology; Hepatitis; Herpes; Immunization and vaccination; Preventive medicine; Protozoan diseases; Syphilis; Urethritis; Viral infections; Warts.

FOR FURTHER INFORMATION:

Biddle, Wayne. *Field Guide to Germs.* New York: Henry Holt, 1995. This comprehensive book is easily accessible to the nonspecialist and includes a discussion of nearly every virus, bacterium, and fungus known to cause human and nonhuman animal disease.

Brodman, Michael, John Thacker, and Rachael Kranz. *Straight Talk About Sexually Transmitted Diseases.* New York: Facts on File, 1993. The senior author, a physician, and his colleagues present information for the general reader about the transmission, effects, and prevention of chlamydia, gonorrhea, genital warts, genital herpes, hepatitis, syphilis, and AIDS. Contains a glossary, a list of resources, and an index.

Eng, Thomas Rand, and William T. Butler, eds. *The Hidden Epidemic: Confronting Sexually Transmitted Diseases.* Washington, D.C.: National Academy Press, 1997. This collection of well-written essays is the recommendation of a sixteen-member expert committee for the prevention and control of STDs in the United States.

Fish, Raymond M., Elizabeth Trupin Campbell, and Suzanne R. Trupin. *Sexually Transmitted Diseases: Problems in Primary Care.* Los Angeles: Practice Management Information, 1992. Written by three physicians, this book describes the effect and treatment of more than fifteen STDs. Contains references to the medical literature and an index.

Little, Marjorie. *Sexually Transmitted Diseases.* Philadelphia: Chelsea House, 2000. This work, designed for students in grades nine and up, provides some historical information on STDs. Little covers both the curable diseases, such as syphilis and gonorrhea, as well as AIDS. Symptoms, diagnoses, treatments, and prevention are discussed.

Murphy, Charles. *What Wild Ecstasy: The Rise and Fall of the Sexual Revolution.* New York: Simon & Schuster, 1997. This book gives a historical context to sexuality and sexually transmitted diseases and discusses contemporary changes in sexual behavior.

Quetel, Claude. *History of Syphilis.* Baltimore: The John Hopkins University Press, 1990. This English edition is translated from a scholarly French history of human experience with syphilis from 1495 to the current day. It is complete with footnotes and an index.

Shaw, Michael, ed. *Everything You Need to Know About Diseases.* Springhouse, Pa.: Springhouse Press, 1996. This well-illustrated consumer reference, compiled by more than one hundred doctors and medical experts, describes five hundred illnesses and conditions, their causes, symptoms, diagnosis, treatment, and prevention. Of particular interest is chapter 11, "Sexual Disorders and Diseases."

SHAKING. *See* TREMBLING AND SHAKING.

SHIGELLOSIS
DISEASE/DISORDER

ANATOMY OR SYSTEM AFFECTED: Gastrointestinal system

SPECIALTIES AND RELATED FIELDS: Bacteriology, gastroenterology, public health

DEFINITION: An intestinal infection caused by *Shigella* bacteria.

Shigellosis accounts for half of the cases of bloody diarrhea in developing countries and a smaller portion of diarrheal illness in the United States. Named after Kiyoshi Shiga, a Japanese scientist who performed much of the original research about it in the aftermath of an 1896 epidemic, *Shigella* is a gram-negative bacillus. The four species that cause shigellosis are *S. dysenteriae*, *S. flexnerii*, *S. sonnei*, and *S. boydii*.

The severity of shigellosis is quite variable, ranging from mild diarrhea to death. The more severe illness, dysentery, is characterized by abdominal cramps, tenesmus (a painful urge to defecate), and a bloody, mucus-filled diarrhea. Most victims of this severe illness are children, with those under age five years being particularly at risk with fatality rates around 25 percent. Poverty, malnutrition, poor hygiene, and overcrowding are associated with this serious disease, which is almost never seen in industrialized countries except in travelers who have visited an endemic area of the world. *Shigella dysenteriae* type 1 is responsible for most of these severe cases.

The pathogenicity (or disease-causing mechanism) of shigellosis is the invasion of the intestinal lining by the bacteria, causing inflammation and ulceration of the intestinal wall. Although *Shigella* bacteria also produce a toxin, the role of this toxin in the infection is less clear and remains a research topic of much interest. In contrast to some other intestinal infections such as cholera, shigellosis produces a relatively small fluid volume loss, making dehydration less problematic. Victims also suffer from fever, malaise, and decreased appetite. Transmission of the *Shigella* bacteria is from person to person; there is no animal reservoir. The diagnosis of shigellosis is made by the growth of *Shigella* in a stool culture. Antibiotic treatment is needed in serious cases, but resistance to antibiotics is a growing problem. Research continues on a possible vaccine.

—Louis B. Jacques, M.D.

See also Bacterial infections; Bacteriology; Diarrhea and dysentery; Gastroenterology; Gastroenterology, pediatric; Gastrointestinal disorders; Gastrointestinal system; Intestinal disorders; Intestines.

FOR FURTHER INFORMATION:

Kabir, Iqbal, et al. "Increased Height Gain of Children Fed a High-Protein Diet During Convalescence from Shigellosis." *The Journal of Nutrition* 128, no. 10 (October, 1998): 1688-1691. The impact of dietary supplementation on catch-up growth was evaluated in sixty-nine malnourished children, ages twenty-four to sixty months, after recovery from shigellosis.

Kelley, William, et al., eds. *Essentials of Internal Medicine*. New York: J. B. Lippincott, 1994. A medical textbook that is particularly useful, with its inclusion of definitions and descriptions of the clinical presentation of the disease, diagnosis, and treatment.

SHINGLES
DISEASE/DISORDER

ANATOMY OR SYSTEM AFFECTED: Nervous system, skin

SPECIALTIES AND RELATED FIELDS: Family practice, internal medicine, virology

DEFINITION: Also known as herpes zoster, shingles is a disease of the central nervous system which is caused by the same virus that causes chickenpox. It is characterized by painful red blisters that join together and rapidly rupture and become crusted. The rash tends to follow one or more of the spinal nerves beneath the skin. Other symptoms include mild chills and fever, mild nausea, abdominal cramps, diarrhea, and aches and pains of the face and chest. Immunity to the disease is usually gained by having chickenpox earlier in life or a prior attack of shingles, but in a few cases, patients have been known to have had more than one attack. Recovery is usually spontaneous after two to three weeks.

—Jason Georges and Tracy Irons-Georges

Shingles

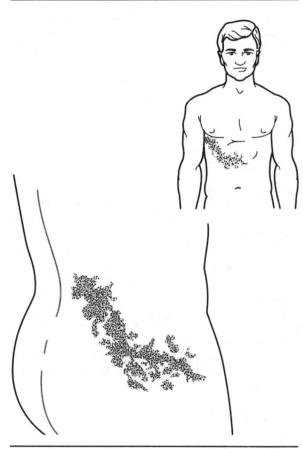

Shingles is characterized by painful red blisters that join, rupture, and become crusted.

See also Chickenpox; Herpes; Nervous system; Neurology; Neurology, pediatric; Rashes; Viral infections.

FOR FURTHER INFORMATION:

Adams, Raymond D., Maurice Victor, and Allan H. Ropper. *Adams and Victor's Principles of Neurology*. 7th ed. New York: McGraw-Hill, 2000.

Siegel, Mary-Ellen, and Gray Williams. *Living with Shingles: New Hope for an Old Disease*. New York: M. Evans, 1998.

Silverstein, Alvin, Virginia Silverstein, and Laura Silverstein Nunn. *Chicken Pox and Shingles*. New York: Enslow, 1998.

Thomsen, Thomas Carl. *Shingles and PHN*. Rev. ed. Cross River, N.Y.: Cross River, 1994.

SHOCK

DISEASE/DISORDER

ANATOMY OR SYSTEM AFFECTED: Blood vessels, circulatory system, heart

SPECIALTIES AND RELATED FIELDS: Critical care, emergency medicine, family practice, internal medicine

DEFINITION: Shock is a life-threatening condition that may occur in response to any circumstance (injury, blood loss, heart attack, toxic substances in the blood) which causes the heart to be unable to pump enough blood to supply the vital organs, which are therefore deprived of oxygen and nutrients and lose normal function; symptoms include rapid, shallow breathing, clammy skin, low blood pressure (weak pulse), dizziness, and unconsciousness.

KEY TERMS:

blood pressure: a measure of how much the fluid in the blood vessels pushes against the walls of the vessels

cardiovascular system: the organ system consisting of the heart and all blood vessels (vasculature)

vasculature: all the blood vessels, including the arteries (blood vessels carrying blood away from the heart), the capillaries (the smallest blood vessels where fluid and nutrients are exchanged), and the veins (blood vessels that return blood to the heart)

vital organs: organs of the body essential to life, usually considered to be the brain, the heart, and sometimes the kidneys

CAUSES AND SYMPTOMS

The primary goal of the cardiovascular system is to provide blood flow, carrying oxygen and other nutrients to all tissues to meet their requirements. The cardiovascular system performs this function by maintaining a blood pressure high enough to push sufficient blood flow through every tissue, especially the vital organs (the brain, heart, and kidneys). To keep the blood pressure up, the heart must pump sufficient amounts of blood even when the demand for increased blood flow to some tissues occurs. The blood vessels also play an important role in maintaining blood pressure. The heart and the blood vessels work in a coordinated manner to maintain blood pressure and blood flow.

A healthy heart is capable of adjusting the strength of its beats and the rate of its beats (the heart rate) to produce enough flow to match the demands placed on it by the tissues of the body. For example, during exercise, the exercising muscles require greater blood flow. If the heart does not pump the increased amount of blood that is necessary, then the blood pressure will fall. Hormones such as adrenaline help the heart beat faster and harder to meet the increased demand for blood by the muscles.

The blood vessels (vasculature) have a special structure and function to help maintain blood pressure. The arteries and veins are elastic in nature and squeeze on the blood like an inflated balloon does to the air inside it. In addition, the walls of blood vessels have special muscle tissue, called smooth muscle, that can contract to make the vessels' internal diameter smaller, which helps keep pressure up. If the vessels' internal diameter becomes too small, however, then the blood flow through them will decrease. The concept of blood vessels getting narrow and making it more difficult to push blood through is termed resistance to flow or vascular resistance. The balance of blood flow produced by the heart (cardiac output) and vascular resistance keeps blood pressure at the proper level. When one or both of these components falter, cardiac output and blood pressure can fall, creating shock.

When the cardiovascular system cannot supply blood flow to the essential organs that is adequate to sustain their function, the body is said to be in shock. A reduction in cardiac output is the primary problem in shock. There are two major ways in which cardiac output can decrease enough to cause shock. First, the ability of the heart to pump may be compromised, which may cause reduced cardiac output. When the heart cannot pump sufficient blood, the resulting condition is termed cardiogenic shock. In the other form of shock, the vascular portion of the cardiovascular system cannot return enough blood back to the heart, so the heart cannot pump adequate amounts. The general term "hypovolemic shock" is used when the heart is not the source of the reduced cardiac output.

Cardiogenic shock may occur in several ways. The most common cause is a myocardial infarction (heart attack). During a heart attack, the heart is damaged, and like any other muscle when injured, does not have the strength to pump much blood. Thus, cardiac output goes down and a fall in blood pressure will follow. Cardiogenic shock is dangerous: About 10 percent of all patients who experience a severe myocardial infarction die of the ensuing shock. After a myocardial infarction, while the heart is still healing, it has a reduced ability to pump blood. Exercise, even light exercise such as walking, must be resumed

gradually. If it is not, the heart may not be able to pump enough blood to supply muscles even though demand for more flow is only slightly increased. Blood pressure may fall, again producing shock and reinjuring the heart.

In cardiac tamponade, another form of cardiogenic shock, the stiff but pliable sac surrounding the heart (pericardium) fills with fluid or swells. This takes up room in the sac, squeezing the heart and prohibiting it from filling adequately from beat to beat. Therefore, the amount of blood pumped decreases, and a drop in blood pressure occurs. Cardiac tamponade can occur for several reasons. It can occur rapidly when the heart is punctured and bleeds into the pericardial sac. Cardiac tamponade occurs much more slowly when excess fluid is produced by the pericardium or when the pericardium becomes swollen. Both of these conditions can be caused by an infection.

A third and less common form of cardiogenic shock is caused by an extremely high heart rate. Normally, the heart beats at a rate between sixty and one hundred beats per minute. When the heart rate exceeds one hundred, the resulting condition is called tachycardia. Occasionally, in some people, the heart rate can go rapidly up to near two hundred beats per minute. The time between beats becomes so short that the heart does not have enough time to refill and cardiac output falls. If this condition lasts for more than a few seconds, the blood pressure may fall, causing shock. When this occurs, the combination of the rapid heart rate and low blood pressure may cause a myocardial infarction.

Shock caused by a problem in the vascular system, not by a primary decrease in heart function, is generally termed hypovolemic shock. It is characterized by a lack of sufficient blood volume returned to the heart by the vascular system. Hypovolemic shock can be caused by a decrease in the body's total blood volume.

Excessive bleeding (hemorrhage) is the most common and striking form of hypovolemic shock. The blood vessels are elastic in nature, and they must remain filled with blood for arterial pressure to be maintained. In addition, enough blood must be in the veins to push it back to the heart, to be pumped through the lungs and back out into the arteries. When blood loss is slight (10 percent or less of the total blood volume), the veins and arteries can contract, thereby maintaining enough pressure and sufficient cardiac output. When enough volume is lost, such as more than 20 percent of the total amount in the body, blood pressure falls.

There are other ways in which blood volume may decrease. When a person is burned severely, plasma (the fluid in which blood cells are suspended) is lost through the burn sites. Enough can be lost to cause hypovolemic shock. Different forms of dehydration can also result in shock. Prolonged diarrhea, vomiting, and sweating can ultimately result in shock if the person does not drink enough liquids to replace fluid lost. All these conditions lead to a loss in blood volume and subnormal return of blood to the heart, and thus reduced cardiac output.

A virtual loss in blood volume may also occur, resulting in shock. Sometimes anesthesia or brain damage can cause the vascular smooth muscle around the arteries and veins to relax. This results in a loss of arterial and venous pressure. Blood tends to accumulate in the veins and is not returned to the heart, and cardiac output falls. An allergic reaction can cause a similar response, called anaphylactic shock. Some bacterial infections can also produce a similar condition. When an infection is the cause of shock, it is called endotoxin shock. All types of hypovolemic shock, actual or virtual, are caused by a loss of blood.

APPLICATIONS

In spite of the different causes of circulatory shock, the symptoms are quite common in nearly all cases of shock. The pulse (heart rate) is usually rapid and feeble. Breathing is generally rapid and shallow. The skin is pale, cool, and sometimes moist. The mouth is dry, and thirst is intense. Blood pressure is diminished. Some of these signs are attributable to the body's attempt to alleviate the problem.

The body has several defense mechanisms to help avoid circulatory shock. Several reflex systems function to maintain cardiac output and blood pressure. The body has sensors in the cardiovascular system that tell the brain what the pressure is in the arteries and the veins. When the brain senses a change in either or both of these pressures, it calls on its defenses.

When the arterial pressure sensors tell the brain that blood pressure is falling, the brain produces several responses. Through the nerves, the brain can make the heart beat faster and with greater force. In addition, the nerves can cause vascular smooth muscle to contract, making the vessels squeeze against the blood and increasing pressure. When the smooth muscle contracts, the veins squeeze blood back to the

heart to enable it to pump more. The brain can also cause the release of adrenaline into the blood. This hormone can also cause the heart to beat harder and faster. The combined actions of this reflex mechanism help return cardiac output and blood pressure to normal during shock.

The sensors in the large veins and atria of the heart can cause a different response. Since most (75 percent) of the blood in the body is in the veins at any point in time, a change in pressure in the veins is an index of how much blood is in the body. If the pressure decreases, it is an indication that blood volume is low. In this condition, the brain causes a release of a hormone called vasopressin into the blood. Immediately (within seconds or minutes), vasopressin constricts the blood vessels to increase both arterial and venous pressure. The increase in venous pressure squeezes more blood back to the heart to improve cardiac output. The squeeze on the arteries raises blood pressure. Over a longer period of time (within hours or days), vasopressin affects the kidneys. The kidneys respond to increased blood levels of vasopressin by decreasing the production of urine. The fluid retained by the kidney is returned to the blood to keep up the vascular volume.

Specialized blood vessels in the kidneys can also initiate a reflex response to a decrease in blood pressure. The kidneys release a hormone called renin into the blood. Renin activates another hormone, angiotensin, which is a powerful constrictor of blood vessels. Angiotensin increases the release of yet another hormone, aldosterone, which helps the kidneys to reabsorb more fluid. All the above reflexes work together to increase blood volume, cardiac output, and blood pressure, and thereby to help alleviate shock. Despite these mechanisms to prevent shock, however, there are mechanisms that work in the opposite direction called decompensatory mechanisms. These mechanisms worsen the state of shock and may eventually cause death.

Some of the important decompensatory factors are heart failure, the production of acid (acidosis), blood-clotting problems, a decrease in the body's bacterial defense system, and a decrease in brain blood flow. If the decompensatory mechanisms become stronger than the compensatory mechanisms, a condition called irreversible shock occurs and blood pressure falls continuously until death results.

When average arterial blood pressure falls below 60 millimeters of mercury (mmHg), the blood flow to the blood vessels supplying the heart (coronary) cannot be maintained. When this occurs in shock, it happens at a time when the heart needs its critical supply of oxygen. In fact, the heart is trying to beat harder and faster, which increases its need for oxygen. As a result, the heart can weaken. When weakened, it pumps less and thus cannot bring the pressure back to normal. The heart becomes weaker and weaker. This condition is termed cardiac failure. In addition to cardiac failure caused by reduced coronary blood flow, the body can produce a hormone called myocardial depressant factor (MDF). This hormone directly causes a weakening of the heart that is independent of coronary blood flow. MDF also causes the body's bacterial defense system to function poorly. The maintenance of heart function is important to defend against shock.

Because the blood vessels contract in most of the body during shock, blood flow to nonessential tissues such as skin, muscle, bone, and the intestines is reduced, depriving these tissues of oxygen. These tissues can tolerate short periods of low oxygen supply, but if shock persists for more than a few minutes, these tissues revert to other energy sources. The end products of these alternative energy sources are acids, which can begin a process of tissue damage. If this process is not controlled or reversed, tissues can die. If a critical amount of tissue in an organ dies, the organ cannot function and may fail. Acid produced by other tissues gets into the blood and can directly decrease the function of the heart and its ability to respond to beneficial reflex signals. Acid production makes it more difficult for the body to fight shock.

Derangements in blood clotting can occur during shock. Blood clots can form in the early stages of shock, blocking small vessels. This causes a loss of oxygen that results in acid production. Increased acid in the blood can increase the rate of formation of blood clots. Thus, the clotting system can start a vicious cycle which increases the severity of shock.

Even when shock is not bacterial in origin, the body needs its bacteria-fighting systems. During shock, the bacterial defenses are weakened. Normally, bacteria from the intestines constantly enter the blood and are rapidly neutralized. If this does not occur, endotoxin shock can intensify the already existing shock. Therefore, a capable bacteria-fighting system is important in defending against shock.

In shock, the blood vessels of the heart and brain are spared the constriction experienced by all other

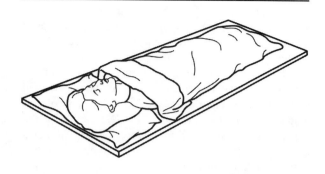

Victims of shock must be kept warm with a blanket and legs slightly elevated; emergency medical attention should be sought immediately.

tissue blood vessels. In fact, arteries in these organs relax to permit as much blood flow as possible, maintaining oxygen supply to these vital organs. Even so, when very low blood pressure persists (less than 50 mmHg), the brain's function decreases. At this point, the brain sends fewer of the beneficial reflex signals to the heart and blood vessels. The final result is a continuous decline in blood pressure and death. Maintenance of brain blood flow is a very important factor in surviving shock.

TREATMENT AND THERAPY
Emergency procedures in response to circulatory shock entail contacting emergency service providers such as paramedics and keeping the victim warm and prone, with slightly elevated legs. The victim must get medical attention immediately.

Treatment of shock can vary depending on the cause. In many cases, most shock can be effectively treated with the appropriate medicines. Some cases require surgical intervention. In all cases, the status of body fluids must be monitored and treated. The body's blood volume is one of the most important things to maintain.

It is particularly important to optimize blood volume in forms of hypovolemic shock. With hemorrhagic shock, whole blood is given intravenously to replace lost blood. In other forms of hypovolemic shock, different intravenous fluids are usually given. In burn shock, when the blood's plasma weeps from the burn sites, blood plasma is the medicine of choice to restore lost volume. When hypovolemia is caused by excessive diarrhea, vomiting, or sweating, a balanced salt solution is given to replenish lost volume.

In other cases of shock, special drugs are needed to alleviate the symptoms. Shock caused rapidly by a myocardial infarction, with cardiac arrest, can be immediately supported by cardiopulmonary resuscitation (CPR), provided by a trained individual. After resumption of the heartbeat, the heart can be helped with several types of drugs. An effective class of cardiac drugs called digitalis is given. Digitalis helps the weak heart to beat with more force. When strengthened again, the heart can bring a decreased cardiac output back to normal. In the case of paroxysmal tachycardia, a drug such as lidocaine can calm the very rapid heart rate to normal, allowing the heart to fill properly and pump adequate blood. Cardiac tamponade must be reduced to allow the heart to pump usual amounts. If the onset is rapid, as when it is caused by chest trauma, the fluid in the pericardial sac may need to be removed immediately. A needle is placed into the fluid, and the fluid is drawn out of the sac to alleviate the pressure around the heart. If fluid accumulates slowly as with an infection and is recognized early, appropriate drug treatment for the infection (antibiotics) may resolve the problem. In cases of shock in which acidosis is a complication or even a potential complication, bicarbonate, a chemical that can reduce the acidity of the blood, is given. No unique therapy can be used in any type of shock because of the complex forms that may occur. For example, hemorrhage may become complicated by heart failure and/or endotoxin. Each case must be treated in accordance with the patient's existing conditions.

PERSPECTIVE AND PROSPECTS

Chinese writings of more than three thousand years ago indicate that a connection existed between the heart and the blood. Until the second century, it was thought that arteries carried air, not blood. Through the Middle Ages, it was believed that "spirits" were the essence of life or "vitality." This belief encouraged "bloodletting" as a treatment for many ailments, including shock. Leeches were applied to remove the "evil spirit" causing the sickness. This was not a very successful mode of therapy.

It was not until the seventeenth century that blood transfusions were tried, with the first experiments conducted by Richard Lower. In the 1660's, Jean-Baptiste Denis administered lamb's blood to a sixteen-year-old boy who was very weak and who had a high fever (perhaps in shock with endotoxin complication). The condition of the boy, who had been bled several

times, improved for a short period of time. Others continued to experiment with transfusion as the remedy for loss of blood, but until the discovery of blood typing at the turn of the twentieth century, most attempts were of limited success.

In the eighteenth century, William Withering published observations on the effect of foxglove (digitalis) tea. He showed that the leaves of the foxglove plant could relieve dropsy, an illness known to be caused in part by heart disease. Digitalis slows the heart and can increase the force of its contraction. Digitalis was the first and is still one of the most important medicines used in treating heart disease.

The practice of giving transfusions greatly increased after the discovery of blood types in 1901 by Karl Landsteiner, who won the 1930 Nobel Prize in Physiology or Medicine for his work. By 1920, blood could be transfused from a bottle, since Luis Agote had discovered that citrated blood would not clot after being removed from the body. Blood banking was established in the 1920's by Russian scientists who discovered that citrated blood could be stored at 40 degrees Fahrenheit.

Little more has been added to heart and blood treatment of shock since that time. Synthetic medicines similar to digitalis have become much more specific in their action. Synthetic blood substitutes have been developed. The challenge is to develop solutions that can carry as much oxygen as blood without complications associated with bloodlike clotting and the transmission of diseases such as acquired immunodeficiency syndrome (AIDS). Hemoglobin solutions free of blood cells have been developed. Fluorocarbon solutions, a synthetic solution which has a high capacity for oxygen, are available but have not totally replaced well-matched blood for resuscitation from shock.

—*J. Timothy O'Neill, Ph.D.*

See also Allergies; Bites and stings; Bleeding; Burns and scalds; Critical care; Critical care, pediatric; Electrical shock; Emergency medicine; Heart attack; Heart failure; Hemophilia; Necrotizing fasciitis; Resuscitation; Septicemia; Transfusion; Unconsciousness.

FOR FURTHER INFORMATION:

Ackerknecht, Erwin H. *A Short History of Medicine.* Rev. ed. Baltimore: The Johns Hopkins University Press, 1982. One of the most complete and readable texts on the general history of medicine.

Asimov, Isaac. *The Human Body: Its Structure and Operation.* Rev. ed. New York: Penguin Books, 1992. This text provides an understandable overview of all the body's organ functions, with a good presentation on the circulatory system.

Avraham, Regina. *The Circulatory System.* Philadelphia: Chelsea House, 2000. This text explains the function of the circulatory system in reasonably simple terms. Provides historical development of knowledge about the heart and blood vessels.

Barrett, John, and Lloyd M. Nyhus. *Treatment of Shock: Principles and Practice.* 2d ed. Philadelphia: Lea & Febiger, 1986. This text presents a complete overview of reasonably current treatments of shock. Unfortunately, it relies on medical terminology.

Mower-Wade, Donna M., et al. "Shock: Do You Know How to Respond?" *Nursing* 30, no. 10 (October, 2000): 34-39. This work presents ways to recognize three types of shock and discusses how to respond appropriately to them. These include hypovolemic, septic, and cardiogenic shock.

Shock therapy

Procedure

Anatomy or system affected: Brain, nerves, nervous system, psychic-emotional system

Specialties and related fields: Neurology, psychiatry

Definition: A psychiatric treatment where chemical, electrical, or other measures are used to induce a coma, convulsions, or seizure in the brain, altering its chemistry and relieving psychiatric distress.

Key terms:

anesthetic: any of a variety of drugs used to cause a patient to become unconscious and amnesic for a brief period of time; electroconvulsive therapy is conducted under the influence of very short-acting anesthetics, such as methohexital, thiamylal sodium, thiopental sodium, and etomidate

convulsion: an instance of high-frequency and amplitude-random electrical activity in the brain; electroconvulsive therapy causes a convulsion in the brain, which is believed to be related to its mechanism of action

electrocardiogram: a recording of the electrical activity of the heart; used during electroconvulsive therapy to monitor changes in heart rate, rhythm, and conduction, any or all of which may be temporarily affected by this procedure

electroencephalogram: a brain wave trace used to monitor the onset, termination, and duration of the convulsion or seizure

mood disorders: any of a number of mental conditions characterized by a primary disturbance of mood as distinct from thinking or behavior

muscle relaxant: any of a number of medications used to paralyze the muscles of the patient temporarily before delivering the electrical stimulus; the main medication used for this purpose is succinylcholine

organic brain syndrome (organicity): changes in memory, orientation, and perception that occur as a side effect of electroconvulsive therapy

psychotic disorder: a psychiatric condition in which an individual's mental state is out of touch with reality, as displayed by abnormal and bizarre perceptions, thoughts, behavior, judgment, and reasoning

seizure: used interchangeably with the term "convulsion"

Indications and Procedures

Shock therapy, also known as shock treatment, is an intervention that has been used for many years to treat severe psychiatric conditions, such as life-threatening depression and psychotic disorders. Many methods of shock treatment exist, ranging from chemically induced shock (via substances such as insulin) to electrically induced shock (from an electrical current). What all the methods share is the purpose of inducing a temporary loss of consciousness, convulsions, and/or seizure in an effort to disrupt brain activity and reset it to a healthier state.

Insulin shock therapy was developed in 1933 by Manfred Sakel. He found that intramuscular administrations of insulin were able to induce a coma that appeared effective for treating severe cases of schizophrenia. By and large, this approach was replaced with other methods of shock therapy, predominantly electroconvulsive therapy (ECT); however, it is still used today when other methods of shock therapy or intervention are judged to be less appropriate. Modern-day procedures are superior to what was originally done in shock therapy approaches. The impact of the shock on the body is better able to be controlled, and the shock treatment itself is more refined in its application. In fact, some newer methods such as transcranial magnetic stimulation (TMS) may be able to provide a similar adjustment to brain activity without the use of electric current or chemically induced shock.

Historically though, shock therapy has been equated with ECT. Formerly called electroshock or shock therapy, it is a very powerful treatment for psychiatric conditions such as mood disorders and psychotic disorders. It is based on the idea that electrically induced convulsions change the chemistry of the brain in a way that relieves the symptoms of severe mental illness, in which depression, mania, or both become debilitating.

In most situations, electroconvulsive therapy involves the participation of the psychiatrist providing the treatment and an anesthesiologist, who anesthetizes the patient for the procedure. The patient is instructed to take nothing by mouth for eight hours prior to the treatment, so that the stomach is empty for the induction of general anesthesia. The danger of having food or liquid in the stomach is that it might be aspi-

rated into the lungs, where it could cause pneumonia, respiratory obstruction, or death. An intravenous needle is placed in an arm vein. The patient is then connected to a number of monitors, including a blood pressure cuff, electrocardiogram, and pulse oximeter (to measure the level of tissue oxygenation). The patient is then anesthetized with a short-acting intravenous drug (usually methohexital, also known as Brevital). This is followed by the administration of a short-acting muscle relaxant (usually succinylcholine). Ventilation is controlled by mask, using 100 percent oxygen. As soon as it is determined that the muscles are paralyzed, a mild electrical current is administered to the patient's brain. The duration of the stimulus is two seconds or less. There is a brief contraction of the muscles of the face, followed by a generalized seizure, which is monitored on the electroencephalo-

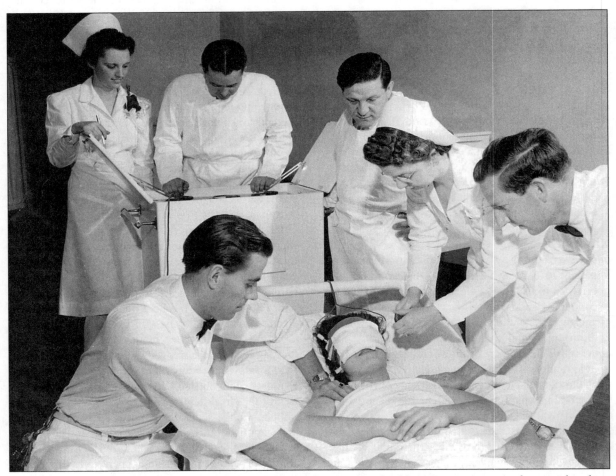

A patient is given electroconvulsive therapy in 1942 to treat bipolar disorder. Many improvements in the procedure have been made since that time, including anesthesia. (AP/Wide World Photos)

gram. Small amounts of physical movement may be seen in the face, feet, or hands. These movements are not nearly as severe as those that occurred before the advent of muscle relaxants. The anesthesiologist continues to ventilate the patient until the effects of the muscle relaxant have worn off and spontaneous respiration is reestablished (three to five minutes). There is a period of confusion and disorientation that rapidly follows the treatment; it clears quickly. With each successive treatment, the patient is left with an ongoing loss of memory which will gradually clear after the course of therapy is finished. The average patient requires between six and twelve treatments. They are administered two or three times per week.

The decision to conduct electroconvulsive therapy usually comes after there has been failure in other forms of treatment, including medication and psychotherapy. Since there are so many medications and combinations of medication that can be used, however, ECT arguably cannot be thought of as a treatment of last resort, as it was in earlier decades. The idea of administering ECT generally arises when it is critical that the patient improve as rapidly as possible. This consideration is often punctuated by frustration on the part of the patient, the family, and/or the psychiatrist with the slowness of response to current therapeutic modalities. In the 1980's, ECT began to be considered earlier rather than later in the course of treatment. It is realistic to say that if one or two medications are not successful, it is unlikely that others will be successful. Yet there are always those cases in which a sudden and complete remission in mood and psychotic disorders occurs without the use of ECT.

Mood and psychotic disorders tend to recur. When treating a patient for the first time, the doctor cannot know whether the effect of ECT will last for a week, months, or years. Some people need only one course of ECT in a lifetime; others will respond well and remain symptom-free for many years, requiring further ECT when symptoms recur. For many patients who develop devastating symptomatology with their illnesses, the early initiation of a course of ECT is warranted. Those who have responded well to only ECT in the past will forgo medication trials in favor of starting ECT as soon as the symptoms reappear. For those patients who respond well to ECT but who have recurrences within weeks or months, maintenance ECT may be a reasonable option. With this regimen, a single treatment is given every four to twelve weeks in order to prevent a recurrence of psychiatric distress. The actual frequency of treatment is based on each patient's particular clinical course and history. For many patients, maintenance ECT has been a way of preventing multiple and frequent hospitalizations. Very little cognitive impairment is associated with low-frequency maintenance ECT, and patients go on to live very productive lives while being maintained in this way.

The following case is an example of the uses of electroconvulsive therapy in clinical practice: A seventy-five-year-old white, widowed female was referred by her psychiatrist for evaluation for electroconvulsive therapy. She had been well until two years prior to this evaluation. At that time, a month following the death of her husband, she began to experience a variety of symptoms, including loss of appetite with a ten-pound weight loss, decreased interest in her friends and the ordinary activities of life which she had found enjoyable, and sleep disturbance characterized by difficulty falling asleep and early morning awakening. The sleep difficulty was responsive to the use of triazolam, a sleep-inducing drug. Additionally, she began to experience episodes of dizziness that were made worse by antidepressant medications. She was not actively suicidal, but she did experience a wish to die and join her husband, who she believed was waiting for her. She had been treated with tricyclic antidepressants (nortriptyline and desipramine) with lithium augmentation, but the side effects of constipation and dizziness made these medications intolerable. Her depression did not improve, and she began to exhibit medical signs of dehydration and malnutrition. The treating psychiatrist believed that electroconvulsive therapy was indicated and that it should be instituted as rapidly as possible as a lifesaving measure.

The patient was given a course of seven unilateral ECT treatments over the period of a month. She responded to the treatments with an elevation in her mood, an improvement in sleep and appetite, and increasing engagement with hospital staff and family. When she was discharged from the hospital, she showed evidence of mild memory impairment. In the weeks following her treatment, her memory improved, and she became brighter and resumed her normal activities with vigor. She was started on a small dose of fluoxetine (Prozac), an antidepressant known to have a milder side effect profile than the medications she had taken previously. After one year of follow-up, she was still doing well.

Electroconvulsive therapy continues to be widely

practiced in the United States and abroad. There is consensus within the field of psychiatry that it is a valuable tool in the psychiatric armamentarium. Patients, patient advocates, and clinicians alike, however, continue to be concerned about its ethical and appropriate use. Practitioners support efforts of the lay community to ensure the proper and ethical use of ECT as long as it does not obstruct access to the treatment for those who require it.

USES AND COMPLICATIONS

Electroconvulsive therapy is used for a variety of psychiatric conditions, including major depressive disorder, depressed bipolar disorder, manic bipolar disorder, mixed bipolar disorder, schizophrenia, manic excitement, and catatonia. Before starting electroconvulsive therapy, all patients are screened for medical illnesses, for two reasons. First, a variety of medical illnesses are associated with depression or mania; the list is long and includes occult cancer, hypothyroidism, vitamin deficiencies, endocrine abnormalities, and brain tumors or infections, among many others. If there is a treatable cause for depression, it must be found and treated before the decision to perform electroconvulsive therapy is made. Once it is clear that the psychiatric illness is not being caused by something else, ECT may be used. It is important to note that there are certain untreatable medical causes for depression or mania in which the disorder may respond to ECT. For example, depressed patients with Alzheimer's disease may respond to ECT, showing significant improvements in mood. Brain-injured patients with depression may, in some circumstances, respond to electroconvulsive therapy.

The second reason for screening the patient is to establish that it is safe to proceed with ECT. A routine evaluation should include a medical history and physical examination, psychiatric history, mental status examination, blood count, blood chemistries, urinalysis, and electrocardiogram. Other tests may be done if they seem important to rule out other possible illnesses. Such tests might include a computed tomography (CT) scan, a magnetic resonance imaging (MRI) scan, an electroencephalogram (EEG, or brain wave study), or tests for antidepressant drug levels.

There are no absolute reasons not to perform electroconvulsive therapy. There are certain conditions, however, that produce a significant increase in risk with ECT. Cerebral aneurysm may increase the danger of electroconvulsive therapy. An aneurysm is a balloonlike swelling of an artery, which may cause severe brain damage if it bursts. The high blood pressure associated with ECT may cause a cerebral aneurysm to burst. Patients who have recently experienced a heart attack are at increased risk of dying with ECT. Electroconvulsive therapy should be delayed for six months, if possible, following a heart attack. Other illnesses that increase risk include emphysema, multiple sclerosis, and muscular dystrophy.

Despite these risks, electroconvulsive therapy is considered by many to be the safest of the somatic treatments available in psychiatry. The death rate from ECT itself is one patient in ten thousand—much lower, for example, than the death rate for patients taking antidepressant medications; the death rate from suicide in depressed people is much higher. Electroconvulsive therapy may be done safely with patients representing a broad range of age and physical condition. For the elderly, malnourished patient, it is clearly safer and more effective than medication. Prior to the use of muscle relaxants, broken bones and vertebrae were a considerable problem with ECT. This is no longer the case. Complications such as uncontrolled hypertension, stroke, and heart attack rarely occur; they are extremely unlikely, because the patients are medically screened prior to beginning the treatment.

In each situation, the risk of doing ECT must be weighed against the risk of not doing the treatment. If the patient is imminently suicidal—so that he or she cannot be left alone—ECT may be indicated even though the risk is high. Similarly, patients who are starving to death as a result of their illness may require immediate treatment. Patients with manic excitement or delirium, who are completely out of control and require seclusion, may require ECT despite increased risk.

The most disturbing and severe side effect of ECT is memory loss. It is believed that this side effect is attributable to the electricity that is passed through the brain. The postseizure state may also have some effect. What seems to be clear is that this memory deficit is not the result of physical damage to the brain. Some memories, especially those of events that occur around the time of the treatment, may be permanently lost. Many patients will lose their memory of the periods of most severe depression or mania. The ability to learn new information may be temporarily lost. Most people return to reasonable function within the first month and to complete function after six months.

In the News: Transcranial Magnetic Stimulation

The 1990's saw the development of an alternative stimulatory procedure to the use of electroconvulsive therapy (ECT) as a standard treatment for severe depression. Transcranial magnetic stimulation (TMS) utilizes a magnetic coil to deliver a pulse to specified areas of the brain, generally in the region of the prefrontal cortex above the temple. The stimulating coil is held close to the scalp so that the field is focused and can pass through the skull. Rapid-rate TMS can deliver up to fifty stimuli per second. When stimulation is delivered at regular intervals, it is termed repetitive TMS (rTMS). TMS therapy can be used on an outpatient basis, reducing the necessity to hospitalize the patient (and providing cost relief for both the patient and the hospital). Unlike with electroconvulsive therapy (ECT), no side effects such as vomiting, fatigue, or memory loss are seen with TMS. The use of TMS is also being studied in connection with movement disorders, epilepsy, bipolar disorder, anxiety disorders, developmental stuttering, Tourette's syndrome, and schizophrenia.

—*Richard Adler, Ph.D.*

There are a number of ways to gauge the response of a patient to ECT. It is a complicated process that has to take into account and weigh three factors: the improvement of the mood of the patient, the number of treatments or total seizure seconds, and the amount of confusion and/or memory loss that is produced. Additionally, it is important to gauge the emotional response of the patient and the family to the changes being brought about by the treatment.

With each successive treatment, the patient's mood should get better. If the patient has been depressed, there should be a decrease of the depressive symptoms. Appetite and sleep patterns should improve. There should be an increased level of activity, and social engagement should get better. These changes may first be noticeable to the family and hospital staff. Very often, the improvement becomes apparent to the patient later. Occasionally, the improvement will not be obvious until there has been a chance for the confusion and memory loss to resolve. If the patient is manic, there should be an improvement in symptoms of hyperactivity, grandiosity, irritability, and inability to organize activity and behavior. The response of mania to ECT is often very rapid, and the results may be quite gratifying.

If confusion occurs too early in the course of ECT and it is clear that more treatment needs to be done, decreasing the frequency of treatment from three times a week to once or twice a week may be indicated. Ultimately the decision to stop ECT is based on balancing the above-mentioned factors in an optimal way. This determination is made by the clinician with the input of the patient and all the others (psychiatrist, family, and staff) who know the patient best. If the patient does not seem to be improving and is not having memory difficulty, ECT should be continued. Some patients may need as many as twenty treatments to achieve resolution of psychiatric distress.

Electroconvulsive therapy is the most effective treatment for major mood disorders and for psychotic disorders with a mood component. The likelihood of success depends on the specific diagnosis as well as the accuracy of the diagnostic assessment. Patients who have not responded to adequate trials of medication are less likely to respond to ECT than are those who have not been treated with medication. This would seem to reflect the idea that treatment-resistant psychiatric distress is less likely to respond to any form of treatment.

PERSPECTIVE AND PROSPECTS

Electroconvulsive therapy was discovered as a therapy of mental illness in 1938. It was first used by Ugo Cerletti and Lucio Bini in Italy. The basis of its use was the observation that patients with epilepsy did not suffer from schizophrenia. It was believed that there was something about brain seizures that either prevented or was protective against schizophrenia. While that clinical observation was not accurate, it became the impetus for research into the curative effects of electrically induced seizures.

The first electrical convulsions were induced without the benefit of general anesthesia. Patients had violent seizures and often suffered broken bones and teeth. They were held down in order to keep the seizures from causing excessive physical harm. The responses to ECT in certain patients were quite dramatic. Symptoms such as depression and mania could often be eliminated. Agitated behavior associated with schizophrenia could be mitigated and patients suffering from catatonia would often become animated as a result of a course of electroconvulsive therapy. The therapy was soon brought to the United States, where it enjoyed frequent use until the early 1950's.

At that time, antipsychotic and antidepressant medications for the treatment of psychiatric illnesses became available. The drugs chlorpromazine and imipramine were shown to be effective in managing the symptoms of schizophrenia and mood disorders. As a result, electroconvulsive therapy was used less frequently and then only in severe, treatment-refractory cases. The political climate of the 1960's and 1970's and films such as *One Flew over the Cuckoo's Nest* (1975) portrayed ECT as a tool of the repressive and oppressing psychiatric establishment to exert behavioral and mind control over an unwitting public. Laws were passed in many jurisdictions, making it more difficult for patients to obtain ECT. There were efforts to outlaw ECT. Now, however, even the most powerful patient advocacy groups accept the appropriate use of this treatment.

Electroconvulsive therapy has been utilized with increasing frequency for a number of reasons: recognition of its efficacy, the safety of electroconvulsive therapy in medically ill patients, the increased safety of anesthetic techniques, improved diagnostic criteria, an improved process of informed consent, and disappointing efficacy and side effects of medication in certain patients.

One of the reasons for the renewed interest in ECT is the improvement in informed consent procedures. Physicians no longer adopt as authoritative an attitude toward patients as they did in the past. In the early years of ECT, patients were not informed of all the potential side effects of the treatment. They were often not told that they had alternatives and what the risks and side effects of the alternatives were. The result was that they experienced complications and side effects for which they were not prepared. They became disappointed and angry. Modern informed consent procedures allow the patient to participate as fully as possible in the decision to take any particular form of therapy. The patient is cognizant of the fact that there are choices and alternatives. The patient is also aware that he or she may decide to discontinue treatment at any time if there is no benefit and the side effects are intolerable. Accurate descriptions of side effects and complications are given to the patient. The patient is apprised of the fact that the treatment may fail and that the treatment is being done this time because it is the one that is most likely to help at this juncture. The patient learns that the choice is simply the best choice, not the only one. Both patients and doctors have benefited from such an enlightened approach to informed consent.

—Frank Guerra, M.D.;
updated by Nancy A. Piotrowski, Ph.D.

See also Bipolar disorder; Brain; Depression; Emotions: Biomedical causes and effects; Epilepsy; Memory loss; Nervous system; Neurology; Psychiatric disorders; Psychiatry; Psychiatry, child and adolescent; Psychiatry, geriatric; Schizophrenia; Seizures; Sleep disorders.

FOR FURTHER INFORMATION:

Abrams, Richard. *Electroconvulsive Therapy.* 3d ed. New York: Oxford University Press, 1997. A textbook on electroconvulsive therapy that presents a complete picture of all aspects of treatment, from the scientific to the clinical.

American Psychiatric Association. *The Practice of Electroconvulsive Therapy: Recommendations for Treatment, Training, and Privileging.* Washington, D.C.: American Psychiatric Press, 1990. This book is the result of the work of a task force on electroconvulsive therapy in the American Psychiatric Association. It shows how psychiatrists have worked to make the practice of ECT as ethical and safe as possible. Argues for the importance of this form of treatment to psychiatric patients.

Endler, Norman S. *Holiday of Darkness.* New York: John Wiley & Sons, 1982. This book documents the clinical depression of the author, a psychologist, who responded well to electroconvulsive therapy. A very important work that many patients who are contemplating the possibility of ECT may find comforting and useful.

Endler, Norman S., and Emmanuel Persad. *Electroconvulsive Therapy: The Myths and the Realities.* Toronto: Hans Huber, 1988. Another good text on electroconvulsive therapy written by a psychologist who experienced the treatment for his own depression. He has gone on to become a much-honored and internationally recognized teacher and researcher in the field of psychology.

Fink, Max. *Convulsive Therapy: Theory and Practice.* New York: Raven Press, 1979. This book continues to be an excellent introduction to electroconvulsive therapy by the leading practitioner and researcher in the United States. A classic text.

George, Mark S., M.D., and Robert H. Belmaker, M.D., eds. *Transcranial Magnetic Stimulation in Neuropsychiatry.* Blackwood, N.J.: American Psychiatric Press, 1999. Compares the effects of transcranial magnetic stimulation (TMS) and ECT in animal models of depression, showing that their similarities may further support the potential role of TMS as an antidepressant treatment.

Kellner, Charles H., et al. *Handbook of ECT.* Washington, D.C.: American Psychiatric Press, 1997. This source describes the procedure, its pros and cons, and how it works and is used in contemporary medicine.

SHUNTS

PROCEDURE

ANATOMY OR SYSTEM AFFECTED: Abdomen, brain, circulatory system, gastrointestinal system, head, liver, nervous system

SPECIALTIES AND RELATED FIELDS: General surgery, neonatology, perinatology, vascular medicine

DEFINITION: Surgically inserted tubes that are used to bypass blocked vessels that normally allow fluid to move from one region of the body to another.

KEY TERMS:

anesthesia: the use of drugs to inhibit pain and alter consciousness

catheter: a tube passed into the body for fluid transport

incision: a cut made with a scalpel

portacaval: referring to a type of shunt used to carry blood from the portal vein to the inferior vena cava, allowing blood to bypass the liver

ventriculoperitoneal: referring to a type of shunt used to carry cerebrospinal fluid from the brain to the abdominal cavity

INDICATIONS AND PROCEDURES

The surgical placement of shunts is performed to reduce fluid pressures when the vessel that normally carries the fluid is blocked. Two of the major types of shunts are ventriculoperitoneal and portacaval. Ventriculoperitoneal shunts are used to remove excess fluid from the brain in hydrocephalus. Shunts used to decrease blood pressure in the portal veins are known as portacaval shunts.

Hydrocephalus is a condition characterized by an excessive amount of cerebrospinal fluid in the brain caused either by too much cerebrospinal fluid production or by the blockage of its flow. Hydrocephalus can occur at birth or be caused by head trauma, infection, or brain hemorrhage. If it occurs at birth, the main signs are an enlarged head that continues to grow more rapidly than normal. An infant's skull bones have yet to fuse, and the fluid pressure causes them to expand. The infant may have seizures, vomiting, abnormal reflexes, and other neurological signs. If hydrocephalus occurs in an adult, when the skull bones cannot expand, the pressure on the brain causes headaches, mental deterioration, loss of consciousness, and, if not treated, death.

Physicians use computed tomography (CT) scanning or magnetic resonance imaging (MRI) to find the blockage. The patient is then prepared for surgery to have a shunt inserted to drain the accumulating fluid. After the individual is anesthetized, the head is prepared for the operation. An incision is made through the skin of the head and a hole drilled into the skull, a procedure called craniotomy. A catheter that is part of the ventriculoperitoneal shunt is inserted into the ventricles of the brain and passed under the skin into the abdominal cavity, which is lined by the peritoneum. The peritoneum is a large membrane capable of absorbing the excess cerebrospinal fluid.

Portacaval shunts are used to reduce the blood pressure in the veins carrying blood from the digestive tract to the liver. Patients with abnormally elevated blood pressure in these veins have portal hypertension. This pressure reduces blood flow from the esophagus, stomach, and intestines, which leads to a pooling of blood and an engorgement of these vessels that may lead to their rupturing. Fluid leaking from the portal vein accumulates in the abdominal cavity, a condition known as ascites.

The most common cause of portal hypertension is cirrhosis of the liver, in which the liver is diseased and scar tissue forms. This scar tissue can block blood entering the liver from the portal vein and lead to portal hypertension. Occasionally, a thrombus (blood clot) will form in the portal vein and cause portal hypertension when the liver is not diseased. The patient may have ruptured vessels that bleed into the digestive tract, causing the feces to appear black.

If the physician suspects portal hypertension, he or she will perform an ultrasound and arteriography to view the vessels.

A portacaval shunt operation may be necessary to reduce the pressure in the portal vein if other treatments have failed. In this surgical procedure, the patient is anesthetized and prepared for a major abdominal surgery called a laparotomy. An incision is made into the abdominal cavity, and the portal vein is exposed. The surgeon must then carefully place a catheter between the portal vein and another large abdominal vein. The latter vein is the inferior vena cava, which helps return blood to the heart from the lower body and the abdominal cavity. Another surgical option is for the surgeon to connect part of the portal vein to the inferior vena cava directly without the use of a catheter. The portacaval shunt diverts some of the blood that normally goes to the liver directly into the inferior vena cava, thus reducing the pressure within the portal vein.

USES AND COMPLICATIONS

The major problem associated with the ventriculoperitoneal shunt is the fact that it will need to be replaced as the infant grows. It is also possible for this tube to become blocked or infected. If the shunt remains in place for a long period of time, it may spontaneously penetrate an abdominal organ.

Portacaval shunt operations reduce the high blood pressure in the portal vein and help prevent bleeding. Unfortunately, they do not significantly improve liver function in most patients and may even cause further liver damage.

PERSPECTIVE AND PROSPECTS

Early detection and treatment of increased intracranial pressure (pressure on the brain) in hydrocephalus and increased blood pressure in portal hypertension are important to the long-term health and survival of the patient.

Early treatment of hydrocephalus with shunt placement prevents further neurological damage and, if the increase in brain pressure is rapid, may even be necessary to prevent death. Drugs such as acetazolamide that inhibit the formation of cerebrospinal fluid may, in certain cases, prevent the need for shunt operations. These agents will likely prove most effective in patients with mild disease.

Physicians may try to stop bleeding from ruptured vessels that is caused by portal hypertension by injecting a solution into the veins to seal them (sclerotherapy). Dietary restriction of salt (sodium) and diuretic drugs may be tried to reduce blood pressure, vessel engorgement, and ascites fluid accumulation.

—*Matthew Berria, Ph.D.,*
and Douglas Reinhart, M.D.

See also Abdomen; Brain; Brain disorders; Bypass surgery; Catheterization; Cirrhosis; Craniotomy; Fluids and electrolytes; Hydrocephalus; Hypertension; Liver; Liver disorders.

FOR FURTHER INFORMATION:

Clayman, Charles B., ed. *The American Medical Association Encyclopedia of Medicine.* New York: Random House, 1994. A concise presentation of numerous medical terms and illnesses. A good general reference.

Schwartz, Seymour I., ed. *Principles of Surgery.* 7th ed. New York: McGraw-Hill, 1999. A standard textbook on the topic. Intended for practicing surgeons, but valuable to general readers for its details.

SIBLING RIVALRY
DISEASE/DISORDER

ANATOMY OR SYSTEM AFFECTED: Psychic-emotional system

SPECIALTIES AND RELATED FIELDS: Family practice, pediatrics, psychology

DEFINITION: A common form of competition between brothers, sisters, or a brother and sister that is considered normal if it is outgrown and/or does not become destructive to individuals or the family.

KEY TERMS:

developmental milestones: the specific achievements accomplished in the normal development of a child (such as motor, cognitive, self-help, social, and communication skills); a child's developmental level affects the expression of sibling rivalry

extended family: a type of family that goes beyond the traditional model of parents and children to include other generations or more distant relatives

family constellation variables: the collection of characteristics that describe the makeup of an individual family, including number of family members, ages, birth order of siblings, gender, and inclusion of any extended family members

interpersonal skills: the social and communication skills that begin developing in childhood; sibling relationships significantly influence the development of these skills *sibling:* a general term for brothers and sisters who share the same set of parents. Siblings that share only one parent are called half sisters or half brothers

stepsiblings: siblings who have no relation through biology or adoption except that a parent of one is married to the parent of the other; varied family forms complicate further the traditional rivalry between siblings

CAUSES AND SYMPTOMS

Sibling rivalry is the competition or jealousy that develops between siblings for the love, affection, and attention of either one or both parents. The concept of sibling rivalry has been discussed for centuries, and it is considered a universal phenomenon in families. Although sibling rivalry is generally described in terms of its negative aspects, healthy competition between brothers and sisters can be useful in the individual development of necessary social, communication, and cognitive skills.

While the dynamics of the ways in which brothers and sisters relate to one another cannot be reduced to specifics of age, birth order, gender, and family size, these family constellation variables are important in the development of sibling rivalry. While each element will be discussed separately, it is important to take into account all the relevant factors when looking at causes of sibling rivalry.

The ages of siblings and their birth order are significant factors that have been related to sibling competition. There are many stereotypes associated with being the oldest, youngest, and middle child in the family. For example, typical firstborn children tend to be highly organized and responsible, while youngest children are likely to benefit from more experienced, relaxed parenting and may be more affectionate and spontaneous. Middle children are often more difficult to characterize. They may be at more risk than other children for receiving less attention, and they tend to develop stronger relationships outside the family. Using these stereotypical characteristics as guides for assessing a particular child, it is possible to speculate on the relevance of birth order and age in the development of sibling competition.

The effects of spacing between children has also given rise to a number of theories. It is generally accepted that the closer siblings are in age, the more similar their life experiences are likely to be. As they may have more in common, siblings close in age are also more likely to struggle with each other more frequently. For this reason, siblings who are close in age may engage in more competition with each other than siblings who are separated by more than a few years.

The gender of siblings is also a variable in the development of sibling relationships, including sibling competition. Siblings help each other discover some of the basic characteristics of male and female roles. Growing up with all brothers or all sisters can teach a child much about dealing with one gender. Having a sibling of the opposite sex can offer a child valuable initial information about the opposite sex. The attitudes of parents regarding gender roles also influence the relationships between siblings. Parents who display favoritism toward children based on gender may contribute to sibling jealousy and competition.

For a wide variety of reasons, specific children may be more emotionally vulnerable to feelings of jealousy than their siblings at a given time. For example, in a family with a child who has a disability, other siblings may feel that they do not receive as much attention or the child with special needs may feel different and unwanted.

Emotionally vulnerable children are frequently found in families experiencing high levels of stress. There is evidence that the emotional climate within the family is directly linked to the quality of sibling relationships. It then follows that sibling rivalry may be more problematic in families where there are stressors such as marital conflict, chronically ill family members, or unwanted extended family involvement.

The competition that emerges between siblings can be for material resources such as toys or space within the household. For example, it is not uncommon for an older child to resent having to share a room with a younger brother or sister. Frequently, the competition for material resources stems from a child's uncertainty regarding his or her status in the family. Children may interpret the need to share space as an indication of their lesser importance to parents.

Jealousy can develop when a child perceives favoritism on the part of a parent. This jealousy results from a lack of equality in treatment. Not only is the less favored child at risk for feeling jealous, but the parental favorite often does not perceive the extra attention as pleasant or comfortable. The challenge in parenting is trying to achieve equality when children are each exceptional beings with their own individual needs. In her book *Dr. Mom's Parenting Guide* (1991), Marianne Neifert recommends loving children

2084 • SIBLING RIVALRY

"uniquely," giving each child the message that his or her place in the family is a special one. A parent who consistently favors one child over another through the amount of love and attention shown is encouraging unhealthy rivalry between the children.

Sibling rivalry can manifest itself in a variety of ways. When a new sibling is born, an older child may be either openly or passively hostile to the new baby. This hostility can be displayed in the form of direct verbal or physical attacks on the baby. Sometimes children request that parents return the infant to the hospital or give it away. In other cases, a child may act up or demand attention when the parent is busy with the infant. Serious abuse by siblings is rare, but even mild incidents need attention by parents.

Some children react to a new sibling by displaying regressive behavior such as bed-wetting, asking to be carried, thumb-sucking, excessive crying, or talking baby talk. Other negative behaviors associated with sibling jealousy are lying, aggressiveness, or destructive behaviors. It is also typical for the child to vent frustration or anger on other individuals, pets, or toys when feeling jealous of a sibling. In older children, sibling rivalry may be exhibited by taking the younger child's toys or demanding more parental attention. Another example of rivalry in older children includes a drive to outperform the other sibling in academic or athletic settings.

Unless managed effectively by parents, feelings of jealousy and competition among siblings can undermine a child's development and may continue into adult relationships. Sibling rivalry can be minimized by the active involvement of parents in setting appropriate rules for dealing with conflicts.

TREATMENT AND THERAPY

The negative impact of sibling rivalry can be minimized through parental education and attention to the conditions that intensify sibling competition. Attending to the development of a relationship between siblings is an ongoing process which parents can enhance through their involvement in helping children develop good interpersonal skills.

The foundation for dealing effectively with sibling rivalry is an awareness and understanding that sibling competition is a normal, healthy part of family life. Rivalry develops between siblings in nearly every family, and it only becomes problematic when taken to extremes or when ignored and allowed to escalate.

The common behavior problems associated with sibling rivalry occur in the context of many interacting factors: parental expectations; the child's developmental level; the temperament of a particular child; parental discipline; family constellation characteristics such as age, gender, and spacing of children; and the presence of extended family members. There is growing evidence regarding the importance of obtaining assessments and information from family members (including extended family) and other sources such as school or day care personnel when identifying a problem of sibling rivalry.

One of the situations in which parents express the most open concern regarding sibling rivalry is when a new baby is expected or an adoption of a child is imminent. When a new sibling is expected, the other children can be invited to be actively involved in the preparation. Age-appropriate discussions with each child about pregnancy or adoption are good preventive measures. Parents should be available to answer questions regarding the changes to be expected with the arrival of the additional child. An open, direct discussion with older children can minimize the adjustment difficulties and address initial concerns. Children need regular verbal and demonstrated assurances that they will continue to be loved following the arrival of a new sibling.

Parents can involve an older child in the care of a baby as a means of acknowledging the unique contributions of that child. Expecting an older child to be a regular caretaker, however, may create additional problems and place unnecessary stress on the older brother or sister.

While some older children exhibit negative behaviors associated with the arrival of a baby, others respond positively by becoming more mature and autonomous. Focusing on the individual contributions of an older sibling can minimize the feelings of jealousy when a new child enters the family.

Parents should avoid making either overt or subtle comparisons between siblings and instead focus on the special qualities and achievements of each child. As Neifert suggests, "honor the individual in every child." This is sometimes difficult to accomplish, as many times parents anticipate that subsequent children will be similar to their firstborn. For example, if a first child is successful in sports, a parent may anticipate that the younger sibling will also be athletically inclined. Such unrealistic expectations can foster unhealthy competition and put needless pressure on a younger sibling.

Jealousy between brothers and sisters seldom ends with the adjustment of a new family member and the acknowledgement that an "only" child now has to share parental attention. Balancing the emotional needs of two or more children of differing ages continues to be an important concern of parents as children move through different developmental stages.

The negative behaviors associated with sibling rivalry can stem from other sources as well. Sometimes siblings fight because they are bored or have few appropriate alternatives to taunting a sibling. Sometimes the behavior can be a reaction to stressors outside of the home, such as problems at school or socialization difficulties. A parent's reaction to negative behavior will have a large impact on whether the behavior continues. Parents who can model effective interpersonal skills themselves are likely to influence the development of these same skills in their children.

When jealous behaviors are displayed by siblings, parents need to be sensitive to the source of the feelings. The cause of the competition or rivalry should be the focus of parental interventions, rather than the negative behavior itself. Children should be encouraged to talk about their feelings openly, and parents need to be willing to acknowledge and validate those feelings for each child. After allowing children to express their feelings and showing appreciation for the difficulty of the problem, parents can encourage siblings to work toward a mutual resolution.

One of the common manifestations of sibling rivalry is the expression of anger and, sometimes, the physical or verbal abuse that accompanies the anger. While common, violent displays of anger are not appropriate. Helping children learn to handle anger responsibly is an important task for parents.

In handling fighting between children, parents must assess the level of conflict and intervene appropriately when necessary. Normal bickering between siblings that does not include verbal abuse or threats of physical abuse rarely requires parental involvement. If the situation worsens, however, the following steps can be useful for parents: acknowledge the angry feelings of each child, then reflect each child's point of view; describe the problem from the position of a respectful bystander, without taking sides on the issue; and express confidence that the children can come up with a reasonable solution.

Parents need to be actively involved in promoting a system of justice within the family which includes age-appropriate rules and consequences for behavior.

Examples of ways that parents can manage the behavior are separating siblings when a situation appears dangerous and redirecting children's activities when aggression is likely to occur. Parents can also take responsibility for encouraging and rewarding cooperative play and providing children with appropriate, nonaggressive models for resolving conflict.

Teaching children conflict resolution strategies is an important way for parents to intervene in sibling rivalry problems. Developing the ability to express one's feelings is a valuable step toward conflict resolution. Children should be encouraged to put their feelings into words in appropriate ways. Young children may need help in doing so through the use of statements such as, "You don't like it when I spend so much time caring for your baby sister, do you?" Granting a child permission to fantasize about a given situation may also help in diffusing angry feelings. Encouraging children to verbalize what they wish would happen allows them to address emotions in an honest way. Children should be taught from an early age to develop creative ways to vent their anger. Children can be taught to use physical exercise, write feelings in a journal, or go to their rooms to cool down as appropriate ways to manage anger.

Managing sibling conflict is complex in any family, but even more so in situations where there is a single parent or a blending of families through divorce and remarriage. Because sibling competition stems from a child's anxiety about sharing parental attention, the presence of a single parent can intensify the feelings of insecurity about one's position in the family. Single parents need to be careful not to turn a child into a spouse substitute, instead viewing each child as a unique individual who deserves to be able to mature at his or her own pace. Extended family members, including grandparents, aunts, and uncles, may be useful in helping a single parent meet the individual needs of each child in the family.

When parents remarry, children are required to make adjustments in their relationships and to include new people into their family. Children need to be allowed to express their ambivalent feelings regarding stepsiblings and half siblings, as these feelings are a normal part of this adjustment process. Parents need to accept and tolerate each child's feelings, as long as guidelines of justice and safety are recognized.

Despite the abundant research available on the topic of sibling rivalry, there is still much that is unknown regarding the complex relationships between brothers and sisters. While it is possible to look at generalizations regarding the issues important in sibling rivalry, it is not possible to predict adjustment or maladjustment in a particular child. Information must be gathered from a number of sources and evaluated for each child when planning a course of action to address concerns about sibling rivalry.

PERSPECTIVE AND PROSPECTS

Through the ages, people have assumed that jealousy and rivalry were unavoidable characteristics of sibling relationships. Sibling rivalry has been a common theme in several classic stories. In the Bible, the competition between brothers Cain and Abel and the jealousy which developed between Joseph and his brothers over issues of parental favoritism are but two accounts of sibling rivalry. Such accounts support the assertion that jealousy among siblings is a common phenomenon.

Sigmund Freud's theory of socialization was one of the first to address the concept of sibling rivalry from a scientific perspective. According to Freud, sibling rivalry, with its struggles and controversy, is inherent in all brother-and-sister relationships. Much of what Freud hypothesized regarding sibling competition was grounded in a personal understanding of his own relationships with his siblings. Freud was the oldest child in a family which included five younger sisters and a younger brother.

Competition for parental attention was a dominant theme in Freud's description of the sibling relationship. He emphasized the negative emotions associated with sibling relationships and concluded that, although these feelings diminished as children matured, the rivalry persisted into adulthood. Few of his remarks about sibling relationships addressed gender differences, as Freud described relationships from his own perspective as a male.

Another theorist who addressed the issue of sibling relationships was Walter Toman. In 1961, Toman published the book *Family Constellations: Its Effects on Personality and Social Behavior*. He suggested that birth order, gender, and spacing were significant factors in the development of personality and strongly influenced the nature of personal relationships both within and outside the family of origin. Toman detailed eight sibling positions, such as oldest brother of brothers, youngest sister of brothers, and so on. While the generalizations presented in Toman's work have significance as a basis of comparison, there are too many intervening variables and complexities in family life to use birth order theories as complete explanations for sibling relationships and family roles. Birth order, gender, and spacing are several of the many significant factors that shape the connections between siblings.

Sibling relationships play an important role in each child's development. Since the works of Freud and Toman were published, researchers have expanded their studies of sibling rivalry to include the broader context of the family. There is growing evidence that the emotional climate of the family is directly related to the quality of the relationship of siblings. The parental relationship, factors of vulnerability in specific children, parental expectations, and family constellation variables each contribute to the development and intensity of sibling rivalry between brothers and sisters in a given family.

—*Carol Moore Pfaffly, Ph.D.*

See also Anxiety; Bed-wetting; Domestic violence; Psychiatry, child and adolescent; Psychoanalysis; Stress.

FOR FURTHER INFORMATION:

Boer, Frits, and Judy Dunn, eds. *Children's Sibling Relationships: Developmental and Clinical Issues*. Hillsdale, N.J.: Lawrence Erlbaum, 1992. This volume is based on presentations from the First International Symposium entitled "Brothers and Sisters: Research on Sibling Relationships, Therapeutic Applications" in 1990.

Franck, Irene M., and David M. Brownstone. *Parenting A to Z*. Rev. 2d ed. New York: HarperCollins, 1996. A unique encyclopedia and resource book for parents which includes a wealth of information on a wide range of personal, educational, medical, social, and legal matters.

Goldenthal, Peter. *Beyond Sibling Rivalry: How to Help Your Children Become Cooperative, Caring, and Compassionate*. New York: Henry Holt, 1999. Clinical and family psychologist Goldenthal believes that sibling rivalry is far more complex than jealousy and competition between children of the same family. Often it reflects poor communication between the parents.

Greydanus, Donald E., and Mark L. Wolraich, eds. *Behavioral Pediatrics*. New York: Springer-Verlag, 1992. This outstanding text summarizes contemporary concepts of pediatric mental health science in a very readable form. Although written primarily for health care providers and clinicians, this book provides straightforward information on a wide variety of common behavioral and emotional problems in children.

Kramer, Laurie, and Chad Radey. "Improving Sibling Relationships Among Young Children: A Social Skills Training Model." *Family Relations* 46, no. 3 (July, 1997): 237-246. The authors describe the results of their experiment in which sixty-four families used a method for helping siblings create positive relationships.

Leder, Jane Mersky. *Brothers and Sisters: How They Shape Our Lives.* New York: St. Martin's Press, 1991. This well-written book examines the assumptions that have shaped the way in which sibling relationships have been viewed in the past. The author describes the foundation of the original theories on sibling rivalry and details the characteristics long associated with the development of sibling competitiveness.

Mendelson, Morton J. *Becoming a Brother: A Child Learns About Life, Family, and Self.* Cambridge, Mass.: MIT Press, 1990. A case study of the transitions that occurred in one family following the birth of a second child. This personal account of the adaptations that followed the addition of a family member encompasses a family systems perspective regarding family changes and includes a chapter on sibling rivalry.

Neifert, Marianne E. *Dr. Mom's Parenting Guide: Commonsense Guidance for the Life of Your Child.* New York: E. P. Dutton, 1991. This well-written book provides supportive and reassuring answers to important questions commonly asked by parents. Each chapter offers realistic advice for dealing with common parenting issues. One chapter is devoted to a discussion of sibling rivalry, including specific strategies for minimizing or eliminating negative behaviors resulting from competitiveness between siblings.

SICKLE-CELL DISEASE
DISEASE/DISORDER

ANATOMY OR SYSTEM AFFECTED: Blood, cells, kidneys, lungs, spleen

SPECIALTIES AND RELATED FIELDS: Genetics, hematology

DEFINITION: A genetic disorder that includes a group of red blood cell disorders in which illness is attributable to the dysfunction of hemoglobin.

KEY TERMS:

anemia: a deficiency of red blood cells, hemoglobin, or total blood volume

aplastic crisis: a sudden decrease in the bone marrow release of red blood cells, associated with very severe anemia

hemoglobin: the substance within red blood cells that transports oxygen and carbon dioxide

infarction: death in a tissue or organ caused by the obstruction of blood flow

CAUSES AND SYMPTOMS

Sickle-cell disease results from the inheritance of the sickle-cell gene from both parents. Sickle hemoglobin has the unfortunate tendency to condense as rods in red blood cells when the oxygen is removed, which occurs during each heartbeat-controlled cycle of blood flow from the lungs to the tissues. These rods distort the cells, making them stiff, rigid, and crescent-shaped. This shape causes obstruction (vasocclusion) of small- and medium-sized blood vessels because of damage to the endothelial inner lining of the vessels (sickle vasculopathy), thereby resulting in tissue death (necrosis) from insufficient blood supply (ischemia). The anemia associated with sickle-cell disease is caused by the rapid destruction of the red blood cells as they circulate because of a shortened peripheral cell survival time of less than 30 days (normal is 120 days).

Sickle-cell disease is marked during the first two decades of life by intermittent episodes of acute painful illnesses interspersed with periods of clinical quiescence and relative well-being. The common, acute complications during childhood are septicemia (a bacterial blood infection), meningitis (a bacterial brain infection), recurrent sickle-cell pain crises, acute chest syndrome (often termed pneumonia), severe upper respiratory tract infections, aplastic crises, an overactive spleen (hypersplenism) with splenic sequestration crises, bone infarctions, priapism (a painful erection of the penis not associated with sexual desire), and pyelonephritis (infection of the kidney).

An increased incidence of invasive infections caused by the bacteria *Streptococcus pneumoniae* is found in children with sickle-cell disease who are between the ages of four months and five years; this is thirty to one hundred times that which would be expected in a healthy population of the same race and age. Blood infections in infants and young children with the disease are associated with a rapid elevation

Sickle-Cell Disease

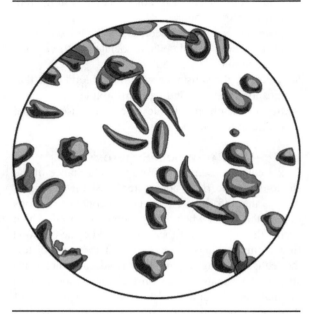

The red blood cells are sickle-shaped rather than round, which causes blockage of capillaries.

of temperature, often to 104 degrees Fahrenheit, and the patient becomes even more anemic. In the untreated patient, death occurs within eight to twelve hours.

Acute painful episodes—particularly in the older child, adolescent, or adult—are the hallmark of sickle-cell disease. A sickle-cell crisis often begins with pain in the abdomen or extremities and joints. A painful crisis in the young child is usually precipitated by an acute fever, with excruciatingly tender swelling of the hands and feet caused by microscopic infarctions of the small growing bones of the hands and feet. Approximately 25 percent of patients have endless and repeated painful episodes requiring frequent hospital care. About 50 percent of the episodes of acute pneumonia-like illness in these patients are related to vasocclusion of the pulmonary blood vessels, or sickle crisis of the lung.

Chronic major organ failure in sickle-cell disease is the direct consequence of sickle vasculopathy. Vascular damage begins years before the overt clinical symptoms are apparent. The spleen is the first organ to be destroyed, usually by five years of age. During young childhood (three to ten years of age), 10 percent of children with this disease will have strokes,

with resulting severe brain damage. Strokes cause paralysis and weakness of the extremities and difficulties in learning. This devastating complication in young children often makes functioning in school or living as self-sustaining adults difficult. Transfusion therapy with normal red blood cells can prevent further progression of brain damage and disability. Sickle vasculopathy eventually culminates in young adulthood as end-stage kidney failure (glomerulosclerosis), sickle chronic restrictive lung disease, intracranial hemorrhages and brain damage, retinopathy with blindness, disabling leg ulcers, and generalized osteonecrosis of many of the bones of the body. Specialized medical care is required for the diagnosis and management of these chronic, irreversible complications.

TREATMENT AND THERAPY

Most acute complications of sickle-cell disease can be treated successfully so that the patient can attend school, be involved in social activities, and have a pleasant childhood and adolescence. Intensive care units with sophisticated monitoring equipment that are dedicated to infants and young children can manage and maintain the vital function of the children during severe illness episodes.

The institution of appropriate immunization programs for children with sickle-cell disease has substantially decreased their mortality and morbidity throughout the world. The importance of preventing the usual childhood infectious diseases such as hepatitis, whooping cough (pertussis), red measles (rubeola), rubella (German measles), diphtheria, tetanus, mumps, polio, and *Hemophilus influenzae* septicemia cannot be overstated. In addition to the usual recommended immunizations for normal children, 23-valent pneumococcal vaccine is used to prevent pneumococcal septicemia. The use of prophylactic antibiotics such as penicillin during young childhood (four months to five years) decreases the incidence of invasive pneumococcal blood infections. Salmonella contamination of chicken is still a major source of septicemia and osteomyelitis (bone infection) in children with sickle-cell disease.

Over time, children with this disease and their families begin to recognize the things that may precipitate a painful sickle-cell crisis. Severe episodes require hospitalization and analgesic treatment, often with narcotic agents in addition to intravenous fluids. Adolescents must learn for themselves those factors that increase the risk of painful episodes.

PERSPECTIVE AND PROSPECTS

Sickle-cell disease is the prototypical molecular disease. The causative gene modifying the chemical structure of the hemoglobin β chain (β^A to β^S)—replacing the amino acid glutamic acid with valine—originated in Africa. The disorder was transmitted to the United States, Arabia, Europe, and South and Central America as part of the slave trade. At that time, healthy persons carrying the sickle-cell gene, who are said to have sickle-cell trait, survived the rigors of a slave ship. As persons carrying the sickle-cell trait migrated throughout the North and South American continents and Europe, genetic drift occurred, accounting for the 15 percent of patients with the various forms of sickle-cell disease who are not phenotypically African in appearance.

Improvements in acute medical care during childhood and in the social and environmental situation for patients, as factors taken together, have made it possible for most children with sickle-cell disease and β^O thalassemia, and essentially all children with β^+ thalassemia, to survive childhood. In the United States, Great Britain, and most European countries, umbilical cord blood diagnosis or peripheral blood sampling of newborns has been in effect since the 1980's. Thus, in the United States, most children with sickle-cell disease are diagnosed at birth and can be provided responsive, knowledgeable medical care.

The focus of new clinical investigations must be the prevention of the tissue destruction that is induced by the repeated endothelial damage caused when sickled red blood cells obstruct blood vessels. Such prevention requires lifelong medical treatment. Drugs that can modify the rate of hemoglobin polymerization in red blood cells have been found to be useful in treating sickle-cell disease. Hydroxyurea, cytosine arabinoside, 5-azosididine, and other agents can increase the amount of fetal hemoglobin in red blood cells. By increasing the fetal hemoglobin, the rate of polymerization of hemoglobin S is modified so that there is less propensity for insoluble rods to be formed. The membrane of red blood cells becomes more flexible, allowing the cells to transverse the microvasculature and thereby decreasing the damage to blood vessels. These powerful chemotherapeutic agents were originally identified for the treatment of cancer. These bone marrow suppressants also cause kidney and liver damage, however, and must be monitored carefully to maintain a therapeutic balance between the toxicity of a drug and its benefits. The next generation of similar-acting drugs should have less toxic potential and be safer to administer to children.

Bone marrow transplantation with a normal bone marrow (normal red blood cells) from a donor with identical human leukocyte antigens (HLAs) is the only cure now available for sickle-cell disease. Bone marrow transplantation is limited by the paucity of HLA-compatible sibling donors who do not have sickle-cell disease.

Gene therapy holds the promise of a cure but has yet to be used successfully in patients with sickle-cell disease. The advantage of gene therapy is that no HLA-compatible donor is required and that stem cells from the cord blood of normal infants could be used for this procedure.

—*Darleen Powars, M.D.*

See also Anemia; Blood and blood disorders; Fatigue; Genetic diseases; Hematology; Hematology, pediatric; Pain management; Thalassemia; Transplantation.

FOR FURTHER INFORMATION:

Edelstein, Stuart J. *The Sickled Cell: From Myths to Molecules.* Cambridge, Mass.: Harvard University Press, 1986. The basic principles of genetics and the biochemistry of the hemoglobin molecule are presented in a very understandable manner.

Embury, Stephen H., et al., eds. *Sickle Cell Disease: Basic Principles and Clinical Practice.* New York: Raven Press, 1994. Following an introductory chapter, the volume is divided into seven sections: sickle hemoglobins, cellular abnormalities, pathophysiology, natural history, diagnosis of sickle-cell syndromes, clinical considerations, and therapeutic considerations.

Reid, Clarice D., Samuel Charache, and Bertram Lubin. *Management and Therapy of Sickle Cell Disease.* 3d ed. National Institutes of Health, National Heart, Lung, and Blood Institute. NIH No. 96-2117, December, 1995. Discusses therapies for the various types of sickle-cell disease, including hemoglobin SC disease and beta-thalassemia. Includes bibliographical references and an index.

Serjeant, Graham R. *Sickle Cell Disease.* 2d ed. New York: Oxford University Press, 1992. Discusses such topics as sickle-cell disease distribution, nomenclature and genetics, diagnosis, pathophysiology, and screening.

Tapper, Melbourne. *In the Blood: Sickle Cell Anemia and the Politics of Race.* Philadelphia: University of Pennsylvania Press, 1999. "Race" is a concept that has occupied a prominent place in American culture for centuries. In spite of being conceptually vague, the use of race in health research has a long and sometimes disturbing history.

SIDS. *See* SUDDEN INFANT DEATH SYNDROME (SIDS).

SINUSITIS
DISEASE/DISORDER
ANATOMY OR SYSTEM AFFECTED: Nose, respiratory system

SPECIALTIES AND RELATED FIELDS: Family practice, otorhinolaryngology

DEFINITION: Sinusitis is the inflammation of the lining of the nasal sinuses; it occurs most frequently as a complication arising from the common cold. Nasal congestion, with a thick greenish-yellow discharge, produces a feeling of pressure inside the head. As normal sinus drainage is obstructed, intense headaches and eye pain may occur. Other symptoms include postnasal drip, coughing, disturbed sleep, and fever. The causes of sinusitis vary from a bacterial infection, initiated by a cold or other upper-respiratory infection, to irritation of the nasal passages by environmental contaminants. Acute cases can be resolved by the administration of antibiotics and through inhalations of steam. Chronic sinusitis may require surgery to drain the sinuses.

—*Jason Georges and Tracy Irons-Georges*
See also Allergies; Bacterial infections; Common cold; Ear infections and disorders; Hay fever; Headaches; Multiple chemical sensitivity syndrome; Nasopharyngeal disorders.

FOR FURTHER INFORMATION:
Norback, Craig T., ed. *The Allergy Encyclopedia*. New York: Penguin Books, 1981.

Smith, Lendon H. *The Encyclopedia of Baby and Child Care*. Rev. ed. Englewood Cliffs, N.J.: Prentice Hall, 1980.

Young, Stuart, Bruce Dobozin, and Margaret Miner. *Allergies*. Rev. ed. New York: Plume, 1999.

SKELETAL DISORDERS AND DISEASES. *See* BONE DISORDERS.

SKELETON. *See* BONES AND THE SKELETON.

SKIN
ANATOMY
ANATOMY OR SYSTEM AFFECTED: Nerves, nervous system

The Major Sinuses

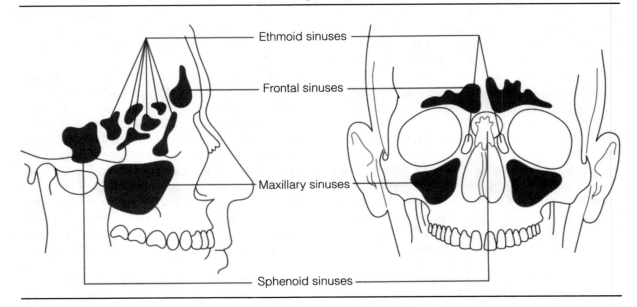

- Ethmoid sinuses
- Frontal sinuses
- Maxillary sinuses
- Sphenoid sinuses

Specialties and related fields: Dermatology, neurology, oncology, plastic surgery

Definition: The largest organ of the body, which is vital to the survival of an organism for its protection against dehydration and abrasion, regulation of body temperature, and sensory reception.

Key terms:

basal cell carcinoma: the most common type of skin cancer; it grows slowly and seldom spreads beneath the skin

collagen: a fibrous protein found in the connective tissue, including skin, bone, ligaments, and cartilage

contact dermatitis: a common skin allergy characterized by inflamed skin; it occurs when skin comes in contact with substances such as poison ivy or allergenic cosmetics

dermatologist: a physician who treats the skin, including its structures, functions, and diseases

dermis: the layer of skin beneath the epidermis, consisting of dense connective tissue and blood vessels

epidermis: the outermost part of the skin, composed of four or five different layers called strata

keratin: an extremely tough protein that is the chief constituent of the epidermis, hair, nails, and tooth enamel

melanin: the dark pigment of the skin or hair that accounts for variations in skin color

melanoma: a cancer arising from a pigmented mole; it tends to spread to internal organs if left unchecked

psoriasis: a chronic skin disease characterized by red, scaly patches overlaid with thick, silvery gray scales

STRUCTURE AND FUNCTIONS

The anatomy of the skin consists of two major parts: the outer epidermis and the underlying dermis. The epidermis is composed of a particular kind of tissue called stratified squamous epithelium. Epithelium consists of cells that are packed together very tightly, a feature that is most important to an organ that must cover and protect the rest of the body. It is called squamous, which means "flat" in Latin, because its cells are flat and fit together like tiles. The word "stratified" describes the dozens of layers of cells that are piled up to create the epidermis. These cells form four or sometimes five strata, with their own characteristics and roles to perform.

The stratum basale, or basal layer, lies on a thin piece of tissue called the basement membrane, which is next to the dermis. The basal layer cells divide continuously throughout life, supplying new cells called keratinocytes for all the layers above the basal layer. About one-fourth of the stratum basale cells are called melanocytes because they produce the pigment melanin. As the keratinocytes are pushed up, they acquire a spiny shape; for this reason, the layer above the basal layer is called the stratum spinosum. While in the spiny layer, the upward-moving cells begin to produce the protein fibers that will eventually become waterproof keratin. As the spiny cells are moved further upward, they begin to flatten out. The layer that they form at this point is called the stratum granulosum because the keratin being formed is visible here, under the microscope, as large clumps or granules. Langerhans cells, which are very important in immunity and protection from disease, are also found in the granular layer. Only in thick skin, such as that found on the palms of the hands and the soles of the feet, do some of the migrating cells form a transparent layer of dead cells full of a shiny substance called eleidin. The shininess of this fourth layer earned it the name stratum lucidum.

The outermost part of the epidermis, the stratum corneum, is what most people think of as "the skin"—dead, dry cells that are completely waterproof because they are packed with keratin. The twenty-five layers of corneum cells form an efficient barrier to water loss and to the entrance of microorganisms. The epidermis has no blood vessels. The living, reproducing basal-layer cells must be nourished by nutrients passed from blood vessels in the dermis. Nerve endings that pick up the sensations of touch and pain extend upward into the epidermis, while those that sense pressure, heat, and cold extend only into the dermis.

Directly beneath the epidermis's basement membrane is the dermis. The dermis extends in a wavy or vertical tonguelike fashion into the epidermis to anchor it. The top of the dermis, which is called the papillary layer, thus forms ridges that account for one's fingerprints and toe prints. There are small blood vessels and fibers scattered throughout the papillary layer. The larger, lower part of the dermis is called the reticular layer. This thicker dermal layer has many more elastic and collagen fibers than does the papillary layer, and it is the location of oil glands, sweat glands, fat cells, hair follicles, and large blood vessels.

Directly under the skin, which is often called the cutis, is the jellylike, fat-filled subcutaneous layer. This packaging material provides heat insulation and

The Structure of the Skin

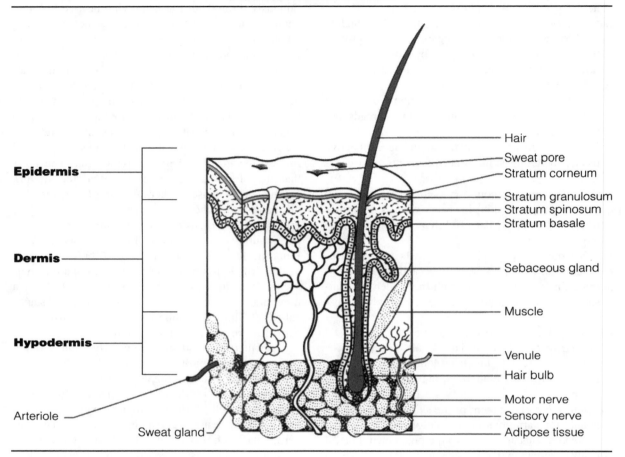

Epidermis

Dermis

Hypodermis

Arteriole

Sweat gland

Hair

Sweat pore

Stratum corneum

Stratum granulosum
Stratum spinosum
Stratum basale

Sebaceous gland

Muscle

Venule

Hair bulb

Motor nerve
Sensory nerve
Adipose tissue

energy storage, and it serves to attach the skin to the muscles and organs below.

The anatomy of the skin makes it able to perform a variety of functions. All these roles have one major purpose: to enable the skin to maintain homeostasis—that is, to keep the body relatively stable inside, in spite of constantly changing conditions outside.

The intact skin acts as a barrier to invasion by the multitude of microorganisms that come into contact with its surface. The waterproof keratin in the epidermis prevents all substances that are able to dissolve in water from entering the body through the skin. The presence of the pigment melanin enables the skin to absorb harmful radiation from the sun safely, up to a point. Too much exposure to the sun causes sunburn, drying of the skin, a loss of elasticity, and wrinkling. More important, every sunburn increases the risk of skin cancer. Inheritance determines the amount of

melanin possessed; although all races have the same number of melanocytes, people of different races differ greatly in the amount of melanin that their cells produce. The more melanin present, the darker the skin. The absence of a certain gene prevents melanin synthesis, causing those persons without the gene to be albinos. Skin color also varies because of the yellow pigment called carotene, which is found in the upper layers of the epidermis, and because of the red blood that is visible through the dermis of light-skinned people.

A very important function of skin is its role in temperature regulation. The body rids itself of excess heat by sweating. Excess heat passes from blood vessels into sweat glands, which conduct heat and perspiration to the surface. A large amount of heat can be lost as the sweat evaporates, thus maintaining normal body temperature. At other times, skin conserves heat by tightening blood vessels and reducing sweat secretion. Simultaneously, shivering, which is the involuntary contraction of skeletal muscles, releases internal heat to counteract excessive heat loss from the body. Only certain sweat glands—namely, those in the armpit and groin—produce the type of sweat that gives rise to an odor.

The waterproof quality of the skin prevents most substances from being absorbed through it into the body. Among the materials that can be absorbed are oxygen; vitamins A, D, E, and K; steroids such as cortisone cream; and, unfortunately, poisons such as insecticides.

The skin is able to produce a form of vitamin D that becomes active and useful to the body after passing through the kidneys. This synthesis requires a small amount of sunshine—far less than that necessary to cause a sunburn. If the skin does not produce enough vitamin D to enable the body to use calcium correctly, then vitamin D is needed in the diet.

Two very specialized accessory structures of the skin have their own particular functions. One of these skin derivatives is the pili, or hair. Except for the palms, soles, lips, and eyelids, the entire body contains hair. Each hair consists of a hair shaft that grows beyond the skin surface and a hair root lying inside a hair follicle. The follicle itself consists of epidermis that has grown downward into the dermis. Each hair follicle has an associated sebaceous gland that produces sebum, an oily substance, to lubricate the hair. Scalp hair protects the scalp from overexposure to the sun and from cold weather; eyelashes and tiny hairs inside the nose and ear canals help keep foreign material from entering.

The other important skin accessory is the nails. Each nail consists of a nail plate attached to a nail bed. Nails contain modified, highly keratinized cells from the stratum corneum. The basal cells that reproduce to make the nails grow lie under the cuticle at the base of the nail. Nails help to protect fingers and toes and enable humans to pick up tiny objects more efficiently.

DISORDERS AND DISEASES

The complex anatomy of the skin allows for the development of many possible defects and diseases. Three disorders that modern medical science attempts to understand and alleviate are psoriasis, cancer, and the many varieties of contact dermatitis.

Psoriasis, one of the most common of all skin conditions, is said to afflict about 3 percent of the American population. It commonly runs in families and affects both sexes equally. It may develop in childhood or old age but typically appears in the second or third decade of life. It most frequently occurs as scaly patches, or plaques, on the elbows, knees, and scalp but may appear on the back, belly, buttocks, and legs. Many people with psoriasis experience itching; surprisingly, some do not.

Human epidermis cells usually take about twenty-eight days to move from the stratum basale, where they are produced, to the top of the stratum corneum, whence bathing removes them. This means that the cycle of normal epidermal cells in transit through the skin is accomplished in a month or more, allowing the cells time to mature. In psoriasis patients, this transit period is as short as four days. The reproducing basal cells divide five to ten times too rapidly, and the epidermis thickens enormously, but in patches. The skin cells of psoriasis patients are so abnormal that the patients' immune systems form antibodies that attack and destroy them, further damaging the ruptured, scaly surface. There is a notable tendency for psoriatic lesions or sores to form at sites of childhood injuries such as sunburns, scratches, scrapes, and areas where chicken pox was particularly widespread. These lesions often become pus-filled abscesses that contain enormous numbers of white blood cells. The epidermal cells no longer die at the stratum granulosum, and even the granules themselves are lost. The outermost corneum layer, which is usually dead, dry, and protective, is full of living but abnormally functioning cells. In the dermis below, large, dilated, thin-walled blood vessels appear, and the epidermis directly above them is disproportionately thin. Scratching or picking at the plaques causes bleeding.

The exact cause of psoriasis is not yet known. Genetic factors play a role in its development, since one-third of all patients have a family member who is also afflicted. In addition to the physical discomfort and damage to self-esteem caused by this very obvious skin condition, it can lead to heat loss, fever, severe arthritis, heart failure, and even death.

The many forms of skin cancer can also cause great disfigurement and even death. Two frequently observed types are basal cell carcinoma and malignant melanoma. Basal cell cancers, which may begin in the hair follicle epithelium, are the most common skin cancers, accounting for almost 70 percent of all cases. Fortunately, they are also the most easily treated. They are most often found where sunlight strikes the hardest, on the neck, scalp, face, and shoulders. Basal cell cancers often start as small bumps but grow wider and more elevated, usually with a cavity in the center. Although their surface is shiny and filled with tiny blood vessels, their color may still be like that of normal skin. If left untreated, basal cell carcinomas may develop a crust or an ulcer that cannot heal. Although they seldom metastasize, shifting or spreading through the bloodstream to another part of the body, they often do great damage to the tissues and structures directly under them. Those that grow near ears and eyes can cause loss of function of those organs.

In almost all cases, the appearance of basal cell carcinomas is directly related to sun exposure. A few seem to be related to previous scars, burns, tattoos, or exposure to arsenic. It is important to be aware of the warning signs of basal cell carcinomas. Some can be felt as well as seen as reddish or dotted lumps; others look like open sores caused by scratches or insect bites that do not heal. Because these cancers, which often grow for two years before detection, have such varied appearances, they can be diagnosed accurately only by biopsy.

The most dangerous skin cancers are the malignant melanomas. They begin in the pigmented cells called melanocytes but usually and quite rapidly invade deeper tissue. Severe sunburns early in life seem to be their usual cause. Many start as small dark brown growths similar to moles, although they may become white, blue, or reddish and irregular in shape as they grow. Often they will bleed if rubbed. People who have acquired one hundred or more moles by young adulthood are considered genetically predisposed toward these dangerous melanomas; such people should use sunscreens every day all year long. It should be noted that half of all melanomas arise from apparently normal skin that has no moles. The malignant melanomas are much more dangerous than the basal cell carcinomas because they tend to release cancerous cells into the bloodstream that latch on to and grow into numerous internal organs.

Seldom life-threatening, contact dermatitis can still be very uncomfortable for a patient. Dermatitis is an inflammation of the skin that usually is a result of an allergic reaction and may include redness, swelling, blistering, crusting, and scaling among its symptoms. In all its many varieties, it probably forms the bulk of a dermatologist's practice. Contact dermatitis results from coming into contact with a causing substance, such as poison ivy, poison oak, or poison sumac. The sap from these plants contains urushiol, a substance to which 70 percent of all people are allergic.

Large numbers of persons are allergic to the metal nickel and can develop inflammations from wearing nickel rings, watches, earrings, or other jewelry. Nickel zippers and clothing snaps, eyeglass frames and sewing needles, and even coins can cause a reaction.

The chemicals in permanent hair dyes cause terrible swelling and itching of the face and neck in some people. Oddly, the scalp under the dyed hair is often unaffected. When dermatitis seems to result from hair dyes, it is often because the affected person has simultaneously been using certain sunscreens, the pain reliever benzocaine, or one of many other common medicines.

The chemical potassium dichromate is found in many detergents. People who experience dermatitis caused by detergent use should also avoid other chromate-containing products. These include inks, paints, bleaches, and spackling, to name only a few.

Other people contract dermatitis caused by a formaldehyde allergy. Permanent-press clothing and sheets are made wrinkle-proof by the use of a formaldehyde-based substance. Individuals with a formaldehyde allergy must also avoid many paper products, cosmetics, and disinfectants that contain formaldehyde derivatives.

Susceptibility to contact dermatitis from rubber products is widespread. Surprisingly, it often appears long after the exposure and is most common in manufacturing workers.

In modern society, with its heavy reliance on over-the-counter drugs, cleaning products of all kinds, deodorants and cosmetics, insecticides and weed-killers, and innumerable other chemical products, the potential causes of contact dermatitis have been and will continue to be multiplied.

Perspective and Prospects

Research in dermatology both borrows from and sheds light upon many other branches of medical science. Immunology, endocrinology, biochemistry, surgery, and oncology are just a few of many.

Diseases of the skin can reveal the presence of many otherwise unseen internal disease conditions. Shiny, thin, reddish-yellow patches on the shins may be a sign of diabetes. Prediabetics are also susceptible to repeated yeast and fungal infections of the skin and have poor wound-healing ability.

Too little thyroid hormone causes coarse hair; thickened, dry, cool skin; and rough plaques on the shins. Too much thyroid hormone causes thin hair, excessive sweating, and, surprisingly, identical rough plaques on the shins.

Abnormally dark skin can be a sign of drug side effects, the presence of heavy metals, poor adrenal gland output, or pituitary tumors. Skin may also darken from excess iron intake or, very noticeably, from a widespread malignant melanoma.

Various bowel diseases may also cause skin conditions. The small intestine defect involving a flattened, malfunctioning lining can produce severely itchy blisters on the limbs and the back. Ulcers in the large intestine often produce deep, dirty-looking skin ulcers.

The presence of cancer in the breast, bowel, or lungs may precipitate thousands of external wartlike growths or flat, waxy-surfaced growths. Similarly, the gradual appearance, usually on the legs of the elderly, of fishlike skin may reveal the early presence of cancer of the lymph glands.

Alcoholism reveals itself in spider telangiectasia, webs of dilated capillaries on the skin surface. The presence of hepatitis, a serious viral infection of the liver, is indicated by the yellowing of the skin known as jaundice.

Two other links among dermatology, immunology, and oncology are the search for a vaccine against skin cancer and a new treatment called photopheresis. Since the late 1960's, there has been an ongoing attempt to develop a vaccine to prevent a recurrence of malignant melanoma. This is a particularly important pursuit because those who have survived one case of melanoma have a high risk of developing future ones.

Photopheresis patients take a drug called psoralen. Two hours later, their blood is drawn and exposed to ultraviolet light. The interaction between the psoralen and the light destroys abnormal white blood cells, after which the blood is returned to the body. Since 1987, photopheresis has been used to treat a cancer of the immune system that begins in the skin. Researchers hope eventually to use psoralen to treat arthritis and lupus, and to prevent the rejection of organ transplants.

For many years, drugs for internal conditions could be administered only orally or by injection. In both methods, the circulating amount may be too high to be safe immediately after it is given and too low to be effective as the hours go by. Dermatologists have greatly advanced medical science by developing transdermal patches. These patches enable a steady supply of a drug to enter the bloodstream by absorption through the skin. By 1989, patches had been developed to treat angina, high blood pressure, motion sickness, menopausal symptoms, and nicotine addiction.

One of the greatest traumas skin can suffer is a widespread burn. Although surgeons have had great success in transplanting many internal organs, they are unable to permanently transplant skin from another person. In 1981, they developed a marvelous technique to produce artificial skin. It uses animal skin protein seeded with a few skin cells taken from the patient. From this small patch, a large enough piece of skin can be grown to cover the wounds until the gradually healing skin replaces it.

From the earliest simple salves for skin rashes to the great discoveries of transdermal patches and artificial skin, dermatologists have done and continue to do their share in advancing medical science.

—*Grace D. Matzen*

See also Abscess drainage; Abscesses; Acne; Acupressure; Acupuncture; Age spots; Albinos; Allergies; Arthropod-borne diseases; Athlete's foot; Biopsy; Birthmarks; Bites and stings; Burns and scalds; Candidiasis; Cell therapy; Cells; Chickenpox; Corns and calluses; Cradle cap; Cryotherapy and cryosurgery; Cyst removal; Cysts; Dermatitis; Dermatology; Dermatology, pediatric; Dermatopathology; Diaper rash; Eczema; Edema; Electrical shock; Electrocauterization; Face lift and blepharoplasty; Fifth disease; Frostbite; Fungal infections; Glands; Grafts and grafting; Hair loss and baldness; Hair transplantation; Hand-foot-and-mouth disease; Heat exhaustion and heat stroke; Hives; Host-defense mechanisms; Itching; Impetigo; Jaundice; Keratoses; Laceration repair; Laser use in surgery; Leishmaniasis; Leprosy; Lice, mites, and ticks; Lower extremities; Lupus erythematosus; Malignant melanoma removal; Measles; Moles; Necrotizing fasciitis; Numbness and tingling; Pigmentation; Pimples; Pityriasis alba; Pityriasis rosea; Plastic surgery; Poisonous plants; Porphyria; Psoriasis; Radiation sickness; Rashes; Ringworm; Rosacea; Roseola; Rubella; Scabies; Scarlet fever; Sense organs; Shingles; Skin cancer; Skin disorders; Skin lesion removal; Smallpox; Stretch marks; Styes; Sunburn; Tattoos and body piercing; Touch; Upper extremities; Warts; Wrinkles.

FOR FURTHER INFORMATION:

Goodman, Thomas, and Stephanie Young. *Smart Face*. Englewood Cliffs, N.J.: Prentice Hall, 1988. An easily understood explanation of skin structure, problems, and care, with special emphasis on delicate facial skin. Contains an extensive appendix of consumer product information.

Lamberg, Lynne. *Skin Disorders*. Reprint. Philadelphia: Chelsea House, 2001. This brief volume is an introduction to the study of skin problems. Contains a very helpful glossary, a bibliography, and a list of organizations to contact for more information.

Mackie, Rona M. *Clinical Dermatology*. 4th ed. New York: Oxford University Press, 1997. Written for dermatology students but useful to general public for more precise and detailed information than that contained in popular works. Illustrated in color.

Siegel, Mary-Ellen. *Safe in the Sun*. New York: Walker, 1995. Presents information from research of leading dermatologists and ophthalmologists showing the relationship between sun exposure and damage to skin and eyes. Easily understood by the general public. Contains an extensive glossary and many pages of helpful further sources of information.

SKIN CANCER

DISEASE/DISORDER

ANATOMY OR SYSTEM AFFECTED: Lymphatic system, skin

SPECIALTIES AND RELATED FIELDS: Dermatology, environmental health, immunology, oncology

DEFINITION: Malignancies of the skin (and sometimes spreading to the internal organs) caused by the ultraviolet radiation in sunlight.

Cancer is the common term used to describe the large class of diseases called neoplasms. Neoplasms, which occur only in multicellular organisms, develop and function in an autonomous way that does not abide by the biological mechanisms that govern the growth and metabolism of the individual cells and the reactions that take place in a living organism. When such neoplasms grow at a rate faster than the tissues from which they arise, while at the same time invading those tissues, they are called malignant and are commonly described as cancerous. Benign neoplasms, which do not invade surrounding tissues, are not as abnormal and as dangerous as malignant ones.

Sun radiation is life-sustaining, but the higher-energy part of the sunlight spectrum brings the danger of skin cancer. When living tissue is irradiated, its molecular structure is disrupted, thus initiating a chain of reactions, many of which are not the usual ones associated with the living organism. Therefore, a change in the chromosomal composition and the development of unwanted cells is likely to occur. Such changes take place because of the formation of free radicals in the deoxyribonucleic acid (DNA) molecules that constitute the genetic code. The result is skin cancer, the most common form of cancer in both men and women in the United States.

Types of skin cancer. Skin neoplasms may be benign or malignant, acquired or congenital, although the majority are benign and acquired. The common mole (the medical term for which is melanocytic nevus) is a neoplasm of benign melanocytes which is often present at birth and is known as a birthmark. Such moles are generally harmless unless they are large in size, in which case they may have up to a 10 percent chance of becoming malignant. Other melanocytic nevi are strawberry hemangiomas and port-wine stains, which are of vascular origin.

The most common forms of skin cancer are the basal cell and squamous cell carcinomas, which arise from the corresponding part of the keratinocytes of the epidermis and are caused by the cumulative effects of ultraviolet radiation on the skin. They are generally localized, however, and rarely metastasize. These cancers are easily identified as persisting sores or crusting patches that grow mostly on sun-exposed parts of the body such as the hands, neck, arms, and nose. They can be treated with routine surgical procedures.

A malignant melanoma is formed from the pigment-forming melanocyte and almost certainly undergoes metastasis. It should therefore be removed surgically at the earliest possible stage. If the melanoma is detected at a later stage, chemotherapy and irradiation are the techniques usually applied. A malignant melanoma appears as a lesion that increases in size and turns several colors, such as black, blue, white, and brown. Symptoms such as itching, bleeding, and pain are not as common at first but are encountered at the later stages of development.

There are two skin malignancies that may be fatal: mycosis fungoides and Kaposi's sarcoma. Mycosis fungoides is a skin lymphoma that may be confined to one location for ten or more years before it metastasizes to internal organs, with death following. As a result, it is difficult to track this skin cancer, both clinically and histologically, and several biopsies (skin histological examinations) may be required to ascertain its presence. On the other hand, Kaposi's sarcoma occurs either as lesions (commonly among older Mediterranean men) or as skin abnormalities in HIV-infected people. The sarcoma is derived from skin blood vessels and appears as violet patches or lesions. As long as it is contained only in the skin, it is not fatal. Once the inner organs are affected, however, death is imminent, even though the lesions may be treated with irradiation and chemotherapy.

The effects of sunlight on skin. Extensive skin exposure to sunlight, such as at the beach, leads to the polymerization of skin chemicals (known as catecholamines) and the subsequent formation of different types of epidermal pigmentation (the melanins), which are responsible for tanning. Tanning occurs only if there is gradual exposure to sunlight; otherwise, a sunburn will arise. Photoprotection is believed to be one of the major biological functions of the melanin pigment. It appears that melanin formation can participate effectively in reducing the harmful effects of sunlight by an array of photoinduced chemical reactions, which result in the consumption of scavenging active oxygen species such as the superoxide anion and hydrogen peroxide. It has been determined that in biological systems, superoxide and hydrogen peroxide are formed in small quantities during normal processes. Both species are known to produce several biological effects, most of which are harmful to tissues. It should be pointed out, however, that although melanin may act as a free radical scavenger, it may also become energetically overloaded and may change to a toxic state. Evidence exists that melanin increases the radiative damage to cells, which leads to sunlight-induced skin cancer. In other words, melanin formation is good only when moderate exposure to sunlight occurs.

In the atmosphere 12 to 48 kilometers above the earth's surface lies a small layer of ozone. Although this layer does not contain much ozone—it is estimated to be about 3 millimeters thick under normal conditions of temperature and pressure—it has a profound effect on life. The ozone layer absorbs the harmful ultraviolet radiation from the sun, thus providing the mechanism for the heating of the stratosphere. A reduction in the ozone layer would lead to a large increase of ultraviolet rays intruding into the atmosphere, thus increasing the incidence of skin cancer.

F. S. Rowland and M. J. Molina declared in 1974 that the presence of the volatile chlorofluorocarbons would eventually reduce the ozone layer. Some measurements done by scientists in 1979 showed a decrease in the layer, which led to the action taken by several governments to decrease and replace the chlorofluorocarbons commonly used in aerosols. As the average life span steadily increases, the incidence of skin cancer will increase as well. The development of effective sunscreens and sunglasses with high ultraviolet blocking are recommended for people who are exposed to large amounts of sunlight, such as sunbathers and hikers.

—*Soraya Ghayourmanesh, Ph.D.*

See also Cancer; Carcinoma; Chemotherapy; Dermatology; Dermatopathology; Kaposi's sarcoma; Lymphadenopathy and lymphoma; Malignancy and metastasis; Malignant melanoma removal; Moles; Radiation therapy; Skin; Skin disorders; Skin lesion removal; Sunburn; Warts.

For Further Information:

Arnold, Harry L., Richard B. Odom, and William James. *Andrews' Diseases of the Skin: Clinical Dermatology.* 8th ed. Philadelphia: W. B. Saunders, 1990. Includes discussion of AIDS, Haber's syndrome, oral hairy leukoplakia, and neutrophilic dermatosis malignancy.

Lookingbill, Donald P., and James G. Marks. *Principles of Dermatology.* Philadelphia: W. B. Saunders, 1986. Text and illustrations show common complaints and discuss differential diagnosis, biopsy, treatment, and complications.

Rook, Arthur, et al., eds. *Textbook of Dermatology.* 6th ed. 3 vols. Oxford, England: Blackwell Scientific, 1998. This multivolume work offers a thorough overview of skin disease. Illustrations illuminate the text.

Siegel, Mary-Ellen. *Safe in the Sun.* New York: Walker, 1995. This comprehensive and up-to-date book describes the benefits that are still possible from the sun, the risks of exposure and how to protect the skin, and how damage that has already occurred can be treated or reversed.

Skin disorders
Disease/disorder
Anatomy or system affected: Skin
Specialties and related fields: Dermatology, family practice, occupational health

DEFINITION: Diseases and conditions that affect the skin, ranging from harmless to life-threatening.

KEY TERMS:

benign: in reference to a neoplasm, having a nonmalignant character

dermatology: the study of the skin, its chemistry, physiology, histopathology, cutaneous lesions, and the relationships of these lesions to systemic disease

malignant: in reference to a neoplasm, having the property of uncontrollable growth and dissemination, recurrence after removal, or both

melanin: dark brown or black molecules of pigment that normally occur in the skin, hair, pigmented coat of the retina, and pupil of the eye and in selected cells of the brain

metastasis: the shifting of a disease, or its local manifestations, from one portion of the body to another; in cancer, the appearance of neoplasms in parts of the body remote from the primary tumor

ANATOMY OF THE SKIN

The skin is the largest organ of the body. It provides a barrier between the external world and the internal world: It protects against external contamination and helps to maintain the sterility of the internal body. The skin also assists in temperature regulation; humans can survive only within a narrow temperature range. The skin has nerve receptors that supply the brain with information, providing an interface with the world. There are specialized receptors for touch, temperature, vibration, and position in space (proprioception).

Appendages to the skin are fingernails, toenails, and hair. They are mainly of psychological importance. Nails protect the tips of fingers and toes in humans but are not needed for protection as claws are in lower animals. Hair is analogous to feathers. In birds, tiny muscles attached to the base of each feather cause them to be ruffled; this creates air pockets and allows birds to conserve heat and keep warm. The same muscles persist in humans, causing "goose flesh," but they do not serve any other function. The main importance of these appendages is cosmetic. For example, people spend billions of dollars on hair care products each year. The motivation for this activity is psychological.

The two main layers in skin are the epidermis and dermis. The epidermis is the upper or outermost layer, and cells are continually formed at its base. As new cells are formed, existing cells are pushed toward the surface of the skin. These cells gradually lose their watery central contents, causing them to dry out (desiccate) and become flattened. This process normally spans approximately a month. Thus, the surface of the body is largely composed of dead cells that have become flattened. These cells are normally lost on a continual basis and create dandruff when shed from the scalp. On other parts of the body, sloughed cells provide excellent conditions for bacterial growth, accounting for the unpleasant odors that accompany poor hygiene habits.

Two other important types of cells are found in the epidermis: melanocytes and Langerhans' cells. Melanocytes contain melanin and provide all the variations of pigmentation found in the human species. They multiply when stimulated by the ultraviolet radiation in sunlight. This causes the skin to become darker, a protective mechanism against damage from ultraviolet radiation. Langerhans' cells contain surface receptors for immunoglobulins. They play a central role in allergic reactions of the skin, such as contact dermatitis or delayed hypersensitivity reaction.

The dermis is an inner layer of skin located beneath the epidermis. Its main function is protection. Within the dermis are highly specialized cells containing microscopic filaments. These cells impart tensile strength to the skin in much the same way that fibers strengthen fiberglass or reinforcing steel mesh strengthens concrete. Because they are so dense, they also serve as a barrier to the entry of most pathogens and many chemicals. Eccrine sweat glands are found in the dermis throughout the entire body. These produce a salty secretion (essentially salt water) that assists in thermoregulation through evaporative cooling. They are also sensitive to emotional stress. Apocrine sweat glands are primarily in the armpits (axilla) and groin and produce a milky secretion. When these secretions are broken down by bacteria on the surface of the skin, a characteristic odor is produced. The bases of hair follicles are also found in the dermis. The small sebaceous, or oil-secreting, gland associated with most hair follicles has the function of softening and moisturizing the hair.

Hair is found on most surfaces of the body; exceptions are the palms of the hands, the soles of the feet, and the glans penis in men. The texture and length of the hair vary with location on the body, gender, genetic heritage, and age. Dramatic increases in the growth and distribution of hair occur at puberty. With increasing age, hair is typically lost from the scalp and other body parts. It also changes color, assuming a gray or white color because of the loss of melanin at the base of the hair follicle.

COMPLICATIONS AND DISORDERS

When normal skin anatomy and physiology are upset, several common diseases or disorders result. When the barrier provided by the skin is broken, bacteria, viruses, fungi, and other pathogens can invade the body, leading to infections. Locally, these infections can cause inflammation (redness and pain) of the skin; if widespread, they can lead to systemic infections. When the cells and other substances found in the skin become irregular or are abnormal, skin disorders or conditions result.

Skin disorders and conditions. Pigmentation of the skin results from the presence of melanocytes, cells that manufacture and contain melanin. Most humans have pigmentation over their entire bodies; the degree of pigmentation varies with different racial and ethnic groups. Local areas of increased color have a range of names depending on the size of the pigmented area. A freckle is small and discrete. A nevus is a larger area of hyperpigmentation. These conditions are attributable to underlying variations in the distribution of melanocytes. They are genetic in origin and permanent; they are also accentuated by exposure to sunlight. Melasmas are irregular, flat, light brown areas on the neck, cheeks, or forehead. They are caused by hormonal changes associated with pregnancy or contraceptive pills and by exposure to sunlight. Melasmas fade with the reduction of excess hormones. There are also color changes in the labia

Common Skin Disorders

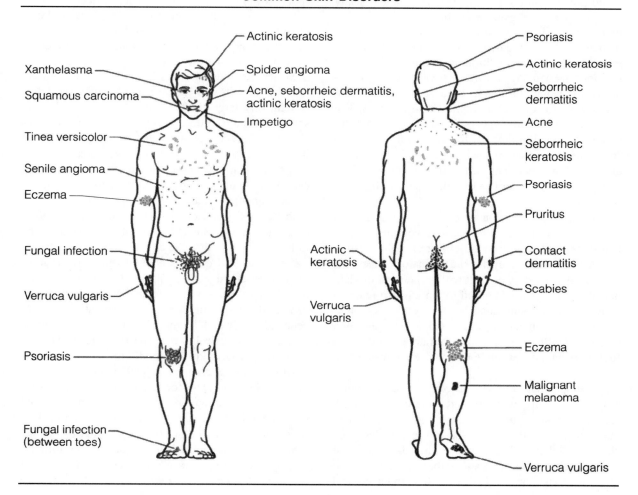

of females during pregnancy; these changes are both harmless and permanent.

Generalized increases in skin coloration can occur with some metabolic diseases. Addison's disease involves an increase in melanocyte-stimulating hormone. This leads to an overall bronzing of the body, with accentuation in creases of the palms and soles. The condition subsides with treatment of the underlying cause of the disease. Similar pigment increases are associated with some forms of lung cancer, hemochromatosis, and chronic arsenic exposure. The latter two conditions are caused by the deposition of iron (hemochromatosis) and arsenic in the skin.

Generalized decreases in skin coloration can also occur. If melanocytes fail to migrate to the skin during embryologic development, hair follicles will lack color, resulting in a condition called piebaldism. Characteristically, this is a white patch in the hair of the forehead. Vitiligo is caused by an immunologically mediated loss of melanocytes. Individuals with phenylketonuria (PKU) experience a generalized depigmentation of hair and eye color, in addition to mental retardation, if the condition is not adequately and promptly treated. An individual totally lacking melanocytes is called an albino; because melanin is also responsible for eye color, albinos have red eyes. The loss of hair is called alopecia. It can occur because of aging, sustained pulling on the hair with some hairstyles, and genetics. Women do not usually experience much alopecia until after the menopause. Conversely, some men start to lose their hair during their twenties.

Skin diseases. Eczema or dermatitis is a general term that describes a skin disease involving vesicles that ooze fluid. These conditions are usually characterized by a rash; they are inflammatory reactions, commonly caused by contact with a chemical or plant material. They can be caused by an adverse reaction to a drug or by sunlight. Bacteria, yeasts, or other fungi on the skin can cause eczema. Most rashes itch or burn; they can be spread by scratching. Athlete's foot is a common example of an eczematous dermatitis.

Maculopapular diseases encompass several common skin conditions, such as red measles (rubeola), German measles (rubella), and scarlet fever. Viruses that land on the skin cause these diseases. They are characterized by relatively large, localized areas of changed skin color (macules) that are also raised (papules) but not fluid-filled. After their clinical course is run, they disappear without leaving a scar. The more dangerous toxic shock syndrome also belongs to this group of diseases; it is caused by toxin from the bacteria *Staphylococcus aureus*.

Thickening of the skin and the formation of red to purple areas having sharply defined borders characterize papulosquamous skin diseases. The most common example is psoriasis. Other examples are pityriasis and ichthyosis. The pathology responsible for psoriasis is an alteration in the normal development of skin cells. In individuals with psoriasis, new skin cells develop and migrate to the surface in only five days instead of the usual thirty. This fact alone explains the flaking (rapid cell turnover), redness (thinner skin and a rich blood supply for new skin), and pain and itching (less protection for sensory nerve endings) experienced. Pityriasis includes a group of different conditions caused by different viruses. Patches or large spots develop on the skin. They usually resolve within a few weeks. Aside from being locally photosensitive, they usually are not serious. Ichthyosis describes a group of genetic conditions characterized by extreme scaling of the skin.

Vesiculobullous diseases have fluid-filled blisters that can vary in size from relatively small (vesicles) to relatively large (bullae). Insect bites, herpes, and some bacterial infections lead to the formation of vesicles or bullae. Such conditions are attributable to an immune reaction that leads to the formation of blisters at the junction between epidermis and dermis. They can be accompanied by intense pruritus (itching); scratching often leads to scarring.

Pustular diseases of the skin include acne, folliculitis, and candidiasis. They are characterized by the inflammation of hair follicles caused by surface bacteria or yeasts. Adequate personal hygiene is the most effective method of prevention. These diseases are usually not serious, but prolonged or repeated attacks can result in scarring and disfigurement. The sebaceous glands, which secrete oil at the base of hair follicles, can increase in size. The subsequent increase in oil output worsens the condition.

Clogged sweat glands can lead to acne. While this is primarily a problem for teenagers, it can affect individuals of any age. Exposure to cutting oils and other hydrocarbons such as gasoline and paint thinners can cause a similar condition called chloracne, which is inflammation in the base of hair follicles found on exposed skin in areas such as the nape of the neck, forearms, and face. The inability to sense temperature and regulate body heat through sweating is called anhydrosis, a condition that can cause shock and potentially death.

Other diseases that can affect the skin. Five such diseases are worthy of mention: leprosy, scleroderma, lupus, atherosclerosis, and diabetes mellitus. Leprosy, or Hansen's disease, is caused by infection by *Mycobacterium leprae*, a relative of the bacteria that cause tuberculosis. In leprosy, the causative organism accumulates in the skin and peripheral nerves. This causes disfigurement and loss of sensation, the latter being similar to that experienced by an uncontrolled diabetic. Disfigurement is responsible for the stigma associated with leprosy since ancient times: loss of fingers and toes, as well as mutilation of the nose and ears. Leprosy is caused by long-term association with the organism and can be adequately treated with appropriate antibiotics.

Scleroderma (literally, "hard skin") is an uncommon disease characterized by fibrosis of the skin and involvement of visceral organs. The skin involvement can range from an isolated, hardened patch to a life-threatening, generalized condition described as an ever-tightening case of steel. The skin becomes stretched tightly over the underlying skeleton. Skin tone is lost with restriction of movement.

Systemic lupus erythematosus is a disease of unknown etiology that is characterized by inflammation in many different organ systems. The skin is usually involved, as nearly all individuals with lupus develop a characteristic butterfly-shaped rash on their faces. This red coloration covers the cheeks and nose. Persons with lupus are also sensitive to sunlight and many develop alopecia. Most of those affected are female. The disease waxes and wanes; treatment depends on the particular organs involved.

Atherosclerosis and diabetes can block the arteries supplying the nerves of the skin, leading to a loss of sensory input. When the patient is unable to experience pain, cuts and other abrasions on the skin are not noticed. Untreated, these lesions can lead to gangrene, sometimes requiring amputation of a body part.

Skin cancer. The most commonly diagnosed form of cancer is that involving the skin. It is not the most fatal form, but millions of cases are discovered annually. The origin of most skin cancers can be traced to excessive exposure to radiation from the sun. They can occur on any surface of the body, although they are more common on areas that are usually exposed to the sun, such as the face, the backs of the hand,

and the neck. Skin cancers can arise in the epidermis or dermis. The majority are noncancerous, or benign. Epidermal nodules are characterized by local thickening of the epidermis, often accompanied by scaling of the skin in the affected area. Nodules in the dermis may appear as lumps with no alteration of the epidermis above them.

There are three malignant forms of skin cancer. Basal cell carcinoma arises from cells deep in the epidermis. This form of tumor rarely spreads (metastasizes), but it can be extensive and destructive locally. Squamous cell carcinoma is less common but can be invasive (involving adjacent tissues) and can metastasize. Melanoma is relatively uncommon but can grow extremely rapidly; it has the potential to be fatal in a matter of months. It involves the uncontrolled growth of melanocytes. Melanomas have irregular borders and color or pigmentation. Any pigmented lesion or suspicious change in the skin should be evaluated by a medical professional in a timely manner.

Prevention is the preferred method of dealing with skin cancer. When outside, loose-fitting clothing can provide protection from the sun, and a hat can protect the head. When exposure is unavoidable, a product with a sun-blocking agent will reduce exposure. Limiting the time of exposure to the sun until the body has reacted by producing additional melanocytes (tanned) is recommended.

Prolonged exposure to the sun also accelerates changes in the skin associated with aging. Collagen fibers provide the characteristic firm feel to the skin of a young person. With aging the skin becomes less firm, losing some of its tone, and begins to sag. Inadequate moisture also contributes to the loss of skin tone. Excessive exposure to the sun hastens both of these processes.

—*L. Fleming Fallon, Jr., M.D., Ph.D., M.P.H.*

See also Abscess drainage; Abscesses; Acne; Age spots; Aging; Albinos; Allergies; Birthmarks; Bites and stings; Carcinoma; Chickenpox; Corns and calluses; Cradle cap; Cyst removal; Cysts; Dermatitis; Dermatology; Dermatology, pediatric; Dermatopathology; Diaper rash; Eczema; Fifth disease; Grafts and grafting; Hair loss and baldness; Hand-foot-and-mouth disease; Herpes; Hives; Impetigo; Inflammation; Itching; Keratoses; Leprosy; Lupus erythematosus; Malignant melanoma removal; Measles; Moles; Necrotizing fasciitis; Neurofibromatosis; Pigmentation; Pimples; Pityriasis alba; Pityriasis rosea; Poisonous plants; Psoriasis; Rashes; Ringworm; Rosacea;

Scabies; Skin; Skin cancer; Skin lesion removal; Stretch marks; Styes; Sunburn; Tattoo removal; Tattoos and body piercing; Warts; Wrinkles.

For Further Information:

Burns, Tony. *Lecture Notes on Dermatology.* 7th ed. London: Blackwell Science, 1997. This is a core text in dermatology that will appeal to professionals and members of the general public who want a concise introduction to the subject. The aim of the book is to integrate basic science with clinical practice.

Frankel, David H. *Field Guide to Clinical Dermatology.* Philadelphia: Lippincott, Williams & Wilkins, 1999. Frankel, a noted internist and dermatologist, has enlisted widely respected and talented colleagues to help in the production of this book. It is a uniquely organized and easily readable field guide complete with 220 pages of excellent color illustrations.

Goldsmith, Lowell A., Gerald S. Lazarus, and Michael D. Tharp. *Adult and Pediatric Dermatology: A Color Guide to Diagnosis and Treatment.* Philadelphia: F. A. Davis, 1997. This book provides excellent pictures to accompany good descriptions of dermatologic diseases.

Grob, J. J. *Epidemiology, Causes, and Prevention of Skin Diseases.* London: Blackwell Science, 1997. This well-written book presents data on large groups of people. The sections on skin cancer are especially noteworthy.

Kenet, B. J., and P. Lawler. *Saving Your Skin: Prevention, Early Detection, and Treatment of Melanoma and Other Skin Cancers.* Chicago: Four Walls Eight Windows, 1994. Skin cancer is the focus of this title, which reviews the early symptoms of melanoma, its causes, and its treatment. Very few skin care titles do more than offer a chapter on the problem.

Rassner, Gernot, and Walter H. Burgdorf. *Atlas of Dermatology.* 3d ed. Philadelphia: Lea & Febiger, 1994. This new edition of a classic book features a greatly expanded text, with the illustrations integrated so that readers can immediately view the described changes.

Sams, W. Mitchell, Jr., and Peter J. Lynch, eds. *Principles and Practice of Dermatology.* 2d ed. London: Churchill Livingstone, 1996. This is a new edition of a dermatology reference guide and text emphasizing accurate diagnosis by succinct discus-sions in eighty-five presentations featuring color photographs.

Skin grafting. *See* **Grafts and grafting.**

Skin lesion removal
Procedure

Anatomy or system affected: Arms, hands, nose, skin

Specialties and related fields: Dermatology, general surgery, oncology, plastic surgery

Definition: The removal of cancerous and precancerous skin lesions under local anesthesia with a curette or scalpel, an electric needle, or liquid nitrogen.

Indications and Procedures

Actinic (or solar) keratoses and skin cancers affect more than 500,000 Americans each year. Actinic keratoses, warty lesions that are considered to be premalignant, are often removed as a precaution. Among skin cancers, basal cell carcinoma is the least harmful. The lesion may appear on the skin surface as a small, flesh-colored or pale pink spot, usually with a raised edge that has a translucent, pearly appearance. It grows slowly and will rarely spread (metastasize) to other parts of the body. Squamous cell carcinoma is more dangerous. It appears on the surface as a small, firm, scaly tumor with an indistinct margin. Untreated squamous cell malignancies may metastasize. Malignant melanoma, called black cancer, is the most dangerous of the three types. Melanoma lesions may resemble a mole with an irregular shape and can be red, blue, black, brown, gray, or even white. Melanoma rapidly invades nearby tissue and can mestatasize readily to other parts of the body.

The method of treatment will depend on the type of lesion and its location and size. Most are treated in the dermatologist's office under local anesthesia. More widespread lesions may be removed in the hospital under general anesthesia.

The site is cleaned with a germicidal swab, and a local anesthetic injected under the skin. The lesion is scraped away with a curette, an instrument with a small, scoop-shaped cutting head. An electric cautery kills any remaining lesion cells and seals off small blood vessels.

The curette is used on basal cell carcinomas that are less than 1 or 2 centimeters in diameter. Larger lesions are removed with a scalpel, and stitches close the incision. Cancers on the eyelids, tip of the nose, or near facial nerves may be removed with radiation (using X rays or another source). If the area treated is large, cosmetic or reconstructive surgery is performed to restore the patient's physical appearance.

USES AND COMPLICATIONS
There is about a 95 percent cure rate for treated basal cell carcinomas. The cure rate for squamous cell carcinomas is only slightly less, especially if the lesion has been treated at an early stage. The cure rate for malignant melanomas is low unless they are diagnosed and treated early.

—*Albert C. Jensen, M.S.*

See also Biopsy; Cancer; Carcinoma; Cryotherapy and cryosurgery; Dermatology; Dermatopathology; Electrocauterization; Grafts and grafting; Keratoses; Laser use in surgery; Malignant melanoma removal; Oncology; Pigmentation; Plastic surgery; Skin; Skin cancer; Skin disorders; Warts.

FOR FURTHER INFORMATION:
McKee, Phillip. *A Concise Atlas of Dermatopathology.* New York: Gower Medical, 1993.

Mehregan, Amir. *Pinkus' Guide to Dermatohistopathology.* 6th ed. Norwalk, Conn.: Appleton-Century-Crofts, 1995.

Vasarinsh, P. *Clinical Dermatology: Diagnosis and Therapy of Common Skin Diseases.* Boston: Butterworth, 1982.

SLEEP DISORDERS
DISEASE/DISORDER

ANATOMY OR SYSTEM AFFECTED: Brain, nervous system, psychic-emotional system

SPECIALTIES AND RELATED FIELDS: Geriatrics and gerontology, neurology, psychiatry, psychology

DEFINITION: Any abnormal pattern of sleep which threatens normal function, including conditions that cause too much as well as too little sleep, and which may be both organic and nonorganic in origin.

KEY TERMS:

circadian rhythm: a physiological process which occurs in twenty-four-hour cycles; examples include the sleep-wake cycle and the maintenance of body temperature

hypersomnia: a group of disorders in which the patient complains of excessive daytime sleepiness or of an inability to stay awake during the day

insomnia: the complaint of poor-quality sleep, which can be caused by a difficulty in falling asleep or a difficulty in maintaining sleep; the most common sleep disorder

narcolepsy: a disorder in which sufferers experience an overwhelming need to sleep during the day; other characteristics include sudden muscle weakness, hallucinations, or sleep paralysis

parasomnias: disorders, occurring primarily in children, in which the patient exhibits abnormal behavior during sleep; examples are sleepwalking and night terrors

periodic leg movements: a disorder in which muscle spasms in the legs partially awaken the sleeper, preventing the proper staging of the sleep cycle

polysomnogram: a collection of physiological information regarding brain waves, breathing, muscle movements, and blood oxygen levels used to diagnose sleep disorders

rapid eye movement (REM) sleep: the period of sleep in which intense brain activity can be measured; the stage of sleep in which dreaming occurs

sleep apnea: a cessation of breathing during sleep, which interrupts the normal sleep cycle; the patient must partially awaken in order to resume breathing

CAUSES AND SYMPTOMS
Sleep is more than the absence of wakefulness. While a person sleeps, the brain continues to be quite active—indeed, this activity is essential for human survival. Brain activity can be measured in sleeping subjects and has been used to classify sleep into stages 1 through 4, where stage 1 is the lightest sleep and stage 4 is the deepest. A sleeper moves from stage 1, through stages 2 and 3, and to stage 4, and then back through stages 2 and 3 to stage 1. This cycle occurs every ninety to one hundred minutes throughout the night. During the latter part of the sleep period, stage 1 sleep is associated with brain activity that is as intense as that seen in waking subjects. During these periods of intense brain activity, rapid eye movements (REMs) are observed, and as a result these periods are referred to as REM sleep, and the other sleep stages are referred to as non-REM sleep. Although the precise function of sleep is still hotly debated in scientific circles, most people can verify from experience that adequate sleep has a major impact on their ability to function effectively and on their emotional stability. For those who suffer from a sleep disorder, life can become a daily struggle, of-

The Sleep Cycle

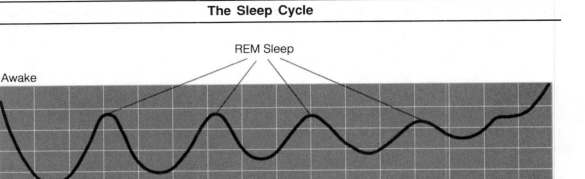

Over an eight-hour sleep period, depth of sleep fluctuates, punctuated by periods of "rapid eye movement" (REM), which appear necessary for restful sleep.

ten with severe physical, financial, and social consequences.

Patients who are having difficulty with sleeping usually complain of insomnia, feeling sleepy during the day, or abnormal behaviors during sleep. Sleep disorders have been divided into four broad categories by the Association of Sleep Disorders Centers: the insomnias, or disorders of initiating or maintaining sleep; the hypersomnias, or disorders of excessive sleep; disorders of the sleep-wake cycle; and the parasomnias, or disorders of partial arousal such as sleepwalking and night terrors. Of these, the most common complaint are the insomnias.

Insomnia is a subjective complaint of nonrefreshing sleep. Patients believe that their ability to function during the day is impeded by short or poor-quality sleep. Since most people experience transient insomnia at various times in their lives, chronic insomnia is defined as insomnia lasting longer than three months. Individuals with insomnia have a variety of sleep patterns: Some may require a long period to fall asleep, some wake up after a few hours and cannot fall asleep again, and some may not know that they have awakened briefly hundreds of times during the night. The sleep patterns of the insomniac can vary from night to night, which increases the anxiety of the patient. Electrical monitoring of brain activity shows that most insomniacs have only a slightly reduced total sleep time, with few changes in sleep stages. Physiologically, poor sleepers have been shown to maintain a higher body temperature during sleep than normal sleepers, which may reflect a higher level of arousal. Insomnia is not a disorder in itself; instead, it can be a symptom of a large number of underlying disorders. These can be physiological, psychological, or behavioral in nature, or they can be a normal part of the aging process.

Insomnia can be caused by medical problems that interfere with breathing, such as sleep apnea, in which patients have multiple episodes each night when they stop breathing. A single episode can last ten seconds to two minutes, and in some severe cases, up to 50 percent of sleep time can be spent without breathing. Sleep apnea is often seen in obese men and women because of obstruction of the air passage. Clinical signs include irregular snoring and daytime sleepiness. Insomnia can also be caused by neurological problems, muscular problems, or conditions that cause pain. Periodic leg movement can (but does not always) cause multiple awakenings during the night, as can a related disorder called restless leg syndrome, which is characterized by a creeping sensation in the legs. Psychiatric research has demonstrated that insomnia can be a symptom of clinical depression. Surveys have shown that insomniacs have a higher level of stress, tension, and anxiety than normal sleepers. In addition, insomnia can occur when behavioral patterns do not encourage sleep. The use of caffeine or engaging in arousing activities just prior to bedtime can contribute to poor sleep. The normal aging process usually causes a decrease in total sleep time and in stage 1 sleep and an increase in fragmented sleep, resulting in drowsiness and sometimes depression in the elderly.

In addition to all these causes, there are some individuals who complain of insomnia in which no abnormalities can be found. When comparing subjective reports from the patient to sleep recordings in the laboratory, there is a tendency for such insomniacs to report wakefulness even though the sleep recording indicates that the patient is sleeping normally. It appears that there are other sleep abnormalities that contribute to the quality of sleep which remain unknown.

The hypersomnias are defined by excessive daytime sleepiness (EDS) and include the group of patients who are unable to stay awake during the day. Several external circumstances can contribute to EDS, such as jet lag, shift work, medications, or some of the disorders underlying insomnia listed above. In addition, narcolepsy, a central nervous system disorder, is characterized by the overwhelming need to sleep several times a day. These sleep attacks often occur without warning. Narcoleptics can also experience cataplexy, or sudden muscle weakness when in emotionally charged situations that cause anger, laughter, or fear. They may also experience hallucinations when sleep begins or sleep paralysis upon waking that can last for several minutes. Narcolepsy affects 0.05 percent of the population and causes significant hardship to those afflicted. It can pose a danger if the person falls asleep while operating a car or when in a dangerous environment.

The daily cycle of wakefulness followed by a prolonged sleep period is controlled by circadian rhythms. People who travel across time zones or who work rotating shifts are often forced to sleep at a time when their circadian rhythm supports wakefulness and work when their circadian rhythm supports sleep. Other individuals have defects in the mechanisms that regulate circadian rhythms and may experience delayed or advanced sleep phase syndrome in which there is a shift of the normal twenty-four-hour cycle. If they follow their circadian rhythm, these patients will sleep for a normal amount of time; however, the social consequences of retiring at 7:00 P.M. or awakening at noon are prohibitive. Internal desynchronization between the sleep-wake cycle and the closely related circadian temperature cycle can also contribute to poor-quality sleep.

The parasomnias, or disorders of arousal, include sleepwalking and night terrors. Both of these disorders occur predominantly in childhood, although they can be experienced by adults. When brain activity is characterized by an electroencephalograph (EEG), there are elements of both wakefulness and REM sleep, often in the deepest stages (3 and 4). This finding dispels the myth that sleepwalkers are acting out dreams, since dreaming occurs during REM sleep. Sleepwalking activity can vary in length. The person usually has his or her eyes open, can respond verbally, and can move about normally. Sleepwalkers are usually aware of the environment at some level, although their judgment is impaired and they can sometimes injure themselves. Night terrors involve signs of panic such as shrieking, sweats, and frenzied movements and can be distinguished from nightmares, which involve little movement and more extensive memory. Both sleepwalking and night terrors are usually not recalled, and there is little connection between these syndromes and psychiatric disease. Both may be exacerbated by sleep deprivation, stress, fever, or medications.

TREATMENT AND THERAPY

One of the difficulties in diagnosing insomnia or one of the other sleep disorders is that there is much individual variability among normal sleepers in sleep needs and amount of sleep logged each night. Therefore, what may be adequate sleep for one person might cause another to report poor sleep. To determine the causes of poor sleep, a person is usually referred to a sleep clinic. There, a detailed history of the problem as well as a description of the patient's sleep habits, lifestyle, and psychological state is recorded. Often, a description of behavior during sleep from someone who shares the bedroom can provide additional important information. Next, a polysomnogram, in which the sleeping patient is monitored with electrodes, is performed so that information on brain waves, breathing, muscle movements, and blood oxygen levels can be obtained. Sometimes this test is administered in the sleep center, and sometimes it is done in the more natural sleep environment of the person's home using ambulatory monitoring devices. From this information, a diagnosis can usually be made and the appropriate therapy determined.

When insomnia is associated with an underlying psychiatric or medical problem, treatment usually begins with the primary problem rather than with the symptom of poor sleep. When the primary problem is solved, the sleep pattern usually returns to normal.

Symptomatic treatment of the insomnia itself is provided only when the cause of the sleep disturbance cannot be treated. There are two major approaches: treatments that emphasize the use of drugs or technical aids and treatments that emphasize a change in behavior.

Although over-the-counter aids cannot improve sleep, large numbers of prescription drugs can affect sleep patterns and influence alertness during waking hours. Historically, barbiturates were administered for insomnia, but in 1970, benzodiazepines were introduced; they are now the most commonly prescribed drugs for sleeplessness. These drugs are usually taken about thirty minutes before bedtime, causing drowsiness and thus decreasing the amount of time it takes to fall asleep. Benzodiazepines alter the stages of sleep, decreasing the amount of stage 1 and REM sleep and increasing the amount of stage 2 sleep. The significance of these changes is not understood. When used alone, benzodiazepines are very safe and have few side effects; if they are combined with other drugs, however, there can be a toxic interaction. Although most people can tolerate these drugs and report no daytime grogginess, some impairment of function may exist upon waking. There is strong evidence to suggest that benzodiazepines be used for only a short period of time. With continued use (longer than thirty days), patients usually find that the drug becomes less effective unless the dosage is increased to an unsafe level. When the drug is discontinued, the original symptoms of insomnia usually recur and often a "rebound insomnia," which is even more severe than before the drug treatment began, may be present for a brief period. Because of these limitations, these "sleeping pills" are usually given when an acute but temporary situation exists. To treat insomnia that is caused by periodic leg movements, a muscle relaxant is sometimes used. For patients whose sleep apnea is not resolved by weight reduction, mechanical devices that hold the air passage open during sleep are usually employed. Orthodontic aids or tongue retainers may provide relief, and other patients wear a mask which holds the air passage open, providing a continuous airflow during sleep.

Since insomnia is often caused by poor habits that condition the sleeper to remain awake, the problem can sometimes be solved by a simple commitment to avoid naps, reduce caffeine and alcohol intake, eat light meals in the evening, reduce noise in the sleep environment, and establish a regular bedtime. Many insomniacs are so preoccupied with the fear that they will not sleep well that they become tense as bedtime approaches. These fears may sometimes be put to rest by the knowledge that sleep needs vary greatly from

In the News: The Effects of Sleep Deprivation

The 2000 Omnibus Sleep in America Poll completed by the National Sleep Foundation found that 43 percent of Americans reported that they are sleepy during the day and that the sleepiness was enough to interfere with daily activities. Richard Gelula, the executive director of the National Sleep Foundation, concluded that the consequences of sleep deprivation are more severe than most people realize and affect metabolism, endocrine functions, memory, mood, and reaction time. The average adult sleeps about an hour less than the eight hours per night recommended by sleep experts. During the work week, only 33 percent of adults get the necessary eight hours of sleep. Forty-three percent of the adults in the survey reported that they often stay up later than they should because of watching television or surfing the Internet. Also, 58 percent of adults experienced the symptoms of insomnia, and 15 percent experienced restless leg syndrome. The factors most often identified for disrupting sleep were stress and pain. Fifty-one percent of Americans reported driving while drowsy, and one in five said they have actually fallen asleep at the wheel. Sleep deprivation has also negatively impacted work performance for 27 percent of adults. The list of work-related problems included being late for work, making errors, reductions in quality of work, lower productivity, diminished concentration, and suffering injuries. Forty-seven percent attempted to remedy sleep problems through the use of herbal remedies, alcohol, and over-the-counter medications. But only 20 percent of adults ever initiated a discussion about sleep problems with a physician.

—*Frank J. Prerost, Ph.D.*

individual to individual. In some cases, people may not physiologically require a "normal" amount of sleep but have been convinced that they have a sleep disorder by spouses who do. Another commonly held misperception that contributes to tension is the notion that, once sleep is lost, it can never be recovered. Studies have shown that sleep-deprived humans are able to return quickly to normal sleep patterns, and therefore a few nights of poor sleep is no cause for alarm.

For those whose anxiety about sleep persists, techniques that teach people to relax their muscles or meditation to decrease mental activity may reduce this anxiety and promote sleep. Patients who experience better sleep when away from their normal sleeping location may have "learned" to associate the bedroom environment with wakefulness. To overcome this problem, stimulus control is used to try to strengthen the bedroom as a cue for sleep. This method requires that patients use the bedroom only for sleeping and go to bed only when sleepy. Most important, if they do not fall asleep within ten minutes of lying down, they should get up, go into another room, and engage in a mundane activity, coming back to the bedroom only when sleepy. This may be done several times, but the main goal is to associate the bedroom with falling asleep quickly. Regardless of the length of sleep, patients should always get up at the same time and not nap during the day. This regimen may need to be continued for several weeks in order to overcome the previous habit and requires perseverance from the patient; however, the advantage of behavioral therapy lies in the absence of the side effects caused by medication.

Excessive daytime sleepiness is usually diagnosed by a polysomnogram followed by a Multiple Sleep Latency Test. In this test, patients are allowed to fall asleep several times a day, and if sleep occurs within five minutes multiple times during the day, the diagnosis is positive. EDS is treated in different ways depending on its cause. If the cause is sleep apnea or periodic leg movements, the disorder is handled as described above. In other cases of sleep fragmentation, medication is used to prevent arousal during the night. The excessive daytime sleepiness found in narcoleptics is usually treated with drugs that act as central nervous system stimulants. Other symptoms of narcolepsy are usually treated with antidepressant drugs that suppress REM sleep. Of these, gamma hydroxybutyrate has been shown to be effective and to cause limited side effects. Short naps taken throughout the day seem to prevent many of the symptoms associated with sleep attacks.

Problems with the circadian rhythms of the sleep-wake cycle are usually not helped by medication. Instead, chronotherapy may be effective in resetting the biological clock. Over the course of two weeks, the patient's bedtime is gradually moved forward or backward around the clock until the desired bedtime is reached. Similar effects may be seen using strong light to shift the sleep period.

PERSPECTIVE AND PROSPECTS

The field of sleep research is still in its infancy. For most of history, sleep was not studied at all because it was difficult to characterize the process without interrupting it. Early scientists such as Lucretius, however, made observations and suggested that the motions of sleeping animals might reflect their dreams. In the early 1800's, sleep was viewed simply as the absence of waking, and the treatment of lethargic patients with damage to the brain stem led doctors to postulate that this area of the brain had two centers—a waking center and a sleeping center. These two centers were thought to function and communicate with each other using chemical signals. As the field of neurobiology advanced, it became possible to measure the electrical properties of the brain using an electroencephalograph. By the 1930's, numerous studies had shown that the brain remains active during sleep and that the different stages of sleep have different patterns of electrical activity. REM sleep was first observed in 1953 and was linked to dreaming. Additional brain structures in the midbrain and pons were identified that controlled REM and non-REM sleep. An understanding of the neurotransmitters, or chemical substances involved in sleeping and waking, began in the 1960's when it was discovered that neurons in the pons contained serotonin and norepinephrine. Another neurotransmitter, acetylcholine, was found in neurons that were active during REM sleep.

It is only recently that the study of sleep disorders has been recognized as a legitimate pursuit. Most of the sleep disorders mentioned here were discovered in the 1960's and 1970's, and public opinion regarding those who complain of tiredness and fatigue is only gradually shifting from disdain to understanding that there might be a real physiological cause. The increase in the number of sleep centers and laboratories that are studying sleep and its accompanying disorders has grown tremendously. These sleep centers have been instrumental in elucidating the primary disorders of sleep and in educating the general public concerning sleep management and the safety risks that result from abnormal sleep. Research laboratories are investigating the anatomical, chemical, and physiological mechanisms of sleep and sleep abnormalities. Some of the most interesting areas of current research include genetic studies that determine whether sleep disorders are inherited. There appears to be a significant genetic component to several sleep characteristics, including bedtime, sleep duration, insomnia, narcolepsy, snoring, and sleep apnea. It is expected that, as scientists come to understand more about the nature and mechanisms of the brain and normal sleep, further understanding of the causes and treatments for sleep disorders will be forthcoming.

—*Katherine B. Frederich, Ph.D.*

See also Aging; Anxiety; Apnea; Chronobiology; Depression; Hallucinations; Memory loss; Narcolepsy; Nightmares; Paralysis; Phobias; Sleepwalking; Stress.

FOR FURTHER INFORMATION:

Carskadon, Mary A., ed. *Encyclopedia of Sleep and Dreaming*. New York: Macmillan, 1993. An extremely important and comprehensive resource which provides well-written articles on all facets of sleep and sleep disorders.

Dement, William C., and Christopher Vaughan. *The Promise of Sleep*. New York: Random House, 1999. Over this book's four sections, the authors cover the basics, such as "Daily Sleep Need," "Alternative Therapies," and "Sleeping Pills." Gives sleep, one of human beings' greatest basic needs, the attention it deserves.

Dotto, Lydia. *Losing Sleep: How Your Sleeping Habits Affect Your Life*. New York: William Morrow, 1990. Discusses the physical and social consequences of sleep disorders, with an emphasis on sleep loss. In an easy-to-read style, the author reports on the effects that a modern, frenetic lifestyle has on sleep and its ramifications for waking hours as well.

Hobson, J. Allan. *Sleep*. New York: Scientific American Library, 1995. This beautifully illustrated volume provides an overview of past and contemporary sleep research. The author draws upon neurology and psychology to provide an interdisciplinary approach to his topic.

Montplaisir, Jacques, and Roger Godbout, eds. *Sleep and Biological Rhythms*. New York: Oxford Univer- sity Press, 1990. This collection of articles highlights the role that biological rhythms play in sleep, wakefulness, and psychological well-being. One chapter is devoted to explaining a possible mechanism for insomnia, and another discusses drugs that are used in the treatments for restless leg syndrome and narcolepsy.

Reite, Martin, and John Ruddy, and Kim E. Nagel, eds. *Concise Guide to Evaluation and Management of Sleep Disorders*. 2d ed. Washington, D.C.: American Psychiatric Press, 1997. Gives an overview of the symptoms and treatments available for different types of sleep disorders.

SLEEPING SICKNESS
DISEASE/DISORDER

ANATOMY OR SYSTEM AFFECTED: Brain, lymphatic system, nervous system

SPECIALTIES AND RELATED FIELDS: Public health

DEFINITION: Common to tropical Africa, sleeping sickness is an infectious protozoan disease transmitted through the bite of a tsetse fly. The parasite *Trypanosoma brucei* multiplies and spreads through the bloodstream, heart, and lymph nodes. Symptoms include fever and lymph node swelling. The parasites eventually reach the brain, causing headaches, fatigue, and a general sleepy look in the victim. If the disease goes untreated, coma and death may occur. The parasite that causes sleeping sickness can be spread from person to person, or from animal to person through subsequent bites of infected and noninfected people or animals. Sleeping sickness can be treated with medication, although brain damage may be permanent if the disease reaches the brain.

—*Jason Georges and Tracy Irons-Georges*

See also Arthropod-borne diseases; Bites and stings; Parasitic diseases; Protozoan diseases; Sleep disorders; Tropical medicine.

FOR FURTHER INFORMATION:

Busvine, James R. *Disease Transmission by Insects: Its Discovery and Ninety Years of Effort to Prevent It*. New York: Springer-Verlag, 1993.

_____. *Insects, Hygiene, and History*. 3d ed. London: Athlone Press, 1983.

Liese, Bernhard H., Paramjit S. Sachdeva, and D. Glynn Cochrane. *Organizing and Managing Tropical Disease Control Programs: Case Studies*. Washington, D.C.: World Bank, 1992.

Snow, Keith R. *Insects and Disease.* New York: John Wiley & Sons, 1974.

SLEEPWALKING

DISEASE/DISORDER

ALSO KNOWN AS: Somnambulism

ANATOMY OR SYSTEM AFFECTED: Brain, musculoskeletal system, nervous system, psychic-emotional system

SPECIALTIES AND RELATED FIELDS: Neurology, psychology

DEFINITION: Repeated episodes of arising from bed during sleep and walking about, without being conscious of the episodes or remembering them.

KEY TERMS:

electroencephalogram (EEG): a report of brain wave activity, achieved through attaching conductors to the scalp

parasomnia: normal waking behavior appearing within sleep (including sleepwalking) that is not caused by psychiatric illness

sleep stages: the division of sleep into rapid eye movement (REM) sleep, in which dreaming occurs, and non-REM sleep divided into four progressive levels, the first two being drowsiness and light sleeping and the last two involving deep sleep

CAUSES AND SYMPTOMS

Sleepwalking occurs during stages 3 and 4 of non-REM sleep and most frequently between one to four hours after falling asleep. Electroencephalograms (EEGs) indicate that children usually make a sudden transition into lighter sleep at the end of the first period of deep sleep. Some children do not make the transition rapidly and engage in parasomnia, or a simultaneous functioning of deep sleep and waking known as sleepwalking. An episode lasts from a few minutes to about an hour.

An estimated 40 percent of children ranging from six to sixteen years have reported sleepwalking, with twelve being the age of prevalence. While sleepwalking before the age of four is rare, partial wakings can affect toddlers and infants. Although sleepwalking usually ends around the age of seventeen, it can continue on into the early twenties. It is slightly more common in boys. Although most children sleepwalk infrequently, some sleepwalk frequently and for a period of five years or longer.

Sleepwalkers may have blank, staring faces and remain unresponsive to the attempt of others to communicate with them. They can be awakened only through great effort. Although sometimes sleepwalking children possibly see and walk around objects during their episodes, their behavior may involve leaving the bed violently and running without regard for obstacles. Partial awareness of their environment may be evident in their ability to negotiate hallway turns or objects on the floor. Some children stumble on stairs, crash into glass windows or doors, or walk out of the house into traffic. Serious injuries have occurred. While memory of these episodes is often absent, there may be a dim recall of the need to escape.

During sleepwalking, aggression toward others or toward objects in the vicinity is rare. The activity may be accompanied by sleeptalking that is characterized by poor articulation. Sleepwalkers also have increased incidence of other sleep disorders associated with non-REM sleep, such as night terrors.

Hormones or other biological factors may affect the character of these nighttime arousals. Statistics show that as many as 50 percent of sleepwalking children have close relatives with a history of similar phenomena. Although sleepwalking in very young children is developmental, many older children exhibit both a biological and an emotional predisposition for frequent sleepwalking. Some children who struggle to avoid expressing their feelings develop sleep problems.

TREATMENT AND THERAPY

Ensuring adequate sleep and providing a normal schedule are the best ways to treat partial wakings in young children. Although these remedies can help, some parents may have to learn to live with their children's sleepwalking. Understanding what is happening will prevent the parents from intervening by attempting to awaken or question children or returning them to bed immediately. Instead, parents should talk quietly and calmly to sleepwalking children. If the children spontaneously awake after the episode, parents should avoid negative comments and treat the event matter-of-factly. In the case of agitated sleepwalking, restraint merely intensifies and increases the length of time of the episode. One should approach the child only to prevent injury, thus allowing the sleepwalking to run its course.

The child's environment should be made as safe as possible to prevent accidental injury. Floors and stairs should be cleared, and hallways should be lit. For young children, gates may be installed at their bedroom doors or at the stairs, and should they attempt to leave the house, chain locks above their reach should be affixed to the doors.

Dr. Richard Ferber, director of the Center for Pediatric Sleep Disorders in Boston and author of *Solve Your Child's Sleep Problems* (1985), believes that older children whose sleepwalking may involve both psychological and inherited factors will benefit from psychotherapy. They may find it very difficult to express their feelings, especially if they are involved in situations in which things are happening outside of their control. In the event of changes, losses, or an absence of warmth or love within a family, Ferber believes that children are often quite angry about the circumstances but do not express it outwardly. Psychotherapy or counseling will encourage children to believe that their feelings are not dangerous and will help them express these feelings. Medication is prescribed reluctantly—only to prevent self-injury—and is decreased as the benefits from psychotherapy increase.

PERSPECTIVE AND PROSPECTS

As late as the 1960's, sleepwalking was believed to be a neurotic or hysterical manifestation or an acting out of a dream. Contemporary studies have confirmed that sleepwalking is a sleep disorder that is not caused by psychiatric illness and is not a walking dream state.

Fortunately, sleepwalking can be outgrown by adulthood. Meanwhile, investigations into the nature of sleep, sleep and waking patterns, and biological rhythms continue to provide the best insight into this distressing family problem.

—*Mary Hurd*

See also Nightmares; Psychiatry, child and adolescent; Sleep disorders.

FOR FURTHER INFORMATION:

Ferber, Richard. *Solve Your Child's Sleep Problems*. New York: Simon & Schuster, 1985. This concise volume is illustrated and includes an index.

Parkes, J. David. *Sleep and Its Disorders*. London: W. B. Saunders, 1985. This volume is aimed at the medical professional and includes illustrations, bibliographical references, and an index.

"Sleep Walking Disorder." In *Oski's Pediatrics: Principles and Practice*, edited by Frank A. Oski et al. 3d ed. Philadelphia: J. B. Lippincott, 1999. A chapter in a text which offers clear descriptions of diseases and illustrations.

SLIPPED DISK
DISEASE/DISORDER

ANATOMY OR SYSTEM AFFECTED: Back, bones, ligaments, musculoskeletal system, spine

SPECIALTIES AND RELATED FIELDS: Orthopedics, physical therapy

DEFINITION: Slipped disks, also known as herniated or ruptured disks, are characterized by a sudden or gradual break in the supportive ligaments surrounding a spinal disk. This break causes the soft tissue between disks to herniate through the outer ring and bulge into the spinal canal. Slipped disks are caused by sudden injury or by chronic stress from constant lifting or obesity. If the rupture occurs in the lower back, the symptoms include severe pain (generally to one side) in the low back and the back of the leg, buttock, or foot. Weakness and numbness of the affected leg may occur. If the slipped disk occurs in the neck, the symptoms include pain, weakness, and numbness in the neck and shoulder and down one arm. In both cases, pain worsens with movement. Slipped disks are generally treated with a few weeks in bed or, if necessary, surgery.

—*Jason Georges and Tracy Irons-Georges*

See also Numbness and tingling; Orthopedic surgery; Orthopedics; Spinal cord disorders; Spine, vertebrae, and disks.

FOR FURTHER INFORMATION:

Cyriax, James Henry. *The Slipped Disk*. London: Gower, 1970.

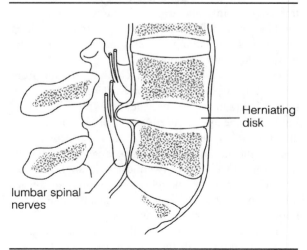

Slipped Disk

Herniating disk

lumbar spinal nerves

Faye, Leonard, and Lydia Encinas. *Good-bye Back Pain: The Safe and Easy Guide to Total Back Recovery.* New York: Berkley Press, 1992.

Fernando, C. Kumarlal, and Rana Weiss. *Fight Back: The Intelligent Person's Guide to Care of the Back.* Downers Grove, Ill.: Forest Hill Institute for Back Pain, 1984.

Manlapaz, Jesse S. *You and Your Slipped Disc.* Danbury, Conn.: Jesman, 1982.

Postacchini, Franco. *Lumbar Disc Herniation.* New York: Springer, 1999.

SMALLPOX

DISEASE/DISORDER

ANATOMY OR SYSTEM AFFECTED: Immune system, respiratory system, skin

SPECIALTIES AND RELATED FIELDS: Microbiology, public health, virology

DEFINITION: A highly contagious disease caused by one of two viruses, variola minor or variola major; it has been eradicated worldwide.

The incubation period for smallpox was about twelve days, and the disease took an additional two to four weeks to run its course. The first symptom was a high fever with the chills, headache, vomiting, and complete physical exhaustion that are often associated with fever. The symptoms increased in severity until the third day, when patients began to feel better. Next, they developed a sore throat and a cough, which could transmit the virus to anyone who shared the same air as the infected person. The next symptom was a rash of pustules (pimplelike eruptions), which broke open and formed scabs. As the scabs fell off, they left deep scars or pockmarks, called pox, in the skin. Smallpox was also spread by contact with flakes of scab or even contaminated clothing.

There was no cure for smallpox—up to 30 percent of its victims died from the disease. Those people who survived a case of smallpox, however, had an immunity that usually kept them from contracting it again. The main treatment for smallpox involved supportive measures, such as keeping the patient as comfortable as possible and preventing secondary infections from invading the body.

An important step in the elimination of this deadly disease was the development of a vaccine that would make humans immune to the variola virus that causes smallpox. The first attempts at immunization began

in the eighteenth century. Doctors in England and colonial America tried to immunize people by exposing them to a small amount of the virus that causes smallpox. It was hoped that only a mild case of smallpox would occur and that the recipient would then be immune to smallpox. Unfortunately, the doctors could not keep these mild cases from developing into full-blown smallpox. A second strategy involved vaccination with a virus that is similar to the smallpox virus, yet relatively harmless to humans. The virus that was used is the cowpox virus, which causes a minor disease in dairy cows.

The discovery of the cowpox vaccine was attributable to the clever detective work of an English doctor, Edward Jenner (1749-1823). He noticed that milkmaids and others who worked around cows seemed to be immune to smallpox. Upon further study, Jenner discovered that all these immune dairy workers had been exposed to cowpox. Vaccination with the cowpox virus gave the desired immunity to smallpox. Between 1967 and 1980, the World Health Organization waged a worldwide campaign of early detection, isolation of infected individuals, and vaccination. This campaign resulted in the complete eradication of smallpox; the last reported case was in 1980. Samples of the variola virus are now kept in medical laboratories for experimental purposes.

—*Steven A. Schonefeld, Ph.D.*

See also Childhood infectious diseases; Immunization and vaccination; Rashes; Viral infections.

FOR FURTHER INFORMATION:

Anderson, Kenneth N., ed. *Mosby's Medical, Nursing, and Allied Health Dictionary.* Rev. 5th ed. St. Louis: C. V. Mosby, 1998. Offers a basic presentation of medical terms and concepts.

Brock, Thomas D., ed. *Microorganisms: From Smallpox to Lyme Disease.* New York: W. H. Freeman, 1990. A collection of readings from *Scientific American.* The book includes a collection of accounts of the history of major infectious diseases. Divided into sections dealing with medical histories, methods of prevention, and means of transmission. Each section includes an introduction that summarizes the material.

Neus, Elizabeth. "U.S. Will Stockpile a Defense Against Smallpox." *USA Today,* October 11, 2000, p. D6. Vaccination against smallpox has existed for almost two centuries. Edward Jenner's first foray into protecting people against contagious diseases in the late 1700's was a crude immunization against smallpox.

Shepherd, H. R., and Peter J. Hotez. "Return of a Vanished Virus." *The Washington Post*, September 27, 2000, p. A23. The United States is dangerously underprepared to combat bioterrorist attack using smallpox. Few individuals have been vaccinated against smallpox since 1972, when eradication allowed immunization to be discontinued.

SMELL

BIOLOGY

ANATOMY OR SYSTEM AFFECTED: Nervous system, nose

SPECIALTIES AND RELATED FIELDS: Neurology, otorhinolaryngology

DEFINITION: One of the five special senses; chemicals interact with receptor sites in specialized structures of the nasal cavity, and the resulting nerve impulses are classified as certain kinds of odor.

KEY TERMS:

anosmia: a loss of the ability to detect aromas; general anosmia describes a lost ability to detect or identify any odors, while specific anosmia describes a lost ability to detect or identify a specific class of odors

Bowman's glands: one of three sources of the olfactory mucus that moistens the membranes of the olfactory center, thereby allowing odoriferous molecules to adhere to the olfactory hairs; glands that are located between olfactory supporting cells

chemoreceptors: in olfaction, specific structures in the nasal cavity upon which odoriferous, gaseous molecules adhere; this attachment induces a neural response that the brain interprets as smell

olfaction: the sense of smell; a process in which nerve impulses caused by chemicals interacting with chemoreceptors in the nose arrive in the olfactory center of the brain and are classified as certain kinds of odor

olfactory adaptation: the relatively quick response to and subsequent fatigue of the sense of smell that allows the presence of odoriferous chemicals to be recognized quickly and then become less and less noticed until they are soon ignored

olfactory bulb: an extension of the brain located below the frontal lobes of the cerebrum and above the ethmoid bone (extending back from the nose); one of a pair of gray masses into which the olfactory nerves terminate, thus serving as the first synaptic sites in olfactory neural pathways

olfactory epithelium: the surface covering of the olfactory region of the nasal cavity from which tiny, hairlike projections monitor the external world; a mucus-coated layer made of olfactory cells, supporting cells, and basal cells

olfactory hairs: the small, cilia-like projections extending from olfactory knobs into the conchae of the nasal cavity; at these projection sites, odoriferous molecules may interact chemically with the hairs to cause a nervous impulse to be sent to the brain

olfactory knobs: unmyelinated, tiny, rounded nerve endings of the sensory cells found at the mucus-coated olfactory membrane; each knob has five to eight extensions, called olfactory hairs, that branch out into the nasal cavity and monitor the environment

olfactory receptor cells: bipolar nerve cells surrounded by supporting cells in the olfactory epithelium; each cell body has one dendrite that terminates as an olfactory knob with hairlike projections

olfactory tract: the canal running posteriorly from the nose into the primary olfactory area of the cerebral cortex of the brain; the tract that houses large, myelinated olfactory nerves

STRUCTURE AND FUNCTIONS

Smell, one of the five special senses, plays an important role in both conscious and subconscious thought. While the loss of smell (anosmia) is troublesome, in isolation it is not a life-threatening problem. Nevertheless, anosmia is frequently an indication of an underlying pathology in either the olfactory or related organs; some of these pathologies may be life-threatening.

Of the special senses—gustation (taste), sight, olfaction (smell), audition (hearing), and equilibrium (balance and direction)—smell is the most primitive. As such, the organs that compose the olfactory system in humans are essentially identical to those found in other animals, including lampreys, cats, or dogs. The olfactory region of the nose is a very discriminating organ. Humans are able to classify smells according to at least seven agreed upon, although vague, classifications of primary odors: camphorlike, musky, floral, minty, ethereal, pungent, and putrid. Other categories that have been suggested are woody, spicy, and burned.

Within each odor category, the olfactory nerves and the brain are able to identify specific aromas with precision. For example, within the category of pungent, smells of onion, garlic, or skunk spray are easily discerned as similar, yet different, odors. Within the floral category, the human mind can readily distinguish among rose, lavender, and gardenia. The human olfactory sense can even distinguish between "left-handed" or "right-handed" molecules. In other words, the olfactory system can identify mirror-image molecules, in which one molecule is the spatial reverse of the other. An example is the substance carvone: When a person sniffs one form of carvone, the smell is spearmint; a sniff of the other form of carvone smells of caraway seed.

While studies of the anatomy and physiology of olfaction have not been finalized, the most accepted model of olfaction depends on the concept of odoriferous molecules attaching to olfactory receptor sites; the size and shape of both the odor molecules and the receptor sites are essential elements in currently adopted theories and descriptions of the mechanics of olfaction. Molecules of an odor-emitting substance chemically interact at receptor sites within specialized structures of the nasal cavity. The olfactory dendrites that are in contact with the external environment are directly linked to the neural centers of the brain. The olfactory tract connects these nerves directly to the hypothalamus region of the brain, which is associated with basic instinctual responses including fight-or-flight cues, food intake, or sexual curiosity and drive. This direct link to the brain causes a rapid and powerful response in animals to odor stimuli.

Because there is no physical barrier to protect olfactory receptors from the outside world, these nerve endings have a certain vulnerability to harm or damage. Olfactory nerves constantly regenerate in about a twenty-eight-day cycle; they are the only nerves that are capable of readily regenerating themselves and returning to full function. Nevertheless, it is esti-

The Sense of Smell

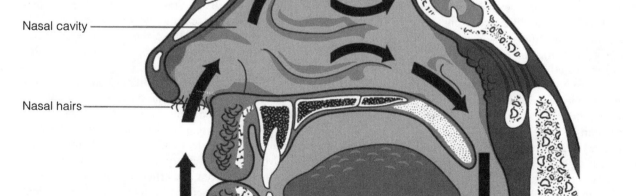

Humans detect odors by a complex series of interactions—some only theoretical—involving receptors in the nasal cavity that interact with odor molecules to send nerve impulses to the brain through the olfactory nerve.

mated that about 1 percent of all olfactory receptors in an individual die each year because of externally induced damage and general wear. Therefore, the sense of smell becomes less sensitive in older adults, which can minimize or repress the desire to eat and result in malnutrition.

The nasal cavity has two roles, one associated with respiration and the other with the sense of smell. The region that is dedicated to olfaction is small and evenly divided between the two septa of the nose. Within each nostril are folds called conchae. Humans have three conchae pairs— lower, middle, and upper. The specialized sensing structures for olfaction are found inside the middle and upper conchae. It is currently believed that olfactory receptors are regions of specialized molecular architecture located on cilia-like fibers called olfactory hairs. Olfactory hairs are extensions, or branches, of the olfactory sensing cells. The hairs, which are actually made of microfilaments, are dispersed over the surface of the olfactory sensing region of the nasal cavity.

While the size of the olfactory region of the nasal cavity is small (about the size of a dime), its surface area is comparatively large because of the many olfactory hairs coating the surface, or epithelium, of the olfactory cleft. It is estimated that humans have between 10 and 40 million olfactory receptors. The number of receptor hairs varies among species; dogs have about 1 million receptors on their olfactory cleft and are far more sensitive to specific odors than are humans. This feature explains why dogs can be trained for hunting game, finding missing persons, and locating drugs or explosives. A person can smell a pot of soup cooking and know it is soup, but a dog smelling the same pot of soup smells each ingredient of the soup, not the scent of the mixture. Nevertheless, among the senses, the sense of smell in humans is second only to vision in terms of number of receptors per unit of surface area.

The olfactory hairs are surrounded by a thick, brown-colored mucus and are partially covered and partially exposed. Thus, the mucosal lining on the epithelium of the olfactory region is a thin and poor protective barrier for the specialized structures that it coats. The mucus on the olfactory epithelium has three structures of origin: Bowman's glands, the goblet cells of the respiratory regions of the nose, and the supporting cells of the olfactory epithelium. Most of the mucus around the olfactory hairs is secreted from Bowman's glands, and only the Bowman's secretions

contain the brown pigment that colors the mucus. It is known that, in other species, pigment is connected to olfactory ability; for example, albino pigs, which are lacking all pigments, are unable to smell toxic plants and often die from ingesting native plants that are poisonous to their species. The true significance of the brown pigment in humans, however, remains unclear.

The significance of the olfactory mucus itself is not in question. Odoriferous molecules must be trapped by the mucus so that they can travel to chemoreceptor sites on the olfactory hairs. The interaction between the odor molecules and the chemoreceptors of the olfactory hairs requires a mutual attraction, originating from small electrostatic forces. The shape, size, and polarity or nonpolarity of molecules causing odor are important factors in the creation of a smell stimulus.

From the olfactory hairs in the membrane structure, the odor molecules travel through the cribriform plate and into the olfactory tract, which leads directly to the hypothalamus in the brain. The olfactory hairs extend from the olfactory knobs, unexposed sensory cell endings completely covered by brown mucus. Five to eight hairs extend from each knob; electron micrographs show that the hairs are actually dendrites extending from the cell body into the external environment, while the axons of the cells carry nerve impulses toward the brain.

The sensory cells are found about midway in the olfactory epithelium. Other cells in the epithelium are the supporting cells and the basal cells. The supporting cells provide a scaffolding for the sensory cells and also contribute fluids to the mucus layer. Basal cells are able to assist in the replenishment of receptor cells.

The cribriform plate, often described as a wafer-thin structure, is an important separation point between unmyelinated sensory nerves, which are in touch with the environment, and the myelinated nerves that direct the tiny electrical impulses of smell to the brain. Myelinated olfactory nerves are large and function with great speed and efficiency in comparison to the unmyelinated sensory cells. Thus, the original nerve signal prompted by an odoriferous molecule is slow, but this time is more than recovered in the myelinated nerve fibers. Working together, the unmyelinated and myelinated nerve bundles detect, transmit, and deliver nerve impulses of smell in fractions of a second, aided by the relatively short path between the nasal cavity and the hypothalamus.

The hypothalamus is located under the thalamus in the brain. It is the center into which nerve impulses originating at the sensory organs of sound, taste, smell, and the somatic senses are delivered. The activity of this portion of the brain is closely linked to the activity of the pituitary gland. This association is important in the sense of smell and sexual maturation, which is triggered by hormones released by the hypothalamus. In addition to these attributes, the hypothalamus is essential to regulating the autonomic nervous system, body temperature, and food intake.

DISORDERS AND DISEASES

Loss of the ability to sense all smells is called anosmia. Hyposmia (a decrease of smell function), dysosmia (an altered sense of smell), and anosmia can manifest themselves in numerous ways.

Most people are well acquainted with the inability to smell during a heavy cold. This condition is a temporary one caused by the presence of excessive mucus. The presence of a cold virus causes the respiratory region of the nose to respond by producing excessive volumes of cleansing mucus from goblet cells. Unfortunately, there tends to be so much mucus that the olfactory region becomes flooded; instead of swimming in mucus, the olfactory hairs are drowning. A thick coating over the hairs prevents odoriferous molecules from reaching the chemoreceptors. The sense of smell is lost until partial recovery decreases the mucus levels and once again allows the olfactory hairs to be partially exposed to the exterior world. The ability to sense odors fully returns once recovery from the head cold is complete.

Because it is uncommon to lose the ability to smell all odors, true anosmia is a rare condition. Furthermore, anosmia is seldom a problem found in isolation. Often there are simultaneously occurring symptoms such as a loss of taste (gustatory) function, undeveloped ovaries and testes, or head injury. In diagnosing possible causes of anosmia or dysosmia, a physician must obtain a complete medical history and perform a thorough physical exam. Special attention is given to the nasal cavity, the head and neck area, and, perhaps surprisingly, to genital maturation and function. Smell function is measured by passing vials containing increasing concentrations of an odoriferous chemical under a patient's nose until a scent can be detected. It is also important to assess whether the patient can properly identify the smell; if not, further studies must be done.

Olfactory problems can originate in one of the three structures that are involved in olfaction: in the sensory receptors, which convert chemical signals arising from odor molecules into electrical impulses; in the sensory nerve cells, which transmit these electrical impulses to the brain; and in the brain, which interprets the incoming electrical signals.

Abnormalities in the nasal cavity that can modify or destroy olfaction may include nasal polyps, a tumor located in an olfactory bulb, or allergic rhinitis (irritated and swollen membranes of the nose). Other olfactory maladies may be of an indirect origin, such as nutritional abnormalities or the presence of a toxic trace metal. Endocrine imbalances can be particularly pertinent in olfaction function.

An example of an endocrine imbalance that can influence the olfactory sense is seen in the cooperative workings of the hypothalamus and the pituitary gland. The hypothalamus receives impulses from olfactory nerves. It also lies just above the major endocrine gland, the pituitary gland. The pituitary gland receives regulating chemicals from the hypothalamus that either stimulate or inhibit the anterior portion of the gland. The anterior region of the pituitary gland monitors the levels of steroid hormones circulating in the body. Steroid hormones are essential to complete sexual maturation in both males and females. A congenital defect that affects both the nose and sexual maturation is Demorsier's olfactogenital dysplasia. Individuals with this malady are anosmic as a result of underdeveloped olfactory lobes. Low levels of gonadotropic hormones are also found in afflicted persons, resulting in undeveloped ovaries or testes. A somewhat similar (but not congenital) problem can be seen in Kohn's syndrome. In this syndrome, the ovaries or testes are underdeveloped and the olfactory nerves are abnormally formed, halting the sense of smell.

Olfaction is believed to play a role in the timely onset of sexual maturation in puberty. It seems that both male and female pheromones, oily scents that subconsciously cause sexual excitement in a species, can assist in or accelerate the events of sexual maturation. Although researchers are still exploring the role of pheromones in the human species, it appears that smell is relevant to the onset of menstruation in pubescent girls. Scents also contribute to sexual arousal in males.

An altered sense of smell can occur with pregnancy because of the resulting changes in hormone levels. For some pregnant women, formerly pleasant aromas may become repugnant, sometimes contributing to the feeling of nausea that some pregnant women experience. In addition, the increased mucus production that occurs with pregnancy works to block full smell function.

Brain tumors or lesions can sometimes account for anosmia, hyposmia, or dysosmia. Head injury is another possible cause because nerves or the hypothalamus itself can be crushed or otherwise damaged. Tumors, lesions, and neural damage can be detected using positron emission tomography (PET) scanning or magnetic resonance imaging (MRI). Some neurological diseases may be considered when diagnosing these olfactory disorders since the sense of smell requires only organs found in the nervous system.

Treatment of olfactory malfunctions vary greatly depending on the origin of the problem. Surgery may be needed to remove tumors. Allergies may be treated by shots; corticosteroids may be used to prevent the inflammation of nasal mucous membranes. Drugs may be administered to either inhibit or activate nerve conduction. Treatment often results in the recovery of olfaction, but not in all cases.

PERSPECTIVE AND PROSPECTS

The sense of smell has been recognized as one of the most primitive attributes of the human species, and it once held a high position in the hierarchy of skills required for species survival. Olfaction has long been a topic of intrigue in intellectual circles. The Greek philosopher Democritus of Abdera (384-322 B.C.E.) proposed his theory of the atom in a time when modern science and scientific methods did not exist. Democritus incorporated his description of atoms into an explanation of olfaction. He presumed that the sense of smell in humans resulted from some kind of connection that formed when atoms of odor-emitting substances entered the nose. Different odor sensations, he proposed, would result from differences in the texture and shape of these atoms. The anatomy of the nose and brain was not considered in his philosophy. Democritus's idea of atoms was largely rejected in Greek circles of thought, however, and the concept of atoms combining to form molecules would not appear for hundreds of centuries. Modern understanding of the sense of smell is largely a more advanced, more informed, and more technical description of the very ideas imagined by this great Greek philosopher.

Another Greek contemplating the subject of smell was the physician Galen of Pergamum (129-c. 199 C.E.), who proposed an insightful description of the neuroanatomy of olfaction which also proved to be validated, with some alterations, centuries later. Whether he accepted the notion of atoms or not, Galen believed that particles actually tunneled into what are now called olfactory bulbs, thereby causing an odor to be detected. Galen also believed that these olfactory bulbs were extensions connected directly to the brain. Living in an era when microscopes and the scientific method did not exist, Galen could only describe what he saw with the unaided eye and reason intuitively. It is fascinating, therefore, to learn that his belief that the olfactory bulbs were extensions of the brain has been proven correct.

As the most primitive, and thus less evolved, of the five special senses, smell is associated with basic instincts, reactions or responses to external stimuli that aid an individual organism. Smell influences instincts of aggression when odors are released in fighting or battle through sweat and perhaps blood. These odors may inspire fight-or-flight responses in the brain and body. Social groups, such as a street gang, a group of soldiers, or a den of lions, can learn to recognize the scent (or the absence of scent) of its members in training or other group activities, helping to identify safe and unsafe groups in darkness or battle when other cues may be masked. Thus, while it is a subtle form of recognition often registered in the subconscious, smell apparently plays a role in modern survival tactics as well.

Another basic instinct that utilizes the sense of smell is the "mothering" instinct. For example, new mothers are better able to identify their newborns by scent than by sight only hours after delivery. This sense seems adaptively helpful to the exhausted mother—who may have been in labor for days and is likely to be suffering from general exhaustion and diminished energy—in locating and feeding her baby. In a primitive human culture, this ability would help mothers identify babies if a flight from danger or a search for food or water caused a temporary separation of the mother-child pair. In addition, a nursing baby is guided to the mother's nipple by the scent released from the sweat glands surrounding the nipples.

Mate selection is believed to be linked to scents and olfactory appeal. There is some evidence that even the most heavily perfumed person of modern society emits pheromones that are sexually alluring to some and repulsive to others. This allure or repulsion seems to occur in the subconscious mind, or the limbic region of the brain.

On a more conscious level, the sense of smell is sometimes useful as a warning of a health problem; thus odors can be helpful in either describing or diagnosing a disease. For example, some people with epilepsy, days or only minutes before the onset of an epileptic seizure, have olfactory hallucinations—they smell odors in the absence of any stimulating molecules. The odor is usually described as either a scent of decay, as at a fish market, or a chemical, such as ether or petroleum. The sweet smell of acetone on a person's breath can indicate a diabetic who is in danger of coma, or who is already in a coma and cannot ask for help. Vincent's angina can be suspected if a foul breath odor is present, while diphtheria causes a sweet scent.

Because of the unique regenerative capacity of the olfactory neurons, neurologists and other researchers are actively attempting to understand the mechanisms that allow these nerves to be so efficient and effective in nerve regeneration. Such research may have an impact upon the understanding and treatment of a variety of neurological disorders that are not directly affiliated with olfaction.

—*Mary C. Fields, M.D.*

See also Allergies; Aromatherapy; Common cold; Nasal polyp removal; Nasopharyngeal disorders; Otorhinolaryngology; Respiration; Rhinitis; Rhinoplasty and submucous resection; Sense organs; Sinusitis; Taste.

FOR FURTHER INFORMATION:

Atkins, Peter. *Molecules.* New York: Scientific American Libraries, 1987. The chapter "Taste, Smell, and Pain" contains simple, but intriguing, examples of molecular shapes that cause a certain odoriferous chemical to be perceived as belonging to one of the primary odor categories. The molecular interactions at the chemoreceptors are briefly described.

Engen, Trygg. *The Perception of Odors.* New York: Academic Press, 1982. Designed for the beginner, this text describes the anatomy, physiology, and psychology behind olfaction. Provides detailed explanations of the classification of odors, odor theories, and the tests that are used to assess olfactory function.

Hole, John W., Jr. *The Essentials of Human Anatomy and Physiology.* 6th ed. Dubuque, Iowa: Wm. C.

Brown, 1993. Chapter 12, "The Somatic and Special Senses," contains a section devoted exclusively to the sense of smell. Other related topics, such as the anatomy and organization of the brain and nervous system, are described in exquisite detail. Although this academic textbook is more advanced than an introductory biology book, it uses definitions and excellent diagrams and drawings to assist the reader.

Schmidt, Robert F., ed. *Fundamentals of Sensory Physiology.* Translated by Marguerite A. Biedermann-Thorson. Rev. 3d ed. Berlin: Springer-Verlag, 1986. Chapter 9, "Physiology of Olfaction," addresses the organization of the olfactory system and its relevant connections in the brain.

Tortora, Gerard J., and Sandra R. Grabowski. *Principles of Anatomy and Physiology.* 9th ed. New York: John Wiley & Sons, 2000. This text offers a brief treatment of the topic of smell, but perusal of the book will allow the reader to place this special sense within the context of the whole human anatomy.

Whitfield, Philip, and Mike Stoddart. *Hearing, Taste, and Smell: Pathways of Perception.* Toronto: Torstar Books, 1985. The last four chapters of the text describe the complex themes regarding the physiology and anatomy of olfaction with clear, yet thorough, terminology.

Wolfe, Jeremy M. *Sensory Systems: Senses Other than Vision.* Boston: Birkhauser, 1988. Includes eight essays, selected from the *Encyclopedia of Neuroscience*, addressing topics of olfaction in humans and other species. The longest of these essays is only three pages in length, but each article contains much useful information.

SMOKING

DISEASE/DISORDER

ANATOMY OR SYSTEM AFFECTED: Circulatory system, lungs, throat

SPECIALTIES AND RELATED FIELDS: Oncology, pulmonary medicine, vascular medicine

DEFINITION: The inhalation of tobacco in the form of cigarettes or cigars, which poses important health risks; those risks can be significantly decreased by smoking cessation, even in older age.

CAUSES AND EFFECTS

Cigarette smoking has long been known to have adverse effects. Smokers get more wrinkles than nonsmokers, so they tend to look older than their chronological age. They also are more likely to develop gum disease and lose teeth, adding to the changes related to eating, such as alterations in sense of smell and taste, that are normal as people age. Loss of teeth leads to difficulty chewing, which in turn leads to difficulties with digestion. Most people who lose teeth eventually develop loss of the bone that should support their teeth, making it increasingly difficult to fit dentures.

Smokers are ten times more likely to get lung cancer than nonsmokers. Lung cancer is now the number one cause of cancer death in women, as well as in men. In addition to lung cancer, smokers have a higher incidence of cancers of the head and neck, esophagus, colon, rectum, kidney, bladder, and cervix. Smokers are twenty times more likely to have a heart attack than nonsmokers. In older people, the major risk factor for disease of the coronary arteries is hypertension, but smoking is still significant, especially when combined with other risk factors for heart disease, such as diabetes or high cholesterol. Smoking and diabetes are also the two most important risk factors for diseases of the veins and arteries of the lower leg. Those who continue to smoke once these diseases develop are much more likely to require limb amputation than those who quit. Smokers may develop chronic obstructive pulmonary disease (COPD), which includes emphysema and chronic bronchitis, and are eighteen times more likely than nonsmokers to die of diseases of the lungs other than cancer. Older smokers also show decreases in muscle strength, agility, coordination, gait, and balance. The changes in these areas make them seem five years older than their actual age.

Smoking has long been thought to be associated with peptic ulcer disease. In addition, smoking makes the symptoms of many diseases worse or increases the risk of complications in patients with allergies, diabetes, hypertension, and vascular disease. Male smokers are at greater risk of experiencing sexual impotence. Female smokers tend to experience an earlier menopause and are at increased risk for hip fracture than nonsmokers. Smokers are more likely to develop glaucoma than nonsmokers. Studies completed in 1996 indicated an increased risk with smoking for macular degeneration, the leading cause of blindness in older adults. The evidence is mixed on smoking and Alzheimer's disease, but a 1998 study contradicted earlier work and found that the risk is greater in smokers than nonsmokers. Finally, smokers

are at greater risk of death or injury caused by cigarette-related fires.

Cigarette smoking tends to speed up the processes in the liver for breaking down, using, and eliminating medications, both nonprescription and prescription. This means that medications may not perform as expected in the body. Smokers may need to take medications more frequently or in greater doses than nonsmokers, so it is important for health care providers to know that a person smokes. The drugs known to be affected by smoking include sedatives, narcotic and synthetic narcotic painkillers, certain antidepressants, anticoagulant medications, asthma medications, and beta blockers. These changes are of particular concern in the older population for a number of reasons. First, older people (whether smokers or nonsmokers) tend to need more medications than younger people. With each additional drug, the risk of serious drug interaction and other adverse effects increases. Second, changes in body composition and function that alter the metabolism of drugs come with age, making medication use somewhat riskier in older persons, in terms of adverse effects and complications. The additional changes associated with smoking increase these risks significantly.

The dangers of passive smoking are well documented. The effects seem to be more harmful in children than in adults, but adults who are affected are at increased risk for cancer, heart disease, noncancerous lung diseases, and allergies.

TREATMENT AND THERAPY
Numerous studies have shown that smoking cessation has health benefits in as little as one year, such as reducing the risk of heart attack and coronary artery disease. Within two years of smoking cessation, the risks of stroke and diseases of the blood vessels in the lower leg are reduced as well. Even though chronic lung disease is not reversible, those who quit smoking slow the decline in lung function considerably. Risks for cancers also decrease significantly with smoking cessation and are similar to the cancer risk for nonsmokers in ten to thirteen years. These findings indicate that it is worthwhile even for older people to give up smoking.

Because smoking is an addiction, it may be difficult to quit, particularly after years of cigarette use. Most smokers have to stop several times before quitting permanently. Setting a quit date, attending support group meetings, taking it one day at a time, undergoing hypnosis, making a contract with a friend or a health care provider, substituting carrot sticks for cigarettes, increasing exercise (particularly swimming), and breathing deeply all seem to be helpful techniques. Nicotine replacement systems are available in the United States on a nonprescription basis, but it is important for older people, particularly those with health problems or who are taking multiple medications, to consult a health care professional prior to using them. It is also important that anyone using these aids stop smoking completely. It is possible to get a toxic dose, perhaps even a fatal one, by smoking and using nicotine replacement simultaneously.

PERSPECTIVE AND PROSPECTS

Smoking is the main avoidable cause of death in the United States and many other developed nations. More than 10 percent of North Americans over the age of sixty-five smoke cigarettes, putting themselves and those with whom they live at risk for significant health problems. These risks appear to increase both with age and with the number of years of smoking. After World War II, more women began smoking. Because the diseases related to smoking usually take years to develop, it was only in the last part of the twentieth century that rates of smoking-related disease among women began to approach those of men. On the other hand, research indicates that smoking cessation appears to be beneficial, even in a person who has smoked for many years.

—*Rebecca Lovell Scott, Ph.D.*

See also Amputation; Bronchitis; Cancer; Dental diseases; Diabetes mellitus; Emphysema; Eyes; Fracture and dislocation; Gingivitis; Glaucoma; Heart attacks; Lung cancer; Lungs; Macular degeneration; Osteoporosis; Pulmonary diseases; Pulmonary medicine; Respiration; Sexual dysfunction; Skin disorders; Strokes; Teeth; Visual disorders; Wrinkles.

FOR FURTHER INFORMATION:

Christen, William, et al. "A Prospective Study of Cigarette Smoking and Risk of Age-Related Macular Degeneration in Men." *The Journal of the American Medical Association* 276, no. 14 (October 9, 1996). The authors evaluated the relationship between cigarette smoking and incidence of age-related macular degeneration (AMD) among men. It is concluded that cigarette smoking is an independent and avoidable risk factor for AMD among men.

Fiore, Michael C. "The Agency for Health Care Policy and Research Smoking Cessation Clinical Practice Guideline." *The Journal of the American Medical Association* 275, no. 16 (April 24, 1996). Fiore summarizes the Smoking Cessation Clinical Practice Guideline that provides recommendations for three groups of professionals: primary care clinicians, smoking cessation specialists, and health care administrators, insurers, and purchasers

Hales, Diane. "Tobacco Use." In *An Invitation to Health*. 9th ed. Pacific Grove, Calif.: Brooks/Cole, 1999. This helpful resource covers many aspects of health, including mental health, physical fitness, stress management, and preventive medicine.

Hermanson, B., et al. "Beneficial Six-Year Outcome of Smoking Cessation in Older Men and Women with Coronary Artery Disease." *New England Journal of Medicine* 319, no. 21 (November 24, 1988). Smoking cessation lessens the risk of death or myocardial infarction in older as well as younger persons with coronary artery disease.

Ott, A. "Smoking and Risk of Dementia and Alzheimer's Disease in a Population-Based Cohort Study: The Rotterdam Study." *The Lancet* 351, no. 9119 (June 20, 1998). Ott found that smoking is associated with a doubling of the risk of dementia and Alzheimer's disease. Carriers of the apolipoprotein E genotype had no increased risk of dementia, which suggests an interaction between smoking and the genotype in the etiology of Alzheimer's disease.

Seddon, Johanna, et al. "A Prospective Study of Cigarette Smoking and Age-Related Macular Degeneration in Women." *The Journal of the American Medical Association* 276, no. 14 (October 9, 1996). The authors evaluated the relationship between cigarette smoking and incidence of age-related macular degeneration (AMD) among women. It is concluded that cigarette smoking is an independent and avoidable risk factor for AMD among women.

SNAKEBITES

DISEASE/DISORDER

ANATOMY OR SYSTEM AFFECTED: Blood, circulatory system, nervous system

SPECIALTIES AND RELATED FIELDS: Emergency medicine, hematology, serology

DEFINITION: The penetration of skin or flesh by the fangs of a snake. Although a snakebite often involves a poisonous snake, not all bites include venom injection into the bloodstream.

KEY TERMS:

antivenin: an antidote given to snakebite victims to combat the effects of venom that has been injected into the bloodstream

venom: the substance that is often injected into the affected part of the flesh during a snakebite

CAUSES AND SYMPTOMS

A snakebite is a wound that results from the flesh penetration created by the hollow teeth, or fangs, of a snake and sometimes the injection of venom into the bloodstream. Venom is usually encountered in snakes, although other animals and insects use it, often as part of their defense system. In Australia, for example, several creatures are classified as venomous, such as twenty-two types of spiders, four types of ants, two types of beetles, two types of caterpillars, all platypus variations, two types of blue-ringed octopi, seven types of jellyfish, and eleven types of rays.

Venomous snakebites have a different effect based on the size of the victim, the location of the bite, the quantity of venom injected, and the time elapsed between the snakebite and the administration of antivenin therapy. Any part of the body is subject to this injury, but statistically legs, feet, and arms are by far the most commonly affected areas.

The symptoms of a snakebite include swelling or discoloration of the skin, a racing pulse, weakness, shortness of breath, nausea, and vomiting. Other symptoms include dilation of the pupils, shock, convulsions, twitching, and slurred speech. In extreme cases, severe pain and swelling and sometimes paralysis, unconsciousness, and even death may occur.

Common North American Poisonous Snakes

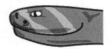

Western diamondback rattlesnake
Location: West, Southwest, esp. arid zones
Color: Brown to reddish
Features: Diamond pattern on skin, rattle on tail

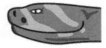

Eastern diamondback rattlesnake
Location: Southeast
Color: Brown
Features: To 8 feet long, diamond pattern on skin, rattle on tail

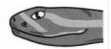

Prairie rattlesnake
Location: Great Plains
Color: Greenish-gray to brown
Features: To 4 feet long, rattle on tail

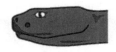

Timber rattlesnake
Location: Forests, swamps, hillsides in Midwest, Northeast
Color: Pale brown with black bands
Features: Rattle on tail

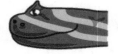

Sidewinder rattlesnake
Location: West, Southwest deserts, arid zones
Color: Pale brown
Features: Hornlike eyelash scales above eyes, rattle on tail

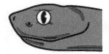

Water moccasin (cottonmouth)
Location: South, Southeast in or near water
Color: Brown with dark crossbands or black
Features: To 5 feet long, opens mouth to show white interior, no tail rattle

Copperhead
Location: East (north to south), South
Color: Russet with dark bands, yellowish head
Features: Vibrates tail when angry

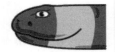

Eastern coral snake
Location: Southeast
Color: Yellow-black or yellow-red recurring ring pattern
Features: To 4 feet long, slender

Snake venom contains an array of substances that are usually proteins in nature and that create tissue damage in several ways. The most important kinds of damage are nerve destruction, in which case the venom is called neurotoxic, and blood and tissue destruction, in which case the venom is hemotoxic. Neurotoxins have the tendency to paralyze the nervous system and lead to heart and respiratory failure. On the other hand, hemotoxins destroy arteries, veins, and blood corpuscles and lead to internal hemorrhaging. Different snakes have various degrees of toxins. Cobra venom is usually neurotoxic, while rattlesnake venom is hemotoxic. The development of gangrene in the location of the snakebite is possible unless the victim is treated promptly.

TREATMENT AND THERAPY

The victim of a snakebite may exhibit mild to severe symptoms. Although the strength of venom of different snakes differs widely, snakebite treatment should be imposed as soon as possible in order to reduce the possibility of a fatality. This treatment should address two points: how to restrict the venom to the smallest body area possible and how to remove as much venom as possible. Thus, all contractions of the body and limb movement should be reduced immediately to a minimum to avoid spreading the venom. This is accomplished by immobilizing the affected area, preferably in a horizontal position and definitely lower than the heart. Any exertion and/or excitement by the bitten person increases the pulse rate and blood circulation, which leads to easier spreading of the venom. This is the same reason that stimulants should be avoided.

Statistically, more than three-quarters of snakebites occur on the lower leg or forearm. Current first aid recommendations do not include ice, any incision, the application of oxidizers such as potassium permanganate, or the administration of aspirin, ibuprofen, acetaminophen, or alcohol. Instead, the bitten part should be wiped, and a relatively tight tourniquet that reduces the lymphatic flow without cutting off the blood supply to the affected area should be applied. A nurse or other emergency medical service employee should check the pulse at the bitten area to ensure adequate blood flow. It is also recommended that the bandage be released every half hour for half a minute. It is also helpful to take the snake, whether alive or dead, to the hospital for proper identification.

If the swelling extends more than 5 inches within the first twelve hours after the bite, antivenin is given through intravenous transfusion in a hospital. Antivenin preparations are extracted by the immunization of animals such as horses, and their efficiency is dependent on the purification and concentration of the substance. Antivenins are usually specific, but some, such as that for tiger snake venom, appear to protect against the venom of more than one snake. If there is no swelling and increasing pain around the bite within thirty minutes, then the wound is one of the approximately one-third of bites by poisonous snakes in which venom is not injected. A notable exception is the bite of the coral snake, in which swelling takes place despite the venom infusion.

After the patient sees a doctor, several nutrients can be taken that appear to relieve pain and symptoms. They include vitamin C (approximately 10,000 milligrams every hour), which serves as a detoxifier and lessens infection; calcium gluconate (500 milligrams every four to six hours), which relieves pain; and pantothenic acid (500 milligrams every four hours for two days), which serves as an antistress vitamin.

PERSPECTIVE AND PROSPECTS

Snakebites have been recorded in history for thousands of years, including such well-known examples as Moses' flight from Egypt and Cleopatra's suicide with an asp. Traditionally, American Indians have had snakebite victims use echinacea, either by chewing the leaves and roots of the plant or drinking it in a tea form. They have also used its pulp placed on the affected area after making an incision and sucking the venom out until blood flows freely.

Approximately one-third of the three thousand snake species are poisonous, and only about three hundred can kill humans. The efficiency of emergency services and the wide availability of antivenins have reduced the death rates from snakebites dramatically. As a result, the number of people killed because of bee, wasp, and scorpion stings in the United States is higher than the deaths attributed to snakebites.

—*Soraya Ghayourmanesh, Ph.D.*

See also Bites and stings; Emergency medicine; Emergency medicine, pediatric; Nervous system; Neurology; Neurology, pediatric; Numbness and tingling; Poisoning; Seizures; Toxicology; Zoonoses.

FOR FURTHER INFORMATION:

Altimari, William. *Venomous Snakes: A Safety Guide for Reptile Keepers*. St. Louis: Society for the Study of Amphibians and Reptiles, 1998. This concise volume covers the handling of poisonous snakes, offering information on snake bites and venom. Includes bibliographical references and an index.

Julivert, Maria Angels. *The Fascinating World of Snakes.* New York: Barron's Educational Series, 1993. Vivid, full-color illustrations provide much detail, especially of predatory activities. Includes a glossary and an index.

Mattison, Christopher. *The Encyclopedia of Snakes.* New York: Facts on File, 1995. This volume discusses aspects of the life cycle of snakes—their biology, history, and taxonomy. Chapter topics include origin and evolution, morphology and function, feeding, defense, and reproduction.

Savage, Jay M. "Squamata." In *McGraw-Hill Encyclopedia of Science and Technology.* 8th ed. Vol. 17. New York: McGraw-Hill, 1997. A chapter in a complete reference for the nonspecialist, which offers thousands of articles written by world-renowned scientists and engineers. It includes many new and revised articles and extensive cross-references and bibliographies and is fully illustrated.

Tu, Anthony T., ed. *Reptile Venoms and Toxins.* Handbook of Natural Toxins 5. New York: Marcel Dekker, 1991. In twenty-four contributed chapters, thirty-seven international specialists describe the latest developments in research on snake venom and summarize what is known to date on Gila monster and frog toxins.

SNEEZING
DISEASE/DISORDER

ANATOMY OR SYSTEM AFFECTED: Chest, immune system, lungs, nose, respiratory system

SPECIALTIES AND RELATED FIELDS: Family practice, internal medicine

DEFINITION: A physiological act in which air is forcibly expelled through the nose via a reflex spasm of chest and pharynx muscles.

CAUSES AND SYMPTOMS

During the breathing process, the lung part of the chest cavity is expanded and air is allowed to flow in. When impulses that cause excitation reach a threshold level in the nasal lining, a message is transferred to the sneeze reflex center of the brain via the sensory nerves. At that point, the stimulus provides the chest muscles with the signal to convulse and therefore squeeze the lungs. The contracted muscles in the pharynx block the exit of the air from the mouth and instead detour it through the nasal cavity and out into the atmosphere. The phenomenon of genuine sneezing cannot be performed voluntarily and, at the same time, cannot be easily suppressed. In fact, suppression may create an increase in pressure in the acoustic part of the body, with occasional serious results.

During inhalation, air is inserted through the nostrils, heated to the body temperature, humidified, and finally filtered of foreign contaminants (such as bacteria and dust particles) before it enters the lungs. When the air contains a large quantity of particles, such as dust or pollen during windy conditions, or is drier or colder than expected, sneezing takes place. The main reason for this reaction is irritation of the nerve endings, which is temporarily relieved by the explosive blowing of air during sneezing. The process is intensified in both children and adults by several nasal disorders, such as congestion attributed to bacterial infection, cold, allergy created by foreign particles, pressure, or a growth inside the nostril.

TREATMENT AND THERAPY

In a way similar to coughing, in which air is expelled through the mouth, sneezing has a protective role in breathing. The hairs inside the nostrils, known as cilia, serve as the filtering device and, when they cannot trap the contaminants, as the instigators for the irritation of the nerve endings. Their presence is therefore instrumental in protecting the windpipe from the solid particles that are suspended in air. Parents may have a young child blow his or her nose in order to remove the trapped particles in the nasal mucus. This action should be performed with the minimum damage of the capillaries, which may collapse and lead to a nosebleed, possibly followed by an infection.

PERSPECTIVE AND PROSPECTS

Sneezing is very important because it serves as the first weapon of the respiratory system's defense against invading foreign particles. The search goes on for inhalers and other medications to relieve the effects of sneezing, as well as for various means to release the pressure created by the common cold and rhinoviruses. The traditional methods of soothing nerve endings with steam and other vaporizers are still dependable and help in avoiding the subsequent spread of the more serious viral infections such as pneumonia and bronchiolitis.

—*Soraya Ghayourmanesh, Ph.D.*

See also Allergies; Common cold; Coughing; Hay fever; Immune system; Nasopharyngeal disorders; Nosebleeds; Otorhinolaryngology; Respiration; Sore throat; Viral infections.

FOR FURTHER INFORMATION:
Karpa, Kelly Dowhower. "The Assault on Allergies: From Diagnostics to Treatments." *Drug Topics* (June, 2000): 12S-16S.
Knight, Allan. *Asthma and Hay Fever: How to Relieve Wheezing and Sneezing.* New York: Arco, 1981.
McCarthy, Robert. "New Approaches to Allergic Rhinitis and Asthma." *Patient Care* 34, no. 19 (October 15, 2000): 108-118.
Ross-Flanigan, Nancy. "Nothing to Sneeze At." *Health* 14, no. 3 (April, 2000): 102-104.
Voelker, Rebecca. "Allergies: More than Just Sniffles and Sneezes." *Business and Health* 18, no. 4 (April, 2000): 19-25.

SOILING

DISEASE/DISORDER

ALSO KNOWN AS: Encopresis

ANATOMY OR SYSTEM AFFECTED: Anus, gastrointestinal system, intestines, psychic-emotional system

SPECIALTIES AND RELATED FIELDS: Gastroenterology, pediatrics

DEFINITION: The passage of fecal material into inappropriate places, usually underclothes.

KEY TERMS:

functional megacolon: the rectal dilatation characteristic of fecal soiling

psychogenic megacolon: fecal soiling as part of a constellation of behavioral disorders

CAUSES AND SYMPTOMS

Some authors use the term "encopresis" to mean the passage of an entire bowel movement into the underwear and reserve the term "soiling" for the seepage of small amounts of semisolid feces. The term "encopresis" was derived by combining the Greek terms *enourein* (meaning "to pass urine") and *kopros* (meaning "feces") to form a term that is analogous to enuresis, which describes bed-wetting.

The term "functional megacolon" is used to describe the rectal dilatation characteristic of this disorder and distinguishes it from congenital aganglionic megacolon (Hirschsprung's disease). In this much less common and far more serious disorder, the failure of development of part of the autonomic nervous

system in the intestines results in a failure of propagation of colonic contractions, which in turn results in distention of the colon. As a general statement, children with Hirschsprung's disease rarely, if ever, have fecal soiling.

The term "psychogenic megacolon" implies fecal soiling as part of a constellation of behavioral disorders. Although behavioral abnormalities occur in children with soiling, most recent studies indicate that they are no more common in soiling children than in normal children and that they tend to be a response to the soiling.

Soiling is caused by chronic constipation in school-aged children. About 1.5 percent of second-graders experience fecal soiling, which is six times more common in boys than in girls. Constipation and its associated complications are common symptoms in young children, accounting for 25 percent of visits to pediatric gastroenterologists. Constipation becomes less frequent with age and usually resolves as puberty approaches. The basis of constipation is slow motility of the colon, usually present in several family members, which allows excessive water absorption from the stool, causing hard stools that are difficult to expel.

Typically, the child will begin having frequent episodes of fecal soiling at ages five to seven. Parents are mystified by this symptom and bring the child to the physician because of the impending forced socialization of beginning school. Upon questioning, a history of infrequent, large-caliber bowel movements, sometimes too large to be accommodated by the plumbing, is often obtained. The size of these bowel movements is evidence of distention of the rectum as a result of long-standing constipation, which is the basis of this disorder.

The rectum normally functions as a sensory organ, responding to rectal distention by alerting the brain that a bowel movement is imminent and that appropriate arrangements should be made. Persistent rectal distention (megacolon) as a result of chronic constipation results in decreased sensitivity of the rectum to acute rectal distention. These children frequently admit that they do not sense an impending bowel movement before or during episodes of soiling, and studies with distention of balloons passed into the rectum bear out this lack of sensitivity to acute rectal distention. Much more air has to be pumped into a rectal balloon before a soiling child can sense it than for a normal child.

In soiling children, the rectum functions as a storage organ, and does so rather poorly. Storage of fecal material in the rectum bypasses the normal mechanisms of continence and leaves the external anal sphincter, a circular muscle holding the anus closed, as the sole mechanism of continence. The external anal sphincter is under voluntary control. In order to keep it closed, the child must keep all the muscles of the pelvic floor contracted. Any distraction or relaxation of the pelvic floor muscles to urinate can lead to leakage of semisolid stool.

TREATMENT AND THERAPY

Since soiling results from rectal distention (megacolon), effective therapy should empty the rectum (catharsis) and keep it empty (maintenance), allowing reversal of the rectal distention and return of normal rectal sensitivity. Several regimens are available, with most using a saline cathartic agent—that is, one that works by pulling water out of the circulation and into the colon, thus flushing out the contents of the colon. Hypertonic sodium phosphate enemas are frequently recommended but carry the risk of dehydration and electrolyte disturbances. In addition, these children are very sensitive to anorectal manipulation. For these reasons, using an oral cathartic is preferable. Such agents include citrate of magnesia, sodium phosphate, and colonic lavage solutions designed for cleaning the colon before an endoscopic examination.

Stool softeners are usually prescribed as maintenance therapy to keep the water content of the stool high. Preparations such as mineral oil, milk of magnesia, lactulose, and sorbitol are generally safe and effective. Stool softeners are safe for long-term use and, unlike stimulant laxatives such as senna and phenolphthalein, do not cause dependence.

The goal of therapy is resolution of the fecal soiling, since this is the only symptom that causes the child to suffer. Constipation is usually benign and self-limiting, and regularity of bowel movements should be seen not as a goal but rather as an indication that the rectal distention is reversing. Even with no treatment, soiling resolves spontaneously around the time of puberty as the underlying constipation resolves.

This therapy is usually very successful if applied consistently, and no child should have to suffer the humiliation of fecal soiling. Many studies indicate that an effort by the child and his or her family to keep track of the episodes of soiling, passage of bowel movements, and dosage of medicine is required for the best outcome. Even if the soiling is re-

solved, however, the tendency toward constipation remains until puberty, and if the problem falls on the family's list of priorities as it resolves, the chance of recurrence is high.

PERSPECTIVE AND PROSPECTS

The demonstration of abnormalities of anorectal function has prompted the use of biofeedback training to resolve those abnormalities. Recent studies show equally good results with less invasive therapy with an initial catharsis followed by maintenance with stool softeners, casting doubt on the importance of these functional abnormalities and the advisability of expensive and invasive techniques.

—*Wallace A. Gleason, Jr., M.D.*

See also Bed-wetting; Constipation; Gastroenterology; Gastroenterology, pediatric; Gastrointestinal disorders; Gastrointestinal system; Hirschsprung's disease; Toilet training.

FOR FURTHER INFORMATION:

Beach, R. C. "Management of Childhood Constipation." *The Lancet* 348, no. 9030 (September 21, 1996): 766-767. Childhood constipation and soiling can be a source of physical and mental anguish. Management of constipation in the early stages without anal manipulation could reduce the numbers requiring more extensive treatment.

Cooper, Candy J., Heidi Murkoff, and Teresa Martinez. "Bye-bye, Diapers." *Parenting* 14, no. 5 (June/July, 2000): 98-105. The authors highlight eight potty predicaments and how to solve them. Some suggestions for picking the perfect potty are offered as well.

Kuhn, Brett R., Bethany A. Marcus, Sheryl L. Pitner. "Treatment Guidelines for Primary Nonretentive Encopresis and Stool Toileting Refusal." *American Family Physician* 59, no. 8 (April 15, 1999): 2171-2178. Six guidelines for managing children with primary nonretentive encopresis, or stool toileting refusal, are outlined. A case study demonstrated the efficacy and simplicity of these guidelines.

Loening-Baucke, Vera. "Clinical Approach to Fecal Soiling in Children." *Clinical Pediatrics* 39, no. 10 (October, 2000): 603. Fecal soiling is common in childhood and can be caused by stool toileting refusal, fecal incontinence due to organic disease, or encopresis due to functional constipation.

McClung, H. J., L. J. Boyne, T. Linsheid, L. A. Heitlinger, R. D. Murray, J. Fyda, and B. U. Li. "Is

Combination Therapy for Encopresis Nutritionally Safe?" *Pediatrics* 91, no. 3 (March, 1993): 591-594. A study was conducted to determine whether, over a six-month period, the current combined therapeutic program of laxatives, lubricants, and fiber has any measurable deleterious effects on the nutritional status of pediatric primary care outpatients and whether a high fiber intake could be sustained in school-age and preschool-age children.

SORE THROAT
DISEASE/DISORDER

ANATOMY OR SYSTEM AFFECTED: Nose, respiratory system, throat

SPECIALTIES AND RELATED FIELDS: Family practice, otorhinolaryngology, pediatrics

DEFINITION: Discomfort and/or pain experienced in the throat, which sometimes indicates the presence of a more serious disorder.

CAUSES AND SYMPTOMS

Sore throat, termed pharyngitis by medical practitioners, is a common cause of patient discomfort and visits to the doctor's office. Though many people equate sore throat with strep throat, in reality there are many infectious and noninfectious causes of this symptom. Sore throat can even be a sign of disease in another part of the body. The sensation, which may be described by sufferers as scratchy, raw, tight, burning, or achy may last from minutes to months, depending on the underlying cause, and may be accompanied by related complaints such as fever, runny nose, hoarseness, or difficulty swallowing.

Most sore throats are caused by infection in the upper-respiratory tract, including the ears, nose, and sinuses as well as the throat and tonsils. Research has demonstrated that more than half of these infections are caused by common viruses. Epstein-Barr virus, which causes mononucleosis, accounts for less than 10 percent. Most of the remainder are caused by various bacteria. Of the bacterial causes, strep, more specifically group A beta-hemolytic *Streptococcus pyogenes*, is the most common pathogen (disease-causing organism). Additional bacterial causes include species of *Staphylococcus, Hemophilus, Mycoplasma*, non-group A streptococcus, and others. More rarely, fungi may account for a larger portion of throat infections in patients with weakened immune defenses.

Noninfectious causes of sore throat are quite varied. Although most are self-limited (resolving over time without treatment), some represent serious illness. These come into consideration especially if the duration of symptoms is longer than usual and if other aspects of the patient's health history suggest the likelihood of secondary causes.

Traumatic causes of throat discomfort include swallowing foreign objects, such as fish bones; thermal injury from a hot beverage; chemical injury from an ingestion, such as bleach; and external force from a blow to the neck. Environmental irritants, such as smoke and solvent fumes or allergies to dusts and pollens, cause symptoms in susceptible, exposed persons. Regurgitated stomach acid causes discomfort, which may be more pronounced when the patient is lying down. Enlargement of the thyroid gland or the salivary glands, cysts arising from embryonic structures such as the thyroglossal duct, or inflammation of lymph nodes can exert local pressure on the throat itself or on adjacent nerves, thereby eliciting symptoms. Cancer is the most ominous cause of sore throat symptoms, and it needs to be considered in patients with risk factors such as smoking and alcohol consumption.

Considering this expansive list of possibilities, which does not include every possible cause of sore throat, it is evident that the expedient diagnosis of sore throat is challenging. Though most sore throats resolve without treatment or complication, the practitioner must consider the possibility of rarer but potentially life-threatening diseases. The initial history and physical examination are sufficient in most cases to separate those patients who are likely to have an infectious cause from those who are unlikely to have one. Since most patients are initially concerned about the possibility of strep throat and the need for antibiotics, clinical algorithms, such as the Centor score, have been developed to assist this process. By tallying associated signs, symptoms, and patient characteristics, the practitioner may increase diagnostic accuracy. In some cases, additional testing, such as a rapid streptococcal antigen throat swab or a culture, is needed.

The search for noninfectious causes often begins when the patient returns with persisting symptoms. Since most throat infections resolve within a week or two, lingering discomfort suggests the need for further evaluation. In many cases, additional historical information from the patient and a follow-up physical examination will significantly narrow the list of possibilities. Clues such as weight loss, hoarseness, and a history of cigarette smoking and alcohol consumption increase the probability of cancer. Occupational information may uncover exposure to noxious dust or vapors. In difficult cases, diagnosis may require examination and biopsy of the throat during a procedure called laryngoscopy.

Treatment and Therapy
The treatments of noninfectious sore throat are as varied as the diagnoses themselves. The treatment of infectious sore throat depends on the underlying cause, ranging from rest, fluids, and analgesics (painkillers) for viruses to antibiotics for certain bacteria and fungi. Penicillin has been the mainstay of strep throat treatment since the mid-twentieth century. Before the discovery of penicillin, throat infection sometimes resulted in serious complications, such as rheumatic fever (which damages the heart valves) and glomerulonephritis (which damages the kidneys). Although group A *Streptococcus pyogenes* has remained remarkably sensitive to penicillin, reports have suggested that the treatment of strep throat is becoming more complex. The presence of other bacteria in the throat, some of which have developed the ability to inactivate penicillin, may actually protect the strep bacteria from the antibiotic. Interestingly, some research suggests that antibiotic treatment very early in the course of disease may even increase the likelihood of subsequent recurrence. Infections by bacteria other than strep or by fungi are treated with other antibiotic and antifungal drugs.

Given this scenario, one may wonder why doctors do not treat everyone with antibiotics, rather than going to the trouble and expense of diagnosing strep throat. Antibiotic treatment is complicated by many factors, including cost, drug interactions, and the potential for fatal allergic reactions. Widespread use has led to the development of antibiotic-resistant strains of "super bacteria," which are very difficult if not impossible to treat.

—*Louis B. Jacques, M.D.*

See also Antibiotics; Common cold; Epiglottitis; Influenza; Multiple chemical sensitivity syndrome; Nasopharyngeal disorders; Otorhinolaryngology; Pharyngitis; Strep throat; Streptococcal infections; Tonsillectomy and adenoid removal; Tonsillitis; Voice and vocal cord disorders.

For Further Information:
Coutts, Cherylann. "A New Way to Treat Tonsil Trouble." *Parenting* 14, no. 10 (December, 2000/January, 2001): 33. If a child's physician determines that a tonsillectomy is required, a promising new procedure may be used. It uses radio-frequency energy to shrink tonsils, allowing for less pain and a much speedier recovery.

Evans, Julie A. "Thirteen Old-Fashioned Cold Remedies That Really Work!" *Prevention* 52, no. 11 (November, 2000): 106-113. Argues that good science is behind Grandma's elixirs for sniffles, sneezes, and other woes. Old-fashioned cold remedies, like honey and lemon for sore throats and chicken soup for a stuffy head, are discussed.

Larson, David E., ed. *Mayo Clinic Family Health Book.* 2d ed. New York: William Morrow, 1996. Perhaps the best general medical text for the layperson, this book covers the entire medical field. While the information is derived from a wide variety of highly technical sources, the articles are written to be easily understood by a general audience.

McIsaac, Warren J., Vivel Goel, Teresa To, and Donald E. Low. "The Validity of a Sore Throat Score in Family Practice." *Canadian Medical Association Journal* 163, no. 7 (October 3, 2000): 811. This study assessed the validity of a previously published clinical score for the management of infections of the upper respiratory tract accompanied by sore throat.

SPEECH DISORDERS
Disease/disorder

Anatomy or system affected: Ears, muscles, musculoskeletal system, psychic-emotional system

Specialties and related fields: Audiology, psychiatry, psychology, speech pathology

Definition: Dysfunction in the brain-coordinated use of speech organs, such as problems with language, vocal quality, articulation, fluency, and dementia.

Key terms:

aphasia: a partial or total loss of the ability to articulate ideas; often results from brain damage

articulation: the act or process of speaking correctly, as a result of appropriate movement and coordination of the speech organs

connective tissue: tissues possessing a highly vascular structure which form support and connecting structures of the body (for example, cartilage, ligaments, and tendons)

dysfluency: another term for stuttering

dysfunction: the disordered or impaired function of a body system or organ

organic: pertaining to, arising from, or affecting a body organ

psychogenic: originating in the mind or in mental conditions and activities

stuttering: a disorder involving speaking with spasmodic hesitation, prolongation, and/or repetition of sounds

CAUSES AND SYMPTOMS

Learning to speak correctly is of great importance to all people. It involves the brain-coordinated use of the mouth, jaws, lips, and tongue, as well as of the vocal cords, lungs, and diaphragm. On average, children learn to talk during their second year by imitating the speech of those persons, mostly family members, with whom frequent and close contact is maintained. Hence, it is important that young children hear correct speech.

The development of speech is viewed as occurring in several distinct stages. First, babies make involuntary noises in response to physical stimuli. Then, they begin to enjoy making these noises at about two months of age. Next, about nine months after birth, they start to imitate the sounds and inflections of the speech of others around them. Beginning at twelve to eighteen months of age, children start to vocalize in a meaningful way, and in due time, they learn to speak.

In many cases, however, a child is quickly found to have some difficulties with the use of speech or with its development to levels viewed as appropriate within expected time spans. Such children suffer from speech disorders including stuttering, lisping, and lack of speech comprehension. They should receive appropriate professional help as soon as possible. Others are born with physical problems, such as cleft palate, which make appropriate speech impossible without medical intervention. Smaller numbers of people develop speech disorders later in life for various reasons, including accidents that damage the brain or the mechanical organs of speech, as well as the physical and mental ravages of advanced age.

Speech disorders fall into three main categories: problems associated with speech production, difficulties of articulation, and dysfunction in the ability to utilize language. These disorders have been known since antiquity and although they are frequently hereditary, the genetic cause is often unclear. In fact, there is often a psychogenic aspect to their origin as well.

Another broad means of categorizing speech disorders is by dividing them into causative organic and nonorganic groups. The term "organic speech disorder" is used to indicate birth defects or later injuries to the brain or the structures, muscles, and connective tissues that are required to produce speech. The disorders for which no such origin can be clearly identified with existing techniques fall into the nonorganic group. Usually, they are attributed solely to psychogenic factors. It is probable, however, that they have subtle organic causes that are beyond present methods of identification.

Speech disorders may be associated with articulation, voice, fluency, language, and dementia. The cures for all these types of speech disorders vary; they include the interactive participation of teachers in school systems and the attention of speech professionals such as audiologists, surgeons, psychiatrists, and physical therapists. Each case must be analyzed carefully and then treated individually. Even so, varied success is obtained from patient to patient, regardless of the disorder, the nature of the therapeutic procedures utilized, and the therapists who are involved.

Articulation disorders are attributable to the inappropriate sequential movement of the jaw, tongue, and related speech structures. Minor, nonpathological differences result in regional differences (accents) in the spoken language within a country. Pathological problems which cause speech that cannot be understood are most often organic in nature. Examples include cleft palate and neurologic dysfunction. Voice disorders include inappropriate pitch, sound quality (for example, hoarseness), lack of audibility, or inappropriate loudness. Fluency disorders are most often identified with stuttering, speech rate problems, and speech rhythm problems. The best-known language disorders are the aphasias, which are characterized by poor language comprehension and childhood language impairment (often resulting from developmental problems). Dementia can impair speech at any age, but it is most common in the elderly, for whom memory, language, and cognitive ability may be greatly impaired.

TREATMENT AND THERAPY

Many viewpoints exist concerning the treatment of speech disorders. All agree, however, that interaction between family, patient, teachers, and various clinicians is essential. Disorders of articulation are quite common and range from mild problems (for example, a lisp) to those which are so extreme that the speech of afflicted individuals becomes unintelligible. Many of the most severe of these speech disorders arise from the organic impairment of motor control in the speech musculature, which may be attributable to stroke, cleft palate, or even the loss of lips or other speech system components.

Frequently, efforts at remediating such problems must include surgical and dental treatment. After any necessary corrective surgery and/or dentistry, many treatment regimens focus on behavior modification. Affected individuals receive instruction regarding the physical basis of their problems and are then trained to overcome them as effectively as possible.

In many cases, the use of psychological and psychiatric counseling is considered to be of great value. Some experts suggest, however, that the main effect of such therapy is to enable afflicted individuals to live comfortably with the imperfections in articulation that remain after all treatments are tried.

Voice disorders occur when the phonatory mechanism is dysfunctional. They range from the consequences of laryngeal, oral, or respiratory disease to the misuse of the phonatory system, which may reflect psychological state. Such functional disorders, if left untreated for too long, may lead to organic damage. In the case of pitch abnormalities, causative factors may include psychological tension, an undersized larynx, misformed vocal cords, and hearing problems, either individually or in various combinations.

Disorders of voice quality likewise have many physical sources, including larynx and vocal cord abnormalities, and ones of psychogenic origin. The disorders associated with loudness range from overly loud voices caused by workplace noise or hearing loss to extremely soft ones that are generally psychogenic. Treatment of all such disorders begins with the disqualification of treatable organic problems. In the case of psychogenic disorders, psychiatric counseling can be extremely helpful. Psychological and medical treatments must be followed, however, by very thorough interaction with speech-language pathologists if optimum results are to be obtained.

Disorders of fluency most often involve stuttering, also called dysfluency, which features spasmodic hesitation and the prolongation or repetition of sounds. In addition, stuttering is often accompanied by tics and other uncontrolled body movements. The basis for the problem is unclear, and different experts point to learned behavior, psychogenic origins, or organic roots. There is no cure for dysfluency, but it (and the accompanying nonspeech problems) can be greatly diminished. Treatment usually involves both psychiatric counseling and behavior and/or speech modification by speech-language pathologists as well as by other related speech professionals. Such therapy varies widely from individual to individual and with the age of the patient.

Language disorders are characterized by the diminished ability to use or to understand spoken language. In children, these disorders are often identified as language delay, or development aphasias. They are most often thought to be attributable to mental retardation, hearing loss, or autism. When lost hearing is not the main problem, the treatments for such language problems often involve behavior modification techniques. In all cases in which hearing loss is an important component, its correction is the first effort; such efforts may work wonders. When hearing problems cannot be remediated entirely, however, the overall treatment will be much less successful because hearing the speech of others is so important to speech development.

True aphasia is very often viewed as speech impairment; it occurs in adults as a result of stroke, accidents that produce severe head trauma, or dementia. It is desirable to begin treatment of afflicted persons as soon as possible after aphasia is observed. Some rapid and spontaneous healing of lost language ability occurs, and this healing can be maximized by the efforts of speech-language pathologists. The continued treatment of aphasias is very important and usually follows careful evaluation of its causes. It is often possible to make progressive, long-term advances in healing aphasias. Complete recovery is rare, however, and the use of sign language or personal computers for interpersonal communication may be necessary.

Perspective and Prospects

For many years, it was thought that speech disorders were caused only by insoluble psychological problems in the very young or by severe head, facial, and brain trauma later in life. It is now clear that they have other causes, ranging from hearing loss to dementia. Furthermore, it is currently understood that speech problems of every type can attack anyone—young children, adolescents, and adults of all ages.

These problems often have disastrous psychological and economic effects on the afflicted person. Young children may be traumatized if speech disorders are not treated early; in severe cases, they may later be unable to enter the workforce in meaningful positions or to receive anything above the most rudimentary education. This is unfortunate because many such problems of childhood, adolescence, and even young adulthood can be almost completely solved by careful medical examination, followed quickly by appropriate corrective action.

There is also help available for older people who develop speech problems because of aging, dementia, or harmful workplace conditions. In all cases, once a sound treatment plan is developed, it is essential that the afflicted person follow it rigorously. Miracles should not be expected; rather, sustained interaction between the treatment team—especially the patient and a speech-language pathologist—must be undertaken. Furthermore, the psychological support of the patient's family and friends has been recognized as a crucial factor in many successful treatment plans.

In the case of the young child, the diagnosis of speech problems by schoolteachers can be another important means to treatment. Once a problem is observed, the child's family can be advised concerning special education available through the school system or local programs. Teachers should be cautioned, however, against attempts to treat the child in question unless they have adequate training. The job of unspecialized teachers should be diagnosis and the recommendation of an appropriate treatment group. When speech disorder therapy results in less-than-adequate treatment of extremely serious problems, the use of sign language, special typewriters, and computer-assisted communication, as well as psychotherapy, should be considered.

Overall, the treatment of speech problems has improved, and its sensible application can enable patients to enter into or return to the workforce at levels commensurate with their abilities, can prevent them from becoming maladjusted, and can enrich society as a whole. Dealing with such problems in the young is particularly important because it may help to prevent neuroses and psychoses from developing. It is hoped that ongoing research will continue to increase the avenues available for the prevention and cure of speech disorders, to identify additional methods for treating them, and to result in their eradication.

—*Sanford S. Singer, Ph.D.*

See also Alzheimer's disease; Aphasia and dysphasia; Audiology; Autism; Cerebral palsy; Cleft lip and palate; Cleft lip and palate repair; Dyslexia; Ear surgery; Ears; Electroencephalography (EEG); Jaw wiring; Laryngitis; Learning disabilities; Lisping; Paralysis; Strokes and TIAs; Stuttering; Tonsillitis; Voice and vocal cord disorders.

FOR FURTHER INFORMATION:

American Psychiatric Association. *Diagnostic and Statistical Manual of Mental Disorders: DSM-IV-TR.* Rev. 4th ed. Washington, D.C.: Author, 2000. This classic text contains diagnostic criteria and other useful facts about a variety of mental disorders, including those associated with speech dysfunction.

Berkow, Robert, and Andrew J. Fletcher, eds. *The Merck Manual of Diagnosis and Therapy.* 17th ed. Rahway, N.J.: Merck Sharp & Dohme Research Laboratories, 1999. Contains useful data on the characteristics, etiology, diagnosis, and treatment of speech disorders and related processes. Although the text is designed for physicians, the material should be useful to general readers as well.

Cole, Patricia R. *Language Disorders in Preschool Children.* Englewood Cliffs, N.J.: Prentice Hall, 1982. This book by an expert speech-language pathologist explains the modalities associated with solving speech-language disorders. Solid and well referenced, it covers language development, disorders, diagnosis, and treatment. Much useful information is offered concerning learning semantics and syntax.

Winitz, Harris, ed. *Human Communication and Its Disorders: A Review, 1987.* Norwood, N.J.: Abex, 1987. This authoritative text covers in detail the prominent disorders of human communications: their occurrence, symptoms, and treatment. Both organic and nonorganic aspects of these communication problems are carefully explored and referenced.

SPERM BANKS
PROGRAMS

ANATOMY OR SYSTEM AFFECTED: Genitals, psychic-emotional system, reproductive system, uterus

SPECIALTIES AND RELATED FIELDS: Biotechnology, ethics, genetics, obstetrics, urology

DEFINITION: The identification of suitable sperm donors and the evaluation, processing, storage and distribution of their semen for use in assisted reproductive technology.

KEY TERMS:

insemination: the process of placing semen in the female reproductive tract; natural insemination occurs during sexual intercourse, while artificial (or donor) insemination is performed with medical instruments in a clinic

semen: the male reproductive fluid consisting of two parts, a liquid called seminal plasma and living reproductive cells called sperm

INDICATIONS AND PROCEDURES

Sperm banks exist to help women with normal adult premenopausal reproductive function to become pregnant. A woman may need this help if she is married to an infertile man, is in a lesbian relationship, or chooses to be a single mother. When a man in a heterosexual relationship produces too few sperm for a pregnancy, sperm from a sperm bank can help the couple become pregnant through artificial (or donor) insemination. A woman choosing artificial insemination will experience pregnancy and birth of a child that has her genes. The woman controls the environmental risks to her fetus, such as chemical exposure (from smoking, drinking, or eating) and physical risks.

A sperm bank makes available the sperm from a number of qualified donors. The primary task of a clinical sperm bank is to identify suitable donors, based upon medical and biological criteria. The sperm bank does a medical physical examination of donor candidates and obtains an extensive medical and family history from them. Special attention is given to semen quality and to the risk of transmitting infectious or genetic diseases.

Semen quality has two major components. The first component is whether the semen has enough fertile sperm to create a pregnancy. The second component is whether enough sperm in the semen survive freezing. Freezing in a special way (cryopreservation) to keep sperm alive is the only way a sperm bank can store its semen inventory. Another important reason for cryopreservation is related to infectious disease testing. For example, a donor is tested for acquired immunodeficiency syndrome (AIDS) at the time he produces the semen, but the test is repeated six months later to increase its certainty. The cryopreservation allows the semen to be stored during this "quarantine" period. Donors are tested for a variety of diseases that can be transmitted through semen: AIDS, gonorrhea, chlamydia, syphilis, trichomonas, and well-known sexually transmitted diseases (STDs), as well as viral hepatitis, cytomegalovirus, and human T-lymphotropic virus (HTLV).

The genetics of a donor is very important. Genes are responsible for each person's positive attributes and negative ones (genetic diseases). There are no genetically perfect persons; there are no perfect donors. There are only a few hundred genetic tests for more than five thousand genetic conditions; therefore comprehensive testing for genetic disease is impractical. Sperm banks usually screen donors routinely for a few very common diseases with a genetic component, such as diabetes, gout, and high cholesterol. Additional tests may be done on donors of certain ethnic backgrounds for diseases linked to specific ethnicities: cystic fibrosis, Canavan disease, Gaucher disease, sickle-cell disease, Tay-Sachs disease. Each sperm bank will have its own list.

Fortunately, both parents determine a child's genetics. The genetic attributes of one often will compensate for the liabilities of the other. A person choosing a donor would be wise to seek the help of a certified genetics counselor. A genetics counselor will help match the genetics of the woman with the genetics of possible donors.

Considering all that is involved in identifying each suitable donor, a sperm bank requires donors to provide many "samples," not only of semen, but also of blood. Additionally, there are annual physical exams, perhaps a psychological exam, and other tests. It is understandable that the bank compensates donors for their time and effort in participating; this is different from "buying sperm." Similarly, sperm banks receive a fee for their efforts in recruiting and evaluating donors plus their work in evaluating, processing, and providing semen to physicians and their patients.

Semen is normally available to a patient through a physician trained in artificial insemination. Sometimes a patient will request to do self-insemination at her home. This is possible with physician authorization, meaning that the physician retains responsibility for mistakes that might occur. The requested semen is delivered frozen by the sperm bank. The shipping container is similar to a thermos. The semen is thawed immediately before insemination.

USES AND COMPLICATIONS

There are many personal decisions to be made regarding artificial insemination. Often there are psychological effects on the woman to be inseminated and her spouse. Usually artificial insemination is done with semen from an anonymous donor, thus preventing any social contact between donor and recipient. The use of an anonymous donor usually conveys full paternal rights and responsibilities on the spouse of the recipient, relieving the donor of any responsibility. Sometimes the recipient or her spouse want to use a donor known to them, a directed donor. Although this is possible, it raises legal and psychological issues that are not fully known. These issues about the kind of donor also have implications for the psychology of the offspring. There are many medical decisions to be made regarding artificial insemination. The procedure must be done at the time of ovulation, an event occurring between menstrual periods. The occurrence of ovulation can be determined in several ways, often by hormonal tests. The physician must decide whether to do one or more inseminations at ovulation. If the timing is off, the patient will not become pregnant. Another attempt can be made on the next monthly cycle.

Although women will become pregnant with semen placed in the vagina at the entrance to the uterus, many physicians prefer to place semen in the woman's uterus. Intrauterine insemination (IUI) requires removing the semen from the seminal plasma, administering substances that cause the uterus to contract strongly, and discharging the sperm into the uterus through a catheter.

Other complications include the possibility of infection or genetic problems. Although the sperm has been properly tested, tests are not perfect. The patient must remember that even when all aspects of insemination are technically perfect, the complex biology of making a baby from a fertilized egg can go wrong.

PERSPECTIVE AND PROSPECTS
Horse breeders may have successfully used artificial insemination as early as the fourteenth century. In 1776, John Hunter, an English surgeon, may have been the first person to successfully artificially inseminate a woman. Cryopreservation of bull semen was developed in England in the early 1950's. An American urologist, Raymond H. Bunge, was the first physician to successfully use cryopreserved human semen. Many sperm banks were established in the early 1980's so that semen could be quarantined to prevent the transmission of AIDS. Sperm banks have expanded to become embryo banks. Future technology will permit cryopreservation of human eggs. These banks will be contributing components of genetic medicine.
—*Armand M. Karow, Ph.D.*

See also Childbirth; Cloning; Conception; Gynecology; Infertility in females; Infertility in males; Obstetrics; Pregnancy and gestation; Reproductive system.

FOR FURTHER INFORMATION:
Pence, Gregory E. *Re-Creating Medicine*. Lanham, Md.: Rowman & Littlefield, 2000.
Schover, Leslie R., and Anthony J. Thomas, Jr. *Overcoming Male Infertility*. New York: John Wiley & Sons, 2000.
Vercollone, Carol Frost, Heidi Moss, and Robert Moss. *Helping the Stork: The Choices and Challenges of Donor Insemination*. New York: Macmillan, 1997.

SPHINCTERECTOMY
PROCEDURE
ANATOMY OR SYSTEM AFFECTED: Anus, bladder, intestines, muscles, musculoskeletal system
SPECIALTIES AND RELATED FIELDS: General surgery
DEFINITION: The surgical removal of a sphincter, a ring of muscle that closes or constricts an opening or passage in the body when the muscles contract, is called a sphincterectomy. In the human body, sphincters can be found in the internal and external region of the anus, in the area that joins the large and small intestine, between the urinary bladder and the urethra, at the lower end of the esophagus, and in the pupil of the eye. Although surgery to correct tears or defects in sphincters is more common than their removal, in cases of extreme damage or disease useless sphincters must be surgically excised. For the removal of internal sphincters, the patient is surgically opened, and the appropriate organs are moved to expose the sphincter in question; external sphincterectomies are performed without incisions in the body cavity. A scalpel is used to dissect the sphincter away from the surrounding tissue. Bleeding vessels are repaired, and the incisions are closed. After removal, an individual will lack the control provided by the sphincter, such as control of defecation or urination, and alternative means of compensating for this loss will be presented to the patient.
—*Karen E. Kalumuck, Ph.D.*
See also Gastroenterology; Gastroenterology, pediatric; Gastrointestinal disorders; Gastrointestinal sys-

tem; Intestinal disorders; Intestines; Muscle sprains, spasms, and disorders; Muscles; Peristalsis; Urinary disorders; Urinary system; Urology; Urology, pediatric.

FOR FURTHER INFORMATION:

Daniel, Edwin E., et al, eds. *Sphincters: Normal Function, Changes in Disease.* Boca Raton, Fla.: CRC Press, 1992.

DiDio, Liberato J. A., and Marion C. Anderson. *The Sphincters of the Digestive Systems: Anatomical, Functional, and Surgical Considerations.* Baltimore: Williams & Wilkins, 1968.

Hunter, J. O., and V. Alun Jones, eds. *Food and the Gut.* Philadelphia: Bailliere Tindall, 1985.

Janowitz, Henry D. *Your Gut Feelings: A Complete Guide to Living Better with Intestinal Problems.* Rev. ed. New York: Oxford University Press, 1994.

SPIDER BITES. *See* BITES AND STINGS.

SPINA BIFIDA
DISEASE/DISORDER
ALSO KNOWN AS: Myelocele, meningomyelocele, lipomeningocele

ANATOMY OR SYSTEM AFFECTED: Bones, brain, nervous system, spine

SPECIALTIES AND RELATED FIELDS: Embryology, neonatology, perinatology, plastic surgery

DEFINITION: A birth defect that results from a mistake early in the development of the spinal cord.

KEY TERMS:

central nervous system: the brain and spinal cord

hydrocephalus: the abnormal accumulation of fluid within the developing brain

neural plate: a layer of tissue in the early embryo from which the brain and spinal cord will develop

neuropore: a small opening into the interior of the brain or spinal cord of the embryo

vertebra: an individual bone in the spine

CAUSES AND SYMPTOMS

The development of the fetal nervous system is the most complicated process during pregnancy. It starts a few weeks after conception and continues until well after birth. The earliest steps are the most crucial, because the basic plan of the nervous system must be established accurately if it is to work properly later.

The central nervous system begins with the formation of a thickened layer of tissue, called the neural plate, along the back of the embryo. The edges of this plate curl up to form ridges, and the whole plate rolls up into a slender tube running from the head to the rump. This cylinder is then covered over by tissues

Types of Spina Bifida

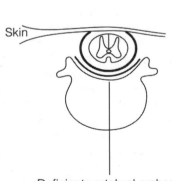

Deficient vertebral arches and dura, associated with minor nerve defects, esp. bladder dysfunction.

Occulta

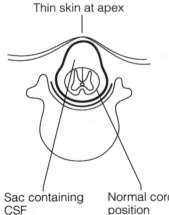

Thin skin at apex

Sac containing CSF / Normal cord position

Meningocele

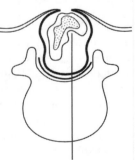

Defective skin, allowing serious infection

Cord displaced into sac, associated with serious nervous deficit, esp. in legs, bladder.

Meningomyelocele

In the News: Folic Acid and Fetal Surgery

One of the most effective measures for preventing spina bifida has been shown to be the daily intake of folic acid. In 2000, *The Chicago Tribune* reported on a folic acid supplement program which took place over a six-year period in South Carolina. During this program, the rate of neural tube defects, including spina bifida, was cut in half due to women taking folic acid supplements daily, before and during their pregnancy.

For babies who develop spina bifida, fetal surgery, which occurs while the baby is still in the womb, has become an option for parents. As reported by *The Philadelphia Inquirer* in 1999, fetal surgery can improve brain malformations, making it unnecessary for many babies to need lifelong shunts—devices that allow drainage of fluid that has accumulated around the brain. Even with the demonstrated benefits of the surgery, however, there is no guarantee that the surgery can correct all neurological functions or that it will be successful for all babies. In fact, it has been shown that fetal surgery increases the risk of a baby being born prematurely, which poses a whole new set of problems.

—Angela Spano and Massimo D. Bezoari, M.D.

that will form the surface of the back. The front end of this tube will soon expand to become the brain, and the rest of the tube will form the spinal cord. In order for these processes to proceed properly, the tube must seal itself along its entire length. If there are any gaps where the tube does not close, it will leak and will not be able to expand and develop properly. Without such expansion, all the later stages of nervous system development will also be prevented from occurring properly.

If the neural tube fails to seal, a small opening called a neuropore will remain at some point along its length. Depending on where the opening is, a variety of abnormalities can result. When the posterior region of the neural tube fails to close, the result is spina bifida. This flaw in the neural tube in turn affects the assembly of the muscle, bone, and skin in this region. In spina bifida, which means "divided spine," the vertebrae of the backbone do not join together properly.

The severity of spina bifida depends on how much damage has been done to the lower spinal cord region. In its mildest form, the only evidence of a problem may be that two of the bones in the spine fail to form quite right. If several vertebrae are involved, the membranes that protect the surface of the spinal cord can bulge outward, forming a ball-like mass in this region. The problems that result depend on how much of the spinal membrane is involved in this bulge. In the most severe cases, the vertebrae fail to protect the spinal cord, so that the nervous tissue itself is also involved and an opening to the outside remains at the base of the spinal cord. Additional problems with nervous system development may result, including improper fluid balances in the brain (hydrocephalus).

Because the brain and spinal column fail to develop properly in spina bifida, a variety of mental, behavioral, and physical symptoms can result. The nerve connections at the base of the spine are likely to be affected, resulting in paralysis in the lower back and legs, problems with bladder and bowel function, and loss of sensation. Because the development of the brain can also be affected, mental abilities may be impaired.

TREATMENT AND THERAPY

Effective measures have been developed to minimize the effects of spina bifida. Often, surgery is performed within twenty-four to forty-eight hours of birth to close any opening in the child's lower back and to reconstruct the spine and other tissues in this area. Problems with feet and legs may also be dealt with surgically. If the child has symptoms of hydrocephalus, the excess fluid will be drained. Bladder and bowel function will be regulated, such as by catheterization. Eventually, prosthetic devices may be fitted to assist the child's movement. Mental health and physical therapy experts will also be involved to assist in overcoming learning hurdles, monitoring physical development and training, and making emotional adjustments.

PERSPECTIVE AND PROSPECTS

Spina bifida has been known since ancient times, but little could be done then to ease the mental and physical damage that it causes. By the 1960's, surgical procedures were being developed that could repair the damage to the spinal cord and other parts of the lower back. Improvements in physical therapy methods, as well as improved prosthetic devices, also began to make physical activity a realistic prospect for these children.

Late in the twentieth century, new insights were gained into the causes of spina bifida. The mutated genes involved were identified, and it was learned why they do not work properly. Studies of neural tube defects in mice revealed how these defects occur and how best to prevent them.

It is now known that the diet of a pregnant woman can influence neural tube development. For example, the vitamin folic acid, if taken starting at the time of conception, can decrease the risk of spina bifida by as much as 75 percent. Other less dramatic effects of diet on spina bifida rates have also been identified.

Support organizations for families can help them cope with the challenges of caring for children with spina bifida. Physical therapy, counseling, and various group activities are available. Thanks to improved treatment and support, it is now possible for children with this condition to lead long and healthy lives.

—*Howard L. Hosick, Ph.D.*

See also Amniocentesis; Birth defects; Embryology; Genetic diseases; Hydrocephalus; Mental retardation; Nervous system; Neurology; Neurology, pediatric; Neurosurgery; Plastic surgery; Spinal cord disorders; Spine, vertebrae, and disks; Stillbirth.

FOR FURTHER INFORMATION:

Bloom, Beth-Ann, and Edward L. Seljeskog. *A Parent's Guide to Spina Bifida*. Minneapolis: University of Minnesota Press, 1988. Designed to assist the parents of children with spina bifida. The book includes chapters on the nature of the disorder and how it is treated, the medical problems associated with spina bifida, and how to help the afflicted child while he or she is growing up.

McLone, David. *An Introduction to Spina Bifida*. Reprint. Washington, D.C.: Spina Bifida Association of America, 1998. A concise report on spinal dysraphism and related disorders. Illustrations illuminate the text.

Nightingale, Elena O., and Melissa Goodman. *Before Birth: Prenatal Testing for Genetic Disease*. Cambridge, Mass.: Harvard University Press, 1990. Offering practical guidance to prospective parents, this volume addresses the question of whether or not to undergo testing, and if elected, how best to use the results.

SPINAL CORD DISORDERS
DISEASE/DISORDER

ANATOMY OR SYSTEM AFFECTED: Bones, musculoskeletal system, nerves, nervous system, spine

SPECIALTIES AND RELATED FIELDS: Emergency medicine, neurology, physical therapy

DEFINITION: Conditions that adversely affect the spinal cord, which normally carries sensory information from the skin and muscles to the brain and returns with information to control movement.

KEY TERMS:

congenital malformation: an abnormal condition that exists at birth; generally not hereditary

lesion: damage to cells, tissues, or organs that results in lost or impaired function; spinal cord lesion usually involves motor and/or sensory nerve fiber tracts

neuroglia: nonneuronal support cells of the central nervous system; oligodendrocytes are one type of neuroglia that myelinate nerve fibers

neuron: a nerve cell, the functional unit of the nervous system, containing dendrite and axon processes specialized for carrying information toward and away from the cell body, respectively

neurotrophic factors: a chemical signal that is required for the normal differentiation and function of neurons; this signal is often produced by neuroglia or by the cells with which neurons form synapses

plasticity: the ability of the nervous system to change its function over time by experience; includes changes in nerve fiber networks

teratogen: a chemical that causes abnormal embryonic development; often an environmental pollutant or something to which the mother is exposed during pregnancy, such as alcohol or other drugs

CAUSES AND SYMPTOMS

Most people take certain basic tasks for granted, such as walking up a flight of stairs, brushing their teeth, or using a personal computer. Motor neurons in the spinal cord control the hundreds of muscle fibers that are involved in each of these activities. At the same time, other neurons of the spinal cord serve as part of the sensory pathways that provide information, regarding body position and motion, that contributes to the coordination of these activities. In amyotrophic lateral sclerosis, also known as Lou Gehrig's disease, the motor neurons in the spinal cord die, leaving patients without control of their muscles. This example of a spinal disorder serves to emphasize the important role that the spinal cord plays as it serves as an interface (input-output system) between the brain and the body.

Similarly, most people have experienced pain in the hand, which is followed by an instantaneous, automatic movement of the hand away from the object causing that pain. Such reflexes represent the simplest of movements, yet they still require the integrative and relay action of neurons of the spinal cord to cause immediate hand withdrawal without requiring the individual to think about the act consciously. Only after the reflex has occurred does the spinal cord activity "inform" the brain that something happened. Therefore, in addition to sensory and motor interface functions for the brain, the spinal cord performs basic integration tasks as it controls reflexes, contributes to the coordination of movement between the left and right sides of the body, and prevents opposing muscle groups from trying to move a joint in opposite directions at the same time. As with any other vital organ of the body, spinal cord damage or defects have serious consequences for the health and well-being of humans.

In the medical research laboratory, paralysis results from complete or partial transection of the spinal cord. In the real world, a fracture or dislocation of vertebrae or damage done by a bullet can cause paralysis in the same fashion. Acute transection of the spinal cord can also result from an inflammatory condition or from any situation in which the spinal cord is compressed, such as by a tumor. The spinal cord is contained within the vertebral column, which is divided into the cervical, thoracic, lumbar, and sacral regions, each of which is associated with a specific set of functions. Transection typically results in the loss of sensory and motor functions below the level of the lesion.

Spinal cord injuries and defects are the result of three basic types of pathological conditions. The first of these conditions is traumatic physical injury to spinal cord tissue, such as the severing of the spinal cord during a car accident. The second condition is a congenital or inherited genetic problem with spinal cord development and function, as illustrated by spina bifida. The third is an acquired condition such as damage caused by a viral or bacterial infection. In each case, the severity of the pathological condition is dependent upon the location and extent of the resultant spinal cord lesion. In the clinical setting, physicians utilize information regarding all aspects of spinal cord function (such as sensory, motor, reflex, and coordination functions), as well as information from a variety of imaging techniques to diagnose pathological conditions and to select appropriate treatments.

Trauma. The neurons of the spinal cord carry out their functions by way of their long nerve processes (axons), which extend to form synapses with, and control, target cells (muscles and other neurons). Some of these nerve processes extend out of the spinal cord to the body, others extend either up to or down from higher-brain regions, and yet others extend from one side of the spinal cord to another. Trauma mainly damages the nerve process of cells and in this fashion disrupts their function in controlling target neurons and muscles. Often, after nerve processes have been damaged, the neuron itself will die because of loss of neurotrophic influences from their target cells. It has been estimated that every year between 10,000 and 12,000 people in the United States are disabled by some degree of paralysis resulting from traumatic injury to the spinal cord.

Congenital defects. Spinal cord defects are not the result of trauma but rather are generally attributed to abnormal events during embryonic development. In particular, most major spinal cord defects arise around the third week of development. During this time, the flattened neural plate is beginning to fold upward as its lateral edges come together and fuse to form the top margin (dorsal aspect) of the neural tube. If this process is incomplete, then the spinal cord remains open and exposed along the embryo's back, accompanied by the failure of the vertebral bones to surround the spinal cord tissue completely. This condition is referred to as spina bifida. Often, rather than simply being exposed, some normal contents of the vertebral canal, including spinal cord tissue, protrude out of the back as a bulge. Spina bifida is most common in the lower lumbar and upper sacral regions of the spine, but more severe cases may involve the cervical and thoracic regions. Depending on the level and extent of the defect, the clinical symptoms of spinal abnormalities range from mild impairment to fatality. This type of neural tube defect often causes some degree of motor and sensory handicap. The cerebrospinal fluid is continuous from the ventricles of the brain to the central canal of the spinal cord. If the spinal defect impairs the normal flow of cerebrospinal fluid, other problems may occur, such as retardation resulting from hydrocephalus (fluid on the brain). Although there is still much to learn about the causes of spinal cord defects, in many cases scientific evidence points the finger at genetic problems (mutations) and the disruptive action of teratogens such as environmental pollutants and drugs.

Infections. Acquired spinal cord lesions are not the result of trauma or developmental problems but rather are related to such conditions as tumor development or viral and bacterial infections. In general, invasion of the spinal cord by viruses or bacteria can produce inflammation known as myelitis. Multiple sclerosis (MS) and amyotrophic lateral sclerosis (ALS) are the two most common nontraumatic disorders of the spinal cord. Many of the nerve fibers of the central nervous system are covered by a myelin sheath produced by neuroglia cells. This sheath contributes to the speed and efficiency of the nerve cells as they carry electrical information. MS involves the destruction of this important myelin sheath, leading to the disruption of motor and sensory nerve pathway functions manifested by such symptoms as abnormal sensations, paralysis, and exaggerated reflexes. Although its cause is not clearly understood, researchers believe that viral infections are involved in some cases, while in others the individual's own immune system might be mistakenly destroying normal myelin tissue (an autoimmune disorder). ALS is a fatal condition that is restricted to the loss of motor neurons. As with MS, there is much speculation regarding the causes of ALS. Acquired immunodeficiency syndrome (AIDS) is a viral infection that can involve the disruption of spinal cord neuron function.

Other infections that can cause spinal cord lesions include tabes dorsalis, poliomyelitis, meningitis, and syringomyelia. Tabes dorsalis involves the degeneration of sensory neurons from the dorsal region of the spinal cord as a result of the invasion of the syphilis spirochete bacterium. The polio virus infects and kills spinal motor neurons in a disease called poliomyelitis; if the disease destroys the brain-stem neu-

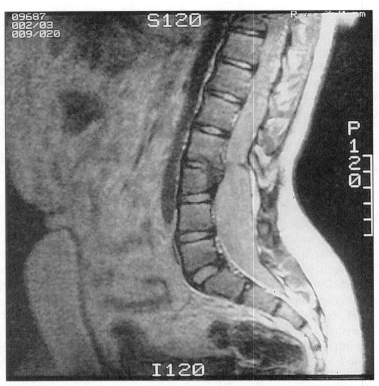

A nuclear magnetic resonance scan of the spine showing the defect spina bifida. (SIU School of Medicine)

rons that control respiration and heart rate, then this condition is fatal. Meningitis is a bacterial inflammation of the layers of cells that cover the spinal cord (collectively referred to as meninges), producing high fever and sometimes inducing a comatose state that can lead to death.

Tumors and cysts. Growths within the spinal cord can also disrupt normal spinal cord function. Syringomyelia is such a condition, in which fluid-filled cysts develop among the neurons of the spinal cord. Cancerous tumors are often the result of uncontrolled growth of the neuroglia cells, which can damage neurons and nerve fiber pathways.

TREATMENT AND THERAPY

Spinal cord defects, either congenital or hereditary, pose serious challenges for the medical community. Surgical intervention is the only option in mild cases of spina bifida, but in severe cases there is no effective treatment. The advent of intrauterine surgery (prior to the birth of the baby) for the correction of minor cases of spina bifida is a major step toward alleviating serious problems. It is believed that better prenatal care may reduce the risk of spinal cord defects. Numerous factors have been implicated in such defects, including alcoholism, drug use, and even environmental pollution. In some cases, genetic screening may provide a method to reduce certain types of defects, while in other cases reduced exposure to risk elements is the most effective preventive action.

Treatments for acquired spinal cord injury involve antiviral and antibacterial drugs that combat infection and in so doing reduce inflammation and cell damage. It is clear that early detection and intervention is an important factor in being able to save as many neurons as possible and to limit the extent of the lesion. Neurotrophic factors are likely to be important therapeutic agents as doctors try to stimulate the maximum recovery of neuronal function. In cases in which the immune system itself may be damaging healthy neurons, as is suspected in some cases of MS, drugs are used to suppress immune function.

PERSPECTIVE AND PROSPECTS

Medical researchers are taking numerous approaches to understand spinal cord development and function, in the hope of utilizing that information to develop new therapies to prevent or treat these clinical conditions. An interesting aspect of the problem is that, unlike most other organ systems, the adult nervous system does not retain stem cell populations after embryonic development. Stem cell populations are groups of cells that divide to produce cells for the growth and regeneration of tissues and organs. Human babies are born with all the neurons in their central nervous system that they will ever have; no new neurons will be produced. The nervous system develops from that point as a result of the maturation of these neurons. As the individual ages, the nervous system becomes more efficient in processing information as neural networks are modified. This modification involves changes in nerve cell connections, a process referred to as plasticity. Researchers hope to utilize information about the biological basis of normal plasticity to help repair damaged or impaired nervous systems.

Modern neuroscience research quickly vanquished the long-held belief that it is impossible to repair neurons damaged by trauma or disease. Experiments with animals and in tissue culture have demonstrated that damaged neurons can survive, regrow nerve processes, and once again carry electrical impulses. In fact, neurons from human spinal cords have been grown in tissue culture under conditions that stimulated them to regrow their axonal process. One of the most important aspects of understanding nervous system development is the fact that the cells communicate with one another not only with neurotransmitters but also with neurotrophic factors. Basic research and clinical trials are being done on neurotrophic factors with the expectation that they will become important parts of therapeutic treatments to stimulate the repair and regeneration of damaged neurons. These neurotrophic factors hold such promise because they are important in stimulating normal cell differentiation during embryonic development and for the subsequent survival of neurons after birth into adulthood. Therefore, clinical treatments are being designed to recreate the embryonic conditions that contributed to normal development. In addition, it is believed that one of the major factors in the lack of a regeneration response in damaged spinal cords is that the neuroglia cells form a scar tissue that is not conducive to nerve fiber regeneration. Therefore, medical researchers are looking at treatments that, in addition to prolonging the life of neurons, reduce the formation of scar tissue.

—*William L. Muhlach, Ph.D.*

See also Anesthesia; Anesthesiology; Bone cancer; Bone disorders; Bones and the skeleton; Cerebral palsy; Chiropractic; Disk removal; Dystrophy; Fracture and dislocation; Head and neck disorders; Kinesiology; Kyphosis; Laminectomy and spinal fusion; Lumbar puncture; Meningitis; Motor neuron diseases; Multiple sclerosis; Muscle sprains, spasms, and disorders; Muscular dystrophy; Nervous system; Neuralgia, neuritis, and neuropathy; Neurology; Neurology, pediatric; Neurosurgery; Numbness and tingling; Osteoarthritis; Osteoporosis; Paget's disease; Paralysis; Paraplegia; Physical rehabilitation; Poliomyelitis; Quadriplegia; Sciatica; Scoliosis; Slipped disk; Spina bifida; Spine, vertebrae, and disks; Spondylitis; Sports medicine; Sympathectomy.

FOR FURTHER INFORMATION:

Carey, Joseph, ed. *Brain Facts: A Primer on the Brain and Nervous System.* Washington, D.C.: Society for Neuroscience, 1990. A publication by the Society of Neuroscience directed at educating the general public about the value of neuroscience research.

Carlson, Bruce M. *Human Embryology and Developmental Biology.* 2d ed. St. Louis: Mosby, 1999. This textbook presents human development in the context of modern scientific and medical research.

Includes a consideration of basic normal spinal cord development, as well as a detailed look at developmental defects such as spina bifida.

Kandel, Eric R., James H. Schwartz, and Thomas M. Jessell, eds. *Principles of Neural Science.* 4th ed. New York: Elsevier, 2000. This massive, comprehensive book serves as the bible for the field of neuroscience. In spite of its tremendous breadth and depth, this book contains excellent basic explanations and illustrations, and thus serves as a valuable reference for people of all academic backgrounds.

Larsen, William J. *Human Embryology.* 2d ed. New York: Churchill Livingstone, 1997. Basic coverage of human embryonic development, including both normal and abnormal spinal cord development.

Spence, Alexander P. *Basic Human Anatomy.* 3d ed. Redwood City, Calif.: Benjamin/Cummings, 1990. An excellent source for adult human anatomy, as well as for definition of anatomical terminology. This text also considers spinal conditions of clinical significance.

SPINAL FUSION. *See* LAMINECTOMY AND SPINAL FUSION.

SPINAL TAP. *See* LUMBAR PUNCTURE.

SPINE, VERTEBRAE, AND DISKS
ANATOMY

ANATOMY OR SYSTEM AFFECTED: Back, bones, musculoskeletal system, nerves, nervous system

SPECIALTIES AND RELATED FIELDS: Alternative medicine, geriatrics and gerontology, neurology, orthopedics, physical therapy, preventive medicine, sports medicine

DEFINITION: The supporting structures of the trunk, from the base of the skull to the end of the tailbone; the vertebrae form a small, central canal for the sensory and motor nerves that constitute the spinal cord.

KEY TERMS:

disk: a soft, cushionlike structure that lies between bony vertebrae from the base of the skull to the sacrum of the pelvis; it has a soft liquid in the center (the nucleus pulposus) and is surrounded by a thickened ligament (the annulus fibrosis)

intervertebral foramina: openings between two adjacent vertebrae to permit the exit of nerve structures from the spinal cord

spinal cord: a cord in the trunk containing nerve cells that transmit impulses to and from the brain

spinous processes: bony projections from vertebrae (horizontally in the neck, tilting downward in the thoracic area, and horizontally in the lumbar area) that are connected to one another by the interspinous and supraspinous ligaments and that control extremes of trunk motion

transverse processes: projections from the sides of vertebrae, to which are attached muscles and ligaments, that assist in motor function by enhancing leverage and limiting extremes of motion

vertebra: a bony structure in the back with a central spinal canal surrounded by an arch; the back part of the arch (the lamina) and the front part of the arch (the pedicle) are joined together by muscles, ligaments, and cartilage for motion, stability, and posture

STRUCTURE AND FUNCTIONS

The spinal column undergoes developmental changes from infancy to the adult state and then degenerative changes with aging. The alignment of the spinal column at birth is in the shape of a C curve, the fetus having been curled up. This forward-tilted curve is retained except in the neck and lower back. As the infant raises its head and attempts to see things, head control and vision gradually require the head to tilt back, resulting in a posterior curve at the neck. As children progress to standing and walking, the lower spine also develops a posterior curve (a normal lumbar lordosis). As individuals increasingly use the predominant upper extremities, these muscles become stronger and increase the pull on that side of the spine, resulting in a lateral curve (a normal scoliosis).

Humans generally have thirty-three vertebrae, but abnormalities can occur in their numbers, shape, alignment, density, and maturation. There are seven vertebrae in the neck or cervical area, twelve in the chest or thoracic area, five in the lower back or lumbar area, five usually joined together in the pelvic region to form the sacrum, and three or four rudimentary vertebrae partially fused to form the coccyx. The typical vertebra develops embryologically from two bone growth centers. The front of one bone growth center becomes the body and part of the arch, while the other bone growth center evolves into the spinous processes, the transverse processes, the articular processes, and the back portion of the arch.

The thirty-three vertebrae of the spine have various

defined parts and characteristics. The oval or round vertebral body has a spongy center surrounded by a dense bone. Above and below it are layers of cartilage. Lack of the mineral calcium reduces the density of the bone, resulting in osteoporosis. This condition may occur in postmenopausal women, causing pain, fractures, and kyphosis (a thoracic humpback). The pedicle portions of this anterior arch have an upper and lower notch called the intervertebral foramen, through which the spinal nerves exit from the spinal canal. At the junction of pedicle and lamina are projections upward and downward that form the articular processes, or joints. The alignment and direction of these joints vary with the spinal region and serve to control spinal motion. The transverse processes assist in the movement of muscles and at the chest level act as links between the ribs. There are generally twelve thoracic vertebrae and twelve ribs. On occasion, an extra cervical rib may be present; this extra rib narrows the exit space at the neck and can pinch the cervical nerves and blood vessels.

The upper two cervical processes are different from all other vertebrae. The first cervical vertebra supports the head and is called the atlas. Instead of a body, it has an enlarged anterior arch and a groove on which the head rests. Its transverse processes are long, but its spinous process is a little knob. The second cervical vertebra is also unique, with an upward projection called the dens that is like a pole fitting into the ring of the first cervical vertebral arch. It represents the body of the first cervical vertebra. This pole and ring permit the head to rotate.

The cervical transverse processes or lateral projections have holes, the transverse foramina, through which the vertebral arteries send blood to the brain. As one progresses downward, the vertebrae become larger and bear more weight. The thoracic vertebrae have their joint surfaces in the frontal plane, and the transverse processes are solid. The ribs share half of the joint surfaces with the adjoining vertebrae, except for the first, tenth, eleventh, and twelfth vertebrae; these vertebrae join only their corresponding ribs. As one continues down the spine, the spinous processes become more slender and project downward, almost touching one another. The lower thoracic vertebrae are closer to the lumbar vertebrae in appearance.

The lumbar vertebrae are more massive, carry more stress, and support the weight of the body. The transverse processes in this region are thinner but longer, increasing the leverage action for muscles. The joint

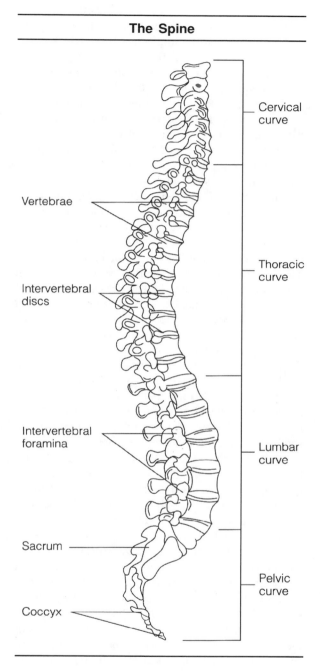

The Spine

Cervical curve

Vertebrae

Thoracic curve

Intervertebral discs

Intervertebral foramina

Lumbar curve

Sacrum

Pelvic curve

Coccyx

surfaces tilt upward, backward, and toward the center, opening the joint space when one bends forward. This action permits side bending, increasing the side pressures on the disks. The five sacral vertebrae are fused, with small ridges representing the sites of fusion. Small openings allow the upper four sacral nerves to exit the spine. The sacrum contributes the back portion of the pelvis. The coccyx, or tailbone, is composed of three or four rudimentary vertebrae, with the first distinct and separate from the other two or three, which are fused. The back of the spine is layered with muscles going to the upper extremities, with long vertical muscles underneath, intermediate-length muscles under these, and the deepest muscle groups closest to the spine and only two or three vertebrae in length.

Vertebrae are separated by washers called disks. The central portion of a disk is a gel-like substance, the nucleus pulposus, which offers hydraulic cushioning and allows some movement. This substance is enclosed in a ligamentous covering called the annulus fibrosis. Disks contribute approximately one-fourth of body length, can add about eight degrees in motion per vertebra, and can alter their shape to accommodate the solid vertebrae when the body is bent. The nucleus pulposus is 70 to 80 percent water, and about 14 kilograms (30 pounds) of pressure must be exerted constantly by ligaments to maintain the shape of the disk. Dehydration, aging, compressive forces, and simply a day of normal activity can temporarily reduce the amount of the watery nucleus pulposus, increase the bulging of the disks, and shorten one's stature.

The spinal cord connects the peripheral structures of the body to the brain and the nerve cells in the spinal cord itself. Until about the third month of life, the spinal cord occupies the entire length of the spinal canal. The vertebrae grow faster than the spinal cord, however, and later in life it occupies two-thirds of the length of the spinal canal (approximately 42 to 45 centimeters) and ends at about the second lumbar vertebra. The coverings on the cord continue as the filum terminale, which is attached to the sacral vertebrae.

There are three coverings of the spinal cord within the spinal canal. The outermost, toughest, and fibrous covering, called the dura, is separated from the bony surfaces by fat and blood vessels. The spinal cord is covered by a thin layer, called the pia, which enters into the spinal cord and separates various portions of the cord. Surrounding the pia is a protective fluid, the spinal fluid, which is held in place by the arachnoid layer; this fluid can be aspirated for analysis, as in a lumbar puncture, or spinal tap. The nerves exiting from the spinal cord are also segmental. There are only seven cervical vertebrae but eight cervical nerves. The eighth cervical nerve exits below the seventh cervical vertebra, and thereafter all roots from the vertebrae leave below the corresponding vertebra. These segmental nerves then join, divide, send messages to

the brain and other organs, and control bodily functions and motion.

Ligaments run vertically in front of the vertebral bodies (the anterior longitudinal ligament) and in back of the vertebral bodies and within the spinal canal (the posterior longitudinal ligament). These ligaments support the vertebrae and disks and limit excessive motion forward and backward. The posterior longitudinal ligament ceases at about the fourth lumbar vertebra, and thus further down the spine the fibrous rings about the disks are weaker, permitting herniations. Such leakages from the disks may press on nerve roots exiting at these levels and cause pain. These ruptures of the disks occur mostly when lifting with the trunk bent forward and sideways. There are additional ligaments between the spinous processes at the tips (the supraspinous ligament) and along the length of the spinous processes (the interspinous ligament). The portion of the arch between the spinous processes and the transverse processes is the lamina. Between the laminae are the ligamentum flavum. The interspinous ligament, ligamentum flavum, and nucleus pulposus have no pain fibers. The laminae and disks may be removed when disk surgery is performed, and pieces of bone from the hip may be used to fuse and reduce motion at this level.

Motion between each vertebra is about eight degrees. Motion is enhanced by the facets, vertical bony projections with joint surfaces. They are structured like the other joints of the body, and thus are subject to irritation and arthritic changes. Flexion of the trunk opens the spaces in the lumbar joints and allows side bending and rotation in the same direction. Extension of the trunk compresses and limits motion in these facets.

The blood supply to the spinal cord and the surrounding tissues diminishes progressively downward. Excessive activity can lead to insufficient circulating blood to these nerves and give rise to symptoms in the lower extremity called intermittent claudication. The front portion of the spinal cord contains motor nerve cells, leading to the trunk and the muscles of the extremities, that can be inhibited or activated by impulses. The lateral areas of the spinal region contain messenger tracts and the autonomic nervous system. The back portion of the spinal cord has sensory structures that carry messages of pain, temperature, position, and touch to the brain. The different levels within the spinal cord connect to different segmental structures of the body. The fifth cervical nerve down

Some Types of Spinal Disorder

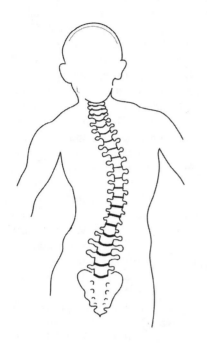

Primary scoliosis
of thoracolumbar
region

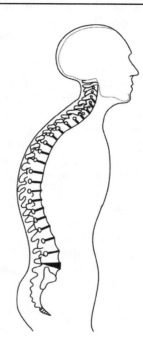

Kyphosis of
thoracic region

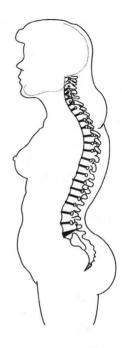

Lordosis of
lumbar region

to the first thoracic nerve connect to the upper extremities, and the second lumbar to second sacral roots connect to the lower extremities. Compression of these nerve roots at the spine may cause symptoms in areas distant from the spine.

DISORDERS AND DISEASES

The anatomy of the trunk regulates the erect, or standing, posture. It is influenced by the structure of the vertebrae and extremities and even by the tilt of the head. It is also influenced by cultural factors, emotion, habits, and occupation. Good posture involves standing straight with the head up, the shoulders back and up, the stomach in, and the hips and knees straight. This position also is most efficient in energy expenditure, since it requires the least amount of muscle activity in order to balance the weights in the front and back of the trunk, as well as the weights on the left and right sides of the body. Looking at the front of the body, the central gravitational, or weight-bearing,

line falls in line with the nose and between the pelvis, knees, and ankles. From the back, the gravitational line follows the center of the head, the spinous processes, the gluteal fold between the buttocks, and between the knees and ankles. The weight stresses should be balanced between the right side and the left side of the body and between the front and the back. The head should be maintained so that the eyes and the labyrinth in the inner ear are level. Any deviations cause imbalance in the trunk, resulting in muscle strain, ligament sprains, pain, and possibly deformities. Abnormalities in posture and gait may be attributable to muscle imbalance, deformities at birth, problems in development, disease, or surgical procedures.

There are several birth defects that affect the spine. Occasionally, during embryonic development, the two bone growth regions that form a vertebra do not fuse together, causing an opening in the arch in the back called spina bifida. Spondylolysis occurs when the articular process remains unattached. Ligaments, muscles, and tendons are unable to attach to these areas securely, and the result is weakness in the vertebra and a reduction in stability. Occasionally, this weakness permits the upper vertebra to slide forward, a condition called spondylolisthesis. The misalignment and narrowing of the spinal canal can compress the nerve structures within it, a condition known as spinal stenosis. The lower cervical and lower lumbar regions, which need more nerve tissue to supply the extremities, are especially vulnerable to pressure symptoms.

Inequality in leg lengths or pain in the lower extremities, upper extremities, abdomen, chest, or neck can lead to compensatory reactions in the trunk. These may then cause misalignment in the spine with side deviations (scoliosis), backward deviations (kyphosis, or humpback, in the thoracic area), and forward deviations (lordosis in the low back). Other contributing factors are overuse, muscle spasm or weakness, birth defects, developmental abnormalities, diseases, aging, and trauma. Some misalignments occur after surgery on the chest, back, or abdomen. Idiopathic scoliosis (scoliosis of unknown cause) may occur in adolescent girls; when it is severe, lung and heart functions can be impaired. Temporarily increased lordosis can occur in pregnancy, to compensate for the extra weight in the abdomen. Lordosis may be permanent because of structural changes in the spine, pendulous abdomen and/or breasts, or poor muscle balance. Therefore, back problems may be caused by poor posture, behavior, occupation, and structural, neurologic, or muscular factors. Pain located only in the back is generally attributable to poor posture, trauma, or inflammation. If pain extends below the knees, the cause may be nerve pressure at the fifth lumbar or first sacral nerve roots. Bladder and rectal sphincter disturbances may indicate sacral nerve or cord involvement and may require immediate surgical care.

The body's center of gravity is in the front portion of the second lumbar vertebra. Thus, the compressive force of body weight is increased when one lifts an object with the arms in front of the trunk. The greater the distance of the object from the center of the body, the greater the need for the back muscles to contract. Lifting a 45-kilogram (100-pound) object may require a 545-kilogram (1,200-pound) muscle pull and compressive force. The posterior longitudinal support for the disks that is provided by ligaments narrows in the sides at the level of the fourth and fifth lumbar vertebrae. Herniations through the fibrous disk ring at these levels are more likely, and a ruptured disk can pinch the nerves exiting at these levels.

Stresses that bear on the spine are categorized as compressive, shearing, elongating, or rotational. Compressive forces may involve the muscles, disks (possible ruptures), vertebrae (fractures), and the facet joints. Shearing stress may lead to forward slippage of the fourth or fifth vertebra from the segment below. This is most common in individuals with incomplete bony union of vertebrae. Rotatory stress may affect the joints, the facets of the spine, the short spine muscles, or the ligaments. On rare occasions, an elongating stretch or traction may strain muscles and sprain or tear ligaments.

Perspective and Prospects

Examinations of the spine usually include the history of the problem: whether it is sudden or gradual and whether it is influenced by certain activities or climates. The physician checks the patient's posture for abnormal curvatures and determines whether they are fixed or functional. Functional curves disappear when the patient is lying down. The gait should be evaluated for symmetry, balance, and deviations. The physician will measure leg lengths for inequalities, the circumference of the chest for rib flare, and the circumferences of extremities for swelling or shrinkage. Next, the trunk's range of motion will be evaluated, followed by palpation to discover tender spots and muscle spasms.

With spinal problems, a full examination of the entire body is indicated since pain can be referred to the back from other organs. Changes in function, sensation, and motor strength can indicate spinal cord or nerve involvement. Simple X rays of the spine will indicate alignment of the vertebrae, bone density, fracture lines, extraneous bone growth, cartilage thickness, and unusual soft tissue densities caused by hemorrhage or calcification. For problems other than bone and cartilage tissue involvement, a computed tomography (CT) scan or magnetic resonance imaging (MRI) may be needed; these techniques provide images of the area to be examined that are at different levels or depths.

—*Eugene J. Rogers, M.D.*

See also Anesthesia; Anesthesiology; Bone cancer; Bone disorders; Bones and the skeleton; Cerebral palsy; Chiropractic; Disk removal; Dystrophy; Fracture and dislocation; Head and neck disorders; Kinesiology; Kyphosis; Laminectomy and spinal fusion;

Lumbar puncture; Meningitis; Motor neuron diseases; Multiple sclerosis; Muscle sprains, spasms, and disorders; Muscular dystrophy; Nervous system; Neuralgia, neuritis, and neuropathy; Neurology; Neurology, pediatric; Neurosurgery; Numbness and tingling; Orthopedic surgery; Orthopedics; Orthopedics, pediatric; Osteoarthritis; Osteoporosis; Paget's disease; Paralysis; Paraplegia; Physical rehabilitation; Poliomyelitis; Quadriplegia; Sciatica; Scoliosis; Slipped disk; Spina bifida; Spinal cord disorders; Spondylitis; Sports medicine; Sympathectomy.

FOR FURTHER INFORMATION:

Faye, Leonard, and Lydia Encinas. *Good-bye Back Pain: The Safe and Easy Guide to Total Back Recovery.* New York: Berkley Press, 1992. A cursory review of the back and the causes of back pain. Tells readers how to diagnose the causes of their back pain and how a physician would diagnose the condition.

Fine, Judylaine. *Conquering Back Pain: A Comprehensive Guide.* Rev. ed. Englewood Cliffs, N.J.: Prentice Hall, 1987. This softcover book summarizes the anatomy of the back, discussing its various structures, types of pain, and areas where pain may be distributed. Also enumerates the treatments, both conservative and surgical, of back pain.

Jenkins, David B. *Hollinshead's Functional Anatomy of the Limbs and Back.* Rev. 7th ed. Philadelphia: W. B. Saunders, 1998. An easy-to-understand and well-illustrated book designed for physical therapy students. It can be useful for those individuals wishing more information about the muscles of the back and extremities, their nerve and blood supplies, and the function of these structures.

Palastanga, Nigel, Derek Field, and Roger Soames. *Anatomy and Human Movement: Structure and Function.* 3d ed. Oxford, England: Heinemann Medical Books, 1998. This large volume (891 pages) contains excellent illustrations, definitions, and indexes and is written to simplify the more complex aspects of anatomy using understandable terms.

SPLENECTOMY

PROCEDURE

ANATOMY OR SYSTEM AFFECTED: Abdomen, lymphatic system, spleen

SPECIALTIES AND RELATED FIELDS: Emergency medicine, general surgery

DEFINITION: The surgical removal of the spleen.

Splenectomy

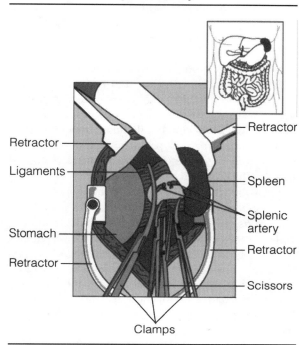

The removal of the spleen is required when the organ has sustained damage from injury or disease; the inset shows the location of the spleen.

INDICATIONS AND PROCEDURES

Splenectomy is often performed after trauma to the upper left abdominal cavity that results in injury to the spleen. When the spleen is damaged in such cases, life-threatening intra-abdominal hemorrhage may occur. Surgical repair of the damaged spleen is sometimes difficult, but the lack of a spleen has relatively few ill effects, as other organs such as the liver and tissues of the lymphatic system compensate for its absence. Therefore, splenectomy is usually the indicated treatment for damage to the spleen.

Patients undergoing splenectomy are first anesthetized by an anesthesiologist. Surgical assistants then prepare the patient by scrubbing the upper abdomen to rid the skin of pathogens. The surgeon than makes an incision in the upper left abdomen or along the midline of the abdomen. He or she will then expose the spleen and tie off blood vessels to the spleen with sutures. The surgeon then cuts the attachments that anchor the spleen in the abdomen and removes the organ. This procedure takes approximately one hour to complete, provided that there are no complications.

Most patients are allowed to leave the hospital after about one week or less. Although surgical infections are rare, they may require the patient to remain hospitalized for a few more days.

USES AND COMPLICATIONS

Splenectomy is also performed to treat patients with certain types of anemia and hypersplenism. Since the normal function of the spleen is to destroy aged or nonfunctional red blood cells and platelets, overactivity of the spleen in hypersplenism results in excessive destruction of these blood cells and leads to anemia and blood-clotting disorders.

Even though splenectomy has few long-term adverse effects, some adult patients have a slightly increased risk of contracting infections. Splenectomy in children, however, results in greater susceptibility, particularly to pneumococcal pneumonia. Physicians often recommend that children who have undergone splenectomy be immunized against this bacterial pneumonia, and many of these patients even receive long-term prophylactic antibiotic therapy to prevent the disease.

—Matthew Berria, Ph.D.,
and Douglas Reinhart, M.D.
See also Abdomen; Abdominal disorders; Anemia; Bleeding; Hematology; Hematology, pediatric; Immune system; Immunology; Internal medicine; Lymphatic system; Metabolism; Pneumonia; Wounds.

FOR FURTHER INFORMATION:

Braunwald, Eugene. *Harrison's Principles of Internal Medicine.* New York: McGraw-Hill, 2000.

Hiatt, J. R., E. H. Phillips, L. Morgenstern, eds. *Surgical Diseases of the Spleen.* New York: Springer, 1997.

Schwartz, Seymour I., James T. Adams, and Arthur W. Bauman. *Splenectomy for Hematologic Disorders.* Chicago: Year Book Medical, 1971.

SPONDYLITIS

DISEASE/DISORDER

ANATOMY OR SYSTEM AFFECTED: Back, joints, spine

SPECIALTIES AND RELATED FIELDS: Rheumatology

DEFINITION: Spondylitis is the inflammation and stiffening of the joints between the vertebrae in the spine. It often results from chronic, progressive diseases of the joints, such as ankylosing spondylitis or rheumatoid arthritis. During the early stages, symptoms include lower back pain and morning stiffness. Later, the pain spreads up the back and into other joints. Diseases that feature spondylitis are often incurable and can lead to congestive heart failure, amyloidosis, gastrointestinal disease, lung disease, nerve compression (causing numbness in the arms or legs), and permanent disability and immobilization.

—Jason Georges and Tracy Irons-Georges
See also Arthritis; Paralysis; Rheumatoid arthritis; Rheumatology; Spine, vertebrae, and disks.

FOR FURTHER INFORMATION:

Dong, Collin, and Jane Banks. *New Hope for the Arthritic.* New York: Ballantine Books, 1990.

Jenkins, David B. *Hollinshead's Functional Anatomy of the Limbs and Back.* Rev. 7th ed. Philadelphia: W. B. Saunders, 1998.

Early- and Late-Stage Spondylitis

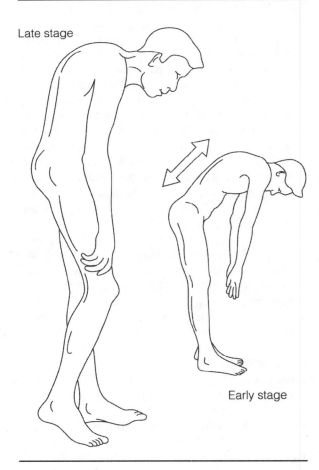

Late stage

Early stage

Palastanga, Nigel, Derek Field, and Roger Soames. *Anatomy and Human Movement: Structure and Function.* 3d ed. Oxford, England: Heinemann Medical Books, 1998.

SPORTS MEDICINE
SPECIALTY

ANATOMY OR SYSTEM AFFECTED: Bones, circulatory system, feet, hands, head, heart, joints, knees, legs, ligaments, muscles, musculoskeletal system, nervous system, spine, tendons

SPECIALTIES AND RELATED FIELDS: Cardiology, emergency medicine, exercise physiology, family practice, internal medicine, nutrition, orthopedics, pharmacology, physical therapy, preventive medicine, psychology, rheumatology

DEFINITION: A medical subspecialty concerned with the care and prevention of athletic injuries, primarily those related to the musculoskeletal system.

KEY TERMS:

joint: a specialized structure in the body where bones come together and motion occurs

ligament: a tough, rubber band-like structure that connects one bone to another and prevents the abnormal motion of these bones in relationship to each other

musculoskeletal: a term used to describe the relationship between bones and muscles within the framework of the body and the way in which they provide stability and locomotion

musculotendinous unit: a structure that consists of a muscle that provides motion of a bone and its attachment to the bone, the tendon, which is a tough, inelastic fibrous structure

orthopedic surgery: the field of surgery that deals with the musculoskeletal system

SCIENCE AND PROFESSION

Sports medicine is a field that has become popular as the number of people who exercise has increased. More than 50 percent of people in the United States exercise on a daily basis. People all over the country are participating in sports, from recreational sports to professional competitive sports. There has been a

Common Sports-Related Injuries

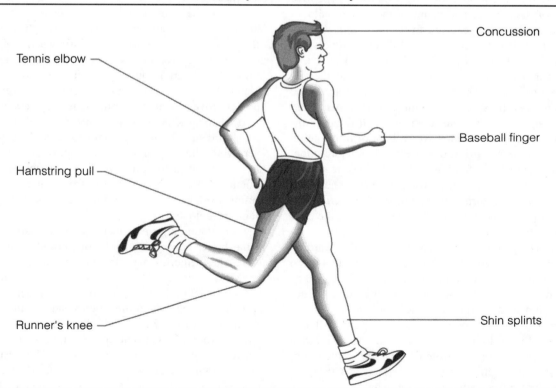

growing trend of participation in exercise as more and more studies have proved that exercise is beneficial to health; however, exercise places people at risk for injuries that a sedentary person would not have. This fact has led to the emergence of sports medicine, with its specially trained health care professionals. These professionals include physical therapists, athletic trainers, nutritionists, exercise physiologists, cardiologists, sports psychologists, family practitioners, internists, and orthopedic surgeons. They all contribute by bringing special knowledge and understanding to the care of athletes and athletic injuries. Such knowledge can relate to nutrition, strength training, cardiovascular conditioning, psychosocial issues, musculoskeletal care, or one or more of many other areas related to the health of athletes. Therefore, sports medicine is a very broad and diverse field that requires a team approach.

Athletic injuries occur with regularity, but very few injuries are unique to sports. Yet treating an injured athlete does not necessarily require the same process as that used to treat an injured sedentary person. The athlete tends to have greater expectations than does the average sedentary person. These expectations usually increase proportionately with the competitive level of the athlete. For example, the athlete with an ankle sprain will spend ten to twelve hours per day performing treatment and rehabilitation supervised by a physical therapist or athletic trainer. The sedentary person, however, might go to physical therapy three times per week. Although the philosophy of the treatment is the same, the number of treatments and the desired outcomes are completely different. Athletes also require an extensive amount of information regarding their injuries, treatment, and rehabilitation. Athletes are not afraid to ask questions regarding their injuries because they want to know when they will be able to return to competition. The average patient, however, is quite uncomfortable asking the physician about an injury or illness.

Sports medicine is a challenging and rewarding profession. It is enjoyable working with patients who have a high level of compliance and motivation. The reward of watching an athlete recover from an injury and compete is exceptional. The sports medicine physician must realize, however, that he or she will also be called upon by the athlete and the athlete's coach and parents to communicate the severity of the injury and its significance—a process which can be quite difficult at times, especially when what the physician has to say is not what anyone wants to hear. Nevertheless, it is the role of the physician to act in the best interest of the athlete. In order for the physician to be prepared to handle this, he or she must fully understand the demands of each and every sport. Attendance at games is usually not enough to achieve this level of knowledge and experience. Observing practice sessions and workouts is often quite useful. With the exception of high-impact collision sports such as hockey and football, most injuries occur during practice and workout sessions. Furthermore, such observation gives the physician an opportunity to be involved in education and injury prevention. Many athletic injuries are witnessed by an athletic trainer or physician who may be called upon to administer first aid in the field or, in some instances, provide treatment for injuries.

By attending practices or competitions, the physician may also have the opportunity to observe the actual mechanism of injury, which can be quite useful in evaluating the type and severity of the injury. Many physicians call the first twenty minutes after an injury has occurred, prior to the onset of swelling and spasm, the "golden period." It is at this time that an accurate and meaningful physical examination can be performed on the injured athlete. The recreational athlete, however, usually will arrive at the physician's office one to two days after the injury, when swelling and spasm are maximal. At this time, examining the injured body part is quite difficult and may not be meaningful. This may result in delays in diagnosis and definitive treatment. For the sedentary person and the occasional athlete, such delays will probably not be significant. The highly competitive athlete, however, would be quite dissatisfied if an injury delayed his or her return to competition. So, although most athletic injuries differ very little from other cases of musculoskeletal trauma, the finer points of managing them are unique.

Most athletic injuries affect one of three structures in the body: bones, ligaments, or musculotendinous units. These injuries may be acute or chronic in onset. Most acute injuries occur as a result of trauma, with presentation being rather soon after the incident. Chronic injuries, which are often insidious in onset, usually result from a change in the athlete or the athletic environment. Chronic injuries tend to be difficult to recognize and treat effectively. The best approach to chronic injuries is prevention. Most acute injuries can be classified as sprains, strains, or fractures, and most chronic injuries can be classified as strains or stress fractures.

Sprains are injuries to ligaments; strains are injuries to the musculotendinous unit. Sprains occur when there is excessive abnormal motion at a joint. This results in overstretching of the ligaments and produces local pain, swelling, limitation of motion, and a sense of instability. Such overstretching can result in partial tears (mild) or complete tears (severe) of the ligament. Strains are usually the result of an abrupt increase in the tension of the musculotendinous unit (for example, they may occur when one lifts weights that are too heavy). This increase may result in partial or complete tears of the muscle, the tendon, or the bone to which the tendon is attached. The most important principle is to realize that strains are not the result of overstretching but occur well within the normal limits of motion. Strains are also graded from mild to severe. Often, there is an obvious deformity at the site of injury because the muscle rolls up into a ball. Fractures are simply breaks in the bones of the body. Stress fractures occur when excessive demands are placed on the bone. Eventually, the bone fails to accommodate these demands and microscopic breaks result.

DIAGNOSTIC AND TREATMENT TECHNIQUES

The initial management of acute injuries is the same in athletics as it is in other musculoskeletal trauma. Treatment should be directed at prevention of bleeding and edema. These conditions usually lead to pain and decreased function of the injured body part, which requires the application of ice, compression, elevation, and rest. There are other methods of treatment used in the professional setting that are also useful in preventing or reducing bleeding and edema. These include electric stimulation, contrast baths, ultrasound, and compression stockings. After the initial phase of bleeding and edema, therapy should be directed at restoring range of motion, strength, and, finally, functional tasks that will ultimately result in the athlete's return to competition. Chronic injuries, however, usually require elimination of the precipitating factors as well as increased rest while the injured body part is allowed to heal. This may require a special taping procedure, a brace, a change in footwear, the alteration of practice sessions, or simply refraining from that activity for a short period of time.

Chronic injuries and overuse injuries are usually caused by change. Change can occur in the athlete, the environment, or the activity. Identifying these changes can be helpful in injury prevention, since the majority of injuries in athletics are chronic. Also, the treatment requires elimination of the offending change and restoration of the proper condition. Strains to the musculotendinous unit can also occur chronically. They tend to result from muscle fatigue, too much training too fast, or poor training conditions. Many of these injuries are called "tendinitis," which means inflammation of the tendon. The most prominent aspect of such an injury is pain. The pain is almost always located in the region of the injured structure. Management is directed at avoidance of painful activity, elimination of the offending factor, and symptomatic relief of pain with ice, ultrasound, injections, electric stimulation, and medicines. Rehabilitation is aimed at restoring strength and flexibility as well as avoiding the initial cause.

Most sprains can be treated with routine physical therapy and rehabilitation, but many severe sprains will require surgery. Average time lost from athletics ranges from seven days (for example, for a mild ankle sprain) to one year (for example, for a severe knee sprain with reconstruction of ligaments). With strains, complete tears of the tendon usually require surgery, while injury to the muscle itself does not. Treatment is similar to that for sprains; rehabilitation should be directed at regaining strength and flexibility. The diagnosis of a fracture can be made only with the aid of an X-ray picture. Treatment of fractures requires immobilization either in a cast, special splint, or brace. Some fractures will require the placement of plates or screws by an orthopedic surgeon. Rehabilitation of fractures involves restoration of motion, strength, flexibility, and proprioception. Proprioception is simply the unconscious awareness of where a body part is in space (for example, a person can tie his or her shoes with eyes closed because the brain knows where the hands are in space). The treatment of stress fractures is different from treatments of other fractures in that immobilization is almost never necessary. Adaptation of activity and relative rest are usually all that is required. Return to competition averages three to six weeks but may be longer.

Sports medicine personnel also provide education and guidance to coaches, athletes, and parents. They make themselves available to provide the best and most efficient care possible. It is the responsibility of the sports medicine physician to coordinate this care. This all begins with the preseason screening history and physical exam.

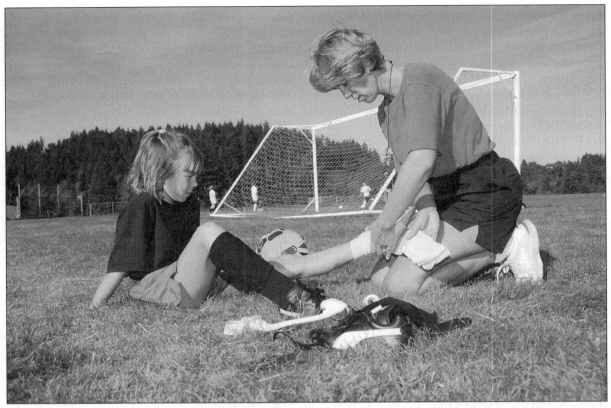

Doctors seek to ensure that injuries sustained during childhood do not interfere with developing bones and muscles. (PhotoDisc)

Prior to the commencement of each athletic season, athletes are usually required to provide a medical history and undergo a physical examination. The requirements of such examinations vary from state to state, college to college, and professional league to professional league. The purpose of these examinations is to identify athletes who may have potential problems in the sport in which they have chosen to compete.

For example, Johnnie is a thirteen-year-old high school freshman trying out for the football team. The doctor listens to his heart and lungs and hears a small heart murmur. The physician recommends that Johnnie see a cardiologist prior to beginning football practice. A further workup by the cardiologist reveals that Johnnie has a condition in which the arteries that supply his heart are abnormal. The cardiologist recommends that Johnnie not participate in athletic activity that requires stress on the heart. Although this scenario is uncommon, it is a perfect example of the benefits of preseason history and physical exams.

Johnnie could have died as a result of his condition if it had gone unnoticed.

The preseason screening also identifies athletes who are at risk for developing strains and sprains because their flexibility is lower than normal. Identifying these athletes allows the athletic trainer to work with them on a stretching program intended to reduce the number and severity of such injuries. It is during the preseason that the athletes are at greatest risk for injury, since the workouts are long and numerous and most athletes are not yet in shape. Injuries may occur at any time during practice or a game. Most injuries occur during practice, however; and especially at the end of the session, because athletes are tired and their concentration level is low.

Dean is a twenty-year-old junior college soccer player who is kicked in the side during a slide tackling drill. He is taken out of practice by the coach and then sent to the training room to see the athletic trainer. The athletic trainer astutely examines Dean's urine and finds blood in it. Also, he finds that Dean's blood pressure is somewhat low and that his heart rate is mildly elevated. Because of this, the trainer is concerned about injury to Dean's kidney or spleen. He promptly phones the team physician, who advises that they meet him in the emergency room at the hospital. After being evaluated by the team doctor, Dean is brought to the operating room by a surgeon, who removes Dean's extensively damaged spleen. Dean recovers quickly and returns to exercise within six weeks but is not allowed to play soccer until the following season. Without the aid of the trainer and prompt attention by the team physician, Dean might not have had such favorable results.

Mary is a fifteen-year-old high school all-state cross country runner. She is now entering her junior year and is expected to compete on the national level. Mary is also an excellent student with a grade-point average of 3.6. She has always been an overachiever. Six weeks into the fall season, Mary's times begin to fall off slightly. When asked about her performance, she states that she has been experiencing pain in both her shins, particularly the one on the right, for two weeks. Her coach, because of her concern, asks Mary to see her family doctor, since Mary's school does not have an athletic trainer or team physician. Mary's doctor, who is not trained in sports medicine, simply tells Mary that she has shin splints and that she should rest. Mary does not accept this, because everyone is counting on her to win for her school. She continues to run against his advice. In the next race, Mary finishes dead last. The pain has become quite unbearable. Mary is finally referred to a sports medicine physician, who discovers several relevant facts. Mary has not been eating well and has in fact been forcing herself to vomit for a number of days prior to each race. Also, Mary has not experienced her first menses, and her secondary sexual characteristics are somewhat immature. X rays of Mary's right leg reveal a stress fracture that is quite severe. Mary is referred to several people, including an orthopedic surgeon who places her in a cast, a nutritionist and a psychologist who evaluate and treat her eating disorder, and a gynecologist who proceeds with a workup for her late development. After several months of treatments from all three doctors, Mary begins retraining on a bicycle under the direction of an athletic trainer and a physical therapist. She moves on to compete in the spring season of track and field and becomes a national champion. Without the aid of the sports medicine team, Mary might have continued to have difficulty and

might not have been evaluated properly until it was too late. This is a quite common scenario among adolescent athletes. The pressures placed upon them by friends, coaches, and parents can become detrimental to their emotional and physical well-being.

Henry is a fifty-five-year-old businessman who spends five days a week playing tennis at the local health club to stay in shape. After buying a new racket, he begins to experience pain in his right elbow. He is seen by an orthopedic surgeon in town who specializes in sports medicine. After speaking with Henry and examining his elbow, the doctor recommends anti-inflammatory medication, a special forearm strap, and use of the old racket. Henry's condition, which is called tennis elbow, or lateral epicondylitis, is quite common. After several weeks of the initial treatment, Henry does not feel any better. His doctor, therefore, injects him with a medicine to ease the pain and calm the inflammation. Henry is instructed to rest his arm for a week prior to starting tennis again. Henry follows the doctor's instructions carefully. He begins to play tennis again and feels fine for about a month, after which he begins to experience the same discomfort. This time, the doctor recommends surgery for Henry's elbow. Three months after the surgery, Henry is free of pain.

These examples have demonstrated how sports medicine can be beneficial to athletes. Each scenario differs in type of athlete, location, diagnosis, and treatment.

PERSPECTIVE AND PROSPECTS

Sports medicine is assuming a significant role in the medical profession today. Sports medicine was first recognized in the days of the early Olympics. It was not until the final decades of the twentieth century, however, that it emerged into a field of its own. Sports medicine training programs have been developing at an exponential rate. Interest in sports medicine can be pursued in various ways. Most sports medicine physicians undergo a one-year fellowship after either a five-year orthopedic residency training program or a three-year family practice residency training program. Athletic trainers must pass a national examination for certification. Most have master's degrees, and all have some form of bachelor's degree. Their expertise is in the prevention, treatment, and rehabilitation of athletic injuries. These are the primary caregivers of the sports medicine world. Certified athletic trainers are being hired at all major universities, many high schools, and many health clubs across the country. Various types of sports medicine centers are continually being developed. These centers offer a wide range of services to both professional and amateur athletes. As more and more people begin to exercise, the need for sports medicine professionals will increase.

Athletes' needs and goals are different from those of most other people. Although the injuries that they experience are not unique to sports, the rapidity with which they recover is of utmost importance. This identifies them as a distinct group of people with special demands for medical care. It is because of this and because of the growing number of people who exercise on a daily basis that sports medicine has evolved into a viable medical field. Sports medicine will continue to grow and will play an important role in preventing many of the injuries that afflict people in the United States.

—*Paul Freudigman, Jr., M.D.*

See also Acupressure; Anorexia nervosa; Arthroplasty; Arthroscopy; Athlete's foot; Biofeedback; Bones and the skeleton; Cardiology; Critical care; Eating disorders; Emergency medicine; Exercise physiology; Fracture and dislocation; Fracture repair; Glycolysis; Head and neck disorders; Heat exhaustion and heat stroke; Hydrotherapy; Kinesiology; Muscle sprains, spasms, and disorders; Muscles; Nutrition; Orthopedic surgery; Orthopedics; Orthopedics, pediatric; Oxygen therapy; Physical examination; Physical rehabilitation; Physiology; Preventive medicine; Psychiatry; Psychiatry, child and adolescent; Spine, vertebrae, and disks; Steroid abuse; Steroids; Tendon disorders; Tendon repair.

FOR FURTHER INFORMATION:

Garrick, James G., and David R. Webb. *Sports Injuries: Diagnosis and Management.* 2d ed. Philadelphia: W. B. Saunders, 1999. This book explains how to diagnose and treat injuries.

Roy, Steven, and Richard Irvin. *Sports Medicine: Prevention, Evaluation, Management, and Rehabilitation.* Englewood Cliffs, N.J.: Prentice Hall, 1983. A simple, easy-to-read text that is invaluable as a reference guide.

Scuderi, Giles R., Peter D. McCann, and Peter J. Bruno, eds. *Sports Medicine: Principles of Primary Care.* St. Louis: C. V. Mosby, 1997. This text covers all types of athletic injuries and offers useful illustrations. Includes a bibliography and an index.

Southmayd, William, and Marshall Hoffman. *Sports Health.* New York: Quick Fox, 1981. Easy reading for the average person who has an interest in sports injuries and related topics.

Sullivan, J. Andy, and William A. Grana. *The Pediatric Athlete.* Park Ridge, Ill.: The Academy, 1990. A readable text designed to deal with issues related to the young athlete. Requires a small amount of knowledge to understand and is applicable to the general public.

SPRAINS. *See* MUSCLE SPRAINS, SPASMS, AND DISORDERS.

SQUAMOUS CELL CARCINOMA. *See* SKIN CANCER.

STAPHYLOCOCCAL INFECTIONS
DISEASE/DISORDER

ANATOMY OR SYSTEM AFFECTED: All

SPECIALTIES AND RELATED FIELDS: Bacteriology, emergency medicine, internal medicine, toxicology

DEFINITION: Staphylococcal infections consist of a wide variety of infections caused by staphylococcus bacteria. These bacteria can cause boils, abscesses, pneumonia, bone infections, and infections in other tissues or organs. Infection occurs when staphylococcal bacteria are not cleared away from a tissue site. When bacteria enter the bloodstream because of contamination from a skin irritation, complications such as arthritis and bone disease may occur. Toxic shock syndrome has been linked to invasion of the bloodstream by staphylococcus bacteria. Symptoms include fatigue, muscle pain, severe nausea and vomiting, diarrhea, high fever, a mild cough, and a pus-filled nasal discharge. Staphylococcal infections are treated with antibiotics, as well as with the intravenous infusion of nutrients.

—*Jason Georges and Tracy Irons-Georges*

See also Abscess drainage; Abscesses; Antibiotics; Arthritis; Bacterial infections; Blisters and boils; Bone disorders; Infection; Pneumonia; Septicemia; Toxemia.

FOR FURTHER INFORMATION:

Biddle, Wayne. *Field Guide to Germs.* New York: Henry Holt, 1995.

Finegold, Sydney M., and William J. Martin. *Bailey and Scott's Diagnostic Microbiology.* 6th ed. St. Louis, Mo.: C. V. Mosby, 1998.

Joklik, Wolfgang K., and Hilda P. Willett, eds. *Zinsser: Microbiology.* 20th ed. East Norwalk, Conn.: Appleton and Lange, 1992.

Pelczar, Michael J., Jr., E. C. S. Chan, and Noel R. Krieg. *Microbiology.* 5th ed. New York: McGraw-Hill, 1986.

Stem cell research

Procedure

Anatomy or system affected: All

Specialties and related fields: Biochemistry, biotechnology, cardiology, cytology, embryology, endocrinology, ethics, genetics, hematology, immunology, neurology, oncology, pulmonary medicine, vascular medicine

Definition: Stem cells are unspecialized cells derived from embryos, fetuses, or adults that retain the capacity to develop into specialized cells and regenerate themselves. Scientists manipulate and study stem cells in the hopes of using these cells to cure diseases.

Key terms:

cell: the fundamental unit of a living organism

differentiation: the process by which unspecialized cells develop into cells with highly specific form and functions

multipotent: referring to stem cells derived from adults that may develop into one specific type of tissue

pluripotent: referring to stem cells that have the capacity to develop into most of the specialized tissues of the body, but not an entire individual

tissue: specialized cells organized to form a specific function; tissue is further organized into organs

Indications and Procedures

Stem cells are unspecialized cells that develop into the specialized tissues and organs of the body. An egg fertilized by a sperm is a totipotent stem cell, in that this single cell will develop into all the specialized structures that make up an individual. Stem cells found in human embryos are pluripotent because they can develop into most, but not all, of the specialized structures needed for the embryo to develop into an adult. Embryonic stem cells do not form the placenta, a structure necessary for an embryo to develop into an independently living individual. Adults also harbor several types of stem cells. These adult cells continually regenerate themselves, as well as differentiate into a specific tissue. For example, skin stem cells are constantly differentiating into mature skin cells, intestinal stem cells continuously regenerate the lining of the intestines, and hematopoetic (blood) stem cells provide the diverse array of cells found in blood.

Because of their capacity to regenerate themselves and their ability to differentiate into specific tissue types, scientists are isolating and studying stem cells in the hope of understanding diseases such as cancer, as well as using stem cells as potential treatments for a host of diseases. Embryonic stem cells are isolated from one of two sources: embryos donated with informed consent by couples who have undergone in vitro fertilization, that are in excess of their fertility needs and would otherwise be destroyed or unused, or fetal tissue available from pregnancies terminated before the first trimester, again with informed consent.

Uses and Complications

By studying the processes by which stem cells differentiate into specific cell types, scientists will gain a greater understanding of normal cell development. Understanding normal development will provide insight into the mechanisms of abnormal growth and development, such as the cellular basis of cancer and birth defects. This understanding may lead to the discovery of new ways to prevent and treat these disorders.

Stem cell cultures will also be useful in pharmaceutical development. During their development, new drugs could be tested for both beneficial and toxic effects in stem cell cultures, thus reducing the numbers of animals used in testing and the number of human clinical trials needed, speeding the drug to market for general use.

The third and most exciting use of pluripotent stem cells would be in the direct treatment of disease. For example, heart muscle cells grown from human stem cells could be transplanted into a failing heart to assist in heart function. In Type I diabetes, the islet cells of the pancreas are disrupted, producing less insulin than is needed by the body. If stem cells are directed to form islet cells, the newly formed, healthy islet cells, when introduced into the pancreas, would potentially cure the diabetes. Many other types of tissues potentially could be generated and used to cure disease, such as neurons to cure Parkinson's disease and other neurological disorders, skin cells to heal burns, and blood cells to cure blood disorders.

Potentially, stem cells could be manipulated so that the surface markers are hidden, and the cells would not be rejected as "nonself" when transplanted into a person. Alternatively, adult human stem cells isolated from a patient could differentiate into a needed cell type that is genetically identical to the patient, thus eliminating the possibility of rejection when the cells are transplanted.

PERSPECTIVE AND PROSPECTS

Much of what is known about stem cells has been derived from studies on mouse embryonic stem cells. In 1981, researchers first isolated stem cells from mouse embryos, grew the cells in cultures, and treated them with various growth factors to stimulate development of a particular cell type. For example, cells treated with a vitamin A derivative differentiated into nerve cells. All types of blood cells and cardiac (heart) cells have been generated in similar fashions, and in 2000 scientists from StemCells, Inc., produced mature liver cells from hematopoetic stem cells of mice.

In November, 2000, neuroscientists at The Johns Hopkins University announced the successful reversal of paralysis in rats and mice by injecting them with embryonic stem cells. The stem cells migrated to a region of the spinal cord which contains motor nerve cells. Half of the rats regained movement in their hind feet. Researchers feel that this is a first step in curing human neurological disorders such as amyotrophic lateral sclerosis (Lou Gehrig's disease) and spinal muscular atrophy.

Human pluripotent stem cells were isolated for the first time by scientists Michael Shamblott and James Thomson, working independently, in early 1998. In 2000, scientists were successful in isolating stem cells from human cadavers and directing their development from bone marrow stem cells into nerve cells. Also in 2000, it was reported that bone marrow stem cells from patients with the autoimmune disease lupus were reinserted into their bone marrow after their existing immune cells were neutralized. Six of the seven patients appeared to be cured.

In April, 2001, a study published in the journal *Tissue Engineering* reported that researchers working with human fat extracted by liposuction from patients' hips and thighs were able to create different cell types. The team processed the fat to leave behind a mixed population of cells that could multiply and replenish itself in the laboratory for at least a year. This cell population had the ability to produce muscle, cartilage, bone, or fat cells, depending on the chemicals added. The scientists did not show that all these cell types developed from the same precursor cell; each type may have emerged from its own precursor cell

instead of from a common primordial fat stem cell.

Research on stem cells provides a powerful promise of cures for currently intractable diseases by replacing worn, diseased tissue with healthy tissue generated from stem cells.

—*Karen E. Kalumuck, Ph.D.*

See also Abortion; Amyotrophic lateral sclerosis; Animal rights vs. research; Autoimmune disorders; Cells; Clinical trials; Diabetes mellitus; Embryology; Ethics; Fetal tissue transplantation; In vitro fertilization; Lupus erythematosus; Paralysis; Spinal cord disorders; Transplantation.

FOR FURTHER INFORMATION:

Campbell, Neil A., Jane B. Reece, and Laurence G. Mitchell. *Biology.* 5th ed. Menlo Park, Calif.: Benjamin-Cummings, 1999.
Pedersen, Roger A. "Embryonic Stem Cells for Medicine." *Scientific American* 280, no. 4 (April, 1999): 68-73.
Quesenberry, Peter J., et al., eds. *Stem Cell Biology and Gene Therapy.* New York: Wiley-Liss, 1998.
Thomson, James, et al. "Embryonic Stem Cell Lines Derived from Human Blastocysts." *Science* 282 (November 6, 1998): 1145-1147.
Zuk, Patricia A., and Min Zhu et al. "Multilineage Cells from Human Adipose Tissue: Implications for Cell-Based Therapies." *Tissue Engineering* 7, no. 2 (2001): 211-228.

STERILIZATION

PROCEDURE

ANATOMY OR SYSTEM AFFECTED: Abdomen, genitals, reproductive system, uterus
SPECIALTIES AND RELATED FIELDS: Family practice, general surgery, gynecology, urology
DEFINITION: The surgical prevention of pregnancy, as performed on males through the cutting of the vas deferens (vasectomy) or on females through the blockage or cutting of the Fallopian tubes, the removal of the ovaries, or the removal of the uterus (hysterectomy).

KEY TERMS:

contraception: the prevention of pregnancy
corpus luteum: a yellow cell mass produced from a graafian follicle after the release of an egg
endometriosis: a disease of the female reproductive system that occurs when cells of the uterine lining (endometrium) grow outside the uterus and cause severe pain

Fallopian tubes: the two tubes that connect the ovaries to the uterus and through which an egg travels during ovulation

graafian follicle: any of the ovarian follicles that produce eggs

hormone: a substance made by a body organ and carried through the blood to a second (or target) organ in order to optimize the operation of that target organ

hysterectomy: a surgery that removes part or all of the uterus

laparoscopy: a surgical procedure in which a small incision is made near the navel and the organs of the abdominal cavity, including the uterus and Fallopian tubes, are viewed with a lighted tube called a laparoscope

ovariectomy: the removal of the ovaries

peritoneal cavity: the abdominal cavity that contains the visceral organs

INDICATIONS AND PROCEDURES

Sterilization, of either a woman or a man, is a permanent method of surgical contraception that is used to render a couple incapable of conceiving children. Female sterilization involves the blockage or removal of the Fallopian tubes, the ovaries, or the uterus. Male sterilization involves the interruption of the vas deferens, the pathway of sperm from the testicles. The vas deferens may be reconnected, while many of the sterilization procedures performed on women are considered irreversible. Although the most frequently utilized types of female sterilization possess the potential for reversal at a later date, attempted reversals are often unsuccessful. Therefore, a woman choosing this type of contraception should be quite sure that she does not want another child.

Far more women than men choose to be sterilized. In 1993, it was estimated that more than one hundred million women had elected to be sterilized, worldwide, and that more than one million American women elected to be sterilized each year. One reason that female sterilization is a popular form of contraception with women is because it represents a one-time effort that is usually both simple and the cause of only mild side effects. Another advantage of sterilization over the use of birth control pills is its high success rate: Less than a tenth as many sterilized women will become pregnant (as a result of improperly performed or incomplete procedures) as will women who rely on birth control pills for their con-

traception. The use of condoms, diaphragms, and all the other manual pregnancy prevention devices are even less effective than birth control pills.

Before considering the various aspects of sterilization, it is useful to describe the female reproductive system and its biological operation. This organ system consists of two ovaries connected to paired Fallopian tubes that open up into the uterus. The entire system passes through a monthly menstrual cycle that is controlled by the female hormones progesterone and the estrogens. During each menstrual cycle, an ovary produces one egg (sometimes more) in a graafian follicle. The egg then enters one of the Fallopian tubes, which carries it to the uterus. If an egg is fertilized, it then implants in the endometrial tissue that lines the interior of the uterus and subsequently develops into an embryo.

Egg formation and uterus preparation for implantation are controlled by the female hormones. Once an egg implants, the uterus is kept in a state that optimizes pregnancy with the production of progesterone and related hormones, first by the corpus luteum (originally the graafian follicle that yielded the egg) and then by the placenta that forms from commingled uterine and fetal tissue. In the absence of fertilization, the menstrual cycle continues, most of the endometrium breaks down into the monthly menstrual flow, and the process begins over again.

Menstruation stops between forty-five and fifty-five years of age in most women, causing them to undergo a process called the menopause. After hundreds of repeated menstrual cycles since puberty, the graafian follicles stop producing eggs. Cessation of the menstrual cycle means that female hormone production stops almost entirely. Therefore, the menopause is accompanied by gradual atrophy of the sex organs and possible related symptoms, including hot flashes, depression, and irritability. When ovariectomy or hysterectomy is performed to achieve sterilization, these symptoms of the menopause may be induced prematurely.

For pregnancy to occur, then, a woman must have at least one functional ovary that produces eggs, an intact and operational Fallopian tube to transport the egg, and a functional uterus. The surgical methods that are used for sterilization must, therefore, make one of these reproductive organs nonfunctional. Most often, sterilization cuts and then blocks or removes the Fallopian tubes. Such interruption of the Fallopian tubes is the preferred form of female sterilization surgery for three reasons. First, these operations are relatively minor surgical procedures and are unlikely to be very risky. In addition, premature menopausal symptoms are not produced because the menstrual cycle continues. Finally, when carried out appropriately, interruption of the Fallopian tubes can sometimes be reversed if the patient changes her mind as a result of altered marital arrangements, lifestyle, or financial circumstances.

In many cases, a 1-centimeter to 1.5-centimeter section in the middle of each Fallopian tube is removed surgically or burned away via electrocoagulation. Alternatively, plastic or metal clips are used to close off each tube, or similar tube closure is effected by making a loop in each Fallopian tube and closing it off with a tight plastic ring or band.

Very frequently, the method that is used to damage the Fallopian tubes is a form of surgery called a laparoscopic procedure. The patient is given a general anesthetic, a very small incision is made close to the navel, and a flexible lighted tube—a laparoscope—is inserted into the incision. The laparoscope is equipped with fiber optics and enables an examining physician to see into the abdominal (peritoneal) cavity. Visibility of the Fallopian tubes and the other abdominal organs with laparoscopic examination is enhanced by pumping harmless carbon dioxide gas or nitrous oxide gas into the abdomen, to distend it. This process is called pneumoperitoneum.

After laparoscopic examination identifies the operation site in the peritoneal cavity, the surgical tools for cauterization, cutting, banding, and other aspects of interrupting the Fallopian tubes are passed through the laparoscope, and the chosen surgical interruption procedure is carried out. An entire laparoscopic procedure often takes less than thirty minutes, which is one of the reasons for its great popularity. In addition, women who choose to undergo such surgery can usually go home in a few hours and are fully recovered after only one to two days of postoperative bed rest, followed by a week or so of curtailed physical and sexual activity.

Despite the popularity of the laparoscopic procedure for sterilization, some physicians prefer to carry out sterilization by use of a larger surgical incision through which the tubes are altered directly. Despite the larger size of the incision, the physicians who use this method believe that it is safer and more sure of success and that it has a greater potential for reversibility.

Other methods for sterilization through Fallopian tube surgery are culdoscopy and chemical means. Culdoscopy, in which an optical instrument and surgical tools reach the Fallopian tubes through the uterus, has a somewhat lower success rate than do the laparoscopic procedure and the direct method. Chemical methods for tubal closure have also been attempted and are not viewed as viable because of a low success rate and frequent, serious postoperative complications.

The other avenues available for sterilization are ovariectomy (removal of the ovaries) and hysterectomy (removal of the uterus). Both of these types of sterilization surgery are much more serious and risky. In addition, ovariectomy and hysterectomy are totally irreversible. Ovariectomy, a more complicated procedure than the one inactivating the Fallopian tubes, is usually utilized only when both ovaries are diseased. This procedure produces an early menopause because most of a woman's female hormones are made by the ovaries' graafian follicles.

Hysterectomy is the most uncommon form of female sterilization because it requires even more extensive surgery and can have fatal complications. While the operation is sometimes carried out when a woman has completed her desired family, most hysterectomies are curative. They are performed in cases of very severe and widespread endometriosis and in the presence of other serious gynecological problems.

An alternative available to couples is sterilization of the male partner. This type of surgery, a vasectomy, is quite simple, brief, and relatively painless and only rarely results in physical or psychological complications. In addition, after vasectomy only one-tenth of a percent of involved couples experience undesired pregnancies. Vasectomy has no effect on sexual desire or male hormone production. It is also relatively easy to reverse such surgery, if so desired later in life. Consequently, the method has become quite popular. In the United States, for example, it was estimated in 1993 that 250,000 to 350,000 men would undergo this sterilization surgery each year.

Vasectomy involves the surgical interruption of the tube—the vas deferens—through which sperm leave the testicle. Vasectomy is carried out after identifying the position of each tube and injecting it with a local anesthetic. A 1-inch-long incision is made in the scrotum, each tube is cut near its middle, a small piece of the tube is removed to keep the cut ends apart, and all the ends are closed with sutures, by cauterization, or with metal or plastic clips.

Vasectomy has a short recovery period and does not stop ejaculation during postoperative intercourse. It is important to note, however, that azoospermia (a lack of sperm in the ejaculate) is achieved only after six to fifteen postoperative ejaculations. Therefore, to ensure sterility, it is critical that the condition of azoospermia has been achieved before the patient carries out intercourse without using condoms or other protective measures. After two consecutive sperm counts indicate azoospermia, unprotected intercourse is deemed safe.

USES AND COMPLICATIONS

The most popular method of female sterilization is to block or damage both Fallopian tubes so that eggs cannot pass through them to the uterus. In some cases, the tubes are removed completely. While removal ensures successful sterilization, it is irreversible and considered too drastic by women who might someday wish to reverse the operation. Several popular alternatives to removal are the methods that interrupt the tubes, retaining the potential for reversal at a later date. Women undergoing this type of surgery are warned, however, that such reversal may be impossible.

When the Fallopian tubes are damaged but not entirely closed off, they may reconnect and cause an ectopic pregnancy, in which a fertilized egg implants in one of the tubes and begins to grow into a fetus. Ectopic pregnancy can be fatal to the pregnant woman, and when identified, it is corrected by surgical removal of the fetus. Although the cause of this problem is not clear, there is some thought that alteration of the interior wall of the tube or slowed passage of an egg through the tube may be the causative agent. Fortunately, ectopic pregnancy is relatively uncommon.

Whether the laparoscopic method or the direct approach is utilized, the best time to carry out female sterilization is at the end of a menstrual cycle; at this time, early pregnancies cannot be compromised. It is advised that the patient discontinue intercourse and the use of birth control pills for at least a month prior to the surgery. The cessation of intercourse eliminates the chance of unexpected pregnancy at the time of surgery, while stopping the use of birth control pills decreases the possibility of blood-clotting problems.

The complications of all types of Fallopian tube surgery can include internal bleeding, blood-clotting problems, injury to the intestines and the other abdominal organs, and abnormal postoperative menstrual cycles. It is estimated, however, that these complications occur in less than 1 percent of patients. A more frequent problem is the difficulty of restoring fertility by reconnecting the Fallopian tubes (with only a 20 to 40 percent success rate).

Hysterectomy is never a highly recommended female sterilization operation. Rather, it is used mostly in those cases where other uterine health problems are sufficiently severe to make the process sensible. These problems may include recurrent and heavy vaginal bleeding, severe endometriosis, and chronic pelvic inflammatory disease (PID). This extensive surgery results in a high rate of complications and a significant number of deaths.

A woman may seek sterilization when she is having an abortion or soon after giving birth to an undesired child. Such a decision, perhaps made hastily at a time of intense emotional stress, is not advisable. It is essential that a sterilization operation be performed only after careful reflection. Divorce or the death of a spouse and subsequent remarriage may cause a sterilized woman regret should she desire more children.

Severe psychological problems for both the patient and her family may accompany female sterilization. Therefore, it is highly recommended that these women, their families, and both partners in married couples consult a gynecologist and a psychological counselor before proceeding with female sterilization surgery.

In contrast to the complications associated with female sterilization, with vasectomy a day of bed rest and a week of avoidance of all strenuous physical activity usually produce complete recovery. Health complications occur in less than 5 percent of vasectomy patients. In addition, these problems are usually minor and almost never lead to fatalities. Skin discoloration, swelling, and oozing of clear fluid from the scrotum incision are common symptoms immediately following the surgery, but they spontaneously disappear as the healing process continues. Less frequently, inflammation and a condition called sperm granuloma can occur when sperm leak out of the cut portion of the vas deferens closest to the testicle. A granuloma produces severe inflammation, pain, and swelling. When this condition does not subside spontaneously, the granuloma must be removed surgically.

PERSPECTIVE AND PROSPECTS

While surgical sterilization was first described in the nineteenth century, it was not widely available for contraception until the 1920's, nor did it become popular immediately. Though voluntary sterilization began slowly in the 1950's, its use accelerated until it became a popular form of fertility control in the industrial and developing nations of the 1970's.

A source of discontent with the sterilization techniques that are available is their total or poor reversibility when fertility reinitiation is desired later in life. This discontent has occurred because, with passing time, an unexpectedly large segment of sterilized men and women have come to regret their decisions regarding sterilization. All hysterectomies and Fallopian tube removals are forever irreversible, and a low reversibility rate is seen even in the two most popular—and potentially reversible—sterilization methodologies: Fallopian tube interruption and vasectomy.

Consequently, the development of sterilization surgery has been directed toward devising methods that will enable much larger incidences of reversibility, where desired. One direction has been to expand the understanding of Fallopian tube and vas deferens anatomy and functionality. Particularly useful results obtained include the realization that destruction of the nerves that control the operation of these organs can make the recovery of fertility incomplete or impossible even when excellent corrective surgery reverses the original interruption of continuity. This discovery has led to the development of more sophisticated interruption surgery that is less likely to damage the vas deferens or Fallopian tube nerve integrity. Some improvement of the reversibility of these operations has been obtained in this manner, but the overall results are still far from satisfactory.

Consequently, many other surgical techniques have been attempted, including the placement of removable plugs in the Fallopian tubes or of tiny, faucetlike valves in the vas deferens that allow or stop the ejaculation of sperm. Other useful methods to ensure reversible sterilization may include hormones, vaccines against eggs and sperm, and chemical treatments. It is hoped that improved antifertility methodologies will be developed that combine more reversible surgical sterilization, vaccines, chemicals, and various contraceptives.

—*Sanford S. Singer, Ph.D.*

See also Conception; Contraception; Estrogen replacement therapy; Gynecology; Hormone replacement therapy; Hysterectomy; Laparoscopy; Menopause; Menstruation; Pregnancy and gestation; Reproductive system; Tubal ligation; Vasectomy.

FOR FURTHER INFORMATION:

Harper, Michael J. K. *Birth Control Technologies: Prospects by the Year 2000.* Austin: University of Texas Press, 1983. This text, written by a physician, is valuable to the general reader because of its many useful topics and references. The chapter on sterilization delineates facts and figures about complications and various surgical techniques that are unavailable in other sources.

Mastroianni, Luigi, Jr., Peter J. Donaldson, and Thomas T. Kane. *Developing New Contraceptives: Obstacles and Opportunities.* Washington, D.C.: National Academy Press, 1990. This book on contraceptive measures other than sterilization by surgery also contains considerable useful information on sterilization practices and legalities. Provides useful insights and allows the reader to consider other effective, long-term methods of contraception, excluding surgery.

Sherwood, Lauralee. *Human Physiology: From Cells to Systems.* 4th ed. Belmont, Calif.: Wadsworth, 2001. This college text provides details about the menstrual cycle, hormones, and the endometrium. Many useful definitions, diagrams, and glossary terms are included.

Van Keep, Pieter A., Kenneth E. Davis, and David de Wied, eds. *Contraception in the Year 2001.* New York: Elsevier Science, 1987. This conference proceeding covers many important issues in fertility control. Included are demographics of contraception need; a discussion of male and female contraception via hormones, vaccine sterilization, and mechanical methods; and predictions for the future.

Wigfall-Williams, Wanda. *Hysterectomy: Learning the Facts, Coping with the Feelings, and Facing the Future.* New York: Michael Kesend, 1986. Discusses sterilization as a motive for hysterectomy, in addition to severe endometriosis. Offers guidelines for the choice of a physician or surgical procedure and explores possible aftereffects, such as depression and changes in sexual function.

STEROID ABUSE
DISEASE/DISORDER

ANATOMY OR SYSTEM AFFECTED: Circulatory system, endocrine system, heart, muscles, psychic-emotional system, reproductive system

SPECIALTIES AND RELATED FIELDS: Exercise physiology, psychiatry, psychology, sports medicine

DEFINITION: The use of illegal anabolic steroids to

increase athletic performance, with negative side effects on physical and psychological health.

CAUSES AND SYMPTOMS

Steroids provide many valuable medical benefits for conditions such as asthma, spastic colon, and other common medical conditions. Unfortunately, however, steroid abuse, particularly of anabolic steroids, continues to be an important problem.

A lack of social acceptability around steroid abuse has resulted partially from the more than seventy side effects associated with steroid use, including such immediate problems as rage, depression, and highly aggressive behavior. Reports have included findings of teenagers committing acts as brutal as murder, without any prior history of criminal or aggressive behavior, while under the influence of steroids. While such acts are rare, the connection between steroids and out-of-control rage is well known. In addition, steroid abuse has been linked with such long-term problems as heart attacks, strokes, and changes in the reproductive system. It is likely that increasing attention will be focused on these kinds of long-term effects, both in research and in terms of problem reporting. Increases in the access to anabolic steroids are also partly responsible for an increase in the visibility of and attention to such problems.

Social research also has demonstrated important findings related to steroid use in college students and in athletes. One study, for example, demonstrated that college students consistently rated anabolic steroid-using athletes more negatively than drug-free athletes. In fact, students tended to evaluate anabolic steroid-using athletes just as negatively as they would an athlete who was using cocaine. In another study, researchers demonstrated that steroid use is not only physically reinforcing but also psychologically reinforcing. Specifically, in interviews with thirty-five male self-reported anabolic steroid users, lower levels of anxiety related to the perception of one's physique and higher levels of satisfaction with one's upper body were demonstrated, relative to the control subjects. There was a psychological gain associated with the steroid use that was directly related to the shorter-term physical benefits of their use.

PERSPECTIVE AND PROSPECTS

Recent estimates suggest that about 1.1 percent of college athletes are using anabolic steroids. A 1997 report by the National Collegiate Athletic Association (NCAA) demonstrated that this was a decrease from the 4.9 percent of student athletes who reported using steroids in 1989. Nationwide, according to the NCAA, collegiate football players were reported to have the highest rate of use, at 2.2 percent. The survey suggested, however, that this lowered rate may reflect underreporting. Factors such as the illegality of the drug use or a lack of social acceptability in acknowledging such personal behavior may be responsible. Such assertions of underreporting also are based on other reports that 5 to 12 percent of male high school students and 1 percent of female high school students have used anabolic steroids. Further, among athletes not in college, reported rates are much higher. Ninety-five percent of weight lifters report use, followed by 99 percent of power lifters, 80 percent of track-and-field athletes, 70 percent of football players, and 40 percent of sprinters.

Future work in this area will likely explore these psychological factors and focus on how to intervene effectively. Additionally, it is likely that social interventions will be explored. Athletics remains competitive and financially lucrative, so special attention will need to be paid to the social context in which steroid abuse occurs.

—*Nancy A. Piotrowski, Ph.D.*

See also Addiction; Exercise physiology; Hormones; Hypertrophy; Muscles; Psychiatry, child and adolescent; Puberty and adolescence; Sports medicine; Steroids.

FOR FURTHER INFORMATION:

Craig, Charles R., and Robert E. Stitzel. *Modern Pharmacology.* 5th ed. Boston: Little, Brown, 1997.

Lin, Geraline C., and Lynda Erinoff, eds. *Anabolic Steroid Abuse.* Rockville, Md.: U.S. Department of Health and Human Services, Public Health Service, Alcohol, Drug Abuse, and Mental Health Administration, National Institute on Drug Abuse, 1990.

Wilson, Jean D., and Daniel W. Foster. *Williams Textbook of Endocrinology.* 9th ed. Philadelphia: W. B. Saunders, 1998.

STEROIDS

BIOLOGY

ANATOMY OR SYSTEM AFFECTED: Endocrine system, glands

SPECIALTIES AND RELATED FIELDS: Biochemistry, endocrinology, pediatrics, pharmacology, sports medicine

DEFINITION: Organic compounds, both natural and synthetic, that enhance specific activities of the body and that can be used as therapeutic agents in the treatment of many clinical disorders.

KEY TERMS:

anabolic steroids: a class of steroids that stimulate body reactions to build up more complex molecules and structures from simpler molecules; most are synthetic derivatives of testosterone

cholesterol: a fatlike steroid alcohol that is found in animal fats, oils, and tissues; most of the body's supply is manufactured in the liver, while some is absorbed from the diet

corticosteroids: the group of steroid hormones produced by the adrenal cortex, which includes the classes of mineralocorticoids, glucocorticoids, and sex steroids

glucocorticoids: steroid hormones that regulate the metabolism of glucose and other organic molecules

mineralocorticoids: steroid hormones that regulate the body levels of sodium and potassium

sex steroids: steroid hormones such as androgens and estrogens that influence the activity of sexual organs and activity

steroid nucleus: the molecular arrangement of four carbon rings that makes up the backbone of all steroids

sterol: a steroid that has long side chains of carbon compounds attached to it and contains at least one hydroxyl group; cholesterol is one type of sterol

STRUCTURE AND FUNCTIONS

Steroids are a group of organic compounds that are distinguished by a unique molecular arrangement of seventeen carbon atoms situated in four adjacent rings. This set of four rings is referred to as the steroid nucleus and is common to all steroid compounds. Three of these rings are hexagonal six-carbon rings arranged in a bent-line fashion to form what is called a phenanthrene group. The fourth group or ring contains only five carbon atoms. Steroids vary with the nature of the attached groups, the position of a given attached group, or some alteration to the configuration of the steroid nucleus. Small chemical differences in the structure of steroids can reflect very great differences in specific biological effects. Steroids are included in the lipid category of biological molecules because they are nonpolar and insoluble in water.

Any steroid that contains a hydroxyl group (-OH) is called a sterol. This term comes from a Greek word meaning "solid"; sterols were so named because they were among the earliest compounds that were found to be solid at room temperature. Once chemical structures were determined, then other compounds with similar structures were given the name steroid, which means "sterol-like." The suffix "-oid" comes from the Greek and means "similar to."

Chemists have isolated hundreds of different steroids from plants and animals; additionally, thousands have been made by chemically modifying natural steroids or by synthesizing the entire molecule. The parent compound for steroids is acetic acid. Assisted by a variety of enzymes, acetic acid is altered and transformed into several other compounds before cholesterol is formed. Cholesterol serves as the parent, or precursor compound, for bile acids and for the steroids that are biologically important to the body.

Cholesterol is the most common steroid in the human body, as it is a structural component of cellular membranes. The prefix "chole-" comes from the Greek word for liver bile, which is a digestive fluid manufactured by the liver and secreted into the intestines. The name is appropriate since the bile contains a considerable amount of cholesterol. Bile is stored in the gallbladder and becomes concentrated there. Cholesterol is not very soluble, and if it accumulates in great enough quantities, it will form small crystals in the bile. These crystals may join together to form larger particles that can block the narrow duct that leads from the gallbladder to the intestines. These aggregations of particles are called gallstones and are composed of almost pure cholesterol. The blockage can result in a buildup of pressure and cause much pain. Often, a surgical operation is required to remove the obstruction.

Cholesterol is also an important molecule because it is the precursor or parent molecule for the steroid hormones produced by the gonads and the adrenal cortex. The gonads, a collective term referring to the testes and ovaries, secrete the sex steroids. These sex steroids include estradiol and progesterone from the ovaries and testosterone from the testes. The adrenal cortex secretes the corticosteroids, which include cortisol and aldosterone as well as other steroid compounds. Most of the steroid hormones are specialized in their function and do not produce general effects on metabolism. The sex hormones influence reproduction by acting on sexual organs to stimulate their development and function, by influencing sexual behavior, and by stimulating the development of secondary sex characteristics. Some of the steroids secreted by the adrenal cortex have more general effects on the metabolism of carbohydrates and proteins in many tissues.

Steroid hormones combine with specific receptors that are located in the cytoplasm of the responsive tissues. Since these hormones are lipid-soluble, they pass readily through cell membranes, which are largely composed of lipids. Inside the cytoplasm, a steroid-specific protein receptor will bind to the hormone. Upon binding, the hormone-receptor complex becomes activated or transformed and is then translocated to the nucleus. In the nucleus, the activated steroid receptor complex binds to the chromatin, or genetic material, causing an activation of a certain set of genes. Gene activation results in the production of messenger molecules which induce the production of specific proteins that are either used by the cell or secreted elsewhere.

The steroid hormones of the adrenal cortex fall into three categories, each having separate actions and sites of actions. Aldosterone is the principal mineralocorticoid and plays an important role in regulating body levels of sodium and potassium. Cortisol, the major glucocorticoid, regulates carbohydrate metabolism. Adrenal androgens are also produced, but they have only weak activity and play a minor physiological role under most conditions. All adrenal steroids are derived from cholesterol.

Mineralocorticoids are the adrenal steroids that regulate levels of potassium and sodium in the body. Aldosterone, the most potent mineralocorticoid, is secreted by the adrenal cortex at the rate of about 0.1 milligram per day. Mineralocorticoids affect the distal tubules of the kidney by stimulating the excretion of potassium and the reabsorption of sodium. The net effect of these actions is to increase the volume of body fluids.

Glucocorticoids are the adrenal steroids that regulate glucose metabolism. In humans, cortisol is responsible for most of the glucocorticoid activity. It is secreted by the adrenal cortex at the rate of about 20 milligrams per day and metabolically affects tissues throughout the body. Cortisol is regulated by the central nervous system and by permissive or stimulatory messenger molecules of the body. Generally, glucocorticoids stimulate the production of glucose and enhance the use of fat and protein as energy sources.

Androgens are steroid hormones that are secreted primarily by the testes but also by the adrenal glands and ovaries. Testosterone is the principal androgen that is secreted by the testes; it regulates the development and function of male sex accessory organs. Increased testosterone secretion during puberty is required for the growth of the seminal vesicles and prostate. Removal of androgens by castration results in these organs undergoing atrophy.

Androgens stimulate growth of the larynx and cause lowering of the voice. They increase hemoglobin synthesis, which is higher in males than females, and affect bone growth by causing the conversion of cartilage to bone. Androgens also promote protein synthesis or anabolic activity in skeletal muscle, bone, and kidneys. As a class of compounds, androgens are reasonably safe drugs, since they have a limited and relatively predictable set of side effects. In human males, testosterone is synthesized by the testes at the rate of about 8 milligrams per day.

Estrogens and progesterones are primarily produced in the ovaries of nonpregnant adult women. In pregnancy, the placenta is the major site of estrogen and progesterone production. Smaller amounts of estrogen synthesis involve the liver, kidney, skeletal muscle, and testes. Estrogens cause the growth of the female reproductive organs and are responsible for the expression of female secondary sex characteristics, such as breast enlargement, female body contours, skin texture, and distribution of body hair. Estrogens are thought to protect against atherosclerosis and heart attacks since occurrence of these health problems in mature women is much lower than in males of similar ages.

USES AND COMPLICATIONS

When cortisone was initially discovered, it was labeled a "wonder drug" and was thought to possess widespread effectiveness in many areas of medicine. Although these expectations have not been realized, a variety of steroids are found to be effective in medical practice and treatment. Steroids are commonly prescribed to serve as replacements for those persons whose bodies are unable to produce specific steroid hormones in adequate quantities. Steroids are effective as anti-inflammatory agents, reducing inflammatory reactions in a variety of body tissues. They are also prescribed for patients who have undergone an organ transplantation or have highly sensitive allergies because they inhibit the responsiveness of the immune system.

The primary therapeutic use of androgens is for testicular deficiency in which the induction and maintenance of male secondary sex characteristics are desired. In these cases, supplemental doses of androgens are given to stimulate and enhance the development of sexual and accessory sex characteristics. Androgens are effective also in the therapy of some anemias when persons have reduced levels of red blood cells. Androgens are used to treat osteoporosis, which is a decrease in bone or skeletal mass. Androgens are given to women in the treatment of breast cancer and are effective about 20 percent of the time. They are used to treat the abnormal growth of endometrial tissue in the peritoneal cavity of women, a disease called endometriosis, and are effective in that role.

Steroids also have anabolic activities that are manifested by stimulating increases in protein production, by enhancing the uptake of amino acids into cells, and by inhibiting the glucocorticoids from breaking down proteins. They influence embryonic development, especially the differentiation of the central nervous system and the male reproductive tract. The excitatory function of androgens occurs at puberty, during which the reproductive organs are activated to produce sex cells. Androgens also maintain the body's sexual characteristics in the adult. Thus, in cases of androgen deficiency there is a regression of male sexual behavior, libido, and reproductive function; this regression is reversible with treatment.

It should be noted that anabolic steroids are frequently abused because of these kinds of effects. Athletes and body builders in search of accelerated muscle building or physical definition are two groups in which such abuse has been seen. A complication has been that the stimulatory effects of the anabolic steroids make the drug administrations reinforcing and therefore loaded with addiction potential. As such, frequent users of anabolic steroids should be aware of conditions such as dependence, as well as withdrawal and other problematic side effects of heavy steroid use. Such effects may include increased periods of sleep disturbance, paranoia, anger and agitation, mood swings or instability of mood, violence or other impulsive behavior, and concentration and memory disturbance. Physical problems may include severe acne, jaundice, excess water retention, decreased sperm count, high cholesterol, liver problems, and difficulty with blood sugar control.

Addison's disease is caused by a failure of the adrenal gland to secrete adequate amounts of both glucocorticoids and mineralocorticoids. The symptoms of this disease are imbalances of body levels of sodium and potassium, dehydration, reduced blood pressure, rapid weight loss, and generalized weakness. A person with Addison's disease will die if not treated with corticosteroids because of the severe electrolyte imbalance and dehydration.

Cushing's syndrome results when the adrenal gland secretes corticosteroids in excessive quantities. Symptoms include high blood pressure, alterations in protein and carbohydrate metabolism, high blood sugar concentrations, and muscular weakness. This syndrome is often caused by a tumor in the adrenal gland that promotes the secretion of corticosteroids. Surgical intervention is often used to remove the portion of the gland that is malfunctioning. Symptoms similar to those seen in Cushing's syndrome are found in people with inflammatory diseases who receive lengthy treatments with corticosteroids in order to reduce the inflammation.

Adrenogenital syndrome results from an excessive level of sex steroids, usually caused by hyperactivity of the adrenal gland. Androgen is the major sex steroid involved in this clinical condition, which causes a premature puberty and enlarged genital sex organs when it occurs in young children. Other characteristics are increased amounts of body and facial hair as well as deepening of the voice.

The greatest use of estrogens as therapeutic agents is in oral contraception, or "the pill." This method is convenient, reversible, and relatively inexpensive; its use is worldwide and includes 25 percent of American women of childbearing age. Most oral contraceptives are active combinations of estrogen and progesterone. Users take a daily pill containing both steroids for twenty or twenty-one days of the menstrual cycle and then a placebo for seven or eight days. Withdrawal bleeding occurs two to three days after discontinuing the pill. The mechanism for the effectiveness of these steroids involves inhibiting the release of hormones that would normally stimulate ovulation.

Antiandrogens are substances that prevent or depress the action of androgens, or testosterone, on the body. They are of value in the management of patients whose bodies are producing abnormally high levels of androgens, who are undergoing a premature puberty, or who are affected with acne, hirsutism (excessive hairiness, especially in women), and certain tumors or neoplasms. Potentially, these drugs can be utilized to cause sterility in males.

Natural body androgens stimulate the growth of the prostate gland in males and enhance the proliferation of many prostate cancers. Treatment of abnormal growths, malignant cancers, or benign tumors in the male prostate gland has frequently used either natural or synthetic steroids. Estradiol, a form of the female sex steroid estrogen, is used to control the advancement of prostate carcinoma in some males and can induce remission in 50 to 80 percent of the cases of prostate tumors. Estrogens exert their effect by interfering with androgen production or by inhibiting the function of androgen-responsive tissues. Thus in some cases estrogens inhibit abnormal cellular growth. A manufactured synthetic drug, cyproterone acetate, is also used in the treatment of benign prostatic enlargement in men. Cyproterone acetate is very effective in treating prostate cancers and tumors, and it does not have the feminizing side effects of the estrogens; however, it does cause inhibition of sperm production and loss of sexual drive.

Perspective and Prospects

The use of steroids as therapeutic agents began in the early 1930's. At that time, Philip Showalter Hench, who was working in the Mayo Clinic, noticed that the symptoms of arthritic women were alleviated when they became pregnant. He suggested that increased secretions from the adrenal cortex may be the responsible agents. Later, clinical trials were conducted to test the role of corticosteroids in treating acute arthritis. With the use of adequate dosages, the clinical response was impressive. The 1950 Nobel Prize in Physiology or Medicine was awarded to Hench and his coworkers for their finding that cortisone was effective in treating arthritis.

Pharmaceutical firms have manufactured numerous steroid derivatives, all of which have different effectiveness levels as glucocorticoids, mineralocorticoids, or sex steroids. Organic chemists synthesize analogs of adrenal steroids in order to create compounds that produce heightened biological effects with a minimum or lack of side effects. As a consequence, hundreds of different steroids are available. Most of these are characterized according to their biological effectiveness, such as their ability to reduce inflammation or to inhibit the immune system. When determining a course of treatment, a physician chooses a particular steroid that enhances the effects that are desired and has minimal effects in related areas. Some pharmaceutical derivatives of adrenal steroids are very poorly absorbed by the skin. These derivatives are especially useful to apply to the skin when a maximal local effect is desired without a generalized effect on other body regions.

Steroids, however, can also have negative, and sometimes dangerous, effects on the body, whether they are ingested (cholesterol) or injected (anabolic steroids).

Evidence indicates that high blood cholesterol levels are associated with an increased risk of atherosclerosis, a clinical condition in which localized plaques (or atheromas) build up in the walls of arteries, reducing blood flow. Atheromas serve as locations for blood clot formation, which can further block the blood supply to a vital organ such as the heart, brain, or lung. High blood cholesterol may result from a diet rich in cholesterol and saturated fat, or it may result from an inherited condition in which affected individuals have extremely high cholesterol concentrations, regardless of their diet. These persons usually suffer heart attacks during their childhood.

Cholesterol is found in foods that are based on animal products. Cholesterol-rich f.oods include most meats, eggs, and dairy products such as cheese, cream, and butter. Humans readily absorb cholesterol from dietary sources. Most Western diets contain 400 to 600 milligrams of cholesterol per day, of which about 75 percent is readily absorbed into the bloodstream from the dietary tract. Cholesterol is carried to the arteries by proteins in the blood plasma called low-density lipoproteins (LDLs). A given cell may engulf the LDLs and use the cholesterol for different purposes. The LDLs in a given location may stimulate other cells to secrete growth factors that either begin or contribute to the development of an atheroma. Thus the risk of atherosclerosis is greatly increased. Most people can significantly lower their blood cholesterol levels through controlled exercise and diet. Since saturated fat raises blood cholesterol levels, foods such as fatty meat, egg yolk, and liver should be eaten sparingly so that fat contributes less than 30 percent to the total calories of a diet.

The use and abuse of anabolic steroids to increase muscle mass and strength are widespread in both amateur and professional sports. Although those promoting steroid use claim increases in muscle mass, strength, and endurance, controlled clinical trials show minimal, if any, enhancement of muscle mass and strength. Testosterone may also enhance training efforts by promoting aggressive behavior. Use of these compounds poses ethical questions and increases the risk of serious toxicity because of the extremely high doses that are administered, often as much as one hundred times the usual therapeutic dosages.

—Roman J. Miller, Ph.D.;
updated by Nancy A. Piotrowski, Ph.D.

See also Cholesterol; Contraception; Cushing's syndrome; Endocrine disorders; Endocrinology; Endocrinology, pediatric; Estrogen replacement therapy; Glands; Growth; Gynecology; Hormone replacement therapy; Hormones; Hypercholesterolemia; Metabolism; Muscles; Pain management; Pharmacology; Prostate cancer; Prostate gland; Puberty and adolescence; Reproductive system; Sports medicine; Steroid abuse.

FOR FURTHER INFORMATION:

Craig, Charles R., and Robert E. Stitzel. *Modern Pharmacology*. 5th ed. Boston: Little, Brown, 1997. This college-level pharmacology text contains easy-to-comprehend sections on steroids, including their chemistry, synthesis, physiological activity, and pharmacological activity.

Guyton, Arthur C. *Human Physiology and Mechanisms of Disease*. 6th ed. Philadelphia: W. B. Saunders, 1997. Guyton is a nationally recognized authority on medical physiology, having written and edited numerous college-level and medical school textbooks on the subject. His writing style is flowing and understandable to the nonmedical specialist and student.

Montgomery, Rex, Thomas W. Conway, and Arthur A. Spector. *Biochemistry: A Case-Oriented Approach*. 5th ed. St. Louis: Mosby, 1990. Surveys the field of biochemistry, examining steroids and steroid hormones in that context. A major section describes the essential role of cholesterol in the body, as well as in the synthesis of other steroids.

Mulvihill, Mary L. *Human Diseases: A Systemic Approach*. 5th ed. Norwalk, Conn.: Appleton & Lange, 2000. This well-written and interesting book uses a case-oriented approach to explore the essential concepts of physiology and health. Numerous examples of pathologies relating to steroids or steroid hormones are illustrated.

Tortora, Gerard J., and Sandra R. Grabowski. *Principles of Anatomy and Physiology*. 9th ed. New York: John Wiley & Sons, 2000. This popular college-level undergraduate anatomy and physiology text contains well-written sections on major biological

molecules such as steroids, as well as longer sections on steroid hormones and their specific effects.

Wilson, Jean D., and Daniel W. Foster, eds. *Williams Textbook of Endocrinology*. 9th ed. Philadelphia: W. B. Saunders, 1998. The definitive upper-level text that discusses the biological and clinical aspects of endocrinology in detail. Contains several chapters dealing with steroids and steroid hormones.

STILLBIRTH
DISEASE/DISORDER

ANATOMY OR SYSTEM AFFECTED: Psychic-emotional system, reproductive system, uterus

SPECIALTIES AND RELATED FIELDS: Embryology, obstetrics, psychology

DEFINITION: "Stillbirth" is the term used when a fetus has died in the womb and is born after the twenty-eighth week of pregnancy. There are many different causes for stillbirth, ranging from terminal deformities, to maternal disorders, to oxygen deprivation, to infectious diseases contracted by the mother during pregnancy. One-third of stillbirths are of unknown cause. Because of advances in obstetrics and an increased understanding of prenatal care, the occurrence of stillbirth has dramatically decreased since the mid-twentieth century. Parents of a deceased baby often experience depression, guilt, and other feelings associated with the loss. Counseling and the support of friends and family are helpful in parental recovery.

—Jason Georges and Tracy Irons-Georges

See also Birth defects; Childbirth; Childbirth complications; Death and dying; Depression; Ectopic pregnancy; Grief and guilt; Miscarriage; Obstetrics; Postpartum depression; Pregnancy and gestation; Premature birth.

FOR FURTHER INFORMATION:

Douglas, Ann, and John R. Sussman. *Trying Again: A Guide to Pregnancy After Miscarriage, Stillbirth, and Infant Loss*. Dallas, Tex.: Taylor, 2000.

Ewy, Donna Hohmann, and Rodger Frank Ewy. *Death of a Dream: Miscarriage, Stillbirth, and Newborn Loss*. New York: Dutton, 1984.

Gonik, Bernard, and Renee A. Bobrowski. *Medical Complications in Labor and Delivery*. Cambridge, Mass.: Blackwell Scientific, 1996.

Lanham, Carol Cirulli. *Pregnancy After a Loss: A Guide to Pregnancy After Miscarriage, Stillbirth, or Infant Death*. New York: Berkley Books, 1999.

STINGS. *See* BITES AND STINGS.

STOMACH, INTESTINAL, AND PANCREATIC CANCERS

DISEASE/DISORDER

ANATOMY OR SYSTEM AFFECTED: Abdomen, gastrointestinal system, intestines, pancreas, stomach

SPECIALTIES AND RELATED FIELDS: Gastroenterology, immunology, oncology

DEFINITION: Malignant tumors of the small intestine, stomach, or pancreas, the latter two types being difficult to detect and treat.

KEY TERMS:

carcinogen: anything that initiates cancer

endoscope: a long, flexible fiber-optic tube used to examine the gastrointestinal tract; the tube's accessories can also remove tissue or stones

gastric: pertaining to the stomach

jaundice: a yellowing of the skin and eyes from an excess of bile pigment caused by a blocked duct or injured liver

metastasis: the dispersal of cancer cells from a tumor to other parts of the body, where they begin secondary tumors

pancreas: a secretory organ behind the stomach and connected to the duodenum; it produces enzymes to digest food and insulin to metabolize sugar

small intestine: the region of gut between the stomach and the colon that comprises the duodenum, jejunum, and ileum; also called the small bowel

tumor: a mass of new cells growing independent of surrounding tissues; either benign (noncancerous) or malignant (cancerous)

CAUSES AND SYMPTOMS

The section of the gut from the esophageal sphincter in the upper stomach to the ileocecal valve at the end of the small intestine digests food taken into the body and absorbs its nutrients. This vital function also exposes the gut and its organs, the liver and pancreas, to ingested toxins that can initiate cancer and to materials that damage the gut lining, also potentially leading to cancer. Because diet greatly influences the chances for contracting these cancers, it is understandable that stomach cancer is the world's most common type. Surprisingly, however, cancers of the small bowel are rare. Pancreatic cancer is the most lethal of these cancers and one of the most difficult to detect before irreversible damage has been done: Few patients live long after diagnosis. These facts and the large number

of suspected carcinogens make the stomach and pancreatic cancers a pressing challenge for physicians and public health.

Broad similarities characterize the types of cancers throughout the upper gastrointestinal (GI) tract. The majority, adenocarcinomas, grow in and mimic gland tissue, but possible as well are cancers of the lymph tissue (lymphoma), hormone-secreting cells (carcinoid tumors), and the muscle wall of the bowel (sarcoma). Early symptoms tend to be vague and do not necessarily point specifically to cancer: abdominal pain, loss of appetite, weight loss, and perhaps diarrhea or vomiting.

While diet is a major factor in stomach cancer, its role in pancreatic and intestinal cancers is not as clear. A diet consisting mainly of pickled, smoked, or salted food with few fruits and vegetables, especially those containing vitamins A and C, is thought to be risky. In fact, countries with the highest rates of gastric cancer, such as Japan, are those that have long relied on such chemical preservation techniques rather than on refrigeration. It is probably no coincidence that the stomach cancer rate in the United States declined sharply after refrigeration became widespread in the 1930's; moreover, Japanese immigrants to the United States have sharply fewer gastric cancers than do their relatives in the homeland.

The presence of nitrites in the diet, alcohol consumption, radiation exposure, chronic gastritis (inflammation of the stomach lining), and cigarette smoking have also been suspected as gastric carcinogens. Hereditary susceptibility may sometimes play a role, although it is also possible that family members, living under the same conditions, are simply exposed to the same carcinogens and that no genetic susceptibility is involved. Finally, chronic stomach infection with the bacterium *Helicobacter pylori* has been linked to gastric cancer development.

Risk factors for the pancreas and small intestine are much less clear. Chronic pancreatitis, gallstones, and cirrhosis (scarring) of the liver pose some danger of initiating pancreatic cancer, and smokers and diabetics are twice as likely to develop it than others. Chemists and others who work with organic solvents and petrochemicals also run a slightly higher risk. Intestinal cancer becomes more likely after the immune system has been damaged or late in the course of chronic intestinal diseases, such as Crohn's disease and sprue.

Risky foods, diseases, or occupations do not inevitably lead to cancers. Tumor growth requires at least three factors: some agent that initiates a change in a cell's genetic structure so that a new type of cell is created, called a mutation; an agent that enhances the cell's response to the initiator, encouraging it to reproduce; and the failure of the immune system to destroy the abnormal cells. Most small bowel and gastric cancers probably result from long-term overstimulation of the glands or mucosa. This overstimulation occurs when the body fights chemical irritants that have been ingested with food, drink, or air; the body's defense mechanisms lead to inflammation in the damaged area. Chronic inflammation and continually stimulated cell division to repair damage eventually is likely to produce a mutated cell. If adapted to the harsh environment that produced it, the cell can multiply unchecked, overwhelm the immune system, and invade normal tissue; eventually, it may metastasize. A potentially lethal cancer can grow for months or

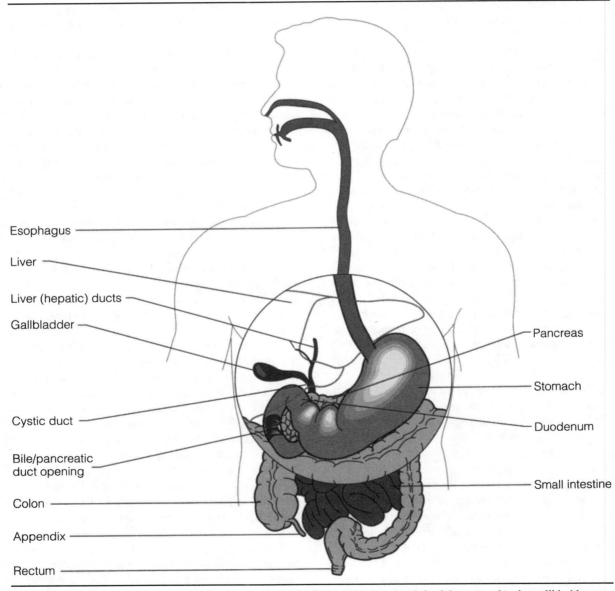

Esophagus

Liver

Liver (hepatic) ducts

Gallbladder

Cystic duct

Bile/pancreatic duct opening

Colon

Appendix

Rectum

Pancreas

Stomach

Duodenum

Small intestine

The magnified section shows the stomach, the pancreas (which lies behind and to left of the stomach), the gallbladder, part of the liver, and the midsection of the large colon.

years before its victim notices any definite changes in particular body functions or general health.

Eventually, however, danger signs begin. After initially complaining of abdominal pain, loss of appetite, and difficulty keeping food down, stomach cancer patients may have black, digested blood in the stool, weight loss, general weakness, bouts of vomiting blood, a swollen abdomen, a noticeable mass in the stomach, and iron-deficiency anemia. When the disease is well advanced, metastases become increasingly common, invading the lymph nodes, bile ducts, and liver and eventually spreading to the lungs, bones, and brain. The cancer becomes symptomatic relatively quickly. On average, patients go to their doctors about six months after noticing symptoms.

Pancreatic cancer is much less likely to cause early symptoms, and by the time patients seek medical help, the cancer is usually too far advanced to cure. Physicians suspect pancreatic adenocarcinoma when a patient complains of food aversion, progressive weight loss, and abdominal and back pain, especially when accompanied by vomiting, diarrhea, and jaundice. A rare form of pancreatic cancer (less than 5 percent of cancers in the pancreas) develops from the insulin-producing cells of the organ and makes abnormally high amounts of insulin; in this case, the symptoms are attributable to low blood sugar (hypoglycemia) and include weakness, loss of energy, dizziness, chills, muscle spasms, double vision, and, in extreme cases, coma.

Adenocarcinomas, lymphomas, carcinoid tumors, and sarcomas may form in the small bowel, and most of these grow slowly. Intestinal adenocarcinomas show up primarily in the jejunum or duodenum of elderly patients. Often, they first become apparent when they clog the bowel or bleed. Usually appearing in the stomach, lower jejunum, or ileum, lymphomas are suspected when the patient has fever, night sweats, weight loss, and abdominal pain. Intestinal carcinoid tumors may actively secrete hormones. If they metastasize, release of the hormones sometimes causes a bizarre group of symptoms that are collectively known as carcinoid syndrome: diarrhea, flushing, itching, low blood pressure, and heart disease. Intestinal sarcomas can occur anywhere in the small bowel and reveal themselves by bleeding.

TREATMENT AND THERAPY

Since other diseases also cause the weight loss, abdominal pain, and nausea common to these cancers—

for example, pancreatitis, malabsorption, inflammatory bowel disease, and gastritis—the diagnosis of cancer requires specific evidence from chemical tests, imaging, endoscopic procedures, or surgery. Suspecting stomach cancer, the physician may send the patient for an upper GI barium study. For this procedure, the patient drinks a mixture containing barium sulfate; the radio-opaque barium coats the stomach and under X-ray photography can be seen to outline a tumor if one is present. Tests to check for anemia and blood in the stool may also be ordered. If imaging and tests support a diagnosis of cancer, a gastroenterologist, inserting an endoscope through the patient's mouth, will obtain biopsies of the tumor so that a pathologist can determine if the tumor is malignant. Since biopsies remove such small samples and can miss a cancerous portion of a tumor (especially a lymphoma or sarcoma), surgical biopsy may be necessary to settle the diagnosis beyond doubt.

Similarly, initial tests for pancreatic and intestinal cancer rely on imaging and chemical assays. A barium X-ray study of the small bowel, a computed tomography (CT) scan, or ultrasonography may locate the tumor. Again, endoscopic or surgical biopsy alone can verify the diagnosis of malignancy. Tumors in the small bowel usually lie beyond the reach of endoscopy, so when a barium study reveals a tumor, surgical biopsy is most often necessary to obtain tissue samples; at the same time, the tumor is usually removed to relieve or prevent obstruction of the bowel.

If a tumor has not spread and is well defined, cutting it out provides the best chance of a cure for cancers throughout the stomach, pancreas, and small bowel. Such surgeries are often technically difficult, however, because the patients are typically malnourished and weak and have difficulty enduring the rigors of surgery. When a stomach tumor is single and small, surgeons remove it and a small margin of tissue around its edges. Larger or multiple tumors force the removal of larger portions of the stomach and adjacent lymph nodes. For pancreatic cancer, if more than a single area of the pancreas is involved, the surgeon may remove the entire organ and, depending on the size and location of the tumor, parts of the duodenum and stomach as well. Cancers of the intestines are cut away along with a section of bowel, whose ends are then reconnected by suturing. Chemotherapy and radiation on their own have not proved reliable for shrinking stomach, pancreatic, and intestinal cancers (except lymphomas) and are usually used in conjunction with surgery, especially when a primary tumor has metastasized.

Sometimes endoscopic maneuvers can stop bleeding or relieve pain by clearing out obstructions or, in the case of an obstructed bile duct, by inserting a small perforated tube called a stent to ensure that bile and pancreatic juices flow freely. Pain management, whether with manipulative procedures or with drugs, becomes the primary focus of treatment when surgical cure for a cancer is unlikely. Surgeons do not attempt curative operations if the cancer has metastasized. At this point, surgery, if possible at all, is for relieving pain, preventing blockage, or minimizing blood loss.

PERSPECTIVE AND PROSPECTS

The frequency of these cancers and their distribution in the world vary considerably. Intestinal cancers make up less than 1 percent of all cancers and less than 5 percent of gastrointestinal cancers; pancreatic cancer accounts for only about 3 percent of all cancers. Yet the incidence of both cancers has been rising. In the United States, for example, pancreatic cancer increased about 25 percent from the 1950's to the 1990's and was responsible for 25,000 deaths in 1993. At the same time, stomach cancer decreased dramatically, dropping from the United States' most common cancer in the 1930's to about 2 percent of all cancers in 1990. Yet in Japan, Iceland, and parts of Central and South America and of Eastern Europe, the stomach cancer rate is very high, accounting for most of the nearly 700,000 new cases yearly. In some countries, such as Japan, it is higher than all other cancer types combined. Until the 1990's, men contracted and died from stomach, pancreatic, and intestinal cancers more often than women; thereafter, however, women and men began to die from pancreatic cancer in nearly equal numbers. In the United States, African Americans get these cancers more often than caucasians. Probably because of their diet, poor people develop them more often than middle-class or upper-class people. The peak age group is fifty to fifty-nine years for stomach cancer and seventy to seventy-nine years for pancreatic and intestinal cancer.

The chances for successfully treating or drastically curtailing small bowel cancer are reasonably good; 20 percent of patients with adenocarcinomas in the small intestine survive for at least five years following diagnosis, and patients with carcinoid tumors have lived ten and even fifteen years after surgery. Treatment of small bowel or stomach lymphomas can result in a cure or prolonged survival in a significant percentage of cases. The prospects for pancreatic and stomach adenocarcinomas, however, are another story entirely. Overall, in the United States about 10 percent of gastric cancer patients are alive five years later. Pancreatic cancer is even deadlier, with 90 percent of patients dying in the first year after diagnosis, regardless of treatment. Of those with cancer of the pancreatic duct, only about 4 percent survive three years. Those with cancer in the insulin-producing cells fare better—a 30 percent survival rate—but this is a very rare type of cancer.

Japan has higher survival rates of stomach cancer than does the United States; 50 percent of Japanese patients survive at least five years. The reason is simple. Because gastric cancer is common in Japan, doctors routinely screen patients for it by endoscopy or photofluorography (a type of X ray). Many more cancers are caught early, while they are still surgically treatable. Endoscopic and chemical screenings for pancreatic cancer are also possible, but since the disease is so much less common, doctors do not perform the tests unless they already have good reason to suspect cancer. Avoidance of carcinogens, especially alcohol, remains the most promising way to escape gut cancers.

—Roger Smith, Ph.D.

See also Alcoholism; Cancer; Carcinoma; Chemotherapy; Colon cancer; Gastrectomy; Gastroenterology; Gastroenterology, pediatric; Gastrointestinal disorders; Gastrointestinal system; Gastrostomy; Ileostomy and colostomy; Intestinal disorders; Intestines; Jaundice; Liver cancer; Malignancy and metastasis; National Cancer Institute (NCI); Oncology; Pancreas; Pancreatitis; Radiation therapy; Tumor removal; Tumors.

FOR FURTHER INFORMATION:

Daly, John M., Thomas P. J. Hennessy, and John V. Reynolds. *Management of Upper Gastrointestinal Cancer.* Philadelphia: W. B. Saunders, 1999. This book addresses such topics as surgical management of gastric cancer, gastric lymphoma, esophageal cancer, and the various treatments associated with these and other ailments.

Levine, Joel S., ed. *Decision Making in Gastroenterology.* 2d ed. Philadelphia: B. C. Decker, 1992. This text for physicians contains detailed information about the symptoms and development of cancers. Accompanying charts explain the sequence of examination, testing, and treatment, and dedicated laypersons can glean much of value from them.

Murphy, G., L. Morris, and D. Lange. *Informed Decisions: The Complete Book of Cancer Diagnosis, Treatment, and Recovery.* New York: Viking Press, 1997. This text from the American Cancer Society is intended for the layperson. It is exemplary in its discussion of cancer.

Rustgi, Anil K., ed. *Gastrointestinal Cancers: Biology, Diagnosis, and Therapy.* Philadelphia: Lippincott-Raven, 1995. This book discusses cancer of the digestive organs, as well as the growth and development of the gastrointestinal system. Includes a bibliography and an index.

Sachar, David B., Jerome D. Waye, and Blair S. Lewis, eds. *Pocket Guide to Gastroenterology.* Rev. ed. Baltimore: Williams & Wilkins, 1991. Contains outlines of the medical subspecialty's basics. An invaluable reference for symptoms, tests, and treatments.

Steen, R. Grant. *A Conspiracy of Cells: The Basic Science of Cancer.* New York: Plenum Press, 1993. Thorough, lucid explanations of all physiological aspects of cancer make this book instructive for readers willing to slog through the subject's complexity and terminology.

STOMACH REMOVAL. *See* GASTRECTOMY.

STONE REMOVAL

PROCEDURE

ANATOMY OR SYSTEM AFFECTED: Abdomen, bladder, gallbladder, kidneys, urinary system

SPECIALTIES AND RELATED FIELDS: Gastroenterology, general surgery, nephrology, urology

DEFINITION: An operation that extracts solidified substances (stones) from an organ; typically, these stones block the organ's ability to release fluid.

KEY TERMS:

calculus: an abnormal crystalline formation of a mineral salt; also called a stone

cholecystectomy: the removal of a diseased gallbladder or one that contains many gallstones

cholelithiasis: the formation of gallstones in the gallbladder or the ducts that connect the gallbladder to the liver or small intestine

ureterolithotomy: the surgical removal of a stone in the ureter

ureters: the two muscular tubes that connect the kidneys to the urinary bladder and that serve as conduits for urine

urolithiasis: the formation of stones in the urinary tract

INDICATIONS AND PROCEDURES

Urinary tract stones can occur in the kidneys, ureters, or urinary bladder. These stones, or calculi, are caused by substances that precipitated in the urine. The most common substance that solidifies in the urine is calcium oxalate. Stones referred to as infective, however, are present in about 20 percent of patients with urinary tract stones. These stones typically occur in patients with chronic urinary tract infections. Bacteria in the urinary tract produce ammonia, which combines with calcium or magnesium. Infective stones have the potential to block large areas of the urinary tract.

Patients with urinary tract calculi may experience a variety of symptoms depending on where the stones are located. If a stone is in the ureter, then a sharper pain that extends from the middle of the back to the groin is felt; this pain is called renal colic. Bladder stones are usually not as painful, but they may obstruct the flow of urine from the urinary bladder.

The patient's physician will have the urine examined for the presence of blood (hematuria) and crystals. X rays and/or ultrasound will show the location of the stone. Blood tests may or may not be ordered depending on whether a metabolic disorder is suspected. Hypercalcemia and hyperparathyroidism can be detected by a blood test; both indicate a problem of excess calcium.

If the urinary tract stone is relatively small, the renal colic is treated with bed rest and an analgesic, along with adequate fluid intake to promote passing of the stone. Larger stones, infective stones, or severe obstruction of urinary flow requires surgery to remove the stone. The patient is usually under general anesthesia and has a small surgical scope (a cystoscope for the bladder or a ureterorenoscope for the ureter) passed up the urethra. These scopes give the surgeon the ability to visualize and crush the stones with attachments on the instruments.

The gallbladder, which stores and concentrates bile, also has the potential for stone formation. Gallstones are usually composed of cholesterol and may be found in the ducts that connect the gallbladder to the small intestine or liver. If a stone has obstructed one of

The Removal of Stones

Surgical removal

Lithotripsy

Gallbladder
containing
gallstones

Kidney containing
staghorn calculus

Bladder
containing
stones

The formation of large calcium deposits in the gallbladder and parts of the urinary system such as the kidneys and bladder can cause pain and obstruction of the ureters or bile ducts. In the case of gallstones, treatment may involve the removal of the entire organ, while kidney or bladder stones can be destroyed using lithotripsy, in which shock waves are used to break up the stones.

these ducts, the resulting symptoms can include intense pain known as biliary colic. This pain is usually felt in the upper right side of the abdomen or between the shoulder blades.

Ultrasound scanning of the upper abdomen can almost always detect the presence of gallstones. If the gallstones do not cause symptoms, they may be left alone, or drugs such as chenodiol and ursodeoxycholic acid may be tried to dissolve them. When symptoms are severe, removal of the gallbladder (cholecystectomy) is indicated. This surgery involves an incision under the ribcage on the right side. A laparoscope may be used or a larger incision made for an open procedure. In either case, the liver is gently lifted to expose the gallbladder, and the blood vessels and cystic duct are tied off so that blood and bile do not leak from the excised organ. The wound is then closed, and the patient may return home within a week.

USES AND COMPLICATIONS

Complications from removing urinary tract stones include infections, scarring, bleeding, and anesthesia risks. These complications are rare when the operation is performed by a competent surgical team. An uncommon but significant adverse result from obstruction relief is an excessive amount of urine loss, sometimes greater than 10 liters per day, which places the patient at risk for dehydration. Reducing fluid intake helps the kidney return to normal function slowly. Occasionally, this complication does not resolve. If the obstruction is not removed, however, the patient is at risk for developing chronic urinary tract infections and even renal failure.

The major risk in performing cholecystectomy is damage to the bile duct that leads to the small intestine. If scarring or inflammation occurs in this duct, it may lead to obstruction of the flow of bile from the liver. This in turn may lead to obstructive jaundice, in which pigments normally released into the intestines accumulate in the liver and blood. The patient may have a yellowish tinge to the skin and eyes until the obstruction is corrected.

If there are no complications during the cholecystectomy, then the outcome of the surgery is usually good. Approximately 90 percent of the patients have no further symptoms and recover completely in about three weeks.

PERSPECTIVE AND PROSPECTS

Advances in medical technology have aided physicians in the removal of stones. Kidney and urethral stones now can be broken up using a technique called lithotripsy. An ultrasonic lithotripsy probe can break the stones using externally applied sound waves that penetrate the skin and other soft tissues. For some patients, a noninvasive technique takes advantage of sound waves transmitted through the abdominal cavity

and directed at the stones. This procedure is known as extracorporeal shock-wave lithotripsy. The latter technique is also used to treat some patients with gallstones.

—Matthew Berria, Ph.D.,
and Douglas Reinhart, M.D.

See also Cholecystectomy; Cholecystitis; Cystoscopy; Gallbladder diseases; Kidney disorders; Kidneys; Laparoscopy; Lithotripsy; Nephrology; Stones; Ultrasonography; Urinary disorders; Urinary system; Urology.

FOR FURTHER INFORMATION:

Clayman, Charles B., ed. *The American Medical Association Encyclopedia of Medicine.* New York: Random House, 1994. A concise presentation of numerous medical terms and illnesses. A good general reference.

Novick, Andrew C., and Stevan B. Streem. "Surgery of the Kidney." In *Campbell's Urology*, edited by Patrick C. Walsh et al. 7th ed. Philadelphia: W. B. Saunders, 1998. A chapter in a classic urology text.

Tierney, Lawrence M., Jr., et al., eds. *Current Medical Diagnosis and Treatment: 2001.* 38th ed. New York: McGraw-Hill, 2000. This book is revised annually. Contains chapters entitled "Liver, Biliary Tract, and Pancreas" and "Urology" that address stones. It is an excellent and concise text but is written for professionals.

STONES

DISEASE/DISORDER

ALSO KNOWN AS: Calculi

ANATOMY OR SYSTEM AFFECTED: Abdomen, bladder, gallbladder, kidneys, urinary system

SPECIALTIES AND RELATED FIELDS: Gastroenterology, internal medicine, nephrology, urology

DEFINITION: Hard deposits of material in the body associated with urine and bile.

CAUSES AND SYMPTOMS

Stones may form in the kidneys, ureters, bladder, and gallbladder. Kidney and ureter stones are typically calcium-based, while bladder stones are most frequently composed of uric acid (a by-product of protein metabolism) or struvite (a result of chronic urinary infection). Gallstones contain very little calcium; they are primarily composed of cholesterol.

The symptoms that accompany urinary stone disease are dependent on the location of the stone, the size of the stone, how long the stone has been present, whether infection is associated with the stone, and the degree of obstruction to urinary flow caused by the stone. Urine, which is produced by the kidneys, located beneath the ribs of the back, is collected into a structure just outside the kidney known as the renal pelvis. From the renal pelvis, urine passes into a thin narrow tube called the ureter and travels a relatively long distance to the urinary bladder. It is easy to envision how a stone traveling along such a narrow, long tube can get stuck and dam the further flow of urine.

Stones caught in the renal pelvis, prior to entry into the ureter, generally cause an intermittent, sharp pain in the back or side. Stones that pass into the ureter can cause pain in the back as well as points distant from the urinary system (the groin, the lower abdomen, and the testicle and penis in men); this phenomenon is known as referred pain. Occasionally, stones in the lowest portion of the ureters will cause pain only with urination or produce the desire to urinate frequently but only in small amounts. Often, blood not visible to the naked eye can be found in the urine with a simple chemical dipstick or by looking at the urine under a microscope, both easily accomplished in most doctors' offices.

Several radiological tests can be performed to pinpoint the location of a stone lodged in the urinary tract. An intravenous pyelogram (IVP) is a series of X rays performed following the administration of a dye into the patient's vein. This dye is concentrated in the urine and can be visualized as it travels through the urinary tract. High-frequency sound waves, or ultrasound, can determine if obstruction is present in the kidneys but will frequently miss stones lodged in the ureters. A computed tomography (CT) scan is similar to an IVP but uses advanced computer technology to visualize better all contents of the body. While the CT scan is the most sensitive test for the detection of urinary stones, certain situations may necessitate the use of different tests. Frequently, people with poor renal function cannot receive the X-ray dye because of its potential harmful effects on the kidneys. A CT scan without contrast or ultrasound will frequently be performed in this situation.

Bladder stones are found much less frequently than stones in the kidney and ureter. Perhaps the most famous person to have suffered from bladder stones is Benjamin Franklin, who reportedly stood on his head to urinate. Throughout the world, bladder stones are

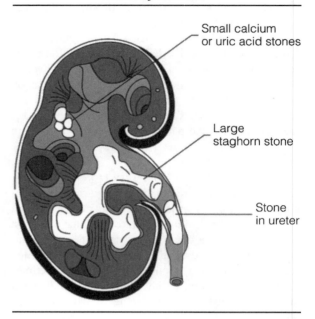

Kidney Stones

Small calcium or uric acid stones

Large staghorn stone

Stone in ureter

almost exclusively a disease of the older, male population. They are most frequently found in association with enlargement of the prostate that obstructs the bladder's ability to empty and allows these stones to crystallize in the urine. Other causes of bladder stone formation should be excluded, such as a narrowed urethra, an abnormal pouching of the bladder, a chronic urinary infection, or a neurologic dysfunction leading to poor bladder emptying.

Symptoms of a bladder stone are pain in the lower abdomen that worsens with movement, intermittent blockage of the urinary stream, a weak urine stream, increased frequency of urination often associated with a strong and urgent need to void, recurrent urinary tract infections, or blood in the urine. Definitive diagnosis of a stone can be made with a simple X ray of the abdomen alone; however, the physician will often need to perform additional tests, including a direct look into the bladder.

Diseases affecting the gallbladder and bile ducts occur commonly in the elderly. By the age of seventy, stones in the gallbladder and bile duct represent the most frequently occurring disorder affecting this organ system. In the late 1990's, it was estimated that 33 percent of the U.S. population over seventy would be diagnosed with gallstones at some point in their lives.

The symptoms associated with stones in the gallbladder or bile duct are numerous and depend on the location and size of the stone and whether there is an associated infection. Frequently, patients complain of pain in the right upper part of the abdomen. This pain often occurs after the consumption of a fatty meal, which causes the gallbladder to contract and release its bile. Fever, sweats, and chills may accompany the pain if there is infection present. Jaundice, a yellowish discoloring of the skin, may occur if the common bile duct or hepatic duct becomes obstructed with a gallstone. As with stones in the urinary tract, it is the blockage of flow of bile from the gallbladder that leads to the symptoms. Elderly patients who appear jaundiced may not always be suffering from gallstones, especially if there is no associated pain. Other diseases of the liver and biliary system, such as cirrhosis of the liver or hepatitis, will also cause jaundice and are frequently found in the elderly.

The biliary system stores bile formed in the liver and delivers it to the intestines following a meal, aiding in the digestion of fat and the absorption of certain vitamins. The gallbladder is a blind-ending pouch that comes off of the bile duct as it courses from the liver to the small intestine. After consumption of a fatty meal, its muscle-lined wall contracts to release bile into the intestine. Stones can form in the gallbladder and can cause pain or infection when lodged in the bile duct or common hepatic (liver) duct. If a stone causes blockage and infection, the patient can become very sick and require emergency medical care.

Unlike kidney stones, gallstones are frequently not visible on plain X-ray examination of the abdomen. Despite their hard nature, gallstones contain very little calcium. They are primarily composed of cholesterol, which, unlike calcium, is not dense enough to be visible on an X ray. Ultrasound examination of the liver and gallbladder is almost always the first test ordered by a physician who is suspicious that a patient may have a gallstone. To determine if obstruction of the bile duct is present, a physician can also use nuclear medicine studies, which use a radioactive material concentrated by the gallbladder, similar to the concentration of X-ray dye used in the diagnosis of kidney stones. On occasion, the diagnosis of a gallstone lodged in the bile duct requires the placement of a telescope into the patient's stomach and intestine and direct visualization of the common bile duct's entry into the intestine.

TREATMENT AND THERAPY

Treatment of any stone depends on the location of the stone, its size, the time it has been in place, and any complicating issues such as infection. The methods for treatment are broad, and the specific means by which a stone is removed is often debated among the experts in this field. Some stones—especially if they are small, cause no pain, and are not significantly obstructing—are given a chance to pass on their own, a treatment termed watchful waiting. The most frequent noninvasive means to treat a small stone located in the urinary tract above the pelvic bone is extracorporeal shock-wave lithotripsy (ESWL). This procedure involves the use of high-energy sound waves created by a machine outside the body and focused through the skin onto the stone. These sound waves break the stone into fine sand, which passes in the urine without symptoms. This is frequently the best method to deal with stones in elderly patients who have other medical problems that can make surgical means of removing a stone risky. Endoscopic removal of a stone involves the use of small telescopes passed into the urinary tract either through the urethra or through the back directly into the kidney. Different means of fragmenting the stone into smaller pieces for direct removal are then employed through the telescopes. This method is highly successful and often used for larger stones. Like ESWL, this low-invasive, endoscopic means of removing the stone places minimal stress on the elderly patient with other medical problems.

The development of these minimally invasive procedures for stone removal has led to a significant decrease in the need for open surgery. Nevertheless, there are special situations when an open surgical procedure may be the first reasonable option for the elderly patient with a urinary stone. These situations include abnormal urinary tract anatomy, concurrent urinary tract pathology other than the stone, or the failure of less invasive means to remove the stone.

Treatment of bladder stones is very successful and appropriate for the elderly. As with stones of the kidney and ureter, endoscopic removal of a bladder stone using small telescopes frequently can be performed. Most bladder stones, however, are removed with open surgery. Paramount to the successful treatment of a bladder stone is the treatment of the underlying cause for its formation, which frequently dictates the method of removal. Whether endoscopic or open surgery is chosen, both are generally well tolerated by elderly patients even if significant other medical problems exist.

Treatment of symptomatic gallstones almost always involves surgery using lighted telescopes passed either directly into the abdomen (laparoscopes) or through the stomach and intestine (endoscopes), or open surgery. Unlike the removal of kidney and bladder stones, which most often merely involves the removal of the actual stone and not the kidney, ureter, or bladder, treatment of gallstones usually also involves the removal of the gallbladder itself. The loss of this unpaired organ often does not lead to significant digestive problems, though in the elderly loose, foul-smelling bowel movements may result from the altered digestion of fats.

The choice of surgical approach again depends on whether an infection is associated with the stone, how severe the symptoms are, whether any liver dysfunction is associated with the stone, and the overall health of the patient. Gallstones not causing symptoms are generally not removed. Patients with diabetes mellitus and other complicating medical conditions are dealt with in a more cautious manner and frequently undergo surgery to remove the gallstone and gallbladder even if symptoms do not exist.

PERSPECTIVE AND PROSPECTS

While there is no evidence of increased incidence of urinary stones with increasing age, stones of the biliary tract (cholelithiasis) do increase with age, affecting approximately 33 percent of the U.S. population over seventy years old.

Kidney stones or stones in the urinary tract affect 5 to 10 percent of the general population of the United States. The likelihood of a person to form a stone for the first time in their life decreases with advancing age. In people who have a prior history of urinary stone formation, however, the incidence, recurrence, and severity of urinary stone disease is similar between the geriatric and younger populations. The composition of urinary stones in the older population is no different from that of those found in younger patients; however, the underlying urinary abnormality leading to the stone formation is different. More frequently, urinary stones in the elderly are caused by high uric acid levels and low citrate levels in the urine. Similar difficulties in the disposal of protein metabolites can lead to gouty arthritis.

—John F. Ward, M.D.,
and Prodromos G. Borboroglu, M.D.

See also Cholecystectomy; Cholecystitis; Endoscopy; Gallbladder diseases; Gout; Kidney disorders; Kidneys; Laparoscopy; Lithotripsy; Nephritis; Nephrology; Nutrition; Stone removal; Urethritis; Urinary disorders; Urinary system; Urology.

FOR FURTHER INFORMATION:

Hosking, M., M. Warmer, and C. Lodbell, et al. "Outcomes of Surgery in Patients Ninety Years of Age and Older." *Journal of the American Medical Association* 261, no. 13 (April 7, 1989): 1909. From 1975 to 1985, 795 patients ninety years or older underwent surgery at the Mayo Clinic. The thirty-day, one-year, and five-year mortality rates were 8.4 percent, 31.4 percent, and 78.8 percent, respectively.

Saunders, Carol S. "Urolithiasis: New Tools for Diagnosis and Treatment." *Patient Care* 33, no. 15 (September 30, 1999): 28-44. Noncontrast helical CT has replaced IV pyelography as first-line imaging for suspected acute renal colic, and treatment decisions have been simplified with new guidelines. This and other advances in prevention are discussed.

Walsh, P., A. Retik, E. Vaughan, and A. Wein, eds. *Campbell's Urology.* 7th ed. 3 vols. Philadelphia: W. B. Saunders, 1998. This edition of a classic urology text maintains its encyclopedic approach while following a new organ systems orientation. Halftone illustrations and contributions by multiple authors.

STRABISMUS
DISEASE/DISORDER

ALSO KNOWN AS: Crossed eyes
ANATOMY OR SYSTEM AFFECTED: Eyes, muscles
SPECIALTIES AND RELATED FIELDS: Ophthalmology
DEFINITION: The improper alignment or crossing of the eyes.

CAUSES AND SYMPTOMS

Strabismus affects approximately 5 percent of the population. It may be caused by a problem with the nerve supply to the muscles that move the eye or by poor vision or obstruction of vision in one or both eyes.

The most common type of strabismus is an esotropia (inward deviation) of the eye, which accounts for 75 percent of the cases of crossed eyes. There is also exotropia (outward deviation), hypertropia (upward deviation), and hypotropia (downward deviation) of the eye. When a child with strabismus has a penlight shown in the eye, the light reflected back does not fall on the pupil in the same place. This is referred to as the corneal light reflex test. When the eyes are aligned, the corneal light reflex will be placed symmetrically on the pupil. It is important to identify strabismus and to have it evaluated to prevent amblyopia (dimness of vision) or blindness in the eye that is deviated. It is also important because without input from both eyes, it is difficult to perceive depth.

A condition called pseudostrabismus gives the appearance of having crossed eyes. It occurs because there is a flat bridge of the nose or extra skin near the nose. In this situation, the corneal light reflex will be symmetrical in the pupil.

TREATMENT AND THERAPY
Treatment of strabismus is aimed at avoiding amblyopia and realigning the eyes to restore depth perception. This realignment frequently requires surgery. Some cases can be treated with glasses and bifocals. An ophthalmologist should be consulted for the treatment of strabismus.

—*Sheila J. Mosee, M.D.*

See also Blindness; Eyes; Optometry; Optometry, pediatric; Sense organs; Visual disorders.

FOR FURTHER INFORMATION:
Eden, John. *The Physician's Guide to Cataracts, Glaucoma, and Other Eye Problems.* Yonkers, N.Y.: Consumer Reports Books, 1992.

Flynn, John T. *Strabismus: A Neurodevelopmental Approach: Nature's Experiment.* New York: Springer-Verlag, 1991.

Van Noorden, Gunter K. *Burian-von Noorden's Binocular Vision and Ocular Motility: Theory and Management of Strabismus.* 3d ed. St. Louis: Mosby, 1985.

STREP THROAT
DISEASE/DISORDER
ALSO KNOWN AS: Streptococcal pharyngitis

ANATOMY OR SYSTEM AFFECTED: Ears, heart, joints, kidneys, throat

SPECIALTIES AND RELATED FIELDS: Family practice, pediatrics

DEFINITION: An acute, contagious, bacterial infection of the throat that often spreads to the ears and sinuses and that can seriously damage the heart and kidneys.

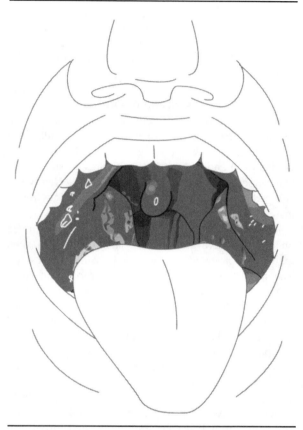

Strep throat may appear with white patches of infection on the tonsils and on the back of the throat.

CAUSES AND SYMPTOMS
Strep throat is caused by a specific strain of streptococcus bacteria. These bacteria are very common and are easily spread by direct, person-to-person contact. Droplets of saliva or nasal mucus from sneezes, coughs, infected hands, and cups or utensils are frequent means of contact. Young children, between the ages of five and ten, are at the highest risk: More than 20 percent of young schoolchildren are carriers.

After a short incubation period, the bacteria produce definite signs and symptoms: a red sore throat with severe pain on swallowing, swollen and pus-filled tonsils, enlarged lymph nodes along the jawline and down the neck, and a high fever. These symptoms may be milder in younger children less than three years of age, and some may show no symptoms at all. Difficulty in diagnosis may arise from distinguishing strep throat from other bacterial or viral infections.

It is critical, however, to make the diagnosis early. Left untreated, strep infections can have serious consequences for the heart and kidneys. More commonly, the throat problem will spread to the sinuses and ears.

TREATMENT AND THERAPY

Strep throat can be differentiated from other throat infections using the technique of sampling (culturing) throat secretions by rubbing the back of the throat with a swab and testing them with special substances that detect this specific strain of bacteria. Newly developed methods can provide results in a few hours, instead of days.

Penicillin and erythromycin are the drugs of choice once a definitive diagnosis of strep throat has been made. Symptoms generally subside within a few days. The most feared complication of strep throat is its spread through the blood to the joints and heart, causing rheumatic fever, and to the kidneys, causing glomerulonephritis. Rheumatic fever can seriously and permanently damage the heart valves, while glomerulonephritis can result in kidney failure. Before the development of antibiotics, many children suffered these complications.

—*Connie Rizzo, M.D.*

See also Antibiotics; Bacterial infections; Childhood infectious diseases; Ears, nose, and throat; Fever; Nasopharyngeal disorders; Otorhinolaryngology; Pharyngitis; Rheumatic fever; Screening; Sore throat; Streptococcal infections; Tonsillitis.

FOR FURTHER INFORMATION:

Biddle, Wayne. *Field Guide to Germs*. New York: Henry Holt, 1995.

Finegold, Sydney M., and William J. Martin. *Bailey and Scott's Diagnostic Microbiology*. 6th ed. St. Louis: C. V. Mosby, 1998.

Pelczar, Michael J., Jr., E. C. S. Chan, and Noel R. Krieg. *Microbiology*. 5th ed. New York: McGraw-Hill, 1986.

Schlegel, Hans G. *General Microbiology*. 6th ed. Cambridge, England: Cambridge University Press, 1986.

STREPTOCOCCAL INFECTIONS
DISEASE/DISORDER

ANATOMY OR SYSTEM AFFECTED: All

SPECIALTIES AND RELATED FIELDS: Bacteriology, emergency medicine, internal medicine, pediatrics, toxicology

DEFINITION: Streptococcal infections are a group of infections caused by the bacteria Streptococcus. In most people, it is common for streptococci to be present in the mouth, throat, and intestines without ill effect. Complications occur when the bacteria enter an already aggravated region of the body. In the throat and respiratory system, tonsillitis, strep throat, otitis media, and pneumonia may be caused by streptococci. In a heart with defective valves, streptococcal infections lead to endocarditis. Urinary tract infections are often caused by streptococcus bacteria. Another form of streptococcal infection called beta-hemolytic infection can lead to scarlet and rheumatic fever, as well as to complications of glomerulonephritis. Antibiotics usually treat streptococcal infections.

—*Jason Georges and Tracy Irons-Georges*

See also Antibiotics; Bacterial infections; Ear infections and disorders; Endocarditis; Glomerulonephritis; Necrotizing fasciitis; Pharyngitis; Pneumonia; Rheumatic fever; Scarlet fever; Sore throat; Strep throat; Tonsillitis.

FOR FURTHER INFORMATION:

Biddle, Wayne. *Field Guide to Germs*. New York: Henry Holt, 1995.

Finegold, Sydney M., and William J. Martin. *Bailey and Scott's Diagnostic Microbiology*. 6th ed. St. Louis, Mo.: C. V. Mosby, 1998.

Pelczar, Michael J., Jr., E. C. S. Chan, and Noel R. Krieg. *Microbiology*. 5th ed. New York: McGraw-Hill, 1986.

Schlegel, Hans G. *General Microbiology*. 6th ed. Cambridge, England: Cambridge University Press, 1986.

STRESS
DISEASE/DISORDER

ANATOMY OR SYSTEM AFFECTED: Immune system, psychic-emotional system

SPECIALTIES AND RELATED FIELDS: Environmental health, epidemiology, family practice, immunology, internal medicine, oncology, psychiatry, psychology

DEFINITION: A psychophysiological response to perceived pressures in the environment, including danger; prolonged stress contributes to hormonal imbalances, immune system collapse, susceptibility to disease, cancer, and death.

KEY TERMS:

alarmone: a type of intracellular hormone which alerts

the cell to various chemical imbalances in the cellular environment

anxiety: a type of stressful condition in which heightened neural activity accentuates an individual's anticipation of a stress-producing event

cellular transformation: carcinogenesis; the biochemical conversion of a cell from a normal state to a cancerous one of uncontrollable proliferation

chaos: a disorderly shift from predictable, linear behavior to nonlinear randomness, a situation which often occurs in stress and homeostatic breakdown

fight-or-flight response: a stressful biochemical reaction in animals, usually involving the adrenal hormone epinephrine, that prepares the animal for confrontation with predators or competitors

homeostasis: the maintenance of constant, linear conditions within a system, such as the maintenance of human body temperature, pH, and hormonal levels at stable states

hormone: a gene regulatory molecule which is produced in one body tissue region and which targets or controls cells in another region

nonlinear system: a process which is unstable and unpredictable in nature; such a process often results from a disturbance to a linear, predictable system

type A behavior: a psychological behavior classification for individuals who exhibit stressful, time-conscious lifestyles

type B behavior: a psychological behavior classification for individuals who exhibit unstressed, relaxed lifestyles

CAUSES AND SYMPTOMS

Stress is a psychophysiological response, within an individual animal, to a perceived danger. Stress involves a complex interplay of nervous and hormonal reactions to internal and external stimuli. All living organisms respond to stimuli, usually by means of gene-regulating chemical messengers called hormones.

Chemistry of stress. Hormones are produced in certain cells within the individual and then target tissues elsewhere in the body; these hormones control by controlling the gene regulation within their target cells. Hormones will activate certain genes within target tissue cells while inactivating other genes. If a hormone activates the control region of a gene so that the gene is "on," then it can be "read" by an enzyme (RNA polymerase), thereby leading to RNA and protein production. The produced protein may affect cel-

lular chemical processes or may affect the expression (the on/off status) of other genes. In the latter case, the protein would be a type of intracellular hormone called an alarmone.

If a hormone inactivates the control region of a gene so that the gene is "off," then RNA polymerase will be unable to read the DNA nucleotide sequence of the gene. Therefore, no RNA and no protein will be produced. In this fashion, a hormone may activate certain genes while inactivating others. Consequently, a hormone controls what happens within the cell.

Such control is critical within complex multicellular organisms such as animals. Different cells specialize to become different tissues and organs (such as eyes, ears, hair, intestines, the heart, and so on) under the specific influence of hormones. Additionally, changes in the development of an organism over time involve changes in gene expression caused by hormones. Critical developmental changes in an individual must occur at precise times when a hormone is produced and acts correctly upon the proper array of genes in target cell tissues. When a hormone does not act correctly or issues incorrect instructions to genes, the homeostatic stability of the organism becomes disrupted. Incorrect proteins are produced in the wrong cells at the wrong times, thereby disturbing development and possibly threatening the organism's survival.

In higher animals, including humans, the body is regulated by hormones and by complex nervous systems that evolved from hormones. Most hormones are produced and secreted from the glands of the endocrine system, including the pituitary, thyroid, and adrenal glands as well as numerous organs, tissues, and cells throughout the body. The nervous system is an array of several trillion nerves concentrated in the brain and spinal cord and extending peripherally to virtually every cellular region of the body. The two systems are tightly interconnected. Both the endocrine and nervous systems at some point involve the secretion of hormones. Nerve tissue secretes hormones called neurotransmitters between electrically conducting cells called neurons.

Physiological responses to stress. Stress is therefore a biochemical response to danger that occurs within animals. The nervous system detects danger from internal or external stimuli, usually external stimuli such as predators, competitors, or life-threatening events. Increased electrical conductivity along millions of nerve cells targets various tissues to prepare the body for maximum physical activity. Among the tissues affected will be the skeletal muscles, the heart muscle, the hormone-secreting glands of the endocrine system, the immune system, the stomach, and blood vessels. Under nerve-activated stress, skeletal muscles will be poised for contraction. The heart will beat faster, thereby distributing more blood and nutrients to body cells, in the process accelerating the breathing rate to distribute more oxygen. Blood vessels will constrict. The stomach and other intestinal organs will decrease their activity, including a decreased production of mucus that protects against acid.

Heightened nerve activity also will trigger the production of various hormones from the immune system, specifically hormones that influence bodily metabolism such as thyroxine and epinephrine (adrenaline). These hormones target body tissue cells to prepare the body for increased output in the face of danger. Massive production of epinephrine will trigger maximum physical readiness and extraordinary muscular output, a phenomenon often referred to as the fight-or-flight response.

These physiological changes within an animal facing danger are important survival adaptations that evolved very early in the history of animal life on earth. Stress is a fact of life for animals because they must eat to survive. Competition for available food resources and avoidance of predators must be faced by all animals, including humans. While predation is of little worry to humans, the struggle for available resources remains. Furthermore, human technology has created stresses of an entirely different character.

The fight-or-flight stress response and other evolutionary stress adaptations endure within the individual for only seconds or minutes. Such natural stresses are to an individual's advantage, ensuring survival. The stresses that humans face are based on these behavioral adaptations. Much human stress is artificial, however, and lasts not for minutes but for hours, days, weeks, months, and years. Such stresses involve the same nervous and endocrine system responses, but they are usually brought about by perceived danger, not true danger.

Human societies impose norms and rules for the behavior of the individuals who compose the society. People must adhere to the societal norms or face punishment. In fast-paced technological societies, increasing bureaucratization and organization place less emphasis on the individual and more emphasis on

process and productivity. People must face deadlines, be on time, produce quotas, generate company profit, and meet the demands of family, colleagues, and administration simultaneously. The result is a continuous fight-or-flight response in which individuals fear losing their jobs and thus the means of supporting themselves and their families.

The physiological manifestations of prolonged stress are devastating. Continued hyperactivity of nerve impulses and overproduction of hormones at incorrect developmental stages lead to the abnormal functioning of internal organs. The stomach undersecretes mucus, thereby leading to ulcers. The heart muscle contracts too rapidly, leading to higher pulse and respiration rates. The blood vessels constrict for lengthy periods of time, thereby causing the heart to pump harder and leading to high blood pressure and heart disease. Hormone overproduction leads to incorrect cell instructions and gene activation/inactivation, causing abnormal tissue functioning and cellular transformation leading to cancer. The immune system weakens under abnormal signaling by hormones, thereby decreasing the body's ability to defend itself from disease.

Stress and disease. A wide variety of human illnesses and disorders have been associated with stress. Heart disease, cancer, stroke, mental illness, allergies, accidents, alcoholism, drug abuse, asthma, chronic fatigue, depression, suicide, and deviant behavior are among the many illnesses and disorders that are considered by scientists to be stress-related illnesses. These stress-related diseases and disorders are responsible for the majority of deaths, hospitalizations, and visits to physicians by people in highly technological societies such as the United States, Japan, and Western Europe. In the United States alone, several billion dollars are spent each year for medications to treat stress-related illnesses that otherwise could be prevented by antistress methodologies.

Before the advent of industrialization in Europe and North America, the leading killers of humans were bacterial and viral diseases, which continue to be the principal killers of humans in the pretechnological and emerging technological countries of the Middle East, Asia, Africa, Latin America, and Oceania. European and North American industrialization has been accompanied by prodigious advances in medical science and the eradication or control of many microorganismal diseases. The psychological demands of fast-paced living and the dehumanized expectations of technological societies, however, have produced a plethora of stress-generated diseases and disorders, some of which had been masked by microorganismal diseases.

There still is some debate concerning the causal relationship between stress and illness, despite overwhelming scientific evidence demonstrating bodily responses to stressful situations. Abnormal nerve hyperactivity and prolonged, abnormal secretions of gene regulatory hormones from various endocrine glands disrupt the balanced homeostasis of many different body systems. Immune system reduction often occurs during stress, thereby making a stressed individual more susceptible to contracting infectious bacterial and viral diseases.

A clear linkage exists between the occurrence of stress in people and their subsequent susceptibility to infectious disease. Furthermore, there is a tendency for strokes, heart attacks, cancer, and sudden death to occur in individuals who recently have experienced major traumatic events in their lives. Too little attention has been given to the effects of everyday living upon the physical well-being of people. Environmental stimuli, nervous and endocrine systems, and physiological rhythms within the body are intricately connected.

Most bodily processes follow a self-regulatory, homeostatic pattern that is rhythmic, linear, stable, and predictable. For example, the beta cells of the islets of Langerhans in the pancreas secrete the hormone insulin in response to elevated blood glucose levels, whereas the alpha cells in these same islets secrete the hormone glucagon in response to low blood glucose levels. Likewise, the body chemically maintains a constant blood temperature (37 degrees Celsius), pH (7.35 to 7.45), calcium levels, and so on. The heart muscle requires an electrical stimulus approximately once per second to trigger a wave of muscular contractions throughout the myocardium via the sinoatrial and atrioventricular nodes.

Linear, balanced physiological rhythms are sensitive to subtle chemical changes in the cellular and organismal environment. An orderly, homeostatic process in the body can collapse into disorderly, nonlinear, and unpredictable chaos because of the slightest disturbance. Stress is a disturbance that imbalances the nervous and endocrine systems, which subsequently imbalance cells and organ systems throughout the human body. Physiological systems become unstable, and disease or cancer may ensue.

TREATMENT AND THERAPY

Psychologists, psychiatrists, physicians, and other medical professionals are becoming more aware of the physiological effects of stress. Psychologists have identified two principal behavioral types among humans: type A behavior pattern and type B behavior pattern. Type A individuals are highly anxious, task-oriented, time-conscious, and constantly in a rush to accomplish their jobs and other objectives. Research indicates that type A individuals may have a higher incidence of heart disease. On the other hand, type B individuals are more relaxed and experience less stress. Nevertheless, it should be emphasized that behavior is a continuum: Different people may exhibit varying degrees of type A and B behavior patterns.

An important focus for health care has become the treatment of stress itself. Health education programs emphasize the importance of physical fitness and stress reduction in everyday living. Stress-reducing methodologies for the individual include time management, peer counseling and support, spending longer amounts of time relaxing, strengthening family bonds, improving self-esteem, and exercise. These approaches greatly enhance an individual's quality of life and help the individual to cope positively with stressful events. All these stress reduction techniques emphasize an individual's personality and the more efficient use of an individual's free time. Relaxation, social interaction, and physical activity help the body to return to normal physiological rhythms following the numerous stressful events that every person faces daily. Individuals in American and Western societies are coming to realize that a slower, more relaxed living pace is essential for reducing stress and the millions of cases of stress-related disease that occur each year.

PERSPECTIVE AND PROSPECTS

Because stress is a major contributor to illness and disease in American and Western societies, a major objective of health care professionals in these countries is the identification of stress initiators and the reduction of stress in the general population. Stress cannot be eliminated entirely in any individual. Humans always will experience stress as a result of their continuous interactions with one another and with the environment. Stress is an important survival adaptation for animal life on earth. Nevertheless, stressful events in an individual's life serve as negative environmental stimuli that hyperactivate the human nervous and endocrine systems to create a fight-or-flight response. When this fight-or-flight response is maintained for abnormally long periods of times, prolonged elevations in nervous and hormonal activity modify body tissues and the developmental gene expression within cells to produce abnormal growths (such as cancers) and abnormal system functioning (such as diabetes mellitus). Breakdown of the human immune system under stress makes the body less capable of fighting spontaneous tumors, cancers, and infectious disease. The net result from physiological stress is illness, disease, rapid aging, and death.

Stress reduction should be a prime focus of medical research and education. The simplicity of educating the public with respect to stress can yield incredible savings in terms of lives saved, quality of lives improved, length of human life spans increased, and money saved. Some researchers propose that stress reduction not only can yield enormous health benefits but also produces greater industrial productivity, happier people, and considerably less crime.

—David Wason Hollar, Jr., Ph.D.

See also Addiction; Alcoholism; Alternative medicine; Anxiety; Cancer; Death and dying; Depression; Domestic violence; Eating disorders; Factitious disorders; Grief and guilt; Hallucinations; Hormones; Hypochondriasis; Manic-depressive disorder; Midlife crisis; Neurosis; Obsessive-compulsive disorder; Panic attacks; Phobias; Postpartum depression; Post-traumatic stress disorder; Psychiatric disorders; Psychiatry; Psychiatry, child and adolescent; Psychiatry, geriatric; Psychoanalysis; Psychosis; Psychosomatic disorders; Schizophrenia; Sexual dysfunction; Sibling rivalry; Stress reduction; Suicide.

FOR FURTHER INFORMATION:

Day, Stacey B., ed. *Cancer, Stress, and Death.* 2d ed. New York: Plenum Press, 1986. This informative work is a collection of scientific survey papers that demonstrate the relationship between stress and disease. The papers are clearly written for both scientific and general audiences.

Finch, Caleb E. "The Orderly Decay of Order in the Regulation of Aging Processes." In *Self-Organizing Systems: The Emergence of Order,* edited by F. Eugene Yates. New York: Plenum Press, 1987. This survey article, written by a leading gerontologist, is a comprehensive survey of factors contributing to aging in humans and other mammals. The author concentrates on hormones and their effects on gene regulation within cells.

Gaudin, Anthony J., and Kenneth C. Jones. *Human Anatomy and Physiology.* New York: Harcourt Brace Jovanovich, 1989. This introductory anatomy textbook for undergraduates provides a basic presentation of human physiology that is understandable to the layperson. Chapter 17, "The Endocrine System," discusses the major human hormones in detail.

Gleick, James. *Chaos: Making a New Science.* New York: Viking Press, 1987. Gleick's outstanding, exciting presentation of an exploding field of scientific research is a must-read for both scientists and laypeople interested in science. He describes the historical development of the study of dynamical systems.

Monroe, Judy. *Coping with Ulcers, Heartburn, and Stress-Related Stomach Disorders.* New York: Rosen, 2000. Designed for students in grades seven and up, this book discusses different types of ulcers, irritable bowel syndrome, food intolerances and allergies of all types, and heartburn and acid reflux.

Newton, Tim, with Jocelyn Handy and Stephen Fineman. *Managing Stress: Emotion and Power at Work.* Thousand Oaks, Calif.: Sage, 1995. This book addresses job stress and offers stress management techniques for coping with it. Includes a bibliography and an index.

Schafer, Walt. *Stress Management for Wellness.* New York: Holt, Rinehart & Winston, 1987. Schafer's textbook is a simple presentation of stress, both positive and negative, for the layperson. He describes how stress affects the body and how it may contribute to illness and death.

STRESS REDUCTION

PROCEDURE

ANATOMY OR SYSTEM AFFECTED: All

SPECIALTIES AND RELATED FIELDS: Alternative medicine, environmental health, immunology, occupational health, preventive medicine, psychiatry, psychology

DEFINITION: A set of procedures with the goal of decreasing bodily and mental tension by increasing rest and coping skills.

KEY TERMS:

palliative treatments: therapies that reduce symptoms without completely eradicating a disorder

psychotherapy: treatment using the mind to remedy problems related to disordered behavior or thinking, emotional problems, or disease

stress: physical, environmental, or psychological strain experienced by an individual that requires adjustment

INDICATIONS AND PROCEDURES

Stress can exacerbate difficulties in daily functioning, slow recovery from mental or physical problems, and impede immunological functioning. Stress reduction techniques represent a cluster of procedures that share the goal of reducing bodily and emotional tension: drug and physical therapies, exercise, biofeedback training, meditation, hypnosis, psychotherapy, relaxation training, and stress inoculation therapy.

The drugs used in stress reduction are designed to provide overall bodily relaxation, to induce rest, or to decrease the anxious thinking that exacerbates stressful experiences. Sedatives, tranquilizers, benzodiazepines, antihistamines, beta-blockers, and barbiturates are examples of such drugs. Similarly, physical therapies and exercise are recommended for these purposes. Baths (hydrotherapy), massages, and moderate exercise can also be part of a stress reduction program.

Psychotherapy is a common treatment for stress implemented by psychiatrists, psychologists, social workers, psychiatric nurses, and counselors. Not only does it help individuals to sort out their problems mentally but it is also an effective stress management strategy. When individuals analyze their lifestyles and life events, stress-inducing behaviors and life patterns can be explored and targeted for modification.

Biofeedback training, meditation, hypnosis, and relaxation training all focus on inducing relaxation or altered consciousness by shifting a person's attention. Biofeedback uses monitoring devices attached to the body to provide visual or aural feedback to the trainee. Such devices include the electromyograph (EMG), which measures muscle tension, and the psychogalvanometer, which measures galvanic skin response (GSR). An EMG involves placing sensors on various muscle groups to record muscular electrical potentials. GSR also relies on sensors, but these sensors record bodily responses caused by sweat gland activity and emotional arousal. The feedback from such devices allows a trainee to learn to control certain bodily processes (for example, muscle tension, brain waves, heart rate, temperature, and blood pressure). Biofeedback training is used to treat headaches, temporomandibular joint (TMJ) syndrome, high blood pressure, and tics, and it can also facilitate neuromuscular responses in stroke patients.

Meditation is a focused thinking exercise involving a quiet setting and the repetition of a word or phrase called a mantra. By blocking distracting thoughts and refocusing attention, meditation reduces anxious thinking. It is useful for mild anxiety, minor concentration difficulties, and daily relaxation.

Hypnosis involves the use of suggestion, concentrated attention, and/or drugs to induce a sleeplike state, or trance. Hypnosis can be induced by a hypnotist or via self-hypnosis. Hypnotic states are characterized by increased suggestibility, ability to recall forgotten events, decreased pain sensitivity, and increased vasomotor control. The ability to be hypnotized varies from person to person based on susceptibility to suggestion and psychological needs. Hypnosis is used as a brief therapy targeting such problems as insomnia, pain, panic, and sexual dysfunction. In addition, hypnosis is sometimes used when drugs are contraindicated for anesthetic use, particularly for dental procedures.

Relaxation training involves three primary methods: autogenic training, which involves such techniques as head, heart, and abdominal exercises; progressive relaxation, which involves becoming aware of tension in the various muscle groups by relaxing one group at a time in a specific order; and breathing exercises. Relaxation training is best learned when a therapist trains an individual in person and then the exercises are practiced independently. Relaxation can be practiced several times daily, as well as in response to stressful events. High blood pressure, ulcers, insomnia, asthma, drug and alcohol problems, spastic colitis, tachycardia (rapid heartbeat), pain management, and moderate-to-severe anxiety disorders are treated with relaxation training.

Stress inoculation therapy is a specific type of psychotherapy involving techniques that alter patterns of thinking and acting. It comprises three steps: education about stress and fear reactions, rehearsal of coping behaviors, and application of coping behaviors in stress-provoking situations. It is useful for treating anxiety disorders related to stress.

USES AND COMPLICATIONS

Individuals should not apply stress reduction procedures without proper consultation; medical conditions that might be causing symptoms should be assessed or ruled out first. Biofeedback training for headaches, for example, would be unwarranted until other, more serious causes of headaches had been eliminated from consideration. Similarly, exercise, drug, and physical therapies could actually worsen conditions such as high blood pressure, alcohol and drug problems, and chronic pain if applied incorrectly. For example, where stress or pain is chronic, drug therapies might encourage the development of drug dependence.

Instead, skilled providers should administer these procedures. Training via self-help materials alone or by an unskilled provider may provide no benefit or create difficulties. Poor training could result in frustration, hypervigilance, heightened anxiety, depression, or pain caused by overattention to symptoms or conflicts. In fact, some individuals are prone to these effects even with good training. Therefore, ongoing assessment is necessary. Finally, interpretation of any memories provoked by hypnosis should be done with caution because of the suggestibility that is characteristic of hypnotic states.

PERSPECTIVE AND PROSPECTS

Stress reduction techniques evolved from ancient meditation practices and simpler methods of pain management predating the development of modern anesthetics. The palliative and preventive effects of these techniques have given these procedures a sure hold in future medical practice, while benefits such as decreased absenteeism and increased feelings of wellness in employees have secured these strategies in the workplace. The expanded use of stress reduction procedures in prenatal care and with the elderly is likely.

—*Nancy A. Piotrowski, Ph.D.*

See also Acupressure; Acupuncture; Alternative medicine; Anxiety; Aromatherapy; Biofeedback; Cardiac rehabilitation; Chiropractic; Electrocardiography (ECG or EKG); Environmental health; Headaches; Hypertension; Hypnosis; Meditation; Occupational health; Qi gong; Stress; Tai Chi Chuan; Temporomandibular joint (TMJ) syndrome; Tics; Yoga.

FOR FURTHER INFORMATION:

Davis, Martha, Elizabeth Robbins Eshelman, and Matthew McKay. *The Relaxation and Stress Reduction Workbook.* 3d ed. Oakland, Calif.: New Harbinger, 1988. Provides guidance for different stress management techniques.

Humphrey, James H. *Stress Among Older Adults: Understanding and Coping.* Springfield, Ill.: Charles C Thomas, 1992. A rich overview of general and geriatric stress management issues and techniques.

Manning, George, Kent Curtis, and Steve McMillenis. *Stress: Living and Working in a Changing World.* Duluth, Minn.: Whole Person Associates, 1999. Road rage and workplace violence are but two of the more obvious symptoms of increasingly stressful times. Manning and his partners have put together this comprehensive manual to show individuals how to manage stress and help managers, counselors, and teachers develop programs that reduce stress.

Newton, Tim, with Jocelyn Handy and Stephen Fineman. *Managing Stress: Emotion and Power at Work.* Thousand Oaks, Calif.: Sage, 1995. This book addresses job stress and offers stress management techniques for coping with it. Includes a bibliography and an index.

Schafer, Walt. *Stress Management for Wellness.* New York: Holt, Rinehart & Winston, 1987. Describes how stress affects the body and how it may contribute to illness and death. Includes tests for identifying high personal stress levels and discusses stress reduction measures.

STRETCH MARKS
DISEASE/DISORDER
ALSO KNOWN AS: Striae
ANATOMY OR SYSTEM AFFECTED: Skin
SPECIALTIES AND RELATED FIELDS: Dermatology
DEFINITION: A whitish line or lesion on the skin caused by excessive stretching or tension on the skin.

CAUSES AND SYMPTOMS

Stretch marks are a type of scar that forms when there is excessive stretching or tension on the skin. This excessive tension can be a result of pregnancy, obesity, growth spurts during puberty, or lifting weights. Stretch marks develop in the skin's middle layer, which is called the dermis. The dermis is an elastic layer consisting of collagen that allows the skin to snap back into shape. When this region is stretched over a long period of time (for example, in pregnancy), the elasticity begins to weaken. Natural processes for the skin's reinforcement cause an increase in the amount of collagen in the overstretched tissue, resulting in the scars called stretch marks.

Stretch marks occur most often around the hips, thighs, buttocks, abdomen, and chest areas. When they first appear, they may be pink in color and can be slightly painful, but as they age, they turn whitish and become painless.

TREATMENT AND THERAPY

Effective measures have been developed to treat the appearance of stretch marks. One of these measures is the use of topical tretinoin, commonly known as Retin A. Applying tretinoin cream to the stretch marks promotes cells, known as fibroblasts, to lay down collagen and elastic fibers at the site. This helps to diminish, if not to completely fade, the appearance of the stretch marks. Tretinoin is known to work best if it is applied while the stretch mark is forming and is still pink, instead of waiting until the mark scars over and turns white. Side effects can occur from the use of tretinoin, including itching, burning, peeling, and redness at the application site.

Another measure that seems to improve the appearance of stretch marks is pulsed dye laser therapy. It is hypothesized that the treatment works by stimulating fibroblast and elastin production, yet no precise mechanism is known.

—*Angela Spano and Massimo D. Bezoari, M.D.*
See also Dermatology; Pregnancy and gestation; Skin; Skin disorders; Weight loss and gain.

FOR FURTHER INFORMATION:

Gutfeld, G., and M. Meyers. "So Long, Stretch Marks." *Prevention* 42, no. 12 (December, 1990): 22.

Kang, Sewon. "Topical Tretinoin (Retinoic Acid) Improves Early Stretch Marks." *Archives of Dermatology* 132 (May, 1996): 519-526.

Moyer, Paula. "Pulsed Dye Laser Seems Effective in Treating Stretch Marks." *Dermatology Times* 17, no. 7 (July, 1996): 66.

STROKES

DISEASE/DISORDER

ANATOMY OR SYSTEM AFFECTED: Blood vessels, brain, circulatory system, head, heart, nervous system, psychic-emotional system

SPECIALTIES AND RELATED FIELDS: Emergency medicine, neurology, speech pathology, vascular medicine

DEFINITION: Stroke, or a cerebrovascular accident (CVA), is the severe reduction or cessation of blood flow to the brain, resulting in a variety of serious and often permanent impairments depending on the area of the brain affected. A transient ischemic attack (TIA) is a temporary, brief loss of blood to the brain, accompanied by temporary impairment of vision, numbness, or other symptoms; it may herald a stroke.

KEY TERMS:

amaurosis fugax: temporary blindness in one eye

angiography: radiological modality to visualize the arteries in the body; involves the placement of a catheter in an artery and the injection of dye

embolus: a small piece of atherosclerotic plaque, thrombus, or other debris that breaks off and lodges in a blood vessel

endarterectomy: a surgical technique in which an atherosclerotic plaque is excised

infarct: tissue death resulting from lack of blood flow

ischemia: lack of blood in a particular tissue

revascularization: procedures to reestablish the circulation to a diseased portion of the body

thrombosis: the aggregation of platelets and other blood cells to form a clot

transient ischemic attacks (TIAs): commonly known as "ministrokes"; associated neurological deficits last less than twenty-four hours and usually only minutes

CAUSES AND SYMPTOMS

Strokes produce damage to portions of the brain as a result of decreased blood supply. Strokes are commonly known as cerebrovascular accidents (CVAs). Symptoms of strokes will vary depending on the part of the brain that is affected. Resulting speech disorders may include aphasia (loss of the ability to speak) or dysarthria (difficulty in speaking). A sudden weakness or numbness of one side of the body is known as hemiparesis or hemiplegia. The eyes can also be involved. A dimness or transient loss of vision, particularly in one eye, is called amaurosis fugax. Occasionally, it can involve the same portion of the visual field in both eyes. Other symptoms of stroke may include dizziness, unsteadiness, sudden falls, headaches, confusion, or stupor. Coma is less commonly involved in a stroke.

Predisposing factors to strokes include hypertension (high blood pressure), diabetes, high cholesterol, smoking, atherosclerotic disease in other portions of the body (such as the heart or legs), and a previous or family history of strokes or transient ischemic attacks. Gender and age are also associated with the incidence of strokes.

In cerebrovascular disease, atherosclerosis affects the arteries that circulate blood to the brain. The brain receives blood from two major sets of arteries. The carotid arteries, in the front of the neck, supply the anterior (front) portions of the brain. The vertebral arteries travel through the transverse processes of the spine and join the basilar artery to provide blood to the posterior (back) portion of the brain. Both circulatory systems are joined within the brain in a structure known as the circle of Willis, a composite of arteries that join to form an anatomical circle. The various arteries supply the necessary blood flow to different areas of the brain. Only 25 to 50 percent of people have a complete circle of Willis; this anatomical variance may be a factor in the severity of the stroke.

In atherosclerotic disease, fat, cholesterol, and calcium deposits are laid down along the walls of the arteries, primarily at sites where arteries divide and natural turbulence tends to occur. These components build up to form plaques, which may cause stenosis (narrowing) and occlusion (closure) of the arterial lumen. Accumulation of platelets and other blood cells can form a thrombus (blood clot) along with plaque buildup, which also may obstruct the arteries. Pieces of plaque or thrombotic material may break off and cause emboli to lodge acutely in the main vessels or their more distant branches.

The most common components of cerebrovascular disease are transient ischemic attacks (TIAs), also referred to as ministrokes. By definition, TIAs last less than twenty-four hours; usually, they last only a few minutes or hours. Most TIAs are produced by emboli. An embolus occurs when a piece of plaque from the lining of a major artery breaks off and temporarily blocks the blood flow to a particular area of the brain. If the symptoms last for more than twenty-four hours, a cerebrovascular accident, cerebral infarct, or stroke has occurred. A reversible ischemic neurological deficit (RIND) is similar to a stroke in that it is an event that lasts for more than twenty-four hours but resolves in about seventy-two hours.

The majority of strokes (63 percent) are the result of impaired blood flow (ischemia) to the brain. Atherosclerosis in the cerebrovascular system will cause similar symptoms of ischemia in other portions of the body. There is increasing narrowing, or stenosis, of blood vessels. Eventually, they will close off completely and become occluded. The development of new, small vessels that bypass a diseased artery is called collateralization. This process requires weeks or months to occur. Collateralization seems to be especially prominent in the cerebrovascular system, since the brain is an organ that requires constant blood flow at all times. Eventual occlusion or thrombosis of a major vessel causes the majority of CVAs,

producing significant ischemia in a portion of the brain.

In certain cases, the blockage is acute, having resulted from an embolus or thrombus that blocks an artery. If collateralization has not developed, the damage to an affected structure is more severe. A thrombus or embolus can also arise from the heart. This is most common in individuals who have had a recent heart attack, who have disease that involves the mitral valve, or who have atrial fibrillation, a variety of irregular heartbeat. Another cause of stroke is

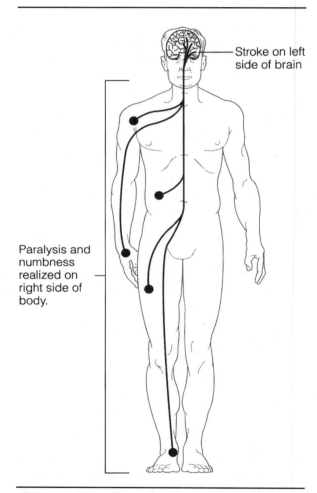

Stroke on left side of brain

Paralysis and numbness realized on right side of body.

A major stroke to one hemisphere of the brain generally results in impairment of motor functions on the opposite side of the body. In addition, because the two brain hemispheres control different mental and autonomic functions, impairments will vary; for example, left-brain stroke is usually associated with some degree of speech impairment, because the speech centers are located in the left brain.

cerebral hemorrhage, or bleeding into the brain, which is also occasionally referred to as apoplexy. Hypertension is the most common cause of intracranial bleeding and accounts for 10 to 15 percent of cases. Other causes of strokes are cerebral aneurysms (5 to 7 percent), tumors that have developed blood supplies (3 to 5 percent), and genetic bleeding tendencies (1 to 2 percent).

A cerebral aneurysm occurs when the wall of an artery becomes weak and enlarges like a balloon. These aneurysms often rupture. With a ruptured cerebral aneurysm and subsequent hemorrhage, by-products of red blood cell degeneration may produce a condition called vasospasm, wherein the arteries will constrict. This often leads to ischemia. One or more thrombi are often formed in an aneurysm. If they break loose, they can become emboli, float until they become lodged in a small blood vessel, block the flow of blood, and cause ischemia. This can ultimately lead to a stroke.

Stroke refers to the disease process that is mainly produced by atherosclerotic changes in the arteries to the brain. Contributing or significant risk factors in the development of atherosclerosis include hypertension (high blood pressure), hyperlipidemia (high levels of cholesterol in the blood), smoking, diabetes mellitus, and a family history of similar incidents. Evidence of atherosclerotic disease in other portions of the body, such as the heart or legs, increases the risk of stroke. Atherosclerosis is a generalized disease process that affects arterial beds throughout the body.

Symptoms of TIAs in structures near the front of the brain, the area supplied by the carotid arteries, include hemiparesis, a numbness or loss of function in half of the body. Hemiplegia, a weakness of an arm or leg (or both), can be attributable to disease in the carotid artery on the side of the body opposite to the affected body part. Another relatively common problem usually caused by disease in the left carotid artery is aphasia, a speech disorder. Disease in either carotid artery can cause amaurosis fugax, or blindness in one eye. Victims often described this condition as a shade being drawn over the eye.

Other, more generalized symptoms are the result of problems in the vertebral arteries or the blood vessels at the base of the brain, which supply the back portions of the brain. Associated symptoms include dizziness, a loss of orientation often produced by decreased blood flow to the brain. Dizziness is frequently caused by abrupt positional changes, in which blood pressure will suddenly fall with rapid standing or sitting, or by cardiac arrhythmias (irregular heartbeats), which prevent adequate amounts of blood flow from being delivered during certain cardiac cycles.

Vertigo is different from dizziness. Individuals suffering from vertigo experience a spinning sensation that may be accompanied by nausea. A common cause for vertigo is a condition known as subclavian steal, in which atherosclerotic disease affects the arteries of the arms just prior to the point where the vertebral arteries branch off. As an arm is used, or with abrupt changes in head position, blood will flow out of the vertebral arteries in a reverse manner (the so-called steal) to aid circulation in the arm (via the subclavian arteries) and vertigo will ensue. In addition, imbalance and other visual disturbances may be associated with problems in the vertebral arteries. These symptoms may also result from cerebrovascular disease in which inadequate blood supply to multiple areas of the brain can produce diverse symptoms.

In the majority of strokes, symptoms last twenty-four to seventy-two hours. Approximately 25 percent of patients will develop permanent deficits that will affect them for the rest of their lives. Approximately 20 percent of individuals who have strokes will experience no symptoms (be asymptomatic) and not know that they have had a stroke. They are unlikely to even develop TIAs. Such unheralded events result from occlusion or thrombosis of the blood vessels in the brain. This causes ischemia that leads to infarction or cell death in a particular section of the brain.

Asymptomatic cerebrovascular disease, however, can often be detected by the presence of a bruit, a French word meaning "noise." Stenosis in arteries can be compared to rapids in a river. Blood will flow very quickly through the narrow area and create turbulence, producing a bruit that can be heard with a stethoscope. Patients with narrowing in the carotid arteries ranging from 20 to 80 percent may possess a bruit. The absence of a bruit does not mean that the carotid arteries are disease-free. Once the stenosis reaches critical proportions, the flow is diminished and turbulence may be negligible, indicating a severe stenosis or an occluded artery. Often, doctors will recommend elective surgery to patients with coronary artery stenosis between 60 and 80 percent in an effort to reestablish blood flow and prevent eventual occlusion and possible stroke. About 75 percent of strokes are caused by ischemia that results from the above process. Crescendo TIAs, in which multiple TIAs occur in a brief period of time, and evolving strokes require immediate medical treatment. Appropriate diagnosis and treatment may prevent a stroke or decrease its severity.

Although disease caused by an aneurysm is a separate entity, it may be associated with atherosclerotic disease in certain cases. Most aneurysms within the brain produce no symptoms. As aneurysms increase in size, the probability of rupture increases; therefore, elective surgery may be recommended. Occasionally, diagnoses of cerebral aneurysms are made during investigations of other cerebral events, such as headaches. Acute onset of severe headaches or stiff neck should mandate immediate medical attention, since rupture of a cerebral aneurysm often manifests itself in this manner.

TREATMENT AND THERAPY

Strokes and TIAs often occur quickly and without warning. The best treatment for them is preventive behavior to avoid the atherosclerotic disease leading to such events. When a stroke or TIA is suspected, however, a complete history and physical examination is usually the first component of diagnosis. Eliciting symptoms and noting significant risk factors and findings upon physical examination will help a physician determine the primary area of the brain affected, schedule the appropriate tests for further diagnosis, and choose the best course of therapy.

Because of the high incidence of death and disability associated with strokes, a variety of diagnostic tests have been developed since the 1950's. One of the oldest noninvasive methods is the directional Doppler test. A Doppler device employs a probe with one or two piezoelectric crystals. An ultrasonic signal using a frequency of 2 to 5 megahertz (MHz) is sent into the body. Movement of red blood cells causes a shift in the frequency of the signal that is transmitted back. The amount of shift is proportional to the speed of blood flow. This device can also be used to determine the direction of blood flow. By listening with a continuous-wave Doppler over a branch of the ophthalmic artery at the corner of the eye and performing certain compression maneuvers on the arteries that supply the face, information regarding possible collateral pathways can be obtained concerning internal carotid artery blockages of greater than 75 percent.

The vascular surgeon William Gee developed another device, called an ocular pneumoplethysmograph (OPG). The OPG utilizes cups placed in the eye to measure the ocular pressure. A vacuum is applied to the eyes, effectively blocking the ophthalmic arteries, which are the first major branches of the internal carotid artery. As the vacuum is released, the blood flow is reestablished and the appearance of arterial pulsations is noted on a strip chart. These pulsations denote systolic blood pressure in the ophthalmic arteries. A pressure difference of 5 millimeters of mercury (mm Hg) between the two eyes or an index of less than 0.66 (comparing the systolic blood pressure in the ophthalmic artery with that in the brachial artery) is consistent with carotid artery blockage of more than 50 to 75 percent.

Both of these methods are indirect tests, in which significant internal carotid artery disease is implied if the test is positive. Deficiencies in the test procedures include quantification of the percentage of carotid artery disease or differentiation of significant stenosis from occlusions. They also may be wrong if the vertebral or basal arteries contribute significant collateral blood flow. The OPG is still used in certain situations as a quick screening tool, but the directional Doppler has lost favor as an accurate diagnostic test.

Duplex ultrasound machines, first employed in the early 1980's, utilize B-mode (brightness-mode) ultrasound to visualize the vessels and type of plaque. In comparison, Doppler ultrasound can audibly evaluate the blood flow in the vessels. Using real-time spectrum analyzers, the Doppler signals are then analyzed in terms of velocity (speed of the blood flow) and waveform characteristics. The greater the velocity, the greater the amount of stenosis. Absence of blood flow will denote occlusions.

Much research has been done in evaluating plaque morphology and its association with the incidence of TIAs, but results have been controversial using the standard gray-scale duplex devices. The use of color duplex ultrasound, in which the Doppler signals are color-coded in terms of flow direction and speed to denote the various flow patterns in normal and diseased vessels, has enhanced the diagnostic accuracies of the examinations. The use of color Doppler in many ultrasound machines is allowing more rapid detection of arterial lesions in blood vessels both inside and outside the skull.

Transcranial Doppler uses a MHz pulsed Doppler probe through various normal anatomic windows (holes) in the skull. Measurements can be made through the side of the head (transtemporal), from the back of the head (transoccipital), and through the eye (transocular). The purpose of the examination is to assess the blood circulation in the circle of Willis. The transcranial Doppler gives information concerning various collateral pathways established when significant disease is present in blood vessels outside the skull. It is also useful when there is stenosis of arteries inside the skull. It is extremely accurate in detecting and monitoring early vasospasm in individuals with bleeding inside the skull. Additional research with this device is ongoing in other areas, such as in the detection of cerebral aneurysms and arteriovenous malformations in which there is an abnormal connection between the arteries and the veins.

Computed tomography (CT) scanning is a radiological technique that provides a three-dimensional picture of the brain and its structures. Occasionally, a contrast medium is also used in this examination. CT scanning is especially useful in the diagnosis of cerebral aneurysms and areas of infarct. Magnetic resonance imaging (MRI) is a nonradiological technique that also provides exceptional three-dimensional images of the soft tissue structures of the brain. MRI can detect cerebral infarcts at an earlier stage than can CT scanning.

Arteriography or angiography is an invasive procedure that is performed in a hospital setting. A catheter is placed in one of the arteries, and dye containing iodine is injected. Multiple X rays are then taken to visualize the circulation. Arteriograms are considered to be standard in diagnosis. The delineation of the blockages and collateral pathways is then used primarily to plan surgical procedures.

Aspirin is often prescribed to alleviate symptoms of TIAs and to help protect patients from strokes or heart attacks. Although it is a powerful drug in decreasing the incidence of embolus formation, a national study has demonstrated that patients with a history of TIAs and carotid artery stenosis of greater than 60 percent should undergo surgical revascularization to protect against major strokes. The chances of having a stroke after suffering a TIA are approximately 40 percent greater. National studies are currently being conducted to evaluate the incidence of strokes in asymptomatic patients with stenosis of greater than 60 percent who take aspirin or who use a combination of aspirin and surgery therapy.

Endarterectomy is a surgical technique in which the inner wall and part of the middle wall of the ca-

rotid artery are excised, effectively scraping out atherosclerotic plaques. Although used in other arterial segments, endarterectomy is the most common surgical procedure used to revascularize the carotid arteries. Occasionally, procedures are performed to bypass diseased segments of the cerebral vessels. Long-term research has shown that they have limited effectiveness. Consequently, many have been abandoned.

Other techniques for intervention have been developed. Percutaneous balloon angioplasty involves placing a balloon catheter in the diseased segment during an angiogram. When the balloon catheter is inflated, it opens up the area of stenosis or small segment of occlusion. This method has been employed in the coronary arteries as well as in the vessels leaving the aorta, the iliac arteries, and arteries in the lower extremities. It is not used often in the treatment of atherosclerotic plaques in the cerebral circulation because of the possibility of emboli traveling to the more distant blood vessels of the brain or eye. Some success in the use of balloon angioplasty has been reported in the treatment of vasospasm.

New drugs that dissolve clots may be used alone or in combination with balloon angioplasty or surgery. Although effective in the treatment of coronary artery and peripheral vascular disease, their use in the cerebral circulation has been restricted because of the risk of embolus formation or bleeding complications.

PERSPECTIVE AND PROSPECTS

Stroke is the third-leading cause of death in the United States, with approximately 155,000 deaths annually. There are 400,000 strokes annually, and about one-fourth of all nursing home patients are permanently impaired from strokes. These statistics have a great impact on the amount of money spent annually on care for victims of strokes.

Since the 1960's, the death rate from strokes in the United States has decreased significantly, by about 50 percent. Control of blood pressure and diet, the development of new drugs and diagnostic techniques, and the advent of cardiovascular surgery in the early 1950's have contributed to these results. Unfortunately, strokes are still prevalent given the extent of atherosclerotic disease in the American population, which is largely attributed to a high-fat diet. Autopsies of U.S. soldiers killed in the Korean and Vietnam Wars demonstrated evidence that atherosclerosis begins at a very early age, often by age eighteen. Atherosclerosis is more prevalent in males. Females have more protection until the onset of the menopause. Within five years of the menopause, however, the stroke and death rates of men and women tend to equalize.

High-salt diets, which contribute to hypertension, also contribute to the development and progression of atherosclerosis, as well as hemorrhagic strokes. Ethnic African and Asian populations appear to be at greater risk in this respect. Since the 1960's, however, extensive education of the American public concerning diet and the control of blood pressure has had a favorable impact. More recently, the increase in individuals who have stopped smoking and who have undertaken regular exercise has helped to lower stroke rates further.

Since the 1950's, a number of both noninvasive and invasive procedures have been developed to diagnose atherosclerotic disease. Cardiovascular surgical techniques were developed in the 1950's. The first bypass surgery (arterial autograft) probably occurred during the Korean War. The development of ultrasound devices in the 1950's initiated the research into using these noninvasive devices to diagnose cerebrovascular disease. The duplex devices introduced commercially in the late 1970's and early 1980's have spurred the development of new diagnostic devices for detecting atherosclerotic disease. These devices allow for visualization of plaque morphology (composition of the plaque, such as thrombus, calcium, hemorrhage, and other particulate matters) and blood flow characteristics for a better understanding of the disease process. Future developments in the field of ultrasound include holographic imaging for the three-dimensional visualization of plaques. These noninvasive technologies will also allow physicians to monitor the effects of new drugs and techniques in the treatment of atherosclerosis. Advances in digital subtraction and computer enhancement of angiographic techniques, along with new contrast media, have made arteriograms safer and more accurate.

Color duplex devices are utilizing low-frequency probes to visualize and produce color scans of blood vessels that lie inside the skull. By analyzing the blood flow direction and velocity in the circle of Willis and within the blood vessels of the skull, physicians will come to a better understanding of the formation of collateral pathways and will learn how to detect other pathological conditions that lead to cerebrovascular disease. Magnetic resonance imaging is also being utilized to measure actual flow in individual arterial segments of the body.

Carotid endarterectomies, which lost favor for a period of time, have become the preferred therapeutic treatment for individuals with episodes of TIAs and severe atherosclerotic plaques in the carotid arteries. Additional studies will further delineate which other patient populations may benefit from this surgery. Aspirin still remains a potent drug in the treatment of TIAs in patients with lesser degrees of disease and in postsurgery patients. Recognition and prompt treatment of symptomatic cerebrovascular symptoms remain the key to better survival rates.

—*Silvia M. Berry, M.Sc., R.V.T.;*
updated by L. Fleming Fallon, Jr.,
M.D., Ph.D., M.P.H.

See also Angiography; Angioplasty; Aphasia and dysphasia; Arteriosclerosis; Brain; Brain disorders; Bypass surgery; Cholesterol; Circulation; Congenital heart disease; Edema; Embolism; Endarterectomy; Heart attack; Heart disease; Heart failure; Hyperlipidemia; Hypertension; Ischemia; Numbness and tingling; Paralysis; Speech disorders; Thrombolytic therapy and TPA; Thrombosis and thrombus; Vascular medicine; Vascular system.

FOR FURTHER INFORMATION:

Frye-Pierson, Janice, and James F. Toole. *Stroke: A Guide for the Patient and Family.* New York: Raven Press, 1987. Written by a leading neurological nurse clinician and a prominent neurologist, this practical guide addresses the questions raised by stroke patients and their families and offers suggestions to aid in rehabilitation.

Ouriel, Kenneth, and Robert B. Rutherford. *Atlas of Vascular Surgery.* 4th ed. Philadelphia: W. B. Saunders, 1998. This is a definitive textbook for the understanding, diagnosis, and treatment of vascular disorders.

Rao, Paul R. *Managing Stroke: A Guide to Living Well After Stroke.* Washington, D.C.: ABI Professional, 2000. The staff of the National Rehabilitation Hospital in Washington, D.C., has created an instructional guide for those who have suffered a stroke.

Wiebers, David O., Valery L. Feigin, and Robert D. Brown. *Handbook of Stroke.* Boston: Little, Brown, 1997. Based on extensive experience at the Mayo Clinic, this book provides a concise and easy-to-read guide for the evaluation and management of stroke. It is filled with algorithms that put pertinent information at the reader's fingertips.

STUTTERING
DISEASE/DISORDER
ANATOMY OR SYSTEM AFFECTED: Nervous system
SPECIALTIES AND RELATED FIELDS: Family practice, neurology, pediatrics, speech pathology
DEFINITION: Breaks in the smooth flow of speech.

CAUSES AND SYMPTOMS
Stuttering is usually recognized as a child develops enough language skill to speak in complete sentences, beginning around three years of age. Typically, the child repeats the beginning sounds of a word, or whole words, before continuing with the sentence, as in, "I l-l-l-like to p-p-p-pet my ca-ca-cat." True stuttering must be differentiated from developmental dysfluency and dysfluency caused by unusually severe environmental or social pressures. Developmental dysfluency is normal, occurring in the three- or four-year-old child whose brain works faster than his or her mouth. This child may repeat parts of words, words, or parts of phrases, especially when excited. When a child feels significantly anxious, language may become dysfluent, or broken up and difficult to understand. This is not true stuttering, and treatment should be aimed at alleviating the anxiety or stress.

True stuttering is less common than the two dysfluencies just described, and it occurs more often in boys. Frequently, the true stutterer is consistently dysfluent on the same sounds or words. There is consistency in repetitions, prolongations, pauses, grammatical forms, and rate of emission of dysfluency. Often, the child will overcome a verbal hurdle by using certain actions such as eye blinking, finger snapping, or foot tapping.

TREATMENT AND THERAPY
Treatment of true stuttering by a competent speech pathologist is imperative, and the prognosis, although variable, can be good. Parents and teachers should be alerted to alleviate any emotional stress that is unusual or severe. Absolutely essential is the ability of all adults to deal with the stuttering child without calling attention to the speech patterns or mannerisms. Practicing reading aloud, especially poetry, and singing—all in the privacy of the company of a caring adult—may help.

PERSPECTIVE AND PROSPECTS
The great ancient Greek orator Demosthenes was dysfluent and allegedly practiced talking with pebbles in his mouth until he could speak clearly. Stuttering does not preclude a person becoming successful in any endeavor. Modern speech therapy and understanding adults can be of great benefit to a child who stutters.

—*Robert W. Block, M.D.*

See also Anxiety; Lisping; Phobias; Psychiatry, child and adolescent; Speech disorders.

FOR FURTHER INFORMATION:
Cole, Patricia R. *Language Disorders in Preschool Children.* Englewood Cliffs, N.J.: Prentice Hall, 1982.
Egland, George O. *Speech and Language Problems.* Englewood Cliffs, N.J.: Prentice Hall, 1970.
Eisenson, Jon, and Mardel Ogilvie. *Speech Correction in the Schools.* 4th ed. New York: Macmillan, 1977.
Winitz, Harris, ed. *Human Communication and Its Disorders: A Review, 1987.* Norwood, N.J.: Ablex, 1987.

STYES
DISEASE/DISORDER
ALSO KNOWN AS: Hordeolums
ANATOMY OR SYSTEM AFFECTED: Eyes, glands
SPECIALTIES AND RELATED FIELDS: Family practice, ophthalmology, optometry, pediatrics
DEFINITION: Styes are small abscesses of the sebaceous, hair follicle glands in the eyelid, sometimes involving the eyelashes and the conjunctiva (the white of the eye). Styes are typically caused by staphylococcus bacteria that produce redness, swelling, warmth, tenderness, and/or pain on the edge of the top or bottom eyelid. Applying warm-water packs relieves the pain and hastens healing. Doctors may prescribe antibiotic eyedrops, oral antibiotics, or topical antibiotic ointments, such as erythromycin or bacitracin.

—*Alvin K. Benson, Ph.D.*

See also Abscesses; Antibiotics; Bacterial infections; Eyes; Glands; Staphylococcal infections; Visual disorders.

FOR FURTHER INFORMATION:
Goodman, Thomas, and Stephanie Young. *Smart Face.* Englewood Cliffs, N.J.: Prentice Hall, 1988.

Novick, Nelson Lee. *Saving Face*. New York: Franklin Watts, 1986.

Paslin, David. *The Hide Guide: Skin Problems and How to Deal with Them*. Millbrae, Calif.: Celestial Arts, 1981.

SUBSTANCE ABUSE. *See* ADDICTION.

SUDDEN INFANT DEATH SYNDROME (SIDS)

DISEASE/DISORDER

ANATOMY OR SYSTEM AFFECTED: All

SPECIALTIES AND RELATED FIELDS: Neonatology, pediatrics, psychiatry, psychology

DEFINITION: The abrupt and inexplicable death of any infant or young child, and the most common cause of infant death between the ages of two weeks and one year; postmortem examination fails to demonstrate a definitive cause of death.

KEY TERMS:

apnea: absence of breathing

bradycardia: slowness of the heartbeat

hyperthermia: environmentally influenced elevated body temperature

hypothermia: environmentally influenced lower-than-normal body temperature

hypoxemia: subnormal oxygenation of arterial blood

neonatal: the period of time succeeding birth and continuing through the first twenty-eight days of life

prone: lying face-downward

supine: lying face-upward

tachycardia: rapid beating of the heart

thermolabile: unstable when heated

CAUSES AND SYMPTOMS

The distribution of sudden infant death syndrome (SIDS) is worldwide. Incidence rates vary from 0.12 to 3.0 for every thousand live births. In the United States, rates range from 1.6 to 2.3 for every thousand live births, with considerable ethnic variation: 0.5 among Asians, 1.3 among whites, 1.7 among Latinos, 2.9 among African Americans (5.0 for those of low socioeconomic status), and 5.9 among American Indians.

Cultural practices may make the incidence rate vary. In England, a Birmingham study found that 22 percent of Asian babies were put to sleep on their backs, compared with 3 percent of white babies. Sleeping prone is significantly more common in infants dying of SIDS than in controls. In the same study, 98 per-

cent of Asian babies slept in the same room as their parents for the first year, 34 percent in the same bed. Only 65 percent of white infants slept in the same room as their parents. Perhaps the risk of sudden infant death increases in proportion to the amount of time an infant spends asleep out of parental earshot. In Zimbabwe, SIDS practically does not exist. According to English pediatrician Duncan Keeley, who served in that country for two years, black Zimbabwean infants almost invariably sleep with their mothers, at least until they are six months old and often until they are a year old.

The cause of sudden infant death syndrome is unknown, but a variety of genetic, environmental, and social factors have been associated with an increased risk of SIDS. Besides sleeping in the prone position, other associations include cold weather, overheating, the hours of the day from midnight to 9:00 A.M., and poor socioeconomic conditions, including overcrowding. The young, unmarried mother, especially if she has had no prenatal care, is more likely to have an infant with SIDS. So is the mother who smokes (either before or after the birth), is anemic, or ingests narcotics. Prematurity, especially with a history of apnea or damage to the immature lungs from elevated levels of inspired oxygen while on a respirator, also increases the risk.

Males are at a higher risk for SIDS than are females; so are the brothers and sisters of infants with SIDS. Likewise, a previously aborted episode of SIDS (that is, a "near miss") increases risk. On average, Apgar scores (a measure of infant health immediately after birth) are lower in infants with SIDS than they are in surviving peers. In a family that has lost an infant to SIDS, the risk for the next or subsequent child is about five times the usual risk. Most risk factors, however, are associated with only a twofold or threefold elevation of incidence. Therefore, predicting which infants will die unexpectedly is extremely difficult. Recent immunization is not a risk factor. Breast-feeding is not associated with a decreased risk, as was originally thought. Although the peak incidence of SIDS is around three months of age and coincides with normally low levels of circulating immunoglobulins, the syndrome is not associated with any known pathogen.

Pathologists report a wide variety of findings in their postmortem reports—especially changes in the brain and other parts of the body that suggest chronic or intermittent hypoxemia. Yet pathologists also fail to find an increase in the number of cells in tissue of the carotid bodies, a chemoreceptor that responds to decreases in blood oxygen tension; such a finding weighs against the presence of chronic hypoxia.

Like many other aspects of this disease, the mechanism or mechanisms of death in SIDS are unknown. Does the infant stop breathing, or does some cardiac irregularity occur? An immature cardiorespiratory control mechanism involving the nervous system is the most common hypothesis.

D. P. Davies and Madeleine Gantley of the University of Wales College of Medicine believe that an important mechanism underlying SIDS is failure of respiratory control at a vulnerable stage of development—more a physiological syndrome than a disease in the accepted sense. These doctors hypothesize that the disturbance to this delicate equilibrium might upset the regulation of breathing, sometimes leading to death. Epidemiological risk factors, such as an upper-respiratory infection (which is not uncommon), are somehow linked with destabilizing influences to breathing. By avoiding or modulating these factors, the risk of death can be reduced.

Although the pathogenesis of SIDS remains unclear, Anne-Louise Ponsonby and her colleagues at the University of Tasmania in Australia propose that SIDS be considered as a biphasic event, with the first set of factors operating to predispose the infant and the second set of factors acting as loading factors that operate at a critical stage of the infant's development. The Australian doctors believe that a warm environment could lead to sudden infant death by direct hyperthermia; a thermolabile, sudden fall in blood pressure leading to a diminished oxygen supply to the brain; impaired respiratory control; altered sleep state; or depressed arousal. An asphyxial mode of death would also be more likely, particularly in heavily dressed infants found prone (face down).

Concern for the confusion of SIDS with child abuse should not be ignored, nor should the efforts of the National Sudden Infant Death Syndrome Foundation to provide information about psychosocial support groups and counseling for families of SIDS victims.

TREATMENT AND THERAPY

Since the causes and mechanisms of death from SIDS may continue to be unknown, strategies that might reduce the incidence of this syndrome seem imperative. Cold weather and the hours of midnight to 9:00 A.M.

bring increased risks for SIDS. A closer look explains that other risk factors are involved. Overheating as a response to cold weather and leaving the infant alone at night (particularly in Western countries) may be more important. Babies sleeping alone might lose external sensory stimulation that may help stabilize breathing patterns. Davies and Gantley, citing experimental work with mothers and infants co-sleeping in sleep laboratories, have shown how patterns of breathing may interact. They say that the alertness of the babies' caregivers to early symptoms of illness might also be important.

French doctors studied the seasonal variation of death from SIDS in their country for a two-year period in the early 1980's. They concluded that for babies born in the spring, the third month of age was not necessarily associated with the highest SIDS risk. Babies born during other seasons, however, exhibited a normal pattern of increasing risk between the first and third months. Age was an especially critical factor among babies who reached three months of age during the winter months. If they reach this age in July or August, they are less susceptible to SIDS.

This finding, then, leads to a consideration of the risk of overheating. Explanations for the association between cold weather and SIDS include hypothermia, increased viral illness, and indirect hyperthermia. New Zealand doctors looked at the role of thermal balance in SIDS by investigating the death scene. They found that infants who died of SIDS were significantly more likely to be overdressed for the room temperature at the death scene and in the prone position, when compared to control infants. They also suggest that parents may have responded to infections in their babies by increasing the amount of clothing and bedding or by otherwise warming the infant.

The government of New Zealand initiated a program of education for parents recommending that the prone sleeping position be avoided, that mothers not smoke, and that breast-feeding be encouraged. (Most experts believe that breast-feeding itself does not reduce risks for SIDS. Rather, closer and more frequent contact with mothers is the operative factor.)

A similar education program for parents in Avon, England, was initiated, but it omitted advice on breast-feeding and included suggestions to avoid overheating after a retrospective case-control study that suggested a nearly ninefold relative risk for SIDS from infants sleeping prone. New Zealand and Avon both reported fewer deaths from SIDS after their parental education programs were introduced. The Department of Health extended Avon's campaign nationally.

In an editorial note in 1986, the National Center for Health Statistics acknowledged that "the rapid decline of infant mortality rates in the 1970's has been attributed largely to the advent of medical technology in the area of premature and other clinically ill newborns." Yet, "in the 1980's, this decline has slowed considerably—partly because of a lack of progress in primary prevention of conditions which lead to infant death." Undoubtedly, the United States would benefit from a massive, national program of education for parents. For example, cigarette packages carry a warning of the harmful effects of smoking on the fetus; perhaps they should also include a warning about the dangers to infants of maternal smoking. Another possibility for intervention exists in the area of infections: Pertussis (whooping cough) could be prevented by the immunization of infants under six months of age. In the long term, all nations should work toward improving the socioeconomic status of the poor and health care.

Finally, improved medical technology will be less important over the long haul than will efforts to educate parents in infant care practices. The ability of parents and other members of the household to monitor infants and respond appropriately to both true and false alarms is crucial, as is appropriate training in infant CPR (cardiopulmonary resuscitation) and the proper use of monitory equipment. Even if all SIDS is eliminated in at-risk children, there will continue to be cases among children not known to have been at risk.

PERSPECTIVE AND PROSPECTS

The term "sudden infant death syndrome" was popularized by Dr. Abraham Berman's book on SIDS in 1969, which grew out of a conference on that subject. Since then, recognition of the syndrome has led to the creation of organizations dealing with it. The Sudden Infant Death Foundation merged, on January 1, 1991, with the National Center for the Prevention of SIDS to form one organization, the Sudden Infant Death Alliance.

In dealing with SIDS, one factor looms most important: Education of parents makes all the difference. In 1991, for example, England's Scarborough district reported a 50 percent fall in the SIDS death rate after parents were advised not to overwarm their small infants. That same year, four other districts in England reported a similar reduction after parents were advised not to let their infants sleep in a prone position. The Foundation for the Study of Infant Deaths and the Department of Health recommend both procedures: a supine sleeping position and prevention of overwarming.

These successes raise two issues: the overall decline in rates of SIDS worldwide in industrial countries and parental guilt. For a number of years, the incidence of SIDS was generally falling. This decline

In the News: Tracking the Causes of SIDS

SIDS is the leading cause of death in infants under twelve months of age, yet the cause of SIDS is unknown. Researchers have identified factors that increase the risk of SIDS, one of which is infants' sleeping on their stomachs. Results of a recent study carried out at the Memorial Hospital of Rhode Island provide some evidence for why stomach sleeping increases the risk of SIDS. It appears that when infants sleep on their stomachs, their capacity to breathe may be compromised. The research team, led by Dr. Vivender Rehan, found that the muscles of infants' diaphragms were shortened and thickened when infants were lying on their stomachs, compared to when they were lying on their backs. These muscle changes could cause infants' breathing to be weakened, leading to higher rates of respiratory distress associated with stomach sleeping.

Another recent study by a team at the University of Milan, Italy, led by Dr. Peter Schwartz, has demonstrated a new link between infants' abnormal heartbeats and SIDS. The team measured the electrical activity that controls infants' heartbeats, and found that infants who had longer QT intervals (the time between electrical signals that produce a heart muscle contraction) were at a higher risk for SIDS. This result suggests that early cardiac screening may help prevent some cases of SIDS.

—*Virginia Slaughter, Ph.D.*

slowed considerably in the 1980's. How much, then, did the parental education programs actually lower the incidence rate in these English districts? No one can say with certainty, but one thing is clear: If doctors make recommendations regarding sleeping positions and warming, they run the risk of inducing guilt in parents who have not followed their recommendations—or, alternatively, who have followed the recommendations but have still lost an infant to SIDS. Parents who have lost a child to SIDS are grief-stricken. They are not prepared for such a tragedy, and their grief is compounded by guilt, because no definitive cause for SIDS has been identified and, as a result, parental behavior seems to be implicated. Investigations conducted by police, social workers, or others who become involved only add to this guilt. Parents may be confronted by questions of whether they positioned their infant correctly or overdressed the child. Regardless of these behaviors, however, the factors causing the death may not have been under the parents' control.

SIDS will continue to occur until the exact etiologies of the syndrome, its mechanisms, and its correct treatment—based on fact, not simply risks alone—are identified. Until that time, it is expected that incidence rates will continue to go down, based on what is now known of the risk factors and recommendations against prone sleeping positions and overwarming.

—*Wayne R. McKinny, M.D.*

See also Apnea; Death and dying; Grief and guilt; Hyperthermia and hypothermia; Neonatology; Premature birth; Respiration.

FOR FURTHER INFORMATION:

Behrman, Richard E., ed. *Nelson Textbook of Pediatrics.* 16th ed. Philadelphia: W. B. Saunders, 2000. This standard pediatric textbook has been around for years and deservedly so. Its excellent chapter on sudden infant death syndrome is a thorough review of the disease.

Berger, Edward C., ed. *SIDS and Sleep Disorders: A Review of the Literature.* St. Paul, Minn.: Aequitron Medical, 1990. This thorough review of the literature brings together much useful information. The results of cited studies are presented in easy-to-grasp charts and lists.

Berkow, Robert, and Andrew J. Fletcher, eds. *The Merck Manual of Diagnosis and Therapy.* 17th ed. Rahway, N.J.: Merck Sharp & Dohme Research Laboratories, 1999. Published since 1899, this classic medical book covers SIDS thoroughly and is easy to read.

Southall, D. P., and M. P. Samuels. "Reducing Risks in the Sudden Infant Death Syndrome." *British Medical Journal* 304 (February 1, 1992): 265-266. These acknowledged experts in SIDS have written a thoughtful, thorough review on reducing the risks of SIDS. They strongly suggest that current interventions and socioeconomic factors need monitoring.

SUFFOCATION. *See* ASPHYXIATION.

SUICIDE
DISEASE/DISORDER

ANATOMY OR SYSTEM AFFECTED: Psychic-emotional system, all bodily systems

SPECIALTIES AND RELATED FIELDS: Geriatrics and gerontology, psychiatry, psychology

DEFINITION: The deliberate taking of one's own life, usually the result of a mental disorder, although sometimes deliberated in the face of life-threatening physical illness.

KEY TERMS:

"no suicide" contract: an agreement, verbally or in writing, that a suicidal person will not act on these urges

psychosomatic: referring to physical symptoms caused by psychological problems

rational suicide: suicide to avoid suffering when there is no underlying cognitive or psychiatric disorder

ritual suicide: a formal, ceremonial, and proscribed form of suicide performed for social reasons in Japanese history

serotonin: an abundant chemical nerve signal in the brain which is involved in modulating aggression

suicide cluster: the occurrence of several suicides immediately following a much-publicized suicide

suicide gesture: a superficial suicidal action in which the intention is not to die but to solicit help

CAUSES AND SYMPTOMS

Suicide is the deliberate taking of one's own life. Most often, suicidal individuals are trying to avoid emotional or physical pain that they believe they cannot bear. Suicide is seen as a solution to an otherwise insoluble problem. Each year, there are about 30,000 suicides in the United States, with 200,000 family survivors. Women attempt suicide more often than men, but men complete suicide more often than women because men tend to use more lethal means, such as a gun. Adolescents and the elderly are two high-risk groups.

When an individual contemplates suicide to avoid the physical pain of a terminal illness and does not have a mental disorder, that form of suicidal thought is called "rational" suicide. This does not imply that this form of suicide is appropriate, moral, or legal but merely that the suicidal thoughts do not arise from a mental disorder (nonrational). Social views on rational suicide vary by culture. For example, many Dutch people consider rational suicide to be acceptable, whereas most Americans do not.

Most suicidal people encountered by physicians, psychologists, social workers, and other mental health professionals experience suicidal thoughts as a result of a mental disorder. The suicidal thoughts and impulses are seen as symptoms of the underlying disorder and require treatment just as any other symptom. The treatment may involve protecting the person against his or her suicidal actions, even to the point of involuntary commitment to a mental hospital.

The rationale behind society's willingness temporarily to deny suicidal individuals' usual civil rights by involuntary commitment is that they are considered to be not "acting in their right mind" by virtue of their mental illness. Thus, they deserve the protection of society until their illness is treated. In fact, suicidal thoughts usually do abate when suicidal patients are treated. The vast majority of these individuals are appreciative afterward; they are glad that they were prevented from killing themselves, as they no longer wish to do so.

The most common mental illness that causes suicidal thoughts is depression. In fact, suicidal thoughts are considered to be a symptom of clinical depression. Other mental disorders associated with suicidal ideation include panic disorders, schizophrenia, alcoholism and other substance abuse disorders, and certain personality disorders.

Although suicide may occur at any time of the year, there is a seasonal variation in its peak incidence. Suicides are most common in both men and women in May; women have a second peak around October and November. This seasonal variation may be attributable to seasonal differences in the incidence of depression.

Why people commit suicide appears to have a multifactorial etiology. There are biological, psychological, and social factors that interact in a complex way to contribute to the causes of suicide in a given individual.

These biological factors include genetic contributions to the development of mental disorders such as clinical depression. In addition, studies have shown that suicidal people have an abnormality in a biochemical nerve communication system within the brain. This system involves a common neurotransmitter, serotonin, which is released at the end of one nerve, travels across a gap to the adjacent nerve, and attaches to that nerve. When the serotonin attaches to the adjacent nerve at a specialized receptor site, it initiates changes within the nerve. In this manner, one nerve communicates with its neighbors. In suicidal patients, the metabolites of serotonin that are found in spinal fluid are present in unusually low quantities. Therefore, it is assumed that inadequate amounts of serotonin exist in the brain at those times. Serotonin is thought to be involved in those areas of the brain that control aggression. Low serotonin levels may increase aggressive urges. In a depressed patient, the aggression is turned inward and the person has thoughts of taking his or her own life.

There is also evidence, although not as strong, that low levels of another neurotransmitter, dopamine, may predispose an individual to suicide. The simple loss of brain cell mass also increases the risk of suicide. This loss occurs with many forms of dementia and to a minor degree from normal aging. It is known that the elderly have an increased risk of completed suicide.

Alcohol and addictive drugs may also cause suicidal ideation. Such thoughts may occur while the individual is intoxicated or during withdrawal. Paradoxically, suicidal thoughts may also arise while the patient is taking antidepressant medications. Fortunately, this side effect is uncommon, arising in approximately 1.5 to 6.5 percent of patients. It does not appear that any one antidepressant is more likely to cause this reaction than another.

Psychological factors contributing to suicide include a depressed and/or anxious mood, hopelessness, and a loss of normal pleasure in life activities. Chronically depressed people often have diminished problem-solving skills during periods of depression and can see no way out of their difficulties; suicide is seen as the only solution. There are also personality characteristics that contribute to suicide. In women, borderline personality disorder is often associated with suicide attempts. This disorder is characterized by widely fluctuating moods, rages, feelings of emptiness or boredom, and unstable relationships.

The social factors involved in suicide include cultural acceptance or rejection of suicide. Japanese people have accepted ritual suicide within their culture and sanction suicide as a response to a severe loss of face or social esteem. The Dutch government has legalized rational suicide, while American society generally has a more negative view of the suicide act. Other social factors that increase the likelihood of suicide include social instability, divorce, unemployment, immigration, and exposure to violence as a child. In the United States, European Americans commit suicide more often than African Americans. Native Americans have a high incidence of suicide. In general, good social support reduces the risk of suicide.

Some patients engage in suicidal gestures; that is, they say they want to kill themselves and take actions such as swallowing some pills or superficially cutting their wrists, but there is no real intention to die. They act this way as a cry for help. For some, this may be the only way to receive attention for what troubles them. Unfortunately, the suicide gesture may go awry and unintended death may occur. Anyone who speaks of suicide or engages in what may appear to be a gesture should be taken seriously.

Most people who are suicidal have ambivalent feelings: Part of them wants to die, part does not. This is one of the reasons that the majority of suicidal people tell others of their intention in advance of their attempts. Most have visited their personal physician in the months prior to the suicide. Adolescents sometimes hint at their wish to die by giving away their prized possessions just prior to an attempt.

Anyone experiencing suicidal thoughts should be thoroughly evaluated by a professional trained in the assessment of suicidal patients. If the risk of suicide is considered to be high enough, the patient will have to be protected. This may require hospitalization, either voluntary or involuntary. It may mean removing suicidal means from that person's environment, such as removing guns from the home. Having someone stay with the patient at all times may be required. These steps should be individualized, taking into account the patient's situation.

Treatment of the underlying cause of the suicidal ideation is very important. Depression and anxiety can be treated with medications and/or psychotherapy. There are treatment programs for alcoholism and drug abuse. Usually, successful treatment of the underlying mental disorder results in the suicidal thoughts going away.

While they await the resolution of the suicidal ideation, patients need to be offered support and hope. Sometimes, a "no suicide" contract is helpful. This is simply a commitment on the part of the patient not to act on any suicidal thoughts and to contact the health professional if the urges become worse. While this contract may be written down, it is usually verbal.

Suicide prevention includes the early detection and management of the mental disorders associated with suicide. Because social isolation increases the risk of suicide, patients should be encouraged to develop and actively maintain strong social supports such as family, friends, and other social groups (such as church, clubs, and sports teams).

It may also be helpful to provide counseling to teenagers after an acquaintance has committed suicide, as this may prevent social contagion and suicide clusters. A suicide cluster is when several teenagers commit suicide after learning of the suicide of an acquaintance or a person who is attractive to them, such as a music or film star. Suicide clusters have increased among the young.

Family members of a suicide victim often go through a grieving process which is more severe than that which occurs after death from other causes. The stigma of suicide and mental illness is strong, and surviving family members often have greater feelings of both guilt and abandonment. Family survivors also have increased psychosomatic complaints, behavioral and emotional problems, and risk of suicide themselves. Referral to a suicide survivor group may be helpful.

TREATMENT AND THERAPY

An understanding of the causes, detection, and treatment of suicide has led to the development of a number of suicide hotlines and suicide prevention centers. There is evidence that, after these support groups are introduced into a community, the suicide rate for young women decreases. It is not yet known if they have any effect on other groups, such as young men or the elderly.

Most people who contemplate suicide do not seek professional treatment even if they tell people around them of their suicidal ideas. Thus, it is important for physicians, clergy, teachers, parents, and mental health workers to remain alert to the possibility of suicidal thoughts in those in their care. Someone who is depressed or very anxious should be asked about suicidal thoughts. Such a question will not plant the idea in his or her head, and the person may feel relieved after being asked. Once someone with suicidal ideation is identified, evaluation and treatment should proceed quickly. The following sample composite cases illustrate the application of the concepts described in the overview.

Mary is a seventeen-year-old senior in high school. She is from a broken home and was severely abused by her father prior to her parents' divorce ten years ago. Her teachers think that she is a bright underachiever who has a rather dramatic personality. Her friends see her as moody and easily angered. Her relationships with boyfriends are intense and always end with deep feelings of hurt and abandonment. Her mother is best described as cold, aloof, and preoccupied with herself.

Mary is brought to the school counselor by one of her friends when Mary threatens to kill herself and superficially scratches her wrists with a safety pin. The counselor learns that Mary has just broken up with her boyfriend, a young man at a local junior college. She is devastated. When she tried to tell her mother about it, her mother seemed uninterested and said that Mary always makes too much of such little things. It was the next morning that she scratched herself in front of her friend.

While more information is needed, this case illustrates a suicide gesture. In this case, Mary does not want to die but instead wants someone to realize how distressed she is. She feels rejected by her boyfriend and then by her mother. One can suspect a gesture rather than a serious suicide attempt by the superficial, nonlethal means (scratching with a safety pin) and by the likelihood of discovery (done in front of a friend).

Tom is a forty-eight-year-old accountant. He is separated from his wife and three children and lives alone in an apartment. He has no real friends, only drinking buddies. Like his father and two uncles, Tom is an alcoholic. Each day after work, he stops at his favorite bar and drinks between eight and twelve beers.

He is brought to the emergency room of the local hospital by the police, who found him sitting on the steps of a church sobbing. He threatened to kill himself if his wife did not take him back. The emergency room doctor noted the strong odor of alcohol on his

breath and ordered a blood alcohol test, which showed that he was legally intoxicated. Tom insisted that he would kill himself by running in front of a moving bus if he could not be with his family. The emergency room doctor had Tom's belt, pocketknife, and potentially dangerous items taken from him and arranged for a staff member to sit with him until he was sober. Six hours later, his blood alcohol had returned to near zero. Tom no longer felt despondent and had no more suicidal thoughts. He was embarrassed by his statements a few hours before. An alcoholism counselor was called, and outpatient treatment for his alcoholism was arranged.

This case illustrates suicidal ideation caused by alcohol intoxication. As often happens, the suicidal ideation resolves when the patient becomes sober. The primary treatment is for the underlying addictive disorder.

Sally is a fifty-three-year-old married mother of two. She is a part-time hairdresser and normally a very active, happy person. For the past three weeks, however, she has gradually lost all interest in her job, her children, her home, and her hobbies. She feels irritable and sad most of the time. Although she is tired, she does not sleep well at night, waking up very early each morning, unable to return to sleep. She is worried by the fact that she is having intrusive thoughts of killing herself. Sally imagines she could end all this dreariness by overdosing on sleeping pills and never waking up. She is a strict Catholic and knows it is against her religion to commit suicide. She calls her parish priest.

After a brief conversation, her priest meets her at the office of a psychiatrist who acts as a consultant for the diocese. The psychiatrist diagnoses major depression as the cause of Sally's suicidal ideation. She has a good social support network, so the psychiatrist decides to treat her as an outpatient and has her agree to a "no suicide" contract. Sally is also started on antidepressant medication, which gradually lifts her depression over a period of two to three weeks. Simultaneously, her suicidal thoughts leave her.

This case illustrates suicidal thoughts caused by depression. If Sally had been more depressed or her suicidal urges stronger, she would probably have needed hospitalization. If she had required hospitalization and had refused to go voluntarily, the psychiatrist could have had her committed according to the laws of the state where he practiced. Most states require a signed statement by two physicians or one physician and a licensed clinical psychologist. They must attest that the patient is a danger to himself or herself and that no less restrictive form of treatment would suffice.

Harry is a sixty-seven-year-old resident of a hospital, where he has been for the past two years. He has a serious neurological disorder called amyotrophic lateral sclerosis (also called Lou Gehrig's disease). It has caused progressive weakness such that he cannot even breathe on his own. Harry is permanently connected to a respirator attached to a tracheotomy tube in his throat. He has few visitors and mostly stares off and thinks.

Harry tells his nurse that he is "sick of it all" and wants his doctors to disconnect him from the respirator and let him die. His neurologist requests a psychiatric evaluation. The psychiatrist confirms the patient's wish to die. There is no evidence of dementia or other cognitive disorder, nor is the patient showing any evidence of a mental illness. Subsequently, a meeting is called of the hospital ethics committee to make recommendations. Membership on the committee includes physicians, nurses, an ethicist, a local minister, and the hospital attorney.

This case illustrates a difficult example of rational suicide. The patient has a desire to die and is not suffering from any mental disorder. In this case, he is requesting not to take his own life actively but to be allowed to die passively by removal of the respirator. Some people do not consider this to be suicide at all. They make a distinction between passively allowing a natural process of dying to occur and actively taking one's own life. If this patient requested a lethal overdose of potassium to be injected into his intravenous tubes, such action would be considered suicide and ethically different. In either event, these matters are more ethical, social, and legal than psychiatric.

PERSPECTIVE AND PROSPECTS

Throughout history, there have been numerous examples of suicide. In Western culture, early views on the subject were mainly from a moral perspective and suicide was viewed as a sin. Mental illness in general was poorly understood and often thought of as weakness of character, possession by evil spirits, or willful bad behavior. Thus, mental illness was stigmatized. Even though society now has a better medical understanding of mental illness, there is still a stigma attached to mental illness and to suicide. This stigma contributes to underdiagnosis and undertreatment of

suicidal individuals, as many sufferers are reluctant to come forth with their symptoms.

Suicide remains an important public health problem, as it is the ninth most common cause of death in the United States (although it is third for adolescents and second for young adults). There are about thirty thousand known suicides in the United States annually. The actual incidence may be higher because an unknown number of accidental deaths or untreated illnesses may actually be undiagnosed suicides. Suicide is more common among young adults and the elderly, with a relative sparing of the middle aged. The rate of suicide is rising among teenagers. The lifetime prevalence of suicide attempts among American adults is about 2.9 percent.

As most cases of suicidal ideation never come to the attention of health professionals, a high index of suspicion should be maintained. Those people who express suicidal thoughts should be taken seriously and thoroughly evaluated. Increased levels of awareness of suicide may help to improve detection and treatment of this potentially preventable cause of death.

—*Peter M. Hartmann, M.D.*

See also Addiction; Alcoholism; Anxiety; Death and dying; Dementias; Depression; Euthanasia; Grief and guilt; Hypochondriasis; Midlife crisis; Neurosis; Panic attacks; Phobias; Postpartum depression; Posttraumatic stress disorder; Psychiatric disorders; Psychiatry; Psychiatry, child and adolescent; Psychiatry, geriatric; Psychoanalysis; Psychosomatic disorders; Puberty and adolescence; Schizophrenia; Stress; Terminally ill: Extended care.

FOR FURTHER INFORMATION:

DePaulo, J. Raymond, Jr., and Keith R. Ablow. *How to Cope with Depression.* New York: McGraw-Hill, 1989. This book was written by two physicians; DePaulo is a national authority on depression. Contains a full chapter on suicide and depression.

Ericksen, Corey. *Depression Is Curable.* Edited by J. A. Blanchard and Victoria Fairham. Clackamas, Oreg.: Rainbow Press, 1986. A good review for the layperson written by a family doctor. Includes a helpful discussion of suicide.

Hafen, Brent Q., and Kathryn J. Frandsen. *Youth Suicide: Depression and Loneliness.* 2d ed. Evergreen, Colo.: Cordillera Press, 1986. An excellent review of all aspects of teenage suicide, with practical suggestions for helping the suicidal young person.

Jamison, Kay Redfield. *Night Falls Fast: Understand-

ing Suicide. New York: Alfred A. Knopf, 2000. Jamison, a distinguished psychologist and academic, brings a rare combination of personal and academic experience to bear in this monumental work on suicide.

Lester, David. *Making Sense of Suicide: An In-Depth Look at Why People Kill Themselves*. Philadelphia: The Charles Press, 1997. This book may be helpful for beginning counselors and family members or friends interested in learning more about suicidal behavior.

Peck, M. Scott. *Denial of the Soul: Spiritual and Medical Perspectives on Euthanasia and Mortality*. New York: Harmony Books, 1997. This book discusses controversial issues related to euthanasia and suicide.

Sunburn
Disease/disorder
Anatomy or system affected: Skin

Specialties and related fields: Dermatology, emergency medicine, family practice, oncology

Definition: An inflammation of the skin produced by excessive exposure to the sun, sunlamps, or occupational light sources.

Causes and Symptoms
Sunburn is caused by overexposure to ultraviolet light coming directly from the sun or from artificial lighting sources, as well as from reflected sunlight from snow, water, sand, and sidewalks. Scattered rays may also produce sunburn, even in the presence of clouds, haze, or thin fog. Symptoms include red, swollen, painful, and sometimes blistered skin; chills; and fever. In severe cases, nausea, vomiting, and even delirium may be present. Depending on the severity of the burn, tanning and peeling may occur during recovery.

Treatment and Therapy
In order to reduce the heat and pain of sunburn, towels or gauze dipped in cool water can be carefully laid on the burned areas. Once the skin swelling subsides, cold cream or baby lotion can be applied to the affected areas. If the skin is blistered, a light application of petroleum jelly prevents anything from sticking to the blisters. Nonprescription drugs, such as acetaminophen, can be used to relieve pain and reduce fever. If necessary, a medical doctor can prescribe other pain relievers or cortisone drugs to relieve itching and aid healing.

Perspective and Prospects
A number of risk factors can greatly intensify the affects of sunburn, including such genetic factors as fair skin, blue eyes, and red or blonde hair; the use of certain drugs, particularly sulfa drugs, tetracyclines, amoxicillin, or oral contraceptives; and exposure to industrial light sources, such as arc welders. For outdoor activities, a sunscreen or sunblock preparation should be applied to exposed areas of the body. Baby oil, mineral oil, or cocoa butter offer no protection from the sun. Brilliant colored and white clothing that reflect the sun into the face should be avoided. If tanning is a must, sun exposure should be limited to five to ten minutes on each side the first day, adding five minutes per side each additional day. Severe sunburn in childhood can lead to skin cancer later in life.

—*Alvin K. Benson, Ph.D.*

See also Cancer; Dermatology; Dermatology, pediatric; Skin; Skin cancer; Skin disorders.

For Further Information:
Grob, J. J. *Epidemiology, Causes, and Prevention of Skin Diseases*. London: Blackwell Science, 1997.

Kenet, B. J., and P. Lawler. *Saving Your Skin: Prevention, Early Detection, and Treatment of Melanoma and Other Skin Cancers*. Chicago: Four Walls Eight Windows, 1994.

Siegel, Mary-Ellen. *Safe in the Sun*. Rev. ed. New York: Walker, 1995.

Supplements
Treatment
Anatomy or system affected: All

Specialties and related fields: Alternative medicine, family practice, internal medicine, nutrition

Definition: Chemical compounds, concentrated into pills, powders, and capsules, that are taken to prevent or treat diseases.

The Role of Supplements
Adequate nutrition is the foundation of good health. Everyone needs the four basic nutrients: water, carbohydrates, proteins, and fats. It is important to choose the proper foods to deliver these nutrients and, as necessary, to complement the diet with supplements.

Health-conscious adults have heard the message repeatedly that they can get the vitamins they need from the foods they eat, but surveys have shown that people in many countries fail to eat adequate amounts of fruit, vegetables, whole grains, and low-fat dairy foods. Should public health officials or registered dieticians recommend that people take supplements to compensate for poor eating habits? The answer to this question can be found in a discussion of vitamin supplements.

The 1990's brought to light much new information about human nutrition, its effects on the body, and the role that it plays in disease. The fuel for the body's engine comes directly from the food that one eats, which contains many vital nutrients. Nutrients come in the form of vitamins, minerals, enzymes, water, amino acids, carbohydrates, and lipids (fats). These nutrients provide people with the basic materials that human bodies need to sustain life.

One of the latest types of dietary supplements are nutraceuticals. These supplements are obtained from naturally derived chemicals in plants, called photonutrients, that make the plants biologically active. They are not nutrients in the classic sense: They are what determine a plant's color, ability to resist disease, and flavor.

Nutritionists have discovered that fruits and vegetables, grains, and legumes contain other healthful nutrients called phytochemicals. Researchers have identified thousands of phytochemicals and have the ability to remove these chemical compounds and concentrate them into pills, powders, and capsules. Phytochemicals are believed to be powerful ammunition in the war against cancer and other cellular mutations. Cancer is a mutation of body cells through a multistep process. Phytochemicals help to fight that disease by stopping one or more of the steps that lead to cancer. For example, a cancer process can be kindled when a carcinogenic molecule invades a cell, possibly from foods eaten or from air breathed. Sulforaphane, a phytochemical commonly found in broccoli, activates an enzyme process and removes the carcinogen from the cell before harm is done.

Researchers and pharmaceutical companies sell concentrated forms of various phytochemicals found in such vegetables as broccoli, brussels sprouts, cauliflower, and cabbage. Several thousand phytochemicals have been identified. Because no single supplement can possibly compete with nature, some nutritionists recommend a shopping basket full of fruits and vegetables, as opposed to using expensive bottled supplements. Tomatoes, for example, are believed to contain

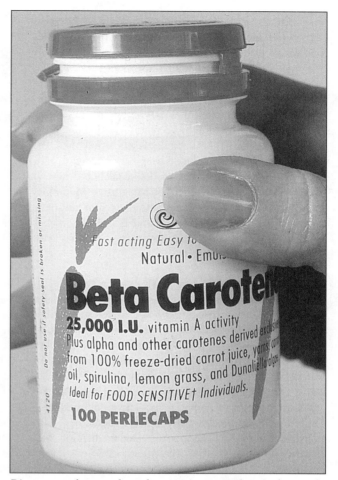

Dietary supplements have become increasingly popular in the United States, despite a lack of government regulation regarding safety and claims. (SIU School of Medicine)

an estimated ten thousand different phytochemicals.

Natural food supplements can be high in certain nutrients. Examples are aloe vera, bee pollen, fish oils, flaxseed, primrose oil, ginseng, ginkgo biloba, garlic, and oat bran. In general, natural food supplements are composed of by-products of foods that can provide a multitude of health benefits.

THE PROMISE OF ANTIOXIDANTS
No discussion of supplements would be complete without mention of antioxidants. They are a group of vitamins, minerals, and enzymes that help to protect the body from the formation of free radicals. Free radicals are groups of atoms that can cause damage to cells and thus impair the immune system. This damage is also thought to be the basis for the aging process.

Free radicals are believed to be formed through exposure to radiation and toxic chemicals such as cigarette smoke, as well as overexposure to the sun's rays.

Some common antioxidants are vitamin A and its precursor, beta carotene; vitamin C; and vitamin E. Zinc and the trace mineral selenium are thought to play an important role in neutralizing free radicals. Each vitamin or mineral has a recommended daily allowance (RDA). A higher supplementation dose of antioxidants is recommended by pioneering researchers in the field of alternative medicine such as Andrew Weil, founder of the Center for Integrative Medicine in Tucson, Arizona. Weil recommends four antioxidant supplements—vitamins C and E, selenium, and mixed carotenes—to protect a person's immune system further.

PERSPECTIVE AND PROSPECTS
The use of supplements is based both on modern research and development and on discoveries by mainstream scientists about the benefits of various substances such as garlic and aloe vera. Natural supplements have been used for centuries in many parts of the world as alternative medicines.

—*Lisa Levin Sobczak, R.N.C.*

See also Aging; Alternative medicine; Antioxidants; Digestion; Food biochemistry; Herbal medicine; Malnutrition; Nutrition; Osteoporosis; Self-medication; Vitamins and minerals.

FOR FURTHER INFORMATION:
Balch, James F., and Phyllis A. Balch. *Prescription for Nutritional Healing: A Practical A to Z Reference to Drug-Free Remedies Using Vitamins, Minerals, Herbs, and Food Supplements.* 3d ed. Garden City Park, N.Y.: Avery, 2000.
Frank, Robyn C., and Holly Berry Irving, eds. *Directory of Food and Nutrition Information for Professionals and Consumers.* 2d ed. Phoenix, Ariz.: Oryx Press, 1992.
Hendler, Sheldon Saul. *The Doctors' Vitamin and Mineral Encyclopedia.* New York: Simon & Schuster, 1990.
Machlin, Lawrence J., ed. *Handbook of Vitamins: Nutritional, Biochemical, and Clinical Aspects.* 2d ed. New York: Marcel Dekker, 1991.
Weil, Andrew. *Eight Weeks to Optimum Health: A Proven Program for Taking Full Advantage of Your Body's Natural Healing Power.* New York: Alfred A. Knopf, 1997.

SURGERY, GENERAL
SPECIALTY
ANATOMY OR SYSTEM AFFECTED: All
SPECIALTIES AND RELATED FIELDS: Anesthesiology, radiology
DEFINITION: A field of medicine that involves a wide range of surgical procedures, from the simple removal of warts and bunions in the doctor's office to complex organ transplantation requiring a large staff in the operating room.
KEY TERMS:
aseptic techniques: procedures that allow surgeons to operate in a germ-free environment
excision: the surgical removal of an organ or tissue

SCIENCE AND PROFESSION
In all probability, surgery has been practiced as long as humans have had cutting tools. Ample reports of battlefield amputations exist almost from the beginning of reported time. Historians tell of rough field surgery, the hacking off of wounded limbs and the sealing of the wounds by searing the lacerated flesh. There are even suggestions that ancient civilizations, such as that of the Egyptians, practiced trepanning, cutting into the skull to operate on the brain.

Until the latter half of the nineteenth century, surgery was a brutal, dirty, and dangerous practice. About this time, the relationship between microorganisms and diseases was first enunciated, a relationship which explained why so many surgery patients sickened and died. It was also at this time that anesthetics were developed, which for the first time allowed the surgeon to deaden the patient's pain.

Surgery today is one of the most respected medical specialties, requiring full training in the disciplines of medicine, as well as years of extensive work in surgical procedures. After becoming physicians, candidates for surgery spend years working under established surgeons learning the techniques that they will use in practice. They are subjected to intensive examination and receive certification only when their peers are convinced that they can perform their duties capably.

The tools and techniques of surgery that the surgical candidate must master present multiple challenges. In their training phase, surgeons learn to become skilled in the manipulation of all the basic instruments used in surgery, such as the various designs of scalpels, scissors, retractors, forceps, and sutures. The training surgeon learns a wide variety of stitching techniques and the materials used in suturing. Most challenging perhaps is mastery of the many new techniques and instruments that modern surgeons use.

After training and certification, some surgeons elect to practice general surgery. As the term implies, this field covers such diverse areas of the body as the stomach, gallbladder, liver, intestines, appendix, breasts, thyroid gland, salivary glands, main arteries and veins, lumps under the skin, hernias, and hemorrhoids. Other surgeons choose to specialize in disciplines that require still more training, such as heart surgery, bone (or orthopedic) surgery, and eye (or ophthalmic) surgery, to name some of the more prevalent specialties.

Modern surgery is a far-ranging practice involving all body structures and systems. It is also a practice that sees constant advancements and improvements in operating techniques, in instrumentation and tools, and in high-tech equipment. Microsurgery, in which the surgeon uses a microscope to view the operating field and manipulates tiny instruments to repair or ex-

A Typical Operating Room

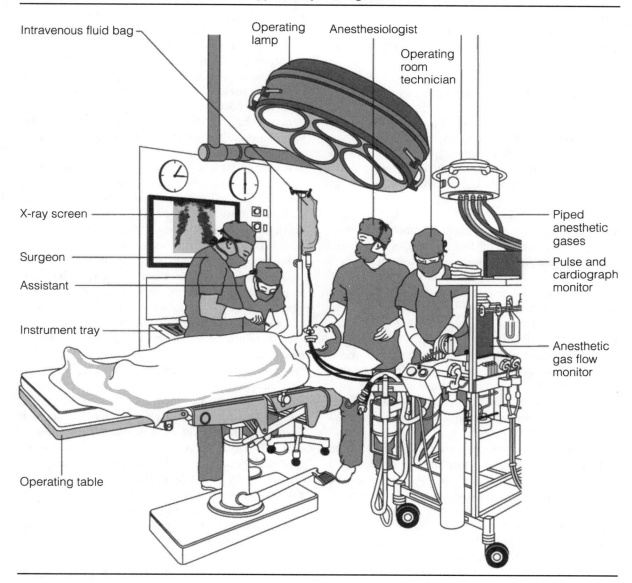

Intravenous fluid bag

Operating lamp

Anesthesiologist

Operating room technician

X-ray screen

Surgeon

Assistant

Instrument tray

Operating table

Piped anesthetic gases

Pulse and cardiograph monitor

Anesthetic gas flow monitor

cise tissue, was virtually unheard of at the middle of the twentieth century. It is now common practice in virtually every surgical facility in the United States. At one time, a severed limb could never be reconnected, largely because it was impossible to repair severed nerves. Now, because of microsurgery, arms, legs, hands, digits, and other severed body parts can be stitched back on to the body, often with much of their mobility restored.

Much minor surgery takes place in the physician's office or clinic. These procedures are generally simple, involving the excision of skin growths such as warts or cancers, hemorrhoids, and other surface conditions. Emergency surgery in the office, clinic, or emergency room may be necessary to open an airway for a patient whose breathing is impaired or to remove obstructions.

Major surgery usually requires a hospital stay, and its main characteristics are anesthesia and aseptic technique. Anesthesia may be local, regional, or general. For local anesthesia, anesthetic is injected into the site of the operation. The patient is usually fully awake during the surgery but feels no pain in the affected area. In regional anesthesia, a whole part of the body is anesthetized, such as a leg or an arm. As with local anesthesia, the patient is awake during the procedure but may be sedated for comfort. In general anesthesia, the patient is put to sleep and immobilized, usually by injections, and inhaled anesthetics are administered throughout the course of the operation.

To create an aseptic, germ-free environment, the operating room and everything in it are subjected to rigorous sterilization. Surgeons and all operating room staff scrub with antiseptic soaps. They don complete uniforms of sterilized cloth or paper: caps, masks, gowns, gloves, and foot coverings. Avoiding transmission of disease in the operating room can be said to be as important as the operation itself. It is vital that the patient be made safe from infection by the staff and from pathogenic organisms in the ambient atmosphere of the hospital.

It is equally important that staff be protected from infection by the patient. Operating room personnel are particularly vulnerable to blood-borne infections, such as hepatitis B and human immunodeficiency virus (HIV). Surgery can be a bloody procedure. In some operations, copious blood spurts are common, and the likelihood of staff being spattered is high, as is the possibility of disease transmission. It is possible that there will be a cut or tear in the staff's protective clothing and that the patient's blood or other body fluids can make contact with an abrasion on the body or even land on mucous membranes of the mouth, nose, and throat, where they can infect the caregiver. This has happened so often that the U.S. government has issued rigorous guidelines to high-risk health care personnel—particularly operating room staff—detailing specific procedures to follow to avoid disease transmission.

DIAGNOSTIC AND TREATMENT TECHNIQUES

The surgeon is rarely the first physician whom the patient sees. Usually, a primary care physician makes a diagnosis and may confer with or send the patient to a specialist for confirmation of the diagnosis. When surgery is recommended, the surgeon confers with the primary care physician and/or the consulting specialist and is fully apprised of the patient's condition. He or she reviews the patient's history and inspects all relevant documents and diagnostic reports, such as X rays, computed tomography (CT) scans, and other information that he or she needs to plan and perform the procedure.

For the most part, surgeons deal with their patients only in the immediate context of the operation. They meet before the operation, and surgeons look in on patients afterward to check their progress and recovery. In some cases, follow-up visits to the surgeon are required.

In the operating room, the surgeon assembles the staff needed for the particular procedure. There will be an anesthesiologist, perhaps other specialized surgeons, and various general and specialized operating room nurses. The surgeon or the staff will also order everything needed for the procedure. There is an enormous range of specialized equipment that surgeons can use in their procedures. Cardiac surgeons use heart-lung machines, which take over the task of circulating the patient's blood and allow the surgeon to open and enter the heart itself. The neurosurgeon may operate through specialized microscopic instruments.

A catalog of specialized endoscopes is now available to surgeons, many of which allow them to operate through a tiny hole in the patient's skin, rather than having to make massive cuts with a scalpel. Pulmonary surgeons use a bronchoscope to look down into the patient's bronchial tubes, where they can perform such surgical operations as removing obstructions and excising cancerous tissue. Gastrointestinal surgeons use a gastroscope both to investigate conditions in the stomach and to take small tissue samples for biopsy. Colon and rectal surgeons use a colonoscope to remove polyps from the colon and rectum, a major step in the prevention and treatment of colon cancer. Major surgery, however, still involves cutting the patient open to repair what has gone wrong inside the body. Fortunately, this procedure is now safer and more specialized than it has ever been before.

Management of disease in the United States has reached the point where there are surgical specialties to cover virtually all parts of the body individually. Some surgeons specialize in individual organs, such as the heart, lungs, brain, eyes, and ears. Some surgeons specialize in body systems such as bones or circulation. Furthermore, many surgeons hone their skills in certain specialized surgical techniques and become so adept that they are recognized as experts in highly complex and critical procedures, such as repairing detached retinas, performing heart transplants, correcting slipped disks, or sealing brain aneurysms.

Surgeons are major inventors and designers. Much of the instrumentation and many of the surgical tools that are used in the operating room were invented by surgeons. They often direct the fabrication of specialized tools and instruments to help them in their work. Most of the metal and plastic prostheses implanted to replace damaged internal structures were designed by surgeons. Orthopedic surgeons design prosthetic hips, knees, and other implants. Ophthalmic surgeons design corneal implants. The specialized surgeon knows his or her area of the body better than anyone else does and can visualize what sort of equipment or device is needed to improve the patient's condition.

Surgeons are also at the forefront of major technical innovations that reach across the entire surgical field. They are adept at recognizing potential applications for new technology and adapting it to surgery. For example, fiber-optic science has been applied in surgical endoscopes. Cryosurgery, a technique of freezing tissue, is used in a wide range of procedures, from the removal of hemorrhoids to the reattachment of retinas.

Laser technology is employed in hundreds of surgical procedures. The laser is used for making incisions, for repairing tissue, and for excising diseased tissue, among other applications. One of the major areas that can benefit from the unique advantages of laser use is eye surgery. Ophthalmic surgeons use lasers to relieve diabetic retinopathy, glaucoma, macular degeneration, cataracts, and certain tumors, as well as to reattach torn retinas.

One of the critical qualities of the competent surgeon is judgment. No matter how thoroughly a surgeon may prepare for a procedure, there may be some surprises on the operating table. The surgeon learns the patient's history and status and also reviews all the appropriate diagnostic documents, X rays, and other visualizations, but unforeseen complications may arise during the operation. The surgeon must have the experience and competence to deal with the unexpected.

PERSPECTIVE AND PROSPECTS

Up to the mid-nineteenth century, surgical procedures were probably responsible for as many deaths as cures. Today, surgery extends the lives of millions: heart disease victims, cancer patients, and victims of infection and accidents. Surgery helps improve the quality of life for patients with arthritis and rheumatism, gastrointestinal problems, lung disorders, and circulation problems.

Furthermore, surgery is entering new areas of medicine. For example, operations can now be performed in the uterus to correct anomalies in unborn fetuses. Many more such procedures are predicted for the future.

New areas of surgical expertise are opening constantly; new techniques, instrumentation, and equipment are making many old procedures obsolete. Practicing surgeons face a constant challenge in keeping abreast of what is happening all over the world and deciding what avenues to explore for the benefit of their patients.

—*C. Richard Falcon*

See also Abscess drainage; Adrenalectomy; Amputation; Anesthesia; Anesthesiology; Aneurysmectomy; Appendectomy; Biopsy; Bone marrow transplantation; Breast biopsy; Breast surgery; Bunions; Bypass surgery; Cataract surgery; Catheterization; Cervical procedures; Cesarean section; Cholecystectomy; Cleft lip and palate repair; Colon and rectal polyp removal; Colon and rectal surgery; Corneal transplantation; Craniotomy; Cryotherapy and cryosurgery; Cyst removal; Cystectomy; Disk removal; Ear surgery; Electrocauterization; Endarterectomy; Endometrial biopsy; Eye surgery; Face lift and blepharoplasty; Fistula repair; Ganglion removal; Gastrectomy; Grafts and grafting; Hair transplantation; Hammertoe correction; Heart transplantation; Heart valve replacement; Heel spur removal; Hemorrhoid banding and removal; Hernia repair; Hydrocelectomy; Hypospadias repair and urethroplasty; Hysterectomy; Kidney transplantation; Kneecap removal; Laceration repair; Laminectomy and spinal fusion; Laparoscopy; Laryngectomy; Laser use in surgery; Liposuction; Liver transplantation; Lung surgery; Malignant melanoma removal; Mastectomy and lumpectomy; Myomectomy; Nail removal; Nasal polyp removal; Nephrectomy; Neurosurgery; Ophthalmology; Orthopedic surgery; Parathyroidectomy; Penile implant surgery; Periodontal surgery; Phlebitis; Plastic surgery; Prostate gland removal; Rhinoplasty and submucous resection; Sex change surgery; Shunts; Skin lesion removal; Sphincterectomy; Splenectomy; Sterilization; Stone removal; Surgery, pediatric; Surgical procedures; Surgical technologists; Sympathectomy; Tattoo removal; Tendon repair; Testicular surgery; Thoracic surgery; Thyroidectomy; Tonsillectomy and adenoid removal; Tracheostomy; Transfusion; Transplantation; Tumor removal; Ulcer surgery; Vagotomy; Varicose vein removal; Vasectomy.

FOR FURTHER INFORMATION:

Horton, Edward, et al., eds. *The Marshall Cavendish Illustrated Encyclopedia of Family Health.* 24 vols. London: Marshall Cavendish, 1986. The surgical listing covers a wide range of topics from anesthesia and aseptic techniques to surgical tools and sutures.

Larson, David E., ed. *Mayo Clinic Family Health Book.* 2d ed. New York: William Morrow, 1996. This book covers the surgical aspects of medicine admirably, with clear and concise descriptions of surgical procedures.

Lewis, Howard R., and Martha E. Lewis. *The People's Medical Manual.* Garden City, N.Y.: Doubleday, 1986. The section on surgery discusses many aspects of surgical procedures, as well as some of the problems that both surgeons and patients face today.

Schwartz, Seymour I., ed. *Principles of Surgery.* 7th ed. New York: McGraw-Hill, 1999. A standard textbook on the topic. Intended for practicing surgeons, but valuable to general readers for its details.

SURGERY, PEDIATRIC
SPECIALTY
ANATOMY OR SYSTEM AFFECTED: All
SPECIALTIES AND RELATED FIELDS: Anesthesiology, general surgery, neonatology, pediatrics

DEFINITION: The surgical correction of medical conditions of infants and children.
KEY TERM:
congenital defect: an anatomic defect present at birth; it is not necessarily hereditary

SCIENCE AND PROFESSION

A pediatric surgeon is a general surgeon who has received additional training in operating on infants and children. The full course of training includes four years of medical school, followed by five years of general surgery residency and two years of pediatric surgery residency. Pediatric surgeons generally practice in large referral hospitals or children's hospitals. The relatively small number of American training programs in this specialty are all located at major teaching hospitals.

Children are not simply small adults. They experience some different surgical disorders than adults, especially congenital defects. Their ability to withstand the stress of surgery is less than that of an older person. Also, many of their surgical problems require years of follow-up care by a surgeon who understands child growth and development.

In the first half of the twentieth century, when pediatric surgery was developing as a specialty, the pediatric surgeon was trained to operate on all parts of the child's body. As the specialty matured, however, the pediatric surgeon came to perform only general surgical procedures on infants and children. This trend was made possible by the development of pediatric subspecialties in the other surgical fields, such as neurosurgery and cardiac surgery. In addition, pediatric surgeons work closely with pediatricians. As a team, they share in evaluating the patient and in providing preoperative and postoperative care.

To a degree, pediatric surgeons differ from general surgeons in their point of view. Infants and children change constantly as they grow, and common surgical diagnoses also change with the age of the patient. Additionally, the ability of a child's body to cope with disease and with surgery alters with age. It is therefore necessary for the pediatric surgeon to understand child growth and development.

Although a disorder may be surgically corrected in infancy, the child may continue to have postoperative difficulty for many years. An example is the removal of a large amount of intestines, which must sometimes be done with premature infants. It takes considerable patience and expertise to follow this sort of patient for years, adjusting the child's diet and treatment to achieve as nearly normal growth as possible. The pediatric surgeon is specially trained to provide this care.

The organs and tissues of an infant or child are much smaller than those of an adult. The pediatric surgeon must develop expert skills to perform surgery on these small structures. Also, the pediatric surgeon is trained to work rapidly when performing surgery. It is important to complete procedures quickly to minimize stress on the pediatric patient.

Congenital defects are, fortunately, relatively uncommon. The pediatric surgeon treats relatively more of these conditions than a general surgeon would and therefore has greater experience in caring for them. Examples of congenital defects treated by pediatric surgeons include defects of the abdominal wall and diaphragm and the obstruction or absence of a part of the intestinal tract.

Because the patient is a child, the pediatric surgeon must also deal with the patient's family. This specialist is trained to build a supportive relationship with parents and to teach them about their child's disorder so that they can be informed participants in decisions regarding the patient's care. Especially with chronic diseases, the parents must be kept aware of their child's progress and changing needs so that they can participate fully in the child's recovery.

DIAGNOSTIC AND TREATMENT TECHNIQUES
The pediatric surgeon's day is split between the operating room and the clinic. This specialist spends relatively more time in the clinic than does a general surgeon. Surgical correction is only one step in pediatric surgery: Careful evaluation and planning must precede any procedure. Afterward, extended follow-up care is often necessary, sometimes for years. This type of care requires patience and an interest in long-range planning on the surgeon's part.

The pediatric surgeon relies heavily on history taking and physical examination of the patient. This information, plus knowledge of the incidence of specific disorders at different ages, leads the surgeon to the most likely diagnosis. Specific laboratory and radiographic tests are ordered to aid in the diagnostic process.

The pediatric surgeon works very closely with the anesthesiologist, the physician responsible for keeping the patient anesthetized and his or her vital functions stable during surgery. The needs of a child are different from those of an adult during surgery. Many hospitals with pediatric surgeons are also staffed with pediatric anesthesiologists.

Like other surgeons, the pediatric surgeon also performs minor surgery on children, often in the clinic. Examples of minor procedures are the suturing of lacerations, the drainage of small abscesses, and the excision of small benign growths under the skin.

PERSPECTIVE AND PROSPECTS
Pediatric surgery began in the United States as an offshoot of general surgery in the first half of the twentieth century. For decades, the specialty met resistance from general surgeons. The American Academy of Pediatrics was first to recognize the value of pediatric surgeons and, following a meeting by the academy in 1948, established a surgical section. C. Everett Koop, the surgeon general under President Ronald Reagan, was a vigorous advocate of pediatric surgical education and a developer of new surgical techniques for children from 1946 through the 1990's. He was an important proponent in the eventual recognition of pediatric surgery as a surgical specialty. It was not until 1973, however, that the Board of Pediatric Surgery certified the first specialists in the field.

In 1995, there were twenty-eight training programs for pediatric surgeons in the United States. Because of the limited number of graduates of these programs, pediatric surgeons will continue to be in great demand.

—*Thomas C. Jefferson, M.D.*

See also Abscess drainage; Adrenalectomy; Amputation; Anesthesia; Anesthesiology; Aneurysmectomy; Appendectomy; Biopsy; Bone marrow transplantation; Cardiology, pediatric; Catheterization; Cleft lip and palate repair; Craniotomy; Cryotherapy and cryosurgery; Ear surgery; Electrocauterization; Endocrinology, pediatric; Eye surgery; Fistula repair; Gastroenterology, pediatric; Genetic diseases; Genetics and inheritance; Grafts and grafting; Heart transplantation; Heart valve replacement; Hernia repair; Hydrocelectomy; Hypospadias repair and urethroplasty; Kidney transplantation; Laceration repair; Laparoscopy; Laser use in surgery; Lung surgery; Nasal polyp removal; Nephrectomy; Nephrology, pediatric; Neurology, pediatric; Neurosurgery; Ophthalmology; Orthopedic surgery; Orthopedics, pediatric; Parathyroidectomy; Pediatrics; Plastic surgery; Pulmonary medicine, pediatric; Shunts; Splenectomy; Surgery, general; Surgical procedures; Surgical technologists; Sympathectomy; Tattoo removal; Tendon repair; Thoracic surgery; Thyroidectomy; Tonsillectomy and adenoid removal; Tracheostomy; Transfusion; Transplantation; Urology, pediatric.

FOR FURTHER INFORMATION:

Cockburn, Forrester, et al. *Children's Medicine and Surgery*. New York: Oxford University Press, 1996. This volume discusses the basics of pediatrics and features illustrations and an index.

Koop, C. Everett. "Pediatric Surgery: The Long Road to Recognition." *Pediatrics* 92 (October, 1993): 618-621. The history of pediatric surgery is discussed. Some believe that pediatric surgery would never have gotten off the ground without the development of pediatric anesthesiology.

O'Neill, James A. *Pediatric Surgery*. 5th ed. St. Louis: Mosby-Year Book, 1998. This is a new edition of a classic textbook of pediatric surgery. It is the most comprehensive text available on the subject, a must for all practicing and aspiring pediatric surgeons. Perhaps a bit too comprehensive for non-pediatric surgeons looking for a simple reference book to keep on their shelf.

SURGICAL PROCEDURES

PROCEDURE

ANATOMY OR SYSTEM AFFECTED: All

SPECIALTIES AND RELATED FIELDS: Anesthesiology, general surgery, nursing, plastic surgery

DEFINITION: The treatment of diseases or disorders by physical intervention, which usually involves cutting into the skin and other tissues.

KEY TERMS:

anesthesia: the use of drugs to inhibit pain and other sensations

hemostasis: the control of bleeding

incision: a cut made with a scalpel

suture: a thread used to unite parts of the body

INDICATIONS AND PROCEDURES

Surgery has progressed as rapidly as other areas of medicine. Early surgeries consisted of gross excision (the cutting out of abnormal or diseased tissue). Today, surgery has been transformed by scientific advances so that surgeons commonly use microscopes, lasers, and endoscopes that allow the surgeon to make small incisions in order to gain access to the surgical site. Modern operations are much more precise and emphasize repair or replacement rather than excision.

When a patient requires surgery, several preoperative procedures are performed to increase the chances of a successful outcome. First, the patient is asked to abstain from eating for at least eight hours prior to surgery. This action reduces the chances of the individual vomiting during surgery and aspirating the gastric contents into the trachea (windpipe). After arriving at the hospital or clinic, the patient removes his or her clothes and puts on a gown, allowing the medical staff easy access to the patient for catheter insertion, intravenous line insertion, monitor placement, and preparation of the surgical site. Next, an intravenous (IV) line is placed in a vein of the hand or arm and connected to a bottle or bag of solution, which is suspended above the level of the patient's arm. The intravenous line gives the physician rapid vascular access for sampling blood and injecting drugs. Just before the actual surgery, the patient is usually given a sedative by an anesthesiologist, and electrocardiogram (ECG or EKG) leads and a blood pressure cuff are applied to the patient to monitor heart rate, heart rhythm, and blood pressure. The anesthesiologist will then anesthetize the patient further while the surgical team begins to prepare the site for the operation. Preoperative antibiotics may be given if there is a significant risk of infection.

The surgery may require either general anesthesia, in which the patient is unconscious, or local anesthesia, in which a specific region of the body is anesthetized. For general anesthesia, the patient will be injected with an intravenous anesthetic and quickly intubated, a procedure in which a tube is inserted into the trachea and attached to a ventilator. This arrangement gives the anesthesiologist the ability to administer gaseous drugs such as nitrous oxide and halothane as well as to control the patient's breathing. Surgical assistants prepare the operative site by cleansing the skin with a disinfectant. A sterile drape is used to cover all areas of the body except the surgical site. Surgeons and assistants must mask themselves and prepare for surgery by thoroughly washing their hands and arms. They then carefully put on a sterile gown and gloves. At this point, they must not come into contact with anything nonsterile.

The surgeon uses a scalpel to make an incision through the skin and any underlying structures in order to gain access to the area of the body needing attention. When blood vessels are cut, bleeding must be controlled by cauterizing, clamping, tying off with

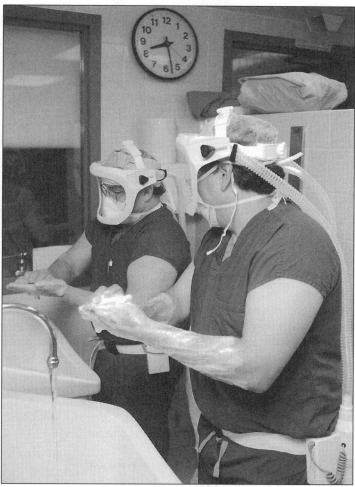

Surgeons scrub their hands and arms before performing an operation. Such procedures are essential to the maintenance of an antiseptic environment. (Digital Stock)

Occasionally, surgery involves damage to healthy tissues, including nerves and blood vessels. Significant intraoperative blood loss may also occur, requiring transfusion. An incision into any part of the body provides an opportunity for bacteria to enter and infect the surgical wound; prophylactic antibiotics help reduce the chance of surgical infection. Rarely, a patient may have an unexpected response to the procedure or drugs, which could result in permanent disability or death. These very infrequent reactions may include a blood clot causing a stroke or heart attack, an abnormal heart rhythm, or severe allergic reactions to medication.

PERSPECTIVE AND PROSPECTS

Modern surgery includes the use of surgical implants, microsurgery, laser surgery, endoscopic surgery, and transplant surgery. Surgery implants are used to replace a part of the body with an artificial implant. These implants include joints, heart valves, eye lenses, and sections of blood vessels or of the skull. During microsurgery, the surgeon uses specially designed instruments and a microscope to perform an operation on minute structures such as blood vessels, nerves, and parts of the eyes or ears. Microsurgery is also being used to reattach severed fingers and toes. Laser surgery utilizes a high-energy, narrow beam that can cut through tissues like a scalpel but that also cauterizes blood vessels during the incision. Lasers can be used on the retina, skin blemishes, and even tumors. Recovery from endoscopic surgery, in which a fiber-optic tube is inserted into the body to view the surgical site, is generally faster than from conventional operations because a smaller incision is made and less tissue damage results. Endoscopes are used to remove stones from the urinary tract and gallbladder and to remove or repair damaged cartilage in joints. With the availability of drugs that suppress tissue rejection, damaged organs can now be surgically replaced by donated organs. The most common examples are the heart, lungs, liver, kidneys, and bone marrow.

—Matthew Berria, Ph.D.,
and Douglas Reinhart, M.D.

sutures, or applying direct pressure to the vessel; this process is known as hemostasis.

After the surgery, the incision sites are closed with sutures, and the anesthetic is reversed. The patient is then taken to a recovery room to be monitored closely. Routine care of the patient recovering from anesthesia includes repeated evaluation of body temperature, pulse, blood pressure, and respiration. Postoperative pain medication (such as meperidine, morphine, or fentanyl) is given as needed.

USES AND COMPLICATIONS

Complications from surgery can result from surgical errors, infections, and abnormal patient reactions to the procedure or medications (idiosyncratic reactions).

See also Anesthesia; Anesthesiology; Biopsy; Bypass surgery; Catheterization; Cervical procedures; Colon and rectal surgery; Craniotomy; Cryotherapy and cryosurgery; Cyst removal; Electrocauterization; Eye surgery; Fistula repair; Ganglion removal; Grafts and grafting; Hernia repair; Laparoscopy; Laser use in surgery; Lung surgery; Neurosurgery; Orthopedic surgery; Periodontal surgery; Plastic surgery; Shunts; Surgery, general; Surgery, pediatric; Surgical technologists; Thoracic surgery; Tracheostomy; Transfusion; Transplantation; Tumor removal.

FOR FURTHER INFORMATION:

Clayman, Charles B., ed. *The American Medical Association Encyclopedia of Medicine.* New York: Random House, 1994. A concise presentation of numerous medical terms and illnesses. A good general reference.

Schwartz, Seymour I., ed. *Principles of Surgery.* 7th ed. New York: McGraw-Hill, 1999. A standard textbook on the topic. Intended for practicing surgeons, but valuable to general readers for its details.

SURGICAL TECHNOLOGISTS

SPECIALTY

ANATOMY OR SYSTEM AFFECTED: All

SPECIALTIES AND RELATED FIELDS: Anesthesiology, emergency medicine, general surgery, nursing

DEFINITION: Surgical team members whose primary functions are to prepare surgical instruments and hand them to the surgeon as needed and to prevent infection by maintaining a sterile field in the operating room.

KEY TERMS:

analgesia: the absence of pain

anesthesia: the absence of sensation; anesthesia may be achieved systemically (general anesthesia) or in a specific region of the body (regional or local anesthesia)

aseptic techniques: the standard procedures that help prevent wound contamination during the performance of surgical procedures; contamination may be followed by infection or death

circulator: the worker in the operating room whose responsibility is to keep records and to open sterile supplies for the team members wearing gowns and gloves

inpatient procedure: a surgical procedure performed on a patient who comes from a room in the hospital and who will return to a room in the hospital

operating room: a room in which surgical procedures are performed

outpatient procedure: a surgical procedure performed on a patient who comes from outside the hospital and who will most likely leave the hospital after a short stay in the recovery room

prep: a short form of the word "prepare"; to prep means to wash and shave the surgical area and to clean the skin surface immediately before a surgical procedure

recovery room: the room where a patient returns to full consciousness after a surgical procedure; in an outpatient facility, patients can change clothes in the recovery room, which may serve double duty as the preoperative waiting room

scrub: to wash one's hands and forearms in preparation for donning gown and gloves, which protect the patient from the surgical technologist and protect the surgical technologist from the patient

sterile field: an area where only sterile supplies may be placed and that only those wearing sterile gowns and gloves may touch; includes the surgical wound, the surgical drapes, and the extra tables

surgical team: the people working together in the operating room during a surgical procedure, including the surgeon, first assistant, surgical technologist, anesthesiologist and/or anesthetist, and circulator

SCIENCE AND PROFESSION

Surgical technologists work as part of the surgical team in an operating room, so they must be familiar with many aspects of patient care. The surgical team typically includes at least one of each of the following: a surgeon, a first assistant, a surgical technologist, an anesthesiologist and/or anesthetist, and a circulator. As a member of the surgical team, a surgical technologist anticipates the needs of the surgeon, prepares the instruments to be used for surgery, hands instruments to the surgeon, promotes efficiency, and at the same time helps prevent infection by maintaining the sterile field. A surgical technologist may also be referred to as a scrub nurse, a surgical assistant, a private scrub, or simply a scrub.

Surgical technologists work in many types of operating rooms, so their training must be fairly extensive. Courses may be taken at community colleges in one-year or two-year programs. Some of the two-year programs are accredited by the Association of Surgical Technologists. The courses taken include medical terminology, anatomy, and physiology. Classes specifically focused on surgical technology may include surgical conscience and ethics, the organization of an operating room, principles of microbiology, sterilization and disinfection, aseptic techniques, preoperative preparation and care of the patient, anesthesia, medications used during surgery, proper positioning of a surgical patient, preparation of the surgical site, methods of closing the surgical wound, surgical routines, the supplies found in the operating room, and the legal aspects of surgery.

A surgical technologist may work in one or all of many surgical services, so coursework must provide information about general surgery; obstetrical and gynecological surgery; plastic and reconstructive surgery; ear, nose, and throat procedures; surgery on the mouth and face; orthopedic surgery; neurosurgery; open-heart surgery; lung surgery; pediatric surgery; and surgery on blood vessels not located in the chest.

Students are required to gain experience in an operating room, which is usually done under supervision at a local teaching hospital. At such a hospital, a student gains experience in appropriate operating room procedures and learns the universal precautions against the transmission of infectious diseases.

Although the surgical technologist may work in any of the available medical services, some hospitals require their surgical technologists to specialize—that is, to rotate through different services so that they will gain familiarity with many operative procedures. At other facilities, the surgical technologist will work primarily in one area. For example, if the facility is a plastic surgeon's clinic, only these types of procedures will be performed.

A surgical technologist who has gained some experience may gain a specific area of interest within a broader field and decide to become a specialist. Common areas in which to specialize include eye surgery, neurosurgery, orthopedics, and plastic surgery. If this is the case, the technologist might be invited to work for a certain doctor or may find a number of (perhaps unaffiliated) doctors with whom to work. Working as a private scrub offers a different way to practice in the field. The surgical technologist works directly for the surgeon, instead of working for the hospital or surgical facility, and can usually expect to charge and earn more. There is also the possibility of greater camaraderie with the physician and more trust of the surgical technologist by the physician. Concentrating in a specific area may offer greater remuneration to

the surgical technologist, greater rapport with a familiar surgeon, and a more regular schedule, with no requirement for working on the weekends.

DUTIES AND PROCEDURES

Surgical technologists typically work in many areas, both inside and outside the operating room. Within the operating room, they may be either scrubbed or not scrubbed. After washing his or her hands, the surgical technologist dons a gown and gloves, which provides a sterile surface to reduce the possibility of transmission of infection, either from the patient to the surgical technologist or from the surgical technologist to the patient. When scrubbed, surgical technologists perform many duties. They assist surgeons during surgical procedures by handing them instruments, following routine procedures. They promote efficiency by keeping the instrument tables neat and organized. They must anticipate the needs of surgeons, so it is necessary that they know the steps of a procedure and monitor its progress. A surgical technologist places instruments in the surgeon's hands so that the surgeon does not have to look away from the wound in search of an instrument. Surgical technologists also help prevent injuries to the patient.

When necessary, the scrubbed surgical technologist may be asked to act as a first assistant for a procedure. In this capacity, it may be necessary for the surgical technologist to hold tissue out of the way (retract it), so that the surgeon can reach deeper tissues. Surgical technologists may also be required to sponge blood out of the wound or to rinse the surgical site to promote visibility of the tissues. They may also cut sutures. Surgical technologists help count sponges, needles, and instruments when such counts are required; items must be counted so that none are left behind in the patient. These items are counted before, during, and after the surgical procedure, in a specified and orderly manner. It is also the responsibility of the scrubbed surgical technologist to keep track of surgical specimens, pieces of tissue removed from the patient that will be sent to the laboratory for analysis. Many specimens may be taken from a particular procedure, so the surgical technologist must hand them off the sterile field to the circulator and make sure that the circulator labels the specimens properly. Specimens must also be handled and treated properly. Some are sent to the laboratory in preserving solutions, some are sent in salt water, and some are sent dry. It is important to keep track of specimens, to identify them, and to put them in the proper container for transportation to the laboratory.

When the surgical technologist is working in the operating room and is not scrubbed, a registered nurse must be immediately available in case there is an emergency. A registered nurse must also be present if medications are needed on the sterile field. A surgical technologist who is not scrubbed may function as a circulator. The circulator opens sterile supplies onto the operative field. Supplies are wrapped in many different ways, and the circulator must be able to pass the contents of a sterile package to the scrubbed surgical technologist without dropping them. Expiration dates must be checked on all supplies opened. Once the patient for a particular procedure is brought into the operating room, the circulator will help position the patient on the surgical table. The surgical technologist knows the position necessary for the particular procedure. Safe positioning methods prevent injury to patients. Once the patient is on the surgical table, the circulator washes the area with specified soaps and solutions and, if necessary, will shave the area around the surgical wound so that the area can be cleaned for the incision. The circulator ties the gowns of the scrubbed surgical technologist as well as the surgeon and other scrubbed assistants. If the anesthesiologist or anesthetist asks for help, the circulator provides that help, which may include holding, informing, or reassuring the patient.

It is the function of the circulator to connect tubings and electrical wires from instruments that may be needed on the sterile field, including power cords for cautery units, special lights, and drills, as well as fluid lines and suction cords. The circulator may need to focus or aim the surgical lights. With the scrubbed surgical technologist, the circulator performs the count of the items that need to be counted, including the suture, sponges, and instruments. The circulator keeps the official legal record of the procedure, the operative report. On this document, the circulator records the particulars of the procedure, including the counts, what was done, and the medications that were given. It is the responsibility of the circulator to receive surgical specimens from the surgical technologist, and to record properly where they came from, before they are sent to the laboratory. It might be necessary for the circulator to wipe the brow of any of the scrubbed personnel, so that sweat will not fall onto the sterile field; however, this is a rare event. The circulator handles all the nonsterile equipment

present in the operating room during the surgical procedure. This could involve moving or connecting equipment. In addition, the circulator helps to move the patient from the operating room to the recovery room after the procedure is over.

When not scrubbed for a procedure or functioning as a circulator, a surgical technologist may be asked to perform other duties in the surgery department. Surgical technologists need to be familiar with the protocols for receiving patients in the department. They may be asked to take patients to and from the surgical area or within the surgery department. Surgical technologists may help to order supplies for a department and, when they arrive, may help transport the supplies to the appropriate storage cupboard. Supplies need to be ordered from the central supply department or directly from manufacturers. In the operating room, not only must supplies be restocked but the expiration dates on sterile items must be inspected as well, to ensure that no outdated supplies are present in the operating room and given inadvertently to the patient. Surgical technologists may assist in cleaning instruments and supplies after a surgical procedure and preparing them for sterilization and subsequent reuse. They must be familiar with ways to sterilize instruments and supplies and must know which methods to use for which items. If equipment is working improperly, it is the responsibility of the surgical technologist to make sure that the equipment is repaired or replaced.

Working in an operating room is a very demanding occupation. It requires first of all personal integrity. As with any professional, the surgical technologist must be willing to admit mistakes. Often mistakes can be corrected if they are detected early. For example, the surgical technologist might have to say, "I forgot to sterilize the instruments, so we'll have to wait another fifteen minutes," rather than rush ahead to meet a particular deadline. In addition, a surgical technologist has to be able to handle stress—from providing fast and accurate care to a very sick patient, to having a patient die on the operating room table, to working with individuals with whom one does not get along on a personal level, to changing schedules for emergency procedures, to not being able to take a break to go to the restroom, to standing in one position for a whole day or a whole procedure.

No discussion of surgical technology would be complete without some mention of its legal aspects. As of the early 1990's in the United States, no state had licensed or defined the practice of surgical technology. Therefore, the surgical technologist has only the common rights of a citizen on the street. If the profession develops definite standards of education and skill levels, this situation may change. One thing is certain: The surgical technologist is not allowed to practice medicine or nursing.

Since surgical technologists are not physicians, they may not diagnose or treat disease, inject medicine into the human body, or pronounce death. These actions are limited to physicians, and in some states, a physician may not delegate certain actions (such as suturing, cutting or penetrating the human body, and clamping) to a surgical technologist. Similarly, since the surgical technologists are not nurses, they may not administer medications, which is a practice relegated to the field of nursing. At one time, only registered nurses were permitted to act as circulators. Many hospitals now allow surgical technologists to circulate, with a registered nurse standing by for emergencies. When circulating, however, a surgical technologist must remember that only nurses may select and measure medications, a right that cannot be delegated to someone without a license.

Surgical technologists must obey the laws in the performance of their duties. They can be prosecuted for breaking a law or for failing to perform a proper job. Surgical technologists must pay attention to laws involving the respecting of property rights, both of patients and of hospitals. In addition to not exceeding the scope of practice, there is another area of concern for surgical technologists: negligence. Any act of carelessness is called negligence, which is legally defined as "the failure to exercise the care that a reasonably prudent person would exercise under similar circumstances." Although negligence itself is not a crime, surgical technologists must remember that carelessness could endanger the safety of the patient.

The most common areas of negligence (and subsequent malpractice lawsuits) that affect surgical technologists involve the following: proper positioning of side rails and patient supports, abandonment of the patient, surgical consent, patient identification, loss of items inside the patient, specimen collections, burns, and explosions. Carelessness involving side rails could result in an anesthetized patient falling on the floor. Abandonment refers to the careless act of leaving an incompetent patient alone. The patient must sign a consent, in which he or she agrees to the surgical procedure; this detailed legal document must

be present before the procedure is begun, and the procedure may not wander from the permission given. Sponges, instruments, and needles are counted many times before, during, and after the surgical procedure, which helps to reduce the possibility of leaving anything inside the patient. Burns could be caused by the improper grounding of electrical devices used in the operating room, by the application of the wrong soap to the wrong area, or by the use of recently sterilized instruments, which may be too hot to be placed directly in contact with the patient. Explosions are less likely now than they used to be, because explosive medications are no longer used for general anesthesia. Nevertheless, the presence of oxygen in tanks and tubing increases the possibility of explosion and fire. In summary, there are many things about which the surgical technologist must be careful in order to avoid legal complications and injuries to patients.

PERSPECTIVE AND PROSPECTS

Historically, surgical technology began during World War II, when medical and nursing personnel in the armed forces trained men and women to assist in surgery in order to increase the availability of surgical procedures for the wounded. At that time, workers in this area were called operating room technicians. The name has gradually evolved to reflect the many areas where surgical procedures now take place—not only in hospitals but also in outpatient clinics, delivery rooms, and doctors' offices. In the beginning, surgical technologists had to work directly under the supervision of a registered nurse, who was legally required to be present in the operating room at all times.

The Association of Surgical Technologists (AST) began as a wing within the Association of Operating Room Nurses, but it later broke away to become the Association of Operating Room Technicians before later changing its name to the current one. Its headquarters are located in Littleton, Colorado. The AST provides many services for its members. It is a private organization that provides a certificate to those surgical technologists who pass a national examination. Certification, however, has little legal significance. States may not delegate their power to provide licenses to a private organization. The certified surgical technologist has demonstrated a level of skills and knowledge; however, one does not have to be certified in order to work as a surgical technologist. The AST also provides continuing education credits, insurance programs, and a magazine, as well as other services.

Working as a surgical technologist can be very demanding, but satisfaction, as in any profession, comes from working with a team in a complex situation in order to achieve a goal. There is satisfaction in a job well done, in being able to work well in stressful situations. There is great satisfaction in seeing the human body in all its complexity and in helping restore it to health. There is satisfaction in knowing in advance what the surgeon is going to use and having it ready at the moment it is needed. It is the excellent surgical technologist who can give the surgeon what is needed and not what is asked for.

—*William F. Taylor*

See also Allied health; Anesthesia; Anesthesiology; Education, medical; Malpractice; Nursing; Surgery, general; Surgery, pediatric; Surgical procedures.

FOR FURTHER INFORMATION:

Caruthers, Bob. *Surgical Technology for the Surgical Technologist: A Positive Care Approach.* Albany, N.Y.: Delmar, 2000. Includes bibliographical references and an index.

Fuller, Joanna R. *Surgical Technology: Principles and Practice.* 3d ed. Philadelphia: W. B. Saunders, 1994. An accessible work that functions as a textbook for surgical technologists. Fuller has assembled a wealth of practical clinical information about caring for patients in surgery.

Gruendemann, Barbara J., and Margaret Huth Meeker. *Alexander's Care of the Patient in Surgery.* St. Louis: C. V. Mosby, 1983. The bible of surgical techniques and practices. A detailed reference work of the most common surgical procedures.

Kohn, M. L., and L. J. Atkinson, eds. *Berry and Kohn's Introduction to Operating Room Technique.* New York: McGraw-Hill, 1986. Another accessible textbook. This one contains much practical information about what goes on in the operating room.

Miller, Benjamin Frank, and Claire B. Keane. *Encyclopedia and Dictionary of Medicine, Nursing, and Allied Health.* 6th ed. Philadelphia: W. B. Saunders, 1997. A comprehensive work which contains much information about the full spectrum of allied health.

SYMPATHECTOMY
PROCEDURE
ANATOMY OR SYSTEM AFFECTED: Back, neck, nerves, nervous system, spine

SPECIALTIES AND RELATED FIELDS: General surgery, neurology

DEFINITION: Sympathectomy is the surgical interruption of part of the sympathetic nerve pathway. The autonomic nervous system controls the involuntary internal environment of humans, and the sympathetic nerves increase energy expenditures by accelerating the heart rate, increasing the metabolic rate, and constricting and dilating blood vessels, among other actions. Occasionally, the proper regulation of vascular constriction or dilation goes awry, and the sympathetic nervous system causes prolonged and inappropriate constriction of the blood vessels to an area, such as the hand. The symptoms that may result from this lack of blood flow include cold and clammy skin, areas of gangrene, and painful fibrous growths and infections. After the specific nerves are located, the patient is prepared for surgery and opened in the location of the nerves—typically the neck or back area. Organs are moved or adjusted as needed. The offending region of nerve is clipped from the remainder and removed. The organs are replaced or repaired, and the incisions are closed. Normal vascular dilation will return rapidly and with it warmth to the area and healing of the infections, fibrous tissue, and areas of gangrene. Potential hazards include those common to all major surgeries.

—*Karen E. Kalumuck, Ph.D.*

See also Circulation; Nervous system; Neuralgia, neuritis, and neuropathy; Neurology; Neurosurgery; Vascular medicine; Vascular system.

FOR FURTHER INFORMATION:

Ernst, Calvin B., and James C. Stanley, eds. *Current Therapy in Vascular Surgery.* 4th ed. St. Louis: Mosby, 2000.

Hershey, Falls B., Robert W. Barnes, and David S. Sumner, eds. *Noninvasive Diagnosis of Vascular Disease.* Pasadena, Calif.: Appleton Davies, 1984.

Rutherford, Robert B., ed. *Vascular Surgery.* 5th ed. Philadelphia: W. B. Saunders, 2000.

SYNCOPE. *See* DIZZINESS AND FAINTING.

SYPHILIS
DISEASE/DISORDER
ANATOMY OR SYSTEM AFFECTED: Abdomen, brain, genitals, nervous system, reproductive system

SPECIALTIES AND RELATED FIELDS: Bacteriology, gynecology, public health, urology

DEFINITION: Syphilis is a serious, often sexually transmitted disease that causes widespread tissue destruction and, potentially, death if left untreated. The disease is passed through sexual contact in its contagious form and to newborns of infected mothers in its congenital form. After an incubation period of two to six weeks, a hard, painless sore (or chancre) may develop on the genitals in either sex or on the mouth or anus. A second stage of syphilis features enlarged lymph glands, headaches, rash on the genitals and mouth, and fever. Months or years later, a third stage arises, causing heart disease, mental deterioration, and loss of feeling or shooting pains in the legs. Syphilis can be cured with penicillin; however, incomplete treatments may only suppress symptoms temporarily.

—*Jason Georges and Tracy Irons-Georges*
See also Antibiotics; Bacterial infections; Birth defects; Genital disorders, female; Genital disorders, male; Gonorrhea; Neonatology; Pregnancy and gestation; Sexually transmitted diseases.

FOR FURTHER INFORMATION:

Brodman, Michael, John Thacker, and Rachael Kranz. *Straight Talk About Sexually Transmitted Diseases.* New York: Facts on File, 1993.

Eng, Thomas Rand, and William T. Butler, eds. *The Hidden Epidemic: Confronting Sexually Transmitted Diseases.* Washington, D.C.: National Academy Press, 1997.

Fish, Raymond M., Elizabeth Trupin Campbell, and Suzanne R. Trupin. *Sexually Transmitted Diseases: Problems in Primary Care.* Los Angeles: Practice Management Information, 1992.

Quetel, Claude. *History of Syphilis.* Baltimore: The Johns Hopkins University Press, 1990.

SYSTEMS AND ORGANS
ANATOMY
ANATOMY OR SYSTEM AFFECTED: All
SPECIALTIES AND RELATED FIELDS: All
DEFINITION: Groups of tissues and organs dedicated to particular functions, all of which must work together to perform efficiently.
KEY TERMS:
atrium: the chamber of the heart where veins terminate; the atrium receives blood returning to the heart and delivers it to the ventricle
bronchi: the airways conducting air from the mouth to the depths of the lungs

carbon dioxide: the gas produced by the body from the use of oxygen; carbon dioxide and the hydrogen ions it can create may become toxic if not excreted by the body
foodstuffs: the basic components of food that the body can use—carbohydrates (which break down to sugars, primarily to glucose), proteins (which break down to amino acids), and fat
hormone: a chemical released by a tissue to signal another tissue to modify its function
ions: small chemical substances that have a positive or negative charge; the most important ions with a positive charge are sodium, potassium, hydrogen, and calcium, while the most important negative ion is chloride
ventricles: the large chambers of the heart that pump blood into the arteries; the left ventricle pumps blood into the aorta, and the right ventricle pumps blood into the lung's arteries

STRUCTURE AND FUNCTIONS
There are essentially nine systems in the human body: the nervous, cardiovascular, respiratory, gastrointestinal, renal, endocrine, reproductive, thermoregulatory, and skeletomuscular systems. All these systems are essential to sustain life, and many work together to perform their functions efficiently. All the other systems need the nervous system to operate or to coordinate their functions. The first six of these systems will be discussed in this article.

The nervous system is composed of the central nervous system (the brain) and the peripheral nervous system (the spinal cord and nerves extending to every part of the body). The brain receives information from the body by way of the sensory nerves. It then evaluates all the information and sends out the appropriate signals to respond. For example, the ears send information to the brain that there are noises coming from behind; the brain tells the head to turn in the direction of the sounds. The eyes send the signals that the noises are coming from, for example, a gorilla. The brain must decide to run, fight, or stand and try to reason with the gorilla. Meanwhile, the brain tells the heart to beat faster and harder. It also tells the stomach and intestines to stop digestion and reduce its blood flow because blood may be needed by the muscles for running. This is called the "fight or flight" response to stress, which the nervous system controls.

Sensory information can come from any of the five

senses—sight, smell, hearing, touch, or taste—but it can also come from other sensors. Sensory nerves send the brain information on pain, temperature, blood pressure, and what is going on in the stomach and intestines (hunger or a full feeling). The brain receives millions of signals each second from every part of the body and must constantly decide how to respond. Humans can choose not to respond instinctively as animals do. For example, humans often eat when they are not hungry.

Different areas of the brain are dedicated to specific functions. The upper portion of the spinal cord and lower portion of the brain (the brain stem) are dedicated to controlling involuntary functions such as breathing, the maintenance of blood pressure and heart rate, and the responses to hot and cold. The middle portion of the brain coordinates movement. The middle brain also coordinates information from upper portions of the brain and generates emotions. The uppermost and outermost portions of the brain (the cerebrum) process the information from the senses and generate responses, such as telling the body to move. The cerebrum also performs such intellectual functions as reasoning.

The cardiovascular system is composed of the heart and blood vessels. Its job is to pump blood containing oxygen and foodstuffs (sugars, proteins, and fat) to every part of the body. Blood is composed of red and white blood cells suspended in plasma, a pale yellow fluid which flows through the cardiovascular system. Red blood cells are the carriers of oxygen, the main source of energy for the body. White blood cells help fight disease and are delivered to parts of the body that are hurt or diseased. The plasma contains platelets that help blood to clot when necessary. Blood also transports wastes produced by the body from tissues to organs that can dispose of them. For example, carbon dioxide is produced by the tissues when oxygen is used for energy. Blood carries carbon dioxide back to the lungs to be removed from the body in exhaled air.

Blood is pumped by the heart in a circuit in the cardiovascular system (also called the circulatory system). The heart has four chambers, two atria and two ventricles. Blood enters the heart through the left atrium, a small pocket of muscles that help pump blood into the left ventricle. The ventricle is a larger chamber with a thick wall of muscle that can pump very hard; it pushes blood into the arteries. The left ventricle pumps blood into the main artery of the

body, the aorta. The aorta branches many times into smaller arteries, which in turn branch into capillaries. Every part of the body has millions of tiny capillaries just big enough for a blood cell to pass through them; in fact, blood cells must fold to get through some capillaries. In capillaries, oxygen and foodstuffs leave the blood, and then carbon dioxide and other waste products enter the blood to be taken away. Blood flows from the capillaries into small veins, which join to make larger and larger veins. The largest veins, the venae cavae, empty into the heart, in the right atrium. The blood is pumped from the right atrium to the right ventricle. Blood is then pumped by the right ventricle through the lung and back into the left atrium to start its journey again.

The lungs are the major organ of the respiratory system. The function of the respiratory system is to bring fresh air into the lungs, getting it very close to the blood, and to expel used air. Air enters the respiratory system through the nose and mouth, which connect to the main windpipe, the trachea. The trachea branches into smaller airways called bronchi. Bronchi in turn branch into smaller airways, bronchioles. The ends of bronchioles form many rounded sacs (alveoli) that resemble a bunch of grapes. These sacs of air have very thin walls that are shared with the walls of the lung's capillaries. This close arrangement of air and blood provides a minimal distance for oxygen to travel into the blood and for carbon dioxide to leave the blood.

Air is moved into the lungs when the muscles of respiration contract and expand the lungs. The diaphragm is a large sheet of muscle which separates the chest from the abdomen. When the diaphragm contracts, it pulls the lungs down. At the same time, muscles on the chest wall contract, pulling the lungs up and out. This expansion of the lungs causes air to be sucked into and fill the air sacs. During exhalation, the respiratory muscles are relaxed, the lung collapses somewhat, and air rushes out, carrying carbon dioxide with it.

Blood, specifically red blood cells, is specialized to carry large amounts of oxygen and carbon dioxide. Red blood cells contain hemoglobin, a special substance that attaches to these gases. When the amounts of oxygen and carbon dioxide in the plasma increase, they tend to leak back into the air sacs or tissues, respectively. These gases are effectively removed from the fluid by hemoglobin, allowing more gases to enter the blood without leaking back out. Hemoglobin also coordinates the release of these gases— oxygen to the tissues and carbon dioxide to the lungs—at the correct time.

The gastrointestinal system is a multiorgan system that breaks down food to be absorbed into the blood. Initially, food is broken down by chewing and by mixing with saliva. Then it is swallowed into the esophagus, a tube which travels through the chest to empty into the stomach. The stomach adds acid and other chemicals to the food, which breaks it down further. The food, now called chyme, passes into the upper small intestine (the duodenum). The pancreas adds enzymes; a chemical called bicarbonate, which neutralizes the acid added by the stomach; and the hormones insulin and glucagon. Insulin is the major hormone secreted by the pancreas. It is absorbed into the blood by the intestine and signals the body to get ready to receive the products of digestion, primarily sugar (glucose). Bile is also added to the contents of the upper duodenum by the liver. Bile helps to break down fat to be absorbed into the blood. As the intestinal contents move along the small intestine, from the jejunum to the ileum, water and mucus are added to help move it along, and carbohydrates are absorbed in their smallest form, glucose. Enzymes attached to the wall of the intestine break up proteins to be absorbed as their component parts, amino acids. Water in chyme is constantly being reabsorbed. Finally the colon, or large intestine, absorbs most of the remaining water. The remaining solids are excreted through the rectum.

Food is moved through the gastrointestinal system by a special type of muscle called smooth muscle. The walls of the gastrointestinal tract are composed of muscle arranged in circular fashion around the tube and along its length. Initially, a circular group of muscles contracts, narrowing a short segment of intestine. This process is called segmentation. The contraction spreads down the muscles arranged lengthwise, squeezing the contents down the length of intestine. Movement of chyme is aided by relaxation of the muscles ahead of the contraction. This motion is called peristalsis. Peristalsis is coordinated by the nervous system, but the intestines have their own set of nerves. These intestinal nerves can control the motion of the intestine without help from the central nervous system.

The kidneys are the primary organs of the renal system. It is the function of the kidneys to regulate both the amount and the composition of the fluid in the body, in spite of wide variations in the human environment and in an organism's intake of food and water. Since blood circulates everywhere in the body, the kidneys can change the composition and amount of plasma, and the other fluids of the body then equalize with it. Therefore, the kidneys can regulate all body fluids. The body has sensors for both the amount of fluid in the blood and the concentration of the important elements in the blood, such as sodium, hydrogen, and potassium.

The kidneys regulate plasma volume and composition by filtering the plasma and returning only the appropriate amounts of fluid and substances back to the blood. Arteries entering the kidneys rapidly branch into capillaries. Approximately 20 percent of all plasma flowing into the kidneys leaves the capillaries and is collected in the capsules that surround them. This fluid is funneled into specialized tubes.

Substances are taken out and put into the fluid in the tubes in order to regulate fluid volume and composition. In the beginning of the tube (the proximal tubule), most of the salt, water, glucose, and amino acids are taken back into the blood. The next sections (the loop of Henle, distal tubule, and collecting ducts) help to regulate the final amount of water excreted in urine. The collecting ducts join to form the ureter, which carries the remaining fluid, urine, to the bladder, where it is stored. From the bladder, the urine is expelled through the urethra.

The endocrine system is another multiorgan system that helps to control and modify the function of almost all other systems. Endocrine glands produce chemicals and release them into the blood to direct the functions of cells and tissues elsewhere in the body. There are three classes of hormones: amines, peptides and proteins, and steroids. Adrenaline is an example of the amine group, insulin is a protein hormone, and estrogen is a steroid hormone. Each of these is produced by a different gland.

The adrenal glands, small glands located near the kidneys, make several hormones. The outer portion, the cortex, produces three types of steroid hormones referred to as corticosteroids: glucocorticoids, mineralocorticoids, and small amounts of androgenic hormones. The major glucocorticoid, cortisol, regulates the production and use of glucose, fats, and amino acids by many cells and tissues. It also plays a helper role for other hormonal actions, such as making them more potent during stress, and it helps prevent inflammation and swelling. The major mineralocorticoid, aldosterone, can modify the kidneys' excretion of sodium, potassium, and hydrogen. A person unable to produce mineralocorticoids will die in a few days without treatment but can be saved by aldosterone therapy. Therefore, these steroids are said to be life-saving. The androgenic steroids can cause the development of adult male sexual characteristics, the same effect as the male sex hormone, testosterone.

The interior portion, or medulla, of the adrenal glands makes catecholamines, such as adrenaline (epinephrine). Adrenaline helps the cardiovascular system during exercise and stress. It is the hormone that stimulates much of the "fight or flight" response, making the heart beat faster and harder. Adrenaline also helps to increase blood flow to muscles, in case flight is the action of choice.

The pituitary gland, also known as the hypophysis, is located at the base of the brain and produces many hormones with a variety of actions. The pituitary is divided into two areas: the anterior lobe (also known as the adenohypophysis) and the posterior lobe (also known as the neurohypophysis). The anterior pituitary produces growth hormone, a protein that has a major influence on all metabolic activity. It causes the body to store carbohydrates, to make proteins for growth, and to use fat for energy. The other anterior pituitary hormones cause other glands to increase their production of hormones. The glands stimulated by distinct pituitary hormones are the thyroid, adrenal cortex, ovaries, testicles, and mammary glands. The posterior pituitary produces the peptide hormones antidiuretic hormone (also known as vasopressin) and oxytocin. Antidiuretic hormone (ADH) decreases the amount of water that the kidneys can excrete, which keeps the body from dehydrating. ADH can also cause the blood pressure to rise, which helps if fluid is lost as a result of bleeding. Oxytocin causes the uterus to contract during the birthing process, and it also stimulates the production of milk in new mothers. The pituitary has direct regulating control over many glands and tissues, and it regulates nearly all tissues and organs indirectly by way of its stimulating hormones. This gland is regulated in a similar fashion by the hypothalamus, a small part of the brain just above the pituitary.

The thyroid gland is located in the neck around the voice box, or larynx. The parathyroid glands are located next to the thyroid gland. Thyroid hormones (peptides) cause almost all tissues in the body to increase the use of foodstuffs for the production of pro-teins, aiding in growth. In addition, the thyroid gland produces calcitonin. Calcitonin and the parathyroid hormones regulate the amount of calcium in the blood. Parathyroid hormone acts by freeing calcium from bone when more calcium is needed in the blood, while calcitonin causes the opposite action. Therefore, when the level of one of these hormones goes up, the other must go down.

The sex organs are also endocrine glands. The ovaries make estrogen and progesterone, while the testes produce testosterone. These steroid hormones cause the body to develop primary and secondary sexual characteristics. When a woman is pregnant, the placenta (the part of a woman's uterus that nourishes the fetus) produces hormones that prepare her body for childbirth and breast-feeding.

DISORDERS AND DISEASES

The body has control mechanisms to ensure that its systems function properly. Many systems use what is called negative feedback to fine-tune their functioning. An example of negative feedback is the control of blood pressure. Sensors in the arteries allow the brain to monitor the body's blood pressure level. When pressure is too high, the brain tells the cardiovascular system to decrease pressure by slowing the heart and opening the blood vessels and tells the kidneys to excrete fluid. Thus, when blood pressure is high, the feedback that the brain provides is negative, because it causes a response that is opposite to the unwanted change from the normal state.

The endocrine system uses negative feedback to regulate many hormones. The simplest endocrine feedback system involves insulin and glucose. When blood glucose increases, insulin secretion increases, which in turn decreases blood glucose. A decrease in blood glucose tells the pancreas to slow down the secretion of insulin. The failure of this system results in diabetes mellitus, a disease in which the ability to regulate blood sugar is lost. When this control is lost, other systems are damaged as a result, such as the renal and cardiovascular systems.

There are also much more complex feedback control systems. The regulation of the adrenal hormone cortisol serves as an example of such a system. Cortisol secretion is controlled by secretion of the pituitary hormone adrenocorticotropic hormone (ACTH), also called corticotropin. The secretion of ACTH is controlled by a hypothalamic hormone called corticotropin-releasing factor (CRF). Stress causes

CRF to be released, which causes the release of ACTH and in turn stimulates the secretion of cortisol. In general, when the level of any of these hormones becomes too high, the release of one of the others can be shut down. High levels of cortisol turn off CRF and ACTH secretion. High levels of ACTH can turn off the secretion of the hormone that triggers its secretion, CRF. It is also thought that CRF can provide feedback to its organ of origin, the hypothalamus, and halt its own secretion. Thus, if one of the control systems fails to function, a backup system guards against total malfunction.

The systems and organs of the body are dedicated to specific functions, but each needs the others to function properly. In addition, each system requires the coordination from the central nervous system to perform efficiently. The lungs bring vital oxygen to the cardiovascular system, and all systems need the nutrients brought to them by the cardiovascular system. Some organs of the endocrine system, such as the adrenal glands, are essential to life. The kidneys keep the blood clean and maintain the body's fluid volume. The reproductive system is essential to maintaining the existence of a species. All these systems must perform their functions for the body to work well. If one system malfunctions, frequently other systems become involved and may malfunction as well.

An example of one system malfunction that causes the failure of many others is renal failure. Kidney failure can be caused by a malfunction of the cardiovascular system such as clogging of the capillaries, which prohibits the kidneys from doing their job. As a result, hydrogen and potassium ions will accumulate. The effects of high levels of hydrogen and potassium ions on the cardiovascular system are a weakened heart and lower blood pressure. The nervous system can sense the increase in hydrogen ions and will tell the respiratory system to breathe faster and deeper to rid the body of carbon dioxide and its hydrogen ions. The increase in breathing helps to lower the hydrogen ion levels in the blood but cannot completely compensate for the kidney malfunction; in fact, the increase in work by the respiratory muscles can produce more hydrogen ions. When levels of hydrogen become too high, the brain begins to malfunction. The patient may experience dizziness, have seizures, or lose consciousness. If these symptoms are not reversed, the malfunction of each system will aid in the deterioration of other systems. The

brain will be irreversibly damaged, and the heart will stop.

There are several ways to treat renal failure to avoid multiple-organ sickness. Treatment of infections with antibiotics before they become severe can help to avoid early and mild kidney failure. In severe, long-term kidney failure, kidney transplantation may become necessary. The damaged kidney (or kidneys) is removed and replaced with an organ from a deceased donor or from a living donor (a person can live a normal life with only one functioning kidney). Kidneys, even from deceased donors, are rare, and many people in need of a transplant must wait for years to receive one that will not be rejected by the body's immune system. For such patients, dialysis is necessary for survival. Dialysis is the use of a machine to perform some of the functions of the kidneys. Patients with total kidney failure must be hooked up to an artificial kidney machine for several hours several times per week. Even with this treatment, they will still be very sick because the machine cannot perform all functions of the kidneys.

PERSPECTIVE AND PROSPECTS

In the Middle Ages, it was believed that "spirits" were the essence of life or "vitality"; thus, the treatment for many ailments was bloodletting, the application of leeches to remove the "evil spirit" causing the sickness. It was not until the seventeenth century that William Harvey discovered that blood circulated from arteries to veins in both the lungs and the rest of the body. Oxygen was discovered at the end of the eighteenth century by Joseph Priestley. Knowledge of chemistry, biochemistry, and physiology grew in the nineteenth century, but most of the information about systems and organs contained in this article was revealed in the twentieth century.

Many discoveries have been in the area of how the body's systems and organs interact with and influence one another. New anatomical techniques of investigation have revealed the minute structures of many organs and tissues. As a result, the presence of previously unknown nervous and other tissue parts has been recognized; their functions are under investigation. Chemical techniques have revealed many new hormone and hormonelike substances through which one tissue or organ can influence another. Research into the molecular structure of some of these biochemical signals is helping to explain how they work.

In addition, the events that occur inside a cell or group of cells have been described in greater detail. How a group of cells produce unified organ function and how this function is altered is currently under investigation. Studies into how a cell can change its function in conjunction with surrounding cells have added to the knowledge of how systems and organs can fine-tune their functions. This research involves information regarding how the genes inside cells carry messages and how these messages in turn are expressed in unified physiological functions.

—*J. Timothy O'Neill, Ph.D.*

See also Brain; Circulation; Ears; Eyes; Gastrointestinal system; Glands; Heart; Immune system; Kidneys; Liver; Lungs; Lymphatic system; Nervous system; Pancreas; Reproductive system; Sense organs; Skin; Thyroid gland; Urinary system; Vascular system.

FOR FURTHER INFORMATION:

Asimov, Isaac. *The Human Body: Its Structure and Operation.* Rev. ed. New York: Penguin Books, 1992. Asimov offers an easy-to-understand overview of all the body's organ functions.

Guyton, Arthur C., and John E. Hall. *Human Physiology and Mechanisms of Disease.* 6th ed. Philadelphia: W. B. Saunders, 1997. This physiology text deals with the function of the body in considerable detail. Excellent advanced reading for the physiology student.

Kittredge, Mary. *The Human Body: An Overview.* Reprint. Philadelphia: Chelsea House, 2001. This text explains the general workings of the human body. Provides background to the historical development of medical knowledge and addresses many of the pathologies that can arise in the body.

TAI CHI CHUAN
PROCEDURE

ANATOMY OR SYSTEM AFFECTED: All

SPECIALTIES AND RELATED FIELDS: Alternative medicine, preventive medicine

DEFINITION: This ancient Chinese martial art, which means "supreme ultimate power," consists of flowing meditative movements. Its major focus is to enhance the C'hi, or life force, which is balanced in healthy individuals. While the movements of Tai Chi Chuan evolved from forms used in combat, as it is practiced for health benefits it is largely a moving meditation. The traditional form consists of 128 movements and requires approximately thirty minutes to perform in a slow motion; shorter versions are also taught. The gentle movements of Tai Chi Chuan are particularly useful for increasing flexibility and for reducing stress by calming and focusing the mind and body. When performed quickly, and with exercises in addition to the traditional form, it is an excellent method to increase oxygen consumption and heart rate and to improve stamina. It is frequently prescribed for the elderly and infirm because regular practice helps blood flow and lymph circulation and decreases fatigue. Treating the body and mind as one also has positive psychological effects on many people.

—*Karen E. Kalumuck, Ph.D.*

See also Alternative medicine; Circulation; Holistic medicine; Meditation; Qi gong; Stress; Stress reduction.

FOR FURTHER INFORMATION:

Jacobs, Jennifer, ed. *The Encyclopedia of Alternative Medicine: A Complete Family Guide to Complementary Therapies.* Rev. ed. Boston: Journey Edition, 1997.

Pelletier, Kenneth R. *Holistic Medicine.* New York: Delacorte Press, 1979.

Salmon, J. Warren, ed. *Alternative Medicines.* New York: Tavistock, 1984.

TAPEWORM
DISEASE/DISORDER

ANATOMY OR SYSTEM AFFECTED: Gastrointestinal system, intestines

---

Parts of a Tapeworm

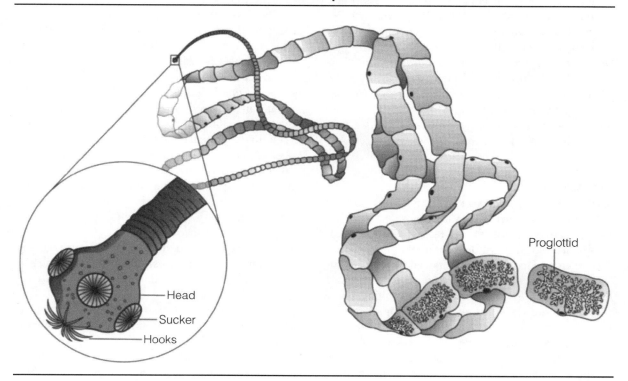

Head
Sucker
Hooks
Proglottid

SPECIALTIES AND RELATED FIELDS: Gastroenterology, internal medicine, pediatrics, public health

DEFINITION: Tapeworms are intestinal parasites that are also called cestodes. Humans become infected with these worms by eating improperly cooked or raw pork, beef, or fish or by being bitten by a larva-carrying flea. In most cases of tapeworm infestation, the victim experiences few or no symptoms. As the number of worms attached to the walls of the small intestine increases or as the size of the worm increases, the infected person may experience upper abdominal pain, diarrhea, unexplained weight loss, symptoms of anemia, and bowel movements containing worm body parts and eggs. Left untreated, embryonic worms pass into the bloodstream and form cysts in the muscles, brain, and other organs. Cysts in the brain often cause epilepsy. Tapeworms can be treated with a single dose of an antihelminthic drug.

—*Jason Georges and Tracy Irons-Georges*
See also Food poisoning; Intestinal disorders; Intestines; Parasitic diseases; Worms.

FOR FURTHER INFORMATION:

Buchsbaum, Ralph, et al. *Animals Without Backbones.* 3d ed. Chicago: University of Chicago Press, 1987.

Despommier, Dickson D., Robert W. Gwadz, and Peter J. Hotex. *Parasitic Diseases.* 4th ed. New York: Springer-Verlag, 2000.

Donaldson, Raymond Joseph, ed. *Parasites and Western Man.* Baltimore: University Park Press, 1979.

Klein, Aaron E. *The Parasites We Humans Harbor.* New York: Elsevier/Nelson Books, 1981.

Smyth, James D. *The Physiology of Cestodes.* San Francisco: W. H. Freeman, 1969.

TASTE

BIOLOGY

ANATOMY OR SYSTEM AFFECTED: Gastrointestinal system, mouth, nervous system, nose

SPECIALTIES AND RELATED FIELDS: Gastroenterology, neurology, nutrition, otorhinolaryngology

DEFINITION: One of the five special senses; chemicals interact with receptor sites in specialized structures of the tongue, and the resulting nerve impulses are classified as certain kinds of taste.

KEY TERMS:

chemoreceptors: specific structures upon which tastant molecules (chemicals that cause a taste sensation on the tongue) adhere; it is presumed that taste receptors have some structural uniqueness because "sweet," "salty," "sour," and "bitter" can be distinguished there

facial nerve: the seventh cranial nerve pair, which relays signals from the face and the front region of the tongue up to the pons of the brain stem; conducts impulses related to taste, salivation, and facial expression

filiform papillae: the small, rounded projections that form the tough, yet velvetlike, texture of the tongue surface; lacking any chemoreceptors, these papillae do not function in taste

foliate papillae: the folded papillae found on the soft edges of the rear of the tongue and just ahead of the V shape formed by the vallate papillae; although found in the regions that detect bitter or sour tastes, foliate papillae are not specific receptors for bitter or sour tastes

fungiform papillae: the papillae scattered about the tongue surface, in no specific array, that are responsive to tastant molecules; these do not exhibit specificity for a particular type of taste

glossopharyngeal nerve: the ninth cranial nerve, which relays signals pertaining to or controlling salivation; sends neurological information to and from the posterior region of the tongue to the medulla oblongata of the brain stem

gustation: the ability to taste, which is independent of smell (olfaction) or textural and temperature enhancements; ageusia, or apogeusia, is the loss of taste sensation

gustatory stimulation threshold: the minimal quantity of tastant molecules that must be present in a water or saliva solution for a neural response at the taste cell to be initiated and the "correct" taste perceived; below this threshold, taste is either absent or identified incorrectly

taste bud: a special sensing structure for taste found on taste-responsive papillae; taste buds are made of three cell types—gustatory or taste cells, supporting cells, and basal cells

taste cell: the cellular compartment of a taste bud that contains chemoreceptors; taste hairs, one type of chemoreceptor, are found at the taste pore, or entry point, of a taste cell

vagus nerve: the tenth cranial nerve, which carries taste messages from the limited number of taste buds located in obscure sites such as the palate, epiglottis, uvula, and other structures at the entrance of the esophagus; also sends important information from the thoracic and abdominal viscera to the brain

vallate papillae: the seven to ten papillae mounds arranged in a V shape, which can be seen when the tongue is fully extended; these taste sensors lack taste specificity

STRUCTURE AND FUNCTIONS

For many people, the thought of biting into a lemon causes a puckering or a tingling sensation in the mouth. A real taste sensation is evoked even though the actual taste stimulus, a lemon, is absent. This kind of response indicates the power of the sense of taste. Taste is also called the gustatory sense, a term derived from the Latin word *gustatus*, meaning taste. This sense evolved to aid animals in the selection of safe, nontoxic foods. Although loss of the ability to experience taste (apogeusia) is not a life-threatening condition, it may indicate the presence of other maladies, some of which are life-threatening. A diminished or absent ability to taste may account for loss of appetite or weight loss in some ill persons; for these persons, sufficient and proper nutrition can become a critical issue.

There are five special senses of the human body: gustatory, olfactory (smell), visual, auditory (hearing), and equilibrium. The organs associated with the special senses take in information from the environment in the form of chemical, light, sound, or mechanical energy and convert that energy into nerve impulses. Nerve impulses are tiny electrical signals that are carried by the peripheral and central nervous systems to the brain, where the information is integrated in order to assess how dangerous or secure an individual may be in any given environment. Taste is a primitive sense, meaning that it need not be taught; it evokes instinctual responses or reactions.

Although taste is not as essential to survival as the sense of vision, it is an important sense for a variety of organisms. Taste preferences can be observed in humans, elephants, monkeys, fish, and even some microorganisms. Yet not all organisms respond equally to the same tastant; one example is sugar. Cats lack taste receptors for sugar; therefore, if a cat eats a sweet food, it does so for other flavors. Just as a cat does not taste sweetness, however, a human might not notice a tastant that a cat recognizes. A tastant is any food or chemical (such as soap) that causes a taste sensation.

Taste is a nerve impulse that is interpreted by the brain. (In organisms lacking a brain, taste is inter-

The Sense of Taste

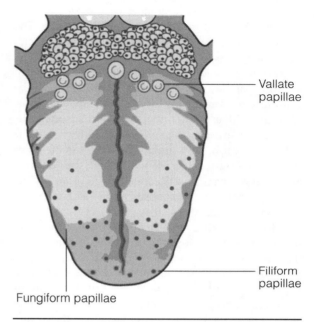

Special receptors on the tongue send nerve impulses to the brain that are registered as various tastes, such as bitter, sweet, salty, and sour.

preted by some other structure that serves as the center of integration and coordination.) For humans, and for many of the larger land animals, taste sensations begin upon the intake of food or other substances into the mouth. This signal is prompted by the interaction of tastant molecules or ions and chemoreceptors located in specialized regions within taste buds.

Composed mostly of muscle fiber, the tongue not only serves as a receptor site for taste stimuli but also is responsible for the refined and coordinated movements that produce speech—an important form of communication in the human species. Different sections of the tongue are in contact with specific nerves that allow coordinated and specialized movements of the tongue. The palatine section of the tongue is easily seen when the tongue is fully extended from the mouth; it constitutes the front two-thirds of the tongue. The back one-third is the pharyngeal section; the palatine and pharyngeal sections are visibly, but subtly, separated by a transverse groove.

The surface of the palatine section of the tongue is coated with small, closely spaced projections called papillae. These structures give the tongue the dual properties of being rough and textured while remaining velvety smooth. Papillae are arranged, from the tongue's tip to the back, in more or less parallel rows that run along the medial groove of the tongue. The medial groove divides the tongue lengthwise into equal halves that are independently coordinated by nerves and muscle working together.

Most papillae covering the tongue are of the filiform type. Unlike the other three papillae forms, filiform papillae do not contain taste buds and thus are not responsive to tastants. Instead, filiform papillae aid in the tearing and grating of food particles. Although filiform papillae are not barbed, they do have a rasping mechanical action that aids in cleansing the body through licking (as observed in cats) and moving food particles about in the mouth.

All other papillae—the fungiform, the foliate, and the vallate—are actively involved in tasting, even though they are not present in great abundance or distributed uniformly over the tongue surface. Fungiform papillae, whose projections are shaped like a mushroom cap, are widely scattered on the tip and lateral sides of the tongue. Foliate papillae mimic the texture and appearance of smooth, folded leaves; they are located on both sides of the tongue, flanking the vallate papillae. The vallate papillae make a semicircular pattern (or a V shape) at the back of the tongue. Located on the palatine region just before the pharyngeal segment of the mouth, vallate papillae resemble rounded, soft cushions. Humans have between seven and twelve of these projections, making the vallate papillae the least abundant form of papillae.

Four tastes are commonly recognized by humans: sweet, salty, sour, and bitter. These tastes are strongly registered in specific zones of the tongue. Much to the frustration of scientists, however, the recognition of taste is not specific to any particular type of taste-responsive papillae (fungiform, foliate, or vallate). Sweet receptors are plentiful at the tip of the tongue, while salty receptors are grouped together on either side just beyond the tip. Sour sensations are detected more strongly along the middle sides of the tongue, and bitter sensations are detected at the rear.

Since the vallate papillae are located in the region where only bitterness is tasted and the fungiform papillae are located in the regions sensitive to sweetness, one may assume that a match between papillae structure and taste type exists. Scientific studies, however, prove this to be a false correlation. A simple relationship between kind of taste and type of papillae

does not exist, nor is there a complete explanation of the anatomy and physiology of the gustatory sense.

Taste-responsive papillae seem to respond to all tastants that enter their taste buds, whether they are classified as sweet, salty, sour, or bitter. The distinguishing factor seems to be a variation in the intensity of the neural message that a tastant induces. The variable levels of nervous impulses caused by a tastant constitute what is called a taste profile. Taste profiles are mixed neural codes that a taste bud receives from certain tastants.

A tastant molecule causes a nervous impulse to be sent to the brain for interpretation. It has been learned that all three taste-sensitive papillae are "fired," to a greater or lesser extent, by all tastant molecules. A neural response is triggered when tastant molecules arrive at specialized sites on the taste buds. Then there is a certain ratio, or "firing pattern," that is interpreted as sweet, salty, sour, or bitter. Oddly, this kind of mixed signal can be misread in the brain. For example, if a sweet solution of table sugar and water (tasted and properly identified as sweet) is greatly diluted with very pure water, the sugar solution may be erroneously classified in the brain as salty. The taste sensation is simply able to recognize when something has interacted with a taste chemoreceptor; a weak stimulus may cause a misinterpretation to occur.

Taste buds are relatively large, bulbous-shaped structures located on the tips of fungiform papillae and in the grooves of the foliate and vallate papillae. It is within the taste bud structure that "sweet," "salty," "sour," or "bitter" begin the journey of becoming distinguished taste sensations. A taste bud is not a wholly sensing bundle; it can be divided into at least three distinct parts—taste (or sensing) cells, support cells, and basal cells.

The number of taste buds in humans ranges from two thousand to nine thousand. About half of these are located in the grooved edges of the seven to twelve vallate papillae, making this a very sensitive taste area of the tongue. Taste buds are abundant in infants and children, but a continuous decline is observed from adolescence throughout adulthood. This explains why adults often like to add rich sauces, gravies, and seasonings to foods; adults need to enhance food so that a greater range of taste sensations is triggered in each mouthful. Children tend to shun sauces and spices because they may experience almost overwhelming taste sensations when they consume adult-prepared foods. In the elderly, low numbers of taste cells can contribute to poor eating habits or food selection, putting them at risk during the most vulnerable stage in adult life. It is often recommended that foods be made readily available and prepared in colorful and aromatically pleasing ways to entice the elderly to eat properly.

Tastant particles must dissolve in saliva in order to cause a taste response that can be identified properly. The minimum amount of tastant that must be present for it to be identified correctly is called the gustatory stimulation threshold. The requirement that a tastant be soluble in saliva is particularly true of sweet molecules (sugars and carbohydrates) or sour and some salty ions (salts and acids can release charged groups of atoms called ions when dissolved in saliva). Bitter substances seem to adhere to lipid sites on the papillae, and thus could be thought of as fat-soluble molecules. Sweet, salty, and sour chemicals are generally hydrophilic ("water-loving"), while bitter chemicals tend to be hydrophobic ("water-hating").

Whether hydrophilic or hydrophobic, tastant molecules or ions must get through the entry point on at least some taste cells located on taste buds. At the entry point of a taste cell, a tiny pore has small taste hair projections that are believed to be the true sensors of taste. The basic premise, according to current theory, is that the ions or molecules of the tastant substance enter the pore and then physically or chemically interact with specialized regions of the taste hairs. This interaction causes an action potential (a nerve impulse) to occur as the permeability of the nerve fibers innervating the taste cell is altered. An action potential will cause a "wave" of permeability changes all the way up the nerve fibers and into the brain. The medulla oblongata is the first site of the brain to receive the action potentials that will be registered as taste.

The exposure of taste cells to the environment renders them at risk to potential damage. Fortunately, new taste cells are regenerated every seven to ten days; regeneration occurs within the basal cells of the taste buds. It is important to note, however, that this is a regeneration of the taste cells, not of the nerves that innervate them. Olfactory nerves are the only nerve cells in the human body that can regenerate.

DISORDERS AND DISEASES

In the medical sciences, gustatory problems are generally not a cause but an effect. A diminished sense of taste (hypogeusia), an alteration of taste (dysgeusia), or the complete absence of the sense of taste (ageusia, or apogeusia) is generally a symptom of an underlying pathology. It is rare for true apogeusia to be an isolated symptom of a malady; it is even rarer for true apogeusia to exist as an isolated physical malady. Yet apogeusia does, in fact, exist in human populations. Among the descendants of the Ashkenazi Jews, for example, a double recessive genetic code mandates that taste papillae will not develop; direct descendants of this group have congenital apogeusia.

In discussing when or how noncongenital apogeusia, hypogeusia, or dysgeusia can become a problem, it is important to review the critical components of a taste message. Three discrete structures are involved: taste cells, which contain taste hairs at their pores; nerve fibers, which connect the chemoreceptors (taste hairs) to the brain; and the brain itself. Alterations in the ability to taste can originate in any or all three of these discrete steps along the path.

Some pathologies that can cause a miscommunication at the receptor sites include actual physical or chemical damage to the taste buds, such as a burn that covers the tongue's surface or the ingestion of lye; accidental or therapeutic exposure to radiation; lingual (tongue) or palatal (palate) carcinomas; tumors or lesions of the tongue surface; or a leukemic infiltrate of the tongue surface.

The ability to taste may be altered or lost if damage occurs to certain cranial nerves. Specifically, damage to any of these cranial nerves may be responsible for taste disorders: the facial nerve (the seventh cranial nerve), which carries sweet and salty messages from the front of the tongue; the glossopharyngeal nerve (the ninth cranial nerve), which carries bitter and sour signals; and the large vagus nerve (the tenth cranial nerve), which carries taste sensations from the throat and epiglottis. Damage to these nerves may occur if they are crushed, severed, or pinched or if tumors, lesions, or neural disease interferes with normal function.

Finally, a head injury or malady can account for apogeusia, hypogeusia, or dysgeusia. Regions of particular concern include damage to the medulla oblongata, the thalamus, or the gustatory cortex, which is located in the parietal lobe of the brain. Lesions, tumors, or head injuries resulting from sudden or severe impact can give rise to true taste pathology. In these cases, the brain can either no longer identify tastes properly or no longer receive or interpret taste impulses.

Indirect impairment of taste may occur as a result of an imbalance in body chemistry. Such imbalances may result from exposure to or ingestion of trace metal poisons or other toxins, insufficient dietary intake to allow for cellular repair or development, incomplete intake of essential vitamins or minerals, or metabolic imbalances, such as hypothyroidism (an underactive thyroid gland). In addition, taste-modifying pathologies, whose origins are not directly associated at the chemoreceptor sites, can involve allergic or drug reactions.

Other taste disorders that can be clinically assessed include cacogeusia, the alteration of once-pleasant tastes to ones that are repulsive (for example, the perception that all foods taste rotten); phantogeusia, the presence of a taste sensation in the absence of any tastant; heterogeusia, a distortion of tastes for all foods (for example, sweets may taste salty, salts may taste bitter, and so on); and parageusia, an unusual taste distortion of one taste type that does not cause a repulsive taste response (for example, bitter foods may taste salty).

In diagnosing a taste disorder, the physician must first obtain a full medical history from the patient and perform a physical examination. Because of the anatomy involved in taste function, special attention will be given to the head and neck area. General laboratory analysis of kidney, liver, and endocrine function must be performed, as well as a complete blood study. Also, tests may be administered to determine the possible role of allergies in a given pathology.

The issue of taste disorder is often complicated by the common use of terms that have specific meaning in a clinical setting. Three of these troublesome terms are "taste," "flavor," and "palatability." Taste means, quite literally, the chemoreceptor response of taste cells embedded in taste buds (located on the papillae), which is caused by tastant molecules. The interaction between the tastant and the chemoreceptors produces a nerve signal that travels from the taste receptor site to the brain. In stringent use of the term "taste," other factors, such as aroma, texture, or color, should not be considered in the assessment of this sense.

Flavor generally means the response of the olfactory and gustatory systems, working in unison, to assess the pleasure or displeasure prompted by a tastant. Smell is fundamentally integrated with taste to the point that people generally salivate more when exposed to an appealing odor, especially if the aroma is associated with a particularly pleasing food, such as freshly baked bread. A common exercise used to demonstrate the close connection between the olfactory and gustatory systems is a blind study in which the subjects close their eyes, pinch their noses shut, and sample uniformly sized cubes of solid foods kept at room temperature. Under such circumstances, most humans cannot distinguish between raw potato, raw onion, white cheese, or peeled fresh apple. Taste-testers may be shocked to discover that raw onions seem much the same as raw apples without visual or aromatic cues. This exercise speaks strongly to the significance of how humans integrate all of their senses in gathering data from the environment.

A loss or a decrease in the ability to smell greatly alters one's sense of flavor, even though there is no true loss of the ability to experience taste. A common example of this interrelationship between ability to smell foods or beverages and the connected ability to enjoy flavor has been experienced at first hand by anyone who has ever suffered from a severe head cold. When the nasal passages are coated with thick mucus, as generally occurs during a viral cold, eating is no longer pleasurable; foods are generally described as tasting "flat" or "bland." The cold virus does not in any way interrupt the mechanics of the taste cells, nor does it disrupt the neurons associated with the taste cells. What is disrupted during a cold is the ability to smell and, therefore, enjoy the flavor of foods and beverages. Thus, a head cold alters the ability to experience fully all the sensory aspects of the foods or beverages that create a complete food sensation.

Palatability describes the association of taste with texture, temperature, and feeling. If a slice of bread is expected to be warm, soft, and sweet but what is ingested is cold, hard, and salty, then palatability is greatly diminished. If a person is truly hungry, however, then the lack of palatability, or even flavor, may be overruled by the greater need for nourishment. In the absence of the ability to see or to smell food (as in blindness or anosmia, respectively), texture and temperature take on heightened importance in the consumption of foods and beverages.

Taste disorders can be quantitatively assessed through various stimuli tests to measure the extent and type of taste disorder present. In addition, magnetic resonance imaging (MRI) and computed tomography (CT) scanning can be used to identify problems that may originate in the central nervous system. Positron emission tomography (PET) scanning can also be used to determine if brain lesions are responsible for a taste disorder. Treatments are as highly varied as the pathologies that cause taste disorders. Those disorders that arise from tumors may be treated by the surgical removal of the tumor. For certain metabolic imbalances, supplements rich in zinc ions may be administered. Some cases require simply restoring the patient to a healthy and balanced diet, while some rare disorders are untreatable.

PERSPECTIVE AND PROSPECTS

Tasting is an inborn sense; it requires no training or skills. "Acquired" tastes are attained by adults mainly as a result of the declining population of taste cells, a natural aspect of the aging process. Because adults cannot sense food as fully as children, they may seek out heightened taste sensations, consuming salty foods such as caviar, drinking strong beverages such as whiskey, or enjoying spicy foods such as curry or hot peppers. Given their divergent taste responsiveness, it is reasonable to expect children to have natural aversions to certain foods, as compared to adults. A child is simply more aware of the mixed flavors of a given food, some of which may be bitter or sour relative to the way in which an adult senses the same food.

Like their primitive ancestors, modern humans let the tip of the tongue sample a new food before actually ingesting it. It is believed, therefore, that sweet receptors evolved to occupy the tip of the tongue to help humans seek out and consume safe foods in nature. Sweet foods, such as carbohydrate-rich vegetables, fruits, and (to some extent) proteins, are generally safe and nourishing. Therefore, humans tend to seek sweet flavors, especially in the infant stages, over salty, sour, or bitter ones. This instinctual drive may account for the powerful attraction many people have for sweet desserts and candies.

Bitterness is detected in the mouth nearer the esophagus. This location seems to prevent humans from naturally seeking bitter foods. Furthermore, it allows for the rejection of a bitter food before it enters the esophagus, where the food would be well on its way to digestion and absorption. This adaptation to the environment aids in human survival. Many naturally bitter substances are poisons or potential toxins. Included in the list of bitter taste sources are caffeine-containing tea leaves and coffee beans, cocaine, nicotine, almond bitters, and lye (sodium hydroxide).

Taste is a special sense that facilitates the ability of an organism to survive in or interact with an environ-

ment. More than this, however, taste provides the body with great sensory pleasure. Serving as both a tool to survive and as a pleasure-seeking sensor, taste is a unique and enriching sense.

—*Mary C. Fields, M.D.*

See also Aging; Digestion; Food biochemistry; Food poisoning; Malnutrition; Nervous system; Nutrition; Otorhinolaryngology; Poisoning; Sense organs; Smell; Toxicology.

FOR FURTHER INFORMATION:

Atkins, Peter. *Molecules*. New York: Scientific American Libraries, 1987. A truly entertaining book supported by pleasing photographs and sketches of some of nature's most intriguing molecules. Includes a chapter entitled "Taste, Smell, and Pain."

Hole, John W., Jr. *Essentials of Human Anatomy and Physiology*. 6th ed. Dubuque, Iowa: Wm. C. Brown, 1993. An academic textbook that goes into greater detail about the human body than an introductory biology book. Chapter 12, "The Somatic and Special Senses," has a section devoted exclusively to the sense of taste.

Schmidt, Robert F., ed. *Fundamentals of Sensory Physiology*. Translated by Marguerite A. Biedermann-Thorson. Rev. 3d ed. Berlin: Springer-Verlag, 1986. A succinct treatment of the anatomy and physiology of taste is provided in chapter 8, "Physiology of Taste."

Tortora, Gerard J., and Sandra R. Grabowski. *Principles of Anatomy and Physiology*. 9th ed. New York: John Wiley & Sons, 2000. This text offers a brief treatment of the structure of taste cells and the stimulation of receptors.

Wolfe, Jeremy M., ed. *Senses Other than Vision*. Vol. 2 in *Sensory Systems*. Boston: Birkhauser, 1988. Composed of readings selected from the *Encyclopedia of Neuroscience*. Four essays address the sense of taste: "Taste," "Taste: Psychophysics," "Taste and Smell Disorders," and "Taste Bud." Each essay is brief (no longer than two pages) but effective in presenting the topic described. An excellent resource for specific information and details.

TATTOO REMOVAL

PROCEDURE

ANATOMY OR SYSTEM AFFECTED: Skin
SPECIALTIES AND RELATED FIELDS: Dermatology, general surgery

DEFINITION: The use of lasers to break up tattoo ink under the skin.

INDICATIONS AND PROCEDURES

Application of a tattoo is relatively easy, although the process is painful. A design is drawn on the skin. Needles are used to push the ink down into the skin. When the skin heals from the multiple punctures, the design remains permanently in place. Attempts have been made to remove tattoos since the first one was applied. Scrubbing with sandpaper or table salt has been tried to scour the surface of the skin and remove the tattoo. The results have usually been disfigurement or scarring.

A ruby laser can be used to remove most tattoos. The laser emits a brief pulse of intense red light. The tattoo ink that has been previously imbedded absorbs the pulse of energy. The laser energy causes the tattoo ink to break up into fragments that can be removed by cells of the immune system.

The treatment feels like a rubber band snapping against the skin. Local anesthetics may be used when attempting to remove large tattoos. Each pulse of energy from a laser covers an area about the size of a pencil eraser. Immediately after the laser treatment, the treated area turns white and may swell slightly. The whiteness usually fades within an hour. Over the next few days, blisters may form. They are usually followed by a scab or crust that eventually drops off. Within seven to ten days, the skin looks normal once again.

USES AND COMPLICATIONS

The number of treatments required to remove a tattoo depends on several factors: the color of ink, the amount of ink, the depth of the tattoo, and the location of the tattoo.

Dark colors of ink such as black, green, and blue are the easiest to remove because they absorb laser energy. Red and yellow inks are more difficult to remove; they often require more treatments. Professional tattoos may require five or more treatments. These laser sessions are spaced one to two months apart to allow the body's immune system to remove the maximum amount of ink between treatments. Amateur tattoos typically require a total of two to four treatments. Tattoos applied by amateurs often contain less ink than those applied at professional tattoo parlors. The smaller amount of ink means that fewer exposures are normally needed to remove the tattoo.

Tattoos that penetrate to deeper layers of the skin require more energy to break up the ink into fragments. Some locations on the body are difficult or dangerous to approach with lasers, such as the genitals and parts of the face.

Side effects may occur with laser treatments. Individuals with darker complexions may experience a temporary lightening of the skin in the area treated by the laser. Over the course of several months, the normal color returns.

In the United States, the Food and Drug Administration (FDA) has approved the use of ruby laser treatment for removing tattoos. Infrared lasers are also used to remove tattoos without destroying pigmentation in the skin. They are totally ineffective, however, for green tattoo ink.

—*L. Fleming Fallon, Jr., M.D., Ph.D., M.P.H.*

See also Dermatology; Laser use in surgery; Pigmentation; Skin; Skin disorders; Tattoos and body piercing.

FOR FURTHER INFORMATION:

Camphausen, Rufus C. *Return of the Tribal: A Celebration of Body Adornment: Piercing, Tattooing, Scarification, Body Painting.* Rochester, Vt.: Park Street Press, 1997.

Graves, Bonnie B. *Tattooing and Body Piercing.* Mankato, Minn.: LifeMatters, 2000.

Hewitt, Kim. *Mutilating the Body: Identity in Blood and Ink.* Bowling Green, Ohio: Bowling Green State University Popular Press, 1997.

Vale, V., and Andrea Juno, eds. *Modern Primitives: An Investigation of Contemporary Adornment and Ritual.* San Francisco: Re/Search, 1989.

Wilkinson, Beth. *Coping with the Dangers of Tattooing, Body Piercing, and Branding.* New York: Rosen, 1998.

TATTOOS AND BODY PIERCING

PROCEDURE

ANATOMY OR SYSTEM AFFECTED: Muscles, skin

SPECIALTIES AND RELATED FIELDS: Dermatology, plastic surgery, public health

DEFINITION: Piercing of the skin to implant devices or make designs.

KEY TERMS:

dermis: the deepest skin layer

epidermis: the outer skin layer

mortification: self-induced physical pain

proof of ordeal: a painful surgical procedure that leaves a scar, design, or skin mutilation

tattooing: piercing of the skin with pigments or dyes

INDICATIONS AND PROCEDURES

Tattooing is accomplished by a variety of techniques, usually by persons who are specialists. Traditionally, a shaman or other religious practitioner would create a tattoo by piercing the skin with a sharpened object (such as a bone splinter or a piece of metal) or with a bundle of porcupine quills or ponderosa pine needles, or by passing a colored string on a needle through the skin. The colors were from mineral salts, charcoal, certain plant juices, and even the feces of dogs that had been fed charcoal.

Coloring inks were available from the end of the nineteenth century and are now supplied in liquid forms. They can be applied in either the so-called European fashion, in which the coloring ink is applied over a small surface and an electric vibrating needle impregnates the epidermis and the dermis, or the American procedure, in which the needle contains the desired pigment.

The skin is prepared in a variety of ways, usually by smearing a thin layer of petroleum jelly over the site to minimize the seepage of blood and tissue fluids that would otherwise obscure the artist's view. When the tattoo is completed, the area is washed and then covered with an antiseptic ointment. Tattoos assume various geometric or curvilinear designs and can be executed over all of a person's body or simply within a restricted area. Extensive tattooing may take several years to complete.

The most obvious forms of body piercing, by both males and females, are performed in the ears, nose, nasal septum, tongue, navel, lips, scalp, eyelids, or cheeks. In some cultures, the lips or ears may be grossly distorted by inserting over time increasingly larger objects, such as pieces of horn, bone, wood, and even metal. In some cases, the particular style of body piercing may indicate a person's marital status, group membership, or religious affiliation, or it may simply be cosmetic mutilation. Body piercing may also be performed on male or female genitals. The breasts, particularly the nipples, are a common site for the insertion of either closed or threaded rings. The infamous Prince Albert penal ring has acquired considerable fashion in Western cultures, being inserted in the top or either side of the glans.

USES AND COMPLICATIONS

Tattoos and body piercing of the human body have been practiced by all cultures throughout the world to serve different functions: for religious purposes, as an indication of certain status changes or the accomplishment of culturally significant tasks, as a proof of ordeal, for medical reasons, as body art, as identification marks, to signify membership in either sacred or profane organizations, or to attain visions through mortification of the flesh. Depending on the culture or specific group, men, women, and children may undergo these frequently painful rituals. Various cultures believe that the soul's transition to a life hereafter is facilitated by having certain tattoos and body piercing. Often, the degree of pain experienced during the rituals of tattooing and body piercing, and from the subsequent wounds, not only are a proof of ordeal but also may serve as a physical and spiritual atonement for a person's moral transgressions. Certain groups, such as the Newar of Bhaktapur in Nepal, believe that they may gain a higher incarnation when they sell their tattoos in heaven.

In the United States during the early twentieth century, it became popular for women to be tattooed for eyeliner, cheek blush, and even colored lips. Although tattooing and body piercing were once associated with motorcycle gang members, prisoners, and military personnel, these surgical procedures have become more popular with the general public. Tattooing and self-mutilation by body piercing are gaining popularity as forms of personal expression, particularly with women, who make up approximately 70 percent of the new business.

A concern, however, is the increasing frequency of adolescents engaging in tattooing and body piercing. Today, body piercing in Western cultures is often viewed by teenagers and young adults as a rite of passage, sometimes symbolically in defiance of the established social order. When self-practiced, tattooing and body piercing can lead to infection and even septicemia, particularly when people use instruments and inks that are not sterile. In addition, there has been an increase in the incidence of blood-borne infections such as human immunodeficiency virus (HIV) and hepatitis B and C being transmitted through contaminated needles.

PERSPECTIVE AND PROSPECTS

Some anthropologists believe that the first documented examples of tattooing were practiced in Egypt approximately four thousand years ago. These conclusions are supported by tattooed female mummies and by clay figurines that have puncture "tattoos." Although there is not agreement among scholars, some believe that the practice of tattooing may have diffused from Egypt to other parts of the world.

Perhaps the most artistic and dramatic full-body tattooing was done by the Japanese as early as the fifth century B.C.E. and the Maori of New Zealand; even today, many young male Maori follow this traditional custom. The Maori were noted for facial tattoos, called *moko*, that served to frighten and intimidate their enemies. The word "tattoo," however, comes from the Tahitian word *ta-tau*; it was acquired by eighteenth and nineteenth century European explorers in Polynesia, who introduced tattoos to Europe and America.

A dramatic historical example of body piercing for religious purposes was part of the Sun Dance ritual of many Plains Indian tribes, in which male participants had hard wooden shafts surgically inserted in the pectoral or back muscles. Long thongs were attached to these poles. The participant would then drag heavy bison skulls or would pull away from a pole, causing tearing in the muscles.

—*John Alan Ross, Ph.D.*

See also Acquired immunodeficiency syndrome (AIDS); Dermatology; Dermatology, pediatric; Hepatitis; Plastic surgery; Puberty and adolescence; Skin; Skin disorders; Tattoo removal.

FOR FURTHER INFORMATION:

Brown, Kelli McCormack, Paula Perlmutter, and Robert J. McDermott. "Youth and Tattoos: What School Health Personnel Should Know." *The Journal of School Health* 70, no. 9 (November, 2000): 355-360. Though tattooing has been practiced by various cultures for centuries, this art form has undergone dramatic changes in the past few decades. Today tattoos appeal to diverse populations and mainstream culture.

DeMello, Margo. *Bodies of Inscription: A Cultural History of the Modern Tattoo*. Durham, N.C.: Duke University Press, 2000. Although academic, this book has much to recommend it for general collections. DeMello's major interest is in describing the new community of tattooed people, both men and women, for whom new meanings are being forged from the meeting of skin and ink.

Gard, Carolyn. "Think Before You Ink: The Risks of Body Piercing and Tattooing." *Current Health* 25, no. 6 (February, 1999): 24-25. Tattoos and body piercing seem to be very popular, but teens should consider the risks associated with these trends. Tattoo dyes can cause allergic reactions.

Shields, Sherice L. "Popular Piercing Opens Possibility of Serious Illness." *USA Today*, July, 19, 2000, p. D9. Experts may worry about the health risks associated with body piercing, but lawmakers have focused on the age of consent. The National Conference of State Legislatures says few states enforce health regulations, but twenty-three states have laws regarding piercing minors.

"Support for Body Piercing Checks." *Nursing Standard* 14, no. 30 (April 12-18, 2000): 8. Body piercing outlets should be strictly regulated because piercing can cause blood poisoning, hepatitis, and even death, according to a congress of professional nurses.

TAY-SACHS DISEASE

DISEASE/DISORDER

ANATOMY OR SYSTEM AFFECTED: Nervous system

SPECIALTIES AND RELATED FIELDS: Genetics, neonatology, neurology, pediatrics

DEFINITION: An inherited disorder in which products of fat metabolism (gangliosides) accumulate in and destroy the brain and spinal cord.

CAUSES AND SYMPTOMS

Tay-Sachs disease is a genetic disorder of lipid (fat) metabolism resulting from a missing enzyme. This enzyme normally breaks down special nerve lipids known as gangliosides, which are present in the brain and spinal cord. These substances accumulate and destroy the cells, killing the child by age three or four years.

Several features at birth may raise the possibility of early detection, particularly cherry-red spots on the retina of the eye. Most newborns with Tay-Sachs disease, however, appear normal at birth. Between the ages of three months and six months, the progressive neurologic damage becomes apparent: deafness, blindness, muscle paralysis, and mental retardation develop. By eighteen months, the infant is usually already in a vegetative state, requiring complete care. The child may survive until three or four years of age, dying from complications associated with comatose and bedridden patients, usually infections.

TREATMENT AND THERAPY

Tay-Sachs disease has no cure, and only supportive measures can be used. Feeding tubes for nutrition and fluids, suctioning of throat secretions, meticulous skin care for bed sores, and oxygen to assist breathing are among the types of support needed. Full-time skilled nursing care at home or at a facility is often necessary.

PERSPECTIVES AND PROSPECTS

While Tay-Sachs disease is the most common lipid storage disease, it is rare in the general population. It is nearly one hundred times more common, however, in people of Eastern European Jewish ancestry, occurring in one per 3,600 births. One person in thirty Eastern European Jews is a carrier of the genetic defect. If two such carriers have children, they have a 25 percent chance of having a child with Tay-Sachs disease. Prenatal testing using amniocentesis or chorionic villus sampling can detect affected fetuses. More important is genetic counseling and screening of couples with a family history. A blood test can identify carriers.

Ongoing research is attempting to correct the disease in the developing fetus through the insertion of the missing gene.

—*Connie Rizzo, M.D.*

See also Amniocentesis; Chorionic villus sampling; Coma; Embryology; Enzymes; Gene therapy; Genetic counseling; Genetic diseases; Genetics and inheritance; Lipids; Metabolism; Neonatology; Pediatrics; Screening.

FOR FURTHER INFORMATION:

Gormley, Myra Vanderpool. *Family Diseases: Are You at Risk?* Reprint. Baltimore: Genealogical Publishing, 1998.

Harper, Peter S. *Practical Genetic Counselling.* 5th ed. London: Wright, 1998.

Millunsky, Aubrey. *Genetic Disorders of the Fetus: Diagnosis, Prevention, and Treatment.* Baltimore: The Johns Hopkins University Press, 1998.

TEETH

ANATOMY

ANATOMY OR SYSTEM AFFECTED: Bones, gastrointestinal system, gums, musculoskeletal system, nervous system

SPECIALTIES AND RELATED FIELDS: Dentistry, orthodontics

DEFINITION: Structures that aid animals in processing food prior to swallowing, bringing food into the mouth and grinding; they may also be used for defense, the killing of prey, and displays of either hostility or pleasure.

KEY TERMS:

cementum: the outer covering of the root of a tooth

crown: the portion of the tooth, normally covered with enamel, that is exposed in the oral cavity above the gingiva (gums)

cusp: the conical projection of the chewing surface of the tooth

cuspid: the longest anterior tooth; also called the canine tooth or the eyetooth

dentin: the substance that composes the major portion of the tooth internally

enamel: the tissue that covers the crown of the tooth; the hardest tissue in the body

gingiva: the gum tissue surrounding the neck of the tooth

incisor: one of the front teeth, used primarily to cut or shear food with a scissoring motion

molars: the back teeth used to grind food into smaller portions prior to swallowing

periodontium: those tissues supporting the tooth in the jaws, including the gingiva, the jawbone, and the periodontal ligament that attaches the root of the tooth into the jaw

premolars: the teeth between the cuspids and the molars, used in crushing and grinding food; also called bicuspids

pulp: the internal, living tissue of the tooth, consisting of nerves, blood vessels, and dental cells

root: the portion of the tooth that is below the crown and is embedded in a bony socket of the jaw

STRUCTURE AND FUNCTIONS

Teeth are functional portions of the mouths of animals that assist them in processing food prior to swallowing. They are also primary offensive and defensive weapons for most animals. Many animals have no hands to grasp or capture food, and their teeth become the principal means of grabbing and killing prey. In humans, teeth not only process food but also have a sociological significance in displaying anger, friendliness, and desirability.

A tooth is composed of three basic parts: the crown, the dental pulp, and the root. The crown of the tooth is that portion exposed above the gingiva, commonly called the gums. The outer surface of the crown is covered by a hard, crystalline substance called enamel. Enamel is an almost completely inorganic material, calcium hydroxyapatite, and it is the hardest tissue in the human body. Underneath the enamel, the bulk of the crown is made up of a substance known as dentin. It, too, is quite hard, but it has more organic material, ground substance and nerve fibers, within it. The dentin is honeycombed by small tubules radiating from the dental pulp chamber at the center of the tooth. These tubules carry nerve fibers from the central nerve within the pulp to the junction of the enamel and dentin.

In the center of the crown is the pulp chamber. The pulp contains nerves and blood vessels that give sensations to and nourish the tooth. These nerves and blood vessels enter at the tip of the root, the apex, and arise from nerve trunks and blood vessels that run through the jawbone.

The root is the portion of the tooth joining the crown to the jawbone. The outer surface of the root is covered by a thin layer of bonelike substance called cementum, and it runs from the junction of the enamel of the crown to the apex of the root. Under the cementum, dentin composes the bulk of the root, continuing from the crown to the apex. The root is attached from the cementum to the bony socket in the jaw by the periodontal ligament. This ligament is composed of elastic connective tissue fibers that act not only as part of the attachment apparatus for the tooth but also as a shock absorber from chewing forces. The pulp chamber narrows into a thin, constricted channel from the pulp chamber to the apex; this is known as the root canal. The tooth is surrounded by the tissues of the attachment apparatus called the periodontium, consisting of the gingiva, the periodontal ligament, and the alveolar bone of the jaws.

In humans, there are normally thirty-two adult teeth and twenty deciduous (or baby) teeth. Deciduous teeth start calcifying in the embryo at about five to six weeks of development. Teeth start to form from two types of cells at an interface in the tooth bud, which becomes the dentoenamel junction. The enamel is formed by a cell called an ameloblast, and the dentin is formed by a cell known as an odontoblast. The enamel grows outward and the dentin inward from the interface. The pulp is formed from nerves and blood vessels in the developing jawbone. While the crown is growing, the root starts to form, lengthening as the tooth develops. After the crown is formed,

the ameloblast cells rest on the outer surface of the enamel, while the odontoblasts line the internal cavity of the pulp chamber.

When the tooth erupts through the gum tissue, the ameloblasts are compressed and destroyed. Enamel is one of the two tissues in the human body that cannot repair itself (the other being the cornea of the eye). The odontoblasts can be activated inside the pulp chamber to form a secondary or reparative dentin. This formation of insulating dentin is in response to aging, advancing tooth decay, or trauma to the tooth or in reaction to the placement of restorative materials into a tooth.

The deciduous teeth begin to erupt through the gums in infancy and continue to do so until the full complement of primary dentition has erupted. Most of the adult teeth develop below the baby teeth, and as they push on the roots of the primary teeth, these roots are resorbed from the pressure of erupting permanent crowns. The primary teeth are shed throughout childhood and into adolescence. Other animals have both primary and permanent teeth. Sharks continually develop full sets of teeth, sometimes as many as seven or eight at a time; as their teeth loosen or break off, new teeth replace them. Humans, however, possess only one set of permanent teeth, and they are not naturally

The Structure of a Tooth

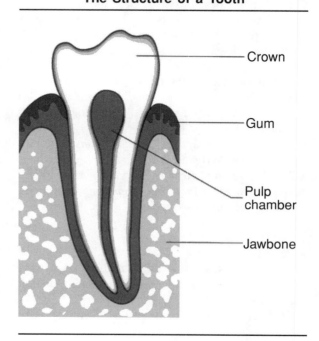

Crown

Gum

Pulp chamber

Jawbone

replaced if they are lost through trauma or disease.

The shape and size of teeth are closely related to their functions. The four front incisor teeth, both upper and lower, are used to shear and cut food. The movement of the mobile lower jaw, the mandible, against the static upper jaw, the maxilla, causes these teeth to work as scissors on food. Horses crop grasses with their large incisors. Cusps are conical projections of the cuspids and posterior teeth. They act as crushing and grinding segments of the posterior teeth, reducing the food into smaller portions that may be swallowed and digested efficiently. The four cuspids, or canines, are conical and pointed. Their primary function is to grasp and tear food. The fangs of a tiger are cuspids, as are those of lions. The eight premolars have two conical cusps that are also used for tearing, but working against the opposing teeth, they also function as a mill, crushing and grinding the food.

The twelve molars are multicusped teeth that grind food into smaller portions; mixed with saliva, the food is then readied for swallowing. The grooves of the occlusal (chewing) surfaces act as sluiceways to channel the food in the oral cavity. The tongue folds the food back onto the surfaces of the grinding teeth until it is chewed sufficiently.

The third molars are commonly called wisdom teeth. These teeth are the last to develop and are more prone to irregular calcification and morphology. In the course of human evolution, the jaws have shortened, and the third molars often do not have enough room in the jaw to erupt in a normal, perpendicular mode. The result is an irregular angle of eruption. When the third molars lock and push against the second molars and are unable to erupt normally, the condition is called impaction. Thus, in many cases, the wisdom teeth must be removed.

Teeth and their supporting tissues are susceptible to disease. The primary disease of the tooth is dental caries, or tooth decay. Caries begins with the decalcification of the enamel crystals by acids. These acids are products of bacteria caught in a sticky film that forms on the teeth called plaque. These bacteria use refined hydrocarbons, principally sugars, for their food. If the plaque is not removed from the surface of the teeth, the acids are kept close to the enamel. Over a period of time, the decalcification of the enamel reaches the internal dentin, and the acid begins to decay the less calcified enamel at a more rapid rate. The acids also can touch the nerve fibers within the dental tubules, causing sensitivity and pain. If this process is not stopped, the decay can penetrate into the pulp and cause infection.

When the pulp becomes infected, it invariably dies. The dead tissues gradually seep through the apex, and bacteria feed on the necrotic material. Inflammatory cells from the blood vessels in the bone try to fight the infection, which can cause swelling, pain, and pus. The result is a periapical abscess.

The periodontium is also susceptible to disease, and again, the bacterial plaque is the chief cause. Surrounding the neck of the tooth is a cuff of gum tissue. The bacteria in the plaque release their waste products into the cuff and irritate the lining. Inflammatory white cells, known as lymphocytes or chronic inflammatory cells, are brought from the blood vessels in the gum tissue to the point of irritation in order to attack the bacteria and their by-products. This disease is called gingivitis, which can be reversed by removing the dental plaque.

If the plaque is allowed to remain on the surface of the tooth, it may calcify into a hard, rough, and porous substance called dental calculus or, more commonly, tartar. This material attracts and entraps more bacteria, and it is abrasive to the soft lining of the gingiva. The gums become further inflamed, bringing more lymphocytes into the area. These cells try to attack the bacteria and dissolve the dead and dying cells of the diseased gingiva.

Over a period of time, the inflammatory cells move deeper into the periodontium, dissolving and detaching the elastic fibers of the periodontal ligament and eroding the crest of the bony socket. This inflammation of the periodontium is called periodontitis. With the destruction of the fibers attaching the gingiva and bone to the root, the cuff of gum tissue deepens into a pocket around the neck of the tooth. The depth of the pocket facilitates the further entrapment of bacteria and makes it more difficult to clean.

If the condition is not corrected, eventually there is enough destruction of the periodontium that the tooth becomes loose. Often, the chronic inflammatory cells at the bottom of a deep pocket are joined by acute inflammatory cells, producing painful swelling and pus. This condition is known as a periodontal abscess. Most extractions of adult teeth are the result of periodontitis.

DISORDERS AND DISEASES

The principal scientific professions requiring knowledge of teeth and their surrounding structures are those of dentistry and dental hygiene. Dentists need to have thorough knowledge of the anatomy and physiology of the teeth and their surrounding structures in the mouth. They must be able to detect and treat diseases of the mouth and all its tissues. Dental caries, infected pulp, diseases of the periodontium, and tooth loss are treated by dentists. Dental hygienists aid dentists by treating and identifying diseases of the mouth. Their principal duty is to remove harmful deposits on the teeth, but hygienists also identify diseases of the teeth and periodontium. Using their anatomical and physiological knowledge of the teeth and surrounding structures, hygienists teach patients preventative techniques that can help prevent or halt the spread of dental disease.

Since the teeth and oral tissues are only a part of the body, knowledge of general human anatomy, physiology, and pathology is a must for dentists. Oral symptomatology discovered by dentists is often the first sign of a serious systemic disease. For example, a certain fruity odor on the breath is a sign of ketosis, which is a symptom of diabetes. Kaposi's sarcoma, a rare type of skin cancer, is often manifested as lesions of the oral tissues; the presence of such lesions may be a strong indication that the patient has acquired immunodeficiency syndrome (AIDS).

The successful treatment of diseases of the teeth and periodontium must be based on a thorough understanding of the anatomy and physiology of these tissues. In order to restore a decayed tooth, the dentist must know how deep to cut into the tooth, the probable location of the pulp, the irritating factors of the restorative material, the possible traumatic chewing forces on the new restoration, and the compatibility between the restoration and the tissues of the periodontium.

The treatment of tooth loss is literally as old as the pharaohs. An X ray of the skull of an Egyptian mummy displayed an attempt to construct a dental bridge using gold wire to secure a tooth between two natural teeth. At present, there are several ways to restore lost teeth. Cemented fixed bridges constructed of metal and porcelain are often the treatment of choice when there are sound teeth to support them. In the case of a partial or total loss of the teeth, removable dentures constructed of plastic or porcelain teeth fixed in an acrylic plastic base are used.

Introduction of newer materials and techniques for the restoration of teeth is a constant challenge for the dental scientist. While the theory of implanting resto-

rations into the jaw to replace teeth is not new, some of the materials are. The recent use of titanium implants into the jaw reinforces the dentist's need to know the anatomy and physiology of the surrounding tissues. It is known that the bone of the jaw attaches to the surface of titanium, a process called osseointegration. Great care must be used, however, in placing correct chewing forces on the supporting bone, and nonirritating restorations must be placed near the periodontal tissues for the implants to be successful.

Special acrylic plastics called composites are sometimes used in restoring lost tooth structure by chemically bonding to the enamel and dentin. Thin films of these materials are placed in the grooves of the newly erupted posterior teeth. This treatment has been shown to prevent decay in the chewing surfaces of the teeth. Laser technology is being explored by scientists to see if the enamel surface might be fused to withstand decay.

While the bone lost as a result of periodontal disease cannot be regenerated, new techniques of grafting the patient's own bone, freeze-dried sterile bone, and other materials show some promise in strengthening the weakened tooth.

PERSPECTIVE AND PROSPECTS

Recorded history and archaeological findings show that humans have tried to treat the teeth and their related diseases probably since the Stone Age. There has been speculation among archaeologists that the practice of trepanning, the surgical opening of the skull, could have been in response to severe toothaches as well as other pain in the head. Mutilation of the teeth by the Incas and Mayans was common in noble families; skulls have been discovered in burial sites of both nations showing the insertion of jade disks in slots filed into the front teeth.

In ancient Greece, Hippocrates wrote of treating a severe tumor of the jaw of a young man. After lancing the lesion, he wrote that the condition was morbid and that the young man would surely die. The Greeks also supposed that tooth decay was caused by small worms that bored into the tooth and ate it from within.

In medieval Japan, dentists were trained to extract teeth with their thumb and forefingers. They practiced on tapered wooden pegs pounded into a board. A soft wood was used at first for easier removal, then successively harder boards and pegs were introduced until the dentist could then remove a tooth from the jaw.

Most of the dentistry in the past was surgical removal of painful teeth. From the Middle Ages to the mid-1800's, barbers performed extractions. Without the benefit of anesthetic, this practice was quite painful. Horace Welles found in 1894 that a patient could be put to sleep with ethyl ether, allowing painless tooth extraction. With the introduction of local anesthetics in the 1920's and later of intravenous drugs, pain during the extraction of a tooth has been virtually eliminated.

In modern practice, the study of the teeth has found new applications. For example, dental forensics contributes to the identification of abusers and criminals who bite their victims. The dental arch and the relationship of the teeth within it are unique, and bite marks are like fingerprints: No two are alike. The forensic scientist can take impressions of the bite marks on the victim's body with an accurate impression material. Plaster casts are formed in the impressions and compared to a cast of the suspect's dental arch. The evidence may either confirm or rule out the suspect's participation in the crime. In addition, dental forensics is used to identify the remains of people who are burned beyond recognition or whose bodies are badly decomposed. The teeth and their dental restorations are often the only way that a deceased person may be identified, especially in a major disaster such as an airplane crash.

The restoration and replacement of diseased teeth is an ongoing challenge, but with the new materials and technology available, humans should have healthier teeth in the future.

—*William D. Stark, D.D.S.*

See also Cavities; Crowns and bridges; Dental diseases; Dentistry; Dentistry, pediatric; Dentures; Endodontic disease; Fluoride treatments; Forensic pathology; Fracture repair; Gastrointestinal system; Gingivitis; Jaw wiring; Nutrition; Orthodontics; Periodontal surgery; Periodontitis; Root canal treatment; Teething; Tooth extraction; Toothache; Veterinary medicine; Wisdom teeth.

FOR FURTHER INFORMATION:

Cook, Allan R., ed. *Oral Health Sourcebook: Basic Information About Diseases and Conditions Affecting Oral Health and Including Cavities, Gum Disease, Dry Mouth, Oral Cancers, Fever Blisters, Canker Sores, Oral Thrush, Bad Breath, Temporomandibular Disorders, and Other Craniofacial Syndromes.* Detroit: Omnigraphics, 1998. This handy reference source, which covers all aspects of dental health, includes helpful statistics on dental disease.

Ferracane, Jack L. "Using Posterior Composites Appropriately." *Journal of the American Dental Association* 123 (July, 1992): 53-58. A discussion of the mechanical properties of acrylic composites, including resistance to wear and the use of bonded seals with this restorative material.

Gray, Henry. *Gray's Anatomy.* Edited by Peter L. Williams et al. 38th ed. New York: Churchill Livingstone, 1999. The definitive book on human anatomy. With 780 illustrations in the text, the interrelationship of nerves, blood vessels, bones, and other anatomical structures of the human body is displayed in a practical manner as a fascinating biological machine.

Moss, Stephen J. *Your Child's Teeth: A Parent's Guide to Making and Keeping Them Perfect.* Boston: Houghton Mifflin, 1977. This book emphasizes the need for home care to prevent dental disease in children and adolescents. Tooth brushing, diet, and visits to the pedodontist and the orthodontist (the latter if necessary) are stressed in clear language.

Vale, Gerald I., J. Lawrence Cogan, and Judy Myers Suchey. "Dentistry in Investigation of the Los Angeles Airport Disaster." *Journal of the California Dental Association* 19, no. 8 (1991): 20. A discussion of the forensic techniques and procedures used in identifying the remains of the passengers and crews involved in the crash of an airliner into a commuter aircraft at Los Angeles International Airport.

Zablotsky, Mark H. "The Periodontal Approach to Implant Dentistry." *Journal of the California Dental Association* 19, no. 12 (1991): 39. An excellent article outlining the important relationships between dental implants and the restorations attached to them and the periodontal tissues.

TEETHING

BIOLOGY

ALSO KNOWN AS: Deciduous dentition, tooth eruption

ANATOMY OR SYSTEM AFFECTED: Mouth, gums, teeth

SPECIALTIES AND RELATED FIELDS: Dentistry, orthodontics, pediatrics

DEFINITION: The eruption of the primary, or deciduous, teeth in infancy.

KEY TERMS:

central incisors: the two center top and two center bottom teeth

cuspids: the teeth on either side of the lateral incisors; also known as the canines or eyeteeth

deciduous teeth: a child's first set of teeth, which will be replaced by the child's permanent teeth; also known as the primary or baby teeth

lateral incisors: the teeth on either side of the central incisors

molars: the grinding teeth located at the back of the mouth

STRUCTURE AND FUNCTIONS

A child's teeth begin to develop about the second month of pregnancy. The first tooth does not usually appear above the gum line, however, until the sixth or seventh month after birth. The tooth is pushed upward through the gum by growth at the base of the tooth. At the same time, the root sheath grows downward toward the jaw. Studies indicate that dental development does not seem to be affected by nutrition, illness, or climate. In addition, there seems to be little difference between girls and boys in their dental development.

Dental development follows a typical pattern. The teeth generally emerge in pairs. Usually, the lower central incisors are the first teeth to erupt, between five and seven months after birth, followed by the upper central incisors at six to eight months. The upper lateral incisors make their appearances between nine and eleven months, followed by the lower lateral incisors at ten to twelve months. The first molars, two upper and two lower, usually emerge between twelve and sixteen months. The cuspids follow next, at about sixteen to twenty months. The final deciduous teeth to emerge are the second molars, at twenty to thirty months. Most children will have twenty teeth, ten on the top and ten on the bottom, by their third birthday. By the time that they are six, most children begin to lose their primary teeth as the permanent teeth emerge.

While this is the typical pattern, there is much individual variation in both the time frame and the order of tooth eruption. Some children do not get the first tooth until their first birthday. On the other hand, children are sometimes born with teeth or have their first teeth erupt in the first month after birth. Those teeth present at birth are called natal teeth, and those that emerge soon after birth are called neonatal. Natal and neonatal teeth have been associated with other oral abnormalities, including cleft palate and cleft lip, although many children with these teeth have no abnormalities. Natal and neonatal teeth can present problems for babies, who may cut their tongues on the teeth, and for nursing mothers, who may experience lacerated nipples.

Although not permanent, a child's primary teeth are important. The primary teeth are necessary for the child to chew solid food. In addition, they are important as space holders and guides for the permanent teeth.

DISORDERS AND DISEASES

Some children have a more difficult time teething than do others. Common symptoms of teething in an infant include wakefulness, excessive drooling, fussiness, refusal to nurse, and finger chewing. An infant's gums may also be swollen and tender. These symptoms have also been observed in animals as their teeth erupt.

Some debate exists over other commonly held beliefs concerning symptoms associated with teething. Historically, fever, diarrhea, and ear pulling have been attributed to teething; however, there is no scientific evidence to suggest that teething causes any of these symptoms. In a 1992 article, "Teething," in the *Journal of Pediatric Health Care*, Patricia T. Castiglia suggests that parents often attribute behaviors such as wakefulness to teething because it alleviates parental worry. She further argues that wakefulness at six to nine months is caused by separation anxiety, not teething.

Those researchers who have attempted to associate teething with disease have found it difficult to do so. The teething period is also the period when babies are no longer fully protected by the mother's antibodies but have not yet built up antibodies of their own, thus rendering them susceptible to disease. Consequently, while diseases may coincide with the teething period, it is difficult to associate teething with disease.

Nevertheless, most pediatricians agree that babies experience some discomfort from teething. Many believe that allowing the child to chew on a cold rubber teething ring or damp washcloth will relieve the pain. While some experts suggest offering frozen teething rings and/or frozen bagels or bread, others argue that neither should be given. They contend that the frozen teething ring can damage the baby's gums, while bits of the frozen bagel can break off, potentially choking the baby. Likewise, there is little agreement about whether acetaminophen should be used.

Most experts discourage using breast-feeding or a bottle to help a teething baby fall asleep. The milk pools around the new teeth, potentially causing decay. Indeed, many pediatricians suggest that a baby's gums and new teeth should be wiped with a clean, damp gauze pad several times a day to remove traces of milk or juice from the mouth.

PERSPECTIVE AND PROSPECTS

Teething has been a concern for doctors and parents for many years. Theorists as early as Hippocrates attributed fever, convulsions, and diarrhea to teething. During the eighteenth and nineteenth centuries, many writers considered teething to be the leading cause of death among infants.

During the last quarter of the twentieth century, however, the use of teething as a diagnosis for diarrhea, fever, and other childhood illnesses diminished among pediatricians, although studies indicated that some pediatricians continued to connect teething with diarrhea during the 1990's.

—*Diane Andrews Henningfeld, Ph.D.*

See also Cleft lip and palate; Cleft lip and palate repair; Dental diseases; Dentistry; Dentistry, pediatric; Neonatology; Pain; Pain management; Pediatrics; Teeth.

FOR FURTHER INFORMATION:

Gorfinkle, Kenneth. *Soothing Your Child's Pain: From Teething and Tummy Aches to Acute Illnesses and Injuries, How to Understand the Causes and Ease the Hurt.* Lincolnwood, Ill.: Contemporary Books, 1998. Aimed at the parents of young patients, this guide includes bibliographical references and an index.

Kump, Theresa. "The Facts About Baby Teeth: From Teething Pain to First Cleanings, Here's What You Do." *Parents* 70, no. 6 (June, 1995): 65-66. Facts surrounding the teething process in babies ages six to twelve months are discussed. Parents can alleviate the pain of teething by offering them teething rings or giving them pain relievers.

Rogoznica, June. "Teething Time." *Parents* 74, no. 3 (March, 1999): 139-140. Babies between the age of one month and one year often become suddenly fussy, finicky, and even slightly feverish because it is teething time.

Shelov, Steven P., et al., eds. *Caring for Your Baby and Young Child: Birth to Age Five.* Rev. ed. New York: Bantam Books, 1998. Offers a comprehensive discussion of the developmental stages of young children.

TEMPOROMANDIBULAR JOINT (TMJ) SYNDROME

DISEASE/DISORDER

ANATOMY OR SYSTEM AFFECTED: Bones, head, joints, mouth, muscles, teeth

SPECIALTIES AND RELATED FIELDS: Dentistry, family practice, psychology

DEFINITION: A disorder that produces pain and stiffness in the joint between the lower jawbone (mandible) and the temporal bone of the skull.

CAUSES AND SYMPTOMS

The exact cause of temporomandibular joint (TMJ) syndrome, or myofacial pain-dysfunction syndrome, is not known. Possible causes include arthritis, bad bite (malocclusion), grinding or clenching of the teeth (bruxism), muscle tension, and psychological stress. X rays and laboratory tests carried out on people with this disorder usually reveal no abnormalities. Another cause of pain and stiffness in the temporomandibular joints at either side of the jaw is rheumatoid arthritis. With rheumatoid arthritis, however, the symptoms are most severe the first thing in the morning, which is not typically the case with TMJ syndrome.

TMJ syndrome affects the temporomandibular joints, producing mild to severe spasms and pain in the jaw muscles that sometimes make it difficult to open the jaw fully. Other symptoms can include blurred vision, sinus problems, and pain that extends into the head, neck, ears, and even as far as the shoulders.

TREATMENT AND THERAPY

If spasmodic pain exists in the jaw muscles, a physician should be consulted. Some type of treatment will usually be arranged to ease the symptoms. Treatment to provide relief varies according to the underlying cause but typically includes local heat therapy, injections or sprays of local anesthetics, and simple analgesics, such as aspirin, ibuprofen, or acetaminophen. Prescribed jaw exercises are also often helpful. Some cases may require dental procedures, and, in the most severe cases, surgery may be necessary to correct the problem.

PERSPECTIVE AND PROSPECTS

TMJ syndrome is fairly common; most people who have spasmodic pain in the jaw muscles have this condition. It is estimated that nearly 25 percent of the population in the United States suffers from some form of TMJ syndrome, ranging from mild to very severe. The majority of cases, however, go untreated.

—Alvin K. Benson, Ph.D.

See also Arthritis; Dental diseases; Muscle sprains, spasms, and disorders; Muscles; Orthopedic surgery; Orthopedics; Orthopedics, pediatric; Pain management; Rheumatoid arthritis; Stress; Stress reduction.

FOR FURTHER INFORMATION:

Bell, Welden E. *Temporomandibular Disorders: Classification, Diagnosis, Management.* Chicago: Year Book Medical, 1990.

Blom, Eric D., Mark I. Singer, and Ronald C. Hamaker, eds. *Tracheoesophageal Voice Restoration Following Total Laryngectomy.* San Diego, Calif.: Singular, 1998.

Myers, Eugene N., Jonas T. Johnson, and Thomas Murry. *Tracheotomy: Airway Management, Communication, and Swallowing.* San Diego, Calif.: Singular, 1998.

Sarnat, Bernard G., and Daniel M. Laskin, eds. *The Temporomandibular Joint: A Biological Basis for Clinical Practice.* Philadelphia: W. B. Saunders, 1992.

TENDON DISORDERS

DISEASE/DISORDER

ANATOMY OR SYSTEM AFFECTED: Back, bones, legs, ligaments, muscles, musculoskeletal system, tendons

SPECIALTIES AND RELATED FIELDS: Occupational health, orthopedics, physical therapy, podiatry, sports medicine

DEFINITION: Inflammation or tearing of the tendons.

Tendons are the tough, white, fibrous cords that connect muscles to movable structures such as bone or cartilage. The presence of tendons allows muscles to act at a distance and concentrates the force of the muscle into a small area. Sometimes tendons can change the direction of a muscle's pull, thus allowing the muscle to act around a joint. The structure of a tendon consists of parallel bundles of collagen fibrils, which makes it extraordinarily strong. A sheath, or vagina fibrosa, surrounds the tendon and is responsible for holding it in place. Between the fibrils and the sheath lie a lymphatic network and a fluid which allow tendon movement without excessive friction. Because of the vital functions of tendons, diseases and injuries to them can be debilitating as well as painful. Damaged tendons tend to heal slower than epithelial tissue, for example, because tendons have a lower blood supply than other soft tissues.

Trauma to tendons usually occurs in conjunction with impact, twisting, overstretching, or the simple overuse of a joint. These actions commonly result in partial or complete tears of the fibrous cord. Only if a tendon has not been stretched more than 4 percent of its original length will it return unchanged to its normal state once the force is released. When it is stretched from 4 to 8 percent of its normal length, the molecular bonds between individual collagen fibers begin to fail and the fibers slide past one another. At 8 to 10 percent strain, the tendon itself is in danger of tearing because individual fibers rupture, placing even more force on the fibers that remain intact. Although Golgi tendon organs send signals to the brain regarding excessive strain on tendons, such tearing usually occurs quickly during physical activities. Pain, swelling, and abnormal motion at the joint follow the damage. Tendinitis is the name given to the inflammation of a tendon.

Tendon disorders of the upper body. Tennis elbow, or lateral epicondylitis, involves the elbow joint and can be attributed to excessive extensor movements in the wrist joint and a sustained gripping of objects such as a tennis racket. There is great diversity in opinion as to the development of this disorder, as well as to its treatment. The latter includes methods such as rest, stretching, icing, heat, ultrasound, bracing, and surgery. Golfers' elbow is less often seen but is a similar tendinitis of the common flexor tendon.

Supraspinatus tendinitis, or swimmers' shoulder, is seen in athletes participating in swimming, tennis, and other activities involving overhead arm movement. Repeated overhead arm swings impinge and sometimes tear the supraspinatus tendon located between the acromion and the proximal end of the humerus. The disorder has also been termed impingement syndrome. Treatments include icing, stretching, modifying stroke technique in swimmers, anti-inflammatory drugs, and surgery.

Bicipital tendinitis usually stems from sports that require throwing or paddling. This type of tendon disorder is similar to the supraspinatus type in that pinching of a tendon is involved. The narrow tendon connecting the long head of the bicep muscle to the scapula lies in a groove and is restrained by a ligament therein. Pain occurring while a physician applies pressure to this groove and moves the patient's arm is diagnostic for this particular tendinitis. Treatments are the same as for supraspinatus tendinitis and are almost always successful.

Vigorous throwing can produce triceps tendinitis. Other tendons prone to injury are those attaching the infraspinatus, teres minor, and teres major muscles. Indeed, any tendon may incur damage depending on the specific activities that an individual undertakes.

Synovitis of the wrist extensor tendons is the result of friction between the tendon, its surrounding sheath, and bone processes. Tenosynovitis brings about a thickening of the tendon sheath, and at times a rubbing sound can even be heard during movement. An aching pain develops and may be relieved by methods applied in tendinitis cases. In addition, ultrasound therapy in water is highly successful. The abductor pollicis longus and the extensor pollicis brevis muscles are most often affected.

Tendon disorders of the lower body. Tendons of the lower body undergo greater stress than tendons of the torso because a greater weight is moved and a more continuous motion is involved. Achilles tendinitis often occurs in people participating in sports involving running and jumping. This type of inflammation has become the most common athletic injury. When great tensile strength is needed, the tendon tends to be long compared with the muscle to which it attaches. The Achilles tendon is long and durable but twists as it descends down the lower leg, making certain areas of the tendon vulnerable to the concentration of stress. Quality footwear with slight heel elevation and heel padding can reduce the tearing effect on this tendon. Stretching the gastrocnemius and soleus muscles before athletic exertion ensures that these muscles will absorb a greater portion of the force that would otherwise be transferred to the tendon.

Jumpers' knee, or patellar tendinitis, is fairly common in basketball and volleyball players; it is often mistaken for arthritis of the knee. Repetitive extending of the leg at the knee causes microtearing in the kneecap tendon; thus, the torn fibers fray and eventually begin to degenerate. More stress than before is then placed on the remaining intact fibers, resulting in the likelihood of their failing as well.

Many other lower body injuries may involve tendons. Groin pull is most frequent in soccer players because of the sudden stresses involved in kicking and changing direction by planting cleats firmly into the ground and jolting the body into a new configuration. Hamstring pull occurs during bursts of sprinting because the hamstring functions in the forward movement of a leg after a stride is completed. During extremely fast running, the hamstring requires great force to keep pace; thus, damage to the connecting tendon and to the muscle itself is likely to occur if attention is not given to proper stretching techniques before the exertion.

The term "shin splints" refers to several painful injuries to the lower leg. Indicative of shin splints are pain and tenderness along the tibia, or shinbone, and the middle one-third of the leg. The condition develops in athletes who do not use sufficient padding in their shoes or who run and play on hard surfaces. Genuine shin splints do not involve tendons directly; fortunately, tendinitis of the tibial muscles can be differentiated from true shin splints because the pain of tendinitis is located higher up on the leg.

Compartment syndrome is most frequently seen in runners. The leg is divided into three compartments, each encompassed by a tight fascial sheath. When injury occurs to muscles or tendons of a certain compartment, swelling accompanied by a cutting off of the blood supply can cause further problems. Even the sudden growth of muscles as a result of physical activity can impair the function of muscles and nerves deeper in the leg.

—*Ryan C. Horst and Roman J. Miller, Ph.D.*

See also Arthritis; Inflammation; Muscle sprains, spasms, and disorders; Muscles; Orthopedic surgery; Orthopedics; Orthopedics, pediatric; Physical rehabilitation; Sports medicine; Tendon repair.

FOR FURTHER INFORMATION:

Józsa, László, and Pekka Kannus. *Human Tendons: Anatomy, Physiology, and Pathology.* Champaign, Ill.: Human Kinetics, 1997.

Stanish, William D., Scott Mandel, and Sandra Curwin. *Tendinitis: Its Etiology and Treatment.* New York: Oxford University Press, 2000.

Weintraub, William. *Tendon and Ligament Healing: A New Approach Through Manual Therapy.* Berkeley, Calif.: North Atlantic Books, 1999.

TENDON REPAIR
PROCEDURE

ANATOMY OR SYSTEM AFFECTED: Bones, feet, hands, joints, knees, legs, ligaments, muscles, musculoskeletal system, tendons

SPECIALTIES AND RELATED FIELDS: General surgery, occupational health, orthopedics, podiatry, sports medicine

DEFINITION: The surgical repair of tendons, the bands of tissue that attach muscle to bone.

INDICATIONS AND PROCEDURES

Tendons are straps of collagenous tissue that attach muscles to bone. They are strong and flexible; a tendon approximately 1.3 centimeters (0.5 inch) thick can support a ton. Tendons are most prominently observed in the hand, where they are associated with the muscles that move the fingers and thumbs, and in the heel, where the Achilles tendon joins the muscles and bones of the foot. The Achilles tendon is the longest and thickest tendon in the body.

Tendon injuries can be of several types. If the hand or foot is badly cut, the slice may enter or sever the tendon, resulting in an inability to move the fingers or toes. Tendons have also ruptured during physical activity; the Achilles tendon is at particular risk during certain running or jumping exercises. The sensation that the patient experiences with initial tear has been likened to a kick. Severance of the Achilles tendon is indicated by an inability to stand on tiptoe.

More often, the Achilles tendon may become inflamed by activity. Such inflammation is usually indicated by pain that develops at the beginning and end of a run but that seems to improve during the exercise. Often, the pain becomes worse at night. Treatment of minor inflammation generally involves rest or cessation of the activity. Corticosteroids may be administered to relieve the inflammation.

If a tendon has been cut or severed, surgery is often required for proper repair. Since tendons are under great tension, they may snap or regress from the site of the injury. The surgeon makes an incision through the affected area, whether hand or foot, and sutures the ends of the tendon together.

USES AND COMPLICATIONS

If carried out properly and quickly, tendon repair is generally satisfactory. The patient may be immobilized for weeks, and some permanent stiffness is common. Because the blood supply to the region of the Achilles tendon is not as extensive as elsewhere in the body, healing may be a problem if the incision is too large.

—Richard Adler, Ph.D.

See also Cysts; Exercise physiology; Ganglion removal; Muscles; Orthopedic surgery; Orthopedics; Orthopedics, pediatric; Physical rehabilitation; Sports medicine; Tendon disorders.

FOR FURTHER INFORMATION:

Garrick, James G., and David R. Webb. *Sports Injuries: Diagnosis and Management.* Philadelphia: W. B. Saunders, 1999.

Roy, Steven, and Richard Irvin. *Sports Medicine: Prevention, Evaluation, Management, and Rehabilitation.* Englewood Cliffs, N.J.: Prentice Hall, 1983.

Scuderi, Giles R., Peter D. McCann, and Peter J. Bruno, eds. *Sports Medicine: Principles of Primary Care.* St. Louis: C. V. Mosby, 1997.

Southmayd, William, and Marshall Hoffman. *Sports Health.* New York: Quick Fox, 1981.

TERMINALLY ILL: EXTENDED CARE
SPECIALTY

ANATOMY OR SYSTEM AFFECTED: All

SPECIALTIES AND RELATED FIELDS: All

DEFINITION: The medical, social, and psychological care of patients who are suffering from a terminal illness, the goal of which is to maintain as high a quality of life as possible for the remainder of a patient's life.

KEY TERMS:

adult day care facility: a facility that offers a temporary daytime setting based on either social, maintenance, or rehabilitative services; often used to give the home care provider some time off

extended care facility: a facility that can be found in several settings, outside the home, where specialized medical care can be rendered under a physician's orders

home care: the provision of outside services to a person living in a home setting

hospice: a program designed to ease the suffering and grief for terminally ill patients and their families; care can be rendered in the home or in a special hospice setting with special emphasis on the relief of pain

nursing home: a type of extended care facility that can be classified as either skilled or intermediate, depending on the type of care; physicians oversee medical care that is rendered around the clock by a nursing staff

ASSESSING THE NEEDS OF THE TERMINALLY ILL PATIENT

Difficult decisions await those trying to care for a patient with a terminal condition. Many families are faced with these decisions soon after the patient leaves the hospital, unable to function alone at home. Physicians and family members are able to choose among several options, depending on the needs and desires of the patient.

The decision process should start when the patient is still in the traditional hospital setting. The decision process should explore all alternatives, based on many factors. The degree of physician involvement is important, since not all doctors make monthly trips to visit patients at other facilities. The possibility of rapid deterioration of health or mental status is a vital concern, and nursing needs and other nonphysician services are also of utmost importance. The patient's desires and the wishes of the family can be addressed through the patient's legal rights to have a living will or durable power of attorney for health care decisions. Both can document, either through the patient's own written directions or through the appointment of a relative as a legal representative, where the patient stands on the issue of being kept alive by artificial means. Specific requests regarding the use of cardiopulmonary resuscitation (CPR) should be made to the physician. These wishes are best discussed long before the patient is near death.

When the terminally ill patient also has a mental illness, such as dementia, the desires of the family members are weighed along with their willingness and ability to care for the person in the home. The problems of mobility, financial constraints, and quality-of-life concerns also enter the picture.

This is a picture that is not clear or easy to visualize. Many questions need to be answered before a suitable arrangement can be made regarding the continued care for a terminally ill person, especially an elderly one. These questions will lead to wiser long-term care decisions.

Extended care includes a wide range of social and support services and can be divided into three categories: in-home services, community-based services, and institutional care. The availability of these long-term care services may vary widely, with differences in eligibility requirements and costs. The choices to be reviewed must fit the family's financial resources. Long-term care should also be based on the medical, personal, and social needs of the patient. Special attention should be paid to the patient's cognitive, psychological/emotional, functional, and economic status. The value system, perspective, beliefs, and goals of the patient are extremely important.

For a terminally ill person, an assessment of the patient's current and potential needs may have to be completed more than once as the illness progresses. A timeline showing the patient's current needs and needs within the next year, or even the next five years, should be made. This long-term planning must address physician involvement; nursing coverage; physical, speech, and occupational therapies; social worker and nutrition consultations; dental care; and the need for medical supplies and equipment. Other services that may be necessary include personal care, preparation of meals, transportation, housekeeping and home maintenance, and assistance with daily living skills. The amount of time for which these services must be available and the necessary financial resources may influence early decisions. Unfortunately, financial considerations often dictate the answer before all options can be explored.

The patient's concerns regarding housing are influenced by such things as the amount of importance that is placed on staying in the present home and questions about living with or near family, friends, and church and about the availability of social activities. When the terminally ill person is elderly, this issue is even more sensitive. Because of the traumatic aspects of moving an elderly person from the home environment, the easiest transition for the patient should be sought. The choices are having a terminally ill patient remain in the home or moving the patient to an extended care facility or a hospice center.

Before family members convene a meeting with the physician to discuss the options, all of them should speak with the patient. The terminal patient should not be given the impression that family members are making decisions for him or her. Such meetings allow patients to inform family members of their wishes, allowing the patient optimum input and providing information that the family may not have. Competent adults, even if they are elderly, have legal rights and privileges that must be honored. Some of these rights present ethical issues to family members trying to decide about long-term care. Unfortunately, such discussions often take place immediately after an older person has an emergency or a patient hears the diagnosis of a terminal illness.

When a patient is in an acute care hospital, the decision process should start before discharge. Many persons within an acute care hospital setting are qualified to assist in these decisions. An attending physician has available many tools to evaluate the patient's needs, especially if the patient is elderly and the doctor has specialized in geriatric care. Questionnaires can determine the daily living needs as well as collect psychological data pertaining to cognitive, emotional, and perceptive functions. The family physician, during the discharge planning, can arrange for the family to speak to the social services area within the hospital.

The family and the patient would be wise to make a checklist to determine the areas of most concern, ranking them by importance so that all persons concerned are able to look at the options more objectively. Although each of the alternative living settings is unique, every person involved in these decisions should visit the actual setting, allowing the patient active involvement to make the transition easier.

OPTIONS FOR LONG-TERM CARE

One of the first options available for a terminally ill patient is to return to his or her own home or to live with relatives. This decision of home health care must be based on the support available from the family: who will help provide care, when, and how. The need for home modifications to make the patient more independent or more comfortable may be a concern. If outside services are needed, such as therapy, family members must determine how they can be obtained. Another difficult question is identifying responsibility for the financial costs of special care.

These questions are difficult to ask and even more difficult to answer. Families may underestimate the additional stress involved in caring for a terminally ill person in the home. Fortunately, services are available to help relieve the additional stresses encountered, such as respite care. Having someone come into the home or having the patient placed in a day care facility can relieve some of the stresses temporarily. One of the first types of stress encountered is one of a physical nature, especially fatigue arising from the additional housekeeping activities of cleaning, laundering, shopping, and cooking. Additional emotional stress results from trying to balance time,

responsibilities, and pressures. Financial worries may also cause stress, even though the costs of home care are often much less than for care in a hospital or other facility.

Home health care does not mean that the family or the patient is alone. Outside professional care, such as part-time nursing or supportive services, can be rendered when a terminal patient is in the home setting. These types of services fall under two headings: skilled care and supportive care. Skilled care involves physicians, nurses, and therapists. Supportive services are those that enable a patient to continue to live independently in the home. These services may meet personal needs (such as bathing and dressing) or involve the performance of chores (such as shopping, meal preparation, and housekeeping). Supportive services may be obtained as often as necessary, but they are not without cost. Moreover, the absence of one needed service may mean that home care is not the best option for this patient, at least at this point in time. Every patient and family member is entitled to make an objective evaluation of which agency is best suited for the homebound patient. An ongoing evaluation should be conducted to ensure that this option remains the best choice. Especially in the case of a terminally ill elder, home care may not remain a viable option for long: As the patient's physical needs change, his or her environment may need to change as well.

One step beyond living independently in the home or with family members would be for the terminally ill patient to arrange for special housing, often called supportive housing arrangements. This option may include continuing care retirement villages, board-and-care homes, domiciliary care, foster homes, personal care homes, group homes, and congregate care facilities. Board-and-care homes provide regular housekeeping and personal care services. This type of care is called assisted living, or even residential care, because the services vary widely, as do the costs. Another possibility is congregate housing, the environment of which is more like an updated version of an old resort hotel, with costs and services greatly variable. Continuing care communities offer independent living arrangements along with twenty-four-hour nursing care. These communities offer what is referred to as life care, with a wide range of services available, a large entrance fee, monthly charges for services, and a lifetime commitment. They usually cost more than board, care home, or congregate housing.

Adult day care, which lies between home care and institutional care, emphasizes either social or medical needs. The three main types of adult day care are social, maintenance, and restorative, with each specializing in addressing the specific needs of the patient. The social model of adult day care emphasizes socialization while also giving families or caregivers some free time. The maintenance model, a mix of social and remedial components, differs from the restorative model, which offers extensive rehabilitation services. These settings may be alternatives to a nursing home. Some specialized adult day care centers, connected to hospitals, teach patients to live independently after discharge, with a special emphasis on daily living skills and the use of community resources.

If extensive care becomes necessary, especially for elderly patients, yet another option would be a nursing home facility, either an intermediate care or a skilled nursing care facility. The skilled nursing home is for the person needing intensive care, twenty-four-hour supervision under a physician's supervision with treatment by a registered nurse. Intermediate care is suitable for those not needing round-the-clock supervision but unable to live alone. This option is expensive, and the costs generally are not reimbursed, placing all the financial responsibility on the patient or on family members. Although nursing homes in the United States are inspected and controlled by the government, the certification status and quality among homes differ greatly. Attention must be given to ensure good medical coverage, provisions for maintaining the patient's individuality and dignity, available activities, nutritious meals, social and recreational activities, and intellectual stimulation.

The hospice setting offers intense medical supervision in comfortable and peaceful surroundings. The philosophy of hospice emphasizes the concept of supportive care and services for the terminally ill and their families in the home or a special center. Although hospices assist in some home health care services and inpatient care, they are designed for terminally ill patients who are no longer being treated for their diseases, with a life expectancy of only weeks or months. Specialized teams composed of a physician, nursing staff, volunteers, social workers, and clergy administer the physical, spiritual, and emotional needs of each patient through the management of medical symptoms and the control of pain. If the patient is not placed into a hospice center, specialized

care from the hospice team is available in the home to meet the needs of terminally ill patients and their families.

PERSPECTIVE AND PROSPECTS

Caring for a terminally ill family member can be a rewarding experience as well as an exhausting one. The location where this care is traditionally given has changed over time and will continue to change in the future. Care in the patient's home or with relatives is the least restrictive and one of the less expensive of the many options available. In fact, care in the home is often the only option because outside care is too expensive. Some family members are motivated to select home care because of a sense of obligation or a fear that no one else can care for the patient as well.

More supplemental resources are available than ever before, allowing home care to be a viable option for some. For many others, however, the additional stresses of responsibility for a terminally ill relative, especially an elderly one, are too high. At this point, tough decisions must be made about where the patient should live. Family members may not be prepared to care for the patient at the home. Despite the high costs of extended care facilities, this option is sometimes the only choice available. An emphasis on quality of life makes placement in the least restrictive environment a common choice. Concerns about pain management and the need for a caring staff may change this choice, however, when the terminally ill face the end of life.

In the United States, the high cost of health care makes such decisions even more difficult. Until some form of national health care reform allows for extensive coverage to assist these families, the financial burden will often dictate placement for the terminally ill. Although many placement options exist, more will be developed in the future because of the increase in the number of older adults. Some will be suitable and some will not, making this decision process a problem for generations to come. While the final decision about where to live remains with the competent patient, the input of physicians and family members and the influence of financial questions will become larger concerns. Societal influences may also come to the surface as the number of elderly people grows. With improving medical technology, the elderly population will have a greater impact on governmental policymakers and will influence national health care provisions. Advances in medicine may also dictate where and how terminally ill patients are cared for.

Resources for this care are available, but they have specific requirements. Possible benefit providers include the federal government through Medicare and the Social Security Administration's supplemental security income (SSI) program. Qualified persons should contact the Veterans Administration. State programs include Medicaid, the Department of Human Resources, and state supplemental programs. In addition to private insurance coverage, financial help could be sought through community agencies, such as municipal or other local support groups. Several health-related organizations offer some assistance for specific groups of patients, such as the American Cancer Society. Many private agencies, both nonprofit and for profit, offer services. The first and best approach for information when seeking care for a terminally ill patient is through family physicians, hospitals, and local health departments.

—*Maxine M. Urton, Ph.D.*

See also Acquired immunodeficiency syndrome (AIDS); Aging: Extended care; Allied health; Cancer; Critical care; Critical care, pediatric; Death and dying; Emergency medicine; Ethics; Euthanasia; Geriatrics and gerontology; Hospice; Hospitals; Law and medicine; Nursing; Oncology; Pediatrics; Pharmacology; Psychiatry; Psychiatry, child and adolescent; Psychiatry, geriatric; Resuscitation.

FOR FURTHER INFORMATION:
Appleton, Michael, and Todd Henschell. *At Home with Terminal Illness: A Family Guide to Hospice in the Home.* Englewood Cliffs, N.J.: Prentice Hall Career & Technology, 1995. This popular work examines hospice care and home nursing for the terminally ill.
Bausell, R. Barker, Michael A. Rooney, and Charles B. Inlander. *How to Evaluate and Select a Nursing Home.* Reading, Mass.: Addison-Wesley, 1988. Explains types of nursing homes and alternatives. Checklists on health and financial status are included, as are addresses and phone numbers for state nursing home licensure offices.
Horne, Jo. *The Nursing Home Handbook: A Guide for Families.* Glenview, Ill.: Scott, Foresman, 1989. Guides the decision-making process through an assessment of patient needs. Offers checklists for facilities and life adjustments, while focusing on quality-of-life concerns.
Levy, Michael T. *Parenting Mom and Dad: A Guide for the Grown-Up Children of Aging Parents.* New York: Prentice Hall, 1991. Discusses common problems, guidelines for financial planning and legal decisions, and health insurance. Outlines how to secure optimal medical care. Special sections cover psychiatric illnesses, dementias, and the deterioration of the body.
Lynn, Joanne, and Joan Harrold. "Preparing for the Inevitable." *The Washington Post*, May 30, 1999, p. X03. Lynn, Harrold, and their colleagues at the Center to Improve the Care of the Dying reveal why the philosophy of palliative care is so important to the debate about the care of the dying.
Portnow, Jay, and Martha Houtmann. *Home Care for the Elderly: A Complete Guide.* New York: McGraw-Hill, 1987. A comprehensive guide covering nutrition, exercise, bathing, grooming, proper environment, bowel and bladder care, and signs of illnesses.

TESTICLES, UNDESCENDED
DISEASE/DISORDER
ALSO KNOWN AS: Cryptorchidism
ANATOMY OR SYSTEM AFFECTED: Genitals, reproductive system
SPECIALTIES AND RELATED FIELDS: Endocrinology, general surgery, pediatrics, urology
DEFINITION: Testicles that neither reside in nor can be manipulated into the scrotum.

CAUSES AND SYMPTOMS
The testicles, or testes, appear in males by seven weeks of gestation; by eight weeks, they are hormonally active. At eleven weeks, they produce testosterone, which is suppressed by maternal estrogens later in the pregnancy. These estrogens decrease before birth, causing a surge in testosterone production that is indispensable for the descent of the testes at about thirty-six weeks of gestation and for future sperm production.

About 3.4 percent of all male infants born after a full-term pregnancy will have undescended testes, or cryptorchidism. Risk factors include being first born or a twin, having a low birth weight, and/or being born prematurely, as well as being delivered by cesarean section. By three months of age, 1 percent of male infants still have undescended testes, a percentage unchanged by one year of age. In premature infants, most testes will descend by three months after the expected date at which the child should have been born (term).

The tissues of descended and undescended testes are the same for the first year. Thereafter, an undescended testis deteriorates and the chance of infertility increases. Rarely will testes descend spontaneously after six months of age.

Cryptorchidism may be isolated or be part of other conditions such as hermaphroditic, genetic, and endocrine disorders. Infertility affects 50 percent of patients with unilateral cryptorchidism. Testicular malignancy is twenty-two times as common in these patients as in the general population; malignancy is six times as common in intra-abdominal testes as in other cryptorchid testes. One-fourth of all cancers occur in the contralateral descended testicle.

TREATMENT AND THERAPY

The American Academy of Pediatric Surgery recommends correction of this condition by the first birthday, thereby decreasing the incidence of infertility and tumors and making the testicle accessible for regular examination. If the testicle is absent, a prosthesis may be inserted for cosmetic purposes. Hormonal treatment is also available, with a success rate of 33 to 90 percent but a 10 to 20 percent chance of recurrence. A pediatric surgeon or a pediatric urologist will evaluate the child and decide what is best for the individual patient.

—*Frances García, M.D.*

See also Endocrine system; Endocrinology; Endocrinology, pediatric; Genetic diseases; Genital disorders, male; Glands; Hermaphroditism and pseudohermaphroditism; Hormones; Orchitis; Premature birth; Reproductive system; Sexual differentiation; Sexuality; Surgery, pediatric; Testicular surgery; Testicular torsion; Urology; Urology, pediatric.

FOR FURTHER INFORMATION:

Montague, Drogo K. *Disorders of Male Sexual Function*. Chicago: Year Book Medical, 1988.

Rajfer, Jacob. *Urologic Endocrinology*. Philadelphia: W. B. Saunders, 1986.

Swanson, Janice M., and Katherine A. Forrest. *Men's Reproductive Health*. New York: Springer, 1984.

TESTICULAR SURGERY

PROCEDURE

ANATOMY OR SYSTEM AFFECTED: Endocrine system, genitals, glands, reproductive system

SPECIALTIES AND RELATED FIELDS: General surgery, urology

DEFINITION: The fixation of a testicle to the scrotum or the removal of a testicle or the veins surrounding a testicle.

KEY TERMS:

orchiectomy: surgical removal of the testicle for benign or malignant conditions

orchiopexy: fixation of the testicle to the internal lining of the scrotum to eliminate the possibility of testicular torsion

testicular torsion: twisting of the testicle in the scrotum, with compromise of the blood supply to the testicle, as a result of spermatic cord rotation

varicocele: an enlarged vein surrounding the testicle as a result of incompetent venous valves; most commonly found surrounding the left testicle

INDICATIONS AND PROCEDURES

Fixation of a testicle may be performed as treatment for torsion (twisting) of the testicle and undescended testicle (cryptorchidism). Removal of a testicle may be required because of infection, traumatic rupture, pain, necrosis (death of the testicle), or the presence of a testicular tumor.

Testicular torsion occurs most commonly in males under twenty-five years of age. Torsion is usually associated with acute testicular pain that is intense enough to produce nausea, vomiting, and severe discomfort. The testicle is usually firm, tender, and displaced upward in the scrotum. It is frequently difficult to examine the gland because of the severe pain. Manual elevation of the testicle may relieve discomfort in some patients with infections of the epididymis, but it has no effect on patients with torsion. Testicular torsion is considered a surgical emergency. Information regarding this condition can be obtained using scrotal ultrasound or radionucleotide scans, but most patients require surgical exploration to identify this condition. It is important to relieve the torsion as quickly as possible to restore blood supply to the testicle. Prolonged delay before surgical intervention can result in a nonviable, necrotic testicle.

Treatment of testicular torsion is by a surgical procedure called orchiopexy. After an incision in the scrotum, the testicle is untwisted under direct vision. If more than six hours have elapsed before surgery, a necrotic testicle may result and orchiectomy may be required. If the testicle appears viable, orchiopexy is carried out. In orchiopexy, the testis is anchored in the scrotum with a row of three or more absorbable sutures through the lining of the testicle and the dartos muscle layer of the scrotal wall. These sutures fix the testicle to the scrotum to eliminate further torsion. A small plastic drain may be placed to limit swelling and enhance drainage during recovery. The skin is closed with absorbable sutures. Because testicular torsion frequently occurs on both sides, the opposite testicle is similarly fixed with orchiopexy.

Undescended testes are located outside the scrotum, usually in the inguinal canal, but they may also be found in the abdomen. Orchiopexy should be performed at one to two years of age to preserve future testicular function. While rare cases require microsurgery, most orchiopexies are performed using a scrotal incision with testicular fixation similar to that described for torsion.

Varicoceles occur in approximately 15 percent of adult males, usually following puberty. Their importance is the association with infertility in some men with low sperm counts. Varicoceles occur primarily on the left side and result from abnormalities in the veins draining the left testicle. While tying off the veins of the varicocele is important in adolescent males with an associated decrease in testicular size, most varicoceles do not require surgery. If low sperm count, persistent infertility, decreased testicular volume, or prolonged pain occur from the varicocele, surgical intervention may be appropriate.

Varicocele surgery can be performed through the abdomen, groin, or scrotum. Most surgeons prefer a high ligation, which involves a small incision just above the groin (internal inguinal ring). The vein draining the testicle is identified beneath the abdominal muscles. It is separated from the vas deferens (sperm tube) and arteries supplying the testicle, is ligated with several sutures, and is divided. This method of treatment is the most direct, least complicated, and most effective for varicocele ligation. The procedure is performed on an outpatient basis. Most patients are able to return to normal activity within seven days. Under certain circumstances, with previous failed high ligations, or very large scrotal varices, a scrotal incision may be selected by the surgeon to remove all dilated veins from around the testicle. This technique is most useful in patients with decreased testicular volume or pain caused by a varicocele.

Orchiectomy, or removal of a testicle, is used to treat an abscess, infection, traumatic rupture, loss of testicular function, prostate cancer, and testicular tumors. Removal of the testicle for testicular tumors is especially important since these tumors are curable if identified and treated early. This procedure is carried out through an incision in the groin and not in the scrotum, a technique that decreases the chance of testicular tumor spread to the scrotum. A small incision in the groin above the scrotum is made, the spermatic cord is clamped, and the testicle is delivered into the incision and inspected. If a testicular tumor is identified, the spermatic cord is tied and the testis removed. The incision is then closed using standard suture techniques. If a testicle is to be removed for other indications such as infection, prostate cancer, pain, or trauma, a scrotal incision is appropriate. The incision, which is similar to that described for testicular torsion, exposes the testicle and spermatic cord and allows for clamping and ligation of the spermatic cord prior to testicular removal. A drain is not usually necessary for orchiectomy.

USES AND COMPLICATIONS

Rapid identification of testicular torsion is paramount, before compromise of the blood supply results in the death of the testicle. Diagnosis of testicular torsion should be within six to eight hours of onset. Episodic torsion can also occur and is associated with preservation of testicular function and anatomy. Varicocele ligation is carried out for associated decreased testicular volume, pain, and most commonly infertility with diminished sperm count or sperm activity.

The complications associated with testicular surgery include infection in the scrotum, bleeding into the scrotum, and scrotal swelling. Pain, which is usually short-lived and localized, may occur with the inguinal incisions used for the removal of testicular tumors. Bleeding is the most common significant complication of testicular surgery and results in enlargement of the scrotum, significant discoloration, and pain. Bleeding is most often identified within six to twelve hours after testicular surgery. Testicular surgery is usually performed using absorbable sutures in the scrotal skin, and suture removal after surgery is unnecessary.

PERSPECTIVE AND PROSPECTS

Surgical procedures for scrotal abnormalities have been common urologic procedures for centuries. New technologies such as radiographic embolization of testicular veins for varicoceles have been tried, but they are not generally accepted as superior to simple surgical procedures. These procedures, which are expensive and have unique complications, are less likely to be effective than more common, simple surgical intervention. Laparoscopy has been widely used for varicocele ligation, but it has little advantage over high ligation and is more expensive and time-consuming. Orchiopexy for abdominal or other high-lying testes can now be treated using microsurgical techniques. The testis can be removed and transplanted to a scrotal location or the spermatic cord rerouted to permit scrotal placement and to avoid orchiectomy.

—*Culley C. Carson III, M.D.*

See also Genital disorders, male; Glands; Hydrocelectomy; Laparoscopy; Orchitis; Penile implant surgery; Reproductive system; Testicles, undescended; Testicular torsion; Urology; Urology, pediatric; Vasectomy.

FOR FURTHER INFORMATION:

Cockett, Abraham T. K., and Ken Koshiba. *Color Atlas of Urological Surgery.* Baltimore: Williams & Wilkins, 1996. Examines both routine and complex procedures, including open, minimally invasive, and endoscopic techniques.

Glenn, James F. *Glenn's Urologic Surgery.* 5th ed. Philadelphia: J. B. Lippincott, 1998. Topics include the adrenal gland, kidney, ureter and pelvis, bladder, prostate, urethra, vas deferens and seminal vesicle, testes, penis, and scrotum. Also addresses urinary diversion, pediatric urology, endoscopy, laparoscopy, and frontiers in surgery.

TESTICULAR TORSION

DISEASE/DISORDER

ANATOMY OR SYSTEM AFFECTED: Circulatory system, genitals, reproductive system

SPECIALTIES AND RELATED FIELDS: Family practice, pediatrics, urology

DEFINITION: A twisting or rotation of the testicle (testis) or spermatic cord on its long axis, causing acute pain and swelling.

CAUSES AND SYMPTOMS

Testicular torsion is most commonly found in infants, adolescents, or young adult males. Roughly half of the cases occur in the early hours of the morning, and cases usually occur on the left side rather than the right. The condition can occur during sleep, rest, game playing, or hard physical activity, but it is more likely to be caused by direct injury. Testicular torsion may also result if the testicle is unusually mobile within its covering in the scrotum because of inadequate connective tissue.

Testicular torsion makes itself known by pain of varying degrees either in the lower part of the abdomen or in the scrotum itself. The pain intensifies rapidly and is occasionally accompanied by nausea as the testicle becomes swollen and very tender and the scrotal skin becomes discolored. A diagnosis can be made by physical examination.

TREATMENT AND THERAPY

Immediate treatment of testicular torsion is necessary. The testicle must be untwisted immediately and blood flow restored to the testicle, the epididymis, and other structures. Otherwise, complete blockage of the blood supply (ischemia) for six hours or more may result in gangrene (tissue death) of the testicle. Even a partial loss of circulation can produce atrophy.

Manual untwisting should be followed by surgery within six hours of the onset of symptoms to ensure that the torsion has been undone successfully and that there is no recurrence. An incision is made in the scrotal skin, and the testicle is secured to the scrotum by small stitches. If irreversible damage exists, removal of the testicle must be performed. The other testicle, which usually remains capable of producing active sperm, is also anchored to prevent torsion on that side. Prompt surgery ensures a complete recovery.

—*Keith Garebian, Ph.D.*

See also Circulation; Genital disorders, male; Glands; Orchitis; Reproductive system; Surgery, pediatric; Testicles, undescended; Testicular surgery; Urology; Urology, pediatric; Vascular system.

FOR FURTHER INFORMATION:

Montague, Drogo K. *Disorders of Male Sexual Function.* Chicago: Year Book Medical, 1988.

Rajfer, Jacob. *Urologic Endocrinology.* Philadelphia: W. B. Saunders, 1986.

Swanson, Janice M., and Katherine A. Forrest. *Men's Reproductive Health.* New York: Springer, 1984.

TESTS. *See* INVASIVE TESTS; LABORATORY TESTS; NONINVASIVE TESTS.

TETANUS

DISEASE/DISORDER

ANATOMY OR SYSTEM AFFECTED: Brain, muscles, musculoskeletal system, nervous system

SPECIALTIES AND RELATED FIELDS: Bacteriology, family practice, internal medicine, neurology, public health

DEFINITION: An often fatal disease of the nervous system characterized by painful, sustained, and violent muscle spasms; it is almost completely preventable through vaccination.

KEY TERMS:

anaerobic: without oxygen; anaerobic organisms grow in an atmosphere free of oxygen

antibody: a protein found in the blood and produced by the immune system in response to contact of the body with an antigen

antigen: a foreign substance (such as a bacteria, toxin, or virus) to which the body makes an immune response

antitoxin: an antibody against a specific toxin; antitoxins can bind toxins and neutralize them

bacterium: a microscopic single-celled organism that multiplies by means of simple division; bacteria are found everywhere; most are beneficial, but a few species cause disease

endospore: a resistant, dormant structure, formed inside bacteria such as Bacillus and Clostridium, that can survive adverse conditions

immunity: a capacity to resist a disease caused by an infectious agent

lockjaw: a popular name for tetanus, derived from a symptom associated with the disease

toxin: a poisonous substance produced by some bacteria that cause certain diseases

toxoid: a form of a toxin that can no longer cause the symptoms of a disease but can cause the body to make antibodies against it

vaccination: inoculation with a specific vaccine in order to prevent or lessen the effect of some disease

CAUSES AND SYMPTOMS

Tetanus is a disease of the nervous system caused by the bacterium *Clostridium tetani* (*C. tetani*). Humans and most species of warm-blooded animals are susceptible to tetanus. This disease is not contagious, meaning it cannot be transmitted from one individual to another. It results from the contamination of a natural or surgical wound by spores (endospores) of *C. tetani*. The bacteria grow in the wound and produce a toxin that spreads throughout the body and causes the symptoms of the disease. Neonatal tetanus is the appearance of tetanus in a child less than one month old; it is usually contracted by the infant directly following birth.

C. tetani is an anaerobic, endospore-forming bacterium. Anaerobic bacteria can grow only in an oxygen-free environment. In harsh environments or at times when oxygen is present, all species of clostridia have the unique ability to form dormant (nongrowing) structures called endospores. These structures develop inside the bacterial cell and serve to protect the genetic material of the cell from harsh environmental stresses that would destroy an actively growing cell. Endospores are very resistant to disinfectants and temperature changes; thus, the bacteria can remain dormant until the surrounding environment becomes better suited for growth. *C. tetani* spores are found throughout the world in soil, human and animal intestines, and especially in soil fertilized with human or animal feces.

A person can get tetanus only if spores from the soil or elsewhere in the environment enter that person under the proper conditions to become living, growing bacteria. The bacteria will grow only if they enter a wound that is free from oxygen, such as a deep puncture wound or a wound that has considerable dead or crushed tissue. There are always a few cases of tetanus, however, that follow no apparent injury. Typical causes of wounds that could be susceptible to tetanus are compound fractures; gunshots; dog bites; punctures caused by glass, thorns, needles, splinters, or rusty nails; "skin popping" by drug addicts; bedsores; outer ear infections; and dental extractions. The most feared form of tetanus, neonatal tetanus, is usually caused by the cutting of the umbilical cord with an unsterile instrument or by improper care of the umbilical stump. In the United States, most cases of neonatal tetanus are found in home deliveries not attended by a health professional.

Spores of *C. tetani* enter the body through a wound or abrasion. In the absence of oxygen, they will germinate (revert from the dormant endospore state to become living, growing cells). The bacteria will grow and multiply but not spread from the initial site of infection. In many cases, the wound hardly appears to be infected at all. As it grows, *C. tetani* produces a toxin called tetanospasmin that can filter through the body. Once the toxin reaches the central nervous system, it binds to nerve cells, causing the beginning stages of symptoms to be seen. Symptoms can appear from one day to several months after infection, with the average incubation period (the time during which symptoms appear after infection) being three to twenty-one days. The wide range of incubation time depends on the amount of time needed for anaerobic conditions to develop and the time required for the toxin to reach the central nervous system.

The tetanus toxin, tetanospasmin, is a simple protein. No one knows why *C. tetani* makes this protein. It has no apparent role in the life of the bacterium, and it is unknown whether this toxin gives the bacterium any selective advantage for survival in the environment. It is unlikely that the bacterium makes this toxin merely to kill people and animals, yet the fact that it does kill them is all that is known about the toxin. Animals vary in their susceptibility to the ef-

fects of tetanospasmin; humans and horses are the most susceptible, while birds and cold-blooded animals are resistant. Tetanospasmin is the second most dangerous known toxin, and it is so powerful that an amount of toxin the size of one period on this page could kill thirty people. One milligram of toxin could kill 200 million laboratory mice.

To understand how tetanospasmin works to cause the symptoms of tetanus, one must first understand how muscles function. Most muscles in the body occur in pairs; one muscle in the pair, when contracted, causes that part of the body to move in one direction, and the opposing muscle in the pair, when contracted, causes that part of the body to move in the opposite

Tetanus

Tetanus is contracted when bacteria enter a wound and produce a toxin, tetanospasmin, that spreads through the body, most often causing death. A program of immunization is nearly 100 percent effective against tetanus.

2246 • <small>Tetanus</small>

direction. Normally, the nerves that control the muscle pairs stimulate one muscle in a pair to contract and signal the opposing muscle to relax. In this way, that part of the body is able to move. For example, in using an arm to lift an object, the nerves send a signal to the muscle in the front of the arm to contract and at the same time send a signal to the back of the arm to relax, so that the arm can bend upward at the elbow and lift the object. If the nerves did not signal the opposing muscle to relax, the contraction of the first muscle would cause the opposing muscle to stretch and trigger the "stretch reflex" in that muscle, causing that muscle to contract and counteract the stretch. Tetanus toxin works by binding to the nerve cells at nerve-muscle junctions and somehow blocking the signal of relaxation to the opposing muscle; therefore, when one muscle in a pair of muscles contracts, both muscles contract. The final effect is called spastic paralysis, in which the muscles are in a state of continuous contraction, pulling against each other, causing rigidity in a normally movable part of the body.

The initial symptoms of tetanus include restlessness, irritability, a stiff neck, and difficulty swallowing. In about half of all cases, the initial symptoms include stiffness or spasms of the jaw muscles, commonly known as "lockjaw." Gradually, the skeletal muscles (muscles of the arms, legs, back, and stomach) become involved. Muscles move through stages of contractions from merely twitching to rigid spasms that are brief but may be frequent, painful, and exhausting. Severe stages of the disease are characterized by tetanic spasms (sustained contractions) of some or all of the muscle groups. The slightest disturbance of the victim may cause spasms, generalized seizures, or both. A typical tetanic seizure is characterized by a sudden burst of tetanic spasm of all muscle groups, causing clenching of the jaw to produce a grimace, arching of the back with the neck back, flexion of arms, clenching of fists on the chest, and extension of the lower extremities. The patient is completely conscious during such episodes and experiences intense pain. Some spasms may be severe enough to cause bones to break. Eventually, the muscles of the cardiac and respiratory systems can be affected. Spasms of the throat muscles and respiratory muscles may lead to suffocation or respiratory arrest. The toxin may affect the circulatory system and heart in such a way as to increase the heart rate, increase blood pressure, and cause constriction of blood vessels. Death caused by tetanus is usually a result of circulatory collapse or respiratory failure.

TREATMENT AND THERAPY

Tetanus is diagnosed mainly on the basis of the symptoms present and the case history of the patient—the vaccination record and the type of injury sustained. A patient with no recent history of tetanus vaccination who receives a puncture or trauma wound is often treated for tetanus with an injection of antitoxin even before any symptoms appear. Antitoxin is quite effective when given to prevent the symptoms from appearing, but less so when given after the symptoms have already appeared. While other diseases are diagnosed after the organism that causes the disease is isolated from the site of the infection, it is very difficult to diagnose tetanus based on the ability to isolate the *C. tetani* bacteria from the wound, for several reasons. First, clostridia are present in almost every wound, but they do not always cause disease, so finding them does not necessarily mean that the bacteria are active. Second, there are many other contaminating bacteria in wounds, which makes it difficult to tell which may be causing disease or whether clostridia are there at all. In addition, the number of *C. tetani* bacteria needed to cause disease is quite small, which makes them harder to isolate. Finally, clostridia, because of their anaerobic nature, are difficult to grow.

Tetanus may take from a few days to several weeks to run its course. Patients who exhibit certain patterns in the course of the disease usually have a poor chance of recovery. These include patients with a short incubation period between the time of the injury and the onset of seizures, patients who exhibit a rapid development from mild muscle spasms to tetanic spasms, patients with injuries close to the head, patients with a high frequency or strong severity of seizures, and patients who are very young or very old. Patients who do recover usually return to a completely normal state after a variable period of stiffness; except for possible damage to the lungs from pulmonary complications or bone fractures, tetanus leaves no permanent damage. Unfortunately, recovery from the disease does not make the patient immune to future attacks, as with other diseases. The amount of toxin needed to kill a person is not even close to enough toxin to stimulate the patient's immune response to make the patient immune to the disease. Only vaccination with a large dose of inactive toxin can give a person immunity to tetanus.

Tetanus is difficult to treat because no one knows exactly what the toxin does. Doctors know only what kinds of symptoms the toxin causes, so the treatment is mainly symptomatic and is directed at preventing the production of more toxin. Antitoxin is given to block the attachment to the nerve cells of any free toxin that might be circulating in the body. Antitoxin has absolutely no effect on toxin that is already fixed to nerve tissue, but it can fully neutralize any free toxin. Originally, doctors used serum from immunized horses as a source of antitoxin, but this caused serious side effects (namely, serum sickness) in patients, so it is recommended that only pooled hyperimmune human globin (purified serum from immunized humans) be used as a source of antitoxin. Second, large doses of an antibiotic such as penicillin are given to kill any remaining bacteria, in order to prevent the bacteria from producing more toxin. If the patient is allergic to penicillin, tetracycline or clindamycin can be given instead. In addition, the wound may need to be cleansed of any dead tissue, to remove the anaerobic environment necessary for growth of the bacteria. Third, the muscle spasms need to be controlled. Mild muscle spasms are controlled with barbiturates and diazepam (Valium), whereas severe spasms need a curare-like agent (D tubocurarine is used to poison the paralyzed muscles so that they do not contract) that completely paralyzes the patient. These various muscle relaxants are used to ease the contractions until the toxin already present at the nerve sites wears out. The patient can be put on a positive-pressure breathing apparatus to maintain respiration. A tracheostomy (an operation in which an opening into the trachea, or windpipe, is made) may be necessary to minimize respiratory complications. Also, patients are often kept in quiet dark rooms that reduce auditory and visual stimuli, in order to minimize the frequency and severity of the tetanic spasms. Even with all these treatment measures, three out of five persons who contract tetanus will die.

The best means of controlling tetanus is prevention. In fact, tetanus is nearly 100 percent preventable with active or passive immunization. Active immunization involves stimulating a person's immune system to produce its own antibody to fight off the disease. An injection of tetanus toxoid is given to immunize actively against tetanus. Tetanus toxoid is purified tetanus toxin that has been treated with formaldehyde to be rendered nontoxic (meaning that it will not cause any symptoms of tetanus) but is still capable of stimulating the immune system to produce antitoxin antibody. Active immunization usually lasts a long time, because the cells that make the antibody can keep making more antibody when the first batch runs out or whenever the person comes in contact with tetanus toxin in the future. The tetanus toxoid is usually administered as part of the DPT vaccine. This vaccine protects against diphtheria (D), pertussis (P), and tetanus (T). In the United States, it is recommended that persons be immunized against tetanus at two, four, six, and eighteen months of age, with a booster at four to six years of age and one every ten years after that. Surveys indicate, however, that more than 50 percent of adults over sixty years of age are not protected against tetanus. It is as dangerous to receive too many booster shots for tetanus as it is to receive too few. With too few shots, a person runs the risk of succumbing to the disease and dying. With too many shots, a person runs the risk of developing a potentially fatal allergic reaction to the vaccine. It is best to keep careful records of all vaccinations and to be certain that one receives a tetanus booster every ten years.

Passive immunization involves giving a person antibodies (made in an outside source) that will protect that person from a disease, instead of stimulating the individual to make antibodies. Patients thought to be at risk for tetanus can be given an injection of antitoxin for protection. This type of protection works only for a short period of time, because once the antibody in the injection is used up, the patient cannot make more. The way to immunize infants passively against neonatal tetanus is to immunize their mothers actively. If one immunizes a pregnant patient with tetanus toxoid, that person will produce antitoxin that is passed on to the baby's blood through the placenta. The baby is then born carrying some antitoxin antibodies in its blood that can protect it from neonatal tetanus.

PERSPECTIVE AND PROSPECTS

As early as the fourth century B.C.E., Hippocrates described tetanus as a common killer of women in childbirth, wounded soldiers, and infants. It was not until 1889, however, that the cause of tetanus, *C. tetani*, was first isolated by Shibasaburo Kitasato. In the early 1900's, W. T. Glenny and Gaston Ramon paved the way for the development of a tetanus vaccine by discovering tetanus toxoid. War-related cases of tetanus were virtually eliminated by vaccinating soldiers. During World War II, only 12 cases of tetanus were recorded among 2,735,000 hospital admissions for wounds and injuries in soldiers previously immunized. This result led most state legislatures in America to pass laws requiring adequate immunization for tetanus before entering school.

Despite advances in treatment, the mortality rate for tetanus is quite high. The United States has about one hundred cases per year, mostly in the very young, who are in frequent contact with the soil, or in the very old, who have weakened immune systems. Many cases in the United States arise from trivial but fairly deep injuries that are thought to be too minor to bring to a physician. Sporadic cases are most frequently seen in the South, the Southeast, and the Midwest.

Tetanus is relatively rare in developed countries, where routine immunizations are not only required but also available; it is, however, a common and uncontrolled disease in the developing world. Tetanus is a health problem in developing countries because of the lack of immunization, unsanitary living conditions, and the performance of common wound-causing procedures (such as ear piercing, tattooing, circumcision, and abortion) in an unsanitary manner. Neonatal tetanus is often caused by mothers or midwives who cut the umbilical cord with an unsanitary instrument. In addition, it is a tradition in many developing nations to apply soil, clay, or cow dung to the cut umbilical cord, which can inoculate tetanus spores right into the wound. Throughout the world, 3.5 million children (mostly under five years of age) die yearly of three infectious diseases for which immunization is available. Two million die of measles, 800,000 die of tetanus, 600,000 die of whooping cough, and another 4 million die of various kinds of diarrhea. In parts of some developing nations, 10 percent of deaths within a month of birth are caused by neonatal tetanus. The World Health Organization is making a concerted effort to reduce the incidence of tetanus—especially neonatal tetanus—in developing nations by providing the personnel and resources needed for vaccination. Strategies for reducing the incidence of neonatal tetanus include providing passive immunity to newborns through the immunization of the mothers. Also important are promotion of safe practices, such as clean deliveries and clean cord cutting, and ensuring that unsanitary substances are not applied to cord wounds.

—Vicki J. Isola, Ph.D.

See also Asphyxiation; Bacterial infections; Childhood infectious diseases; Immunization and vaccination; Muscle sprains, spasms, and disorders; Muscles; Paralysis; Seizures; Toxicology; Wounds.

FOR FURTHER INFORMATION:

Centers for Disease Control. "Diphtheria, Tetanus, and Pertussis: Guidelines for Vaccine Prophylaxis and Other Preventive Measures." *Morbidity and Mortality Weekly Report* 34 (1985): 405-426. Describes the different types of vaccines that are used to immunize against tetanus, when to get which type of vaccine, and the side effects associated with each.

Snider, S. "A Responsibility to Remember: Childhood Vaccines." *FDA Consumer* 24 (September 1, 1990): 19-26. A broad overview of all childhood diseases for which a vaccine is available. This article briefly describes each disease and presents the current U.S. recommendations (by state) concerning when to get inoculated.

Traverso, H. P., et al. "A Reassessment of Risk Factors for Neonatal Tetanus." *Bulletin of the World Health Organization* 69, no. 5 (1991): 573-579. A controlled study on the factors associated with the risk of neonatal tetanus in Pakistan. Gives a good introduction to the problem of neonatal tetanus in developing countries.

Worf, Neil. "Tetanus—Still a Problem." *RN* 63, no. 6 (June, 2000): 44-49. Nurses need to recognize the symptoms of tetanus and how to treat it. Despite widespread availability of an effective vaccine, the disease still occurs today and kills a third of reported cases. A continuing education test for nurses on this topic is offered.

Zinsser, Hans. *Zinsser Microbiology.* Edited by Wolfgang K. Joklik et al. 20th ed. Norwalk, Conn.: Appleton and Lange, 1992. An excellent textbook describing all infectious diseases. Chapter 46, "Clostridium," discusses all diseases caused by species of Clostridium, including tetanus, botulism, and gangrene.

THALASSEMIA
DISEASE/DISORDER
ANATOMY OR SYSTEM AFFECTED: Blood

SPECIALTIES AND RELATED FIELDS: Hematology, serology

DEFINITION: Thalassemia is an inherited form of anemia in which red blood cells contain less hemoglobin than normal. Also known as Mediterranean anemia and hereditary leptocytosis, thalassemia is caused by an inadequate production of hemoglobin A. The severity of the disease varies from mild to severe. In mild cases, the individual experiences either no symptoms or mild anemia. As the severity of the thalassemia increases, the symptoms may include fatigue, paleness, breathlessness, irregular heartbeat, bloody urine, jaundice, leg ulcers, and an enlarged spleen. Frequent blood transfusions are necessary in severe cases. Symptoms can be relieved and controlled; however, the life span of patients with thalassemia is often limited to early adulthood or middle age.

—*Jason Georges and Tracy Irons-Georges*
See also Anemia; Blood and blood disorders; Genetic diseases; Hematology; Hematology, pediatric; Transfusion.

FOR FURTHER INFORMATION:

Leavell, Byrd S., and Oscar A. Thorup, Jr. *Fundamentals of Clinical Hematology.* 5th ed. Philadelphia: W. B. Saunders, 1987.

Lee, G. Richard, et al., eds. *Wintrobe's Clinical Hematology.* 10th ed. Vol. 1. Philadelphia: Lea & Febiger, 1999.

Millunsky, Aubrey. *Genetic Disorders of the Fetus: Diagnosis, Prevention, and Treatment.* Baltimore: The Johns Hopkins University Press, 1998.

Pierce, Benjamin A. *The Family Genetic Sourcebook.* New York: John Wiley & Sons, 1990.

THALIDOMIDE
TREATMENT

ANATOMY OR SYSTEM AFFECTED: Arms, blood vessels, feet, hands, immune system, legs

SPECIALTIES AND RELATED FIELDS: Immunology, oncology

DEFINITION: A drug that previously had been used as a sedative and which then was banned for many years because of its severe effects on the developing fetus, but is now finding application in the treatment of leprosy and different cancers.

INDICATIONS AND PROCEDURES

In 1961, a link was established between the use of thalidomide, a mild sedative, and an increase in the frequency of severe defects in newborn babies in Germany, Great Britain, and other countries around the world where the drug had been in use. The "thalidomide babies" had minor defects of the fingers or toes but had major malformations of the limbs, resulting in incomplete or even missing arms and legs.

The defects resembled those of a rare genetic disorder known as phocomelia ("seal limb"). Following the tragic discovery that thalidomide is a potent teratogen (a substance that causes a birth defect), use of the drug was discontinued.

In recent years, however, it has been discovered that thalidomide may be a useful therapeutic agent in a number of conditions including leprosy, several other dermatologic disorders, different types of cancer, and acquired immunodeficiency syndrome (AIDS). The Food and Drug Administration in the United States has approved thalidomide for use in the treatment of leprosy. Studies have demonstrated that thalidomide can inhibit in vitro angiogenesis, the process of formation of new blood vessels. Since many types of cancers require development of new blood vessels for their continued growth, thalidomide may be especially useful in cases where conventional treatments have ceased to be effective. Its use may be indicated in patients either relapsing after high-dose chemotherapy or who are developing serious side effects and are not able to tolerate additional chemotherapy.

USES AND COMPLICATIONS

Since thalidomide is such a powerful angiogenesis inhibitor, it is being used in disorders requiring antiangiogenic therapy. Successful treatments have been made in cases of ovarian cancer, breast cancer, gastrointestinal carcinoma, renal melanoma, chronic graft-versus-host disease, and multiple myeloma. In some cases, the effectiveness of thalidomide increased when accompanied by other treatments, including immunotherapy, chemotherapy, and surgery.

Thalidomide appears to have few side effects in its new applications, but its return to medical respectability has raised again the specter of "thalidomide babies." Adverse effects noted in a few patients have included lethargy, constipation, and peripheral neuropathy. The potential problems associated with thalidomide causing a new round of severe birth defects may be a more serious consequence.

PERSPECTIVE AND PROSPECTS

The outbreak of thalidomide-related birth defects in the 1950's and 1960's led to the creation of birth defect surveillance programs in many countries. Unfortunately, medical standards and safeguards are not uniformly good, and there already appears to be an increase in birth defects associated with the new applications of thalidomide in South America. It will be necessary to regulate and to monitor closely the prescription, dispensing, and use of the drug. Counseling of patients of childbearing age will be an especially critical component if the tragedy of thalidomide's history is not to be repeated.

—Donald J. Nash, Ph.D.

See also Birth defects; Cancer; Leprosy; Pharmacology; Pregnancy and gestation.

FOR FURTHER INFORMATION:

Patrias, Karen, Ronald L. Gordner, and Stephen C. Groft. *Thalidomide: Potential Benefits and Risks, January, 1963, Through July, 1997, 1495 Citations.* Bethesda, Md.: U.S. Department of Health and Human Services, 1998.

THORACIC SURGERY
SPECIALTY

ANATOMY OR SYSTEM AFFECTED: Chest, heart, lungs, respiratory system

SPECIALTIES AND RELATED FIELDS: Cardiology, general surgery, pulmonary medicine

DEFINITION: The branch of surgery that treats diseases of the chest cavity, especially the heart.

KEY TERMS:

aneurysm: a weakened segment of a heart or blood vessel

balloon catheterization: the use of a balloonlike device on the tip of a catheter to widen blood vessels

cardiac catheterization: the guidance of a catheter into the heart or great blood vessels to measure function, assess problems, and identify solutions

computed tomography (CT) scanning: the use of X-ray computer technology to identify diseases of hard and soft tissues, such as bone and the heart

echocardiography: the use of sound waves to examine heart structures

mitral valve: the valve between the heart's left auricle and ventricle

stenosis: the narrowing of heart valves or blood vessels

SCIENCE AND PROFESSION

The chest, or thorax, lies between the neck and the abdomen, from which it is separated by the diaphragm. Its side boundaries are the ribs and the muscle that surrounds them, which are attached to the spine and breastbone (sternum) in the back and front of the body, respectively. Overall, the thorax is cone-shaped, with its small and large ends bounded by the neck and diaphragm. Inside this airtight cavity, the lungs are suspended on the right and left sides, covered by the membranous pleura. Between the lungs is the heart, with its covering, the pericardium.

Also located in the chest cavity are the trachea (windpipe), which leads to the lungs; the esophagus, which connects the mouth and stomach; the major blood vessels that enter and leave the heart; and nerves. The chest cavity inflates and deflates as a result of diaphragm and rib muscle movement. This action provides the entry of oxygen to the blood that is circulated around the body through the cardiovascular system.

Thoracic surgeons, sometimes called cardiothoracic/cardiovascular and thoracic surgeons, handle a wide variety of surgery associated with these organs. Preeminent in many cases is surgery of the heart and major blood vessels. This precise, exacting surgery requires residency training of six years in general surgery and three years in thoracic surgery. In the United States, thoracic surgeons are certified by the American Board of Surgery and the American Board of Thoracic Surgery. Much of the time of thoracic surgeons is spent in hospitals working with critically ill patients whose lives depend on the prompt use of technical and demanding surgical techniques. Most patients are aged fifty-five to sixty-five.

DIAGNOSTIC AND TREATMENT TECHNIQUES

The diagnostic techniques associated with thoracic surgery are highly refined. They include careful patient histories, laboratory tests, and noninvasive techniques such as echocardiography, computed tomography (CT) scanning, electrocardiography (ECG or EKG), and other types of electrophysiology. Invasive procedures include cardiac catheterization and cineangiography of the heart and surrounding blood vessels with fiber-optic devices. Hence, cardiothoracic surgeons require extensive technical backup and wide expertise. After quick, careful assessment of all information obtained, surgery is carried out. Thoracic surgeons are noted for great surgical dexterity, scientific expertise, and logical, stepwise development of a complete picture that enables them to arrive rapidly at sensible decisions before and during surgery.

Entering the chest cavity, thoracotomy, is required for all thoracic surgery. Patients are given a general anesthetic and concurrently have heart and lung function replaced by a heart-lung machine, which oxygenates the blood and pumps it through the cardiovascular system.

Anterior thoracotomy is used to gain access to the heart and its coronary arteries. First, a vertical incision is made from between the collarbone to the lower end of the sternum, to which the ribs are attached. The sternum is divided with a bone saw and pried apart to expose the surgical area. After surgery, a drain is inserted into the chest, the sternum is wired together, and the muscle and skin are closed.

Lateral thoracotomy uses curved incisions made from between the shoulder blades and around the side of the trunk to just below a nipple. It provides access to the lungs and the great blood vessels. This technique is used by thoracic surgeons, general surgeons, and other specialists who perform lung surgery. After the incision is complete, the ribs are spread apart and surgery is performed. Closure is as with the anterior procedure.

Many different thoracic surgery procedures are carried out on heart and great blood vessels when medical and dietary treatments fail or in cases of congenital and traumatic problems. They can be divided into valve replacement, artery surgery, and heart transplantation. Once, bypass surgery was a major aspect of cardiothoracic surgery. Today, it has been largely replaced by balloon catheterization and related techniques carried out by other specialists.

Three types of important cardiothoracic surgery are heart valve replacement, aneurysm resection, and heart transplantation. Heart valve replacement may be necessitated by severe mitral valve damage, which causes mitral insufficiency or stenosis that can lead to heart failure and death. Aneurysms are weakened portions of the heart or great blood vessels. Heart aneurysms are caused by myocardial infarction (the death of parts of the heart muscle), yielding areas of weak, noncontractile scar tissue. Vessel aneurysms are caused by atherosclerosis or infectious disease. In extreme cases, aneurysms can rupture, and they are always painful and/or life-threatening. They are repaired by resection and replacement with graft materials such as Dacron or Teflon appliances. In the most severe cardiac problems, whole heart transplantation is needed using cadaver hearts. When this is not possible but the heart must be aided, ventricular assist pumps and artificial hearts can be connected temporarily.

PERSPECTIVE AND PROSPECTS

Thoracic surgery was first successful in the United States in the early twentieth century. Development of the New York Thoracic Surgical Society in 1917 began its acceptance as a medical specialty. In the 1930's, the *Journal of Thoracic Surgery* started to describe the area, and treatment methods evolved rapidly. Much impetus came from thoracic injuries that occurred during World War II. By the late 1940's, a Board of Thoracic Surgery was affiliated with the American Board of Surgery. In 1971, it became the independent American Board of Thoracic Surgery, which certifies thoracic surgeons. There are several thousand board-certified thoracic surgeons.

Some firsts in this field were the relief of mitral stenosis, by Elliott Cutler (1923); surgical intervention for cardiac aneurysm, by Ernst Sauerbruch (1931); the successful ligation of an arterial duct, by Robert Gross (1939); the development of a heart-lung machine for humans, by John Gibbon (1954); and the relief of congenital pulmonary defects, by Alfred Blalock (1954).

In current thoracic surgery, the treatment of coronary artery disease, once restricted to surgical bypass, has largely been replaced by techniques performed by cardiologists. Nevertheless, thoracic surgical procedures continue to improve, and the development of ever-better diagnostic tools and appliances is expected, such as a satisfactory artificial heart.

—*Sanford S. Singer, Ph.D.*

See also Aneurysmectomy; Aneurysms; Bypass surgery; Cardiology; Cardiology, pediatric; Chest; Congenital heart disease; Heart; Heart disease; Heart transplantation; Heart valve replacement; Lung surgery; Lungs; Mitral valve prolapse; Pulmonary medicine; Pulmonary medicine, pediatric.

FOR FURTHER INFORMATION:
Berkow, Robert, and Andrew J. Fletcher, eds. *The Merck Manual of Diagnosis and Therapy.* 17th ed. Rahway, N.J.: Merck Sharp & Dohme Research Laboratories, 1999. This is a reference work for physicians, and the nomenclature can be daunting. It is best consulted after more general introductory reading.

Taylor, Anita D. *How to Choose a Medical Specialty.* 4th ed. Philadelphia: W. B. Saunders, 1999. Gives a useful description of many medical specialties. Included are information on residency and certification and on the economics of various types of practice, a personal suitability self-examination, and references.

Way, Lawrence W., ed. *Current Surgical Diagnosis and Treatment.* 11th ed. Norwalk, Conn.: Appleton and Lange, 1998. A reference work on general surgery for physicians, this tome is nevertheless comprehensible to laypersons familiar with medical terminology. Presents succinct overviews of the stoma procedures and their potential complications; contains finely detailed illustrations.

THROAT, SORE. *See* SORE THROAT.

THROMBOLYTIC THERAPY AND TPA
PROCEDURE

ANATOMY OR SYSTEM AFFECTED: Blood, blood vessels, circulatory system, heart, lungs, nervous system, respiratory system

SPECIALTIES AND RELATED FIELDS: Cardiology, critical care, emergency medicine, hematology, pharmacology, pulmonary medicine, vascular medicine

DEFINITION: The use of drugs to dissolve blood clots blocking an artery or vein (often in the heart, lungs, or brain); TPA is one of the best thrombolytic agents and is frequently administered to patients experiencing heart attacks.

KEY TERMS:

embolism: the blockage of an artery by matter (such as a blood clot) that has broken off from another area

fibrinolysis: the breakdown of fibrin, a major component of blood clots, that occurs after the broken vessel wall has healed; fibrinolytic agents are used to dissolve unwanted clots

hemostasis: a physiological response that arrests bleeding; involves the constriction of the injured blood vessel, the clumping of platelets to form a plug, and the activation of blood-clotting elements such as fibrin

occlusion: the blockage of any vessel in the body, which may be caused by a thrombus or other embolus

plasmin: an enzyme present in the blood that can dissolve clots; plasmin is normally found in its inactive form, plasminogen, until needed

platelets: specialized blood-clotting particles that travel in the blood and become sticky when they come in contact with a damaged blood vessel

thromboembolism: the blockage of a blood vessel by a fragment that has broken off from a thrombus in another blood vessel

thrombolytic drugs: a group of drugs that dissolve blood clots by increasing the level of plasmin in the blood

thrombus: a blood clot that has formed inside an intact blood vessel; a thrombus can be life-threatening if it occludes a vessel that supplies the heart or brain

tissue plasminogen activator (TPA or tPA): a substance produced by the body to prevent abnormal blood clots by stimulating the formation of plasmin from plasminogen; can also be administered to dissolve blood clots

THE PHYSIOLOGY OF BLOOD CLOT FORMATION
In an undamaged, healthy blood vessel, blood flows smoothly past the lining of the vessel wall. If a blood vessel wall breaks or there is damage to its lining, however, a complex series of biochemical reactions occurs to stop the flow of blood. The blood vessel spasms (vascular spasm), platelets in the bloodstream clump together to form a plug, and proteins form to cause the blood to clot (coagulate). This process is rapid, localized to the area of injury, and carefully controlled. It involves many clotting factors normally present in blood, as well as specialized clotting particles called platelets and some substances that are released by the injured tissues.

The most immediate response to a blood vessel injury is vasoconstriction, a narrowing of a blood vessel. Vasoconstriction decreases the diameter of a vessel, resulting in a decreased flow of blood at the site of damage. Some factors that cause vascular spasm include direct injury, chemicals released by the cells that line a vessel wall, platelets, and nervous reflexes. When the cells that line the interior wall of a blood vessel are damaged, platelets are attracted to the site. They then swell and become sticky. The platelets adhere to the damaged area and release chemicals called prostaglandins, which attract more platelets to the area. Aspirin, in relatively low doses, is an effective inhibitor of prostaglandin synthesis and therefore an excellent therapy for some individuals who are susceptible to inappropriate blood clotting. The vascular spasm and platelet plug help to stop the bleeding at the injury site. Blood-clotting proteins must be activated, however, in order to seal the damaged area of the blood vessel completely.

Once the platelet plug is formed, coagulation is triggered. Several clotting proteins are produced by the liver and released in their inactive form to the blood. Bacteria within the intestinal tract are responsible for synthesizing vitamin K, which is essential for normal production of the clotting proteins by the liver. Vitamin K is absorbed by intestinal blood vessels and transported to the liver.

The mechanism by which clotting proteins are activated is called a cascade. First, a substance called prothrombin activator is formed. Prothrombin activator converts a protein in the plasma called prothrombin into thrombin, which in turn converts another plasma protein, fibrinogen, into fibrin. Fibrin molecules then combine to form a loose meshwork that fills in the gaps between the cells of the platelet plug, preventing blood loss at the site of injury.

A clot is not meant to be a permanent solution. If the clot completely occludes, or stops the flow of blood to, a tissue, the tissue may die. A process called fibrinolysis removes clots that are no longer needed. Because small clots are continually formed in vessels throughout the body, clot dissolution is essential to reestablishing normal blood flow. Without fibrinolysis, blood vessels would gradually become completely occluded.

One essential component of this natural clot-reducing process is the enzyme plasmin, which is produced when the blood protein plasminogen is activated. A large amount of plasminogen, which binds to fibrin, is incorporated into a blood clot. The plasminogen remains inactive until it receives appropriate signals. Healing of the blood vessel and surrounding tissues will cause the release of a substance called tissue plasminogen activator (TPA or tPA). TPA then converts the plasminogen in the clot to plasmin. It is plasmin that breaks down the fibrin, and thus the clot, through fibrinolysis. Enzymes will quickly destroy any plasmin that escapes into the general circulation. Therefore, most of the fibrinolytic effect of plasmin occurs within the clot itself.

It is important to note that once a clot begins to form, something must limit its growth. A clot that is allowed to grow uncontrollably would eventually fill up all the vessels in the body. Several factors regulate the extent of clot formation. Any tendency toward clot formation in rapidly moving blood is usually unsuccessful because the activated coagulation factors are diluted and washed away, preventing them from accumulating to a concentration necessary for clotting. The second mechanism restricting clot formation is that as a clot forms, almost all the thrombin produced is absorbed into the fibrin. Therefore, fibrin effectively acts as an anticoagulant to prevent enlargement of the clot by holding onto thrombin so that it cannot act elsewhere. Any thrombin that escapes is bound by a substance in the blood called antithrombin III. Antithrombin III can be activated by a substance called heparin, a natural anticoagulant produced by some white blood cells and other undamaged cells that line blood vessels. Heparin acts to inhibit thrombin activity, and thus clotting, by stimulating antithrombin III.

Additional factors prevent clotting in undamaged blood vessels. The factors that normally ward off unnecessary clotting include both structural and chemical characteristics of the lining of blood vessels. As long as the cells lining the vessels remain undamaged, there is no vasospasm, no platelet plug forms, and no clot results. The cells on the wall lining can repel platelets using specialized chemicals on their surfaces. They also secrete heparin and a substance known as prostacyclin, both of which prevent platelet activation.

Despite the body's protective mechanisms to prevent inappropriate blood clots, clotting sometimes does occur. A clot that forms in an undamaged vessel is called a thrombus. If the thrombus is large, it may block blood flow to the tissue beyond the occlusion and starve the tissue to death. This starvation process is called ischemia, and the result is infarction, or cell death. A relatively common site for a thrombus to occlude a vessel is in the heart. If the blockage occurs in a coronary artery, a vessel that supplies the heart with blood, the consequences may be death of this tissue and even death of the affected individual.

A thrombus (or any other type of matter, such as lipids) that breaks away from a vessel and floats freely in the bloodstream is called an embolus. An embolus becomes a problem if it enters a blood vessel that is too narrow for it to pass through. For example, emboli that become trapped in a blood vessel going to the lungs can significantly alter an individual's ability to obtain oxygen. An embolus that occludes a vessel feeding the brain will cause a stroke.

What would cause a clot to form in the body when there is no trauma to a vessel? Several factors are known to cause clot formation even when there is no bleeding. Anything that causes the lining of a blood vessel to become roughened or irregular will allow platelets to gain a foothold and cling to the vessel wall, starting the clotting process.

Arteriosclerosis, in which there is an abnormal accumulation of fatty plaques in the wall of an artery, and blood vessel inflammation are the most common causes of irregularities in the lining of blood vessels.

Anything that causes the flow of blood to slow and pool enhances clot formation. In this case, clotting factors are not washed away and diluted, so they tend to accumulate until their concentrations are high enough to initiate clotting. Conditions in which this may occur include atrial fibrillation, aneurysms, and varicose veins. Atrial fibrillation is the abnormally rapid beating of the upper chambers (atria) of the heart. Because the contractions that normally force blood into the lower chambers (ventricles) are ineffi-cient, blood pools and clots may form. Aneurysms occur when there is a weakening of an artery wall. This causes the blood vessel wall to bulge out and form a pocket where blood can pool. Thus, aneurysms provide a potential site for inappropriate clotting. Varicose veins are relatively common and usually oc-cur in the veins returning blood from the legs. When the valves in a vein weaken, the flow of returning blood slows and the vein swells. As a result, clotting factors may accumulate in the vein and be returned to the heart or forced into the lungs.

INDICATIONS AND PROCEDURES

If inappropriate clotting occurs in blood vessels sup-plying critical tissues, such as the brain, heart, lungs, or kidneys, the resulting tissue damage can be debili-tating or even life-threatening. Fortunately, physicians have a few options in treating patients with clotting problems.

A blood clot in the arteries supplying oxygen and nutrients to the heart can cause numerous symptoms. Sudden pain, pressure, squeezing, and fullness in the chest that last longer than fifteen minutes may indi-cate a heart attack. The pain may be excruciating; it may also be mild, resembling heartburn or indiges-tion. In general, the elderly tend to have less pain during a heart attack. Heart attack pain does not go away with rest and may radiate across the chest to the shoulders (usually on the left side), neck, arms, jaw, or even the middle of the back. Because the pumping mechanism and efficiency of the heart have been im-paired, patients often feel dizzy or light-headed. They may even faint, become nauseated or vomit, have dif-ficulty breathing, or begin to sweat.

A number of drugs are used to prevent undesirable clotting in persons at risk for a heart attack. Aspirin is a common drug whose action blocks the production of chemicals called prostaglandins, which cause plate-lets to adhere to one another. Heparin helps to prevent clot formation. Warfarin is a drug that interferes with

the action of vitamin K in the formation of clotting proteins. If a clot has already formed, some drugs are available that will dissolve clots, including TPA, streptokinase, and urokinase. These drugs are known as thrombolytic agents and are often administered in an emergency room to people experiencing heart at-tacks.

The time period for which thrombolytic agents are effective is relatively brief; the sooner these drugs are given, the greater is the benefit. In order to be effec-tive, these potent drugs must be given before irrevers-ible damage occurs. For heart attack victims, this means within six hours after the onset of symptoms. Most studies indicate that thrombolytic therapy can be given safely and effectively before heart attack victims reach the emergency room and that early treatment reduces the likelihood of death. Therefore, it is important for individuals to contact a physician or emergency medical team promptly after experienc-ing suspicious symptoms that may indicate a heart attack.

USES AND COMPLICATIONS

Most patients who are thought to be experiencing a heart attack are given TPA or streptokinase intrave-nously to reverse or at least halt damage. Like all drugs, however, the thrombolytic agents have poten-tially adverse effects. Because these medications can increase bleeding, patients are not given thrombolytic therapy if they are at high risk for hemorrhage (ab-normal bleeding). Some of the factors that may in-crease the risk of bleeding include surgery within the past six weeks, severe hypertension, diabetic eye dis-ease, recent head trauma, recent stroke, stomach or duodenal ulcers, or recent cardiopulmonary resuscita-tion.

If the thrombolytic drug is administered and bleed-ing becomes a significant problem, a drug called aminocaproic acid can be used to help correct the problem. Aminocaproic acid inhibits the thrombolytic effects of TPA, streptokinase, and urokinase by pre-venting their action and inhibiting plasmin. In life-threatening situations, the physician may have to give the patient blood transfusions or fibrinogen infusions to reverse the effects of thrombolysis. The adverse ef-fects of thrombolytic agents are relatively rare, how-ever, and should not discourage physicians from the appropriate use of these agents.

Thrombolytic therapy is used in nearly 300,000 patients in the United States each year. Tissue plasminogen activator is the fastest-acting thrombolytic agent. It is produced naturally in the body but can be manufactured in large amounts using genetic engineering techniques. Streptokinase, on the other hand, is produced by bacteria and at about one-tenth the cost of TPA. When these two thrombolytic agents were compared in 41,000 heart attack patients, TPA showed a slightly better effectiveness. In a one-month follow-up study, researchers found that there were 14 percent fewer deaths among heart attack patients given TPA and intravenous heparin (to help keep blood clots from reforming) than among heart attack patients treated with streptokinase and heparin.

In addition to their use as therapeutic agents for heart attacks, thrombolytic drugs are also used to treat abnormal blood clots in the blood vessels of the lungs. These clots, known as pulmonary emboli, usually originate in a leg vein, a condition called venous thrombosis. Part or all of the thrombus breaks away, forms an embolus, and travels to the heart, which then pumps it into the pulmonary arteries. If the embolus is large enough to block the main pulmonary artery leading from the heart to the lungs, or if there are many clots, the condition can be life-threatening. Pulmonary embolism is responsible for more than 50,000 deaths in the United States each year.

The symptoms that a patient may experience depend on the size of the obstructing clot. If an embolus is so large that it blocks the main pulmonary artery, an affected individual will die. Smaller emboli may cause severe shortness of breath, rapid heart rate, dizziness, sharp chest pains when breathing, and coughing up of blood.

Physicians treat pulmonary emboli with similar medical therapy as that used for heart attacks. Anticoagulant drugs such as heparin and warfarin are usually administered to reduce the clotting ability of the blood and to reduce the chance of more clots occurring. Thrombolytic agents, including urokinase and streptokinase, can also be used to destroy the clot in much the same way that they are used in heart attack victims.

The third major use of thrombolytic agents is to clear intravenous catheters of blood clots. A catheter may be placed into a person's vein if health care workers need to draw frequent blood samples or administer drugs at frequent intervals. Because the catheter is in direct contact with the blood, it is a site for potential clot formation. Urokinase can be used to reopen an occluded catheter.

Perspective and Prospects

Each year, 1.5 million Americans experience a heart attack. An attack lasts longer than most people realize. It is actually a four-to-six-hour process that starts when one of the arteries supplying the heart muscle becomes blocked, usually by a blood clot. The pain that one experiences is partially attributable to a cramping of the heart muscle from lack of oxygen and an accumulation of waste products. As a result, heart muscle is destroyed, which interferes with the heart's function. If the amount of muscle destruction is severe, it can lead to the patient's death.

Studies show that individuals treated within one to two hours of the onset of heart attack symptoms have significantly less heart damage than those treated later. Yet, half of all heart attack patients wait more than two hours before getting medical attention. The American Heart Association estimates that 300,000 Americans die of heart attacks each year before reaching a hospital. This number could be greatly reduced if people responded more quickly to the symptoms of a heart attack.

Recent studies have shown that women are even less likely to receive initial medical care within the required four-to-six-hour time interval. Women frequently see to other responsibilities such as child or elder care before seeking medical help. Many women believe the myth that they are not likely to have a heart attack. This is true before the menopause, but, within five years of the menopause, women have the same risk of heart attacks as men. In addition, physicians are more likely to misdiagnose heart attack symptoms in women, attributing them to anxiety or stress.

The goal in treating a heart attack is to stop it and, if possible, reverse the clotting process. Treatment with thrombolytic agents helps to minimize or even reverse the damage to heart tissue. As with most diseases, however, it is better to prevent heart attacks entirely. Individuals who exercise regularly, who eat a diet relatively low in fat, and who do not smoke have a low incidence of heart attacks and may never need drug therapy to unclog their arteries. Yet, it is comforting to know that these agents are available if the need ever arises.

Because of the success of thrombolytic agents in the treatment of coronary artery disease, these agents are also being tried in patients showing early symptoms of stroke. Strokes and heart attacks occur for similar reasons. In a stroke, blood clots in the arteries that supply the brain prevent the delivery of oxygen and nutrients to the sensitive nerve cells and cause an accumulation of waste products. As a result, these sensitive brain cells die. As in heart attack treatment, timing is critical. In heart attack patients, agents that dissolve clots work best when given within six hours after the onset of symptoms. For stroke patients, it appears that treatment with a thrombolytic drug must begin within three hours to have maximal effectiveness. Therefore, awareness of the early symptoms of stroke is even more important. These symptoms develop rapidly and depend on the region of the brain that is damaged. Some common symptoms include muscle weakness, loss of touch sensations, speech disturbances, and visual disturbances.

If thrombolytic agents are found to be effective in treating strokes, up to 80 percent of all stroke victims may be helped. As with heart attack patients, these drugs cannot be used in stroke patients with hemorrhagic (bleeding) strokes or other disorders in which the risk of bleeding is greater than the potential benefits from such therapy.

—Matthew Berria, Ph.D.;
updated by L. Fleming Fallon, Jr.,
M.D., Ph.D., M.P.H.

See also Angiography; Angioplasty; Arteriosclerosis; Bleeding; Blood and blood disorders; Brain; Bypass surgery; Cardiology; Catheterization; Circulation; Embolism; Emergency medicine; Endarterectomy; Enzymes; Heart; Heart attack; Heart disease; Heart valve replacement; Hematology; Ischemia; Lungs; Pharmacology; Pulmonary medicine; Strokes; Thrombosis and thrombus; Varicosis; Vascular medicine; Vascular system.

FOR FURTHER INFORMATION:

Becker, Richard C., ed. *Textbook of Coronary Thrombosis and Thrombolysis: Developments in Cardiovascular Medicine.* Amsterdam: Kluwer Academic, 1997. This is an excellent and well-written book. It uses technical language but can be understood by nonmedical readers. Part 4 focuses on thrombolytic agents.

Clayman, Charles B., ed. *The American Medical Association Encyclopedia of Medicine.* New York: Random House, 1994. This encyclopedia lists, in alphabetical order, medical terms, diseases, and medical procedures. It does an excellent job of explaining rather complex medical subjects for nonprofessional audiences.

Hales, Dianne, and Barbara Sayad. *An Invitation to Health: The Power of Prevention.* 8th ed. Redwood City, Calif.: Brooks/Cole, 1999. This book is recommended for anyone who wishes an overview of health topics. Several chapters deal with the function of the heart and how lifestyles influence its health. Chapter 17, which covers cardiovascular disease, includes a description of thrombolytic and surgical therapy modalities for helping heart attack patients.

Katzung, Bertram G. *Basic and Clinical Pharmacology.* 8th ed. Norwalk, Conn.: Appleton & Lange, 2001. This well-written text provides detailed information about thrombolytic and anticoagulant agents. It discusses usage of these drugs, as well as their adverse effects and contraindications.

McCance, Kathryn L., Sue E. Huether, and Clayton Parkinson. *Pathophysiology: The Biological Basis for Disease in Adults and Children.* 3d ed. St. Louis: C. V. Mosby/Year Book, 1997. This book contains a comprehensive presentation of diseases, symptoms, and treatments. The authors have done an excellent job of tying together basic physiological principles with the pathology of various organ systems.

Spence, Alexander P., and Elliott B. Mason. *Human Anatomy and Physiology.* 4th ed. St. Paul, Minn.: West, 1992. An introductory text that describes the structure and function of the human body. In chapter 18, the authors detail blood-clotting mechanisms and the dissolution of clots after blood vessel repair.

Verstrate, M., Valentin Fuster, and Eric Topol. *Cardiovascular Thrombosis: Thrombocardiology and Thromboneurology.* 2d ed. Philadelphia: Lippincott-Raven, 198. This book contains the very latest information concerning thrombolytic agents.

THROMBOSIS AND THROMBUS
DISEASE/DISORDER

ANATOMY OR SYSTEM AFFECTED: Blood, blood vessels, brain, circulatory system, head, heart, lungs, respiratory system

SPECIALTIES AND RELATED FIELDS: Cardiology, hematology, internal medicine, vascular medicine

DEFINITION: Thrombosis is an abnormal blood condition in which blood cells called thrombocytes (platelets) produce clots that move through the bloodstream and eventually clog blood vessels; a thrombus is such a clot.

Key terms:

artery: a blood vessel which transports blood away from the heart to the cells and tissues of the body

clot: a clumping of platelets, blood, fibrin, and clotting factors that normally accumulates in damaged tissue as part of the body's healing process

embolus: an object, air bubble, or other material moving through the bloodstream that is capable of creating a blockage to circulation

fibrin: a critical protein produced by platelets during the clotting process in bleeding, damaged tissue; the fibrin seals openings in damaged blood vessels

myocardial infarction: a condition in which the blood and oxygen supply to the cells of the heart muscle is cut off, thereby causing heart cell death; commonly called a heart attack

shock: a situation in which the body or a region of the body is not receiving an adequate supply of blood and oxygen, thereby leading to collapse of the organism

thrombocytes: white blood cells that secrete the proteins thrombin and fibrin in response to chemical signals from damaged tissue in the body; also called platelets

thrombus: an abnormal clumping of platelets and platelet proteins that moves through the bloodstream and may act as an embolus to block circulation through key arteries

vein: a blood vessel which returns blood to the heart from various regions of the body

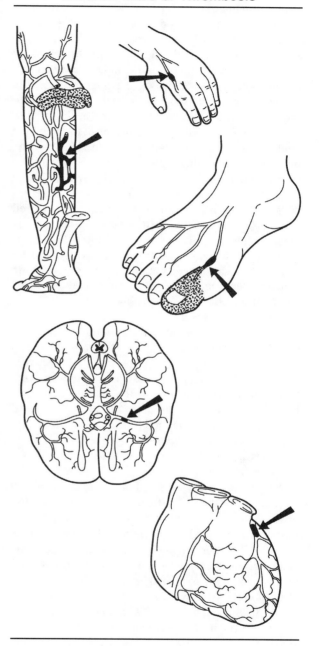

Common Sites of Thrombosis

Causes and Symptoms

Clotting is a critical process in the maintenance of damaged bodily tissue and the prevention of blood loss leading to conditions of shock within the organism. Shock involves the disorientation and collapse of major organ systems within the body when excessive blood has been lost; it can be fatal if it is not treated immediately.

When the body is damaged from a cut or other breach of the body's epithelial and connective tissue defense layers in the skin, chemical signals called chemoattractants stimulate a white blood cell type called a thrombocyte to secrete proteins, leading to the sealing of the damaged tissue region. Thrombocytes, also called platelets, are versatile cells floating in the approximately 10 to 12 liters of blood flowing through roughly 100,000 kilometers of blood vessels within the average human body. There are roughly five hundred thousand thrombocytes per cubic millimeter of blood. Their clotting response to tissue damage is rapid and efficient, although very intricate in the chemical signaling between cells.

Once activated by alarmones, emergency chemical-signaling hormones released from the damaged tissue, the thrombocytes are activated to respond at the site of tissue damage. Each thrombocyte releases the proteins thrombin and fibrinogen. The thrombin modifies the fibrinogen to produce fibrin, the principal sealant protein for the damaged region. The fibrin is secreted massively from thousands of thrombocytes within only a few minutes of the initial tissue damage. Fibrin protein is put down by the cells in intricately connected layers from the outer edges of the cut progressively inward, eventually forming a plug.

Following the sealing of the damaged tissue by the clotting thrombocytes, other white blood cells of the immune system called leukocytes move into the region to immobilize and destroy contaminating bacteria and viruses, as well as to break down damaged cells. Surrounding healthy cells initiate mitotic cell divisions to grow into the damaged region, thereby regenerating the missing tissue. White blood cells such as leukocytes and thrombocytes are termed "white" because they do not produce hemoglobin and hence are not "red." The two white blood cell types work intricately in the maintenance of body tissue primary defense layers.

When the clotting process of thrombocytes and other related cells does not occur properly, problems can arise. Normally, a clot will form at a breach in a blood vessel, whether that vessel is an artery carrying blood away from the heart to the body or a vein returning blood to the heart from the body. Abnormal clotting of thrombocytes and fibrin proteins, however, can form masses that break off from a blood clot and float through the bloodstream. Such a floating blood clot is called a thrombus.

A thrombus is a type of embolism, an object which floats through the bloodstream and which can cause a blockage in small arteries, veins, and capillaries. Emboli can be pockets of air or solid clots such as thrombi. Both air emboli and thrombus emboli can cause serious blockages of important vessels supplying blood to particular body regions. As a thrombus or other embolus flows along with blood, it will eventually float through a vessel which becomes progressively smaller in diameter. The thrombus blocks the vessel so that nothing can pass any further through it—not the thrombus, not blood, and not the oxygen and nutrients within the blood.

As a result, cells downstream from the blockage will be starved for essential oxygen, sugar, and other nutrients necessary for carrying out the cellular chemical reactions of life. Most cells have only about a ten-minute supply of chemical and oxygen reserves needed

for life. These cells depend on a continuous supply of blood to provide oxygen, sugar, and other nutrients and to carry away carbon dioxide and other waste products. The blood clot occludes the artery going to a cell region, thereby preventing blood flow and causing the death of these cells. In many parts of the body, these dead cells cannot be replaced, particularly within the heart, brain, and spinal cord.

The existence of thrombi within the circulatory system is a serious medical condition known as thrombosis. The five principal types of thrombi are agonal, ball, hyaline, laminated, and white thrombi. An agonal thrombus is a type of blood clot which forms from clumping blood cells when a person is dying. A ball thrombus is a spherically shaped blood clot composed of platelets, red blood cells, and fibrin. A hyaline thrombus is a mass of depigmented, hemoglobinless, clumped red blood cells. A laminated thrombus is an array of clumped cell types accumulated at differing times, creating a snowball effect. A white thrombus is a clump of leukocytes of varying types. Regardless of type, all thrombi can seriously impede efficient blood flow and thereby contribute to localized cellular and tissue death, damage that is often irreparable.

Two of the most serious cases of localized cellular and tissue death brought about by thrombi are myocardial infarctions and strokes. A myocardial infarction, also called a heart attack, occurs when the muscular layer of cells within the heart (the myocardium) is starved for oxygen and nutrients, and dies, because of a blockage to one of the branches of the coronary arteries supplying blood to the heart. If only a small branch of the coronary artery is blocked by a thrombus or other occlusion, then only a few hundreds of myocardial cells will die and the heart attack will be mild.

If the thrombus blockage is to a major coronary artery, however, then many thousands of cells in the myocardium will die, and a major heart attack will occur. It should be emphasized that the death of myocardial cells is permanent; they cannot be replaced. Therefore, a thrombus-induced heart attack causes permanent death of a region of heart muscle, whether large or small. In many cases, the heart attack is so severe that the normal, rhythmic contraction of the heart is disrupted, thereby leading to cardiac arrest and death.

In the same manner, a stroke, also called a cerebrovascular accident, occurs when an artery transporting blood to a region of brain cells is blocked by a thrombus or other embolus. Brain cells downstream from the blockage are starved for oxygen and nutrients; they die within minutes. If a small artery or capillary is blocked, only a few brain cells will die and the stroke will be minimal, perhaps not even noticeable to the individual. It is possible that many people have such "microstrokes" repeatedly during the course of their lives, although the effects of these small strokes are cumulative over time. Decreased and impaired neurological and motor functioning throughout the body ensue from damaged brain regions in stroke victims.

If the thrombus-induced blockage is to an artery supplying blood to a large brain cell region, however, then millions of brain cells will die. The stroke is severe, perhaps deadly, if the affected brain region is essential for certain bodily life processes. If the severe stroke victim survives, then the effects will be noticeable as sluggish neuromuscular motor activity on the opposite side of the body from the affected brain region. Heart attacks and strokes are manifestations of the same problem: arteries occluded by thrombi and other emboli.

TREATMENT AND THERAPY

Thrombosis is a problem of major concern for the physician facing patients with certain types of medical conditions and patients who recently have had major internal surgery. Furthermore, individuals with blood-clotting abnormalities, compromised immune systems, and bone marrow abnormalities also are prone to forming thrombi and other solid emboli. Phlebitis is an inflammation of a vein brought about by surgery or prolonged confinement to bed in which blood clots form in deep veins. These blood clots can break off and flow through the general blood circulation, eventually clogging an artery or vein leading to a critical bodily region.

Consequently, thrombi and thrombosis are of major concern to medical doctors because they represent potential complications and side effects from other medical conditions and certain needed surgical treatments. People who have had abdominal or pelvic surgery (such as the removal of certain organs such as the spleen and portions of the stomach because of cancer) or individuals who have been bedridden with leg fractures are prone to forming thrombi and emboli.

The elderly are particularly prone to thrombi because of the gradual decline of the immune system and the breakdown of bone development that accompany the aging process. Moreover, the natural chemical substances in the blood which dissolve floating blood clots are not as prevalent in the elderly. As a result, more cases of thrombi are seen in elderly patients, particularly individuals above the age of seventy.

Once thrombi and other solid emboli have formed, they may float for a long time through an individual's blood vessels. They usually can pass through the heart unimpeded without causing any serious disruptions of cardiac rhythm. Occasionally, large thrombi can become lodged in one of the four valves of the heart, creating an occlusion and triggering a heart attack, but this is very rare. More commonly, the thrombi become trapped in the general circulation in progressively smaller arteries and capillaries going to a localized tissue region.

Within the body, oxygenated blood leaves the left ventricle of the heart through the largest artery in the body, the aorta, and subsequently branches and sub-branches through thousands of successively smaller arteries, arterioles, and capillaries until reaching each of the thousand trillion cells of the body. These cells extract oxygen and nutrients from the blood and deposit carbon dioxide and waste products into the bloodstream. Small capillaries combine to produce small venules that combine to produce small veins, which in turn combine into larger veins. These veins eventually come together into the inferior and superior vena cavae, returning blood to the right atrium of the heart for eventual delivery to the lungs. Once in the heart, blood flows from the right atrium to the right ventricle and then through the pulmonary arteries branching to the tissues of the lungs, where the blood is oxygenated through breathing. Oxygenated blood returns to the left atrium of the heart via the pulmonary veins and then flows through the left ventricle to the aorta to make another trip through the body.

Thrombi can flow through this system repeatedly. They usually become caught, however, in the progressively smaller arteries and capillaries transporting blood to the tissues. The resulting blockage and starvation of cells downstream from the blockage leads to the death and decay of the affected tissue region, resulting in a localized tissue infarction. The two most serious types of infarctions are the myocardial infarction and the stroke, but both of these infarctions can be caused by other types of blockages, including arterial rupture and fatty clogging of arteries from the conditions atherosclerosis and arteriosclerosis. Nevertheless, thrombi are a major contributory factor to the occurrences of strokes and heart attacks, two leading killers in the United States and other stressful, technological Western nations. In both strokes and heart attacks, thrombal blockages to key cellular regions lead to localized cellular death. Heart cells and brain cells cannot be regenerated. The tissue death is permanent, and the resulting physiological effects will remain with the victims for the rest of their lives if they survive the stroke or heart attack.

Another serious thrombal blockage can occur in the pulmonary arteries and arterioles transporting blood to lung tissue for oxygenation. Such blockages lead to the localized death of lung tissue and sudden shortness of breath in affected individuals. About 10 percent of cases of pulmonary thrombosis and embolism end in death, resulting in a fatality figure much smaller than the hundreds of thousands of deaths from heart attacks and strokes in the United States each year.

Scuba divers who spend excessive periods of time at great depths and then ascend rapidly are prone to decompression sickness, in which nitrogen bubbles form emboli that create the same blockages as thrombi in localized tissue spaces. Nitrogen bubble emboli can accumulate in the heart, lung, and brain tissue and are fatal if not immediately treated in a decompression chamber.

PERSPECTIVE AND PROSPECTS

Thrombi and thrombosis are serious problems which can arise in any individual, although the likelihood increases with age and the corresponding decline in individuals' immune systems. Care must be taken with various surgical procedures, particularly abdominal and pelvic surgery and the treatment of leg fractures, to reduce the chances of thrombi forming. Any severe cut has the potential to form thrombi, but the status of an individual's immune system is an important factor in determining whether these thrombi are captured and dissipated.

In many surgical procedures, including open heart surgery, physicians and surgeons will administer anticlotting agents to minimize the risk of thrombi forming during and following the surgery and in the recovery phase of the operation. These anticlotting agents are administered intravenously and diffuse throughout the patient's circulatory system so that any thrombi and other blood clots dissolve before they can occlude various tissue regions. Medical doctors are versed in the science of thrombi and thrombosis

because these conditions often are associated with other medical conditions. Physicians are aware of contributory factors to thrombosis and can take action to guard against thrombal occurrence early in the medical treatment process.

—*David Wason Hollar, Jr., Ph.D.*

See also Arteriosclerosis; Blood and blood disorders; Cardiology; Cholesterol; Embolism; Heart; Heart attack; Heart disease; Hyperlipidemia; Hypertension; Ischemia; Phlebitis; Strokes; Varicosis; Vascular medicine; Vascular system; Venous insufficiency.

FOR FURTHER INFORMATION:

Gaudin, Anthony J., and Kenneth C. Jones. *Human Anatomy and Physiology.* New York: Harcourt Brace Jovanovich, 1989. An outstanding introduction to human anatomy and physiology for the biology or health science major. Chapter 12, "The Central Nervous System," includes a discussion of how thrombi and emboli can contribute to stroke.

Memmler, Ruth L., Barbara J. Cohen, and Dena L. Wood. *Memmler's The Human Body in Health and Disease.* 9th ed. Philadelphia: J. B. Lippincott, 2000. This brief book is an excellent introduction to human anatomy and physiology for the layperson. Excellent definitions, descriptions of processes, and illustrations highlight each short chapter. Chapter 14, "The Heart and Heart Disease," discusses the formation of thrombi, their contribution to heart attacks, and anticlotting thrombolytic drugs.

O'Keefe, Michael F., et al. *Brady Emergency Care.* 8th ed. Upper Saddle River, N.J.: Prentice Hall, 1998. A primer in emergency care for the emergency medical technician (EMT) and paramedic. Offers useful information and illustrated procedures for handling various types of life-threatening emergencies, including strokes and heart attacks.

Wistreich, George A., and Max D. Lechtman. *Microbiology.* 5th ed. New York: Macmillan, 1988. This very detailed work is an outstanding introduction to the sciences of microbiology and immunology. Chapter 17, "Introduction to Immune Responses," discusses the role of thrombocytes and thrombin in the normal immune response.

THUMB SUCKING
DEVELOPMENT

ANATOMY OR SYSTEM AFFECTED: Mouth, teeth
SPECIALTIES AND RELATED FIELDS: Dentistry, pediatrics, speech pathology

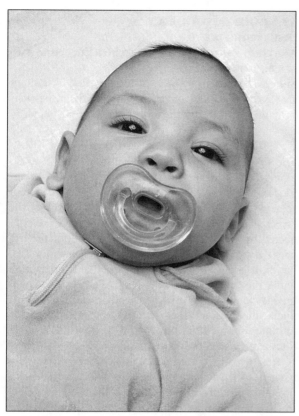

A thumb or pacifier fulfills some infants' strong need for sucking in the early months of life but can become a difficult habit to break. (PhotoDisc)

DEFINITION: A common oral behavior among young children that may cause physical, psychological, and social problems if it is continued past a certain age.

PHYSICAL AND PSYCHOLOGICAL FACTORS

It has been estimated that 45 percent of all two-year-olds, 36 percent of four-year-olds, 21 percent of six-year-olds, and 5 percent of all eleven-year-olds suck their thumbs. As children grow older, by age five, the occurrence of thumb sucking generally begins to fade during the daytime. If children continue to suck their thumbs, it is generally limited to nighttime.

Thumb sucking seems to be reinforcing to children because of its soothing property. For example, it is often observed among children when they are tired, frustrated, hungry, or uncomfortable, such as when teething causes discomfort. Furthermore, thumb sucking tends to increase the level of independence in infants. This becomes evident when observing an infant who is occupied by this self-stimulating behavior.

DISORDERS AND EFFECTS

Although thumb sucking is relatively harmless among children younger than three years of age, problems can develop if the behavior persists. Negative consequences may consist of dental problems, inhibited speech development, and critical peer and negative parental reactions.

One of the main problems associated with thumb sucking is dental problems, especially if this behavior persists after the age of four. Thumb sucking can also inhibit speech development in formal and informal settings at school or day care. For example, when children are sucking their thumbs during formal group activities, they are less likely to respond to adult questions. Also, during free-play time, children who are sucking their thumbs are less likely to speak spontaneously.

In addition to causing problems for speech and physical development, thumb sucking can create social difficulties for children. According to the *Pediatrics* article "Influence of Thumb Sucking on Peer Social Acceptance in First-Grade Children," by P. C. Friman and colleagues, "Social acceptance is lower among children who suck their thumb, and they are viewed by their peers as being less intelligent, happy, attractive, likable, or fun, and less desirable as a friend, playmate, seatmate, classmate, or neighbor." Furthermore, thumb sucking can create negative interactions between the parents and children. Because parents are often troubled by thumb sucking, children are routinely asked to stop. These requests can be positively reinforcing to the child and can increase the frequency of the behavior.

Given the problems associated with thumb sucking, many parents wonder at what point in time a child should be treated for this behavior. In their 1989 article "Thumb Sucking: Pediatricians' Guidelines" in *Clinical Pediatrics*, Friman and B. D. Schmitt provide some guidelines to answer this question. As a simple rule, thumb sucking should not be treated until the potential negative consequences outweigh the benefits, which is seldom before the age of four. When children do suck their thumbs, often it is not frequent enough to warrant treatment. They also point out that at times the potential benefits may outweigh the risks, such as when a child uses thumb sucking as a means of coping with fear, pain, or a significant loss. As suggested by these authors, another indication for treatment is chronic thumb sucking, which they define as occurring "across two or more settings (e.g., home and school) and when it occurs day and night."

PERSPECTIVE AND PROSPECTS

Attitudes toward oral behavior in children have fluctuated over the years. It has been viewed as both indulgent and detrimental. There have been high and low attempts to prohibit the activity. Sigmund Freud and his colleagues did much to draw attention to the oral drive in the first year of life, and over the years many writers have made observations about oral habits and psychological health.

The advent and wide use of pacifiers has done much to neutralize concern over oral behaviors. Pacifiers are generally seen as preferable to the thumb, from a dental perspective. Thumb sucking tends to arouse more anxiety for both parents and medical specialists than does the use of the pacifier.

—*Jay D. Schvaneveldt, Ph.D.*

See also Anxiety; Cognitive development; Dental diseases; Dentistry; Dentistry, pediatric; Developmental stages; Phobias; Psychiatry, child and adolescent; Reflexes, primitive; Separation anxiety; Teeth; Teething; Weaning.

FOR FURTHER INFORMATION:

Friman, P. C., K. M. McPherson, W. J. Warzak, and J. Evans. "Influence of Thumb Sucking on Peer Social Acceptance in First-Grade Children." *Pediatrics* 91, no. 4 (April, 1993): 784-786. The influence of thumb sucking on social acceptance was assessed among forty first-grade children.

Herbert, Martin. *Problems of Childhood: A Complete Guide for All Concerned.* London: Pan Books, 1975. Addresses the emotional problems of children. Includes bibliographical references and an index.

Walker, C. Eugene, and Michael C. Roberts, eds. *Handbook of Clinical Child Psychology.* 3d ed. New York: John Wiley & Sons, 2000. Covers normal and abnormal development, assessment and diagnosis, psychopathology (in three sections encompassing infancy, childhood, and adolescence), and intervention strategies.

Wright, Logan, Arlene B. Schaefer, and Gerald Solomons. *Encyclopedia of Pediatric Psychology.* Baltimore: University Park Press, 1979. Discusses such topics as psychosomatic illnesses, child psychology, and child behavioral disorders. Includes bibliographical references.

THYROID DISORDERS
DISEASE/DISORDER

ANATOMY OR SYSTEM AFFECTED: Endocrine system, glands, neck
SPECIALTIES AND RELATED FIELDS: Endocrinology
DEFINITION: Underactivity (hypothyroidism) or overactivity (hyperthyroidism) of the thyroid gland.

CAUSES AND SYMPTOMS

The thyroid gland normally weighs about 20 to 35 grams and is located in the neck just below the larynx, or voice box. The gland is named for the shield-shaped "thyroid" cartilage that forms the front of the larynx. The thyroid has two lateral lobes that are connected by an isthmus that crosses in front of the trachea. By placing a finger on the trachea below the larynx it is possible to feel the ridgelike isthmus pass under the finger after swallowing. The bilobed (two-lobed) shape of the rest of the gland can be felt just under the skin of the neck on either side of the midline, although its boundaries are normally indistinct except to a trained examiner.

The thyroid produces two major hormones. Thyroxine, a product of the follicular cells, is the major hormone produced by the thyroid that helps regulate metabolism. Within the thyroid are also parafollicular cells that produce calcitonin, an essential hormone in-

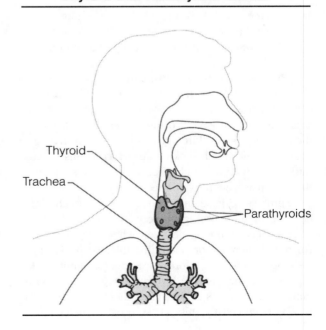

Thyroid and Parathyroid Glands

volved in calcium metabolism. In the tissue of the thyroid are also embedded two pairs of parathyroid glands. The parathyroid glands produce parathyroid hormone, which is required to maintain normal levels of blood calcium. In the case of thyroid surgery, it is important that the parathyroid glands are not damaged or removed; otherwise, there may be life-threatening tetanus—the sustained contraction of muscles, including those needed for breathing.

The normal functioning of the thyroid results from an elaborate physiological control system involving the hypothalamus of the brain, the anterior lobe of the pituitary gland, and the thyroid gland. The hypothalamus produces thyrotropic-releasing hormone (TRH), which is passed by special blood vessels to the anterior lobe of the pituitary, the adenohypophysis. The TRH-stimulated cells in the adenohypophysis produce thyroid-stimulating hormone (TSH), which is released into the general circulation. When it reaches the thyroid gland, it stimulates the gland to produce thyroxine. Normally, thyroxine has a negative feedback effect on its own production; that is, thyroxine can inhibit the activity of the hypothalamus and the pituitary to maintain its concentration in the blood. Various thyroid disorders, which are more common in women than in men, can develop from tumors that either increase or decrease the hormones produced in these three interdependent structures.

The normal thyroid (or euthyroid state) produces mainly thyroxine, which is converted into triiodothyronine in the tissues of the body before it has its effects, which are generally to increase the metabolic rate of the body. Some triiodothyronine is directly produced by the thyroid. The thyroxine molecule contains iodide, the negative ion of iodine; iodine is therefore an essential component of one's diet. If iodine is not available in the diet—as in the case of vegetables grown in geographical areas glaciated in the past, such as mountainous terrain and the American Midwest—then the body cannot produce thyroxine. Industrialized countries have iodine added to table salt to ensure an adequate supply of this element in the diet. A lack of iodine, and therefore a lack of thyroxine, prevents the functioning of the negative feedback effect of thyroxine on the hypothalamus and pituitary, resulting in very low thyroxine levels and high TSH levels in the blood. High levels of TSH cause substantial growth of the thyroid, which will bulge from the neck as a goiter. A person with such a condition would be hypothyroid (that is, have

Symptoms of Graves' Disease

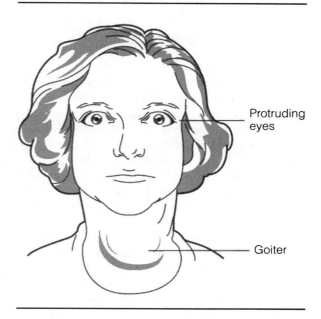

lower-than-normal thyroxine levels in the blood) and may become a cretin (mentally impaired and of short stature) if this condition occurs early in childhood.

Hypothyroidism can arise in other ways as well. Hashimoto's thyroiditis is a common type of hypothyroidism that is caused by an autoimmune reaction whereby white blood cells known as lymphocytes infiltrate the thyroid and gradually destroy its tissue. The presence of antibodies against normal thyroid proteins can be detected with this condition. The usual signs of hypothyroidism are an intolerance of cold, a low body temperature, a lower rate of metabolism, a tendency to sleep longer, a general lack of energy, infrequent bowel movements, constipation, possible weight gain, a puffy face and hands, a slow heart rate, cold and scaly skin, a lack of perspiration, and possible emotional withdrawal and depression.

Graves' disease, the most common type of hyperthyroidism, is an autoimmune disorder in which antibodies mimic the action of TSH and therefore stimulate the thyroid to produce excessive thyroxine. Sometimes, nodules develop in the thyroid that may produce the excessive thyroxine. Although the presence of a nodule in the thyroid may cause a person to suspect cancer, the nodules are usually benign. Hyperthyroidism may be associated with bulging eyes, but this orbitopathy does not always occur. Generally, there is an intolerance of heat, a loss of body weight, a high degree of nervousness, increased or decreased skin pigmentation, more frequent bowel movements, loss of hair, and a very rapid heart rate.

TREATMENT AND THERAPY

Patients suspected of having hypothyroidism or hyperthyroidism will have their blood tested for levels of TSH and thyroxine. Ultrasonography can be used to detect tumors and serve as an anatomical guide for potential surgery. Hypothyroidism patients are prescribed a small oral dose (less than 1 milligram per day) of thyroxine, which is adjusted until a euthyroid state is obtained within a few months. Then the patient is maintained on thyroxine, with perhaps yearly checkups by a physician. For hyperthyroidism patients, several modes of treatment are possible. Antithyroid drugs, such as propylthiouracil (PTU) or methimazole, can be given to inhibit thyroxine synthesis. Radioactive iodine is commonly given to destroy part of the thyroid gland and thus reduce its thyroxine output. Second or even third doses of radioactive iodine may be given if the blood thyroxine levels remain high. Radioactive iodine is not used during pregnancy because damage to the fetal thyroid is likely. Additionally, surgery can be performed to remove enough thyroid tissue to restore normal thyroxine levels. Following any of the treatments, a hypothyroidism may be induced that will require that the patient receive thyroxine supplements. Finally, surgery can be used to reduce the bulging of the eyes caused by hyperthyroidism.

—*John T. Burns, Ph.D.;*
updated by Matthew Berria, Ph.D.

See also Endocrine disorders; Endocrinology; Endocrinology, pediatric; Glands; Goiter; Hormones; Hyperparathyroidism and hypoparathyroidism; Metabolism; Parathyroidectomy; Thyroid gland; Thyroidectomy; Vitamins and minerals.

FOR FURTHER INFORMATION:

Griffin, James E., and Sergio R. Ojeda, eds. *Textbook of Endocrine Physiology.* 4th ed. New York: Oxford University Press, 2000. This textbook of basic endocrinology is used widely in medical schools as well as graduate and undergraduate programs.
Hershman, Jerome M. *Endocrine Pathophysiology: A Patient-Oriented Approach.* 3d ed. Philadelphia: Lea & Febiger, 1988. Discusses diseases of the endocrine glands. Includes bibliographical references and an index.
Surks, Martin I. *The Thyroid Book.* Yonkers, N.Y.: Consumer Reports Books, 1993. This concise volume discusses diseases of the thyroid gland. Includes an index.

THYROID GLAND

ANATOMY

ANATOMY OR SYSTEM AFFECTED: Endocrine system, glands, neck

SPECIALTIES AND RELATED FIELDS: Endocrinology

DEFINITION: A gland found in the neck that secretes the hormones responsible for the synthesis and breakdown of proteins and the metabolism of carbohydrates.

KEY TERMS:

cretinism: a severe hypothyroidism in which infants are born with insufficiently developed thyroid tissue

endocrine system: a series of ductless glands that deliver hormones to target cells directly through the bloodstream

Graves' disease: a common type of hyperthyroidism in which the thyroid gland produces an oversupply of hormone

hormones: chemicals, usually proteins or steroids, that carry messages regulating the body's chemical balance, responses to stimuli, and development

hypothyroidism: a condition in which the thyroid gland produces an insufficient supply of hormone

parathyroid: one of four small endocrine glands physically close to the thyroid that control the calcium balance of the body

pituitary: the endocrine gland responsible for the functioning of the thyroid; along with many other central control activities

thyroid: the endocrine gland that produces hormones which regulate human growth and metabolism

thyroxine: the chief hormone of the thyroid gland, an iodine-containing derivative of the amino acid tyrosine

STRUCTURE AND FUNCTIONS

The human body is, to an extraordinary extent, under the metabolic control of chemical secretions called hormones. These molecules are produced by the ductless, or endocrine, glands and carry messages that regulate the rate of production of necessary substances in remote parts of the organism. The endocrine glands in turn are largely controlled by the nervous system, which also uses chemical messengers to manage the multiple and interrelated systems of the body.

The thyroid gland was one of the earliest glands to be studied in detail. It synthesizes, stores, and secretes two principal hormones, thyroxine and triiodothyronine. These substances stimulate carbohydrate metabolism and protein synthesis or breakdown.

The first description of the thyroid that has been accepted as definite was given by Thomas Wharton in 1656; he also named the gland. In his studies of all the glands, he performed animal dissections and human autopsies. Although his written accounts were widely reprinted, it was more than two hundred years later before any serious further work was undertaken.

Nineteenth century clinical studies of goiter (swelling of the thyroid) and hyperthyroidism (the gland's overproduction of hormones) contributed little to an understanding of the thyroid. An exception is found in the study of the insufficient production of hormone by the thyroid, called hypothyroidism. English and Swiss physicians made discoveries that are considered by some medical historians to be as important as the demonstration that the element iodine is associated with thyroid action.

In the 1870's, the Swiss surgeon Emil Theodor Kocher began to describe the significance of the thyroid gland and its role in goiter formation. He was awarded the 1909 Nobel Prize in Physiology or Medicine for providing a fuller appreciation of the thyroid and associated glands. Kocher was neither a physiologist nor a pathologist by training or disposition, but he recognized that to be an effective surgeon it was essential to understand well the function of the thyroid and its role in the goiters so common in Bern. In this region, 80 to 90 percent of schoolchildren had a malfunctioning thyroid gland and the often-associated goiter. Kocher's drawings in books and papers show that such enlargements are extremely disfiguring and often interfere with normal breathing and speech.

In Kocher's day, little was known about any of the endocrine glands, of which the thyroid is the first to have been studied surgically. Such glands deposit chemical regulatory substances called hormones directly into the bloodstream, which carries them to the sites of their activity.

Later clinical observations provided evidence that the thyroid gland produces some material essential for good health. In 1896, Eugen Baumann made the key discovery that the thyroid contains an unusual amount of iodine. He also showed that this excess iodine is present in a protein that he could decompose with water to yield a new substance. During the next twenty-five years, technical progress was made to the point that the hormone thyroxine could be produced in a pure, crystalline form.

With the new tool of radioactive iodine, a powerful method for the study of thyroid functions and malfunctions became available. For example, overactive and underactive thyroid glands can be easily determined through the ingestion of a tiny amount of one of the radioactive isotopes of iodine and the later determination of the amount of the tracer present in the thyroid.

DISORDERS AND DISEASES

It is possible for the thyroid to produce either too much (hyperthyroidism) or too little (hypothyroidism) of the hormone thyroxine, which plays a role in controlling metabolism and body growth. If an insufficient quantity of it is produced, the condition called Gull's disease results. In children, this condition limits both physical and mental growth and is known as

The Thyroid Gland

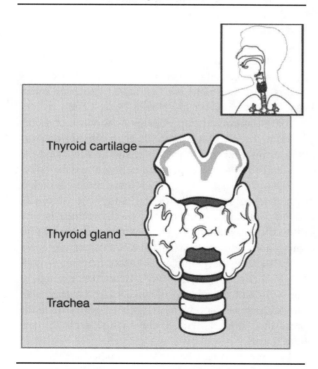

The thyroid is an important gland that produces thyroid hormone, the proper level of which is crucial to health; the inset shows the location of the thyroid gland.

cretinism. In Graves' disease and related conditions, the overactive thyroid gland produces too much hormone. Either of these conditions can produce an enlarged thyroid gland, or goiter. This imbalance existed in many different countries, but physicians designated it by various names, thus causing much misunderstanding and confusion. Emil Kocher's studies presented the first organization of the field in the form of these basic definitions.

In his first 101 operations carried out between 1872 and 1883, Kocher completely removed the thyroid gland in 34 cases. After a report by his colleague Jacques Louis Reverdin indicating that removal of the thyroid was a causal factor in cretinism, Kocher made as detailed a follow-up of these patients as possible. His conclusion was that if the entire gland was removed, cretinlike symptoms almost always appeared. If at least some of the gland was left, it appeared to regenerate itself and supply the required hormone. He vowed never to remove a thyroid completely again except in the case of malignancy.

Only in the twentieth century have reliable diagnoses and treatments become available for thyroid disorders. Because of the variety of these conditions and their causes, accurate diagnosis is indispensable. Modern approaches which supplement radioactive iodine include ultrasound and the needle biopsy.

The principal difficulty in the treatment of a malfunctioning thyroid gland is the several variations often displayed. Hyperthyroidism can occur in forms that appear quite unrelated to the most common form, Graves' disease. For example, there may not be a heredity basis, the condition may not spread over the entire gland, the production of antibodies may not be involved, and there may be no progressive failure of the thyroid.

The causes of hypothyroidism are also less than uniform. The age at which the disorder begins is significantly related to its cause. Newborn children with this condition may have never developed the required amount of thyroid tissue. Others may have inherited a defect which prevents the thyroid from producing sufficient hormone. In developing countries, iodine deficiency remains a problem (although an overabundance of that element in the diet of expectant mothers can lead to infants with hypothyroidism and a goiter). Later in life, infection can be the cause of Hashimoto's disease and the loss of thyroid tissue. Finally, the treatment of an overactive thyroid places a person at risk of later underproduction of hormone.

The most common symptoms associated with thyroid problems are a too rapid or too slow heartbeat, nervousness or a tired and run-down feeling, frequent bowel movements or constipation, and weight loss or weight gain. An excess of the hormones that direct the use of food and the production of energy might reasonably be expected to produce the first of each pair of contrasting observations, while a deficiency would lead to the opposite effects.

The treatment of Graves' disease falls into three distinct classes, and in modified application these techniques are employed with the other forms of hyperthyroidism. Since the early 1940's, a series of antithyroid drugs have been synthesized. They function by preventing the gland from making hormone, and the symptoms lessen in a short time. Unfortunately, only about 30 percent of patients remain well when the medication is stopped after six to twelve months.

If antithyroid drugs fail to control the overactive thyroid, a radioactive isotope of iodine is often successful. Since the iodine goes directly to the thyroid and remains there for a period of time, it is able to irradiate and destroy a portion of the tissue. It is a demanding task to calculate the proper amount of iodine to administer, but a surprising 80 percent of patients find their condition under control after a single treatment.

Surgical treatment of Graves' disease and related hyperthyroid conditions became practical with Kocher's efforts, and it remains the method of choice in many cases. Kocher began his Nobel Prize lecture by describing the crucial importance of the work of Louis Pasteur, Joseph Lister, and others in making the surgery of internal organs possible, and he suggested the future of thyroid research when he examined the effective use of extracts and the search for chemical means of providing substitutes for the gland's secretions.

The standard treatment of hypothyroidism is oral thyroid hormone tablets. Both extracts of animal thyroid glands and more highly purified preparations are available, but the evidence suggests that better control is obtained using tablets that contain only one of the two chief thyroid hormones. As is the case with Graves' disease, good follow-up is essential since the prescribed dosage will likely change with the patient's age.

Two notes should be made in concluding this discussion of malfunctions of the thyroid. First, there is a tendency to believe that iodine prevents and cures goiter. Statements to that effect, found in many general reference books, are both misleading and dangerous. Second, publications for laypersons tend to minimize the importance of thyroid blood tests, which is a serious disservice. Regular and complete physical examinations are essential in maintaining good health.

PERSPECTIVE AND PROSPECTS

Historians of medical history have attributed knowledge of the thyroid gland and the treatment of goiter to nearly everyone of significance. The works of Galen, Paracelsus, ancient Chinese writers, and other classical Roman and Greek authors, as well as medieval manuscripts, have been studied. In the twentieth century, the study of the thyroid and goiter illustrates central themes in the evolution of medical practice; these are shown clearly in the career of Emil Kocher. His being chosen as an early Nobel laureate is prophetic—first for his role in creating modern surgery, with its total reliance on a germ-free environment and its demand for detail, and second for successful synthesis of the roles of clinician and research scientist. He both possessed the necessary surgical skill to develop such a delicate procedure as thyroidectomy (removal of the thyroid gland) and appreciated the importance of understanding the role played by the thyroid in controlling distant and seemingly unrelated functions. Finally, Kocher kept abreast of any new discovery that might, in any way, be of significance to his surgical goals.

The study of the thyroid in many ways unlocked the secrets of other endocrine glands. As in many areas of scientific research, new medical knowledge follows quickly after the discovery of materials and techniques. At the same time, the search for knowledge provides both motivation and information driving the discovery of materials and techniques.

The identification of iodine as an elemental substance by the French chemist Bernard Courtois in 1811 rapidly led to its indiscriminate use as a treatment for goiter, along with a wide variety of related conditions. Important work in the mid-nineteenth century by A. Chatin demonstrated the high correlation between goiter and low levels of iodine in the food and water supplies throughout central Europe. In the 1930's, with the creation of radioactive isotopes, including those of iodine, a vital and productive new phase of thyroid research began.

A similar pattern is seen during World War II, when four independent research groups showed that sulfa drugs were capable of exerting a strong influence on the behavior of the thyroid. All these studies were conducted within a two-year period, and it was less than a year later that the therapeutic use of sulfa drugs was demonstrated.

While much knowledge and technical skill concerning the thyroid has been gained, the number of conferences and publications devoted to endocrinology attests to the continued importance of that general field of study. For example, while malignant tumors are rare in the thyroid, benign lumps or nodules are common. The reasons for this pattern and the role of endocrine glands in the development and spread of cancerous cells warrant detailed and continuing study.

—*K. Thomas Finley, Ph.D.*

See also Endocrine disorders; Endocrinology; Endocrinology, pediatric; Glands; Goiter; Growth; Hormone replacement therapy; Hormones; Metabolism; Systems and organs; Thyroid disorders; Thyroidectomy.

FOR FURTHER INFORMATION:

Bayliss, R. I., and W. M. Tunbridge. *Thyroid Disease: The Facts.* New York: Oxford University Press, 1991. Well written and researched. Provides a wealth of information in a not-too-technical fashion.

Burrow, Gerard N., Jack H. Oppenheimer, and Robert Volpé. *Thyroid Function and Disease.* Philadelphia: W. B. Saunders, 1990. A textbook that offers a detailed understanding of the entire range of the gland and its medical interest to the interested reader.

DeGroot, Leslie J., and John B. Stanbury. *The Thyroid and Its Diseases.* 6th ed. New York: John Wiley & Sons, 1996. Much technical material can be found in this standard textbook, but there are also valuable details to give the reader a greater appreciation of the subject.

Marieb, Elaine N. *Essentials of Human Anatomy and Physiology.* 6th ed. Redwood City, Calif.: Benjamin/Cummings, 2000. This introductory anatomy and physiology textbook, easily accessible to those with little science background, is richly illustrated with diagrams and photographs, which help to illuminate body systems and processes.

Wood, Lawrence C., David S. Cooper, and E. Chester Ridgeway. *Your Thyroid: A Home Reference.* 3d ed. New York: Ballantine Books, 1995. An excellent description of the entire field, with much wise advice for all, including those suffering with thyroid problems. Includes important supplemental information for those seeking further assistance.

THYROIDECTOMY

PROCEDURE

ANATOMY OR SYSTEM AFFECTED: Endocrine system, glands, neck

SPECIALTIES AND RELATED FIELDS: Endocrinology, general surgery

DEFINITION: The surgical removal of a portion of the thyroid gland.

INDICATIONS AND PROCEDURES

The thyroid gland is located at the base of the neck. It is composed of two lobes that straddle the trachea (throat) and a third lobe that is in the middle of the neck. Surgery on the thyroid is usually performed under general anesthesia. The patient's neck is extended, and an incision along a natural fold or crease is made through the skin, platysma muscle, and fascia that lie over the thyroid. The muscle is cut high up to minimize damage to the nerve that controls it.

The thyroid is next carefully freed from surrounding structures (blood vessels, nerves, and the trachea). One at a time, the upper portion of each lobe is freed to allow identification of the veins that take blood from the thyroid. The veins are ligated (tied) in two places and cut between the ties. The ligaments that suspend the thyroid are cut next. It is important for the surgeon to avoid damaging the superior laryngeal nerve. Once the nerve has been protected, other blood vessels are clamped, tied, and cut. A similar procedure is followed for the lower lobes: ligating and cutting veins, protecting the inferior and recurrent laryngeal nerves, and freeing the remainder of the thyroid lobes.

Four parathyroid glands, each about the size of a pea, are imbedded in the thyroid gland. At least one of these must be preserved, as they play a vital role in regulating calcium. Once these glands are identified, the tissue of the thyroid is cut away, leaving the parathyroids intact.

The remnants of the thyroid gland are folded in and sutured to the trachea to control bleeding. A final inspection for bleeding is made. The fascia is sutured closed over the thyroid; any muscles that were cut are sewn back together. Finally, the edges of skin are carefully brought together and sutured with very fine material; occasionally, clips are used. The instruments needed for a tracheostomy are left nearby to cope with any emergency that might occur during the next twenty-four hours.

USES AND COMPLICATIONS

Approximately one week after a thyroidectomy, the patient returns for a postoperative checkup, and sutures or clips are removed. Many, but not all, individuals having this procedure must take a synthetic thyroid hormone to make up for the tissue removed during the thyroidectomy.

Thyroid surgery is not uncommon. In the past, radiation was used to shrink the thyroid, but this procedure led to many cancers and has been discontinued. Laser techniques may reduce the size of the incision, thus reducing the size of the resulting scar in the neck.

—*L. Fleming Fallon, Jr., M.D., Ph.D., M.P.H.*

See also Endocrine disorders; Endocrinology; Endocrinology, pediatric; Glands; Goiter; Hormone replacement therapy; Hormones; Parathyroidectomy; Thyroid gland.

Bayliss, R. I., and W. M. Tunbridge. *Thyroid Disease: The Facts*. New York: Oxford University Press, 1991.

Burrow, Gerard N., Jack H. Oppenheimer, and Robert Volpé. *Thyroid Function and Disease*. Philadelphia: W. B. Saunders, 1990.

Hamburger, Joel J. *The Thyroid Gland: A Book for Thyroid Patients*. Southfield, Mich.: Author, 1979.

Wood, Lawrence C., David S. Cooper, and E. Chester Ridgeway. *Your Thyroid: A Home Reference*. 3d ed. New York: Ballantine Books, 1995.

TIAs. *See* STROKES.

TICKS. *See* LICE, MITES, AND TICKS.

TICS

DISEASE/DISORDER

ANATOMY OR SYSTEM AFFECTED: Brain, muscles, musculoskeletal system, nerves, nervous system, psychic-emotional system

SPECIALTIES AND RELATED FIELDS: Neurology, psychology

DEFINITION: Small, brief, recurrent, inappropriate, compulsive jerking movements or twitches, sometimes called habit spasms, often set off by stressful events and including tic douloureux, involving the trigeminal nerve, and Tourette's syndrome, a life-long disorder associated with a large variety of tics.

KEY TERMS:

neuralgia: pain in one of the peripheral nerves

paroxysm: an uncontrolled spasm or convulsion which may sometimes be violent

psychogenic: psychological in origin; set off by psychologically stressful events

stereotyped: performed exactly the same way from one occasion to the next, or from one individual performer to the next

tic douloureux (trigeminal neuralgia): painful tics of the fifth cranial nerve (trigeminal nerve)

Tourette's syndrome: a neurological disorder characterized by bizarre or unusual tics, compulsive swearing, strange facial gestures, and animal-like noises

CAUSES AND SYMPTOMS

Tics are small, inappropriate, involuntary, compulsive jerking or twitching movements that recur uncontrollably and appear to be nonrhythmic (erratic) in pattern. Tics are stereotyped movements of small portions of the body that last only briefly but may be repeated often. They are often set off by psychologically stressful events. In many cases, tics can be voluntary and temporarily suppressed, but often with the result that the same movements occur more forcefully afterward. The term "habit spasm" is often used for tics that occur among children. A tic is a symptom rather than a disease. Many tics are believed to be of psychogenic origin, and certain others seem to be related to epilepsy, encephalitis, or diseases of unknown origin.

Motor tics commonly involve coarse muscle movements of small magnitude, including movements of the face (such as eye blinks, grimaces, or sniffing movements), shruggings of the shoulders, jerks of the neck, or twitches of the body parts. Many motor tics (and also vocal tics) are easily imitated by others but are performed involuntarily and uncontrollably by the patient. Distracting the patient's attention may stop certain tics. In most cases, the tic does not interfere with the patient's use of the hands or feet, even in delicate movements. Several neurologists distinguish simple motor tics (eye winking, head twitching, shoulder shrugs, or facial grimaces) from complex motor tics using more muscles and requiring coordination. Complex motor tics may include touching oneself or other people, jumping, hitting, or throwing things.

Vocal or phonic tics include the making of sounds, which may include grunts, coughs, sniffs, clearings of the throat, animal noises (especially barking and yelping), or understandable words. The words may simply be repeated utterances of the patient's own words (palilalia), repetition of words spoken to the patient (echolalia), or obscene and offensive words (coprolalia). Although coprolalia is one of the more striking symptoms of Tourette's syndrome and has been vividly portrayed in many popular accounts of this disorder, it is usually a mild or transient symptom that appears in only a minority of cases.

Sensory tics are unusual sensations of pressure, cold, warmth, tickling, or other common sensations that are generally brief in duration. Some otherwise inexplicable movements may be interpreted as actions taken by the patient to alleviate these sensory tics. Sensory tics are reported to be present in about 40 percent of patients with Tourette's syndrome.

Tic disorders can be classified into four types: tic douloureux, transient tic disorder of childhood, chronic tic disorder, and Tourette's syndrome. One of the most common forms of tic is trigeminal neuralgia, also called tic douloureux, a disorder which affects about fifteen thousand individuals annually in the United States. Tic douloureux is a disorder of the trigeminal or fifth cranial nerve, the nerve that supplies motor stimulation to the jaw muscles and sensory innervation to much of the skin of the face. Tic douloureux usually begins with a very brief but very intense, sharp pain, often described as feeling like an electric shock or a stabbing, swiftly spreading in many cases along the course of the affected nerve. The pain is usually accompanied by uncontrolled spasms or paroxysms that last less than a second but continue to recur for several minutes. These episodes may be separated from one another by tic-free periods lasting from weeks to more than a year. The pain and twitching are generally confined to one side of the face, often to one of the three divisions of the trigeminal nerve, usually the maxillary or mandibular division, or, much less often, the ophthalmic division. In addition to the uncontrollable tics, patient suffering from tic douloureux often wince visibly from the pain, and this habit is responsible for the term "tic douloureux," meaning "painful tic."

The immediate event precipitating an attack of tic douloureux is usually a mild stimulation or irritation of a "trigger zone" on or about the face, lips, tongue, or gums. The trigger zone is often a small area that is constant for a particular patient; some patients can trigger an episode by stimulating the trigger zone themselves. The most common locations for the trigger zone are along the cheek or the attached parts of the lips; less common locations include the gums or the floor of the mouth beside the tongue. Some patients suffering an attack of tic douloureux will apply pressure to their faces, but the pain usually goes away by itself. Attacks generally occur during the day rather than at night, and they typically increase in intensity and become more frequent and exhausting to the patient until treatment is sought.

The stimulus that normally evokes an attack of tic douloureux may be an exposure to touch or pressure, to cold, to food in the mouth, or even to a puff of air. Because an attack can be precipitated by touching or otherwise stimulating the trigger zone, many victims of tic douloureux avoid touching the region in which the trigger zone is located. When the trigger zone is on the outside of the face, patients may become very fearful of touching the affected part and men may avoid shaving. Some patients avoid brushing their teeth and remain unwashed for weeks or even months in the vicinity of their trigger area, with social consequences that often contribute to pessimistic feelings and even depression.

When tongue or cheek movements precipitate attacks, patients suffering from tic douloureux may develop the habit of holding the affected side of their face motionless, which sometimes restricts talking, eating, or similar everyday movements. In some cases, certain chewing movements or the presence of food in certain locations in the mouth may precipitate an attack; in these cases, patients are often very careful to avoid eating or chewing on the affected side, and in extreme cases they may so often avoid eating or drinking that they become dehydrated and emaciated. Some physicians advise such patients to modify their diet and drink only liquids, fortified with vitamins, that can be consumed without chewing. Malnutrition and physical inactivity are in many cases reinforced by the social consequences of facial uncleanliness and lack of hygiene, or by the fear of such consequences. The lack of social contact may result in pessimistic or negative feelings, feelings of inadequacy or lack of worth, preoccupation with loss and with past events, feelings of rejection or powerlessness, and other symptoms of clinical depression in many patients.

Dental disease or trauma may sometimes be associated with tic douloureux, but in most cases the tic has no apparent cause. Tic douloureux is more common after the age of forty and is slightly more common in women than in men. Some researchers believe that infection with a herpesvirus (especially herpes simplex) may be causally related to trigeminal neuralgia, but other researchers doubt this connection. Tumors of the trigeminal (Gasserian) ganglion, brain-stem tumors, multiple sclerosis, or localized damage to the brain stem tissue can sometimes give rise to conditions that closely resemble tic douloureux, but the majority of tics occur among patients having none of these conditions.

The remaining forms of tic disorder are considered by at least some researchers to be related to one another, or to form a spectrum of conditions from mild or imperceptible to severe. The mildest types are the tics or "habit spasms" of children. These tics are usually considered psychogenic in origin because they occur more often under conditions of stress or tension. Tics of this kind are more common in boys than in girls. Common types of childhood tics include eye blinks or other facial movements, as well as occasional vocal tics such as throat-clearing noises. In some children—perhaps many—tics of this kind may disappear (or be "outgrown") spontaneously if no attention is drawn to them.

Chronic tics can be of either the motor or the vocal type. Chronic motor tics are uncommon tics in which three or more muscle groups are usually involved at the same time. Chronic vocal tics are also uncommon and consist of uncontrolled sounds that are more often animal sounds than words of articulate speech. Either kind of chronic tic can originate either in children or in adults, even beyond the age of forty. In either case, they usually last for the remainder of the patient's life. The disorder is equally prevalent in both sexes. Some researchers think that these chronic tics, and possibly also the transient habit spasms of childhood, may result from the same (as yet unidentified) cause as Tourette's syndrome, but in much milder form.

Tourette's syndrome is a neurological disorder named for its discoverer, Georges Gilles de la Tourette. The disease is characterized by bizarre or unusual tics, compulsive swearing or cursing, strange facial gestures, and sudden barking or other animal-like sounds. The spectrum of these tics and other symptoms is broad, which has complicated earlier attempts to describe the disease or to find its cause. The disease usually first appears in children between five and ten years of age and continues throughout life.

The variability of symptoms is one of the characteristic features or highlights of Tourette's syndrome. According to the American Psychiatric Association's *Diagnostic and Statistical Manual of Mental Disorders* (4th ed., 1994, DSM-IV), among the diagnostic criteria for Tourette's syndrome are that both motor and vocal tics must occur and that the number, frequency, complexity, severity, and anatomical location of these tics must change over time. The tics must occur many times a day, usually in bouts, and they must recur "nearly every day or intermittently throughout a period of more than one year." The disease must appear before the age of twenty-one to be considered Tourette's syndrome (although in many cases symptoms are so mild as to escape attention).

Associated with Tourette's syndrome are a number of other conditions, including obsessive-compulsive behaviors, attention-deficit disorder, hyperactivity, school phobias, test anxiety, conduct disorders, depression, dyslexia, poor socialization skills, and low self-esteem, though many of these symptoms can also appear by themselves. Several experts consider Tourette's syndrome and attention-deficit disorder to be variable manifestations of a common underlying disorder which may relate to a chemical imbalance in the brain. About half of Tourette's patients also show symptoms of attention-deficit disorder, such as frequent inattention, impulsiveness, and hyperactivity.

The association between Tourette's syndrome and attention-deficit disorder should be regarded as provisional. The two disorders may have an underlying cause in common, such as a common genetic basis. In many cases, however, the motor and vocal tics are made worse by the administration of stimulants such as methylphenidate, which is commonly used for the treatment of the hyperactivity that so often accompanies attention-deficit disorder. Thus it is possible that the presence of Tourette's syndrome in such cases may be attributable not to the attention-deficit disorder, but to the drugs used to treat the disorder. In certain cases, these drugs may have caused a transient or chronic tic disorder to progress to the more severe Tourette's syndrome. Clearly, more research is needed to clarify the exact nature of the relationship between Tourette's syndrome and attention-deficit disorder, both in the presence and in the absence of various drugs.

There are several other aspects of Tourette's syndrome that are being examined. For example, a number of researchers now suspect that the factors which predispose a patient to develop Tourette's syndrome may also predispose male patients to one form of alcoholism. Other researchers believe that the brain disorder responsible for Tourette's syndrome is related to the endorphins, the brain's natural opiates.

Some promising research involves the connection between this disorder and the neurotransmitter dopamine. Neurologists suspect that Tourette's syndrome results from increased sensitivity of certain parts of the brain to dopamine. Some of the evidence for the hypersensitivity of dopamine receptors derives from the observation that drugs such as haloperidol, which is known to inhibit the dopamine receptors, are effective in reducing the symptoms of Tourette's syndrome, while amphetamines and other drugs which enhance dopamine neurotransmission make the symptoms worse. Also, the cerebrospinal fluid of patients with Tourette's syndrome contains reduced levels of homovanillic acid, a breakdown product of dopamine. The corpus striatum in the brain is considered to be the most likely location for the supersensitive dopamine receptors. One researcher has found a total absence of a brain peptide called dynorphin in fibers of the corpus striatum, where this peptide normally occurs. The fibers in question project to the globus pallidus at the base of the cerebral hemispheres.

One theory that attempts to explain the relationship of the several symptoms in Tourette's syndrome is that they all stem from a loss of the inhibition that normally controls involuntary movements. The obscene or offensive words, normally inhibited, are expressed more often than other types of words because the inhibition has been removed. This theory supposes that children who find that they have expressed "bad" words that should not have been said out loud become obsessed with these words and thus (in the absence of inhibitions) say them more often, making the problem worse.

Studies of the families of Tourette's syndrome patients show that there are familial inheritance patterns, with many family members having at least some symptoms of tic disorders, attention-deficit disorders, or both. In many or most cases, the tic disorders of affected family members are so mild that they never caused any problems and were never mentioned to any physician. This finding leads many researchers to conclude that the underlying disorder is variable in the extent of its expression and that it is much more common than medical records show. One expert has even estimated that nearly 1 percent of the population has some form of tic disorder.

If all forms of tic disorder are included, it becomes clear that tics run in families and that Tourette's syndrome is simply one end of a spectrum of variable expression. Studies on identical twins confirm that the trait has a genetic basis. Additional studies of family histories suggest that everyone with the gene experiences symptoms of the disorder. The penetrance of the gene is somewhat greater in males than in females, meaning that more males have symptoms while females are more often symptom-free. Among those family members who have symptoms, the expression of those symptoms is highly variable.

Mimicking some of the symptoms of Tourette's syndrome are the so-called tardive tics that appear during adolescence or adult life. Tardive tics are considered by many researchers to be iatrogenic (drug-induced), arising from the prolonged use of neuroleptic drugs (tranquilizers) such as phenothiazines (Thorazine, Compazine, and Mellaril). Symptoms include isolated, short, quick, uncoordinated jerking movements. The mechanism by which tardive tics appear is unclear, but the same dopamine pathways may be involved as in genuine cases of Tourette's syndrome.

TREATMENT AND THERAPY

Various treatments are available for tic douloureux, both medical and surgical. Partial relief may be afforded by medical treatments, which include carbamazepine (tegretol), trichloroethylene, anticonvulsants such as phenytoin or phenylhydatoin (Dilantin), vasodilators such as tolazoline (Priscoline), analgesic (pain-killing) drugs, vitamin B12, or the repeated injection of 95 percent ethyl alcohol directly into the trigeminal nerve ganglion.

None of these treatments is successful in all cases, however, and some, such as trichloroethylene, have toxic side effects. Surgical treatments include neurotomy (cutting of the affected branch of the trigeminal nerve), decompression of the posterior nerve root, or the cutting of one or more of the trigeminal tracts in the brain stem, either in the midbrain or in the medulla. The most frequently performed surgical procedures include destruction, or partial destruction, of the trigeminal ganglion, either by electrocoagulation, by radio frequency therapy, or by mechanical means. The facial paralysis or partial paralysis that follows

nerve destruction often resembles Bell's palsy except that the damage is usually permanent, with minimal possibility of recovery.

Treatment of childhood transient tic disorders usually consists of psychological intervention to control or reduce the level of stress. Many cases of transient or chronic tic disorder are so mild that they do not require any treatment.

For Tourette's syndrome, haloperidol (Haldol) is most often prescribed, and it is said to be effective in 50 to 90 percent of the cases, depending on the authority consulted. Other drugs occasionally prescribed include clonidine, penfluridol, and pimozide. These drugs can reduce the severity and frequency of tics and may reduce impulsive or aggressive behavior. They also have side effects, however, causing sedation, depression, and weight gain in many patients.

PERSPECTIVE AND PROSPECTS

Because tics are highly noticeable, suggestions regarding their cause have been made throughout history. It was not until the eighteenth century, however, that scientific studies were conducted on patients exhibiting these movements. Thus, while there are indications that tic douloureux was known and recognized in ancient times, James Fothergill (1712-1780) is usually credited with the first modern description of the disorder in 1773.

Georges Gilles de la Tourette (1857-1904) was a French physician who, in 1885, first described the medical syndrome that bears his name. Tourette described the disorder, which he considered to be heritable, on the basis of eight patients whose symptoms included jerking movements, noises, coprolalia, and echolalia. Tourette was shot three times by one of his patients in 1893; he never recovered from the resulting brain injury. Tourette's syndrome was usually ignored or described as a rare disorder until the 1980's, when several researchers studying the families of Tourette's syndrome patients began to notice that many of the family members had mild forms of the same disorder that had previously escaped attention. When they looked more closely for tic symptoms, they discovered that such disorders were much more common than had previously been thought. Connections with obsessive-compulsive disorders and with alcoholism were first noticed from the discovery of these conditions among the relatives of Tourette's syndrome patients.

—Eli C. Minkoff, Ph.D.

See also Anxiety; Attention-deficit disorder; Encephalitis; Epilepsy; Motor neuron diseases; Muscle sprains, spasms, and disorders; Muscles; Nervous system; Neuralgia, neuritis, and neuropathy; Neurology; Neurology, pediatric; Palsy; Seizures; Stress; Tourette's syndrome.

FOR FURTHER INFORMATION:

Adams, Raymond D., Maurice Victor, and Allan H. Ropper. *Adams and Victor's Principles of Neurology.* 7th ed. New York: McGraw-Hill, 2000. A good but somewhat technical source on neurology. Contains a lengthy discussion of Tourette's syndrome.

American Psychiatric Association. *Diagnostic and Statistical Manual of Mental Disorders: DSM-IV-TR.* Rev. 4th ed. Washington, D.C.: Author, 2000. The standard work in the field of psychiatry. Lists the criteria for the presence of Tourette's syndrome in a given patient.

Behrman, Richard E., ed. *Nelson Textbook of Pediatrics.* 16th ed. Philadelphia: W. B. Saunders, 2000. Includes a brief and very readable summary of tic disorders, emphasizing Tourette's syndrome. A bibliography is included.

Chipps, E. M., N. J. Clanin, and V. G. Campbell. *Neurologic Disorders.* St. Louis: Mosby Year Book, 1992. A good, simple reference written for nurses, using everyday language and frequent illustrations. Includes a section on tic douloureux.

Waxman, Stephen G. *Correlative Neuroanatomy.* 23d ed. Stamford, Conn.: Appleton and Lange, 1996. A very readable treatment, balancing basic information with clinical discussions.

TINGLING. *See* NUMBNESS AND TINGLING.

TIREDNESS. *See* FATIGUE.

TOENAIL REMOVAL. *See* NAIL REMOVAL.

TOILET TRAINING
DEVELOPMENT

ANATOMY OR SYSTEM AFFECTED: Bladder, gastrointestinal system, genitals, intestines, kidneys, psychic-emotional system, urinary system

SPECIALTIES AND RELATED FIELDS: Family practice, gastroenterology, pediatrics, psychiatry, psychology, urology

DEFINITION: Toilet use is a complex skill that children usually master within the first four years of life.

KEY TERMS:

encopresis: defecating outside the toilet
enuresis: urinating outside the toilet

PHYSICAL AND PSYCHOLOGICAL FACTORS

Toilet use may seem simple, but it is a complex skill. Children must learn to produce both urine and bowel movements on the toilet, stay dry when not on the toilet, clean themselves, dress and undress, initiate going to the toilet without being reminded, and stay dry while asleep. Most children are fully toilet trained—dry all day and night with complete independence in cleaning and dressing—by the age of four. All successful toilet training methods have three things in common: timing, consistency, and a positive approach.

Two kinds of timing are important. First, training should begin when the child is ready. The child is physically ready when voluntary control over the urethral and anal sphincters is established, usually between twelve and twenty-four months of age. Behavioral signs of physical readiness include a reduction in the frequency of urination. Another sign of readiness is seeking out privacy, often under or behind furniture, before defecating.

The child may indicate psychological readiness by showing awareness of being wet, revulsion or irritation when soiled, or interest in watching parents and older children in the bathroom. Some children show these signs of readiness as early as twelve months of age; others never do. Nearly all children can begin toilet training successfully by twenty-four months of age.

The second type of timing is in visiting the toilet. Children need to use the toilet after meals, every two or three hours between meals, and before bedtime or long car trips, just as adults do. Encouraging the child to sit on the toilet at these times for a few minutes each visit usually produces results.

Consistency is also important. A consistent schedule for meals and visits to the toilet is helpful, as is a consistent place for the child to use the toilet, such as a child-sized toilet, or potty, in the bathroom. Training pants help children to recognize when they are wet and should be worn every day once toilet training starts—although diapers can still be used at night. Finally, parents should respond consistently, showing pleasure every time that the child is successful and remaining calm when accidents occur.

A positive approach includes providing small treats or special activities to celebrate successes, giving children encouragement and affection whether or not they succeed, and discussing toilet use with the child in a calm and encouraging manner. Picture books for toddlers can provide an easy way for parents to talk to their child about toilet use.

DISORDERS AND EFFECTS

Children who have developmental delays or physical disabilities may have difficulty with toilet use. Sometimes, mild developmental delays or health problems are first discovered because of problems with toilet training. Special training methods for these children include positive reinforcement; liquid, food intake, and bathroom trips scheduled to maximize the chance of success; timers to remind children to use the bathroom; and sensors in clothing that trigger an alarm when wet. In some cases of physical malformation or disease, biofeedback, medication, or surgery may be attempted. Even children with very severe disabilities can learn to use the toilet, although they may continue to need reminders or physical assistance.

Toilet use problems of typically developing children include enuresis; fear of the toilet, urine, or feces; encopresis and hiding or playing with feces; retention of feces or urine; and frequent tantrums and accidents. It is normal for children under the age of four occasionally to have any of these problems, stressful as they are for parents. For older children, medical causes should be ruled out. Family therapy directed at both toilet use and discipline problems is often helpful. Nighttime enuresis, or bed-wetting, is the most common toilet use problem experienced by older children and adults. The cause of most cases of bed-wetting is probably developmental immaturity and may be inherited; it is rarely caused by mental illness, as many once believed. Effective treatments are available for this common problem.

PERSPECTIVE AND PROSPECTS

In European history, toilet training recommendations have ranged from sitting the child on the toilet at three months to giving no training at all. Punitive methods such as tying the child on the toilet, forcing food or drink, or hitting the child were common. By the early 1900's, two schools of thought on toilet training had developed. Sigmund Freud, the founder of psychoanalysis, believed toilet training that was too early, punitive, indulgent, or sexualized would cause lifelong personality problems. The behaviorist school of thought held that with the right technique, children could be toilet trained quickly at any age in as little as a day. Neither camp had any direct evidence in support of its position.

Freudian ideas dominated popular advice on child care in the United States from the 1940's through the 1960's, leaving many parents anxious about ruining their children's lives with the wrong toilet training methods. During the 1960's, researchers discovered the variety of actual toilet training practices around the world. They found that toilet training before thirteen months was not effective and that training after thirteen months through age three was typical and rarely led to problems. Often, children who were punished during toilet training not only developed toilet use problems but also had nightmares, tantrums, and discipline problems throughout childhood. In addition, they found that children and adults with disabilities— previously thought to be untrainable—could be toilet trained using positive methods. By the early 1980's, developmental psychologists concluded that consistency, encouragement, and patience produce the best long-term results.

—Kathleen Zanolli, Ph.D.

See also Anxiety; Bed-wetting; Developmental stages; Emotions: Biomedical causes and effects; Motor skill development; Phobias; Psychiatry, child and adolescent; Soiling, Stress.

FOR FURTHER INFORMATION:

Brazelton, T. Berry. *Toddlers and Parents: A Declaration of Independence.* Rev. ed. New York: Seymour Lawrence, 1989. Life with a toddler can be perplexing. Parents sorely need the practical advice Dr. Brazelton offers for surviving— and enjoying— the struggles and triumphs of their child at this age.

Faull, Jan. *Mommy, I Have to Go Potty! A Parents' Guide to Toilet Training.* Seattle: Parenting Press, 1996. Faull's overall tone is one of guiding and teaching, not rigid "training," and is therefore easier on both parent and child. A section entitled "Stories from the Bathroom," which details parents' experiences, will be helpful to any parent attempting toilet training.

Frankel, Alona. *Once upon a Potty.* Woodbury, N.Y.: Barron's, 1987. With over two million books sold, this resource is widely recognized as a premier picture book about toilet training.

Schaefer, Charles, and Theresa Foy DiGeronimo. *Toilet Training Without Tears*. New York: Signet, 1997. For years, parents have turned to the advice of child-care expert Schaefer to help their children reach this developmental milestone in their lives.

"Toilet Training: Is Your Child Ready?" *Health News* 18, no. 3 (June/July, 2000): 8. Most child development experts advocate a child-centered approach to toilet training. Signs that a child is ready to begin toilet training and steps parents can take to encourage their child to become potty-trained are discussed.

TONSILLECTOMY AND ADENOID REMOVAL
PROCEDURE
ANATOMY OR SYSTEM AFFECTED: Lymphatic system, respiratory system, throat

SPECIALTIES AND RELATED FIELDS: General surgery, otorhinolaryngology, pediatrics

DEFINITION: The removal of the palatine tonsils (tonsillectomy) or the palatine tonsils and the adenoids (pharyngeal tonsils), in adenotonsillectomy.

KEY TERMS:
abscess: a painful, localized collection of pus in any part of the body; caused by tissue infection and deterioration

antibody: a blood protein that provides immunity against a disease-causing microorganism

crypt: a pit or cavity in the surface of a body organ (such as a tonsil)

lymphocyte: a white blood cell that produces antibodies

lymphoid tissue: tissue that can make lymphocytes; any portion of the lymphatic system

pharynx: the throat

INDICATIONS AND PROCEDURES

In common use, the term "tonsils" indicates two pinkish palatine tonsils, almond-shaped masses of soft lymphatic tissue located on either side of the back of the mouth. There are two other tonsil types: the lingual tonsils, positioned at the back of the tongue, and the pharyngeal tonsils (adenoids), found in the pharynx and near the nasal passages. Together, the three types of tonsils constitute an irregular band of lymphatic tissue which roughly encircles the throat at the back of the mouth. This tissue band is called Waldeyer's ring. The surface of each tonsil is composed of many deep crypts that, in the case of the palatine tonsils, of-

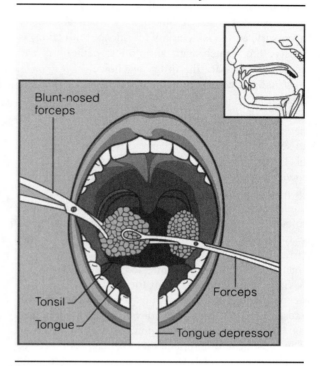

Tonsillectomy

Blunt-nosed forceps

Tonsil

Tongue

Forceps

Tongue depressor

Although this procedure is performed less often than in the past, the removal of the tonsils may still be required by chronic or severe infections; the inset shows the location of the tonsils.

ten become the sites where food debris lodges or sites of bacterial and viral infections. The resulting inflammation of the tonsils is called tonsillitis.

In many cases, acute tonsillitis causes severe throat pain that is easily cured by antibiotic treatment, without recurrence. In others, it returns repeatedly, leading to chronically infected palatine tonsils. Infection of the pharyngeal tonsils (adenoids) causes ear infections and nasal congestion, and it sometimes produces hearing loss as a result of the obstruction of the Eustachian tubes, which lead from the ear to the throat.

Severe, chronic tonsillitis is most often treated by surgery to remove the palatine tonsils. When such surgery is carried out, physicians often elect to remove the infected adenoids as well. This double surgery is called adenotonsillectomy. The lingual tonsils are rarely removed because they do not often become infected. While the exact function of the components of Waldeyer's ring is not clear, they are seen as important to the production of bacteria-killing lymphocytes and antibodies, which protect the throat and digestive system from infection. For this reason, unlike in the past, the tonsils are removed only when absolutely necessary, and tonsillectomy (or adenoid infection) is most often treated with antibiotics; penicillins and cephalosporins are the drugs of choice.

Usually, the onset of acute tonsillitis is signaled by sudden and severe throat pain, high fever, headache, chills, and diffuse pain in the lymph glands of the neck. These symptoms will normally clear up in five to seven days. The most dangerous form of tonsillitis is caused by streptococcal bacteria, usually the *Streptococcus pyogenes* species, which causes strep throat in people whose tonsils have been removed. Associated complications increase with the severity of the infection. In many severe cases, the bacterial infection may spread upward into the nose, sinuses, or ears (from infected adenoids) or downward into the larynx, trachea, and lungs (from infected palatine tonsils).

Especially severe cases of tonsillitis may lead to a deep infection of the throat involving peritonsillar abscess (quinsy). Many cases of quinsy must be treated by lancing the infected region, causing it to drain. The most severe complications of inappropriately or incompletely treated streptococcal tonsillitis are acute nephritis (kidney disease) and rheumatic fever, which may lead to serious heart problems. Both kidney and heart problems are attributable to unsuspected bacterial infection of these organs.

When tonsillectomy is carried out, the adenoids are not removed unless they too cause frequently recurring health problems. The removal of the adenoids alone (adenoidectomy) is sometimes deemed necessary in children when repeated blockages of the nasal passages have caused excessive breathing through the mouth. Prolonged mouth breathing in children can lead to facial deformities because of stress on the developing facial bones.

The tonsils of children are removed under general anesthesia. With adults, local anesthesia is used whenever possible. Tonsillitis in children is much more severe and frequent than in adults because the tonsils decrease in size as one gets older. Similarly, the surgery is more difficult and severe in children because of larger tonsil size.

USES AND COMPLICATIONS

In most cases, tonsillectomy, adenotonsillectomy, and adenoidectomy are simple surgeries with few complications. The entire recovery period from such a pro-

cedure is usually several weeks. Most patients experience severe throat pain during the first few days of the recovery period, but this pain diminishes rapidly with time. It is important for the patient to eat soft food during recovery in order to prevent bleeding, which can become dangerous in some cases. Palatine tonsils do not grow back after surgery, although adenoids may sometimes reappear. The secondary adenoids, however, rarely become troublesome. Tonsillectomy, adenotonsillectomy, and adenoidectomy do not lead to freedom from sore throats. They do usually result, however, in a decreased frequency and severity of throat infections.

—*Sanford S. Singer, Ph.D.*

See also Abscesses; Antibiotics; Bacterial infections; Ear infections and disorders; Hearing loss; Lymphatic system; Otorhinolaryngology; Pediatrics; Quinsy; Sore throat; Strep throat; Streptococcal infections; Tonsillitis.

FOR FURTHER INFORMATION:

Berkow, Robert, and Andrew J. Fletcher, eds. *The Merck Manual of Diagnosis and Therapy.* 17th ed. Rahway, N.J.: Merck Sharp & Dohme Research Laboratories, 1999. This is a reference work for physicians, and the nomenclature can be daunting. It is best consulted after more general introductory reading.

Sabiston, David C., Jr., ed. *Textbook of Surgery: The Biological Basis of Modern Surgical Practice.* 16th ed. Philadelphia: W. B. Saunders, 2001. A standard textbook of surgery.

Tierney, Lawrence M., Jr., et al., eds. *Current Medical Diagnosis and Treatment: 2001.* 39th ed. New York: McGraw-Hill, 2000. This text, updated yearly, is the point of reference for physicians and other health care practitioners. It incorporates each year's biomedical research discoveries that have immediate, relevant, and applicable use for the patient.

TONSILLITIS
DISEASE/DISORDER

ANATOMY OR SYSTEM AFFECTED: Ears, lymphatic system, throat

SPECIALTIES AND RELATED FIELDS: Family practice, general surgery, otorhinolaryngology, pediatrics

DEFINITION: Inflammation, infection, and enlargement of the palatine tonsils, two small masses of lymphoid tissue located on either side of the back of the throat, and frequently of the pharyngeal tonsils, or adenoids, which are located high in the throat above the soft palate.

CAUSES AND SYMPTOMS

Four small pairs of lymphatic tissue called tonsils together form a ring that circles the nasal cavity and mouth. In children, these tonsils help filter and protect the respiratory and alimentary tracts from infection. As children grow, however, this function dwindles and the tonsils shrink. Tonsillitis, or an infection of these tissues, can be either viral or bacterial in origin. Viral infections are more common in children under three, while older children usually suffer from bacterial infections. A throat culture can determine whether bacteria are present, thus indicating antibiotic treatment.

The two pairs of tonsils most often infected and inflamed are the palatine tonsils, which are those removed in a tonsillectomy, and the adenoids. Symptoms of infected and enlarged tonsils include a sore throat, difficulty swallowing, fever, chills, bad breath, and breathing exclusively through the mouth.

TREATMENT AND THERAPY

Viral tonsillitis is self-limiting and typically lasts for five days or less. In these cases, treatment should be symptomatic and includes a soft or liquid diet, warm saltwater or mild antiseptic gargles, throat lozenges, rest, and an analgesic drug such as acetaminophen. If a throat culture indicates bacterial causes, treatment should also include a ten-day course of penicillin and a second culture to determine the effectiveness of the treatment.

Occasionally, tonsillectomy (removal of the palatine tonsils) and adenoidectomy (removal of the adenoids) may also be indicated. Because the tonsils play an important role in the development of the immune system, children under three should not be surgically treated. Before the discovery of penicillin and other antibiotics, a tonsillectomy was the treatment of choice for children who suffered recurrent tonsillitis. Because of the inherent risks of even minor surgery, however, tonsillectomies are now performed only if infected and enlarged tonsils are so problematic that they threaten to obstruct breathing.

—*Jane Marie Smith, M.S.L.S.*

See also Abscess drainage; Abscesses; Antibiotics; Bacterial infections; Immune system; Inflammation; Nasopharyngeal disorders; Otorhinolaryngology; Phar-

yngitis; Quinsy; Sore throat; Strep throat; Streptococcal infections; Tonsillectomy and adenoid removal; Viral infections.

FOR FURTHER INFORMATION:

Baldry, Peter. *The Battle Against Bacteria*. Cambridge, England: Cambridge University Press, 1965.

Berkow, Robert, and Andrew J. Fletcher, eds. *The Merck Manual of Diagnosis and Therapy*. 17th ed. Rahway, N.J.: Merck Sharp & Dohme Research Laboratories, 1999.

Tierney, Lawrence M., Jr., et al., eds. *Current Medical Diagnosis and Treatment: 2001*. 39th ed. New York: McGraw-Hill, 2000.

TOOTH DECAY. *See* CAVITIES.

TOOTH EXTRACTION
PROCEDURE

ANATOMY OR SYSTEM AFFECTED: Gums, mouth, teeth

SPECIALTIES AND RELATED FIELDS: Dentistry, orthodontics

DEFINITION: The surgical removal of a tooth because it is damaged by decay, disease, or trauma; threatening the health of other teeth; or near the site of significant disease.

INDICATIONS AND PROCEDURES

A tooth may have to be extracted for one of several reasons. Impaction is a condition in which a developing tooth is forced into an adjacent tooth, blocking its progress; the impacted tooth can threaten the health and proper alignment of nearby teeth if it is not extracted. The occurrence of crooked or misaligned teeth may also require surgical removal. In tooth decay, dental tissue weakens in a gradual process and can eventually be destroyed. Decay usually begins in the outer layer of the tooth, penetrates to the underlying dentin, and kills the innermost tissue (pulp) of the tooth. Tooth extraction is necessary if this process of decay cannot be halted.

The extraction of teeth is one of the most common procedures in dentistry. Dentists usually perform simple extractions, but they often refer patients needing more complicated procedures to oral surgeons.

In simple extractions, the dentist first applies a local anesthetic to deaden the area surrounding the tooth that is to be pulled. Then, the dentist uses forceps and short levers to loosen the tooth in its socket. The tooth is removed in one piece by breaking the ligaments that hold the tooth in place. Once the tooth has been extracted, the dentist cleans the empty socket and ensures that the blood flowing from the socket is clotting properly. The socket is dressed to protect it and help it heal.

The oral surgeon may use a general anesthetic with a patient needing a complex extraction. The surgeon may need to cut through gum and bone to gain access to the tooth requiring extraction. The tooth may be cut into small pieces before it can be removed. Sutures may be required to close the wound.

The pain caused by extraction usually peaks a few hours after the procedure. Patients are given analgesics (painkillers) and are encouraged to keep the head elevated and to use an ice pack.

—*Russell Williams, M.S.W.*
See also Cavities; Dental diseases; Dentistry; Endodontic disease; Orthodontics; Periodontal surgery; Periodontitis; Root canal treatment; Teeth; Toothache.

FOR FURTHER INFORMATION:

Christensen, Gordon J. "When It Is Best to Remove a Tooth." *Journal of the American Dental Association* 128, no. 5 (May, 1997): 635-636. Christensen describes situations in which removing teeth might be more acceptable than retaining them.

Klatell, Jack, Andrew Kaplan, and Gray Williams, Jr., eds. *The Mount Sinai Medical Center Family Guide to Dental Health.* New York: Macmillan, 1991. Designed for the lay reader, this handbook covers oral hygiene and dental care. Includes an index.

Morant, Helen. "NICE Issues Guidelines on Wisdom Teeth." *British Medical Journal* 320, no. 7239 (April 1, 2000): 890. The routine practice of prophylactic removal of disease-free, impacted third molars should be discontinued, according to the National Institute for Clinical Excellence. The savings could be as much as $8 million.

TOOTHACHE
DISEASE/DISORDER
ANATOMY OR SYSTEM AFFECTED: Gums, mouth, teeth
SPECIALTIES AND RELATED FIELDS: Dentistry
DEFINITION: Toothaches are generally characterized by pain in the teeth or gums. The pain may range from dull, throbbing sensations to more painful, sharp attacks. Toothache can be caused by a variety

of sources, ranging from temperature and a sensitivity to sweet substances (with dental caries and exposed roots caused by receded gum lines) to inflammation of the dental pulp (from an unlined filling) to pressure sensitivity (with injury). Illnesses such as sinusitis can cause pain to be focused in the upper molars. In general, the pain of toothache can be temporarily alleviated with analgesic drugs, but the underlying cause of pain often requires treatment by a dentist.

—*Jason Georges and Tracy Irons-Georges*
See also Cavities; Dental diseases; Dentistry; Endodontic disease; Gingivitis; Periodontal surgery; Periodontitis; Root canal treatment; Sinusitis; Teeth; Tooth extraction.

FOR FURTHER INFORMATION:

Anderson, Pauline C., and Martha R. Burkard. *The Dental Assistant.* 6th ed. Albany, N.Y.: Delmar, 2000.

Cranin, A. Norman. *A Modern Family Guide to Dental Health.* New York: Stein & Day, 1971.

Moss, Stephen J. *Your Child's Teeth: A Parent's Guide to Making and Keeping Them Perfect.* Boston: Houghton Mifflin, 1977.

TORTICOLLIS
DISEASE/DISORDER
ALSO KNOWN AS: Spasmodic torticollis
ANATOMY OR SYSTEM AFFECTED: Muscles, neck
SPECIALTIES AND RELATED FIELDS: Neurology, physical therapy
DEFINITION: A form of dystonia (muscle rigidity) in which the neck muscles contract involuntarily, causing spasms, abnormal movements, and posture of the neck and head backward (retrocollis), forward (antercollis), or sideways (torticollis).

CAUSES AND SYMPTOMS
Torticollis occurs equally in the sexes and may develop in childhood or adulthood. Its causes are unknown, but some cases seem to be genetic, while others are acquired from secondary damage to the nerves affecting the head or neck muscles. Congenital torticollis may be caused at birth by malpositioning of the head in the uterus or by prenatal injury of the muscles or blood supply in the neck. Torticollis results from abnormal functioning of the basal ganglia, situated at the base of the brain, which control all coordinated movements.

The first symptoms may appear gradually as the head tends to rotate or turn to one side involuntarily. Other symptoms may involve asymmetry of an infant's head from sleeping on the affected side, enlargement or stiffness of the neck muscles, limited range of head motion, neck pain, and even headaches.

TREATMENT AND THERAPY

Because the cause of torticollis is unknown in most cases, presently no certain cure exists. Drug therapy is frequently employed, but these medications often produce only unpredictable, short-term benefits. Some patients experience relief when treated by physiotherapists, who may use local moist heat, ice, ultrasonography, or a custom-fitted soft collar. Surgery is not recommended as an initial treatment, but it has proven helpful in cases unresponsive to medication.

PERSPECTIVE AND PROSPECTS

Torticollis is easiest to correct in infants and children and in adults who receive early treatment. With chronic conditions, tingling and numbness may develop as nerve roots in the cervical spine become depressed. Recent innovative surgical procedures are helpful, but they are not a complete cure for chronic spasmodic torticollis. Patients with long-term torticollis will probably retain some degree of head tilt or rotation.

—*John Alan Ross, Ph.D.*

See also Head and neck disorders; Headaches; Muscle sprains, spasms, and disorders; Muscles; Numbness and tingling; Neurology; Neurology, pediatric.

FOR FURTHER INFORMATION:

Clayman, Charles B., ed. *The American Medical Association Family Medical Guide.* 3d rev. ed. New York: Random House, 1994.

Larson, David E., ed. *Mayo Clinic Family Health Book.* 2d ed. New York: William Morrow, 1996.

Moore, Keith L. *Clinically Oriented Anatomy.* 3d ed. Baltimore: Williams & Wilkins, 1992.

TOUCH

BIOLOGY

ANATOMY OR SYSTEM AFFECTED: Nerves, nervous system, skin

SPECIALTIES AND RELATED FIELDS: Dermatology, neurology

DEFINITION: One of the five special senses; nerve endings and specialized structures in the skin and other tissues send the brain data about the organism's environment, both internal and external.

KEY TERMS:

adaptation: a decreased sensitivity to a stimulus, even though the stimulus may still be present, ultimately resulting in an ever-slowing release of nerve impulses until the impulses stop entirely

exteroceptors: sensory receptors generally located on the skin or body surfaces that supply the brain with information about the external environment in which the body is located

mechanoreceptors: sensory receptors that, when mechanically deformed (such as being pressed on), send nerve impulses causing sensations of pressure and touch

Meissner's corpuscles: receptors at which the sense of a light touch or low-frequency vibrations are detected; also called corpuscles of touch

Merkel's disks: sensory receptors located in deeper layers of epidermal (skin) cells; also called tactile disks

modality: the ability to distinguish one sensation from another; the ability to discriminate light or heavy touch, pain, pressure, vibratory, or hot and cold sensations from one another

Pacinian corpuscles: receptors at which the sensations of heavy touch or deep pressure originate; also called lamellated corpuscles

projection: the process whereby the cerebral cortex determines where the point of a stimulus is located

root hair plexus: a network of sensory receptors located at hair roots that generates an impulse when hairs are moved

Ruffini endings: sensory receptors that respond to heavy and continuous touch and pressure; also called type II cutaneous mechanoreceptors or the end organs of Ruffini

STRUCTURE AND FUNCTIONS

An essential attribute of the survival of a species is the ability to detect both the internal and the external environment. This is necessary so that appropriate and life-sustaining actions can be taken at all times. When changes or modifications of these environments take place, many responses can occur within an individual, ranging from rolling over during sleep to restore blood flow to an arm to avoiding contact with a prickly pear cactus. This kind of monitoring occurs within the general and special sense organs or structures found in humans and many other species.

The Sense of Touch

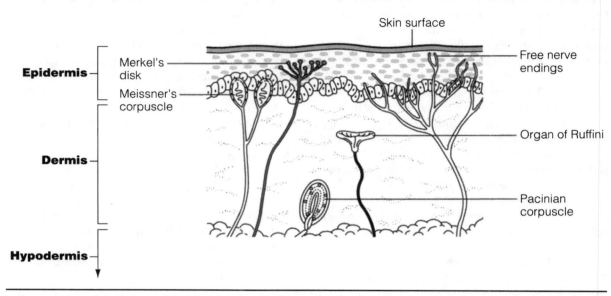

The sensation of touch is produced by special receptors in the skin that respond to temperature and pressure stimuli.

One way in which the body monitors its internal and external environments is through the general senses. General sensations include temperature, pain, touch, pressure, vibration, tickle, and proprioception (internal sensations relating to how one's body is situated in space). Sensations of touch usually originate at or very near the skin surface; some originate from receptors found in deeper, subcutaneous (below-the-skin) layers. Many of the general senses are collectively called the tactile senses, notably those of touch, pressure, vibration, and tickle. In addition, the term "somatic senses" refers to the sensory receptors associated with skin, muscles, joints, and visceral organs. Receptors in the muscles or joints are essential for the awareness of body movement. Visceral receptors play important roles in monitoring changes in body pain, as in stomach pain, hunger, and thirst. The somatic senses provide a means by which the internal and external environments are monitored with regard to touch, pressure, stretch, pain, and temperature. While these terms are not precisely interchangeable, there is overlap in the sensations of touch, pressure, vibration, and tickle with all three categories: general, tactile, and somatic sensations.

Another means whereby a human interacts with the environment is controlled by the special senses. Special senses include taste, vision, smell, hearing,

and body equilibrium in space (or balance). Special senses involve relatively large and specialized structures of the tongue, eyes, nose, and ear and inner ear, in contrast to the general senses, in which the structures are relatively simple but are more widely dispersed throughout the entire body. The neurological pathways are also simplified relative to the neurological events that occur in the special senses' organs and pathways. Combined, the general and special senses form an intricate and elegant system that allows for an individual's survival.

Sensations occur when a receptor receives a stimulus from the external or internal world. The result is a neural impulse that can be utilized in the brain to provide some awareness of the body and its immediate environment. Perception results from the interpretation of the sensory information at a conscious level. Conscious awareness of sensory stimulation generally occurs only when a sufficiently large, or sometimes abrupt, change in the status quo happens in either the internal or the external environment. At that point, the perception of a sense will be registered and noted in the cerebral cortex.

An untold number of sensory receptors are stimulated at any given second, including receptors that note where each body part is placed—from the tiniest portion of each finger and toe, to the position of the body in a chair. Other receptors respond to inhalation and exhalation pressure changes or feel air brushing past. All receptors work simultaneously and in harmony in a healthy person, but most of this activity is on a subconscious level. Only if a sufficient change in either the internal or the external world occurs will a sensation no longer be simply monitored but will cause a conscious response. An example is feeling the hard coolness of a bench when being seated: At first, the perception of the hard and cold surface is pronounced, but this perception will decrease over time until one seemingly "forgets" about being seated on an uncomfortable bench. This kind of decreased sensitivity to a stimulus is called adaptation.

It appears that adaptation prevents the conscious mind from being overloaded with "meaningless" data or data that require no particular response. Adaptation may also allow for new, perhaps more important, stimuli to be noted at the receptor sites. Thus, the adaptation mechanism acts as a "reset" button. Consider the bench example again: In spite of one's "forgetfulness" about the bench being beneath the body, the stimulus is not, in fact, gone. Rather, the mind conveniently elects to ignore the stimulus unless a change occurs that reminds the brain of the bench's presence. This new perception of the bench might recur if a shift in body position causes new receptors to receive stimuli from new contact places between the body and the bench. Eventually, these new sensations will undergo the adaptation process and the bench will once again be "forgotten." (Although thermal equilibrium will be reached between the bench and the person, this process is slow and does not account for the quick rate of adaptation.)

There are four necessary components of sensation: a stimulus, which is generally caused by a change in the environment; a receptor, which can experience a stimulus and produce a generator potential to initiate a nerve impulse; an impulse, which carries the signal from the point of stimulation of the receptor to the brain; and a translation of the impulse within the brain, so that a meaningful interpretation of the kind of sensations experienced, such as a tickle or a floral fragrance, can be made.

All sense receptors are very excitable, but only if stimulated by the specific sensation that they are designed to monitor. This means that sensory receptors are highly specialized in their function. Sense receptors have a low threshold of response to the type of stimuli to which they are designed to respond, while

having a high threshold of response to other kinds of stimuli. (Pain receptors are an exception to this rule, perhaps because of the variety of stimuli that can include a sense of pain.) An example of specialization of the receptors is seen in the fact that certain regions of the body are more susceptible to sensing a tickle than others. Specialization of receptors is attributed to the unique structures of the receptors, even though all sense receptors contain dendrites from sensory neurons.

At a receptor site, a stimulus may induce a generator potential, which sometimes is called the receptor potential. The generator potential is a localized and graded response that may reach its threshold if enough depolarization of the dendrites occurs. In other words, if threshold potential is achieved at the receptor, then a nerve impulse will ensue. This kind of response is an all-or-none response, the landmark characteristic of nerve cells.

The cerebral cortex is essential in the perception (interpretation) of a sensation. All different impulses arriving at the cerebral cortex are chemically the same; the only difference between an impulse carrying a message of a soft touch or of a heavy pounding is where the impulse arrives within the cerebral cortex. Impulses arriving at different locations of the cortex allow the brain to identify, classify, and locate the origins of a stimulus. The ability to distinguish one sensation from another is called modality; the ability to locate precisely the point at which the stimulus is applied is called projection. Modality and projection are functions of the cerebral cortex. In addition, the cortex can prompt many shifts in body position (such as stretching after reading) or body chemistry (such as the release of epinephrine to increase heart rate and blood flow in a crisis) if a response to the stimulus is deemed necessary.

Receptors can be classified according to the location or type of stimuli that cause the receptors to respond. Touch receptors can be classified as exteroceptors by virtue of the fact that these sensory receptors are externally located, mainly on the skin surface. Other classes of somatic receptors are located internally. Visceroreceptors monitor internal organs for data on hunger, thirst, pressure, and nausea. Proprioceptors monitor the muscles, tendons, joints, and inner ear for exacting knowledge of body position and body movement.

Mechanoreceptors are an alternative classification for touch receptors. This label is based on the type of stimuli—a mechanical displacement or disfiguring, for which touch receptors have a low threshold. Light touch is felt when the skin is very gently touched and no indentation or distortion of the skin results. Touch pressure is felt when a heavy touch causes a distortion of the skin surface, either laterally, as in a tugging sensation, or vertically, as in a depression of the skin surface.

Six types of touch receptors have been identified in the human anatomy: root hair plexuses; free nerve endings; tactile disks, or Merkel's disks; corpuscles of touch, or Meissner's corpuscles; type II cutaneous mechanoreceptors, or end organs of Ruffini; and Pacinian corpuscles, or lamellated corpuscles. At these structures, a mechanical stimulus can be transformed into a sensation, provided that the stimulus is sufficiently strong to bring about a threshold potential.

Root hair plexuses are located in networks at the hair roots. On the scalp, these generate a sensation of touch when the hair is being pulled, brushed, or stroked. On the body surface, these receptors are sensitive to movement of the hair, as can occur if a small breeze passes over the skin or if a silk scarf is dragged lightly over the skin hairs. Root hair plexuses are not structurally supported, nor are they protected by any surrounding structure.

Free nerve endings are everywhere on the skin surface and seem to be responsive to many kinds of stimuli. These little dendritic processes of sensory neurons are not protected or supported by surrounding structures.

Made of disklike formations of dendrites, Merkel's disks, or tactile disks, are found in the deeper layers of the skin. Merkel's disks are particularly abundant on the fingertips, palms, soles of the feet, eyelids, lips, nipples, clitoris, tip of the penis, and tip of the tongue. Merkel's disks are particularly suited to receiving stimuli of fine touch and pressure.

Meissner's corpuscles, or corpuscles of touch, are egg-shaped dendritic masses that are sensitive to light touch and vibrations of a low frequency. Found in the hairless portions of the skin, these receptors are also used in making judgments about the textures of whatever the skin may contact. Two or more sensory nerve fibers enter each corpuscle of touch; the nerve fibers terminate as tiny knobs within the corpuscle. In addition, Meissner's corpuscles contain dendritic extensions. The entire mass is enclosed in connective tissue, which offers some support and protection to the disks. Corpuscles of touch are found in the exter-

nal genitalia, tip of the tongue, eyelids, lips, fingertips, palms and soles, and nipples of both sexes.

The end organs of Ruffini, or type II cutaneous mechanoreceptors, are found all over the body but especially in the deep dermis (skin) and deeper tissues below the dermis. These are also called corpuscles of Ruffini and are responsive to heavy and continuous touch and pressure.

Finally, the Pacinian corpuscles are relatively large ellipses that are found in the subcutaneous tissue (below the skin) and deeper subcutaneous tissues. Also known as lamellated corpuscles, these touch receptors are found under tissues that contain mucous membranes, serous membranes, joints and tendons, muscles, mammary glands, and external genitalia. Pacinian receptors are sensitive to deep and heavy pressure and vibrations of low frequency. As such, these receptors detect pulsating, vibrating stimuli. There is an abundance of Pacinian receptors in the penis, vagina, feet and hands, clitoris, urethra, breasts, tendons, and ligaments. Inside each ellipsoid are dendrites from sensory nerves; the bundle itself is wrapped in connective tissue that can serve as a protective support.

DISORDERS AND DISEASES

Loss of tactile senses is a symptom rather than a disease. In general, a lost ability to sense touch, pressure, vibration, or tickle is a result of physical damage to a group of nerves or of a disease of the nervous system. Sensory receptors are not themselves targets of disease, but they can be physically or chemically impaired, especially if the skin is severely damaged.

An example of severe damage to the skin that will cause a loss of tactile sensations is a third-degree burn of the body. Third-degree burns are marked by the total destruction of the full thickness of the skin. This destruction includes the epidermis, the dermis, and any associated skin structures, such as secretion glands, hair, and the general sensory receptors. No pain is sensed when regions of the body that have received a third-degree burn are touched, because the nerve fibers that innervate the touch receptors and the free nerve endings, as well as nerves located in the subcutaneous layers, have been destroyed by the burn. In such cases, total destruction of the nerve fibers and the skin has occurred. Third-degree burns can have a charred, dry appearance or a mahogany or ash-white color. Regeneration of the dermis and the subcutaneous structures is slow and painful as the healing occurs. Although skin grafting can facilitate the regeneration process, it is not uncommon for scarring to result from the rapid contraction of the wounded area as it heals.

The sense of touch is largely lost in scar tissue, since new nerve fibers cannot be formed. (Nerve cells are formed only during gestation and early life and are designed to last a lifetime.) Some tactile senses can return to scarred regions through a process called sprouting. This process involves the branching forth, or the sprouting, of dendritic processes originating in undamaged nerve cells near to, but removed from, the injured site. In this kind of recovery, the healthy nerves assist in restoring tactile senses, to a limited degree, in the damaged regions.

Aside from a total loss of sensation, a sense of numbness can indicate a loss of proper blood circulation to a body region. For example, if one sits or folds oneself into a position so that a leg is receiving pressure from other body parts, the sensation of touch and pressure on the leg will eventually cause a sense of numbness; a form of pain ensues that feels like a tingling sensation that is often described as "pins and needles" all over the leg. The loss of blood circulation to the numbed region actually triggers pain receptors, sending an impulse to the cerebral cortex that warns of an odd feeling. The cerebral cortex will perceive the problem and command responses of the skeletal and muscular systems to change body position. Proprioceptors will sense the new body position and, as blood circulation restores a normal environment, the tingling decreases until it disappears. Numbness can also be a symptom of nerve damage or can result from the use of certain drugs, such as Novocain, which are used in dental and medical applications.

Changing of body position is an important outcome of the touch, pressure, and pain senses. Without the ability to change the position of the body, as can happen in some elderly or quadriplegic persons, damage to the areas on which the whole of the body is resting can occur. Neglect of these persons in home care or in health care facilities will result in bedsores developing at these pressure points. If left unchecked, these bedsores will grow and can lead to gangrene. As a part of their care, such individuals require physical therapy or physical aid in moving body parts and in changing sitting and sleeping positions several times each day.

Damage to the right lobe of the brain may cause abnormalities in the senses of touch and pressure, which in turn can cause a deficit in the ability to lo-cate precisely where a tactile sensation originates on the body surface (the ability to project tactile sensations), making adjustment to and interaction with the external environment challenging. Right lobe damage, therefore, may give rise to a condition called passive touch deficit. Passive touch deficits are revealed by an impaired ability to discriminate touch sensations and by altered thresholds of touch and pressure that cause a sensation to be perceived.

Damage to the right lobe may also lead to deficits in active touch, meaning that such descriptors as size, shape, and texture cannot be readily discerned in touch tests. Generally, right lobe damage also leads to the loss of fine motor control of the fingers, which is especially challenging for piano players, authors, computer operators, painters, surgeons, and others who require exacting motor control of the fingers.

Sometimes, lesions in the right lobe of the cerebral cortex will lead to a condition called tactile agnosia. Tactile agnosia will occur only in the left hand, given the contralateral arrangement of the hands and neurological pathways to the cortex. The symptom of tactile agnosia is the diminished ability, or the inability, to identify common items (such as a key, pencil, or comb) when it is placed in the left hand. Fortunately, this condition is not common.

Another interesting form of loss of touch can occur in an odd behavior called neglect. Again, the problem with this loss of sensation originates from damage to the cerebral cortex, not to the touch receptors of the body. In neglect, lesions of the right parietal lobe are generally present but the contralateral neural pathway results in lost sense on the left side of the body. The ability to perceive a left-side stimulus is lost; patients may not notice anything in the internal or external environments on the left side of the body. In left-side neglect, patients may step into the right leg of a pair of pants but not the left leg and will not know that anything is wrong. Left-side neglect can also result in only right turns being made in walking patterns, and stimuli from the visual, auditory, and tactile sensations are not at all perceived. The sensation is traveling from the point of stimulation, but the cerebral cortex cannot process the sensation.

Finally, the issue of the phantom limb has significance in the medically related aspects of the sense of touch. "Phantom limb" is the term used to describe a sensation that seems to arise from a limb that has been amputated. Patients who have lost body parts to amputation, either surgically or mechanically (as a result of trauma, such as a car accident or an accident while operating a meat-processing machine), often describe sensations of itching, burning, or heat or cold, as well as other general sensations in the limb that is missing.

Although the limb—such as a finger, toe, or part of a leg or arm—may be absent, general sensations seem to arise from these absent body parts because of the neurological pathways that would normally connect the limbs to the cerebral cortex. In addition, a sensation is only as accurate as the cortex's ability to locate and identify the stimulus. This recall is called perception. Perception, however, is not an exact science; it results from experiences and associations that teach the cortex how to sort and analyze sensory data. Much information comes into the brain on common pathways, as if only a few streets led into a special city and all cars wanted to travel those streets to get there. An index finger may have had priority access to the paths during the training days of a young concert pianist. If, however, the pianist loses that index finger, neurological activity along the pathway to which the finger was once connected has not stopped. In fact, during the adjustment and recovery period immediately following the amputation, neurological activity may be heightened. As these sensory receptors and neurons send impulses along the avenues as before, these impulses will now be dominant in the absence of the index finger. Although the conscious mind is fully aware that the finger is absent, the subconscious mind has not yet acclimated itself to the change. Thus, a false association is made before the conscious mind can "correct" the perception and realize that the stimulus must be originating from a place other than the absent body part.

PERSPECTIVE AND PROSPECTS

Responsiveness to different kinds of touch at different locations on the body reveals a relationship between receptor structures and their subsequent function. Specifically, the hands of the human body are exquisitely sensitive to touch. The calculated innervation (number of nerve connections) for touch alone on the palms of the hands is 17,000 units.

On the palms, the most abundant type of touch receptors are Meissner's corpuscles. Accounting for 43 percent of all the touch receptors of the palms, they are responsible for the sensations of texture, light touches, and low-frequency vibrations and clearly play an important role in the human experience. Meiss-

ner's corpuscles are particularly abundant on the tips of all fingers and both thumbs. Although these receptors adapt at a moderately rapid pace, they are not so fast at adapting that the pleasure of stroking a cat or caressing a baby's head is lost.

After Meissner's corpuscles, Merkel's disks are second most abundant on the palms. Constituting 25 percent of the touch innervation density, these cells are suited for fine touch and pressure. Mainly confined to the digits' and thumbs' full length, Merkel's disks are important in tactile pursuits such as painting, drawing, sewing, writing, and dentistry. They are equally important in the expression of loving gestures to other people, animals, and plants via touch. Merkel's disks are slow to adapt; thus, these sensations are somewhat sustained.

Constituting 19 percent of the palms' innervation are the Ruffini endings. These are scattered throughout the palm surface area and are not localized. Ruffini endings are receptive to heavy and continuous touch and are slow adaptors. While a person is carrying a stack of books, for example, these endings are "firing" the nerves that connect to them.

Finally, making up only 13 percent of the palms' innervation to touch are the Pacinian corpuscles. Having a slight clustering in the fingertips, these are very quick at adapting to stimuli. They are receptive to deep and heavy pressure, such as the sensations that can be felt while massaging the hands.

Hairless regions of the skin, such as the palms, soles, penis, and vagina, contain Merkel's disks, Ruffini endings, Meissner's corpuscles, and Pacinian corpuscles. The combinations of receptors within these regions make these body parts acutely aware of and sensitive to light or heavy touch, rough or velvety textures, and pulsating or vibratory stimuli. These areas are also associated with pleasure centers of the body, in part because of their heightened tactile sensitivity.

Hairy skin, such as on the legs, chest, and arms, contains tactile disks, Ruffini endings, root hair plexuses, and Pacinian corpuscles. These body parts are sensitive to vibratory stimuli, breezes and other forms of displacement of body hairs, and pressure and tugging or pulling of the skin.

People are often willing to go to extra lengths to take care of their special sensory organs—the eyes, ears, mouth, and nose—because of their unique and important functions in the human body, but rarely do the general senses receive such attention. In spite of being largely overlooked, the general senses provide humans and other species with something so fundamental to life that it is often forgotten: touch. Offering a means of experiencing the most intimate communication and connection between self and others or between self and the environment, touch is an integral aspect of life.

—Mary C. Fields, M.D.

See also Acupressure; Amputation; Burns and scalds; Grafts and grafting; Nervous system; Neuralgia, neuritis, and neuropathy; Neurology; Neurology, pediatric; Numbness and tingling; Physical rehabilitation; Sense organs; Skin.

FOR FURTHER INFORMATION:

Hole, John W., Jr. *Essentials of Human Anatomy and Physiology.* 6th ed. Dubuque, Iowa: Wm. C. Brown, 1993. An academic textbook designed to give more detail about the human body than an introductory biology book. Chapter 12, "The Somatic and Special Senses," has a section devoted exclusively to receptors and sensations. Related topics, such as the anatomy and organization of the brain and nervous system, are described in exquisite detail.

Schmidt, Robert F., ed. *Fundamentals of Sensory Physiology.* Translated by Marguerite A. Biederman-Thorson. Rev. 3d ed. Berlin: Springer-Verlag, 1986. Chapters 1 through 4—"General Sensory Physiology, Psychophysics," "Somatovisceral Sensibility," "Neurophysiology of Sensory Systems," and "Nociception and Pain"—address the topics of touch sensations. Sketches and postreading quizzes assist the reader in comprehension.

Tortora, Gerard J., and Sandra R. Grabowski. *Principles of Anatomy and Physiology.* 9th ed. New York: John Wiley & Sons, 2000. Provides a treatment of the topic of touch. Entitled "The Sensory, Motor, and Integrative Systems," this chapter gives an excellent introduction to the topic of the general senses.

Wolfe, Jeremy M., ed. *Senses Other than Vision.* Vol. 2 in *Sensory Systems.* Boston: Birkhauser, 1988. Readings selected from the *Encyclopedia of Neuroscience,* addressing topics relevant to touch. Most essays are only one page in length, but some are fairly technical.

TOURETTE'S SYNDROME
DISEASE/DISORDER
ALSO KNOWN AS: Gilles de la Tourette syndrome

ANATOMY OR SYSTEM AFFECTED: Brain, muscles, musculoskeletal system, nerves, nervous system, psychic-emotional system

SPECIALTIES AND RELATED FIELDS: Biochemistry, family practice, genetics, neurology, psychiatry, psychology

DEFINITION: A disorder characterized by recurrent, multiple motor tics and one or more vocal tics that causes stress and impairs social functioning.

KEY TERMS:

coprolalia: involuntary vocalization involving the uttering of obscenities or other socially inappropriate comments

copropraxia: a complex motor tic that involves involuntary, obscene gestures

echolalia: repetition of the words or gestures of others

palilalia: repetition of one's own words

tic: a sudden, rapid, recurrent, irresistible, nonrhythmic, and stereotyped movement; tics may involve motor movements, sudden vocalizations, or a combination of both

CAUSES AND SYMPTOMS

Tourette's syndrome is a disorder marked by multiple motor tics, involuntary vocalizations, and significant impairment of social functioning, often resulting in low self-esteem. For a diagnosis of Tourette's syndrome, the symptoms must persist for a period of at least one year, although they may decrease or subside during that time for brief periods of three months or less. Onset must be prior to eighteen years of age. The motor and vocal tics manifested must not be a consequence of drug use or the result of a previously existing medical condition such as Huntington's chorea.

Definitive causes for Tourette's syndrome remain under investigation. Research in the late 1990's included an exploration of genetic factors that might cause a susceptibility to the disorder and studies of the frequency of the disorder in subsequent generations within families. Studies in brain chemistry were also conducted.

Tourette's syndrome differs from a disease in that sufferers manifest a number of symptoms that occur together. Symptoms may be seen in sequence or in combination. Simple motor or vocal tics are most often first noticed in children between the ages of two and seven, but initial symptoms may be seen in the teenage years. Typically, the first symptoms noticed are simple motor tics such as eye blinking, tongue protrusion, facial grimacing, or other movements in the head area, such as grunting, coughing, throat clearing, or unusual vocalizations.

Complex motor tics include such behaviors as involuntary touching, knee bends, touching of objects in sequence, or other repetitive behaviors. Although many patients first display eye blinks, the anatomical location, severity, and frequency of the tics may change over time. As a youngster matures, the tics may involve other areas of the body, such as the torso or the limbs.

The social implications of this disorder are as important as the physical ones for a child with Tourette's syndrome. Such motor tics as touching inappropriately and involuntary utterances and outbursts can be disastrous to both self-image and social standing. Palilalia, echolalia, coprolalia, copropraxia, and bizarre behaviors brought about by involuntary compulsions cause affected children much anxiety. That their symptoms may mimic or coexist with other disorders is another concern. Although some children may outgrow the disorder in their twenties, generally Tourette's syndrome is a lifelong disorder. Social difficulties abound for those afflicted and for their families. With concentration and relaxation techniques, tics may be delayed or suppressed for brief periods, but they present ongoing problems for those living with Tourette's syndrome.

TREATMENT AND THERAPY

As of the late 1990's, physical treatment for Tourette's syndrome involved a combination of relaxation techniques and medication therapy. Counseling has also proven useful, in conjunction with other treatments, in helping to deal with the social and emotional effects of this disorder. Relaxation techniques such as visualization of a calm setting and a variety of related therapies have proven successful in reducing the number and severity of the tics. Touch therapy and related techniques such as stroking and rocking have been helpful in reducing stress, as have some forms of massage.

Music is another effective means of relaxing the mind and the body. Some researchers have recommended that musical selections with a beat close to one's resting heartbeat are the most effective in reducing stress levels. Musical instruments and other forms of creative expression have proved to be effective tools against stress and associated tics. Hobbies, diaries, written expression, and counseling have all

been used effectively to treat the physical and emotional symptoms of Tourette's syndrome.

A number of medication therapies are also being used. Catapres has been helpful in the treatment of tics, with some side effects. Drugs such as Haldol and Orap have also had success, but with undesirable side effects. Children also suffering from related disorders such as attention-deficit disorder (ADD) have been treated successfully with Ritalin. Drugs such as Anafinil and Prozac have proven useful in treating obsessive-compulsive disorder and other anxiety disorders sometimes seen in conjunction with Tourette's syndrome.

PERSPECTIVE AND PROSPECTS

Treatment and understanding have evolved substantially since 1885 when Georges Gilles de la Tourette first identified Tourette's syndrome, which was thought to be a psychological disorder influenced by environmental factors. Many significant gains have been made since the 1980's in the clinical and scientific understanding of this complex disorder. Research in the late 1990's explored connections between brain chemistry and Tourette's syndrome. The role of genetics in the transmission and manifestation of the disorder was also studied extensively. Promising new medications continued to be developed as well.

—*Kathleen Schongar*

See also Anxiety; Attention-deficit disorder (ADD); Learning disabilities; Motor skill development; Nervous system; Neurology; Neurology, pediatric; Obsessive-compulsive disorder; Psychiatric disorders; Psychiatry; Psychiatry, child and adolescent; Tics.

FOR FURTHER INFORMATION:

American Psychiatric Association. *Diagnostic and Statistical Manual of Mental Disorders: DSM-IV-TR*. Rev. 4th ed. Washington, D.C.: Author, 2000. The bible of the psychiatric community, this is a compendium of descriptions of disorders and diagnostic criteria widely embraced by clinicians.

Cohen, Donald J., and Ruth D. Bruun, et al., eds. *Tourette's Syndrome and Tic Disorders*. New York: John Wiley & Sons, 1988. Covers aspects of Tourette's syndrome, tic disorders, and other diseases of the central nervous system.

Koplewicz, Harold S. "Tourette Syndrome." In *It's Nobody's Fault: New Hope and Help for Difficult Children and Their Parents*. New York: Times Books, 1996. Designed for the lay reader, this volume offers helpful advice to parents. Includes an index.

Shimberg, Elaine Fantle. *Living with Tourette Syndrome*. New York: Simon & Schuster, 1995. Designed for sufferers of Tourette syndrome and their families and friends, this practical guide offers detailed information about diagnosing, treating, and dealing with Tourette syndrome at home, school, and work.

TOXEMIA

DISEASE/DISORDER

ANATOMY OR SYSTEM AFFECTED: Blood

SPECIALTIES AND RELATED FIELDS: Bacteriology, hematology, internal medicine, serology, toxicology

DEFINITION: Often called blood poisoning, toxemia is the presence of toxins in the blood that are produced by bacteria. This poisoning can occur with or without a bacterial infection existing in the body; for example, the bacteria can come from food that is ingested. Toxemia can be caused by infection in one of many places, including the appendix, teeth, sinuses, pelvis, gallbladder, or urinary tract. It may also occur because of an infected wound, abscess, or burn. Symptoms may include shaking chills, a rapid temperature rise, rapid heartbeat, flushed skin, mental impairment, and a drop in blood pressure. Septic shock may occur with very low blood pressure, and death is a possible outcome. In pregnant women, untreated toxemia can cause premature labor, fetal death, and the death of the mother (in rare cases). The condition is usually curable with the use of intravenous antibiotics. Antitoxins are used in some cases.

—*Jason Georges and Tracy Irons-Georges*
See also Abscesses; Antibiotics; Bacterial infections; Blood and blood disorders; Burns and scalds; Infection; Poisoning; Septicemia; Shock; Toxicology; Wounds.

FOR FURTHER INFORMATION:

Avraham, Regina. *The Circulatory System.* New York: Chelsea House, 1989.

Barrett, John, and Lloyd M. Nyhus. *Treatment of Shock: Principles and Practice.* 2d ed. Philadelphia: Lea & Febiger, 1986.

Raven, R. W. *The Treatment of Shock.* Edited by L. Horder. London: Oxford University Press, 1942.

Strand, Calvin L., and Jonas A. Shulman. *Bloodstream Infections: Laboratory Detection and Clinical Considerations.* Chicago: American Society of Clinical Pathologists, 1988.

TOXICOLOGY

SPECIALTY

ANATOMY OR SYSTEM AFFECTED: Blood, brain, cells, immune system, nervous system

SPECIALTIES AND RELATED FIELDS: Anesthesiology, biochemistry, cytology, endocrinology, family practice, microbiology, occupational health, oncology, pathology, pharmacology, public health

DEFINITION: The study of poisons and their effects on the body.

KEY TERMS:

clinical toxicology: the area of medical science dealing with the diagnosis and treatment of disease associated with toxic substances

environmental toxicology: the study of the impact of chemical pollutants on biological organisms; human health is the primary consideration, but the specialty also examines the effects of toxins on nonhuman organisms

epidemiology: the study of common factors related to disease in a community; in the case of toxicology, such studies may be designed to evaluate the health of residents living in an area adjacent to a source of toxic chemicals

forensic toxicology: the branch of toxicology that interacts regularly with the legal community and law enforcement

occupational toxicology: a subspecialty of environmental toxicology that focuses on the effects of chemicals on the health of a workplace population

risk assessment: the process that establishes whether a health risk exists for a population exposed to a toxic substance

therapeutic drug monitoring: the medical term for clinical laboratory measurement of the level of therapeutic drugs in patient blood; this process ensures effective treatment and the avoidance of toxic effects that could result from excessive drug administration

toxicokinetics: the study of the time course of chemical absorption, distribution, metabolism, and elimination of toxic chemicals in the body; when the chemicals considered are therapeutic drugs, the correct term is "pharmacokinetics"

xenobiotics: drugs and chemical compounds foreign to the body; the terms "xenobiotic," "toxin," "drug," and "chemical" are used interchangeably when discussing toxicology, since all substances are poisonous at some concentration

SCIENCE AND PROFESSION

The application of toxicology to human health encompasses a diverse range of activities, including medical emergencies involving drugs or hazardous substances, occupational or environmental exposure to toxic chemicals, and medical investigations of chemical- or drug-induced injury or death. Toxicology has become an increasingly important aspect of medicine and health care as society has become more industrialized and technologically complex. It combines the knowledge of the medical sciences with that of the natural and applied sciences. Certain subspecialties of toxicology, called risk assessment and epidemiology, are also heavily dependent on the mathematics of statistics and probability. Toxicology affects the lives of virtually everyone in the industrialized countries, where millions of dollars are spent each year on the toxicological evaluation of products used by the consumer. In addition, government regulatory agencies and testing laboratories evaluate the toxicity and exposure level of hundreds of chemicals.

The areas of toxicology with the most medical relevance are clinical and forensic toxicology. Clinical toxicology deals with the diagnosis and treatment of the poisoned patient. It has been estimated that roughly 20 percent of all emergency room cases involve exposure to a hazardous chemical, an adverse drug reaction, or a drug overdose. The list of possible toxic drugs and chemicals increases every year. Therapeutic drug monitoring is the most common application of clinical toxicology. Drugs that are prescribed by physicians and may have toxic or lethal side effects can be measured in the blood by a variety of techniques. The results are used by the physician to determine whether the patient's dosage needs to be adjusted to achieve optimal therapeutic concentration.

In an emergency toxicology case, these same analytical techniques can be employed to screen for the presence of these medications. The more routinely a drug is prescribed or is available in a community, the more likely it is that overdose and toxicity problems will appear in the emergency room. The primary problem for hospital-based emergency toxicology testing is one of funding and staff support. Unless the medical facility is an urban-based toxicology center that receives specimens from a large area, it is very expensive to purchase the necessary sophisticated instruments and pay the salaries of laboratory personnel trained to operate such equipment. Cases arrive in an unpredictable fashion at the average hospital, so toxicological testing must be as integrated as possible into the normal clinical routine in order to keep costs low. Fortunately, most emergency toxicology cases are caused by a few predictable substances. Hospitals can usually offer a limited toxicology service that provides for testing of the most common toxic substances encountered in their specific patient populations.

Toxicology testing that will be utilized for legal purposes is called forensic toxicology. The forensic toxicology laboratory is most commonly involved in an after-death investigation in which there is a suspicion that either a drug overdose or underdose was involved. There are between eight thousand and ten thousand drugs that could be present in a patient or suspected overdose case. Most forensic laboratories routinely test for about one hundred fifty. The choice depends on the circumstances surrounding the death and what specimens are available.

Depending on the size of the forensic facility and budgetary considerations, toxicology testing may be done either on all cases as a matter of routine or on only those that have a strong drug-related component. In the former case, the toxicology data make possible a more complete investigation and provide valuable statistical information for evaluating current drug usage and tabulating drugs associated with violent death.

Although the forensic laboratory and the clinical laboratory use some of the same analytical techniques, a forensic laboratory uses a larger variety of analytical instruments and usually employs a full-time staff of specialists. In addition, the analytical approach is different from that used in clinical toxicology. Testing results for a forensic laboratory are rarely needed quickly for medical treatment, as is the case for clinical toxicology. Usually, the analysis is performed after death or used in a court case months or years after the event. The critical goal for a forensic laboratory is that each significant xenobiotic present be identified, its concentration be determined, and the results be defensible in court. All positive findings must be confirmed by at least one, and preferably two, methods that are technologically different from that used for the initial detection.

One area in which the distinction between clinical and forensic toxicology becomes ambiguous is that of drug abuse testing. Such testing can be ordered as part of either a medical or forensic workup. In the medical setting, the information is sought primarily for diagnosis and treatment, but many hospitals and medical referral laboratories also perform such testing as part of an employee drug testing or rehabilitation program. Enormous personal damage to the employee and legal liability to the testing agency can result from punitive action taken on the basis of a specimen misidentification or a false-positive result. All such programs should, therefore, strictly follow forensic rules of sample security, documentation of specimen handling, and confirmation of all positive results by methodology other than that used for initial detection.

In the United States, environmental and occupational toxicology historically have been regulated by government agencies separate from those that regulate health and medical care. The federal government has established the U.S. Environmental Protection Agency (EPA) for environmental regulation and the Department of Health and Human Services (DHHS) to deal with health. The Department of Energy (DOE) regulates the use of and exposure to radiation, although some governmental officials have suggested that such matters should be transferred to DHHS. These divisions usually are maintained at the state level also. As a result, the necessity of performing a risk assessment for the exposure to a particular chemical is often mandated by political pressure or by the eventual accumulation of significant statistical evidence to document an existing health problem.

Data used as the basis for determining the health effects of exposure to toxic chemicals are based on two principal sources: toxicological data derived from animal studies and worker exposure. Unfortunately, each of these sources has major disadvantages when used to calculate the risk of long-term exposure for the workplace or surrounding community. Animal and human reactions to the same toxin can be quite different, and medical histories of acute worker exposures may not provide sufficient information to determine the health effects of long-term, continuous human contact with a toxic chemical. Attempts to compensate for the uncertainty inherent in these main sources of toxicity data are made during the process of risk assessment. This process, besides using analytical data and hypothetical models of worker or community exposure, determines what adjustments in the data (safety factors) are to be used to express the uncertainties of the animal and worker exposure data to human health.

For many chemicals, there are few or no data to provide a comprehensive scientific basis for risk assessment, and there is even less information on the possible health effects of simultaneous exposure to multiple chemicals. The correlation of toxicological data with allowable exposure levels is a very complex process that must be continually updated as new information becomes available.

DIAGNOSTIC AND TREATMENT TECHNIQUES

The problems for the hospital analytical laboratory confronted with a "poisoned" victim have already been briefly discussed. For the physician charged with the care of such a patient, treatment often must begin before the specific identification of the toxic substance is known. Frequently, treatment is based on the physiological "fingerprint": the group of symptoms characteristic of one or a group of toxicologically similar agents. These groups of symptoms are also called "toxic syndromes" or "toxidromes." For example, those drugs that cause symptoms of central nervous system excitation—headache, seizures, hypertension, accelerated pulse, and profuse sweating—fit the pattern of a "sympathetic" toxidrome. For example, patients who have overdosed on amphetamines (uppers) or cocaine would be expected to display these symptoms. Despite the diversity of drugs that could cause this toxidrome, treatment can be based on ameliorating the symptoms of central nervous system excitation. If a toxidrome can be established, the physician can begin lifesaving therapy even when available information is minimal.

Therapeutic drug monitoring is used routinely for most patient medications with the potential for a toxic overdose. Blood levels of antiseizure medications, potentially toxic antibiotics, cardiac medications, and chemotherapeutic agents that have potential toxic side effects are monitored for individuals undergoing treatment.

Phenytoin is a commonly prescribed antiseizure medication. A dosage regimen is prescribed to maintain a blood concentration that is efficacious to the patient but does not exceed the concentration above which toxic effects can occur. Paradoxically, concentrations of phenytoin in the blood that exceed this value can induce seizures rather than suppress them. Phenytoin blood levels can change dramatically on the basis of changes in age, the presence of other diseases, and whether other drugs have been prescribed that may interfere with the disposition of phenytoin by the body. As a result, patient blood samples should be analyzed for phenytoin whenever a toxic reaction is possible and at times of changes in medication or patient health.

A common drug test performed by the laboratory that has both medical and forensic implications is that for ethanol. As the primary legal intoxicant available in the United States, ethanol is associated with a great number of vehicular accidents and criminal activities. Chronic alcoholism is also a major medical problem that leads to heart disease, liver disease, and nervous system disorders. The differences in the operating goals of forensic and clinical laboratories can be best illustrated by describing the routine protocol for ethanol analysis by both types of laboratories.

In the clinical laboratory, ethanol is detected in the liquid portion of the blood called serum. Since serum is the most convenient sample for automated laboratory chemistry analysis, clinical chemistry blood specimens are most often processed to obtain the serum, and the cellular portion is discarded. The physician requesting the alcohol testing is primarily interested in possible ethanol-related medical problems and cannot justify expending extra effort to document specimen handling and patient identification.

When a specimen is collected at the request of a law enforcement official, the judicial issues are of paramount importance. A formal chain of custody is maintained to document all contact with the specimen. Since the legal definition of intoxication is based on the analysis of whole blood alcohol, the testing is performed on whole blood by a special laboratory following a forensic protocol. Test results are generally accepted by the courts with minimal challenge. Although the alcohol testing results of a clinical laboratory can be accepted in legal proceedings, their use may require interpretation and testimony from a physician, a medical technologist, and sometimes the clinical toxicology laboratory director, in order to establish their legitimacy.

Among the groups of drugs commonly analyzed in a forensic laboratory are drugs of abuse, nonprescription pain relievers, anesthetics, toxic gases such as carbon monoxide and cyanide, heavy metals, and common alcohols other than ethanol. Prescription drugs that are commonly abused or that may result in lethal overdose are also likely to be tested. Samples obtained for testing may include not only blood or urine but also vitreous humor (eyeball fluid), bile, gastric fluid, and drug paraphernalia found at the site

of the event being investigated. In addition, tissue samples obtained at the time of autopsy can also be tested.

One of the primary applications of environmental toxicology is the assessment of carbon monoxide exposure, the leading cause of poisoning in the United States, accounting for 3,500 to 4,000 fatalities annually. The principal mechanism of toxicity of carbon monoxide involves its combination with the oxygen-carrying component of blood called hemoglobin. Carbon monoxide binds to hemoglobin with a higher affinity than that of oxygen and lowers the oxygen-carrying capacity of blood.

Exposure to environmental sources of carbon monoxide is very common. The gas is a common environmental pollutant. The body also produces some carbon monoxide endogenously, and cigarette smoking as well as exposure to any combustion process will result in some increase in carbon monoxide levels in the blood.

Inhaling high concentrations of the gas is the most common cause of immediate death in fire victims and is a major occupational hazard to firefighters. Death can occur in minutes. About one-third of all carbon monoxide fatalities are fire related. The remaining two-thirds are caused by exposure to products of incomplete combustion. Continuous inhalation of low concentrations over several hours can be as lethal as acute exposure. Carbon monoxide has no characteristic odor or appearance. The insidious and cumulative toxic effects of the gas can result in unconsciousness leading to death before the victim is aware of the problem. Chronic exposure causes headache, nausea, lethargy, and other symptoms that can easily be mistaken for a case of the winter flu. Faulty home heating systems, kerosene heaters, and the use of charcoal grills and other assorted open-flame cooking devices in closed spaces have all resulted in carbon monoxide poisonings. Treatment of either chronic or acute exposure consists of immediate removal of the victim from the exposure site, followed by the administration of oxygen and respiratory support when needed. The blood level of carbon monoxide can be monitored using a device called a cooximeter.

In terms of tons of pollutants emitted into the air annually, carbon monoxide is one of the top five and accounts for about 52 percent of the total. Its concentration is routinely monitored in major cities as an indicator of air quality. Exposure to levels of carbon monoxide found on the Los Angeles freeways has been shown to induce cardiac abnormalities in motorists with a history of heart disease. These individuals, as well as newborn children, are especially susceptible to toxic effects from this chemical.

Another environmental or occupational source of exposure is paint thinner. Solvents used in this product can be converted to carbon monoxide when inhaled or absorbed by the body. Their use for three or more hours in a poorly ventilated space by patients with preexisting cardiac conditions may result in death.

In summary, carbon monoxide is a toxic gas that may be considered a chemical poison, an industrial toxicant (commonly associated with fires), or an environmental pollutant (emitted by automobile exhausts). While toxicology can be subdivided into a spectrum of separate specialties, the basic physiological, chemical, and biological principles used within those specialties remain the same. Differences occur mainly in the source of xenobiotics of interest, the emphasis on risk assessment, and the regulatory framework.

PERSPECTIVE AND PROSPECTS

Toxicology is an ancient practice that has evolved into a science by combining the ancient knowledge of poisons with the techniques and knowledge of biology, chemistry, mathematics, and physics. Early humans utilized animal and plant toxins as part of the hunting and fighting arsenal—a practice continued even today by primitive tribes.

There are accounts throughout history of the uses of toxic agents. Among the more prominent are hemlock (the execution agent for Socrates), aconite (a Chinese arrow poison), opium (used as a poison and an antidote), and heavy metals such as lead, copper, and antimony. Descriptions of the use of poisons in early Greece and Rome as agents of execution, suicide, assassination, and political intrigue abound in ancient writings. That tradition was apparently continued in Italy and France during the Middle Ages by several experts who sold their knowledge and skill to many ambitious, but impatient, politicians and spousal heirs to family fortunes.

During the later years of the Middle Ages and the Age of Enlightenment, several figures were pivotal in the development of modern toxicology. One of the most influential was Philippus Aureolus Theophrastus Bombast von Hohenheim, better known as Paracelsus. Paracelsus recognized the fact that experimentation was essential in the study of the effects of toxic chemicals and that the difference between a toxic or therapeutic effect of a drug was often simply a matter of dose. Other significant contributors of later centuries were Matthieu-Joseph-Bonaventure Orfila, a Spanish physician in the French court who first used autopsy material and chemical analysis systematically as legal proof of poisonings; François Magendie, who studied the mechanisms of action of a number of toxins, including "arrow poisons"; and Claude Bernard, a student of Magendie who worked on the mechanism of action of carbon monoxide.

Living in the country with the most highly developed chemical industry of its time, German scientists in the late nineteenth and early twentieth centuries contributed significantly to the development of toxicology. Modern toxicology has really flourished as a result of industrialization, world wars, and the technological and analytical developments of the twentieth century. As human health was threatened—often dramatically exemplified by some toxic catastrophe— reformist and legislative action drove toxicology to increased prominence as a distinctive scientific discipline.

Elements of art remain part of the discipline, however, as they do in medicine. While the analytical and fact-gathering activities of toxicology can be considered the more traditional scientific aspects, the hypothesis-forming and risk assessment features of the discipline are its intuitive aspects. It may be a fact, for example, that saccharin in high doses causes cancer in rats or other laboratory animals, but the assertion that this chemical causes cancer in humans is a prediction. Although hypothesis forming involves a higher level of certainty than does speculation, it does not carry the certainty of fact until confirmed experimentally. Many of the controversial facets of toxicology in today's society are the result of mistaking hypotheses for facts. A primary challenge of toxicology is to confirm or refute those hypotheses that form the decision-making basis for determining the risks of exposure to hazardous chemicals.

—*David J. Wells, Jr., Ph.D.*

See also Bites and stings; Blood testing; Botulism; Critical care; Critical care, pediatrics; Dermatitis; Eczema; Emergency medicine; Environmental diseases; Environmental health; Enzyme therapy; Food poisoning; Forensic pathology; Hepatitis; Herbal medicine; Homeopathy; Intoxication; Itching; Laboratory tests; Lead poisoning; Liver; Occupational health; Pathology; Pharmacology; Pharmacy; Poisoning; Poisonous plants; Rashes; Snakebites; Toxemia; Toxoplasmosis; Urinalysis.

FOR FURTHER INFORMATION:

Amdur, Mary O., John Doull, and Curtis D. Klaassen, eds. *Toxicology: The Basic Science of Poisons.* 5th ed. New York: Pergamon Press, 1996. A basic work on toxicology that serves as a text as well as a reference for the basic principles, concepts, and foundations of thought for the discipline. A good summary discussion of the history of toxicology is found in the first chapter.

Baselt, Randall C., and Robert H. Cravey. *Disposition of Toxic Drugs and Chemicals in Man.* 3d ed. Chicago: Year Book Medical, 1989. A condensed toxic substances reference book. All toxins are listed alphabetically rather than by class or mechanism of action. The commonly encountered drugs and chemicals are listed, along with information on toxicokinetics, treatment, analytical techniques, and references for further information.

Crosby, Donald G. *Environmental Toxicology and Chemistry.* New York: Oxford University Press, 1998. With the experienced perspectives of a chemical practitioner, Crosby follows a careful and logical design for sixteen chapters, integrating the fields of environmental chemistry and toxicology in a coherent fashion.

Ellenhorn, Matthew J., et al. *Ellenhorn's Medical Toxicology: Diagnosis and Treatment of Human Poisoning.* 2d ed. Baltimore: Williams & Wilkins, 1997. A classic medical reference book on toxic substances. Drugs, industrial chemicals, animal and plant toxins, household products, and pesticides are discussed with an emphasis on medical symptoms and treatment.

Garriott, James C., ed. *Medicolegal Aspects of Alcohol Determination in Biological Specimens.* Littleton, Mass.: PSG, 1988. This book concentrates on ethanol. Chapters are devoted to discussions of alcoholic beverages and their chemical constituents, the metabolism and disposition of alcohol, methods of analysis, state and federal regulations on drinking and driving, and the reliability of breath and blood alcohol testing.

TOXOPLASMOSIS
DISEASE/DISORDER

ANATOMY OR SYSTEM AFFECTED: Gastrointestinal system, immune system, nervous system, skin

SPECIALTIES AND RELATED FIELDS: Family practice, pediatrics

DEFINITION: A widespread, infectious disease caused by a parasite.

CAUSES AND SYMPTOMS

The parasite *Toxoplasma gondii* that causes toxoplasmosis is fairly common and can infect warm-blooded animals as well as reptiles, but the ordinary house cat is the only known animal that sheds the toxoplasma parasite in its feces. Humans can also be infected by coming into contact with cat feces in a litter box or by eating raw or undercooked meat from infected animals.

The parasite may be acquired or congenital. Both forms seem to have a wide variety of clinical outcomes, ranging from a mild, asymptomatic state to an infection with fatal results. Congenital infection may manifest itself with jaundice, fever, anemia, convulsions, inflammation of the retina (chorioretinitis), an enlarged spleen or liver, and lymphadenopathy.

Acquired toxoplasmosis infection may be mild or severe. The vast majority of people that contract the disease have no or few symptoms, while others may have swollen glands, headaches, or a sore throat. These symptoms generally appear within ten to fourteen days after infection and subside within two to twelve weeks. Severe toxoplasmosis manifests itself by a possible fever, rash, pneumonia, encephalitis, myocarditis, pericarditis, hepatitis, and muscle inflammation (polymyositis).

When toxoplasmosis is acquired during pregnancy, it may badly harm the fetus, even if the mother did not have any symptoms. The degree to which the infection damages the fetus depends upon the stage of pregnancy. The parasite can be passed to the fetus in 15 percent of women infected during the first trimester, in approximately 25 percent infected during the second trimester, and in up to 65 percent of those infected during the last trimester. It is possible for the pregnant woman to suffer a spontaneous abortion or a stillbirth or to deliver a premature or a full-term child in which birth defects are present.

TREATMENT AND THERAPY

Pyrimethamine and sulfa drugs have reduced the complications from toxoplasmosis. When pyrimethamine is given to a pregnant woman during her first trimester, however, birth defects may occur. Physicians will prescribe sulfa drugs alone for infections occurring during pregnancy.

PERSPECTIVE AND PROSPECTS

The sporozoan *Toxoplasma gondii* was first isolated from an African rodent and was eventually described as a new species in 1909. In 1940, it was established as a factor for human disease.

It is possible to prevent toxoplasmosis by feeding cats only well-cooked meat or commercial cat food; keeping cats indoors, so that they cannot hunt and eat birds or mice; staying away from cats and having someone else clean the litter box during pregnancy; washing one's hands after touching uncooked meat; and cooking meat at a minimum of 151 degrees Fahrenheit (66 degrees Celsius).

—*Earl R. Andresen, Ph.D.*

See also Birth defects; Encephalitis; Eyes and visual disorders; Fever; Glands, swollen; Headaches; Hepatitis; Parasitic diseases; Pneumonia; Pregnancy and gestation; Protozoan diseases; Rashes; Sore throat; Zoonoses.

FOR FURTHER INFORMATION:

Buchsbaum, Ralph, et al. *Animals Without Backbones.* 3d ed. Chicago: University of Chicago Press, 1987.

Despommier, Dickson D., Robert W. Gwadz, and Peter J. Hotex. *Parasitic Diseases.* 4th ed. New York: Springer-Verlag, 2000.

Donaldson, Raymond Joseph, ed. *Parasites and Western Man.* Baltimore: University Park Press, 1979.

Klein, Aaron E. *The Parasites We Humans Harbor.* New York: Elsevier/Nelson Books, 1981.

TRACHEOSTOMY

PROCEDURE

ANATOMY OR SYSTEM AFFECTED: Neck, respiratory system, throat

SPECIALTIES AND RELATED FIELDS: Critical care, emergency medicine, general surgery

---

Tracheostomy

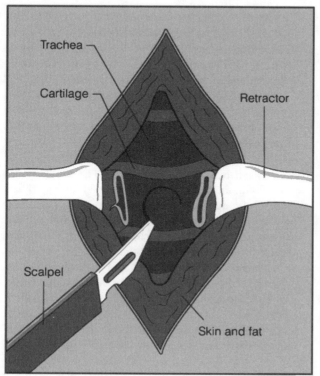

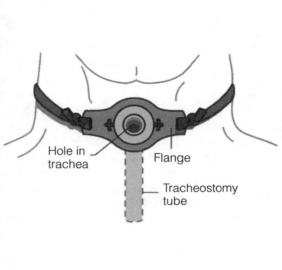

Certain throat disorders and diseases or the emergency need for an open airway may indicate the need for tracheostomy, the creation of a hole in the trachea (windpipe) through which the patient can breathe.

DEFINITION: The creation of a hole in the trachea, thus providing an alternative source for getting air into the lungs.

INDICATIONS AND PROCEDURES

A tracheostomy is the surgical creation of an opening into the trachea through the throat. It is done to relieve upper airway obstruction, decrease the effort of breathing, provide access for mechanical ventilation, and improve patient comfort. It is uncommonly used in an emergency except in the field; the preferred method of establishing an airway is to pass a tube through the trachea via the mouth.

Local anesthesia is used to deaden the skin of the front of the neck. A horizontal incision is made over the space between the second and third tracheal rings. If the thyroid gland is encountered, it is divided. Bleeding must be carefully controlled throughout the procedure. The trachea is entered through an incision which will divide the second and third rings of cartilage. In an adult, a small portion of the third ring may be removed. A previously tested tracheostomy tube with a cuff is inserted within the interior of the trachea. The wound is loosely closed, and a gauze dressing is applied. An X ray is taken after the procedure to ensure that the tube has been correctly placed and that there is no free air in the mediastinum or thorax.

USES AND COMPLICATIONS

Once a tracheostomy has been performed, ambient air in a patient's room must be humidified and warmed. If any secretions develop, the tracheostomy site must be suctioned in a sterile manner. If shortness of breath is observed, the tracheostomy site should be examined for a mucus plug. The tracheostomy tube should be removed and the opening closed at the earliest possible time that is consistent with the condition of the patient.

Some potential problems are associated with a tracheostomy. The most common is bacterial contamination of the lungs or adjacent tissues. Air may enter the space between the lungs and the tissue which lines the cavity containing the lungs, a condition known as pneumothorax. The tube may also become displaced. Attempting to replace the tube blindly can result in obstruction.

PERSPECTIVE AND PROSPECTS

Although dramatic when portrayed on television shows, a tracheostomy is a delicate surgical procedure that requires skill and training. With the invention of modern laryngoscopes, tracheostomies are uncommon, being used primarily in cases of fracture of the anterior neck.

—*L. Fleming Fallon, Jr., M.D., Ph.D., M.P.H.*

See also Asphyxiation; Choking; Critical care; Critical care, pediatric; Emergency medicine; Paramedics; Pulmonary medicine; Pulmonary medicine, pediatric; Respiration; Resuscitation.

FOR FURTHER INFORMATION:

Anderson, Kenneth N., et al., eds. *Mosby's Medical, Nursing, and Allied Health Dictionary.* Rev. 5th ed. St. Louis: C. V. Mosby, 1998.

Kittredge, Mary. *The Respiratory System.* Edited by Dale C. Garell. New York: Chelsea House, 1989.

Parker, Steve. *The Lungs and Breathing.* Rev. ed. London: Franklin Watts, 1989.

TRACHOMA

DISEASE/DISORDER

ANATOMY OR SYSTEM AFFECTED: Eyes

SPECIALTIES AND RELATED FIELDS: Environmental health, family practice, ophthalmology, pediatrics

DEFINITION: An infectious disease of the eyes that causes blindness.

CAUSES AND SYMPTOMS

Trachoma is caused by the *Chlamydia trachomatia* bacteria. It is carried primarily by children throughout the developing world, where water is scarce and washing is difficult. Combined with a general lack of hygiene, blowing dust and smoke from cooking fires provide a perfect environment for *Chlamydia trachomatia* bacteria to take hold.

Flies from refuse areas crawl on faces of children who sleep in crowded conditions. The insects touch those with the bacteria, then infect and reinfect others rapidly throughout an entire village. The eyes become red, painful, and sticky, causing irritation to the underside of the eyelid. Infection easily spreads as children touch the faces of their mothers and other children.

Left untreated, the eyelid and eyelashes turn in, damaging the cornea. The disease becomes more painful and injurious to adults as the eyelashes break off. This bristle-like effect lacerates the cornea and opaque scarring builds (a condition called trichiasis). Blindness is inevitable, usually by the age of forty to fifty.

TREATMENT AND THERAPY

Tetracycline eye ointment, twice a day for six weeks, gets rid of the infection. Face cleansing, especially for children, is the best way to prevent infection, along with environmental improvement and education. After the disease has advanced, the last hope is a surgical procedure to rotate the eyelid to its original position. The procedure is relatively simple. Nurses, medical assistants, and technicians can be trained to perform it at local clinics. Efforts to eliminate *Musca sorbens*, the aggressive flies in Africa and Asia, are also effective in controlling trachoma.

PERSPECTIVE AND PROSPECTS

The World Health Organization (WHO) estimates trachoma has blinded 6 million of the 38 million blind people in the world. Active infectious trachoma affects 150 million children. Areas most affected are Mexico, Brazil, Burkina Faso, Egypt, Kenya, China, Myanmar, and interior Australia.

In 1907, WHO launched a concerted effort to control trachomatous blindness by forming a consortium, the Global Elimination of Trachoma by 2020 (GET 2020). Strategy for GET 2020 is summarized by the acronym "SAFE," which refers to the four field-tested activities for control of trachoma; *s*urgery, *a*ntibiotics (tetracycline), clean *f*aces, and *e*nvironmental change. Trachoma control is one of the most affordable health interventions.

Education of the peoples involved is difficult. Because the disease is not fatal, they have little concern, accepting the disease as a fact of life. Mothers are being educated to find time to retrieve well water for washing their children's faces even when drought and poverty make feeding their families a trial. Mothers are being taught to understand the relationship between dirt on children's faces and the eye diseases making their own eyes red and sore. As such environmental improvement techniques are taught, villages are motivated to cooperate with worldwide and local agencies in the interest of curing trachoma.

—*Virginiae Blackmon*

See also Arthropod-borne diseases; Bacterial infections; Blindness; Childhood infectious diseases; Epidemiology; Eyes; Visual disorders; World Health Organization; Zoonoses.

FOR FURTHER INFORMATION:

Dawson, Chandler. "Flies and the Elimination of Blinding Trachoma." *The Lancet* 353, no. 9162 (April 24, 1999): 1376.
Schachterm, J., et al. "Azithromycin in Control of Trachoma." *The Lancet* 354, no. 9179 (May, 1999): 630.

TRANSFUSION

PROCEDURE

ANATOMY OR SYSTEM AFFECTED: Blood, circulatory system, immune system

SPECIALTIES AND RELATED FIELDS: Critical care, emergency medicine, general surgery, hematology, immunology, neonatology, serology, vascular medicine

DEFINITION: The introduction of whole blood or blood components (such as platelets, red blood cells, or fresh-frozen plasma) directly into the bloodstream.

KEY TERMS:

allogeneic: of the same species; in allogeneic blood transfusion, recipients are transfused with blood from another human being

alloimmunization: immunization by means of antibodies that react against substances from another person (such as blood)

apheresis: the removal of whole blood from a donor, followed by its separation into components, the retention of the desired component, and the return of the recombined remaining elements

autologous: self-derived; in autologous blood transfusion, recipients are transfused with their own blood

plasma: the liquid portion of blood in which the particulate components, such as proteins, are suspended; plasma is the origin of the blood components fresh-frozen plasma and cryoprecipitate

platelets: small, disk-shaped structures in blood that play a key role in blood clotting

red blood cells: blood cells that contain hemoglobin; the role of red blood cells is to transport oxygen

white blood cells: blood cells involved in the defense systems of the body; granulocyte components consist of white blood cells and are used to combat infections

whole blood: blood from which none of the elements has been removed

INDICATIONS AND PROCEDURES

Blood transfusion is the introduction of whole blood or blood components directly into the bloodstream. Human blood has been transfused with success since the early nineteenth century. Modern transfusion therapy, however, is largely the result of scientific advances made during the twentieth century and is, therefore, a young discipline. Blood transfusion plays a critical role in modern medical practice by enabling physicians to provide care, both surgical and non-surgical, which is not feasible in its absence. Until relatively recent times, transfusion options were limited to two items: whole blood and plasma. The introduction of blood component therapy in the 1960's had a major impact on transfusion practice.

Physicians are now able to choose from a large variety of specific blood products. Some products are the result of manufacturing processes that concentrate a portion of blood (blood derivatives), such as factor VIII concentrates for the treatment of hemophilia A. Other products, such as red blood cells or platelet concentrates (blood components), are separated, produced, and distributed by blood collection facilities for transfusion purposes. The cardinal principle of modern transfusion therapy is to administer the specific blood products that patients require. Portions of blood not required by the patient should not be transfused. Therefore, indications for the use of whole blood are very limited and its use is considered, in general, to be wasteful. The two major categories of transfusion are autologous and allogeneic. Autologous transfusion is the infusion of an individual with his or her own blood. Allogeneic transfusion is the infusion of blood collected from a person or people other than the transfusion recipient.

Autologous transfusion. Currently, there are four distinct types of autologous blood transfusion services available; preoperative donation, intraoperative hemodilution, intraoperative blood collection and reinfusion, and postoperative collection and reinfusion.

Patients scheduled for surgical procedures in which blood transfusion is likely are candidates to donate and store their own blood in advance for use at the time of surgery. This is preoperative donation. It may be possible to collect and store multiple units of blood with this technique. Close communication between patient and physician is critical in preoperative donation because the number of autologous units required must be determined and a donation schedule must be established. Usually, the last donation occurs no later than seventy-two hours before the scheduled operation. For surgical procedures in which the likelihood of transfusion is remote, preoperative donation has not proven to be cost-effective.

Intraoperative hemodilution is the removal of one or more units of blood from a patient at the beginning of an operation for reinfusion during or at the end of the procedure. The volume of blood removed is replaced by the infusion of solutions that contain no blood cells and no risk of infection, such as Ringer's lactate or albumin. Intraoperative hemodilution is considered beneficial for a number of reasons. First, this technique lowers blood viscosity (that is, it thins the blood), which may improve blood flow to vital organs. Second, the amount of actual blood loss during the operation is decreased because the patient's blood is diluted at the start of the surgery. Third, a supply of fresh, normal autologous blood for transfusion is available during and at the end of the surgery.

Intraoperative blood collection and reinfusion refers to the collection and return of blood recovered from the operative field or from machines used for the performance of an operation, such as a return of blood from the cardiopulmonary bypass machine used in cardiovascular surgery. Intraoperative autologous transfusion has proven to be an effective form of blood conservation in a number of surgical procedures, including cardiac, vascular, orthopedic, urologic, trauma, gynecologic, and transplantation surgeries.

Postoperative blood collection and reinfusion refers to the collection and return of blood recovered from surgical drains following an operation. This technique has been used predominantly following cardiac or orthopedic surgery. The overall effectiveness of this technique is still being clarified.

The different types of autologous transfusion should not be considered independently of one another. A coordinated approach using multiple techniques offers the greatest opportunity to maximize the value of autologous transfusion and minimize the chance that allogeneic transfusion will be required.

Allogeneic transfusion. This type of therapy begins with blood collection from informed, healthy donors. The allogeneic blood supply in the United States has never been as safe as it is at present. Blood donors are selected according to criteria designed to maximize donor safety and minimize recipient risks. Donor selection criteria are based on a high standard of medical practice and must comply with federal, state, and local regulations concerning blood collection. Facilities that collect and/or process blood and blood components for transfusion must comply with the United States Public Health Service's "Current Good Manufacturing Practice for Blood and Blood Components." These manufacturing practices are defined by the Code of Federal Regulations and are administered by the Food and Drug Administration (FDA). State and local laws often govern blood donor age requirements and the filing of reports, such as to state and county health departments, pertaining to donors whose laboratory tests reveal the presence of infectious diseases.

Blood donor selection starts with education regarding donor qualifications. Prior to every donation, potential blood donors are given information about human immunodeficiency virus (HIV) and acquired immunodeficiency syndrome (AIDS). Information is provided on the potential of HIV transmission to individuals receiving blood and on risk behaviors associated with HIV infection. Potential donors are informed of the absolute necessity of refraining from donation if they are at risk for HIV infection. Honest donor self-exclusion is a critical step in maintaining a safe blood supply.

The next phase of the donation process is the health history interview. Confidential interviews, often consisting of both a self-administered questionnaire and direct questioning, are conducted prior to every blood donation. Prospective donors are also tested for hemoglobin level (to check for the presence of anemia), temperature, pulse, and blood pressure. Some individuals are excluded because it is determined that blood donation poses an unacceptable health risk for the donor. Some exclusions, such as when a donor has a history of infectious disease or risk factors for HIV infection, are designed to protect blood recipients. Prospective donors are allowed to terminate the blood donation process at any time. Prior to the start of the actual blood donation, eligible donors are given the opportunity to ask additional questions and provide additional information. They are then asked to sign an informed consent statement. Some individuals may feel obligated to donate blood despite the realization that they do not qualify as safe donors. In this situation, donors are provided another opportunity to disqualify themselves through confidential unit exclusion (CUE). In CUE, blood donors choose "Transfuse" or "Do Not Transfuse" by marking a form or selecting a bar code label following the blood donation.

Laboratory testing of donor blood is required before whole blood or blood components can be made available for routine transfusion. A blood sample from every donation must pass an FDA-licensed test and found to be negative for hepatitis B surface antigen (HBsAg) and for antibodies to HIV viruses types 1 and 2 (anti-HIV 1/2), hepatitis B core antigen (anti-HBc), hepatitis C virus (anti-HCV), and human T-cell lymphotropic viruses types I and II (anti-HTLV-I/II).

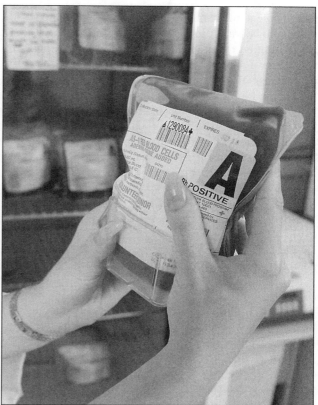

A bag of type A whole blood is stored for transfusion if needed. (Digital Stock)

Other tests routinely performed with every donation include a test for syphilis and a test for liver function called the alanine aminotransferase (ALT) level; these tests must be negative and normal, respectively.

Units of blood collected for "Autologous Use Only" at blood centers are ordinarily tested for syphilis, anti-HIV 1/2, HBsAg, anti-HCV, and anti-HBc. Blood units remain acceptable for autologous transfusion despite positive results in one or more tests. Some health care facilities collect Autologous Use Only blood components for transfusion within the institution. Such blood components drawn, stored, and infused at one facility may have not been tested for all the above-mentioned infectious diseases. If autologous blood donors have been screened and tested in a manner identical to allogeneic blood donors, unused autologous blood may be used for allogeneic blood transfusions. Most transfusion services, however, opt to destroy unused autologous blood.

The transfusion process begins with a physician's assessment of patient need and a formal order, clearly identifiable in the patient record, specifying the blood product to be transfused, the quantity, and any special administration requirements. This order is then transcribed to a special transfusion request form; computer-transmitted requests are acceptable as long as the required information is present. Forms requesting blood or blood components and forms accompanying blood samples from the patient must contain sufficient information for positive identification of the recipient. The first and last name and unique identification number of the patient are required. With the exception of extreme emergencies, such as patients who will bleed to death if there is any delay in transfusion of blood or blood components, the ABO (A, B, AB, or O) and Rh (positive or negative) types of the intended recipient must be determined before blood or blood components are issued for transfusion.

If the patient is to receive whole blood, red blood cells, granulocytes, or platelet components containing more than 5 milliliters of red cells (red cell-containing components), the recipient's serum (plasma lacking coagulation factors) must also be tested for the presence of clinically significant unexpected antibodies and for compatibility with the donor red blood cells. The only expected antibodies in a patient's serum are those directed at the A and/or B groups. Individuals who are in blood group O have antibodies directed toward the A and B groups, those who are in group A have anti-B antibodies, and group B individuals have anti-A antibodies. People who are in group AB do not have antibodies directed toward the A or B groups. There is no anti-O antibody. If the serum of a prospective transfusion recipient contains a clinically significant unexpected red cell antibody, red cell-containing components chosen for transfusion must lack the corresponding antigen (the determinant to which the antibody is directed).

With the exception of emergencies, the recipient's serum is usually tested with red blood cells from the donor prior to the release of red cell-containing components for transfusion. This procedure is known as the major crossmatch, and if recipient serum does not react with donor red cells, the red cell-containing unit is termed crossmatch compatible. It is now acceptable to use properly functioning computer systems to select compatible red cell units for transfusion in the place of a major crossmatch for recipients who do not have clinically significant unexpected antibodies. Blood components that do not contain 5 milliliters or more of red blood cells, such as fresh-frozen plasma,

cryoprecipitate, and most platelet components, do not have to be crossmatched.

Patients should receive blood and blood components of their own ABO group whenever possible. For red cell-containing components, with the exception of whole blood, alternative choices exist when ABO identical components are not available. For red cell-containing components, the donor red cells must be compatible with the recipient's plasma. For example, group A recipients may receive group O red blood cells. When transfusing components that contain plasma (whole blood, fresh-frozen plasma, cryoprecipitate, or platelets), it is best to transfuse blood products that are compatible with the recipient's red blood cells. For example, group A recipients may receive group AB fresh-frozen plasma since the plasma from group AB donors does not contain anti-A. Whole blood transfusion should be ABO identical because donor red cells and plasma must be compatible with the recipient.

For whole blood, red blood cells, platelets, and granulocytes, Rh-identical products should be provided whenever possible. Rh-negative units are acceptable for transfusion into Rh-positive individuals, but Rh-negative units should be reserved for Rh-negative recipients because of the limited supply of Rh-negative blood. The transfusion of Rh-positive blood into Rh-negative recipients will likely result in the formation of antibodies to the Rh antigen and therefore should be avoided in all but emergent situations. Rh type is not a consideration when transfusing fresh-frozen plasma or cryoprecipitate.

When there is a desperate requirement for blood, there may be a need to transfuse uncrossmatched red blood cells. If the recipient ABO group and Rh type are unknown, group O red cells should be transfused, and it is preferable that they be Rh negative. If there has been time to determine the recipient's ABO and Rh types with a current blood sample, then appropriate ABO and Rh type blood can be issued uncrossmatched (that is, uncrossmatched A positive red cells can be provided to a recipient determined to be A positive). Previous records must not be used to determine which blood group to issue, nor may the recipient's blood type be taken from other records such as credit cards, dog tags, or a driver's license.

Whole blood. A unit of whole blood contains approximately 450 milliliters of blood and 63 milliliters of anti-coagulant/preservative solution. All the elements that make up human blood are in whole blood.

Whole blood stored for more than twenty-four hours, however, contains few functional platelets or white blood cells. In addition, the levels of two proteins in whole blood necessary for normal blood clotting, known as coagulation factors V and VIII, decrease with storage. Stored whole blood, therefore, cannot be considered a source of functional platelets, functional white cells, or therapeutic levels of coagulation factors V and VIII. Whole blood provides oxygen-carrying capacity and blood volume expansion. Oxygen-carrying capacity is accomplished through the red blood cells present in whole blood. Red blood cells carry oxygen, which they deliver to vital organs and tissues. The approximately 500-milliliter volume of a unit of whole blood may make a significant addition to the total blood volume of a patient. The maintenance of a normal blood volume is vital to maintaining a proper level of pressure within the vascular system to get blood to and from vital organs and tissues. Patients lacking in blood volume may benefit from the volume provided by whole blood. Whole blood transfusions may be used, therefore, when there is a need for blood volume support combined with oxygen-carrying capacity, such as in patients experiencing severe acute hemorrhage.

For patients requiring oxygen-carrying capacity only, such as patients who have a normal blood volume but are anemic, red blood cell transfusion is recommended. When blood volume support is the sole need, such as in the early stages of acute blood loss when oxygen-carrying capacity has not yet become compromised but the blood volume is diminished, blood volume expanders that pose no risk of infectious disease—for example, normal saline (a salt and water solution)—are favored. Whole blood and other red cell components should not be used in patients with anemias that can be treated safely with specific medications such as iron, vitamin B$_{12}$, recombinant erythropoietin, or folic acid. Coagulation factor deficiencies, such as hemophilia, are more effectively treated with other blood components or derivatives. The storage period for whole blood varies from twenty-one to thirty-five days, based on the type of anticoagulant/preservative solution. As a result of time constraints posed by prerelease testing, whole blood that is less than twenty-four hours old is not routinely available. Whole blood stored less than seven days is often considered a desirable blood product for exchange transfusions in neonates (newborn children).

Red blood cell components. These components are produced when centrifugal or gravitational separation of red cells from plasma in whole blood is followed by the removal of 200 to 250 milliliters of plasma. The storage period of red cells collected and stored in an anticoagulant/preservative solution known as CPDA-1 is thirty-five days. Many red cell components contain a supplemental additive solution in addition to the anticoagulant/preservative. Additive systems in current use extend the storage period for red blood cells to forty-two days. Red cell transfusions increase oxygen-carrying capacity by increasing the circulating red blood cell mass. Increasing oxygen delivery to the body's organs and tissues with red cell transfusions may correct or prevent the manifestations of anemia. Red cell transfusions should be administered to patients with symptomatic anemia when other treatments are unavailable or ineffective and to those patients for whom rapid replacement of red cell mass is of critical importance. A unit of red blood cells contains essentially the same number of red cells as a whole blood unit. The volume of a red cell unit, however, is approximately 50 to 66 percent of whole blood. Thus, the use of red cells allows delivery of more red cells per milliliter transfused than whole blood, and smaller volume transfusions are required to achieve desired increases in oxygen-carrying capacity. When red blood cell components are used for exchange transfusion, it is common to use units that are less than seven days old. Stored red blood cells do not contain functional platelets or white blood cells.

In adults, a hemoglobin value of 7 grams per deciliter or less is commonly used as a guideline for red cell transfusion. (An example of a normal range for hemoglobin is 13.5 to 16.5 grams per deciliter in adult men and 12.0 to 15.0 grams per deciliter in adult women.) This is a useful guideline; however, the decision to transfuse red cells should be based on patient clinical status. Laboratory data should be utilized as part of overall patient assessment and not as a sole indicator for transfusion therapy. Signs and symptoms reflecting a possible need for red cell transfusion include fainting, shortness of breath, a drop in blood pressure when sitting up or standing up, rapid heart rate, chest pain, and transient neurologic deficits. In rapid acute blood loss, the hemoglobin value may not reflect circulating red cell mass. Red cell transfusion decisions in this setting are based on assessments of blood loss, cardiorespiratory status, and oxygen delivery to tissues. Certain diseases compromise oxygen delivery to tissues or the adequate oxygenation of red blood cells, such as heart disease, lung disease, and disease of the blood vessels supplying the brain. Such patients may need to be transfused at higher hemoglobin levels than other patients in order to maintain adequate organ and tissue oxygenation. In summation, the decision to transfuse red cells should be based on patient symptoms, laboratory data, underlying diseases, and the urgency of need for oxygen-carrying capacity.

In neonates, red cell transfusions are usually small in volume (5 to 10 milliliters per kilogram) and administered frequently. The most common indication for red cell transfusion in neonates is to replace blood drawn for laboratory studies. Blood losses caused by laboratory sampling are proportionately large in neonates because of their small blood volumes. Usually, red cells are transfused following the removal of 5 to 10 percent of the estimated blood volume from sick neonates requiring frequent monitoring. Neonates with severe respiratory disease, particularly those requiring oxygen and/or respiratory support, are usually transfused to maintain a hematocrit level (a laboratory test used as a marker for anemia) above 40 percent. An example of a normal range for hematocrit values in children is 40 to 50 percent. Similar transfusion guidelines have been established for neonates with congenital heart disease. In neonates without severe respiratory or heart disease, it has been recommended that red cell transfusions be given to maintain hematocrit levels above 30 percent for infants with shortness of breath, rapid breathing, episodes of no breathing, rapid heart rate, and abnormal heart rhythms. Some physicians advocate red cell transfusions to maintain hematocrit levels above 30 percent for infants experiencing poor weight gain.

Red cell components may be modified by centrifugation, filtration, washing, sedimentation, or freezing/thawing to remove white blood cells. White cell removal procedures must result in a component that contains fewer than 5×10^8 residual white blood cells while maintaining at least 80 percent of the original red cells. Many currently available white cell filters achieve much higher levels of white cell removal. White cell-depleted blood components are used to prevent febrile transfusion reactions (fever), to prevent or delay alloimmunization to white blood cell antigens, to prevent poor responses to platelet transfusions as a result of alloimmunization, and to prevent the transmission of white blood cell-associated viruses, such as cytomegalovirus, by cellular blood components.

Automated techniques are available for the washing of red cell units with sterile saline. This is less effective than filtration for white blood cell removal. The washing of red cells, however, does remove as much as 99 percent of the plasma from the red cell unit. Washed red cells may be indicated for patients requiring minimal plasma exposure. Examples include patients with a disease known as paroxysmal nocturnal hemoglobinuria, patients with IgA antibodies, and patients who have experienced recurrent or severe allergic transfusion reactions. Signs and symptoms of allergic reactions include hives, wheezing, low blood pressure, swelling of the throat, and fluid in the lungs.

Frozen red cells are prepared through the addition of glycerol, a cryoprotective (cold-protecting) agent, to red cells that are usually less than six days old, followed by freezing. The storage period for frozen red cells is ten years from the date that the unit was collected. When needed for transfusion, frozen red cells are thawed and washed with a series of saline-glucose solutions to remove glycerol. The unit is resuspended in sterile saline or a saline-glucose mixture. After thawing, washing, and resuspension, the storage period is twenty-four hours at 1 to 6 degrees Celsius. Frozen/thawed red cells are virtually devoid of plasma, anticoagulant, and platelets. The degree of white cell removal with this procedure is comparable to current filtration methods. Freezing is useful for the storage of rare red cell units and for the long-term preservation of autologous red cells. Because frozen/thawed red cells contain minimal amounts of plasma and white blood cells, they may be used when leukocyte-depleted and/or plasma-depleted red cell units are indicated.

Platelets. Platelet concentrates are prepared from whole blood by centrifugation. Most platelet concentrates contain at least 5.5×10^{10} platelets. The usual storage period for platelet concentrates is five days at 20 to 24 degrees Celsius. Platelets are often administered as a pool of concentrates.

Apheresis platelets are the second type of platelet component available. They are collected from a donor through the use of a blood cell separator in a procedure known as plateletpheresis. Most apheresis platelets contain at least 3×10^{11} platelets. An apheresis platelet (collected from one donor) is the equivalent of six to eight units of platelet concentrates. Apheresis platelets are sometimes beneficial in patients who are not responding satisfactorily to platelet concentrates because of antiplatelet antibodies (alloimmunization). Antiplatelet antibodies often arise in response to human leukocyte antigens (HLAs) present on donor platelets; these antigens aid the immune system in recognizing "self" or "nonself" material. Donors possessing HLAs that are identical or similar to those of the recipient may be selected to provide platelets for transfusion. Such components are known as HLA-matched platelets. Apheresis platelets can be used to decrease the number of blood donor exposures for a recipient and to reduce or delay the development of alloimmunization.

A low number of platelets (less than 50,000 per cubic millimeter) is known as thrombocytopenia; the normal range for platelets is 150,000 to 400,000 per cubic millimeter of blood. Thrombocytopenia may result from disease processes, such as leukemia or aplastic anemia, or from the medical treatment of diseases, such as the use of chemotherapy for the treatment of cancer. Thrombocytopenia can lead to bleeding problems. Patients with functionally abnormal platelets may experience bleeding and have normal platelet counts. Platelet transfusions may be indicated to treat significant active bleeding or to protect against bleeding prior to invasive procedures, such as major surgery, in patients with platelet dysfunction or thrombocytopenia. Prophylactic platelet transfusions are commonly administered to prevent bleeding in patients with thrombocytopenia caused by decreased platelet production, as with cancer therapy. A commonly accepted threshold for prophylactic platelet transfusion in such patients is a platelet count of less than 20,000 per cubic millimeter. Platelet transfusions are usually not effective in the setting of rapid platelet destruction, such as in a condition known as idiopathic (or autoimmune) thrombocytopenic purpura (ITP). Platelets are also not recommended for routine use in a condition known as thrombotic thrombocytopenic purpura (TTP). In the event of life-threatening hemorrhage in ITP or TTP, however, platelet transfusions may be necessary.

Prophylactic platelet transfusions are recommended for all neonates with a platelet count less than 20,000 per cubic millimeter. In the presence of active bleeding or prior to invasive procedures, platelet transfusions are recommended to keep the platelet count above 50,000 per cubic millimeter. In stable premature neonates, prophylactic platelet transfusions are recommended to maintain a platelet count above 50,000 per cubic millimeter. In sick premature neonates, platelet transfusions are given to maintain a platelet count above 100,000 per cubic millimeter.

Fresh-frozen plasma. The fluid portion of whole blood is called fresh-frozen plasma (FFP). It can be separated and frozen at −18 degrees Celsius or colder within eight hours of whole blood collection. FFP may be stored for up to one year at −18 degrees Celsius or colder. It contains all plasma proteins present in normal blood.

FFP may be used to treat isolated deficiencies of coagulation proteins (factors II, V, VII, IX, X, and XI) when more specific components are not available or appropriate. Patients on oral anticoagulant therapy, such as warfarin, may require FFP to reverse anticoagulant effect rapidly prior to emergency invasive procedures or because of active bleeding. Depletion of multiple coagulation factors may occur in patients who have developed a deficiency of vitamin K, in those patients receiving massive blood replacement, or with a condition known as disseminated intravascular coagulation (DIC). The use of FFP may be necessary to treat such problems. FFP may be required for patients with liver disease who are actively bleeding or who face invasive procedures. FFP contains antithrombin III (AT-III), a naturally occurring anticoagulant, and it may be used in patients requiring AT-III. Plasma components, either through simple transfusion or as part of plasma exchange procedures, have become a vital aspect of therapy for TTP.

Indications for FFP in neonates include liver failure, inherited coagulation factor deficiencies, bleeding caused by vitamin K deficiency, the treatment of DIC, protein C deficiency (another naturally occurring anticoagulant), and AT-III replacement therapy.

FFP is not recommended for coagulation abnormalities that can be treated more effectively or safely with specific therapy such as vitamin K (in less serious situations, vitamin K deficiency is treated with vitamin K replacement instead of FFP), cryoprecipitate, or specific coagulation factor concentrates. FFP should not be used as a volume expander or as a nutritional source.

Cryoprecipitate. A concentrated source of certain plasma proteins, cryoprecipitate is a white precipitate that forms when FFP is thawed at between 1 and 6 degrees Celsius. The cryoprecipitate is removed and refrozen at −18 degrees Celsius or colder. A single bag of cryoprecipitate has a volume of 10 to 15 milliliters. Cryoprecipitate has a storage period of one year when stored at −18 degrees Celsius or colder. Several proteins necessary for normal blood clotting are present in cryoprecipitate, including factor VIIIc, von Willebrand factor (vWF), fibrinogen, and factor XIII.

Cryoprecipitate is used in the treatment of hemophilia A (a deficiency or abnormality of factor VIIIc), von Willebrand's disease (a deficiency or abnormality of vWF), inherited or acquired fibrinogen deficiency or dysfunction, and factor XIII deficiency. Cryoprecipitate has been beneficial in some kidney disease patients with abnormal bleeding. It is used to prepare fibrin glue, a material with adhesive and hemostatic properties which has been shown to be of value as a sealant in many operative procedures.

Granulocytes. Units of white blood cells (granulocytes) may be obtained by apheresis or by removal from units of fresh whole blood. Granulocytes collected by apheresis have a volume of 200 to 300 milliliters and should contain more than $1.0 \times 10_{10}$ granulocytes. To maximize therapeutic effect, granulocytes should be transfused as soon as possible following preparation. If storage is necessary, granulocytes may be stored for twenty-four hours at 20 to 24 degrees Celsius.

Granulocyte transfusions have been used to aid treatment of serious infections in patients with dysfunctional or very low numbers of white blood cells who are not responding to conventional therapies. Neonates with blood infections (sepsis) may receive granulocyte transfusion as a supplement to antibiotic therapy.

USES AND COMPLICATIONS

The use of autologous transfusion has increased markedly since the mid-1980's. This increase is largely the result of concerns of patients and physicians about the transmission of certain diseases, such as AIDS and hepatitis. In addition to minimizing the risk of transmitting such diseases, autologous transfusion provides numerous other advantages. Alloimmunization, the formation of antibodies to substances (alloantigens) present in allogeneic blood, will not occur when autologous blood is used. Some patients requiring blood transfusion are already alloimmunized from previous allogeneic transfusion or pregnancy. The provision of compatible allogeneic blood in such patients can sometimes be difficult. Therefore, the availability of autologous blood in these situations, when possible, is advantageous.

A number of transfusion reactions may result from exposure to allogeneic blood—allergic reactions, fever, hemolytic reactions, graft-versus-host disease (GVHD)—that are prevented with autologous blood. Allogeneic blood appears to suppress the immune systems of transfusion recipients. Although there is still much to be learned about this phenomenon, the effect may adversely influence recurrence rates and mortality following some forms of cancer surgery and may lead to increased susceptibility to viral and bacterial infections. Autologous blood usage avoids these potential immunosuppressive effects. The use of autologous blood also leads to the conservation of vital blood resources. In the absence of the availability of autologous blood, transfusion needs must be met through the use of a volunteer allogeneic blood supply. For practical purposes, transfused autologous blood can be thought of as conserving a like amount of allogeneic blood. The availability of autologous blood may also lessen patient anxiety regarding the need for transfusion.

The overall risk of HIV infection from allogeneic blood transfusion is estimated at one in 225,000 per unit of blood (whole blood and blood components). The transfusion-transmitted infection rates for hepatitis B virus, HTLV-I/II, and HCV are estimated to be one in 200,000, one in 60,000, and one in 3,300 per unit, respectively. Although fear of HIV infection is a primary concern of transfusion recipients, transfusion-transmitted HCV infection is the principal infectious disease risk. The incidence of other transfusion-transmitted infections is very low in the United States. The current estimate of risk is less than one in one million per unit for transfusion-transmitted yersiniosis (*Yersinia enterocolitica* infection), malaria, babesiosis, and Chagas' disease (trypanosomiasis).

Transfusion-associated GVHD is a rare but severe complication of transfusion therapy. While patients with underdeveloped or impaired immune systems are at the greatest risk for developing this disease, it can occur in patients with normal immune systems. The transfusion of blood and blood components donated by blood relatives may put a recipient at risk for transfusion-associated GVHD. Gamma irradiation of whole blood and cellular blood components is the only currently acceptable method to reduce the risk. Fresh-frozen plasma and cryoprecipitate have not been implicated in this disease.

It is an absolute necessity that proper identification of recipients be obtained prior to any transfusion procedure. Transfusing facilities must have strict policies to guarantee that the appropriate types of blood or blood components are transfused to the correct patients. Blood and blood components are visually inspected prior to their release for transfusion. If their fitness is questioned upon inspection, they will not be released. Visual abnormalities include hemolysis (evidence of red cell breakage), follicular material, cloudy appearance, or a deviation from the usual color of the blood or blood component. Blood and blood components are prepared by techniques designed to safeguard sterility through their expiration date. Once the seal of a blood component has been broken for any reason, the expiration time is four hours if maintained at room temperature (20 to 24 degrees Celsius) or twenty-four hours if refrigerated (1 to 6 degrees Celsius). All transfusions must be administered through a filter. Transfusion recipients should be observed carefully during the first fifteen minutes of a transfusion. If a life-threatening transfusion reaction occurs, such as from the mistaken transfusion of incompatible red blood cells, it usually develops following the infusion of only a small volume of the blood or blood component. Blood transfusion must be completed prior to the expiration time of the component or within four hours, whichever is sooner. All adverse reactions to transfusion, including possible bacterial contamination or suspected disease transmission, must be reported to the transfusion service.

PERSPECTIVE AND PROSPECTS

The first well-documented transfusion of human blood to a patient was administered by James Blundell on September 26, 1818. For most of the first hundred years of human blood transfusion, blood was transfused from donor to recipient by means of a direct surgical communication between the donor and recipient blood supplies. Numerous transfusion-related fatalities resulted, probably from the infusion of incompatible blood. A landmark event in the history of transfusion medicine occurred in 1901 when Karl Landsteiner published his observations that the sera of some individuals caused the red cells of others to agglutinate (clump). This led to the discovery of the ABO blood group system and set the stage for safe transfusion therapy. Reuben Ottenberg and David J. Kaliski subsequently published their key observations on the importance of pretransfusion compatibility testing in 1913.

Despite these advances, blood transfusion remained a cumbersome technique until the value of blood anticoagulants was noted by multiple investigators in

1914 and 1915. For the first time, blood donation could be separated, in time and place, from blood transfusion. Blood could be drawn and set aside for use at a later time. This led to the development of blood banks for the storage and distribution of blood. The first hospital blood bank in the United States was established at Cook County Hospital in Chicago in the mid-1930's. Blood was collected in glass bottles that were washed, sterilized, and reused following transfusion. The introduction of plastic containers for blood in 1952 led to the development of disposable plastic systems for the collection, separation, and preservation of blood products. The advent of such plastic systems allowed whole blood to be separated easily into multiple blood components, thus setting the stage for modern blood component therapy.

Transfusion medicine has become a vital aspect of modern medical practice. Patients with cancer may be treated more aggressively because of the support provided by blood products. Organ and tissue transplantation (such as liver, kidney, and bone marrow transplants) and other complex surgical procedures have become possible because of blood and blood component therapy.

The use of blood and components is constantly evolving. Continual efforts are being made to maximize the safety and availability of the blood supply. Indications for blood and blood component transfusions continue to be analyzed and clarified. Alternatives to allogeneic blood transfusion, such as autologous transfusion, the use of blood growth factors (such as recombinant erythropoietin), and manufactured blood substitutes (such as oxygen-carrying perfluorochemical solutions), continue to be explored and are expected to receive more widespread application.

—*James R. Stubbs, M.D.*

See also Anemia; Bleeding; Blood and blood disorders; Blood banks; Blood testing; Catheterization; Circulation; Critical care; Critical care, pediatric; Emergency medicine; Hematology; Hematology, pediatric; Immune system; Immunology; Immunopathology; Rh factor; Serology; Surgery, general; Surgery, pediatric; Surgical procedures; Transplantation; Vascular medicine; Vascular system.

FOR FURTHER INFORMATION:
American Association of Blood Banks, American Red Cross, and Council of Community Blood Centers. *Circular of Information for the Use of Human*

Blood and Blood Components. ARC 1751. Arlington, Va.: Author, 1992. This small pamphlet is considered an extension of blood component container labels and as such is a standard informational source on the use of blood and blood components.

McCullough, Jeffrey. *Transfusion Medicine.* New York: McGraw-Hill, 1998. Transfusion medicine, a young science, is continuously growing and changing. The result is a great body of knowledge about the practical aspects of blood collection and transfusion, and an incomparably better understanding of the blood groups and of the unintended effects of transfusion at the molecular level.

Petz, Lawrence D., et al., eds. *Clinical Practice of Transfusion Medicine.* 3d ed. New York: Churchill Livingstone, 1996. Another comprehensive, detailed textbook on virtually all aspects of transfusion medicine. As a reference source, it is comparable to the text edited by Rossi et al.

Rossi, Ennio C., Toby L. Simon, and Gerald S. Moss, eds. *Principles of Transfusion Medicine.* Baltimore: Williams & Wilkins, 1991. A comprehensive textbook that contains detailed discussions on virtually all aspects of transfusion medicine. As opposed to the *Technical Manual*, which is a day-to-day working resource, the value of this text is as a reference source containing detailed information.

Walker, Richard H., ed. *Technical Manual.* 11th ed. Bethesda, Md.: American Association of Blood Banks, 1993. This book is the bible of blood banking and transfusion practice. An indispensable source of information that deserves a place in every blood bank. The chapters are filled with easy-to-understand, practical information on blood banking.

TRANSIENT ISCHEMIC ATTACKS (TIAS). *See* STROKES.

TRANSPLANTATION
PROCEDURE
ANATOMY OR SYSTEM AFFECTED: Blood, circulatory system, eyes, heart, immune system, kidneys, liver, lungs, pancreas, respiratory system, spleen, urinary system

SPECIALTIES AND RELATED FIELDS: Cardiology, emergency medicine, general surgery, genetics, immunology, nephrology, oncology, urology

DEFINITION: The transfer of tissue or organs from one individual to another, usually from cadavers or living related donors.

KEY TERMS:

acute rejection: the rejection of a transplanted organ by cells of the immune system; acute rejection is common days to weeks after cadaveric organ transplants and can usually be treated successfully with antilymphocytic drugs

allotransplantation: the transplantation of tissue or organs between unrelated individuals

chronic rejection: the rejection of a transplanted organ months or years after the procedure because of mechanisms that are poorly understood; most long-term graft losses are caused by chronic rejection, and no effective therapy exists

distributive justice: allocating transplanted organs to recipients based on need

haematopoietic stem cell transplantation (HSCT): transplantation of the bone marrow cells to a recipient

human leukocyte antigens (HLAs): structures located on the surface of each cell that are unique to an individual; also called transplantation antigens

material justice: allocating transplanted organs to recipients based on who would most benefit

orthotopic: the placement of a transplanted organ in the position occupied by the original organ

tissue typing: the process of identifying a person's transplantation antigens

utilitarianism: an ethical theory in which individuals make moral decisions based on the likelihood of benefitting the maximum number of people

vascularized transplant: transplanted tissue or organs that must have blood vessels reattached in the recipient in order to function (such as a kidney); corneal or bone marrow transplants are examples of nonvascularized transplants

xenotransplantation: the transplantation of tissue or organs between different species (such as baboon to human)

THE IMMUNE SYSTEM AND TRANSPLANTATION

Transplantation antigens are proteins expressed on the surface of an individual's cells. Every individual has a unique set of these proteins, called human leucocyte antigens (HLAs), which are encoded on chromosome 6. Each parent contributes one HLA-containing chromosome, and both chromosomes are expressed in the offspring. The purpose of these antigens is to help the body recognize what is "self" and what is not. In this manner, bacteria and other pathogens harmful to the individual can be sensed as "nonself" and destroyed by the immune system.

When an organ is transplanted between unrelated people (allotransplantation), it will not be recognized as self in the recipient's body, and the immune system will start to attack it in a process called "rejection." In the same way, transplants between identical twins, with the same HLA proteins on their cells, will be recognized as self and not be rejected.

White blood cells (WBCs or lymphocytes) are intimately involved in the body's immune response. They protect the individual from invading bacteria, viruses, and fungi. Lymphocytes can be divided into two subsets: B and T cells. The T cell is the main cell involved in the recognition and destruction of allotransplants. Receptors found on the T lymphocyte cell surface are stimulated by the foreign antigens found on allotransplants. With T-cell stimulation, events are initiated that lead to the allotransplant's destruction.

With the knowledge that T cells are responsible for rejection, methods of modulating T cell activity were developed. One of the first approaches was to destroy them using total-body irradiation. This method had only limited success, and the side effects of the radiation were severe. Attention then turned toward drugs that acted directly on T cells.

Azathiaprine was one of the first drugs to be used successfully. By preventing the biosynthesis of essential components of cell growth, azathiaprine inhibits T cells from replicating. Steroids were next found to have immunosuppressive properties. Azathiaprine and steroids at one time were used in combination to prevent rejection in human kidney allografts. Although these drugs were effective, they were not specific for T cells. Other cells were affected, and both immunosuppressive drugs had serious side effects in high doses. In 1978, a T-cell-specific inhibitory drug was tried clinically for kidney allotransplants. This drug, named cyclosporine, has since become the mainstay of immunosuppressive therapy for all vascularized allotransplants. In most transplant centers, patients who have received allotransplants are given a combination of the above three drugs, since each drug works differently on T-cell function. The harmful side effects of these drugs can be minimized by using all three in smaller amounts, thus preventing the side effects from larger doses.

With the advent of cyclosporine, patients receiving kidneys without matching HLAs do almost as well in the short term (one to five years) as those receiving HLA-matched kidneys. Transplanted kidneys with HLAs in common, however, function significantly longer (ten years). Therefore, physicians try to match HLAs between donor and recipient. Most organs available for transplantation are from cadavers. It takes days to tissue-type the cadaver, find a compatible recipient, and transport the organ to him or her. Kidneys are the only organ that can be stored this long and still function. Therefore, only kidneys are matched for HLAs. With the liver, heart, and pancreas, only blood type is matched between donor and recipient. Currently, kidneys may be stored up to three days. The liver and pancreas must be transplanted within eighteen to twenty hours.

INDICATIONS AND PROCEDURES

With the advent of dialysis in 1960, renal failure is no longer fatal and patients can live by having their blood filtered several times per week. Kidney transplantation, however, offers a significant improvement in the quality of life compared with dialysis. Unfortunately, while more than 9,000 patients in the United States receive kidney transplants each year, another 8,500 patients remain on waiting lists. With only 13 percent of potential donors actually being utilized, there is much room for greater success.

Two donor options are available to the recipient awaiting a kidney transplant: living related and cadaveric. The first option involves removing a kidney from a willing family member and transplantation into the recipient. Removing one of two donor kidneys does not significantly affect a healthy individual. The second option is for the recipient to be placed on a waiting list for a cadaveric kidney. When a cadaveric kidney that is of a compatible blood type for a particular recipient becomes available, arrangements are made to admit this patient to the hospital for transplant.

Approximately 25 percent of all kidney transplants are living related. The advantages of a living related transplant are twofold. First, the waiting period for a cadaveric kidney is eliminated, as the operation can be scheduled as soon as the recipient has been evaluated. Second, kidneys from living related donors tend to work immediately, with better long-term results. Because of organ shortages, some medical centers will allow unrelated volunteers to donate a kidney to a recipient. Such transplants usually occur between spouses.

A typical kidney transplant operation takes three hours to perform. Usually, the patient's own kidneys are not removed, and the transplanted kidney is placed in the pelvis. The vessels of the new kidney are sewn into the iliac blood vessels of the leg. After the transplant procedure, patients stay in the hospital ten days before returning home. They must take medications every day to prevent rejection but otherwise are independent.

Orthotopic liver transplantation is now considered the optimal form of therapy for end-stage liver disease in adults and children. Since no machine exists to take the place of the liver, transplantation is the only alternative in patients with liver failure. Cadaveric livers are the source for transplants because individuals have only one liver. Because of a shortage in cadaveric organs, many patients die each year waiting for a liver transplant. For this reason, a few medical centers have experimented with living related liver transplants, usually from parent to child. In this operation, one of the two lobes of the donor's liver is removed and transplanted to the recipient. The remaining liver in the donor will grow back to normal size in one week.

A liver transplant is one of the most difficult operations to perform. Unlike heart operations, there is no machine to take the place of the liver during surgery, and speed is vital. The liver is the largest organ in the body, weighing about 5 pounds in an adult. Because the liver is so large, and its blood supply complex, it is necessary to remove the patient's own liver during the transplant. The average time for a liver transplant varies, ranging from five to thirty hours. The worst complication of liver transplant is failure to function after surgery. The only treatment is to find another liver for transplantation before the patient dies.

Pancreas transplants are done exclusively for patients with complications of insulin-dependent diabetes mellitus (IDDM). Around half of the 15,000 new cases of IDDM per year will develop complications such as renal failure and blindness. There is no way to predict which patients will develop these complications. Currently, combined pancreas-kidney transplants are done for diabetics who experience renal failure. The transplanted pancreas prevents damage from recurring in the new kidney and also makes the individual insulin-independent. Pancreas transplants are not performed for diabetics without complications because the risk of immunosuppression is not worth the benefit of insulin independence.

Unlike with liver transplants, short operative time for pancreas-kidney transplantation is not essential to patient survival. Both the pancreas and the kidney are placed into the pelvis, and the pancreas is anastomosed (sewn) to the right iliac vessels and the kidney to the left. Operative time is about ten hours. As with kidney transplants, the patient's own pancreas and kidneys are left in place because there is no advantage to removing them.

The transplantation of bone marrow, sometimes called haematopoietic stem cell transplantation (HSCT), is less demanding than transplantation of vascularized organs. The bone marrow is composed of stem cells that are primarily responsible for developing into red and white blood cells. A stem cell is any cell from which a whole population of different cells may develop. Transplant recipients, who usually have a blood disease such as leukemia, undergo a process of chemoradiotherapy to destroy their own stem cells. Once it is certain that all their own cells are destroyed, the donor cells are injected into the long bone of the leg. Following HSCT, the recipient may be immunologically incompetent for some time. The functioning of the immune system is vital to the success of this type of transplant. The WBCs begin to reappear in the blood during the second or third week after the transplant. Although many lymphocytes begin functioning as soon as they are generated, the T and B cells do not become active until later. This is primarily due to the suppression of WBC function due to the presence of immunosuppressive drugs. There is evidence from immunologist Katalin Poloczi that bone marrow recipients have normal immune responses and may be vaccinated against various diseases. However, he has also observed that such patients must get booster shots more often than "normal" individuals to maintain immunity.

Fetal tissue transplantation therapy is related to stem cell therapy in that vascularized organs are not transplanted. Fetal tissue cell lines, sometimes called pleuripotent stem cells, have the ability to develop into any cell types found in the adult human body: brain cells for Alzheimer sufferers, pancreas cells for diabetics, heart cells for cardiac patients, and more. There are four sources for pleuripotent stem cells: preimplanted human embryos from in vitro fertilization (IVF), umbilical cord blood, cadaveric human fetal tissue, and human germ cell tumors. Although potentially very valuable, research in this area has become an ethical firestorm due to the embryonic source of the tissues. There is the worry that to obtain these cells researchers may actively begin aborting human embryos. Despite this controversy, the stem cell treatment holds such therapeutic promise that no one has yet abandoned the concept.

Researchers at the University of Wisconsin are presently growing pleuripotent stem cells in culture. Unfortunately, since the sources of those cells were aborted, preimplanted human embryos, there is the ethical question of whether this is tainted research. The funding for these investigations was chiefly private, since the U.S. government has banned funding for research into development of these human cell lines.

Another controversial process is xenotransplantation, the transplanting of organs from one species to another. Xenotransplantation, if successful, could dramatically increase the supply of organs worldwide. Porcine transplants to replace human hearts and kidneys are being considered. Because of fears of transmitting animal diseases into human populations, some researchers have demanded a worldwide ban on such research. It is not clear whether these fears are justified. For example, a 2000 study from Stellan Welin of Göteborg University reported that patients with porcine transplants displayed no signs of porcine endogenous retrovirus. Even if xenotransplants do not transmit diseases, many ethical problems remain. One such problem is whether researchers should genetically modify source animals to change their immunological profiles. The consequences to altered livestock are still not clear. For example, a transgenic pig making bovine growth hormone may grow faster than normal but may be more susceptible to numerous uncharacterized, pathologic changes.

Perspective and Prospects

There are a number of ethical problems connected to organ transplantation. Primary among these is the problem of donor selection. Cadaverous donors sometimes present the problem of whether sufficient permission was given to donate organs. Without full consent of the donor, it is considered unethical to harvest tissues. In cases where the potential donor died without giving consent, very often relatives who knew of their wish will give consent in their stead. In the case of living donors who are donating kidneys or bone marrow, questions will sometimes arise of their ability to give full consent; for example, whether the donor is fully competent and informed of what consent means. These questions of competence will usually arise with the mentally ill, but often arise when the donor potentially has been coerced by physicians or relatives. Coercion on anyone's part eliminates full consent from the donor.

Another recent ethical dilemma is the use of human newborns or late stage embryos as organ donors.

In the News: Xenotransplantation

The shortage of available human organs has led to the consideration of using animal organs as a source of transplants for humans, a process called xenotransplantation. Although its genetic similarity to humans is not as close as that of nonhuman primates, the pig is close enough to represent a potential, and controversial, source of organs. For decades, pig hearts have served as a source of replacement valves in humans with few adverse reactions. However, if pigs are to be seriously considered as subjects for organ xenotransplantation, they would have to be genetically modified to reduce the risk of rejection by human recipients. Such transgenic modifications are theoretically possible and would probably involve relatively few human genes being transplanted into embryonic pigs.

Even if pigs did become available for possible xenotransplants, significant problems remain. Cross-species transplants have rarely been found to be successful. Furthermore, pigs are known to carry a number of endogenous viruses not found in humans. While the chance of transplanting such viruses into the human species is remote, the danger still exists. The cost of xenotransplantation procedures would also be considerable and, under the current health care system, would likely benefit relatively few individuals.

Religious considerations would also have to be factored into the question of the pig as a source of organs. Both Judaism and Islam consider the pig to be an "unclean" animal; use of organs from a pig may be precluded among observant individuals in these faiths.

—*Richard Adler, Ph.D.*

Is it ethically permissible to use a fetus as an "organ farm"? There have been reports in the last several years of parents with a terminally ill child conceiving another child to act only as an organ donor. Although most often these donor infants become family members, they are sometimes aborted because the needed organ can only be obtained in that way. The bioethicist Mary Anne Warren has argued that the mere "potential to become a person"—unaccompanied by awareness, consciousness, and perception—does not entitle one to life compared to that of a person that needs a transplant. Warren finds no ethical objection to killing a fetus, an "entity below the level of personhood," in order to save the life of a grown human being. Whether or not there is abortion involved in the harvesting process, the ethicist Daniel C. Maguire submits that "person" is a relative term and even baby persons are intrinsically related to other persons. Maguire argues that using the uterus as an organ farm or the "objectified" fetus as an organ bank is intrinsically wrong at the level of consent. What right does anyone have to presume the permission of the baby to donate an organ to a sibling or even a parent? He suggests that the privacy and autonomy of the baby be protected until it grows and itself can consent to an organ donation.

Maguire's argument has also been applied to the harvest and use of embryonic stem cells. When the cells are harvested directly from an embryo, whether that embryo was discarded from IVF or conceived for that specific purpose, the question of consent still remains unanswered.

Finally, allocation of transplanted organs has become increasingly difficult in recent years as the number of available organs has become overwhelmed by the number of recipients. A series of ethical questions has arisen in organ transplant allocation. Will the young or old recipient better benefit from a transplant? Should countries limit organ donations from their citizens to non-immigrant aliens? Should organ recipients of particular note, such as film stars and athletes, be moved ahead of "commoners" who are already on the waiting list? Should the location of the recipient affect the decision to provide an organ?

One principle that has been suggested as a guide to allocation is called "distributive justice." Distributive justice suggests that donor organs should go to those most in need. Most countries have now devised rules by which available organs go to those who are the most critically ill. The problem with this selection

strategy is that the patients who are in the greatest need are the least likely to survive long term. If the goal is to maximize the overall benefit to society, as the ethical theory of utilitarianism suggests, then this method reduces the overall advantage to society compared to a system that would donate to patients with a better prognosis.

The opposing theory, called "material justice," suggests that patients who are likely to benefit most from transplantation get the organs first. This would maximize the benefit to society, which is risking less on a recipient with a better prognosis. One interpretation of this principle is that children with longer lives ahead of them would get preference for transplantation over adults or the elderly.

These two principles seem at odds with one another. Although the individual will benefit most from distributive justice, society may suffer, and the opposite might be true of material justice where society will benefit, but the individual may suffer. In order to make allocation as just as possible, the United Network of Organ Sharing (UNOS), the primary body which coordinates organ donors and recipients worldwide, has utilized a point system since August 1995. This point system creates a value for determining the suitability of a recipient for a particular donor based on number of years waiting, rank on the waiting list, HLA tissue mismatches, immune reactivity, and age.

Besides these other factors, very often the geographic profile of the recipient can be problematic. If a potential transplant recipient has come to the United States from the Third World, where organ donors are rare, in the hope of more easily getting a transplant, should he or she be considered a serious candidate? Should that person be placed ahead of native or naturalized citizens on the waiting list? Should an American citizen and potential recipient living in an isolated geographic location be placed lower on a waiting list because of his or her isolation? These questions are difficult to answer because they bring geography and politics into the equation with medicine and human needs. In September, 2000, the U.S. Department of Health and Human Services (DHHS) proposed rules to reduce the importance of geographic and political boundaries on organ allocation. The prime selection criterion—especially in heart and lung transplantation—would be altered by the DHHS primarily to reflect waiting time. Under these criteria, it would not matter where the candidate resided or where they originated. The only basis for selection would be their need and how long they had been waiting for a transplant.

It has been proposed that organ donors be allowed to sell transplanted organs to the highest bidder. This concept has been defended as "allowing the free market economy to flourish" and letting the poor have the right to do with "their bodies as they see fit." One ethical difficulty with the idea of commercializing human organ sales is that those who are richest will tend to receive the "best" organs. Organ allocation would suffer from these sales, and just distribution would become meaningless. No longer would the most needful recipient get an organ, but rather those who could most afford it. Furthermore, the poor would be victimized, become commodities, and be dehumanized as they potentially become organ farms. Legislation was passed by the World Health Organization and the Transplantation Society in 1999 to universally prohibit the sale of organs.

—Edmund C. Burke, M.D.,
and Peter N. Bretan, M.D.;
updated by James J. Campanella, Ph.D.

See also Bone marrow transplantation; Cancer; Cirrhosis; Corneal transplantation; Diabetes mellitus; Dialysis; Eye surgery; Eyes; Fetal tissue transplantation; Grafts and grafting; Hair loss and baldness; Hair transplantation; Heart; Heart transplantation; Hepatitis; Immune system; Immunology; Kidney transplantation; Kidneys; Leukemia; Liver; Liver transplantation; Renal failure; Systems and organs.

FOR FURTHER INFORMATION:

Nora, Paul F., ed. *Operative Surgery: Principles and Techniques.* 3d ed. Philadelphia: W. B. Saunders, 1990. Offers a concise, well-written chapter that summarizes the facts and operative details regarding kidney, liver, and pancreas transplantation. Written by leaders in the field of transplantation.

Sabiston, David C., Jr., ed. *Textbook of Surgery: The Biological Basis of Modern Surgical Practice.* 16th ed. Philadelphia: W. B. Saunders, 2001. An outstanding textbook that details all aspects of transplantation and immunology. The milestones in transplantation history are well covered. The authors of individual sections are all pioneers in the field of transplantation.

Schwartz, Seymour I., ed. *Principles of Surgery.* 7th ed. New York: McGraw-Hill, 1999. A chapter reviewing most aspects of surgical transplantation is provided in this text. The section on transplant im-

munology is particularly excellent, with most of the important terms clearly defined.

Toouli, James, et al., eds. *Integrated Basic Surgical Sciences.* New York: Oxford University Press, 2000. Offers a concise, well-written chapter that summarizes the facts and operative details regarding kidney, liver, and pancreas transplantation. Written by leaders in the field of transplantation.

Trzepacz, Paula T., and Andrea F. Dimartini, eds. *The Transplant Patient: Biological, Psychiatric, and Ethical Issues in Organ Transplantation.* New York: Cambridge University Press, 2000. This excellent book addresses many ethical issues dealing with transplant patients, including specialty transplant populations, psychopharmacology, and assessment of the psychiatric characteristics of transplant patients.

Whitehead, E. Douglas, ed. *Current Operative Urology 1990.* Philadelphia: J. B. Lippincott, 1989. Includes a chapter that reviews kidney transplantation in adults from a practical viewpoint. Gives the reader an understanding of the selection and preparation process of recipients for kidney transplants.

TREMBLING AND SHAKING
DISEASE/DISORDER

ANATOMY OR SYSTEM AFFECTED: Brain, muscles, musculoskeletal system, nervous system

SPECIALTIES AND RELATED FIELDS: Neurology

DEFINITION: Also known as tremors, trembling and shaking are characterized by a series of involuntary, quivering movements which are caused by uncontrolled tightening and relaxing of a group of muscles. Transient or temporary tremors may occur as a result of hunger, cold, physical exertion, fatigue, or excitement. Some trembling and shaking may be hereditary. Several diseases have tremors associated with them, including Parkinson's disease, hyperthyroidism, Wilson's disease, diseases of the cerebellum, and multiple sclerosis. Tremors can also be caused by toxins. Treatment varies depending on the cause of the tremor.

—Jason Georges and Tracy Irons-Georges

See also Multiple sclerosis; Muscle sprains, spasms, and disorders; Muscles; Parkinson's disease; Thyroid disorders.

FOR FURTHER INFORMATION:

Adler, Charles H., and J. Eric Ahlskog, eds. *Parkinson's Disease and Movement Disorders: Diagnosis *and Treatment Guidelines for the Practicing Physician.* Totowa, N.J.: Humana Press, 2000.

Elble, Rodger J., and William C. Koller. *Tremor.* Baltimore: The Johns Hopkins University Press, 1990.

Findley, Leslie J., and William C. Koller, eds. *Handbook of Tremor Disorders.* New York: Marcel Dekker, 1995.

Joseph, Anthony B., and Robert R. Young, eds. *Movement Disorders in Neurology and Neuropsychiatry.* 2d ed. Malden, Mass.: Blackwell Science, 1999.

TRICHINOSIS

DISEASE/DISORDER

ANATOMY OR SYSTEM AFFECTED: Gastrointestinal system, intestines, muscles, musculoskeletal system

SPECIALTIES AND RELATED FIELDS: Gastroenterology, public health

DEFINITION: Trichinosis is an infection caused by larvae of the parasite *Trichina spiralis.* It is contracted by eating uncooked pork or pork products. The larvae develop into adults in the intestines and release fresh larvae into the bloodstream and into other organs, such as the heart and brain, where they form cysts. Symptoms include appetite loss, nausea, vomiting, diarrhea, and abdominal cramps. Later stages include muscle pain, puffy eyelids and face, irritated skin, sweating, and high fever. Untreated cases can lead to congestive heart failure, respiratory failure, and permanent damage to the central nervous system. Thorough cooking of meats kills the parasites and makes food safe to eat. Trichinosis is treated with antiparasite drugs that kill adult worms in the intestines.

—*Jason Georges and Tracy Irons-Georges*
See also Food poisoning; Intestinal disorders; Intestines; Parasitic diseases; Worms.

FOR FURTHER INFORMATION:

Buchsbaum, Ralph, et al. *Animals Without Backbones.* 3d ed. Chicago: University of Chicago Press, 1987.

Despommier, Dickson D., Robert W. Gwadz, and Peter J. Hotex. *Parasitic Diseases.* 4th ed. New York: Springer-Verlag, 2000.

Donaldson, Raymond Joseph, ed. *Parasites and Western Man.* Baltimore: University Park Press, 1979.

Klein, Aaron E. *The Parasites We Humans Harbor.* New York: Elsevier/Nelson Books, 1981.

TROPICAL MEDICINE

SPECIALTY

ANATOMY OR SYSTEM AFFECTED: All

SPECIALTIES AND RELATED FIELDS: Bacteriology, critical care, environmental health, epidemiology, immunology, microbiology, neonatology, nutrition, pediatrics, pharmacology, preventive medicine, public health, virology

DEFINITION: The prevention, diagnosis, and treatment of diseases that are prevalent in tropical regions, particularly those occurring in poor countries with inadequate health care delivery.

KEY TERMS:

arthropod: a member of the phylum Arthropoda, which includes mites, ticks, spiders, and insects

helminths: a general term for roundworms (nematodes) and flatworms (platyhelminths), many of which are parasites of humans and animals

morbidity: in medical statistics, the occurrence of clinical disease, in contrast to mortality (death) and occurrence (which includes subclinical infections)

parasite: an organism whose principal food source is another living organism; in medicine, the term refers to unicellular and multicellular animals

reservoir: an animal population infected with a disease that can be transmitted either to other animals or to humans; also called alternate hosts

vector: an organism, usually an insect or other arthropod, which transmits a disease from one host to another; the vector may itself be a host in which the pathogen multiplies, or it may merely transmit the pathogen mechanically

SCIENCE AND PROFESSION

Humankind evolved in tropical Africa, and it is presumed that many of the diseases and parasites characteristic of the tropical environment were inherited from nonhuman primate ancestors. Over the centuries, tropical diseases have challenged the limited resources of tribal medical practitioners and the more sophisticated medical learning of Chinese and Arab physicians. Western involvement in tropical medicine developed as a consequence of colonial expansion. The great number and diversity of tropical diseases may be grouped according to the nature of the causative agent, the symptoms involved, their mode of transmission, or their geographical distribution. The causative agent is the focus of this entry.

Viral diseases have become the most important infectious diseases in the temperate zone since the introduction of antibiotics. In the tropics, they are important but not preeminent. The principal tropical viral diseases are yellow fever and dengue fever, which are transmitted by arthropods. The transmitted viruses are called arboviruses. Yellow fever and dengue fever are acute illnesses with mortality (death) rates that exceed 50 percent if left untreated. The diseases occur sporadically when mosquitoes transmit the virus from a primate reservoir. There is potential for devastating epidemics to occur if a breakdown in health care delivery prevents prompt immunization of the population in affected areas. Arboviruses are distributed throughout tropical areas of both the New and Old Worlds. Until a massive eradication campaign orchestrated by the World Health Organization (WHO) eliminated smallpox, they exceeded other viral diseases in mortality and morbidity (illness).

Other viral diseases affect tropical regions. Human immunodeficiency virus (HIV), the agent that causes acquired immunodeficiency syndrome (AIDS), is prevalent and spreading in East and Central Africa, as well as in Haiti and Brazil in the New World. Influenza and measles, although not predominantly tropical, have high mortality rates among poor tropical populations. Hepatitis is endemic throughout the Third World. Until recently, poliomyelitis was virtually universal in the tropics, although paralytic cases were infrequent. Rabies claims a small number of victims. Finally, scientists are constantly encountering new viral diseases. Some (such as filoviruses) are exceedingly virulent. Ebola, Marbourg, and Bolivian hemorrhagic fevers are examples. Their distribution is confined to relatively small areas, probably because of the rapidly fatal nature of these diseases.

The Worldwide Prevalence of Malaria

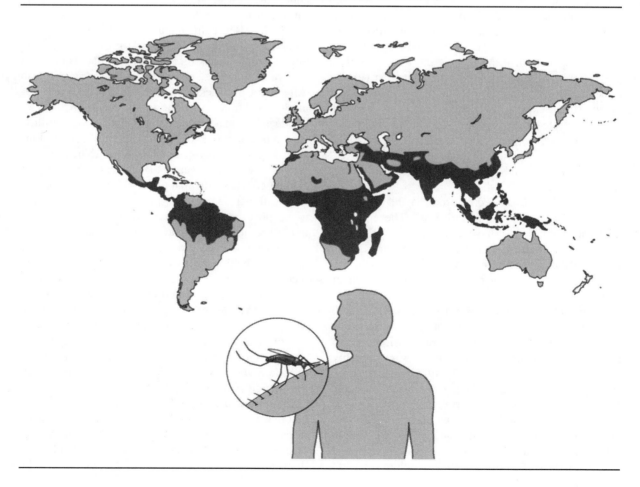

2312 • Tropical medicine

Tropical diseases caused by bacteria include some of the diseases most feared by humanity: cholera, bacillary dysentery, typhoid fever, tuberculosis, leprosy, and bubonic plague. As a result of the lack of safe sources of drinking water, there has been a resurgence of epidemic cholera in urban slums in the Third World. Fortunately, the discovery of inexpensive methods of oral rehydration therapy has reduced mortality from cholera and dysentery. Leprosy is surprisingly common and, because of its low infectivity and slow onset of debilitating symptoms, is not always perceived as a major menace. Bubonic plague occurs in isolated outbreaks within and outside the tropics where rodent reservoirs exist. In the southwest United States, approximately one hundred cases of plague are reported each year. Trachoma, an inflammation of the eyelids, affects large numbers of people—as many as a million in Brazil alone—and is a leading cause of blindness. Vaccines and antibiotics exist for the most prevalent bacterial diseases.

Spirochetes of the genus *Treponema* cause syphilis and yaws, which are chronic, endemic, and degenerative illnesses characterized by skin ulcers and neurological involvement. Yaws was the most common major tropical disease reported by WHO in the 1950's, affecting twelve million people in Southeast Asia alone. The disease is rarely fatal. Since then, aggressive wholesale treatment campaigns employing penicillin have reduced the incidence of yaws considerably in Asia and the Americas. Typhus and relapsing fever, arthropod-transmitted rickettsial diseases, can occur in epidemics.

Parasitic diseases caused by protozoa and helminths constitute the classic tropical diseases. These groups of organisms typically have complex life cycles that involve invertebrate vectors (flies, worms, and amoebas). Since many organisms are intolerant of freezing, human parasites are much more common in tropical areas.

A mosquito-transmitted protozoan causes malaria. Schistosomiasis is caused by a flatworm whose alternate hosts are aquatic snails that inhabit rice paddies and irrigation canals. These two diseases are arguably the greatest threats to human health anywhere in the world today. They affect enormous numbers of people throughout the tropics and warm temperature regions. Both cause chronic infections that may persist for decades, undermining the health and vigor of the host. In poorer tropical nations, malaria, schistosomiasis, and ancylostomiasis (hookworm) affect much of the adult population. These victims are chronically malnourished and may harbor other parasites. Trypanosomiasis—African sleeping sickness and its South American counterpart, Chagas' disease—is caused by insect-transmitted protozoa. Both diseases declined in frequency and geographical distribution following aggressive attempts to eliminate vectors.

Kala-azar is a lethal, disseminated form of the disease leishmaniasis. It is comparatively rare; some experts predict a resurgence because of increases in vector populations and drug resistance. Cutaneous leishmaniasis is widespread throughout the tropics. The organism responsible for amebic dysentery is universal in contaminated water in the tropics; infection is extremely common. Carriers are often asymptomatic; unsuspecting tourists and natives with compromised immune systems contract the most serious forms of the disease. Filariasis, called elephantiasis in its extreme form, is caused by a mosquito-transmitted nematode. It is common in Africa and the Indian subcontinent. In 1998, the pharmaceutical company SmithKline Beecham announced that it would donate its antiparasitic drug albendazole for use by the one billion people at risk for contracting filiarisis until the disease is eliminated completely. Onchocerciasis, also called river blindness, is a parasitic disease found primarily in Africa. It is one of the leading causes of blindness in the world. Approximately one million people become blind each year. Economic limitations and politics have hampered campaigns to treat onchocerciasis. There are many other parasitic diseases, including guinea worm, that occur locally in the tropics.

Nutritional deficiencies primarily result from extreme poverty and parasitic infection but also from ignorance and poor dietary practices. Characteristic of tropical regions is kwashiorkor, a protein deficiency disorder affecting primarily very young children and increasing in regions where modernization encourages early weaning. Children with kwashiorkor are fed carbohydrates but inadequate amounts of protein. Marasmus (wasting) is usually caused by a combination of insufficient total calorie intake and very inadequate intake of protein. It is made worse by dysentery or other parasitic infections and the B-complex vitamin deficiencies beriberi and pellagra.

Diseases caused by other factors are not as prevalent in tropical countries. While severe systemic fungal diseases are predominantly tropical, the total number of cases is not high. Sickle-cell disease, an inherited disorder, is frequent in central Africa because the mild, heterozygous form confers immunity to malaria. Little is known, however, about other genetic disorders in the tropics as a whole. In South Africa, genetic diseases are more common in white than in black populations. Typical so-called diseases of affluence may also pose a particular threat to people who make an abrupt transition from tribal to urban life in developing countries. The urban black population of South Africa is experiencing high rates of obesity and adult-onset diabetes.

DIAGNOSTIC AND TREATMENT TECHNIQUES

Tropical medicine is a vast field in which progress is slow and sporadic, with gains in one area often offset by losses in another. Tropical medicine, especially in developed countries which are located in temperate climates, is hampered at every stage, from research to clinical practice, by the low proportion of resources devoted to basic research in tropical disease etiology and ecology. Pharmaceutical companies often assign low priorities to the development of medicines and therapeutic agents for tropical diseases because of the potentially low returns on their investments. In affected countries, governmental policies are often established that ignore human health consequences. Extreme poverty among affected populations slows efforts to improve sanitation and general health. Explosive population growth and social and political instability slow efforts to improve infrastructures that, in turn, would improve human health. Persistent customs and attitudes in many tropical regions, which may once have been adaptive, are often harmful in modern settings. Finally, health care facilities and professionals are in short supply and unevenly distributed throughout the world and within countries affected by tropical diseases.

All these factors are important. No tropical country enjoys an average life span as long or an infant mortality rate as low as Western Europe, North America, or Japan. Nevertheless, the overwhelming influence of poverty and lack of health care access is well illustrated by contrasting the health status of the populations of Puerto Rico, Okinawa, or Taiwan with the conditions in Central Africa and the Indian subcontinent. In relatively prosperous, politically stable countries, diseases that can be prevented by immunization (such as polio) or easily cured by chemotherapy (such as yaws) are unimportant. Education, better sanitation, and environmental management have dramatically reduced the incidence of the parasites that cause ma-

laria, schistosomiasis, and hookworm. In developed countries, severe malnutrition is rare.

Existing medical knowledge is constantly being refined, and an increased commitment to tropical medical research is needed. It is worth noting, however, that many typical tropical diseases were prevalent in the southeastern United States before World War I. Furthermore, the medical knowledge and governmental agencies available in the 1920's proved effective in combating malaria, yellow fever, hookworm, and pellagra in the United States.

The development of drugs to combat disease is largely the business of a pharmaceutical industry based in developed countries. These companies have been accused of neglecting tropical diseases because of a low potential for profit. WHO has provided incentives in some cases but has also opposed exclusive licensing of drugs developed under its aegis, a potential disincentive. Less than 5 percent of health research worldwide is devoted to the health problems of developing nations.

The pharmaceutical industry has also been implicated in marketing drugs to developing nations that have been banned as ineffective or dangerous in the United States. This practice underscores a wider and growing health threat: multinational corporations exporting pesticides, industrial chemicals, and manufacturing processes that undermine human health to the Third World. Any process resulting in wholesale environmental disruption produces an increase in disease in ways that are unpredictable.

Drug-resistant strains of pathogens are most likely to evolve when large populations are treated with a single therapeutic agent and when treatment is insufficient to cure patients completely. The risk of this pattern occurring is high in tropical countries. Drug-resistant strains of malaria are already increasing and complicate the task of combating this dangerous disease.

Poverty among individuals leads to malnutrition, overcrowding, poor sanitation, lowered resistance to infection, and an inability to avoid exposure to vectors and contaminated water. In many tropical areas, access to medical care ranges from limited to nonexistent. On a regional and national level, poverty leads to political and social instability and an inability to implement public health programs. Political upheaval facilitates the interregional spread of pathogens.

In much of the tropics, efforts to improve infant health and agricultural productivity backfire because social and economic customs favor large families. The resulting population increase exacerbates poverty-dependent variables responsible for disease. Training skilled medical personnel and maintaining clinics are costly. In the Third World, however, this cost is less because labor costs are low.

If market forces alone dictate the allocation of medical resources, health care providers gravitate toward the most prosperous areas. Medically trained Third World nationals frequently emigrate to Europe or the United States. Paramedic personnel, such as the so-called barefoot doctors of China, are effective only to the extent that their training, supervision, and support services are adequate. The number of doctors relative to the population in many tropical countries is too low to provide adequate medical care even without the additional factors of uneven distribution and higher incidence of serious disease.

PERSPECTIVE AND PROSPECTS

The Old World tropics, especially tropical Africa, were dubbed the "white man's grave" because European military personnel and colonists lacked both inherited resistance and customary methods of avoidance to protect themselves from the ravages of malaria, yellow fever, Asiatic cholera, and scores of other life-threatening diseases. Occasionally, disease resulted in the failure of colonial enterprise. In Hispaniola (Haiti), black slaves were successful in their bid for independence after yellow fever killed all but six thousand of the thirty thousand troops sent by Napoleon to quell the rebellion. In Africa, large areas in which sleeping sickness was endemic were inaccessible to European colonization.

The period of maximum European colonial expansion (from 1830 to 1914) coincided with great strides in the understanding of disease causation and prevention, although effective cures lagged until the beginning of World War II. In 1900, Walter Reed, in the course of investigating a devastating epidemic of yellow fever among workers and soldiers digging the Panama Canal, discovered that the disease was mosquito-borne. In 1898, the Italian researchers Amico Bignami, Giovanni Grassi, and Giuseppe Bastianelli, who were also working with malaria, made a similar discovery. These observations paved the way for ef-

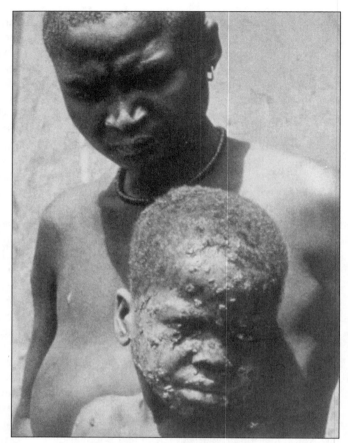

A young boy suffering from yaws. (National Library of Medicine)

fective control through exclusion and eradication of the vectors.

European activities in the tropics have often exacerbated tropical disease problems. The African slave trade introduced a number of tropical diseases into the southern United States, including schistosomiasis, one of the most debilitating and intractable of tropical parasitic infections. Bengalis in India dubbed kala-azar "the British government disease," since road-building and improved communication introduced a previously localized pathogen into large areas, with disastrous results. Dam-building and artificial irrigation dramatically increase the incidence of schistosomiasis in tropical areas. Paradoxically, medical intervention reducing infant mortality and allowing rapid population growth tends to undermine health and increases the incidence of nutritional disorders and parasitic infections. Inadequate sanitation in rural clinics, especially the use of poorly sterilized hypodermic needles, contributes to the spread of disease and has been implicated in the spread of AIDS in Africa.

The examples of Brazil and China, however, illustrate how nationally coordinated efforts within a tropical region of low per capita income can be effective. In China's regimented society, a blanket application of environmental control measures with mobilization of a large rural workforce, mass screening and treatment, education at all levels, and coordinated targeted research have been shown to be feasible. Between 1956 and 1987, the areas in which schistosomiasis occurred and the number of people at risk of exposure were halved. At the same time, the number of infected individuals declined by a factor of ten. In Brazil, the Superintendency for Public Health Campaigns (SUCAM) works in frontier areas where social control is slower and channels for education and communication do not function well. SUCAM relies on the Guarda, a field staff composed of a large number of paraprofessionals trained to recognize symptoms and risk factors in a particular disease and to implement control measures. SUCAM has had notable success against Chagas' disease, which can be controlled by eliminating the insect vector from houses through the use of insecticides and renovation. Egypt, Zimbabwe, and the Philippines have also mounted successful campaigns that have reduced the incidence of parasitic diseases.

Education of women is an important factor in the health of poor populations. Women play a crucial role in maintaining the health of infants and children. They are also more likely to be vulnerable to neglect and ill health than are adult males as a result of cultural attitudes. In the Indian state of Kerala, longevity and infant mortality statistics are now comparable to those of African Americans because the government has devoted a large proportion of resources to universal education and public health. Nearby Bangladesh, which has a comparable climate and per capita income but lacks the commitment to education and health access, has some of the worst statistics on survival and longevity in the developing world.

The net result of improving public health in the developing world has been an increase in average life expectancy of approximately ten years, from fifty to sixty, between 1970 and 1990. Increased longevity results in an increase in diseases of old age and their demands on the health care system. This is most true in China, where life expectancy approaches seventy years and aggressive measures have reduced the birth rate dramatically.

In an age of international travel, virtually any communicable disease has the potential to spread rapidly. The worldwide epidemic of AIDS clearly illustrates this phenomenon. Some medical ecologists view the large AIDS-infected population in Africa as a medical time bomb in which a novel, virulent pathogen, such as the Ebola virus, could gain a foothold. Military incursions and tourism in the tropics expose people from the temperate zone to tropical ailments. These factors should provide an additional impetus for research into tropical diseases and general awareness of them by physicians.

Tropical diseases extract an enormous toll in human productivity that, by perpetuating poverty and hindering all forms of development, contributes to global political instability. The interaction of tropical disease processes and European colonialism was destructive for both Europeans and colonial subjects. Medical science and social policy are a long way from solving the medical problems of the tropics.

—*Martha Sherwood-Pike, Ph.D.;*
updated by L. Fleming Fallon, Jr.,
M.D., Ph.D., M.P.H.

See also Acquired immunodeficiency syndrome (AIDS); Antibiotics; Arthropod-borne diseases; Bacterial infections; Bacteriology; Beriberi; Childhood infectious diseases; Cholera; Diarrhea and dysentery; Drug resistance; Ebola virus; Elephantiasis; Epidemiology; Fungal infections; Immunization and vaccination; Kwashiorkor; Leishmaniasis; Leprosy; Malaria; Malnutrition; Microbiology; Nutrition; Parasitic diseases; Plague; Poliomyelitis; Protozoan diseases; Rabies; Schistosomiasis; Sleeping sickness; Syphilis; Typhoid fever and typhus; Viral infections; World Health Organization; Worms; Yellow fever.

FOR FURTHER INFORMATION:

Busvine, James R. *Disease Transmission by Insects: Its Discovery and Ninety Years of Effort to Prevent It*. Amsterdam: Springer-Verlag, 1993. This interesting history of tropical medicine is complete and relatively easy to read.

Camus, Emmanuel, and James House, eds. *Vector-Borne Pathogens: International Trade and Tropical Animal Diseases*. New York: Annals of the New York Academy of Sciences, 1996. This extensive and highly readable work provides a wealth of information concerning the spread of tropical diseases through commerce and rapid world transportation.

Garrett, Laurie. *The Coming Plague: Newly Emerging Diseases in a World Out of Balance*. New York: Farrar, Straus & Giroux, 1994. This book contains an excellent discussion of many tropical diseases and the efforts of the World Health Organization to eradicate them. The author has a style that is easy to read. This book is highly recommended.

Liese, Bernhard H., Paramjit S. Sachdeva, and D. Glynn Cochrane. *Organizing and Managing Tropical Disease Control Programs: Case Studies*. Washington, D.C.: World Bank, 1992. A summary of the organization, financing, and implementation of public health programs in Brazil; schistosomiasis control programs in China, Egypt, the Philippines, and Zimbabwe; and malaria and tuberculosis control in the Philippines.

Peters, Wallace, and Herbert M. Gilles. *Color Atlas of Tropical Medicine and Parasitology*. St. Louis: Mosby-Year Book, 1995. This handbook provides illustrations and descriptions of symptoms, pathogens, and vectors, with maps of distribution, for serious tropical diseases. It includes those that are widespread and globally important and some that are rare and local, but of interest from a medical standpoint.

Sanford-Smith, John. *Eye Diseases in Hot Climates*. 3d ed. London: Butterworth-Heinemann, 1997. This text devotes an extensive section to onchocerciasis. The disease, attempts to treat it, and problems associated with economic development are discussed.

Sen, Amartya. "The Economics of Life and Death." *Scientific American* 268 (May, 1993): 40-47. This article contrasts the health of nations with the wealth of nations, focusing on areas with low per capita income and comparatively high longevity. The author suggests that longevity and infant mortality are better measures of the well-being of a population than income alone.

Strickland, Thomas, ed. *Hunter's Tropical Medicine*. 7th ed. Philadelphia: W. B. Saunders, 1991. This is a classic textbook written by internationally known experts in the field. Although it uses some technical words, most readers should find the text understandable.

TUBAL LIGATION

PROCEDURE

ANATOMY OR SYSTEM AFFECTED: Abdomen, reproductive system, uterus

SPECIALTIES AND RELATED FIELDS: Gynecology
DEFINITION: A surgical procedure which closes the Fallopian tubes and causes permanent sterilization.

INDICATIONS AND PROCEDURES

Tubal ligations are performed strictly for sterilization of a female patient. While there has been some success with reversing the procedure, it must be considered permanent. The woman must be well informed and certain that she does not want additional children under any circumstances.

The most common technique for tubal ligation is laparoscopy. As an outpatient, the woman receives local anesthetic and a light sedative. A small incision is made in the navel, and gas is used to inflate the abdomen, allowing easy visibility of the patient's Fallopian tubes. An instrument called an intrauterine cannula is inserted through the vagina, and a clamp called a tenaculum is positioned on the cervix. Both are used to manipulate the tubes into position. A laparoscope, a thin tube containing a camera and light, is inserted through the incision in order to view the tubes. An instrument to block the tubes is inserted through the laparoscope. The tubes may be blocked by burning, cutting, or applying rings or clips. The incision is sewn closed.

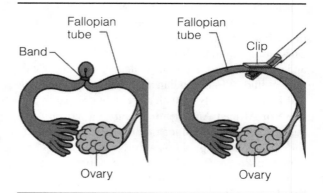

A common means of sterilization for women is tubal ligation, in which the Fallopian tubes through which eggs must pass to reach the uterus are severed or interrupted with clips or bands.

In a minilaparatomy, a small incision is made above the woman's pubic bone. The tubes are brought through the incision and are tied and cut. Tubal ligations can also be performed through a woman's vagina (culdoscopy or colpotomy).

USES AND COMPLICATIONS

The only purpose of tubal ligation is sterilization. It is highly effective (with a 0.2 percent failure rate) and largely irreversible. Depending on the type of blockage used, it is about 30 percent reversible; however, only 10 percent of women become pregnant after undergoing tubal reconstruction. Other forms of birth control are recommended for any patient who is not absolutely certain about the procedure.

Tubal ligations take only thirty minutes to perform, and there is only minor postsurgical pain. A rare complication may be an ectopic pregnancy within the Fallopian tube, which could rupture. Other potential problems are those associated with any abdominal surgery, including unintentional damage to other internal organs, bleeding, and infection.

—*Karen E. Kalumuck, Ph.D.*

See also Contraception; Gynecology; Hysterectomy; Laparoscopy; Pregnancy and gestation; Reproductive system; Sterilization.

FOR FURTHER INFORMATION:

Barnes, Josephine. *Essentials of Family Planning.* Oxford, England: Blackwell Scientific, 1976.

Corson, Stephen L., Richard J. Derman, and Louise B. Tyrer, eds. *Fertility Control.* Boston: Little, Brown, 1985.

Harper, Michael J. K. *Birth Control Technologies: Prospects by the Year 2000.* Austin: University of Texas Press, 1983.

Keith, Louis G., Deryck R. Kent, Gary S. Berger, and Janelle R. Brittain, eds. *The Safety of Fertility Control.* New York: Springer, 1980.

TUBERCULOSIS

DISEASE/DISORDER

ANATOMY OR SYSTEM AFFECTED: Chest, lungs, respiratory system

SPECIALTIES AND RELATED FIELDS: Bacteriology, microbiology, public health, pulmonary medicine

DEFINITION: A chronic, highly infectious lung disease that can destroy tissue.

KEY TERMS:

BCG: a weakened version of *Mycobacterium bovis* that is used in vaccines to protect against tuberculosis

PPD (purified protein derivative): proteins from mycobacteria used in the tuberculin test; exposure to tuberculosis will result in the sensitization of the immune system to these proteins

primary tuberculosis: a form of tuberculosis that often does not produce symptoms and that develops after exposure to tuberculosis-causing bacteria

sanatorium: an institution designed for the treatment of chronic illnesses, such as tuberculosis

secondary tuberculosis: the recurrence of tuberculosis in individuals who chronically carry the bacterium; a more severe form of the disease in which the lungs are usually damaged

tuberculin test: a skin test used to detect exposure to tuberculosis; a useful test in countries in which vaccines against tuberculosis are not routinely administered

tuberculosis bacilli: bacteria that belong to the genus and species *Mycobacterium tuberculosis*; sometimes called tubercle bacilli, these organisms are the causative agents of tuberculosis

CAUSES AND SYMPTOMS

Tuberculosis derives its name from the Latin word *tubercle,* which means "little lump." Tubercles, or small nodules of diseased tissue, are often found in the lungs of infected individuals. In humans, bacteria that belong to the genus *Mycobacterium* cause tuberculosis. In the vast majority of cases, *Mycobacterium tuberculosis,* often referred to as the tuberculosis bacillus or the tubercle bacillus, is the responsible organism. Other species within the genus may also cause tuberculosis or tuberculosis-like diseases. For example, *Mycobacterium avium,* a disease-causing organism, or pathogen, is found in birds and swine; it can cause a tuberculosis-like disease in humans. Before it was common to pasteurize milk, *Mycobacterium bovis,* a pathogen found in cattle, was responsible for cases of human tuberculosis of the digestive tract. In most cases of tuberculosis in humans, the lungs are the major organs affected, but other tissues and organs such as the bones, skin, and digestive tract may also be sites of infection.

Poverty, overcrowding, unsanitary conditions, poor health, and poor nutrition provide ideal conditions for the spread of tuberculosis. It is found at a high frequency in the developing areas of the world, such as parts of Africa, Asia, and Oceania. Immigrants from these countries present a serious public health concern when they enter the United States and other countries. In the United States, the incidence of tuberculosis is still relatively high in African Americans, Asians, Pacific Islanders, American Indians, Alaskan natives, and Hispanics. Other individuals who have a greater risk for developing tuberculosis infection are inmates of correctional institutions, alcoholics, intravenous drug users, the homeless, and the elderly.

People at a particularly high risk of developing tuberculosis after exposure are those whose immune systems are compromised or suppressed, such as cancer patients receiving chemotherapy, organ transplant recipients, or people with acquired immunodeficiency syndrome (AIDS). Diabetics and individuals with a lung condition known as silicosis are also at high risk of developing tuberculosis as a result of exposure to the disease. Silicosis is an occupational disease that develops as a result of exposure to silica. Silica is found in sand and is a crystalline material encountered by miners, tunnel diggers, stone cutters, glassmakers, and those involved in sandblasting operations.

Under a microscope, tuberculosis bacilli appear as straight or slightly curved, rod-shaped organisms. Their widths vary from 0.3 to 0.6 of a micrometer, and their lengths vary from 1 to 4 micrometers. My-

cobacteria have unique properties that appear to be linked to their abilities to cause tuberculosis. The cell wall, a protective layer that surrounds all bacteria, is unique in mycobacteria because it contains some unusual lipids. These lipids, which include mycolic acid, give the bacteria special staining properties. Mycobacteria are the only bacteria that resist decolorization with a solution of acid and alcohol (hydrochloric acid and ethyl alcohol) and are thus termed acid-fast. Acid-fastness is the most important characteristic of mycobacteria because it can be used to differentiate them from other types of bacteria. The acid-fast staining procedure can be used to identify mycobacteria and to visualize them in clinical specimens such as lung tissue and sputum.

Mycobacteria populations grow very slowly compared to other bacteria. Under optimal conditions, typical mycobacteria will divide every twelve to eighteen hours, while many other bacteria will divide in twenty to thirty minutes. Mycobacteria require oxygen for

Development of Tuberculosis

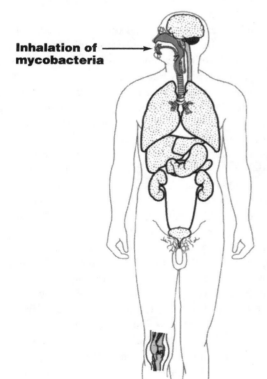

Inhalation of mycobacteria

Primary infection with no symptoms or nonspecific symptoms such as fever, fatigue. Lymph nodes may be involved. Recovery follows, or:

Secondary infection: Death and softening of lung tissue, merging and liquefaction of lesions, spread to other parts of lung, coughing up of sputum, contamination of others and environment.

Miliary tuberculosis: Small lesions (like millet seeds) spread throughout body, especially lymph nodes, nerve and brain membranes (meninges), bones and joints, urogenital system, other internal organs.

growth and are very resistant to drying, most likely because of the lipids in their cell walls. Mycobacteria also resist many chemical and physical agents that would normally kill bacteria. This resistance allows them to survive both in the body and in the exterior environment. Cultures of *Mycobacterium tuberculosis* maintained in a laboratory usually remain viable for many years. These bacteria can also remain viable outside both a laboratory and the human body. They can retain their pathogenic properties in dried sputum for many months. They are sensitive to ultraviolet light, however, and are killed in about two hours after exposure to direct sunlight.

The mycobacteria that cause tuberculosis are found in the droplets released when a person with active tuberculosis coughs, sneezes, or even talks. This mist of tiny droplets can remain aloft for hours. The manner by which a person becomes infected with tuberculosis usually involves the inhalation of these droplets. The tuberculosis bacilli can then be carried to the lungs. It is fortunate that most individuals who are exposed to tuberculosis will not develop the disease. Tuberculosis is less contagious than the common childhood diseases (such as measles, chickenpox, and mumps) and is usually contracted only after long exposure to an infectious individual who has an active case of tuberculosis. Of all newly infected individuals, approximately 5 percent will show symptoms of tuberculosis within a year. The remaining infected individuals continue to have some risk of developing the disease at any time.

When tuberculosis infection does occur, the initial period is referred to as the primary infection. During this period, an infected individual may not experience any symptoms of illness, or the symptoms may be nonspecific, such as low fever and tiredness. Tuberculosis bacilli in the lung become the focus of an attack by the body's immune system. Primary tuberculosis may also involve the lymph nodes and the pleural cavity. This reaction may lead to the accumulation of fluid within the pleural cavity, accompanied by fever or chest pain. As a result of activities of the immune system and the ingestion of tuberculosis bacilli by white blood cells known as macrophages, the primary infection will often spontaneously subside without medical intervention. Yet, although healing occurs, the tuberculosis bacilli can remain in a somewhat dormant state, walled up in the primary lesions. They live within the cells of the immune system but do not divide. The bacilli can remain in this state for years

or decades without producing further symptoms of the disease. Untreated individuals will remain infected throughout their lifetimes even though the disease is in remission.

Most individuals recover from primary tuberculosis. In a small percentage of cases, however, the disease progresses and lung destruction occurs. The reactivation of the disease is referred to as secondary tuberculosis and most frequently occurs when the immune system is weakened. Destruction of lung tissue is a hallmark of this phase of the disease. Much of the damage produced in the lung is the result of efforts by the immune system to destroy the tuberculosis bacilli. Parts of the lung suffer tissue death (necrosis) and soften. These lesions can merge, enlarge, liquefy, and discharge their contents of tuberculosis bacteria into the bronchi. The bacteria can spread to other parts of the lung and be coughed up in sputum, where they contaminate the environment and serve as a source of infectious organisms that will spread the disease. Secondary tuberculosis, if untreated, is a chronic condition in which the symptoms worsen progressively to include fever, fatigue, loss of appetite, and weight loss.

If the bacteria spread to other parts of the body, a condition known as miliary tuberculosis results. Multiple small lesions that resemble millet seeds are found throughout the body. The most common sites in which these lesions are found are the bones and joints, the urogenital system, lymph nodes, the meninges (membranes surrounding the brain and spinal cord), and the peritoneum. Individuals with AIDS are at an increased risk for contracting tuberculosis outside the lungs (extrapulmonary tuberculosis).

TREATMENT AND THERAPY
On a global basis, close to ten million new cases of tuberculosis are diagnosed each year, and 1.5 million deaths are attributable to this disease. Every minute, ten new people become infected with tuberculosis; of these, three will die from it. Since tuberculosis presents a serious public health concern, many countries have employed strategies to prevent its spread. Control of the spread of tuberculosis could decrease the numbers of new cases seen each year. Improvements in living conditions, sanitation, and general standards of living have, in the past, been associated with the decreased incidence of tuberculosis in populations. These goals cannot easily be met in impoverished regions of the world. The medical approaches designed

to inhibit the further transmission of tuberculosis include vaccination, rapid diagnosis, and the development of effective drug treatments.

In the United States after the mid-twentieth century, measures were developed to diagnose tuberculosis and prevent its transmission. This program resulted in a marked decrease in death rates from tuberculosis. Total death rates declined dramatically until the mid-1980's. Prior to this time, most cases of tuberculosis were found in the southeastern part of the country and on Indian reservations. By the 1990's, tuberculosis was once again on the rise, but the distribution pattern of the disease had changed. Tuberculosis began to be seen more in African American and Hispanic patients and in individuals with AIDS. The rate of tuberculosis infection became much higher in patients with AIDS than in any other group in the population. The immunocompromised nature of AIDS patients renders them highly susceptible to tuberculosis. An illustration of the extent of this phenomenon is the fact that all individuals newly diagnosed with tuberculosis are also presumed to have AIDS until laboratory tests prove otherwise.

The tuberculin skin test is a safe and reliable diagnostic test for tuberculosis. When some of the proteins from the tubercle bacilli, in a preparation known as purified protein derivative (PPD), are injected into the skin of an individual who has been exposed to tuberculosis, a characteristic skin reaction will occur. The reaction is characterized by redness and swelling around the injection site, which appears in forty-eight to seventy-two hours. The accumulation and activities of cells of the immune system that recognize the bacterial protein cause this reaction. This type of immune response is referred to as a delayed hypersensitivity reaction and will be seen only in persons who have been previously exposed to these bacterial proteins, usually following infection with tuberculosis bacilli. A positive test does not necessarily mean that a person has an active case of tuberculosis and could therefore be contagious; it merely indicates that at some time, past or present, a tuberculosis infection occurred, even if the individual did not display symptoms of the disease.

The tuberculin skin test is not useful in those parts of the world where many individuals in the population have been vaccinated against tuberculosis with a vaccine composed of bacillus Calmette-Guérin (BCG). The BCG vaccine contains proteins that sensitize the immune system to PPD. After this occurs, a tuberculin skin test will be positive in an individual who has been vaccinated, even though the individual has never been exposed to live tuberculosis bacilli. In the United States, BCG vaccination is not routinely performed because of the great value in tuberculin skin testing as a public health measure. All individuals who may become exposed to tuberculosis, such as medical personnel, are advised to receive the tuberculin skin test at regular intervals. If an individual should have a positive skin test, it is common practice to begin treatment with antituberculosis drugs.

Other methods for the diagnosis of tuberculosis include the detection of acid-fast mycobacteria in sputum, chest X rays to examine the lungs, and the laboratory culture and examination of mycobacteria grown from clinical specimens. The latter procedure may take from four to six weeks because mycobacteria grow so slowly. The growth and examination of these organisms in the laboratory is necessary, however, to confirm diagnosis when tuberculosis is suspected because of the patient's history and the lung damage seen on X ray but microscopic examination fails to show the presence of mycobacteria.

The treatment of tuberculosis changed drastically in the last half of the twentieth century. In the place of quarantine in a sanatorium, a common practice to prevent the spread of the disease, or surgery to remove portions of the diseased lung tissue, tuberculosis patients are now treated with antituberculosis drugs and antibiotics on an outpatient basis. Once treatment is begun, individuals can no longer transmit the disease and are therefore not contagious.

The most effective antituberculosis drugs include isoniazid, pyrazinamide, ethambutol, and the antibiotics rifampicin and streptomycin. The prescribed antituberculosis medications must be used for a long period, usually about nine months, to ensure the destruction of all live tuberculosis bacilli. An ever-increasing problem in the treatment of tuberculosis is the appearance of tuberculosis bacilli that are resistant to drug therapy. These bacteria develop resistance as a result of genetic mutation, and when such drug-resistant bacteria are present in a patient, the disease will not respond to that particular drug. For this reason, most treatment procedures involve the use of three to four different antituberculosis drugs. The probability of the development of two or more separate mutations is much less than the development of a single mutation.

Even though tuberculosis bacilli are less likely to

be resistant to more than one drug, multiple-drug-resistant bacteria are emerging in populations throughout the world. Combined drug therapy is ineffective because these organisms can withstand exposure to several of the antituberculosis drugs at once. Without an effective means of treatment, patients who harbor these multiple-drug-resistant organisms are a continued source of infection to the community unless they are kept in isolation.

Because of the long treatment period, some tuberculosis patients stop taking their medication before the destruction of all tuberculosis bacilli. Some of these patients discontinue their medication because their symptoms have disappeared and they believe that they are cured. A recurrence of the disease is highly probable when the full course of treatment is not followed.

In some countries, the BCG vaccine is widely used as a preventive measure. This vaccine is prepared from live bacteria that belong to a strain of *Mycobacterium bovis* that has lost its pathogenic properties. The effectiveness of the vaccine is not absolute; studies show that in countries where the vaccine is employed, there may be a 60 to 80 percent decrease in the incidence of tuberculosis. The BCG vaccine is not used in the United States because the incidence of tuberculosis in the general population is quite low compared to other countries. In addition, if the BCG vaccine were widely used, it would negate the utility of the tuberculin skin test as a reliable and valuable diagnostic tool.

PERSPECTIVE AND PROSPECTS

Throughout the ages, tuberculosis has been a scourge of humankind. Human fossils, excavated from a Neolithic burial ground dated about six thousand years ago, show evidence of tuberculosis of the spine. Egyptian mummies from 1000 B.C.E. with signs of tuberculosis suggest that the disease was widespread in ancient Egypt. Symptoms of tuberculosis such as fever, excessive weight loss, night sweats, breathlessness, pain in the side and chest areas, and coughing up of sputum and blood are described in the writings of ancient Hindu, Greek, and Roman writers. The widespread nature of the disease appears in accounts from early European history, from the fifth to eighteenth centuries, which refer to a "touching" ceremony that was performed by English and French monarchs and believed to cure scrofula (tuberculosis of the lymph glands in the neck region).

One of the greatest causes of disease and death in the world, tuberculosis has been known by many names, including scrofula, phthisis, and consumption. In writings, it has been referred to as "the white plague" and "the captain of all the men of death." During the nineteenth century, tuberculosis was widespread in Europe. The symptoms of tuberculosis were not thought to represent a disease but rather hallmarks of an especially sensitive personality—the ideal for an artist, musician, poet, or writer. At that time, it was somewhat fashionable to be pale and thin, and to have a slight cough.

Although tuberculosis has been a serious health threat for such a long period of human history, the disease and its cause were poorly understood until the 1880's. Robert Koch is credited with discovering the tuberculosis bacillus. His masterful treatise, published in 1882 and translated under the title "The Etiology of Tuberculosis," presented convincing experimental evidence for implicating a bacterium that came to be known as *Mycobacterium tuberculosis* as the causative agent of tuberculosis. Despite this great breakthrough, a rational effective treatment for the disease could not be found. One type of therapy that became popular was simply rest and fresh air. Edward Livingston Trudeau, an American physician who suffered from tuberculosis, observed that he regained his health when he traveled to Saranac Lake in the Adirondack Mountains in the state of New York. He attributed his recovery to the restful environment and clean air. Trudeau later founded a sanatorium at Lake Saranac that became popular for tuberculosis patients.

It was not until the discovery of the antibiotic streptomycin in 1943 by Selman A. Waksman that a truly potent antituberculosis agent was found. The tuberculosis bacilli, however, proved to be quite resistant to a multitude of other antibiotics and antibacterial drugs. Fortunately, several antibiotics and antibacterial drugs, especially when used in combination and for the full duration of their prescription, can cure many tuberculosis patients.

Today, the major problems presented by tuberculosis are the increasing incidence of the disease, the increasing prevalence of cases that display multiple-drug resistance, and the association with AIDS. These cases of tuberculosis are difficult to treat and further the possibilities for widespread transmission of the disease.

—Barbara Brennessel, Ph.D.;
updated by L. Fleming Fallon, Jr.,
M.D., Ph.D., M.P.H.

See also Acquired immunodeficiency syndrome (AIDS); Antibiotics; Bacterial infections; Bacteriology; Coughing; Drug resistance; Epidemiology; Immunization and vaccination; Lungs; Pulmonary diseases; Pulmonary medicine.

FOR FURTHER INFORMATION:

Daniel, Thomas. *Captain of Death: The Story of Tuberculosis*. Rochester, N.Y.: University of Rochester Press, 1997. This book is written for nonprofessional readers. It is interesting and well researched.

Dormandy, Thomas. *The White Death: A History of Tuberculosis*. New York: New York University Press, 2000. Accessible scientific and sociological history are combined by Dormandy, a consulting pathologist in London, in this account of a tenacious disease that has claimed victims since ancient Egypt.

Lutwick, Larry I. *Tuberculosis: A Clinical Handbook*. Chicago: Chapman and Hall, 1995. This well-written book, intended for general practitioners and internists, provides an account of the disease, its manifestations, and prevention in children, adults, and HIV-infected patients.

Ratledge, Colin, and John Stanford, eds. *The Biology of the Mycobacteria*. 3 vols. New York: Academic Press, 1989. Part of a series written to consolidate the scholarly research on the bacteria that cause tuberculosis and leprosy. The first volume details the physiology, structure, genetics, and biochemistry of mycobacteria; the second discusses the immunological and environmental aspects of mycobacterial disease

Rom, William, and Stuart M. Garay, eds. *Tuberculosis*. Philadelphia: Lippincott-Raven, 1996. A group of experts wrote chapters for this book, which can be easily understood by general readers.

Scharer, Lawrence, and John M. McAdam. *Tuberculosis and AIDS: The Relationship Between Mycobacterium TB and the HIV Type 1*. Amsterdam: Springer-Verlag, 1995. This book considers the relationship between tuberculosis and patients with AIDS. It is written for professionals but contains a wealth of information for general readers.

TUMOR REMOVAL
PROCEDURE
ANATOMY OR SYSTEM AFFECTED: All (primarily brain, breasts, gastrointestinal system, intestines, lungs, respiratory system)

SPECIALTIES AND RELATED FIELDS: General surgery, histology, oncology

DEFINITION: The removal—through surgery, chemotherapy, or radiotherapy—of any neoplasm.

KEY TERMS:

computed tomography (CT) scanning: a medical imaging technique which involves the X-ray observation of cross sections of tissue

magnetic resonance imaging (MRI): a medical imaging technique in which the image is produced by the scanning of a magnetic field

metastasis: the spread of cancer cells from the primary tumor to other sites in the body

neoplasm: an uncontrolled growth of cells which can develop into a tumor; may be malignant (cancerous) or benign

oncogene: a regulatory gene in a cell which, when mutated, may cause that cell to become cancerous

INDICATIONS AND PROCEDURES

The uncontrolled, progressive growth of cells, termed a neoplasm, usually results in a mass or tumor. The tumor may be malignant (cancerous) or benign. Generally, benign tumors remain localized, are often encapsulated, and contain cells that remain well differentiated. Since the cells of a benign tumor do not metastasize, the tumor is usually less of a threat to life. The site of the tumor, however, can be as critical as its malignant or nonmalignant state: Tumors within inoperable portions of the brain may pose a threat regardless of whether they are malignant.

Most tumors are initially observed as localized masses of cells, or lumps. Any symptoms that occur result from tumor growth in this particular tissue. While any tissue or cell is at risk for the development of a tumor, most such forms of uncontrolled growth are found in the female breasts, the colon, and the lungs, the latter a result of the increased use of cigarettes in the twentieth century.

When a tumor is observed, several options exist for its elimination. Surgery remains the method of choice when applicable. This method poses two advantages: Under ideal circumstances, surgery can result in complete removal of the tumor and total cure. In addition, the removal of the tissue allows for proper diagnosis, and subsequent prognosis, of the form of tumor. Surgery may also play a palliative role, allowing for elimination of some of the tumor mass, temporary relief of symptoms, and a greater chance for alternative forms of therapy to effect a cure.

While alternative methods of noninvasive diagnosis were developed during the latter half of the twentieth century, most notably computed tomography (CT) scanning and magnetic resonance imaging (MRI), surgery remains the best method for both tumor diagnosis and cure. The procedure for diagnosis of most tumors is relatively straightforward. When the patient is examined, a complete analysis of symptoms is carried out. The tumor, though not necessarily its prognosis, may be directly observable, such as a lump in the breast. Sometimes, symptoms may be secondary, such as blood in the feces resulting from a tumor in the colon or a cough associated with lung cancer. Biopsy of the material, often in conjunction with surgery, may be necessary to determine whether the tumor is malignant; many tumors are not. If the tumor is determined to be malignant, the material obtained in the biopsy may also be useful in determining the staging of the tumor, a classification system used to identify the extent of the tumor, its degree of spread, and the likely prognosis. Though several methods of staging are used, the most popular is the TNM system. T refers to the size of the tumor (T0 to T4, depending on its size), N refers to the extent of lymph node involvement (N0 to N2), and M indicates whether metastasis has occurred (M0 or M1).

If the tumor is localized, surgical removal remains the best chance for a cure. In general, the patient is anesthetized and the region of the tumor is surgically removed. For a tiny breast tumor, this may involve a lumpectomy (removal of the lump only). For larger tumors, extensive amounts of tissue may have to be excised. Surgery usually involves the use of a knife, though alternative forms such as laser surgery or electrosurgery may be used under specific circumstances. The surgeon will attempt to remove the area of cancer or, when warranted, the entire organ and a margin of adjacent normal-looking tissue, in the event that a few cells have spread beyond the visible tumor. Localized lymph glands may also be removed, both to estimate the chance of metastasis and to improve the chance of removing all the tumor since the local lymph nodes are generally the sites to which cancer cells initially spread.

When the tumor is too large, or if metastasis has occurred, additional forms of treatment to effect tumor removal may be needed. Radiation therapy, the use of beams of high-energy X rays, may be used to reduce the size of a tumor or to eliminate any cancer cells that remain in the vicinity of an excised tumor.

Chemotherapy, the use of metabolic poisons, is often employed when the tumor has spread beyond its initial site.

Tumor removal may also be palliative, a procedure employed for the reduction of symptoms or for the restoration of normal organ function. For example, the removal of a tumor on the colon may reduce pain and restore function temporarily, even if the tumor has spread and the prognosis is poor. Common benign tumors may also cause discomfort, even if not life-threatening. Nearly one-quarter of women over the age of thirty develop fibroid tumors on the wall of the uterus, a condition which is more of a nuisance than dangerous; surgical removal of such tumors may be necessary to eliminate pain or bleeding.

The decision regarding the methodology of tumor removal often depends on the site and extent of the tumor. The biopsy of the material may be immediately followed by surgical removal of the tumor while the patient remains under anesthesia. This is often the method of choice if the tumor is small or confined to a single organ. After surgery, any additional options can be discussed with the patient. If various options exist for tumor removal, the results of the biopsy may first be discussed with the patient, and a decision on specific forms of treatment may follow.

The most convenient procedure for biopsy during surgery is needle aspiration, the insertion of a small needle into the tumor for the removal of a small number of cells. If more tissue is needed, a larger needle may be used. If the tumor is small enough, the entire tumor may be removed at this stage.

When the tumor has been removed, the entire tissue is given to a pathologist. Analysis of this gross specimen allows for a firmer diagnosis of the form of tumor, its staging, and a possible prognosis.

USES AND COMPLICATIONS

Two strategies are associated with tumor removal: First is the attempt to effect a cure. Ideally, complete elimination of a malignant tumor will result in a cure for the disease. The assumption in this case is that metastasis has not occurred. If the tumor is benign, removal should alleviate any symptoms associated with its growth. As indicated above, fibroid tumors of the uterus, while common in middle-aged women, rarely pose a threat to life; it is their very presence that results in discomfort or other symptoms. Likewise, parotid tumors, growths in the salivary gland, may result in unsightly lumps in the region of the jaw, as well as pain or discomfort; on some occasions, there may be facial paralysis. Removal of the tumor, generally through surgery but with radiation or chemotherapy if the condition warrants, may be indicated.

Colon cancer is one of the more common forms of cancer among adults, with more than 100,000 cases per year in the United States. Symptoms include rectal bleeding, diarrhea, loss of weight, and loss of appetite. If a patient complains of such symptoms, the physician will likely recommend a rectal examination, including the removal of tissue for biopsy, generally as part of colonoscopy (the visual examination of the colon with a flexible fiber-optic tube).

Treatment for colon cancer depends on the results of the biopsy and the general health of the patient. Surgical removal, however, is the most common treatment. If the tumor is small and confined, as in the form of a polyp, the removal of the polyp (polypectomy) is usually sufficient to effect a cure. If the tumor is relatively large, both the tumor and surrounding tissue must be removed (wedge resection). The extent of tissue removal depends on the size and stage of the tumor. Complete removal often includes supplementary treatments such as chemotherapy or radiation therapy. Since metastasis has often occurred by the time that symptoms appear, the prognosis for colon cancer is often poor.

Surgical procedures for smaller, more accessible tumors in other parts of the body are more straightforward. In the case of a parotid tumor, diagnosis often includes a CT scan or MRI, along with a biopsy. If the tumor is benign, removal of the lump is relatively simple. In rare instances in which the tumor is malignant, radiation therapy may be included as part of the treatment.

Breast cancer is one of the more common forms of cancer in women. In addition to its life-threatening potential, the disease can result in disfigurement as a result of treatment. Nearly 200,000 women per year in the United States are diagnosed with the disease.

Breast cancer often is first observed as a lump in the breast. If the biopsy shows it to be malignant, several courses of action may be considered, usually associated with surgical removal of the tumor along with healthy surrounding tissue. If the tumor is very small, removal of the lump may sufficient; if the tumor has spread, complete removal of the breast is often the choice (mastectomy). Radical mastectomy, which also involves the removal of surrounding muscle, may

be necessary if the cancer has spread into that tissue. Nearby lymph nodes from the armpit (axillary nodes) are often included in order to evaluate whether the cancer has metastasized.

PERSPECTIVE AND PROSPECTS
The first attempts at the surgical removal of tumors date to as early as 1600 B.C.E. in Egypt. These procedures were obviously crude and limited. Modern surgical treatment for tumor removal is credited to the American surgeon Ephraim MacDowell, who in 1809 removed a 22 pound tumor from a patient. (The patient survived and lived another three decades.) Two complications limited such forms of surgery, even for localized, readily accessible tumors: pain and infection. Though extracts from the poppy and the drinking of alcohol were both used to deaden pain in earlier centuries, it was not until the routine use of ether in the mid-nineteenth century that pain could be eliminated from surgery. In 1846, William T. G. Morton demonstrated the use of ether as a general anesthetic, first in the extraction of a tooth and later in a public demonstration in which a vascular tumor of the jaw was removed from a young patient. The pain-free operation lasted nearly thirty minutes and ushered in the era of general surgery.

Though pain during surgery could now be eliminated, there was still the problem of infection. Tumor removal in the mid-nineteenth century was confined to those of the breast or superficial areas of the body. It remained for Joseph Lister in the 1860's and 1870's to develop the antiseptic procedures necessary to reduce the chances for infection and subsequent mortality associated with surgery as a means of tumor removal.

Surgical procedures continued to improve in the twentieth century. Following the discovery of radioactivity by Wilhelm Conrad Röntgen, the use of X rays was added to the repertoire for the elimination of tumors. By damaging the genetic material of cells, radiation was demonstrated to be capable of reducing the size of tumors or of eliminating localized tumors altogether. The discovery in the mid-twentieth century of chemicals that interfere with the growth or metabolism of cancer cells resulted in the development of chemotherapy as a method of treatment.

Technological advances have resulted in better methods both for the diagnosis of tumors and in their elimination. Both CT scanning and MRI have the advantage of being noninvasive, though surgical biopsy remains the method of choice for diagnosis and staging of a tumor. Along with the development of these techniques have come more aggressive forms of treatment. Until the 1970's, tumor removal generally involved surgery, chemotherapy, or radiation therapy, but not often in combination. It became apparent that the elimination of the tumor was more effective when these procedures were used together: Radiation therapy could be used first to shrink the tumor, allowing for more effective surgical removal. As knowledge of the immunology of cancer (and the immune system in general) developed, physicians began to apply the immune system itself as a form of therapy. Interleukins and other chemicals secreted by the body's immune cells were seen to boost the immune response, aiding in the killing of tumor cells.

Many of the future goals in this medical field center on prevention of tumor formation, as well as their elimination. It is known that certain carcinogens such as cigarette ingredients are involved in the induction of tumors. Reduction in the number of persons smoking would have a significant impact on the prevalence of smoking-related tumors of the mouth and respiratory system. In addition, many tumors have been found to have a genetic basis; specific forms of cancer are associated with oncogenes in the cell. Through periodic screening, it is possible to observe whether such genes have undergone mutation and to remove any tumors that occur while they are still small and before they have undergone metastasis.

—*Richard Adler, Ph.D.*

See also Biopsy; Breast biopsy; Breast cancer; Breasts, female; Cancer; Cervical, ovarian, and uterine cancers; Chemotherapy; Colon and rectal polyp removal; Colon cancer; Colonoscopy; Cryotherapy and cryosurgery; Electrocauterization; Gastroenterology; Gastrointestinal disorders; Gastrointestinal system; Gynecology; Lung cancer; Lung surgery; Lungs; Malignancy and metastasis; Malignant melanoma removal; Mammography; Mastectomy and lumpectomy; Myomectomy; National Cancer Institute (NCI); Oncology; Plastic surgery; Prostate cancer; Prostate gland; Prostate gland removal; Pulmonary diseases; Pulmonary medicine; Radiation therapy; Stomach, intestinal, and pancreatic cancers; Tumors.

FOR FURTHER INFORMATION:

Altman, Roberta, and Michael Sarg. *The Cancer Dictionary.* Rev. ed. New York: Facts on File, 2000. More than simply serving as a dictionary, this book provides an extensive discussion of all major aspects of tumors. Included are descriptions of various forms of tumors, treatments, and terminology. An excellent source for the nonspecialist.

Dollinger, Malin, Ernest H. Rosenbaum, and Greg Cable. *Everyone's Guide to Cancer Therapy.* Kansas City, Mo.: Andrews & McMeel, 1997. An excellent resource on types of cancers, terminology, options, and discussions of topics for cancer patients such as questions to ask, methods of payment, and forms of therapy.

Nuland, Sherwin. *Doctors: The Biography of Medicine.* New York: Alfred A. Knopf, 1988. Though it does not deal with tumors specifically, this book includes a good discussion of the history of surgery. Particularly interesting are the chapters covering the use of anesthesia and the work of Joseph Lister.

Schwartz, Seymour I., ed. *Principles of Surgery.* 7th ed. New York: McGraw-Hill, 1999. A detailed discussion of surgery as a method of tumor removal that requires some knowledge of basic anatomy. A good reference for the reader wanting surgical details.

Way, Lawrence W., ed. *Current Surgical Diagnosis and Treatment.* 11th ed. Norwalk, Conn.: Appleton and Lange, 1998. A compromise between a dictionary and a comprehensive surgical treatise. Contains extensive discussions and diagrams of surgical treatments such as tumor removal. The depth of coverage is appropriate for a basic reference book.

TUMORS

DISEASE/DISORDER

ANATOMY OR SYSTEM AFFECTED: All

SPECIALTIES AND RELATED FIELDS: Endocrinology, histology, internal medicine, oncology, pulmonary medicine

DEFINITION: Abnormal growths of bodily tissues caused by genetic changes within normal cells; tumors may be benign (noninvasive) or malignant (invasive).

KEY TERMS:

benign tumor: a tumor which grows rapidly within a localized area without invading other tissue regions; noncancerous

cancer: a malignant tumor which grows rapidly and uncontrollably, starting with a transformed cell and spreading throughout the affected body, causing organ damage, failure, and death *carcinogen:* a mutagenic substance which triggers cellular biochemical events causing normal cells to become cancerous

cellular transformation: the biochemical process by which a normal body cell becomes tumorous, especially cancerous

differentiation: the physiological event in all multicellular organisms by which identical cells with identical genetic information specialize to become different tissue types

gene regulation: the control of whether a gene is active (that is, encoding messenger RNA and protein) or inactive (that is, not encoding RNA or protein), a process often affected by hormones

malignant tumor: a cancerous mass of cells which invades various body regions, contributing to tissue and organ failure as well as to the eventual death of the entire organism

metastasis: the breaking off and movement of cancer cells from one body tissue region to another, with transport being facilitated by the organism's bloodstream

mutagen: a substance (usually chemicals or ionizing radiation) which penetrates body cells and alters the nucleotide sequence of deoxyribonucleic acid (DNA), thus generating a mutation

virus: an obligate intracellular parasite, composed of genetic information protected by protein, which reproduces within living cells

CAUSES AND SYMPTOMS

Tumors, also called neoplasms, are caused by a variety of factors—including mutations, improper hormonal signaling, viruses, and environmental influences—which cause certain normal body cells to deviate from a genetically determined developmental pattern for that particular organism. Tumors arise in all multicellular eukaryotic organisms, such as animals, plants, and fungi, where colonies of cells are intricately connected and are dependent on one another.

A tumor arises when a mistake is made in the cellular expression of a given gene. At a certain point in the cell's development, a gene may be activated when it should not produce protein, or it may be inactivated when it should be producing protein. In either case, a cascade of subsequent developmental changes within the cell may be initiated. The cell may function inefficiently, die, or start to grow and divide at a faster rate than normal. In this latter scenario, the cell has become tumorous.

Many developmental biologists view the tumorous state as a throwback to the early embryonic development of the organism, when cells are undifferentiated and do not reveal the effects of specific hormonal genetic controls. Therefore, tumors reflect a dedifferentiated state of the cell. Tumors may be benign or malignant. A benign tumor grows as an enlarged tissue region without spreading elsewhere; often, it is only an inconvenience or irritant to the organism without harming the individual. A malignant tumor is invasive, spreading rapidly throughout many tissues, draining the organism of various resources, and eventually destroying key tissues and killing the individual. The breaking off and rapid spread of malignant tumors is termed metastasis.

The changes within genes and the subsequent gene expression or cellular dedifferentiation associated with tumors are brought about by mutations, changes within the nucleotide sequence (the genetic code) of the genes. Mutations can be caused by a number of agents called mutagens. Two major classes of mutagens are chemical mutagens (including benzene, carbon tetrachloride, and diethylstilbestrol) and radiation such as ultraviolet light, X radiation, and gamma radiation. Some mutagens also are carcinogens, causing malignant tumors. Not all mutagens, however, are also carcinogens. Caffeine, for example, is mutagenic but not carcinogenic.

Tumors can arise within cells of any of the five principal tissue types: epithelia, endothelia, connective tissue, nerve, and muscle. Epithelial tissue lines the organs outside and inside the body, including the skin, exocrine glands (such as oil and sweat glands), the digestive tract, and the reproductive organs. Endothelial tissue includes blood cells, blood vessels, and lymph nodes and glands. Connective tissue includes bone, fat cells, and cartilage. Nerve tissue includes the billions of nerves that compose the brain, spinal cord, and peripheral sensory and motor nerves. Muscle tissue includes the heart, more than six hundred skeletal muscles, and tens of thousands of smooth muscles.

Epithelial tissue cancers collectively are called carcinomas; they include adenocarcinomas, basal cell carcinomas, melanomas, malignant melanomas, squamous cell carcinomas, cervical cancer, uterine cancer, prostate cancer, colon and rectal cancer, and lung cancer. Whereas benign tumors of the skin such as freckles, moles, and warts are not serious, cancers of the skin and internal organ membranes can be fatal.

Adenocarcinomas affect glands. Basal cell carcinomas, melanomas, and squamous cell carcinomas are serious cancers of the skin that can arise from prolonged sun exposure. Malignant melanoma is a rapidly invasive skin cancer which can penetrate other body tissues and cause death within two or three months. Cervical and uterine cancers are serious tumors of the female reproductive tract. Prostate cancer is prevalent among males and is a leading cause of cancer deaths. Colon and rectal cancers, believed to be triggered by the lack of roughage in diets, are also relatively common in the United States. Lung cancer may result from exposure of lung tissue to cigarette smoke and air pollution.

Endothelial tissue cancers include leukemias, which affect blood cells, and lymphomas, which affect lymphatic tissue. Most leukemias affect the immune system's white blood cells (leukocytes) or the stem cells from which they are derived. Leukemias include acute lymphoblastic leukemia, acute myeloblastic leukemia, acute monoblastic leukemia, chronic lymphocytic leukemia, and chronic granulocytic leukemia. Lymphatic cancers attack the lymph nodes and glands that serve as blood reservoirs for the circulatory system. Lymphatic cancers include lymphosarcomas, Hodgkin's disease, and Burkitt's lymphoma, which is induced by the Epstein-Barr virus.

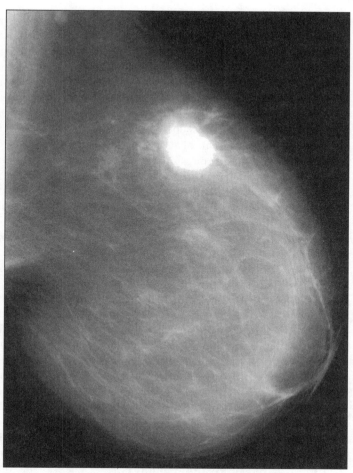

A mammogram showing a tumor in the breast. (SIU School of Medicine)

Connective tissue tumors include benign varieties such as osteomas and osteochondromas affecting bone, chondromas affecting cartilage, and lipomas affecting adipose (fat) tissue. Connective tissue cancers are called sarcomas. Chondrosarcomas are cartilaginous tissue cancers affecting joints. Osteosarcomas are bone cancers. Liposarcomas are fatty tissue cancers that attack a variety of bodily regions. Fibrosarcomas are cancers of the dense, fibrous tissue that holds together many bodily structures, including the skin.

Benign muscle tissue tumors are called myomas, whereas malignant muscle cancers are called myosarcomas. Leiomyosarcoma is a malignancy of smooth, visceral muscle. Rhabdomyosarcoma is a malignancy of cardiac and skeletal muscle.

Benign tumors of the central nervous system are called neuromas and neurofibromas. They include multiple neurofibroma, a condition in which numerous nerve tumors develop throughout the body, thereby causing a severely distorted physical appearance; multiple neurofibroma (or neurofibromatosis) is also known as the "Elephant Man" syndrome after the term used to describe Joseph (or John) Merrick, a nineteenth century Englishman who suffered from this disease. Nervous system cancers include brain cancer and neurogenic sarcoma, glioblastoma, neuroblastoma, and malignant meningioma.

The formation of tumors is probably triggered by many factors. For example, the stress associated with living in a fast-paced technological society causes severe disturbances to the normal homeostatic balance within the body, particularly with reference to the nervous and endocrine systems. The nervous system activates many organ systems and tissues throughout the body. Even more potent in its effects is the endocrine system, which directly controls gene expression in various body cells and tissues via chemical messengers called hormones. When these hormones are hyperactivated by stress, they may activate or inactivate certain genes and their protein products at the wrong time in an individual's development, thereby causing drastic changes in cellular functioning, often accompanied by abnormal growth of tissue into a tumor.

Virus infections may also result in cancer. In 1908, cell-free extracts prepared from leukemia in mice were shown to transmit the disease. In 1910, Peyton Rous discovered that a similar filterable agent would transmit a solid tumor, a sarcoma, in chickens. However, it was felt at the time that cancers in animals represented special circumstances, and that the work was not directly applicable to human cancer. The existence of the Rous sarcoma virus (RSV) was corroborated later by other researchers, culminating in the awarding of the 1966 Nobel Prize in Physiology and Medicine to Rous. Most human cancers are of endogenous (genetic) origin and not associated with viral infection, but there are a number of notable exceptions. Hepatitis B virus infection is associated with a hepatocarcinoma, or cancer of the liver. The Epstein-Barr virus, the etiological agent of infectious mononucleosis, is also the cause of both Burkitt's lymphoma and nasopharyngeal carcinoma.

TREATMENT AND THERAPY

Oncologists and other medical researchers study both benign and malignant tumors. Studies are devoted to the occurrence of these tumors, improved means of diagnosis, and the development of effective treatments. Cancer is the second-leading cause of death in the United States and many Western nations. Stress, viruses, pollution, and an individual's everyday exposure to hazardous materials increase the chance of developing tumors.

Regardless of a tumor's cause, it is important that it be identified and treated. The American Cancer Society's seven warning signs for cancer serve as an important model for tumor and cancer prevention. The warning signs are a sore that does not heal, persistent coughing, a lump anywhere on the body, unusual bleeding, a change in a wart or mole, a change in bladder or bowel movements, and difficulty swallowing.

Tumors may be benign or malignant. Benign tumors are less severe in most cases because they continue to grow within a localized region without invading other tissue regions. Benign tumors may press on critical organs and cause discomfort, however, thereby necessitating their surgical removal or inactivation using lasers, freezing, cytotoxic chemicals, or radiation. Warts represent a good example of a benign tumor. Warts are caused by a papillomavirus which infects skin cells of the dermis and enters a lysogenic phase, where it lays dormant in the host cell DNA but accelerates cell growth into a small tumor. A person can contract a papillomavirus merely by shaking an infected individual's hand; nearly thirty million Americans have this type of tumor. Some warts may become malignant.

Malignant tumors are invasive cancers which multiply rapidly, break off into the bloodstream, and colonize other body regions, where they destroy tissues, organs, and sometimes the entire organism. Malignant cancer cells are immortal in the sense that they reproduce without any developmental barriers. Many malignant colonies can manipulate available blood supplies away from normal tissue, thereby promoting their own growth. Malignant cancers are classified according to tissue type. Any tissue is subject to cancerous growth, given the appropriate stimuli.

Genetic and biochemical research focuses heavily on the study of neoplastic cellular transformation. The prime emphasis is upon gene regulation, the ultimate control point that determines whether a cell will function properly. Mutations in gene regulatory regions, improper hormonal signaling, or viral interference via lysogeny may contribute to abnormalities in cellular growth.

Benign and malignant tumors can be induced and studied in laboratory animals. The application of a chemical mutagen to a localized tissue region in a mouse usually gives rise to a tumor. Female mice infected with the mouse mammary tumor virus pass the virus to their young via milk during suckling; this virus generates grotesquely large tumors which are often as big as the mouse itself. Tumors or sections of tumors removed from humans are studied by biopsy and subsequent biochemical analysis. Human ccells are grown in tissue culture in flasks and roller bottles containing fetal calf serum so that medical researchers can study the nature of the neoplastic tumorous cells.

PERSPECTIVE AND PROSPECTS

The study of tumors is of critical importance to medicine because tumor formation is a major cause of illness in millions of people yearly. An understanding of the genetic mechanisms underlying tumor formation is directly applicable to both the study of cancer and the understanding of mechanisms that regulate cell growth in general.

Critical to understanding the genetic basis of cancer was the discovery of retroviruses, RNA viruses which replicate using a DNA intermediate. These viruses were discovered to carry oncogenes, cancer-causing genes which the viruses originally acquired from the cells they infected. It was discovered that oncogenes actually encode a variety of proteins that regulate cell growth, including growth factors and DNA regulatory proteins. The genetic basis behind most human cancers seems to involve mutations in these genes. The study of the mechanism by which these proteins function may eventually lead to a fuller understanding of how cancers develop.

Since most cancers have a genetic origin, the ability to screen for certain genetic patterns allows clinicians to observe patients most at risk for the disease. For example, women who carry certain forms of the genes BRCA1 and BRCA2 are at greater risk for developing ovarian or breast cancer.

Developing cancers in certain tissues may also secrete unique forms of proteins, allowing for detection of the disease at an early stage. For example, prostate tumors, the leading form of cancer in men, secrete a prostate specific antigen (PSA); elevated levels of PSA in the blood suggest a possible tumor in the prostate.

Oncofetal proteins, normally found on fetal cells, may also be reexpressed by certain tumors. Elevated levels of alpha-fetoprotein and carcinoembryonic antigen in serum may indicate liver or colorectal cancer. The increasing sensitivity of such screening methods holds out the prospect that the most common forms of cancer may be detected in a "curable" stage.

—*David Wason Hollar, Jr., Ph.D.;*
updated by Richard Adler, Ph.D.

See also Biopsy; Bone cancer; Breast biopsy; Breast cancer; Cancer; Carcinoma; Cervical, ovarian, and uterine cancers; Colon cancer; Cysts; Endometrial biopsy; Hodgkin's disease; Keratoses; Leukemia; Liver cancer; Lung cancer; Lymphadenopathy and lymphoma; Malignancy and metastasis; Mammography; Mastectomy and lumpectomy; Mutation; National Cancer Institute (NCI); Neurofibromatosis; Oncology; Ovarian cysts; Prostate cancer; Sarcoma; Skin cancer; Stomach, intestinal, and pancreatic cancers; Tumor removal; Warts.

FOR FURTHER INFORMATION:

Alberts, Bruce, et al. *Molecular Biology of the Cell.* 3d ed. New York: Garland, 1994. This enormous textbook, written by six pioneers of molecular biology, is a presentation of genetics, cellular biochemistry, and developmental biology in a language understandable to the beginning biology student.

Chiras, Daniel D. *Biology: The Web of Life.* St. Paul, Minn.: West, 1993. Chiras's introductory biology textbook is clearly written with numerous examples, detailed sketches and photographs, and guest essays by leading scientists. Chapter 9, "Molecular Genetics," discusses gene regulation and the role of mutation in cellular transformation.

Day, Stacey B., ed. *Cancer, Stress, and Death.* 2d ed. New York: Plenum, 1986. An excellent survey of the relationship between stress, cancer, disease, and death. Essays by leading medical researchers such as Jean Tache and Hans Selye describe the link between stress and the nervous, endocrine, and immune systems of the body.

Gaudin, Anthony J., and Kenneth C. Jones. *Human Anatomy and Physiology.* New York: Harcourt Brace Jovanovich, 1989. This introductory anatomy and physiology textbook provides a wealth of information concerning the human body—its structure, function, and diseases. Chapter 3, "Cell Structure and Organization," provides a thorough but clear discussion of gene regulation and neoplastic cellular transformation.

Hood, Gail Harkness, and Judith R. Dincher. *Total Patient Care: Foundations and Practice of Adult Health Nursing.* 8th ed. St. Louis: Mosby Year Book, 1992. An outstanding introduction to health care for nursing and premedical students. Chapter 9, "The Patient with Cancer," includes extensive information on cancer types.

Joesten, Melvin D., David O. Johnston, John Netterville, and James L. Wood. *World of Chemistry.* 2d ed. Philadelphia: W. B. Saunders College, 1999. This textbook is an excellent introduction to chemistry and biochemistry for those with no previous chemistry experience. The authors emphasize the impact of chemistry on our everyday lives, problems of toxins and hazardous waste in the environment, and basic chemical principles.

Kuby, Janis. *Immunology.* 4th ed. New York: W. H. Freeman, 2000. A detailed examination of the field of immunology. Several chapters deal with subjects of cell regulation apropos to tumor development. Included is an update of tumor specific markers.

Varmus, Harold, and Robert Weinberg. *Genes and the Biology of Cancer.* New York: W. H. Freeman, 1993. Insight into the genetic mechanisms behind tumor formation. Discussions include the roles played by carcinogens, viruses, and oncogenes. Profusely illustrated at a level appropriate for the nonscientist.

TURNER SYNDROME
DISEASE/DISORDER

ALSO KNOWN AS: Gonadal dysgenesis

ANATOMY OR SYSTEM AFFECTED: Cells, endocrine system, reproductive system

SPECIALTIES AND RELATED FIELDS: Endocrinology, genetics, gynecology, obstetrics

DEFINITION: The most common sex chromosome abnormality in females.

CAUSES AND SYMPTOMS

Turner syndrome affects an estimated one out of every 2,000 to 2,500 girls conceived. The disorder is congenital, which means that it begins at birth. Normal males have one X and one Y chromosome. Normal females have two X chromosomes. Females with Turner syndrome have only one X chromosome (an XO pattern) in each of their cells. Although the exact cause is unknown, scientists believe that the disorder may result from an error during the division of the parent's sex cells.

Shortness is the most common feature of Turner syndrome. The average height of a woman with this condition is 4 feet, 8 inches. Other physical features associated with the syndrome include puffy hands and feet at birth, a webbed neck, prominent ears, a low hairline at the back of the neck, and soft fingernails that turn up at the end.

Most patients experience ovarian failure. Since the ovaries normally produce estrogen, girls and women with Turner syndrome lack this essential hormone, resulting in infertility and incomplete sexual development. Cardiovascular disorders are the single source of increased mortality in patients with Turner syndrome.

TREATMENT AND THERAPY

No treatment is available to correct the chromosome abnormality that causes this condition. Nevertheless, injections of human growth hormones can restore much of the growth deficit. Unless they take hormone replacement therapy, women and girls with Turner syndrome will not menstruate or develop breasts and pubic hair. Although infertility cannot be altered, pregnancy may be possible through in vitro fertilization.

PERSPECTIVE AND PROSPECTS

Turner syndrome was first identified by Dr. Henry Turner in 1938. In 1959, Dr. C. E. Ford discovered that a chromosomal abnormality involving sex chromosomes causes the syndrome.

Research is underway to assess the best way to administer female sex hormones that provide maximum bone development and growth in adolescents who need this therapy.

—*Fred Buchstein*

See also Dwarfism; Endocrine system; Endocrinology; Endocrinology, pediatric; Genetic diseases; Genetics and inheritance; Growth; Hormone replacement therapy; Hormones; Infertility in females; Menstruation; Puberty and adolescence; Reproductive system; Sexual differentiation.

FOR FURTHER INFORMATION:

Money, John. *Sex Errors of the Body and Related Syndromes: A Guide to Counseling Children, Adolescents, and Their Families.* Baltimore: Paul H. Brookes, 1994.

Pinsky, Leonard, Robert P. Erickson, and R. Neil Schimke. *Genetic Disorders of Human Sexual Development.* New York: Oxford University Press, 1999.

Rosenfeld, Ron G., and Melvin M. Grumbach, eds. *Turner Syndrome.* New York: Marcel Dekker, 1989.

TWINS. *See* MULTIPLE BIRTHS.

TYPHOID FEVER AND TYPHUS
DISEASE/DISORDER

ANATOMY OR SYSTEM AFFECTED: Gastrointestinal system

SPECIALTIES AND RELATED FIELDS: Bacteriology, emergency medicine, public health

DEFINITION: Acute infectious diseases caused by bacteria or rickettsiae. Typhoid, also known as typhoid fever, is caused by the bacterium *Salmonella typhi.* In contrast, typhus is caused by *Rickettsia prowazekii.* Rickettsias are microorganisms that are smaller than bacteria and larger than viruses.

Typhoid. Thomas Willis was the first to describe typhoid fever in 1643, but the disease was confused with typhus until 1837, when William W. Gerhard distinguished between them and also provided the name typhoid fever to indicate its similarity to typhus. In 1856, William Budd became the first to prove its infectious character via the patient's feces, and Karl Eberth demonstrated the existence of the typhoid bacillus. Thousands of people died because of typhoid fever, especially during the Spanish-American and Boer wars, until a typhoid vaccine was developed. By the end of World War II, the disease was practically eradicated because of improved sanitary conditions, especially in developing countries.

The typhoid bacillus enters the body via the swallowing of infected food, such as raw shellfish, fresh fruit, or vegetables. Once it enters the body, the bacillus accumulates in the Peyer's patches of the lower small intestine, where it multiplies and eventually enters the bloodstream. During the first week, the patient exhibits no symptoms or only mild ones: headache, body pains, and loss of appetite. Ten days after infection, a fever starts and often reaches and stays at 104 degrees Fahrenheit for almost two weeks, while all lymphoid tissues become inflamed. For the next two weeks, the infected person has a very low pulse, a low white blood count, and a bloated abdomen and is often delirious. The development of rose spots, swelling of the spleen, and perforation of the bowel also accompany the disease. Constipation often alternates with the passage of a characteristic stool that resembles pea soup. Complications include intestinal hemorrhage, pneumonia, thrombosis, and laryngitis.

The bacteria can be isolated from the blood during the first ten days and from the feces in the next five weeks. Between 2 and 5 percent of those who recover (usually women) become chronic carriers, as the microorganisms may stay in the gallbladder. The disease leaves the patient with a high number of antibodies, which indicates the presence of the infection and can be detected after the second week. Vaccination with an oral vaccine is generally ade-

Development of Typhoid Fever

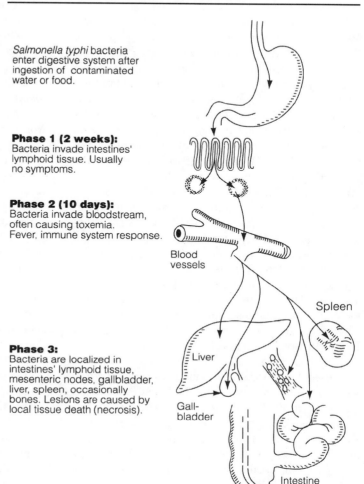

Salmonella typhi bacteria enter digestive system after ingestion of contaminated water or food.

Phase 1 (2 weeks): Bacteria invade intestines' lymphoid tissue. Usually no symptoms.

Phase 2 (10 days): Bacteria invade bloodstream, often causing toxemia. Fever, immune system response.

Blood vessels

Spleen

Phase 3: Bacteria are localized in intestines' lymphoid tissue, mesenteric nodes, gallbladder, liver, spleen, occasionally bones. Lesions are caused by local tissue death (necrosis).

Liver

Gallbladder

Intestine

quate for about three years. The only effective antibiotic is chloramphenicol, which has reduced mortality to less than 10 percent of the total incidence. Carriers of the microorganism can be treated with ampicillin, but if the gallbladder is infected it should be removed. Isolation of the patient, sanitary precautions, frequent bacteriologic testing, and the avoidance of fecal contamination of foodstuffs are essential to prevent the spreading.

Paratyphoid fever is caused by bacteria that belong to the *Salmonella* genus but is shorter in duration and generally less severe than the fever produced by *S. typhi*. Modern clinicians use the umbrella term salmonellosis to cover diseases attributed to food poisoning, localized infection in various organs, and paratyphoid fever.

Typhus. Communicable only via an arthropod and not via humans themselves, typhus can be epidemic (louse-borne, Brill-Zinsser), endemic (flea-borne, murine), or mite-borne (scrub, tropical). The most devastating type in human history is epidemic typhus (also known as ship fever, jail fever, or tabardillo), which is transmitted by the louse *Pediculus humanus corporis*. First documented in Germany during the sixteenth century, it played a significant role in the outcome of the Thirty Years' War (1516-1546), Napoleon's defeat during the Russian invasion (1812), the Crimean War (1853-1856), and World War I (1914-1918). It is estimated that more than three million typhus deaths occurred in Russia between 1917 and 1921. Thousands of people died in the Nazi German concentration camps, and many more died in Japan and Korea after World War II because of typhus. In 1909, Charles Nicolle reproduced the disease in monkeys and Stanislas von Prowazek demonstrated the role of the body louse in transmitting it. Rudolph Weigl prepared a vaccine from louse guts in 1930, and in 1941 Herald R. Cox prepared it in the yolk sacs of embryonated chicken eggs.

The epidemic form of typhus is most common in winter because the carrier, the body and head louse, flourishes in thick winter clothing. The disease lies dormant in chronic human carriers between epidemics and is transferred to the louse via biting. The louse in turn transmits it by depositing its feces after biting a new host. The incubation period is ten to fourteen days and starts with strong chills, a high fever, headache, and a severe abdominal rash. The fever drops, usually abruptly, after two weeks, and the disease is diagnosed positively during the second week by the Felix-Weil blood test. During World War II, all American soldiers were given a vaccine prepared in chicken embryos. Louse insecticides are extremely effective in controlling the spread of the disease, while antibiotics, such as chloramphenicol and the tetracyclines Aureomycin and oxytetracycline (Terramycin), are effective in curing the patient. The Brill-Zinsser disease resembles epidemic typhus but is much milder. It may occur years after the initial attack of the fever and can start an epidemic of the classic louse-borne disease.

The endemic form of typhus is rare in the United States but occurs in the warmer parts of the world. It is much milder than the epidemic form, exists in rats, and is transmitted by the rat flea. Immunization is effective but is not necessary because of effective preventive methods, such as pesticides to kill the rats and decrease the flea population. Murine endemic typhus occurs in rats by *R. mooseri* and is transmitted to humans by means of fleas of the species *Xenopsylla cheopis*.

Scrub or mite-borne typhus is caused by *R. tsutsugamushi* and is indicated by a lesion at the wound site. Although the disease was devastating during World War II, such deaths became rare after 1948 when the massive use of antibiotics was introduced. Prevention involves the use of mite-killing chemicals (such as benzyl benzoate) and mite repellents spread on the skin.

—Soraya Ghayourmanesh, Ph.D.

See also Antibiotics; Arthropod-borne diseases; Bacterial infections; Bacteriology; Bites and stings; Childhood infectious diseases; Fever; Food poisoning; Immunization and vaccination; Lice, mites, and ticks; Microbiology; Parasitic diseases; Salmonella infection.

FOR FURTHER INFORMATION:

Cobelens, F. G., S. Kooij, A. Warris-Versteegen, and L. G. Visser. "Typhoid Fever in Group Travelers: Opportunity for Studying Vaccine Efficacy." *Journal of Travel Medicine* 7, no. 1 (January, 2000): 19-24. This study was designed to describe the epidemiology of typhoid fever in travel groups and to assess whether travel groups can be used for studying the efficacy of typhoid fever vaccines.

Pang, T., C. L. Koh, and S. D. Puthuchear, eds. *Typhoid Fever: Strategies for the Nineties.* Teaneck, N.J.: World Scientific, 1992. This text is based on an Asia-Pacific Symposium on Typhoid Fever, Kuala Lumpur, Malaysia, October 1-3, 1991. Includes bibliographical references.

Pinkowish, Mary Desmond. "Typhoid Fever Is Increasing, Especially in Travelers to India." *Patient Care* 32, no. 10 (May 30, 1998): 146. *Salmonella typhi* remains a scourge in travelers. Officials at the Centers for Disease Control and Prevention (CDC) report that the incidence of this sometimes fatal disease is increasing in certain travelers, as is drug resistance.

"Salmonelloses." In *McGraw-Hill Encyclopedia of Science and Technology.* 7th ed. Vol. 8. New York: McGraw-Hill, 1992. A chapter in a complete reference for the nonspecialist, which offers thousands of articles written by world-renowned scientists and engineers. It includes many new and revised articles, extensive cross-references, and bibliographies and is fully illustrated.

Zinsser, Hans. *Rats, Lice, and History.* New York: Black Dog & Leventhal, 1996. A history of typhus is offered, with an examination of the role of rats and lice as vectors of the disease. Includes bibliographical references.

ULCER SURGERY

PROCEDURE

ANATOMY OR SYSTEM AFFECTED: Gastrointestinal system, intestines, stomach

SPECIALTIES AND RELATED FIELDS: Gastroenterology, general surgery, nutrition

DEFINITION: The removal of areas of the stomach or duodenum that are ulcerated; a procedure often avoided by nonsurgical treatment.

KEY TERMS:

duodenum: the first part of the small intestine

metastasis: the transfer of disease-producing cells to other parts of a body

partial gastrectomy: the removal of part of the stomach

pepsin: a substance in the stomach that breaks down most proteins

peritonitis: inflammation of the peritoneum or stomach lining

pyloric stenosis: a narrowing of the passageway between the stomach and the duodenum

INDICATIONS AND PROCEDURES

Many people who are host to peptic ulcers have no symptoms. As these ulcers—which may occur as single or multiple eruptions having a diameter of from 0.75 centimeter (0.3 inch) to 2.5 centimeters (1 inch) and a depth of about 0.02 centimeter (0.01 inch)—enlarge and multiply, however, symptoms often become apparent. These symptoms include a burning or gnawing pain in the abdominal region, particularly when the stomach is empty. Therefore, people who are asymptomatic during the day, when they are ingesting food at regular intervals, may become symptomatic at night. One way to allay symptoms, particularly those caused by a duodenal ulcer, is to eat, so that the gastric juices feed on the food rather than on the lining of the stomach or duodenum. Symptoms often reappear, however, a few hours after eating.

In some cases, patients experience a loss of appetite. If the ulcer is in the duodenum, however, the opposite may occur, in which case it is best to eat small quantities of food that is not overly spicy. Belching often accompanies ulcer problems, although, in and of itself, this is not categorically indicative of ulcers. People suffering from ulcers sometimes lose weight, largely because they feel bloated and therefore tend to eat less. Nausea and vomiting accompany some ulcer problems.

In extreme cases, an ulcer may start to bleed, in which case the patient may vomit blood. Black, tarry stools are also an indication of bleeding in the stomach, although elements in one's diet, particularly iron, can also produce darkened stools. Where bleeding is profuse, the patient may require a blood transfusion. On rare occasions, an ulcer may eat through the back wall of the digestive tract and involve the pancreas, causing a pain that reaches as far as the patient's back. When ulcers eat through the front of the duodenum, the result may be peritonitis, a life-threatening

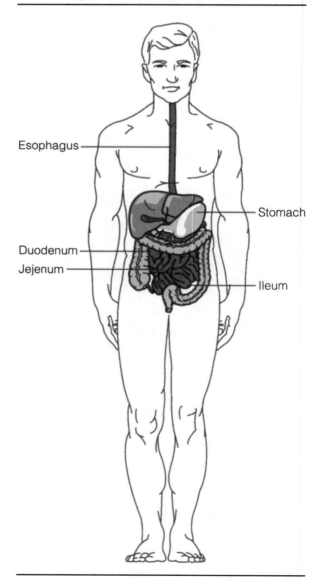

Major Sites of Ulcer Formation

Esophagus

Stomach

Duodenum

Jejenum

Ileum

inflammation of the abdominal lining that requires immediate attention.

If ulcers persist and go untreated, they can cause dangerous scarring of the stomach lining and duodenum. As a result, the passageway between the stomach and duodenum narrows. When this condition, called pyloric stenosis, occurs, patients usually experience vomiting and weight loss.

Some ulcers are malignant (cancerous) and must be removed surgically at once. Follow-up radiation and/or chemotherapy may be indicated in such cases. The surgical removal of ulcers involves making an incision in the abdomen and removing the portion of the stomach or duodenum that is ulcerated. The area affected is then joined and sutured. Large portions of the stomach may be removed if necessary and will, in time, regenerate.

USES AND COMPLICATIONS

Except where a malignancy is suspected, ulcer surgery is a treatment of last resort. Often, changes in diet can control the situation, as can discontinuing smoking and the drinking of alcoholic beverages or beverages that contain caffeine. Aspirin and nonsteroidal anti-inflammatory drugs (NSAIDs) can irritate the stomach and are usually not advised for people with ulcers. Because ulcers occur frequently in people under stress, changes in lifestyle can also result in considerable improvement.

The most common early treatment is with nonprescription antacids or with similar prescription drugs that coat the stomach lining and neutralize the acids that are causing the problem. Ulcer patients are also generally advised to eat several small meals a day rather than two or three large ones. It helps to keep food in the stomach, and even nibbling through the night produces favorable results in some patients.

Because ulcer surgery is major and is usually done under general anesthesia, it carries the risks associated with any major surgery. The recovery rate after ulcer surgery is good, however, particularly as the areas around the excision begin to return to normal through regeneration. Where a malignancy has been detected early and removed surgically, metastasis can usually be prevented, particularly if follow-up radiation or chemotherapy is employed.

PERSPECTIVE AND PROSPECTS

Ulcers were once treated by bed rest and a bland, boring diet, mostly of such soft foods as boiled eggs,

The Removal of a Peptic Ulcer

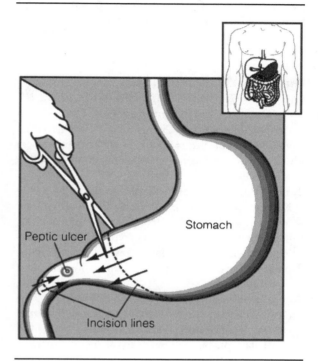

With a severe peptic ulcer, it may be necessary to remove a section of the stomach and join the remaining ends; the inset shows the location of the stomach.

toast, and custards accompanied by plenty of milk, which supposedly lined the stomach and protected it from damage by gastric juices. Such treatment is now generally considered unnecessary. Most ulcer patients can remain active and can eat sensibly but relatively normally. Extremely spicy food, which can irritate an ulcer, should be avoided if ulcer symptoms are present.

In the past, another method of ulcer treatment was to freeze the affected area, which seemed to produce immediate, favorable results. In time, however, many of the ulcers treated in this way returned. This treatment, although appealing for its short-term results, is now uncommon because its benefits do not appear to be lasting.

In recent years, the management of ulcers has become increasingly conservative, with surgery the least frequent and most extreme treatment of all. In the foreseeable future, it is likely that ulcer surgery will become an increasing rarity.

—R. Baird Shuman, Ph.D.

See also Digestion; Endoscopy; Food biochemistry; Gastrectomy; Gastroenterology; Gastrointestinal disorders; Gastrointestinal system; Intestinal disorders; Intestines; Peritonitis; Stress; Stress reduction; Ulcers; Vagotomy.

FOR FURTHER INFORMATION:

Louw, J. A. *The Medical Management of Peptic Ulcer Disease: Cure in Our Time?* Cape Town, South Africa: University of Cape Town, 1997. A concise volume that discusses the treatment of peptic ulcers and gastric acid secretion. Includes bibliographical references.

Swabb, Edward A., and Sandor Szabo, eds. *Ulcer Disease: Investigation and Basis for Therapy.* New York: Marcel Dekker, 1991. Twenty-four contributed chapters in four sections give medical researchers and practicing clinicians a review of the origins, presentations, therapies, and human investigation of ulcer disease.

Szabo, Sandor, and Carl J. Pfeiffer, eds. *Ulcer Disease: New Aspects of Pathogenesis and Pharmacology.* Boca Raton, Fla.: CRC Press, 1989. The latest data on the pathogenesis of ulcer disease is presented in this text, with the emphasis that an understanding of the pathogenesis and etiology of ulcer diseases represents the most rational approach to pharmacology.

Tytgat, G. N. J., ed. *Peptic Ulcer Disease.* Orlando, Fla.: W. B. Saunders, 2000. Discusses conceivable mechanisms by which *Helicobacter pylori* provokes duodenal ulcer disease and the management of gastroduodenal ulcers caused by nonsteroidal anti-inflammatory drugs.

Zakim, David, and Andrew J. Dannenberg, eds. *Peptic Ulcer Disease and Other Acid-Related Disorders.* Armonk, N.Y.: Academic Research Associates, 1991. Discusses gastric acid secretion and digestive system diseases generally. Includes bibliographical references and an index.

Zinner, Michael. *Atlas of Gastric Surgery.* New York: Churchill Livingstone, 1992. This text covers stomach surgery, peptic ulcers, and gastrointestinal diseases generally. Includes an index.

ULCERS
DISEASE/DISORDER
ANATOMY OR SYSTEM AFFECTED: Gastrointestinal system, mouth, stomach

SPECIALTIES AND RELATED FIELDS: Family practice, gastroenterology, internal medicine, nutrition

DEFINITION: Ulcers, specifically those referred to as peptic ulcers, are open sores that develop on the mucous membranes that line the gastrointestinal tract and are caused by excessive secretion of gastric juices, particularly from the pancreas into the intestine.

KEY TERMS:

acid pump inhibitors: a group of drugs that block the stomach cells' mechanism for producing hydrochloric acid

histamine II blockers: the general term used to describe various drugs that block the hormonal stimulation of histamine, one inducer of stomach acid

nonulcerous dyspepsia: a condition that exhibits many of the symptoms of peptic ulcers but does not involve actual lesions in the linings of the stomach or intestines

pepsin: the first component of gastric juice to be discovered, in the 1830's; the term "peptic ulcer" derives from the name of this digestive fluid

prostaglandins: chemical substances in the stomach lining that help fight ulceration by increasing blood flow to the lesion area

Zollinger-Ellison syndrome: a rare condition in which secretions of acid are so sudden and excessive that normal gastric defenses cannot prevent the immediate ulceration of stomach membranes

CAUSES AND SYMPTOMS

In the most general of terms, an ulcer is an open sore that does not respond readily to the normal processes of healing. It may occur on the skin itself or on internal mucous membranes. A corneal ulcer, for example, may occur as a result of infections stemming from local injuries of, or foreign objects lodged in, the eye. Circulatory disturbances associated with varicose veins or long periods in bed without sufficient body exercise can also cause skin ulcers. The latter form is sometimes referred to as bedsores.

The most commonly occurring ulcer, however, is the peptic ulcer, which occurs at various points in the gastrointestinal tract. Specifically, such ulcers affect the lower portion of the esophagus, the stomach (in which case the term "gastric" ulcer may be employed), and two locations in the small intestine: the duodenum and the jejunum. It has been estimated that, by the latter quarter of the twentieth century, approximately 10 percent of the general population in the

United States and Western Europe stood a statistical chance of suffering from peptic ulcers. A substantially higher percentage of the population may suffer from a condition that resembles ulcers in its symptomatic levels of discomfort and pain but that does not actually involve lesions. This condition is called nonulcerous dyspepsia.

When ulceration of the stomach or intestinal tissue advances past a certain stage, internal bleeding usually occurs. Reaction to this stage of deterioration may involve vomiting, in which case the granular bloody material that is expulsed resembles partially digested food and is brownish rather than red in color. This condition stems from the effect of acidic gastric juices on the blood that has been released. If bleeding from ulcers becomes evident through the presence of blood in the stools, the effect is different: The fecal material is black in color, a condition that was referred to in past generations as "tarry stool."

Although modern medical science has identified the hydrochloric acid content of the gastric juice as the corrosive agent that causes ulcer sores in all these regions of the digestive system, the term "peptic ulcer" is still commonly used to refer to all ulcers. This label was first applied following the discovery, in 1836, of the enzyme pepsin, one of the first subcomponents of the gastric juice to be isolated in the laboratory.

In the twentieth century, the original contributions of physicians to the understanding of what ulcers are were combined with equally scientific observations of social and psychological factors that can bring about ulcers. Increasingly, many of these causes were associated with environmental and nervous emotional factors.

The likelihood of ulcers forming in the gastrointestinal tract is increased if an imbalance occurs in the normal functioning of a specific phase of the digestive process. That phase begins when, at the time that foods are taken into the mouth and swallowed, the body secretes gastric juice containing both acid and pepsin. The essential acid in gastric juice is hydrochloric acid, which is highly dangerous in its pure state and poisonous if swallowed directly. Pepsin is an enzyme produced in the lining of the stomach that has proteolytic, or protein-degrading, characteristics. Both these components in gastric juices are essential in the first stages of digestion to break down the foodstuffs in the stomach and to facilitate their passage into the small intestine, where other secretions from the liver and pancreas continue the process of digestion. In the case of the enzyme pepsin, it is secreted in an inactive chemical state; it therefore requires the presence of hydrochloric acid (also secreted in the stomach lining) to convert it chemically to an active state and an optimum degree of acidity (pH 1 to 3) for the digestive function it fulfills. If the chemical conversion of pepsin into an active digestive agent does not make use of all the hydrochloric acid that has been secreted, the excess acid is free to do damage to the sensitive tissue of the stomach or intestinal lining.

Ulcers can occur in any of several areas of the gastrointestinal tract when excessive amounts or imbalanced component proportions of gastric juice are secreted. In recent times, doctors established that a continuing state of nervousness or hostility can cause gastric juice to flow almost continuously. Such hypersecretion will damage the mucous membranes lining the digestive tract unless a more-or-less constant supply of food is taken in by the organism. Thus, the nervous eater who is constantly consuming foods may be unconsciously trying to control the potential development of ulcers in his or her gastrointestinal tract. The side effects on the body of constant nervous eating may be potentially as harmful as the localized effects associated with ulcers.

In essence, what happens when an ulcer begins to form is that the acid and pepsin in the gastric juice begin to digest membrane tissue in the gastrointestinal tract itself. Normally, the stomach has a series of internal defenses to combat localized attacks by active gastric juice against its own sensitive membranes. In the first place, the mucous lining of the internal organs themselves forms a sort of barrier between membrane tissue and the combined food-gastric juice content of the functioning organ.

The cells of the stomach lining also secrete a natural antacid in the form of bicarbonate of soda. If the normal presence of these two protective agents is insufficient to prevent deterioration of the stomach or intestinal lining, a more active struggle ensues in the area where an ulcer has begun to develop. Surface cells begin to constrict to form a more resistant surface area around the nascent lesion. If the process does not proceed too rapidly, damaged cells may be replaced by healthy cells in the immediate area of the lesion.

Even more specialized reactions in the area of ulceration are associated with prostaglandins, which are chemical agents in the stomach lining that stimulate increased blood flow to nourish besieged cells. Prostaglandins can also bring about higher levels of antacid production and mucus accumulation where they are needed most.

With one notable and fairly rare exception, known as the Zollinger-Ellison syndrome (excessive production of acid), almost all cases of stomach ulcers (gastric ulcers) occur as a result of dysfunction in the defensive systems described above. As for duodenal (upper small intestine) ulcers, it appears that only about a third of all cases stem from higher-than-normal secretions of acid.

Doctors are not in full agreement regarding the way in which certain externally introduced substances may cause, or seriously contribute to, ulcers. Most have concluded, however, that a "big three" of clearly abusive substances—cigarettes, alcohol, and some over-the-counter drugs, especially aspirin—play a significant role. Cigarette smoking has been linked with the slowing down of essential body functions that either provide defenses against ulcers or contribute to their healing. One such function is the rate of blood flow itself, which is vital for the nourishment of cells that may be under attack by ulcers. Other side effects of smoking may include reduced production of prostaglandins, which make important contributions to the defensive reaction of the body against ulcerations.

As for the other potentially abusive agents, alcohol and certain over-the-counter or otherwise common drugs, it is the latter that are almost universally condemned for their negative effects on the proper functioning of the gastrointestinal system.

Alcohol, for its part, apparently does nothing to stimulate excessive acid production in the stomach. It does, however, interfere with the healing processes that are so vital in combating ulcers.

Development of an Ulcer

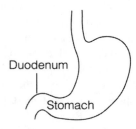

Glands in the stomach lining secrete acid and pepsin to digest food.

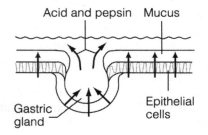

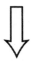

Increased acid secretion, reduced mucus, or irritants (alcohol, bile, bacteria, caffeine, aspirin) may begin road toward an ulcer.

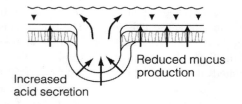

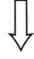

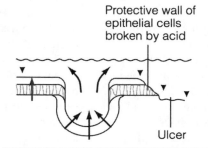

Ulcer forms when these factors lead to breakdown of the lining of the stomach or the duodenum.

While caffeine is not usually considered to be an over-the-counter drug, it is known to be an important stimulator of acid secretions. Some doctors consider it to be second only to aspirin as a negative "foreign agent" affecting the sensitive mechanism of digestion in the stomach and small intestine.

Another common drug, aspirin, shares a dubious reputation in this respect with a number of other drugs classified as nonsteroidal anti-inflammatory drugs (NSAIDs) that are used to treat arthritis and other muscular or joint inflammations.

There is a widespread consensus that the occurrence of ulcers may be linked to external agents that are taken into the body. The simplest evidence of this hypothesis revolves around associations that have been established between the bacillus *Helicobacter pylori* (*H. pylori*) and ulcerous conditions in the stomach and intestines.

Doctors had observed the presence of this bacillus (along with many others) in the human stomach for at least a century. Studies by the Australian researchers Bernard Marshall and J. R. Warner, however, noted that a very high percentage (nearly 100 percent) of patients diagnosed as having ulcers also had substantial traces of *H. pylori*.

TREATMENT AND THERAPY

As the debate over the role of *H. pylori* in causing ulcers took form in the early 1990's, those researchers who wanted to find proof that medicine was on the verge of a major breakthrough organized a full campaign to prescribe drugs that were known to kill the suspect bacillus.

It is now clear that *H. pylori* is a major contributing factor not only in ulcer development but also in the extremely high recurrence rate of relapse in healed patients. Because of the inflammation that the infecting organism causes in the stomach and duodenal linings, normal protective mechanisms break down. Once these barriers that protect the lining from damage by the acid and enzymes used in digesting food are gone, the process of ulceration begins. Even after the ulcer has healed, very high rates of recurrence are found unless the bacterial infection is eradicated.

Because so many people are infected with these common bacteria but not everyone develops ulcers, other contributing factors are clearly present. In the vulnerable patient, a combination of the well-known risk factors along with infection work together to bring about ulcers. It is now a routine treatment to administer antibiotics and stomach acid inhibitors simultaneously. Cure rate times and relapse rates have improved significantly.

Whatever the ultimate explanation concerning the causes of this surprisingly common ailment may be, the medical world remained, at least as late as the first years of the 1990's, devoted to the necessary use of a number of drugs to control the effects of gastric and peptic ulcers by fighting the flow of gastric juices that do the physical damage of ulceration. On the whole, these drugs, which are called histamine II blockers, aim at one objective: to block the formation of stomach acid. A similar effect is produced by several widely used (and markedly expensive) medicines that are prepared under commercial labels: Tagamet, Zantac, Pepcid, and Axid. The new drug class, acid pump inhibitors, such as Prilosec and others, also block stomach acid, but by a different and nearly complete method: They prevent the stomach cells from actually making the acid, in the final step before it is secreted into the stomach. These drugs are effective even in the most difficult cases of ulceration.

Much more complicated than the problem of treating normal cases of ulcers is the technical question of how to guard against the further deterioration of ulcers into different forms of gastrointestinal cancer. New forms of technology were being tested in the 1990's that allowed physicians to examine the inner mucous membranes of the intestines directly. One such device, called the fiber-optic endoscope, consists of a long tube that is passed through the esophagus and stomach to penetrate the upper portions of the small intestine. The fiber-optic endoscope not only views and photographs the surface areas affected by ulcers but also allows the physician to biopsy the tissue at the same time. This and other methods of diagnosis, although not available to all hospitals and clinics, and not mastered by all physicians who were trained in the pre-fiber-optic generation, represent enormous potential advances over the rather basic therapies developed during the previous century.

PERSPECTIVE AND PROSPECTS

Long before modern scientific research techniques provided the medical world with a relatively precise idea of what causes ulcers and how to treat them, an entire literature on the disease had accumulated. It was apparently Hippocrates himself, in the fifth century B.C.E., who first studied the gastric hemorrhaging that can result from a peptic ulcer. Others, including the first century C.E. Roman Celsus, noted the favorable effect of prescribing a nonacid diet to patients suffering from ulcers. It was not until the eighteenth and nineteenth centuries, however, that doctors prepared the first clinical accounts of the effects of ulcers based on pathological studies.

Not much had changed by the early twentieth century regarding the attitude of physicians toward the role of acids in the stage-by-stage degenerative process of ulceration. The American doctor Bertram W. Sippy was often quoted after his famous 1912 statement to medical students that "where there is no acid, there is no ulcer." The question of what caused the presence of excess acid in the intestines aside, medical science would try to come closer to being able to detect the actions of the "culprit at work." To the general public, the advanced process of fiber-optic endoscopy gives the appearance of having been developed overnight in the last decades of the twentieth century. In fact, a number of necessary prestages had been pioneered all over the globe for more than a century.

As early as 1868, nearly thirty years before X rays were discovered, German physician Adolf Kussmaul performed experiments that involved inserting a hollow lighted tube into patients' stomachs. He was actually able to see the interior surface of the stomach with the naked eye. Later, also in Germany, in 1908, a doctor named Hammeter was able to display a gastric ulcer by using barium meal X-ray technology. At a certain point, still well before the advent of fiber-optic endoscopy, a technique called arteriography was employed to explore the extent of ulcer damage when hemorrhaging occurred. This method, which still complemented fiber-optic endoscopy into the 1990's, involves the injection, through a fine tube passing through key arteries, of a dye whose movement in the intestinal tissue is then traced by means of a rapid series of X-ray images.

—*Byron D. Cannon, Ph.D.;*
updated by Connie Rizzo, M.D.

See also Abdomen; Abdominal disorders; Alcoholism; Bacterial infections; Endoscopy; Gastrectomy; Gastroenterology; Gastrointestinal disorders; Gastrointestinal system; Heartburn; Indigestion; Intestinal disorders; Intestines; Ulcer surgery.

FOR FURTHER INFORMATION:

Bennett, J. Claude, et al., eds. *Cecil Textbook of Medicine.* 21st ed. Philadelphia: W. B. Saunders, 2000. The standard medical reference text. Difficult but complete, it covers the disease process from its inception through diagnosis, treatment, and course.

Janowitz, Henry D. *Indigestion: Living Better with Upper Intestinal Problems from Heartburn to Ulcers and Gallstones.* New York: Oxford University Press, 1994. A general text exploring various symptoms of digestive ailments and what causes them. Several chapters are devoted to peptic ulcers.

_____. *Your Gut Feelings: A Complete Guide to Living Better with Intestinal Problems.* Rev. ed. New York: Oxford University Press, 1994. An early, scientifically based contribution to general knowledge of the digestive processes and dangers of imbalances which may exist.

Tierney, Lawrence M., Jr., et al., eds. *Current Medical Diagnosis and Therapy: 2001.* 39th ed. New York: McGraw-Hill, 2000. This text, updated yearly, is the point of reference for physicians and other health care practitioners. It incorporates each year's biomedical research discoveries that have immediate, relevant, and applicable use for the patient.

ULTRASONOGRAPHY

PROCEDURE

ANATOMY OR SYSTEM AFFECTED: Abdomen, bladder, blood, gallbladder, heart, kidneys, reproductive system, urinary system, uterus

SPECIALTIES AND RELATED FIELDS: Cardiology, embryology, gynecology, internal medicine, obstetrics, radiology, urology, vascular medicine

DEFINITION: A technique that directs ultrasonic waves into body tissues and uses the reflections to create visual images, making it possible to view the anatomy of organs and blood vessels and to evaluate the dynamics of blood flow.

KEY TERMS:

Doppler effect: the relationship of the apparent frequency of waves, such as sound waves, to the relative motion of the source of the waves and the observer or instrument; the frequency increases as the two approach each other and decreases as they move apart; also known as the Doppler shift

duplex scan: an ultrasound representation of echo images of tissues and blood vessels combined with a Doppler representation of blood flow patterns

frequency: the number of complete cycles, such as sound cycles, produced by an alternating energy source; sound is measured in cycles per second, and one cycle per second is equal to 1 hertz

oscilloscope: an instrument that displays a visual representation of electrical variations on the fluorescent screen of a cathode-ray tube

transducer (probe): a device designed to transfer ultrasound waves into the body noninvasively, receive the returning echoes, and transform those echoes into electrical voltages

ultrasonic: referring to any frequency of sound that is higher than the audible range—that is, higher than 20,000 cycles per second (20 kilohertz)

INDICATIONS AND PROCEDURES

Sound waves are mechanical pressure waves that can propagate through liquids, solids, and, to some extent, gases. A sound wave is composed of cyclic variations that occur over time; one cycle per second is called 1 hertz (Hz). Ultrasound waves have a frequency of oscillation that is higher than 20,000 hertz, placing ultrasound above the audible range for humans. The useful frequency range for medical diagnostic ultrasound is between 1 and 10 megahertz (10 million hertz), although surgical instruments often use carrier frequencies greater than 20 megahertz.

The basic ultrasound system has two principal components. The first, and perhaps the most important, component is the transducer, or probe. The transducer converts electrical pulses into mechanical pressure (sound) waves that are transmitted into the tissues. It then detects the echoes that are reflected from the tissues and transforms those echoes into electrical voltages. The second component is the audiovisual electronic component, which processes and displays the reflected echoes in the form of an image of internal organs and structures or an image of the movement of red blood cells.

Ultrasound waves are created when the crystalline material within the transducer is excited by an electrical voltage produced by the instrument's oscillator. The application of an electrical charge causes the crystalline particles to expand and contract, producing mechanical waves and pulses. These pulses of sound pass from the face of the transducer into the body, where they strike the organs, bones, and blood vessels. The reflected echoes in turn strike the face of the transducer, again causing the crystalline particles to vibrate and produce an electrical charge. Such crystalline material is said to have piezoelectric (a combination of the Greek word *piesis*, meaning "pressure," and the word "electric") properties.

Ultrasound systems commonly employ sound in two modalities. The transducer uses sound waves to create an echo image of body structures. The audiovisual component uses the Doppler shift theory to analyze the range of velocities over which red blood cells are moving.

To create an echo image, millions of pulses of sound must be transmitted into the body each second.

For each transmitted pulse, one line of echo information is received by the transducer crystal. In order to build up an image rapidly and depict the real-time motion of body structures, the pulses are sent into the body from many angles as the sound beam is moved over the body surface. The depth of the echoes is displayed as a function of time, and a two-dimensional image is created by relating the sound's direction of propagation to the direction of the echo-image trace that appears on the instrument's oscilloscope.

The time required for a sound pulse to travel from the transducer to its target within the body, reflect, and return to the transducer can be used to measure the distance to the target, as radar does. In body tissues, sound travels at a speed of 1,540 meters per second. It takes approximately thirteen microseconds for a sound pulse to travel 1 centimeter into the body and return to the transducer. The depth and orientation of echoes may be determined by using this information.

As a sound beam travels through tissues, it is attenuated, or reduced in amplitude and intensity. Attenuation occurs as the energy from the beam is absorbed by the tissues and transformed into heat. Additionally, a part of the beam may be reflected into the surrounding tissues at an angle away from the incident angle or backscattered as the long wavelength of the sound beam strikes the smaller red blood cells. Only a small fraction of the returning echoes reach the face of the transducer.

Because the attenuation of the sound beam increases as the depth of penetration increases, the echoes that return from the deepest part of the image field will be reduced in intensity when compared to the echoes that return from the structures nearer the skin surface. The echo intensity is dependent on the degree of change and impedance of each tissue through which the echo passes, the strength of the incident sound beam, and the degree of attenuation of the beam. In order to equalize the intensity of the echoes from all depths of the image field, the echoes that travel farthest, and therefore take the longest time to reach the transducer, are amplified over time by using time-gain compensation methods.

For medical imaging applications, the returning echoes may be displayed in several ways. The amplitude mode (A-mode) depicts the returning echoes as deflections on the instrument's oscilloscope; the height of the deflection depends on the strength of the returned signal, and the distance between the deflec-

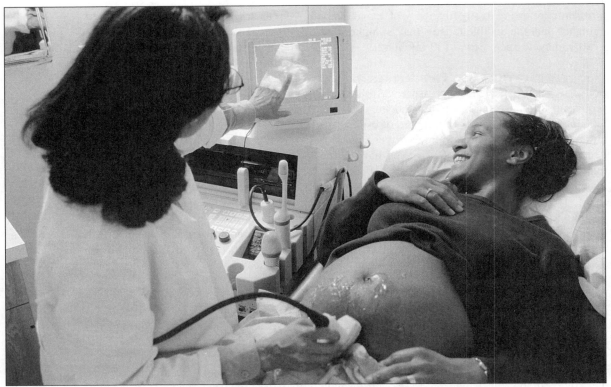

A pregnant woman undergoes ultrasound to check the health of her baby. (PhotoDisc)

tions depends on the depth of the signal. The brightness mode (B-mode) depicts the strength of the echoes as shades of gray, with the strongest echoes appearing the brightest. The B-mode display makes it possible to differentiate tissue texture characteristics. The time-motion mode depicts movement over time by moving the B-mode trace across the face of a high-persistence oscilloscope, showing the depth, orientation, and strength of echoes with respect to time.

The transducer crystal determines the shape and focus of the sound beam and the frequency of the sound waves, features that are important in resolving echo information into complex images. The beam may be divided into three parts: the near field, the focal zone, and the far field. The beam width, close to the face of the transducer, is equal to the width of the transducer. The beam converges as it travels away from the transducer and then diverges at its narrow focal zone. In order for tissue targets to be resolved into discrete image points, both the lateral and the axial planes of the beam must be narrow. The focusing of the beam is facilitated by placing convex acoustic lenses in front of the transducer crystal to shorten the

near field to a narrow focal point, thereby increasing the lateral resolution.

Axial resolution is the ability to distinguish targets along the sound beam. If a single pulse is emitted from the transducer, echo sources lying close together in the axial path of the beam may not be separated. Multiple short bursts of sound are used to separate the echo sources; each echo is captured as a discrete burst. Because axial resolution is inversely proportional to the duration of the ultrasound pulse (and the resonant frequency of the crystal is inversely proportional to its diameter), small-diameter, high-frequency crystals are used to obtain maximum axial resolution.

Ultrasound may be used to determine the velocity of blood flow. This velocity is determined in relation to the frequency of the incident sound beam according to the Doppler theory. Several different techniques may be used to process and display the echoes from moving red blood cells. The ultrasound system's computers may be programmed to perform fast Fourier transform analysis, a complex mathematical method for ranking the speed of the echoes returning over time. The signals may be displayed either as spectral tracings of the range of Doppler frequency shifts, represented in the returned echoes recorded throughout the cardiac cycle, or as color-coded Doppler-shifted signals from within the blood vessels, superimposed on a gray-scale image of the surrounding tissues.

USES AND COMPLICATIONS

High-resolution abdominal ultrasonography is a valuable technique for the visualization of intra-abdominal organs and disease processes. For example, liver conditions such as parenchymal abnormalities, abscesses, hematomas, cysts, and cancerous lesions can be identified easily by means of this technique. B-mode and Doppler color-flow imaging are particularly valuable technologies that can be used to evaluate the tissue characteristics and blood flow patterns of transplanted organs. An ultrasound examination of the gallbladder may reveal gallstones, obstruction of the common bile duct, or inflammatory disease. Ultrasound imaging of the pancreas is used to identify pancreatitis, pancreatic pseudocysts, and carcinoma of this organ. An ultrasound examination of the spleen may reveal splenomegaly, or enlargement of the spleen in response to disease or trauma. Additionally, ultrasonography can be used to evaluate splenic volume and to identify hematomas, congenital cysts, infarctions, and tumors within the organ. The technology is particularly well suited for the study of tumors and abscesses within the abdomen. Ascites and other fluid collections may be recognized, and primary tumors and lymph node metastases within the abdominal cavity may be identified by means of pulse-echo imaging.

Ultrasound has certain characteristics that make it particularly valuable for examining the kidneys and the genitourinary tract. The ability to image both native and transplanted kidneys noninvasively from the longitudinal and transverse planes provides additional diagnostic information in uremic patients for whom the injection of contrast agents is undesirable or may fail to provide sufficient information. Urologic ultrasonography may be used to determine renal size and position or to identify cysts and masses, kidney or bladder stones, obstruction of the ureters, and bladder contour.

Transabdominal scanning of the pelvic organs, which is used to determine the presence or absence of suspected lesions, makes possible the precise localization and quantitative mapping of pelvic abdominal masses, facilitating the determination of disease stages

and the positioning of radiation ports. The technology is used to differentiate cysts from solid tumors and to determine if pelvic tumors are of uterine, ovarian, or tubal origin.

The sonographic resolution of deep abdominal structures is achieved by internal scanning; endorectal or endovaginal approaches are used to reduce the distance between the transducer and the target organ. During these procedures, the transducer probe either is in direct contact with the genital organs or prostate gland or is separated from them by the thin walls of the bladder or rectum. The information obtained with these techniques is thought to be submacroscopic, observed at approximately twenty to thirty times light magnification.

Ultrasonography plays a major role in the evaluation of obstetrical cases. Ultrasonic imaging is used to study early pregnancy and high-risk cases, as well as to confirm ectopic pregnancy (development of the fetus outside the uterus). In cases of spontaneous abortion, ultrasound procedures are used to indicate whether the fetus and placenta have been retained. Ultrasonography is often used to determine fetal growth rate and placental development and to confirm intrauterine fetal death, threatened abortion, and fetal abnormalities. It is the best method for guiding amniocentesis (the sampling of placental fluids).

Echocardiography, the ultrasound evaluation of the heart, is a reliable and useful tool for the study of patients with congenital and acquired heart disease. The role of cardiac ultrasound in the investigation of cardiac dysfunction, tetralogy of Fallot, transposition of the great vessels, and atrial septal defect has been well defined. Echocardiology is used to detect pericardial effusion; is coupled with Doppler ultrasound to evaluate the pulmonic, mitral, tricuspid, and aortic valves; and is used to investigate primary myocardial disease and atrial tumors. Improved resolution of cardiac structures and patterns of blood flow can be achieved by using endoesophageal (transesophageal) imaging and Doppler color-flow technology.

The vascular system of the body can be studied by combining pulse-echo imaging of the blood vessels and Doppler ultrasound detection of red blood cell movement. This combined technology, known as duplex scanning, not only offers information that is relevant to the anatomy and morphology of blood vessels but also—and this is most important—provides the opportunity to evaluate the dynamics of blood flow and the pathophysiology of vascular disease. Duplex technology is used to demonstrate the presence and characteristics of atherosclerotic disease and to define the severity of vascular compromise resulting from the progression of disease or the presence of blood clots in vessels (thrombosis).

Applications of the technology have been extended to the evaluation of arteries and veins of the extremities, the abdomen, and the brain. Advances in computer technology have made it possible to color-code the Doppler-shifted signals returning from moving red blood cells within the vessels. Doppler color-flow imaging has facilitated the investigation of vascular disorders that result in slow or reduced blood flow (venous thrombosis or preocclusive narrowing of vessels) or that affect the vascularity of organs and tissues (tumors or transplanted organs). Therefore, vascular ultrasonography plays a major role in the evaluation of patients with arterial occlusive disease and those suspected of having thrombosis of the deep or superficial venous systems.

PERSPECTIVE AND PROSPECTS

Ultrasonic techniques have assumed a preferred role in the diagnosis of many diseases and have become an essential component of quality medical care. In contrast to the rapid development and use of X-ray technology in medical diagnosis, the application of diagnostic ultrasound has been relatively slow. Progress depended in large part on the development of high-resolution electronic devices and transducers. Early research into medical applications involved the adaptation of instruments that had been designed for industrial or military purposes.

The first attempts to locate objects with ultrasound probably occurred following the sinking of the *Titanic* in 1912. Improvements in the technology led to the widespread industrial and military use of ultrasound for the detection of flaws in metals, for the determination of range and depth information, and for navigation. The first application of ultrasound to medical diagnosis occurred in 1937, when K. T. Dussik attempted to image the cerebral ventricles by measuring the attenuation of a sound beam transmitted through the head. In 1947, Douglas H. Howry pioneered the ultrasonic imaging of soft tissues and constructed a pulse-echo system that utilized a transducer submerged in water. The system utilized surplus Navy sonar equipment, a high-fidelity recorder power supply, and a metal cattle-watering trough in which the patient and the transducer were immersed.

In the 1960's, Howard Thompson and Kenneth Gottesfeld performed obstetric and gynecologic examinations using the first contact scanner, which had been produced in 1958 by Tom Brown, an engineer, and Ian Donald, a professor of midwifery, at Glasgow University in Scotland. The first commercial scanner marketed in the United States was designed by William L. Wright, an engineer at the University of Colorado.

The two-dimensional scanning system was developed in 1953 by John Reid, an engineer, in cooperation with John Wild, a physician who demonstrated that ultrasound could detect differences between normal tissues, benign tumors, and cancers. The collaboration between medicine and engineering has propelled diagnostic ultrasonography forward at a phenomenal rate of development since that time.

The field of echocardiography was pioneered by Inge Edler, who discovered in the 1950's that echoes from the moving heart could be received and displayed by using a time-motion ultrasonic flow detector. Using this technology, Edler diagnosed mitral stenosis, pericardial effusion, and thrombus in the left atrium.

The use of ultrasound to evaluate blood flow was first described by S. Satomura in 1959. This investigator observed that ultrasound could be transmitted through the skin to derive information about the velocity of blood flow by using the Doppler effect to analyze the reflected signals from the moving blood cells. The first transcutaneous continuous-wave Doppler system was developed at the University of Washington in the 1960's. The instrument was first used to detect fetal life by demonstrating the fetal heartbeat. This application of Doppler ultrasound spurred research under the guidance of Eugene Strandness, Jr., that ultimately led to the development of duplex scanners, instruments that combine pulse-echo imaging with analysis of blood flow patterns derived from the Doppler effect. As a result of the efforts of these early investigators and others, diagnostic medical ultrasonography has evolved into a highly useful tool with diverse clinical applications.

—*Marsha M. Neumyer*

See also Abdomen; Abdominal disorders; Abscesses; Amniocentesis; Cholecystitis; Circulation; Ectopic pregnancy; Embryology; Gallbladder diseases; Heart; Heart disease; Imaging and radiology; Lithotripsy; Noninvasive tests; Obstetrics; Pancreas; Pancreatitis; Pregnancy and gestation; Stone removal; Stones; Tumors; Vascular medicine; Vascular system.

FOR FURTHER INFORMATION:

Bernstein, Eugene F., ed. *Noninvasive Diagnostic Techniques in Vascular Disease.* 3d ed. St. Louis: C. V. Mosby, 1985. This bible of noninvasive vascular technology contains chapters written by experts in the field. This important text not only presents up-to-date information on diagnostic vascular ultrasonography but also takes a futuristic look at the clinical applications of this technology.

Hagan, Arthur D., and Anthony N. DeMaria. *Clinical Applications of Two-Dimensional Echocardiography and Cardiac Doppler.* 2d ed. Boston: Little, Brown, 1989. This exceptional textbook correlates normal and abnormal cardiac anatomy with two-dimensional echocardiography and pathophysiology.

Kremkau, Frederick W. *Diagnostic Ultrasound: Principles and Instruments.* 4th ed. Philadelphia: W. B. Saunders, 1993. A well-organized, programmed text for the student of ultrasound. Each chapter contains easy-to-understand information on the physical principles of ultrasound followed by written, self-assessed review exercises.

Mittelstaedt, Carol A. *Abdominal Ultrasound.* New York: Churchill Livingstone, 1987. This superbly written text is the best in abdominal sonography. Mittelstaedt, an outstanding teacher in the field of medical ultrasound, has assembled a wealth of practical clinical information on normal and abnormal anatomy and sonographic techniques.

UMBILICAL CORD

ANATOMY

ANATOMY OR SYSTEM AFFECTED: Blood vessels, skin

SPECIALTIES AND RELATED FIELDS: Neonatology, perinatology

DEFINITION: The cord connecting the developing fetus to the placenta.

STRUCTURE AND FUNCTIONS

The umbilical cord is composed of a thickened fibrous covering over a gelatinous material that protects three blood vessels. Two umbilical arteries carry blood from the baby to the placenta and coil around the single umbilical vein. Blood containing oxygen and other essential nutrients returns from the placenta through the umbilical cord.

At term, the umbilical cord measures approximately 20 inches. The cord may be short if there is little amniotic fluid and if the baby has a muscular weakness, limiting movement inside the uterus. Umbilical cord lengths of less than 14 inches have a high incidence of traumatic separation and fetal blood loss at the time of a vaginal delivery.

DISORDERS AND DISEASES

Normally, the umbilical cord dries rapidly after birth, with most of its fluid content evaporating in two days. The base of the cord is then colonized by bacteria. An immune system response to the bacteria and chemicals released by white blood cells are required for the final shedding of the dried cord. The untreated umbilical cord is shed approximately seven to ten days after birth. Any treatment (such as alcohol) used to dry or delay cord bacterial colonization allows the cord to persist for nearly twice as long as in the untreated condition.

Persistence of an umbilical cord beyond three weeks after drying may be caused by a persistent blood supply and may require evaluation by a pediatric surgeon. Conditions that are associated with a persistent cord blood supply include a hemangioma, a connection from an artery in the skin to the vein of the umbilical cord, a small outpouching of the lining of the abdominal cavity, or retained elements of tissue connected to the bladder.

Once the cord has been fully shed, a reactive overgrowth of tissue may occur at the base of the cord. This is termed an umbilical granuloma and is readily managed by the application of silver nitrate, which cauterizes the tissue. There should be no further drainage from the base of the umbilicus beyond six weeks after birth.

—David A. Clark, M.D.

See also Childbirth; Childbirth complications; Circulation; Embryology; Hernias; Hypertrophy; Neonatology; Pediatrics; Perinatology; Pregnancy and gestation; Vascular medicine; Vascular system.

FOR FURTHER INFORMATION:

Moore, Keith L., and T. V. N. Persaud. *The Developing Human.* 5th ed. Philadelphia: W. B. Saunders, 1993.

Oppenheimer, Steve B., and George Lefevre, Jr. *Introduction to Embryonic Development.* 2d ed. Boston: Allyn & Bacon, 1984.

Patten, Bradley M. *Patten's Human Embryology.* Edited by Clark Edward Corliss. 4th ed. New York: McGraw-Hill, 1976.

UNCONSCIOUSNESS

DISEASE/DISORDER

ANATOMY OR SYSTEM AFFECTED: Brain, head, nervous system

SPECIALTIES AND RELATED FIELDS: Emergency medicine, neurology

DEFINITION: Unconsciousness is a state in which an individual is unaware of either surroundings or self and lacks response to stimuli. Sleep is a common example of such a state. Unconsciousness can be caused by a variety of events or situations, including breathing difficulty, shock, drugs, poisons, or electrolyte imbalances. Often, it results from a lack of oxygen to the brain. Other causes include injury, stroke, seizures, brain tumors, or infection. Unconsciousness can range from fainting to more prolonged states, such as coma.

—*Jason Georges and Tracy Irons-Georges*

See also Asphyxiation; Bleeding; Brain; Brain disorders; Choking; Coma; Concussion; Critical care; Critical care, pediatric; Dizziness and fainting; Electrical shock; Emergency medicine; Epilepsy; Head and neck disorders; Heart attack; Heat exhaustion and heat stroke; Intoxication; Resuscitation; Seizures; Shock; Strokes.

FOR FURTHER INFORMATION:

Bledsoe, Bryan E., Robert S. Porter, and Bruce R. Shade. *Brady Paramedic Emergency Care.* 3d ed.

Upper Saddle River, N.J.: Brady Prentice Hall Education, Career & Technology, 1997.

Handal, Kathleen A. *The American Red Cross First Aid and Safety Handbook.* Boston: Little, Brown, 1992.

Heartsaver Manual: A Student Handbook for Cardiopulmonary Resuscitation and First Aid for Choking. Dallas: American Heart Association, 1987.

UNDESCENDED TESTICLES. *See* TESTICLES, UNDESCENDED.

UPPER EXTREMITIES

ANATOMY

ANATOMY OR SYSTEM AFFECTED: Arms, bones, hands, lymphatic system, muscles, musculoskeletal system, nerves, nervous system, skin

SPECIALTIES AND RELATED FIELDS: Neurology, orthopedics, physical therapy

DEFINITION: The arms (upper arms, forearms, and hands), which are attached to the shoulder blade at the shoulder joint and which consist of muscles, bones, blood vessels, lymph vessels, nerves, skin, and fingernails.

KEY TERMS:

carpus: the wrist

distal: further away from the base or attached end

elbow: the joint between the upper arm and the forearm

forearm: the region from the elbow joint to the wrist; also called the antebrachium

humerus: the bone that forms the structural beam of the upper arm

proximal: closer to the base or attached end

radial: toward the edge of the forearm and hand containing the radius and thumb

radius: the shorter of the two forearm bones, on the thumb side

ulna: the larger of the two forearm bones, forming the principal part of the elbow joint with the humerus

ulnar: toward the edge of the forearm and hand containing the ulna and little finger

upper arm: the region from the shoulder joint to the elbow joint; also called the brachium

A person who is unconscious and breathing freely should be placed in this position, which allows free breathing to continue and prevents fluids from flowing back into airways; if the person is not breathing, the airway must first be cleared and artificial respiration administered. Emergency medical help must be summoned immediately.

STRUCTURE AND FUNCTIONS

The upper extremities consist of the upper arms, forearms, and hands. Each extremity is attached to the shoulder blade (or scapula) at the shoulder joint. The upper extremity is made mostly of bones and muscles, but it also contains blood vessels, lymphatics, nerves, skin, fingernails, and other associated structures. Important directional terms associated with the upper extremity include proximal (closer to the base or attached end), distal (further from the base or attached end), radial (on the same side as the radius and the thumb), and ulnar (on the same side as the ulna and the little finger). Along the forearm and hand, the surface bearing the palm is called palmar; the opposite surface is called dorsal.

The bones and muscles of the shoulder provide support structures for the upper extremity. Beyond the shoulder, the major parts of the upper extremity include the upper arm (or brachium), from the shoulder joint to the elbow; the forearm, from the elbow to the wrist; the carpus, or wrist; and the manus, or hand. Beginning with the thumb, the five fingers of the hand are numbered one through five. Digit two is also called the index finger, digit three the middle finger, digit four the ring finger, and digit five the little finger.

Like other parts of the body, the upper extremity is clothed in skin, or integument. The skin covering the armpit (or axilla) has more hair and also more glands (especially the apocrine sweat glands) than most other parts of the body. The palm of the hand is unusual, along with the sole of the foot, in being completely hairless and in having a very thick outermost layer, called the stratum corneum. The ridges on the palm and fingers form individually characteristic patterns called dermatoglyphics, both fingerprints and palm prints. Each finger also has on its dorsal surface a fingernail; the thin crescent of semitransparent skin covering the base of the fingernail is called the eponychium.

The bones of the upper extremity include the scapula, clavicle, humerus, radius, ulna, carpals, metacarpals, and phalanges. The scapula, or shoulder blade, develops as part of the skeleton of the upper extremity and remains more strongly attached to the upper arm than to the trunk of the body. The outer (superficial) surface of the scapula is marked by a ridge called the spine, perpendicular to the scapular blade; the outer tip of this blade is called the acromion. The sculpted area above the spine is called the supraspinous fossa; the larger sculpted area below the spine is called the infraspinous fossa. The flat undersurface of the scapula is the subscapular fossa. The superior border of the scapula is marked by a hooklike coracoid process. At the shoulder joint itself, the scapula has a nearly spherical glenoid cavity into which the head of the humerus fits. The clavicle, or collarbone, runs from the upper end of the sternum (the manubrium) to the edge of the glenoid cavity of the scapula. It strengthens the shoulder region and provides additional support to the upper extremity.

The humerus runs from the shoulder joint to the elbow. At the shoulder joint, it attaches to the scapula by means of a rounded head which fits into the glenoid cavity of the scapula. The head is flanked by two protruding structures, the greater and lesser tuberosities, to which various muscles attach. At the elbow joint, the humerus attaches to the ulna by means of a pulleylike structure called the trochlea. The humerus also attaches to the radius by a smaller, rounded structure called the capitulum. Areas for muscle attachment on the lower end of the humerus include the lateral epicondyle (on the outer side) and the medial epicondyle (on the inner side).

The forearm contains two bones, the radius and ulna. The ulna is the larger of the two and forms the principal attachment with the humerus by means of a semilunar notch. Part of the ulna extends proximally beyond this semilunar notch to form a projection called the olecranon process (the hard structure on which one rests the elbows). The smaller of the two forearm bones is the radius, which articulates loosely with the humerus and more strongly with the wrist and hand.

The carpus, or wrist, includes two rows of small bones. The proximal row includes (in order from the radial side to the ulnar) the scaphoid, lunate, cuneiform (triquetrum), and pisiform bones. The distal row includes the trapezium, trapezoid, capitate, and hamate bones, also in order from radial to ulnar. The trapezium supports the thumb, the trapezoid supports the index finger, the capitate supports the middle finger, and the hamate supports the two remaining digits. An important ligament called the transverse carpal ligament (or flexor retinaculum) runs across the palmar side of the wrist, forming a tunnel through which the tendons of the flexor muscles run. A similar ligament, the dorsal carpal ligament (or dorsal retinaculum) crosses the back of the wrist, forming a similar tunnel through which the tendons of the extensor muscles run. Beyond the wrist, the palm of the hand is supported by five bones called metacarpals, numbered one through five. The thumb contains two finger bones, or phalanges; each of the remaining fingers contains three phalanges.

The muscles of the upper extremity are divided into extensors (which straighten joints) and flexors (which bend joints). The shoulder muscles attaching the upper extremity to the trunk of the body include the trapezius, pectoralis major, pectoralis minor, deltoideus, coracobrachialis, subscapularis, supraspinatus, infraspinatus, teres major, teres minor, and latissimus dorsi. Of these, the trapezius, deltoideus, and supraspinatus are extensors; the coracobrachialis, latissimus dorsi, and the two pectoralis muscles are flexors; and the remaining muscles are primarily responsible for rotational movements. The trapezius originates from the cervical and thoracic vertebrae, including the adjoining ligaments and the adjacent part of the skull; its fibers converge mostly onto the spine and acromion of the scapula, but some also insert onto the clavicle. The pectoralis major is triangular in shape; it originates from the sternum, costal cartilages, and a portion of the clavicle, from which its fibers converge toward an insertion on the greater tuberosity of the humerus. The pectoralis minor originates from the third through fifth ribs and inserts onto the coracoid process of the scapula. The deltoideus is a triangular muscle which originates from the clavicle and from the spine and acromion of the scapula; its fibers converge to insert by means of a strong tendon onto the shaft of the humerus. The coracobrachialis runs from the coracoid process to an insertion along the shaft of the humerus. The subscapularis originates from the subscapular fossa and inserts onto the lesser tuberosity of the humerus. The supraspinatus originates along the supraspinous fossa and inserts onto the greater tuberosity of the humerus. The infraspinatus originates from the infraspinous fossa and inserts onto the greater tuberosity of the humerus. The teres major and teres minor originate from the lower (inferior) border of the scapula; the teres major inserts onto the lesser tubercle of the humerus, and the teres minor inserts onto the greater tubercle. The latissimus dorsi is a broad, flat muscle that originates from the lower half of the vertebral column (and part of the ilium) by way of a tough tendinous sheet (the lumbar aponeurosis); it inserts high on the humerus.

The major flexors of the upper arm include the biceps brachii and the brachialis. The biceps brachii originates in two heads, one from the coracoid pro-

The Bones of the Hand

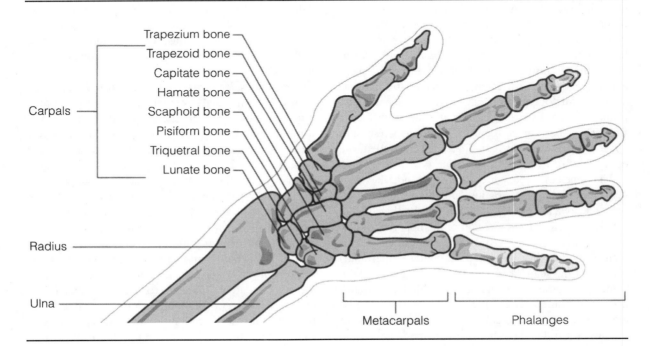

Trapezium bone
Trapezoid bone
Capitate bone
Hamate bone
Scaphoid bone
Pisiform bone
Triquetral bone
Lunate bone

Carpals

Radius

Ulna

Metacarpals

Phalanges

cess of the scapula and one from the capsule of the shoulder joint. Both heads insert by means of a strong tendon onto a raised tuberosity of the radius. The brachialis originates from the shaft of the humerus and inserts high on the ulna.

The major extensor of the upper arm is the three-part triceps brachii, but a smaller anconeus and an epitrochlearis are sometimes present as well. The long head of the triceps originates from the scapula just below the armpit; the other two heads originate along the shaft of the humerus. All three heads insert onto the olecranon process by means of a strong tendon. The anconeus (or subanconeus) is not always present; its fibers run directly from the shaft of the humerus to that of the ulna. The epitrochlearis (or dorsoepitrochlearis), also variably present, may be viewed as a connecting band of muscle tissue from the latissimus dorsi onto the triceps brachii.

Flexors of the forearm include the flexor carpi radialis, palmaris longus, flexor carpi ulnaris, pronator teres, flexor digitorum superficialis, flexor digitorum profundus, flexor pollicis longus, and pronator quadratus. Many of these muscles have long, thin tendons that run in the tunnel formed beneath the transverse carpal ligament. The first five of these muscles originate from the medial epicondyle of the humerus. The pronator teres runs at an angle and inserts onto the shaft of the radius. The flexor carpi radialis inserts by a long, thin tendon onto the base of the second metacarpal. The palmaris longus ends in a broad tendon which spreads out over the palm of the hand to form the palmar aponeurosis, a sheet which sends tendinous branches into the fingers. The flexor carpi ulnaris inserts by a tendon onto the pisiform bone; the tendon then continues onto the hamate bone. The flexor digitorum superficialis originates from parts of the radius and ulna as well as the humerus; its strong tendon passes beneath the transverse carpal ligament, then divides into four branches to each of digits two through five. Each of these branches splits and then reunites to allow a tendon of the flexor digitorum to penetrate. The flexor digitorum profundus originates mostly from the shaft of the ulna; it gives rise to four strong tendons that run beneath the transverse carpal ligament, separate from one another over the palm of the hand, run into the second through fifth fingers, penetrate through the openings in the tendons of the flexor digitorum superficialis, and insert onto the base of the terminal phalanx of each finger except the thumb. The flexor pollicis longus arises from the ra-

dius alongside the previous muscle; its tendon runs beneath the transverse carpal ligament and inserts onto the base of the distal phalanx of the thumb. The pronator quadratus consists of a muscular sheet running between the distal portions of the radius and ulna.

The more superficial (shallower) extensors of the forearm include the brachioradialis, extensor carpi radialis longus, extensor carpi radialis brevis, extensor carpi ulnaris, extensor digitorum communis, and extensor digiti minimi. The brachioradialis originates from a ridge on the shaft of the humerus and inserts onto the radius at its distal end. The extensor carpi radialis longus originates from the shaft of the humerus; its tendon passes beneath the dorsal carpal ligament to insert near the base of the second metacarpal. The next four muscles originate together from the lateral epicondyle of the humerus. The extensor carpi radialis brevis gives rise to a tendon which passes beneath the dorsal carpal ligament to insert onto the base of the third metacarpal. The extensor carpi ulnaris gives rise to a tendon which passes beneath the dorsal carpal ligament and inserts onto the base of the fifth metacarpal. The extensor digitorum communis gives rise to four tendons that pass beneath the dorsal carpal ligament, then diverge to run into each finger except the thumb, where they each insert onto the base of the second phalanx, the base of the terminal phalanx, and a tendinous sheath covering the first phalanx. The extensor digiti minimi gives rise to a tendon which runs beneath the dorsal carpal ligament and unites over the first phalanx of the fifth finger with the tendon to that digit of the extensor digitorum communis.

The deeper extensors of the forearm include the supinator, abductor pollicis longus, extensor pollicis brevis, extensor pollicis longus, and extensor indicis. The supinator originates mostly from the proximal end of the ulnar shaft, but some of this muscle also originates from the capsule of the elbow joint and from the lateral epicondyle of the humerus. Its fibers spiral toward the midline of the body and insert onto the shaft of the radius. The abductor pollicis longus originates beneath the supinator from the shaft of the radius; it inserts by means of a tendon onto the base of the first metacarpal. The extensor pollicis brevis originates from the shaft of the radius and inserts by means of a tendon onto the base of the first phalanx of the thumb. The extensor pollicis longus originates from the middle portion of the shaft of the ulna; it gives rise to a tendon which runs beneath the dorsal carpal ligament to insert onto the base of the distal phalanx of the thumb. The extensor indicis arises beside the preceding muscle from the shaft of the ulna; its tendon passes beneath the dorsal carpal ligament and eventually attaches to the tendon going to the index finger from the extensor digitorum communis.

The flexor muscles that are "intrinsic" to the hand—that is, those confined to the hand—include the flexor pollicis brevis, abductor pollicis brevis, adductor pollicis, opponens pollicis, palmaris brevis, flexor digiti minimi, abductor digiti minimi, opponens digiti minimi, the lumbricales, and the interossei. There are no intrinsic extensor muscles in the hand.

The upper extremity can move in various ways. At the shoulder joint, possible movements include extension (or protraction) of the shoulder, which raises the arms; flexion (or retraction) of the shoulder, which lowers the arms; adduction of the arms, bringing them closer together; and abduction of the arms, pulling them further apart. The two movements possible at the elbow joint are extension (straightening) and flexion (bending). Two special movements are possible within the forearm: Pronation is an inward rotation of the radius upon the ulna in such a way that the palms face downward; supination is an outward rotation of the radius upon the ulna in such a way that the palms face upward. Various movements are possible at the wrist, including flexion (bending), extension (straightening), hyperextension (bending the hand upward), radial abduction (twisting the hand toward the thumb side), and ulnar abduction (twisting the hand toward the little finger side). Movements of the phalanges include flexion (bending), extension (straightening), abduction (spreading the fingers), and adduction (bringing the fingers back together).

Blood vessels of the upper extremity include both arteries and veins. The brachial artery is the major continuation of the subclavian and axillary arteries into the upper arm; as it approaches the elbow, it divides into the radial and ulnar arteries, which supply most of the forearm. Near the wrist, each of these last two arteries divides into a branch that runs closer to the palm and another that runs closer to the back of the hand. The two palmar branches then connect with each other to form a loop called the palmar digital arch; the other two branches also connect, forming a loop called the dorsal digital arch. From these two digital arches arises a secondary digital arch running

into each finger, connecting in each case to the palmar arch at one end and to the dorsal arch at the other end. This type of arrangement, called collateral circulation, uses multiple alternate routes to permit blood flow even if one of the routes is temporarily blocked.

There are several important veins draining the upper extremity. Several of these run just beneath the skin: the cephalic vein, running along the radial margin of the forearm and upper arm; the median antebrachial vein, draining the palmar surface of the hand and forearm; and the basilic vein, continuing the median antebrachial vein along the inner side of the upper arm. The deep veins of the arm all drain into the brachial vein. As it flows into the shoulder, the brachial vein joins with the basilic vein to form the axillary vein, which then becomes the subclavian vein when it reaches the rib cage.

The major nerves to the upper extremity arise from a series of complex branchings known as the brachial plexus, originating mostly from the fifth through eighth cervical nerves and the first thoracic nerve. The major nerves of the brachial plexus are a lateral cord (formed from branches of the fifth, sixth, and seventh cervical nerves), a medial cord (formed from branches of the last cervical and first thoracic nerves), and a posterior cord (formed from branches of the sixth, seventh, and eighth cervical nerves). The major nerves of the arm include a musculocutaneous nerve arising from the lateral cord, an axillary nerve and a radial nerve arising from the posterior cord, an ulnar nerve and a medial antebrachial cutaneous nerve arising from the medial cord, and a median nerve arising from both the lateral and the medial cords. The musculocutaneous, ulnar, and median nerves constitute the main nerve supply to the flexor muscles of the arm and hand, while the axillary nerve supplies the deltoid muscle and the radial nerve supplies the remaining extensor muscles. In addition, the radial nerve supplies sensory branches to the skin of the dorsal side of the forearm and hand (except for the fifth finger and part of the fourth), while the musculocutaneous and medial antebrachial cutaneous nerves supply sensory branches to the skin over the palmar or flexor side of the arm and forearm. The median nerve sends sensory branches to the skin over most of the palmar surface of the hand from the thumb up to the middle of the fourth finger, while the ulnar nerve sends sensory branches to the skin on both the palmar and dorsal sides of the fifth finger and the ulnar half of the fourth. At the elbow, the ulnar nerve passes around the olecranon process just under the skin, where it is easily subject to accidental pressure; the tingling that results from such pressure is the source of the term "funny bone."

DISORDERS AND DISEASES

Many types of medical conditions and disorders can affect the upper extremities. For example, many types of contact dermatitis, from poison ivy to "dishpan hands," are first noticed on the surface of the hands and forearms. Other medical problems of the upper extremity include animal bites, injuries, and an assortment of neuromuscular disorders.

Neuromuscular disorders involving the upper extremity include nerve paralyses, uncontrolled shaking (choreic) movements, muscular atrophies, and muscular dystrophies. Nerve paralyses may arise from traumatic injury, but the most common type of paralysis is cerebral palsy. Cerebral palsy is actually a group of paralytic disorders that begin at birth or in early childhood. The extent of the paralysis may vary, often involving large groups of muscles while sparing others. In addition to the lack of muscular control of the limbs, other symptoms may include spasms, athetoid (slow, rhythmic, and wormlike) movements, or muscular rigidity. Some types of cerebral palsy may result from injuries received at birth or in early infancy.

Uncontrolled, purposeless, and irregular shaking movements of the extremities are called choreic movements. These disorders, which involve the upper extremities more often than the lower, include both Sydenham's chorea and Huntington's chorea. Sydenham's chorea (true chorea) typically begins in children and young adults, with maximum disability occurring two to three weeks after symptoms begin. Choreic symptoms typically diminish and disappear in a few months, but they may recur at a later time. The movements can be controlled with drugs. Huntington's chorea, also called Huntington's disease, seldom begins before the age of forty. It typically begins with uncontrolled choreic movements of the hands. The disease progressively worsens and ultimately causes death about fifteen years after onset. The disease is caused by a single dominant gene.

Muscular atrophies are a variety of diseases in which muscle tissues become progressively weaker and smaller, usually beginning between forty and sixty years of age. Spastic movements may sometimes occur. The small muscles of the hands are usu-

ally affected sooner and more severely in comparison to the large muscles of the arms and shoulders. Amyotrophic lateral sclerosis (ALS), commonly called Lou Gehrig's disease, is a progressive muscular atrophy that usually begins with weakness and deterioration of the hand muscles. The disease proceeds to affect the rest of the extremities, then other parts of the body; it is usually fatal within three to five years after onset. A more rare type of atrophy, myelopathic muscular atrophy (or Aran-Duchenne atrophy), also begins in the small hand muscles and slowly spreads to the arms, shoulders, and trunk muscles, in that order. A degenerative lesion of the gray matter in the cervical region of the spinal cord is usually responsible. Weakness and wasting of the muscles of the hands and forearms also characterize syringomyelia, a disorder of the glial cells in the cervical region of the spinal cord. Impairment of the cutaneous senses often occurs with this disease and frequently results in burns and other injuries to the hand when the patient, unaware of a threat, fails to withdraw or take other countermeasures.

Muscular dystrophy is an inherited disease—actually several related diseases—that usually begins in early childhood and affects males more often than females. The most common type, Duchenne muscular dystrophy, is believed to be caused by a sex-linked recessive trait. Spastic movements do not occur, and the disease affects the large muscles of the shoulder, arm, and thigh more than the small muscles of the hand. The affected muscles become very weak but remain approximately normal in size or increase as fatty and fibrous tissue replaces muscle. Progressive weakening makes walking impossible, but patients can live for decades with proper care.

Repetitive motion injuries of the upper extremity may occur at the elbow joint (tennis elbow) or in the vicinity of the wrist. Some repetitive wrist movements are capable of producing carpal tunnel syndrome, an injury of the tendons running through the tunnel beneath the transverse carpal ligament.

PERSPECTIVE AND PROSPECTS

The first well-illustrated anatomical texts were produced by Andreas Vesalius (1514-1564); they showed the major muscles and bones of the upper extremities. An accurate medical understanding of the circulatory system began with the studies of the Renaissance physician William Harvey (1578-1657), who examined the veins in the arms of many patients. Harvey noticed the valves in the veins and was able to prove that the blood circulates outward from the heart, throughout the body, and then back again to the heart.

Injuries to the arm are generally treated surgically. Whenever possible, broken bones are set in place, immobilized in a cast, and then allowed to heal. Torn muscles (or tendons) must be sewn together, and nerve endings must be placed in their former positions for them to grow back correctly. If the whole hand is severed at the wrist, many tendons and blood vessels must be reattached; such an operation is very difficult. When a portion of the upper extremity must be amputated, the stump is generally covered with a flap of skin. Sometimes an artificial hand is attached to the muscles that are still usable.

—*Eli C. Minkoff, Ph.D.*

See also Amputation; Arthritis; Arthroplasty; Arthroscopy; Bone disorders; Bone grafting; Bones and the skeleton; Carpal tunnel syndrome; Fracture and dislocation; Fracture repair; Frostbite; Grafts and grafting; Lower extremities; Marfan syndrome; Muscle sprains, spasms, and disorders; Muscles; Nail removal; Orthopedic surgery; Orthopedics; Orthopedics, pediatric; Osteopathic medicine; Rheumatoid arthritis; Rheumatology; Warts; Wounds.

FOR FURTHER INFORMATION:
Agur, Anne M. R., and Ming J. Lee. *Grant's Atlas of Anatomy.* 9th ed. Baltimore: Williams & Wilkins, 1999. Includes excellent, detailed illustrations of the human body.

Gray, Henry. *Gray's Anatomy.* Edited by Peter L. Williams et al. 38th ed. New York: Churchill Livingstone, 1995. A classic, with the most thorough descriptions of anatomical structures. Most of the excellent color illustrations offer considerable, realistic detail, and others provide well-selected highlights.

Rosse, Cornelius, and Penelope Gaddum-Rosse. *Hollinshead's Textbook of Anatomy.* 5th ed. Philadelphia: Lippincott-Raven, 1997. A thorough, modern, and detailed reference with good descriptions and illustrations.

URETHRITIS
DISEASE/DISORDER
ANATOMY OR SYSTEM AFFECTED: Abdomen, bladder, urinary system

SPECIALTIES AND RELATED FIELDS: Gynecology, urology

DEFINITION: Urethritis is the inflammation or infection of the urethra; it is caused by a bacterial infection. In women, urethritis is associated with bacteria that enter the urethra from skin around the genitals and anal area. In men, the infection can reach the urethra through the bloodstream from the prostate gland or through the penis. In both sexes, bacterial infections that cause urethritis can be contracted through sexual intercourse with a gonorrhea-infected person or through irritation associated with sexual intercourse. Symptoms include painful urination with cloudy discharge, frequent need to urinate, painful sexual intercourse, temporary impotence in males, and dribbling of urine in males over fifty. Treatment varies with the cause of the urethritis.

—*Jason Georges and Tracy Irons-Georges*

See also Bacterial infections; Cystitis; Glomerulonephritis; Gonorrhea; Reproductive system; Sexual dysfunction; Urinalysis; Urinary disorders; Urinary system; Urology; Urology, pediatric.

FOR FURTHER INFORMATION:
Boston Women's Health Book Collective. *Our Bodies, Ourselves for the New Century.* New York: Simon & Schuster, 1998.

Gorbach, Sherwood L., John G. Bartlett, and Neil R. Blacklow, eds. *Infectious Diseases.* 2d ed. Philadelphia: W. B. Saunders, 1997.

Stamm, W. E., and T. M. Hooton. "Current Concepts: Management of Urinary Tract Infections in Adults." *New England Journal of Medicine* 329 (October 28, 1993): 1328-1334.

Thompson, F. D., and C. R. J. Woodhouse. *Disorders of the Kidney and Urinary Tract.* Baltimore: Edward Arnold, 1987.

URETHROPLASTY. *See* HYPOSPADIAS REPAIR AND URETHROPLASTY.

URINALYSIS
PROCEDURE
ANATOMY OR SYSTEM AFFECTED: Bladder, kidneys, urinary system

SPECIALTIES AND RELATED FIELDS: Biochemistry, microbiology, nephrology, toxicology, urology

DEFINITION: The chemical, microscopic, and/or physical examination of urine.

KEY TERMS:

dipstick: a chemically treated paper strip used for the chemical analysis of urine *ketones:* the by-products of fat metabolism; their presence may be indicative of diabetes mellitus

pH: a value which represents the relative acidity or alkalinity of a solution; values below pH 7 are acidic, while values above pH 7 are basic

specific gravity: the density of a solution relative to that of water; abnormal values can be indicative of elevated sugar or protein levels in urine

INDICATIONS AND PROCEDURES

Urinalysis is one of the oldest and most useful of noninvasive clinical tests. In addition to aiding in the diagnosis of urinary tract or kidney disease, the procedure may be applied to the analysis of most metabolic by-products that pass through the kidneys. Thus it may be applied to observations of kidney or liver abnormalities and metabolic diseases such as diabetes mellitus.

For routine analysis, approximately 10 to 15 milliliters of urine are collected in a clean jar, though larger volumes are preferable. Initial examination involves the physical appearance of the urine sample: color, turbidity, and possible odor. Normal urine is generally pale yellow in appearance, though variation from such color is not necessarily abnormal. Bacteria may cause alterations in this color, as can simple by-products of the diet. Normal urine is generally clear, though as with color, turbidity (cloudiness) may be associated with a variety of causes. Fresh urine also has a characteristically mild odor.

The specific gravity of the urine may be analyzed at this time, though the usefulness of this test is limited to those circumstances in which the water intake of the patient is known. Generally, the only specimen of use for this test is one utilizing the first urine output of the day. The pH is most accurately determined using a pH meter, though dipstick pads impregnated with colored pH indicators can be used when frequent (or inconvenient) monitoring is necessary.

Hematuria, the presence of blood in the urine, is never normal, though its detection need not indicate a significant pathology. Hemoglobin may be detected using a dipstick method, with follow-up necessary to determine the specific cause.

The microscopic examination of urine consists of centrifugation of a volume of urine under specified conditions, followed by resuspension of the sediment in a standard volume of liquid. The presence of blood cells, bacteria, yeast, or other types of sediment can be applied to analysis of the urine.

Chemical analysis can be utilized for determination of the presence of a wide variety of chemicals or drugs. Routinely, chemical procedures are used to detect sugar, protein, or by-products of fat metabolism such as ketones. Dipsticks are available for routine analysis.

USES AND COMPLICATIONS

Diagnosis of urinary or metabolic problems cannot necessarily be made from a single abnormal test result, as a variety of factors have a potential impact on test results. Rather, analysis of a combination of tests is often necessary in diagnosis of a problem.

Urinalysis involves the physical, chemical, and microscopic analysis of urine. Physical examination centers on the color, turbidity, and odor of urine. A pink or red color can be indicative of the presence of blood, though microscopic or chemical examination is needed for confirmation. (For example, a red color may simply indicate that the patient recently ate beets.) An increase in turbidity can result from the presence of yeast or mucus, indicating infection, or from diet by-products such as lipids. Likewise, abnormal odors can result from urinary tract infection (elevated levels of ammonia) or certain metabolic diseases; however, ingestion of asparagus may also result in unusual odors.

Chemical analysis of urine ranges from the determination of pH to the detection of any of a variety of chemicals. On a routine basis, this usually involves examination for sugar, protein, or ketones. Normal urine is usually acid (pH 6), though the patient's diet will often affect such values as well. A high pH may be indicative of urinary tract infection; microscopic detection of microorganisms may be used to confirm this diagnosis.

Small quantities of protein in the urine are normal. Elevated levels of proteinuria, however, can result from kidney disorders, particularly those associated with glomerular damage, or from urinary tract disease. Likewise, small quantities of sugar in the urine are generally of no clinical significance. In the case of diabetes, however, with resultant high levels of glucose in the bloodstream, significant quantities of glucose may be found in the urine. Persons with severe diabetes are unable to remove and utilize glucose from the blood; metabolism in such individuals will switch to the utilization of fat, with resultant breakdown products such as ketones being secreted in the urine. Such products are volatile and may disappear from urine if the sample is not analyzed within sufficient time. Since fat metabolism is employed as a source of energy in the absence of carbohydrates, severe dieting may also result in the excretion of ketones.

PERSPECTIVE AND PROSPECTS

Analysis of urine for diagnosis of disease was among the earliest of medical procedures. Greek physicians at the time of Hippocrates observed the color of urine and its taste. Pouring urine on the ground to see if insects were attracted to it could be used to test for sugar.

Until the mid-twentieth century, chemical tests on urine utilized a variety of liquid reagents. The introduction of dipsticks significantly improved the efficiency of such analysis, in addition to their convenience. The dipstick consists of a thin strip of plastic with a cellulose pad attached. Impregnated in the pad are the chemicals necessary to carry out the specific test. For example, the dipstick used in the analysis of pH contains an indicator which will change color depending on the degree of acidity or alkalinity.

Instrumentation is becoming available that will allow the analysis of a combination of tests simultaneously, much as a blood sample can be analyzed. Either the dipstick or the urine sample itself may be inserted into a machine for urinalysis. For simple home analysis in which only a single test is necessary, commercial production began in the 1980's of analogous materials for detection of urinary chemicals. For example, home pregnancy kits are available, and, in theory, similar kits could be used for the detection of any substance in urine.

—*Richard Adler, Ph.D.*

See also Cystectomy; Cystoscopy; Cytology; Cytopathology; Laboratory tests; Noninvasive tests; Pathology; Pregnancy and gestation; Urethritis; Urinary disorders; Urinary system; Urology; Urology, pediatric.

FOR FURTHER INFORMATION:

Boston Women's Health Book Collective. *The New Our Bodies, Ourselves.* New York: Simon & Schuster, 1998. Contains in-depth discussions of topics covered in this article. This book was written by women for women and is one of the best reference works available on this subject for the general reader.

Kelley, William, et al., eds. *Textbook of Internal Medicine.* 3d ed. New York: Lippincott-Raven, 1997. A medical textbook that is particularly useful, with its inclusion of definitions and descriptions of the clinical presentation of the disease, diagnosis, and treatment.

Simon, Harvey. *Staying Well.* Boston: Houghton Mifflin, 1992. A description of various diseases, their causes and symptoms. Much of the book deals with methods of prevention, including the importance of proper nutrition and exercise. A portion of the text covers screening for urinary tract infections.

URINARY DISORDERS

DISEASE/DISORDER

ANATOMY OR SYSTEM AFFECTED: Abdomen, bladder, kidneys, urinary system

SPECIALTIES AND RELATED FIELDS: Gynecology, nephrology, urology

DEFINITION: Diseases or pathologies associated with any organs of urine production or secretion, such as the kidneys, ureters, urinary bladder, and urethra.

KEY TERMS:

bacteriuria: the presence of bacteria in the urine

cystitis: inflammation of the urinary bladder, often characterized by pain and dysuria

dysuria: painful or difficult urination, often the result of urinary tract infection or obstruction

urethra: the tubular structure that drains the urine from the bladder

urethritis: inflammation of the urethra, often characterized by dysuria

urinary bladder: the muscular organ that stores urine to be discharged through the urethra

urinary tract infection: infection involving any organs associated with the urinary system

CAUSES AND SYMPTOMS

Diseases of the urinary tract represent one of the most common forms of infection by microorganisms. In the United States, the prevalence of urinary tract infections is a reflection of both gender and age. By the age of five, bacteriuria is found in approximately 4 to 5 percent of girls, which is about ten times the rate among boys. Infections are far more common among female adolescents and young women than among men, with a yearly prevalence of approximately 20 percent of American women in the age group of sixteen to thirty-five years accounting for approximately six million reported cases each year. The prevalence of infection among both men and women rises sharply among the elderly, often reflecting problems with aging, including enlargement of the prostate in men. Most infections are self-limiting, particularly among the young. If not treated properly, however, such infections have the potential to be more serious.

Normally, urine is free of microbial contamination. The much higher incidence of urinary tract infections in women reflects, to a large degree, the anatomical differences between males and females. In women, the close proximity of the urethra to the rectum permits relatively easy access of intestinal flora to the urinary tract. Not surprisingly, most urinary infections are caused by enteric bacteria. The most common infectious agent, *Escherichia coli*, represents approximately 80 percent of the acquired infections of the urinary tract. Other bacterial genera of importance include *Enterobacter, Klebsiella,* and *Proteus. Proteus* infections may be of particular significance because colonization by that organism may lead to the deposition of urinary calculi (stones). Less often, *Streptococcus faecalis* or *Pseudomonas aeruginosa* may be involved; the latter can be a particular problem because of its high level of drug resistance.

Urinary tract infections usually begin with entry of the organisms into the distal end of the urethra; the migration of microorganisms into the vagina may occur in a similar manner. Most bladder infections result from ascending movement of the microbial agents along the urethra into the urinary bladder. Inflammation of the urethra (urethritis) or urinary bladder (cystitis) results from a combination of microbial colonization and the host's immune response to the infection. Often, such inflammation may be the first symptom of these infections.

Various factors appear to predispose certain individuals to urinary tract infections. Strains of *E. coli* that colonize the urethra appear to have a greater ability to adhere to the surface tissue. In particular, those strains that frequently ascend into the ureters or kidneys often possess unique types of fimbriae (filamentous structures), which promotes adherence to the epithelial cells that line the surface of the urinary tract; this bacterial structure may be of particular importance to the course of the infection, since the flushing action of urinary flow is a mechanism by which the body maintains the sterility of the urinary tract. Likewise, anything with the potential to interrupt micturition (urination), such as the presence of calculi or tumors, may predispose an individual to a urinary tract infection. Enlargement of the prostate gland in

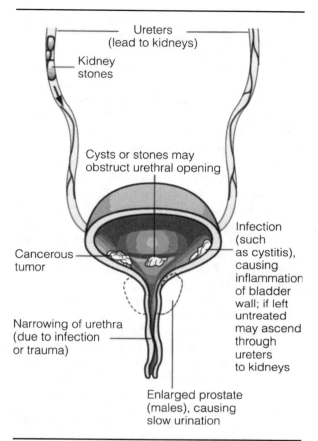

In addition to the variety of infections that may attack the urinary system, urinary disorders may be caused by cancerous tumors, cysts, stones that cause obstruction, reactions to trauma, and in males pressure from an enlarged prostate.

older men is a frequent cause of such problems. Among children, congenital abnormalities at the site of ureter entry into the bladder may result in a vesicoureteral reflux, or urine backflow, which may interfere with normal urine flow. Such abnormalities, which are not uncommon, are found in equal numbers among both young boys and girls; they frequently disappear naturally by the time of puberty. Nevertheless, such problems may contribute to infections among those in this age group.

Certain forms of birth control, in addition to the act of intercourse itself, may contribute to urinary infections. The term "honeymoon cystitis" is often applied, reflecting the bacteriuria often found following intercourse. The colonization of *E. coli* may be associated with the use of diaphragms or spermicides. The reasons for this connection are unclear, but both appear to represent an alteration in the normal flora of the periurethral area and vagina.

Clinical manifestations of urinary tract infections vary with age and are often nonspecific. The infiltration of leukocytes (white blood cells), resulting in inflammation, account for many of the symptoms. Among children, abdominal pain is often present, accompanied by fever and sometimes vomiting. Among adults, cystitis and urethritis are often accompanied by difficulty in urination (dysuria), including painful urination and frequent urination, particularly in women. A sensation of abdominal heaviness or lower back pain, in addition to low-grade fever, is often observed. The urine may be bloody or turbid, reflecting a mixture of microbial agents and white blood cells. Bacteriuria is detected by the collection of a sample of voided urine and inoculation of an appropriate culture dish; the presence of at least 100,000 colony-forming units per milliliter of sample constitutes "significant bacteriuria."

Infection of the urinary tract may also result from a variety of sexually transmitted organisms. Chlamydial infections are common in both males and females, and they represent one of the most commonly observed forms of sexually transmitted disease (STD). *Chlamydia trachomatis* causes urethritis in both males and females; though many chlamydial infections are asymptomatic, they can lead to severe complications. Urethritis may also result from other microbial STDs, both viral and bacterial.

The use of catheters, particularly among hospitalized elderly persons, is a frequent cause of urinary infections. An estimated 40 percent of nosocomial (hospital-acquired) infections result from use of catheters. Despite attempts to maintain sterility through the use of closed, sterile drainage systems, by two weeks after catheterization 50 percent of both men and women have developed a urinary tract infection, and with longer or permanent catheterizations, nearly all persons will develop some degree of infection. In most cases, these infections are inapparent, but such persons remain predisposed to cystitis or urethritis.

The urinary tract is also subjected to other disorders, including cancer. The most common form of neoplasm of the urinary tract is bladder cancer. Such cancers tend to be highly aggressive, often occur as multiple growths, and are difficult to cure once metastasis has begun. Approximately two-thirds of cases

of bladder cancer are diagnosed in men, perhaps in part a reflection of risk factors. Exposure to both cigarette smoke and carcinogens, particularly those used in the petrochemical industry, has been linked to an increased incidence of bladder cancers. The symptoms of bladder cancer resemble those of urinary tract infections: dysuria, cystitis, and the frequent need to urinate. If the tumor is diagnosed early enough, electrosurgery or resection may be sufficient to remove the lesion. If the tumor has begun to infiltrate the bladder tissue, complete removal of the bladder may be necessary. Radiation and chemotherapy are also commonly used in the treatment of certain forms of urinary tract cancers.

TREATMENT AND THERAPY

Standard treatment for urinary tract infections consists of a regimen of antimicrobial drugs. Ideally, the antibiotics of choice are secreted in the urine over a prolonged period, rather than achieving high concentrations in the blood serum. In this manner, the drug is directed at the infection itself, with minimal effect on the normal flora elsewhere in the body.

Depending on whether the infection is limited to the lower urinary tract (urethra or bladder) or has spread to the upper tract (ureters or kidneys), the period of regimen may last for several days or up to two weeks. Generally, infections of the upper urinary tract require more prolonged treatment and may be subject to recurrence.

Standard therapy of conventional lower-tract infections routinely consists of a three-day regimen of trimethoprim-sulfamethoxazole (TMP-SMX), or TMP alone. Since most of the drug combination is excreted in the urine, there is a minimum of side effects and little danger to the normal flora within the body. The short duration of treatment also minimizes the chances of encouraging the growth of resistant populations of bacteria. Elderly patients or persons with diabetes mellitus may require longer treatment. If the person shows evidence of upper-tract infection, treatment is generally given over a two-week period.

If there is evidence of kidney involvement or inflammation (pyelonephritis), the patient is often hospitalized in order to monitor treatment, which usually involves a fourteen-day course of TMP-SMX. Severe illness or evidence of spreading may require more intensive therapy with other antibiotics.

Since the flushing action of urine is itself a nonspecific means of removing bacteria from the bladder or urethra, patients are usually advised to drink as much water as possible. In this manner, weakly adherent or nonadherent bacteria may be flushed from the site of infection, reducing the number of bacteria and supplementing the course of antimicrobial therapy. In some cases, this action is sufficient to relieve symptoms or even cure the infection.

In situations in which the infection is asymptomatic, unless the situation warrants treatment (such as impending surgery), antimicrobial therapy may not be necessary, as the infection is self-limiting. Given the large proportion of persons, particularly women, who develop bacteriuria, forgoing therapy may minimize the chances for the artificial selection of resistant strains. In individuals with heart disease, renal failure, or diabetes, however, such therapy may be necessary as a preventive measure for later problems.

Bacteriuria during pregnancy represents a special situation. During early pregnancy, from 4 to 7 percent of women develop bacteriuria, which is probably related to such physiological changes as the dilation of the bladder and uterus, along with vesicoureteral (bladder and urethra) reflux. Even though the infection may be asymptomatic, urinary tract infection is associated with increased risk of both pyelonephritis and loss of the fetus; about one-third of women with untreated bacteriuria during pregnancy develop infections within the upper urinary tract by the third trimester. For this reason, it is generally recommended that pregnant women be screened for such infections and undergo treatment if bacteriuria is present. Pregnant women generally undergo a three-day treatment regimen, though with alternative antibiotics considered safer in the presence of a developing fetus: ampicillin, nitrofurantoin, or cephalexin. Patients should be monitored at intervals during the pregnancy to prevent recurrence. If pyelonephritis should develop, the woman is routinely hospitalized to allow close monitoring of both the mother and the fetus during therapy.

Bacteriuria associated with catheterization is generally treated only when it is symptomatic, since recurrence of the infection is common; long-term treatment presents no advantage and may select for antibiotic resistant strains. Since the catheter may harbor bacteria, it usually is removed at the start of therapy.

The treatment of sexually transmitted diseases follows much the same pattern. Fortunately, most STDs can be treated or controlled. Both chlamydial infections and gonorrhea are generally treated with doxycycline, a derivative of tetracycline.

PERSPECTIVE AND PROSPECTS

Urinary tract infections are notoriously difficult to prevent. Because in most cases the associated etiological agents are the normal intestinal flora, vaccination or prophylactic use of antibiotics would be impractical. Proper hygiene appears to be the most effective means of prevention among young adults.

STDs as a source of urinary tract disease represent a class in itself. Either a decrease in sexual promiscuity or more effective use of physical barriers (such as condoms) is necessary to reduce the level of such forms of infection. While vaccines against some of the more prevalent forms of STD (gonorrhea, chlamydia) remain a possibility, antibiotic therapy continues to be the most reliable means to treat urinary infections within the individual.

Catheter-associated infections represent an important source of infection among the elderly, particularly those who are hospitalized. Since a single catheterization results in infection among less than 1 percent of patients, limiting catheterization, or avoiding it entirely, would appear to be the most effective preventive measure. The use of closed drainage systems has also reduced significantly the incidence of such infections. Antiseptic solutions and ointments have had limited success in the prevention of urinary tract infections. The use of antibiotic therapy has been effective in the short term, but over time such therapy may simply select for resistant mutants among the microorganisms. Development of catheters that do not lend themselves to microbial colonization, or that actively inhibit microbial growth (such as silver-impregnated catheters), may reduce the chances of such types of urinary tract infections.

—*Richard Adler, Ph.D.*

See also Abscess drainage; Abscesses; Adrenalectomy; Bed-wetting; Candidiasis; Catheterization; Cystectomy; Cystitis; Cystoscopy; Cysts; Dialysis; Endoscopy; Fistula repair; Genital disorders, female; Genital disorders, male; Glomerulonephritis; Hypertension; Incontinence; Internal medicine; Kidney disorders; Kidney transplantation; Kidneys; Laparoscopy; Lithotripsy; Nephrectomy; Nephritis; Nephrology; Nephrology, pediatric; Renal failure; Reye's syndrome; Sexually transmitted diseases; Stone removal; Stones; Ultrasonography; Urethritis; Urinalysis; Urinary system; Urology; Urology, pediatric.

FOR FURTHER INFORMATION:

Boston Women's Health Book Collective. *Our Bodies, Ourselves for the New Century.* New York: Simon

& Schuster, 1998. An updated discussion of topics related to women's health. A compendium of material relevant to a wide variety of issues, the book contains a well-written section dealing with urinary tract problems.

Dollemore, Doug, et al. *Symptoms: Their Causes and Cures*. Emmaus, Pa.: Rodale Press, 1994. A reference guide to health problems. The authors have cataloged symptoms, methods of home relief, and perhaps most important, a discussion of when to visit a physician. A section of the book is devoted to urinary tract problems.

Gorbach, Sherwood L., John G. Bartlett, and Neil R. Blacklow, eds. *Infectious Diseases*. 2d ed. Philadelphia: W. B. Saunders, 1997. A textbook dealing with the general topic of infectious disease. The section covering urinary tract infections provides a thorough discussion of the subject. An excellent source for someone interested in such material in depth.

Kelley, William, et al., eds. *Textbook of Internal Medicine*. 3d ed. New York: Lippincott-Raven, 1997. A medical textbook containing a section on urinary tract infections that is thorough in its analysis of the subject. This source is particularly useful, with its inclusion of definitions and descriptions of the clinical presentation of the disease, diagnosis, and treatment.

Simon, Harvey. *Staying Well*. Boston: Houghton Mifflin, 1992. A description of various diseases, their causes and symptoms. Much of the book deals with methods of prevention, including the importance of proper nutrition and exercise. A portion of the text covers screening for urinary tract infections.

Stamm, W. E., and T. M. Hooton. "Current Concepts: Management of Urinary Tract Infections in Adults." *New England Journal of Medicine* 329 (October 28, 1993): 1328-1334. The authors present a moderately detailed overview of the types and management of urinary tract disease. Offers a good synopsis of the most common infectious agents involved. A useful reference for anyone interested in a brief survey of these forms of illness.

Wallace, Robert A., Gerald P. Sanders, and Robert J. Ferl. *Biology: The Science of Life*. 4th ed. New York: HarperCollins, 1996. A text covering general biology. The section on the urinary tract is concise and clearly written using a nonclinical approach. Clear diagrams and illustrations are included.

URINARY SYSTEM

ANATOMY

ANATOMY OR SYSTEM AFFECTED: Abdomen, bladder, kidneys

SPECIALTIES AND RELATED FIELDS: Nephrology, urology

DEFINITION: A system, composed of the kidneys, ureters, urinary bladder, and urethra, that removes body waste, maintains the proper amount of body water, and regulates the acid-base balance of the blood.

KEY TERMS:

glomerular filtration: the first step in urine formation; passive filtration in which fluids and solids dissolved in the fluid (solutes) are forced through a membrane, resulting in the filtration of the blood

nephron: tiny blood-processing units located in the kidneys that carry out the processes that form urine; each kidney contains approximately one million nephrons

tubular reabsorption: the process of returning important solutes that were filtered out of the blood back into the blood; these important solutes include glucose, amino acids, vitamins, and most ions

tubular secretion: the process of tubular reabsorption in reverse; important solutes moved from the filtrate to the urine include hydrogen and potassium ions, organic acids, ammonia, and creatine

ureters: slender, expandable tubes that carry urine from the kidney to the urinary bladder

urethra: a muscular tube which transports urine from the urinary bladder out of the body

urinary bladder: a stretchable, muscular sac that functions to store urine

STRUCTURE AND FUNCTIONS

The urinary system consists of two kidneys, two ureters, a urinary bladder, and a urethra. The kidneys function to remove metabolic waste from the blood, maintain proper water balance for the body, and maintain the proper acid-base balance in the blood. The ureters, urinary bladder, and urethra are involved in the moving of the urine formed in the kidneys to the external environment. The kidneys play the major role in the function of the urinary system.

Most people have two kidneys, located at the lower end of the rib cage and lying against the back of the body wall. Typically, the right kidney is positioned a little lower than the left kidney because the right kidney is pushed down by the liver. An adult kidney is about 12.5 centimeters long, 7.5 centimeters wide, and 2.5 centimeters thick and is shaped like a kidney bean. Each kidney is surrounded by a thick layer of fat, which is important for holding the kidneys in their normal body position.

Inside each kidney is a lighter outer region called the renal cortex. Deep in the cortex is a darker layer called the renal medulla. Within the cortex and medulla are found tiny structures called nephrons. Each kidney contains approximately one million nephrons, most of which are in the renal cortex. Nephrons are the functional units of the kidney, as they carry out the processes involved in urine formation.

Each nephron consists of two main parts, the glomerulus and the renal tubule. The glomerulus is composed of a knot of capillaries that fit inside the Bowman's capsule, the cup-shaped head of the renal tubule. The rest of the renal tubule is about 2.5 centimeters long. The neck of the renal tubule undergoes a high degree of coiling and twisting just before it makes a hairpin loop. This part of the renal tubule is called the proximal convoluted tubule. The hairpin loop of the renal tubule is termed the loop of Henle. After coming out of this loop, the renal tubule again undergoes a high degree of coiling and twisting and is called the distal convoluted tubule. The distal convoluted tubule then enters another tube, the collecting duct. Surrounding and encasing the renal tubule is the peritubular capillary bed.

Urine formation occurs in the nephron and is the result of three processes: glomerular filtration, tubular reabsorption, and tubular secretion. The glomerulus acts as a filter. This process of glomerular filtration occurs as a result of the capillaries in the glomerulus being somewhat leaky as compared to other capillaries in the body. This process of filtration is a passive process that does not require any metabolic energy. High pressure in the glomerular capillaries causes the formation of a filtrate that consists primarily of blood, except that it lacks the red blood cells and blood proteins. (Both red blood cells and blood proteins are too large to pass through the leaky glomerular capillaries.) The filtrate contains the metabolic waste as well as the many useful substances found in the blood, including glucose, amino acids, vitamins, and water. This filtrate will be continually formed as long as the systemic blood pressure is normal.

The filtrate that is formed is caught in the Bowman's capsule of the renal tubule. From here, the filtrate will pass into the proximal convoluted tubule.

Rather than losing the useful substances in the urine, the nephron works to put them back into the blood through the process of tubular reabsorption. Tubular reabsorption begins as soon as the filtrate enters the proximal convoluted tubule. Cells within the tubule take up needed substances from the filtrate and pass

The Anatomy of the Urinary System

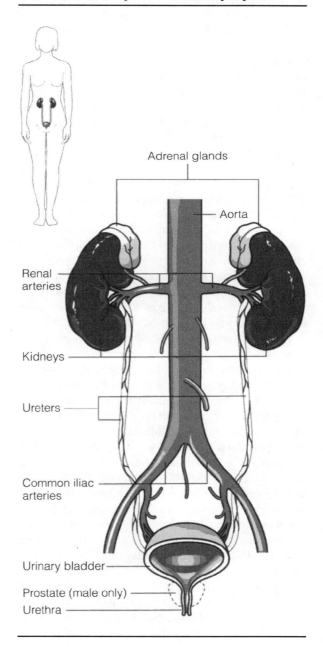

Adrenal glands

Aorta

Renal arteries

Kidneys

Ureters

Common iliac arteries

Urinary bladder

Prostate (male only)

Urethra

them out to the space between the proximal convoluted tubule and the surrounding peritubular capillaries. Once these useful substances are brought into this space, termed the extracellular space, they can be absorbed back into the blood contained within the peritubular capillaries. Some of this reabsorption is passive, not requiring any metabolic energy; water is an example of a substance that is reabsorbed passively. Most substances, however, depend on membrane transporters to carry them out to the extracellular space. These membrane transporters require metabolic energy in the form of adenosine triphosphate (ATP). There are a large number of membrane transporters for those substances that need to be reabsorbed and few if any transporters for those substances that do not need to be transported. This imbalance helps to explain why substances such as glucose and amino acids are almost completely reabsorbed back into the blood while metabolic waste products such as urea and uric acid are not.

The process of tubular secretion occurs in the loop of Henle and is essentially opposite to that of tubular reabsorption, with substances taken from the blood and put back into the filtrate. Some substances that are secreted from the blood and into the filtrate include hydrogen and potassium ions, ammonium ions, and certain drugs (for example, penicillin). It is the process of tubular secretion that allows the kidneys to remove toxins and drugs from the body, as well as to maintain the acid-base balance of the blood.

The regulation of the volume of urine secreted is controlled by the distal convoluted tubules and the collecting ducts to which they attach. After the filtrate has gone through the proximal convoluted tubules and the loop of Henle, it is fairly concentrated and therefore does not contain a large amount of water. The distal convoluted tubule and collecting duct are impermeable to water when a substance called vasopressin, or antidiuretic hormone (ADH), is present, in which case the filtrate will contain little water and the final urine volume will be small. If ADH is not present, the distal convoluted tubule and collecting ducts become permeable to water and, because the concentration of solutes is higher in the distal convoluted tubule and collecting duct, water enters into these two structures from the blood. The result is a dilution of the filtrate, with an increased water content, and a large volume of urine. The role of ADH in determining urine volume can be seen with the ingestion of alcohol or coffee, both of which inhibit ADH

release from the pituitary gland: The distal convoluted tubule and collecting duct become permeable to water, and the urine volume and the frequency of urination increase. It is by this mechanism that the kidneys regulate the body's water balance.

Once the urine is formed in the kidney, it will flow into a tube, the ureter. The ureters, one for each kidney, are passageways that carry urine from the kidney to the urinary bladder. Because the ureters run downward from the kidney, it might seem that the movement of urine to the urinary bladder is created by gravity. In reality, the ureters, which are stretchy and muscular tubes, contract at a rate of one to five times per minute to force the urine toward the bladder, a process termed peristalsis (the same type of contractions that move food through the digestive system). Where the ureters enter the urinary bladder, small, valvelike folds prevent the backflow of urine from the urinary bladder toward the kidneys.

The urinary bladder is a muscular, collapsible sac located in the pelvic cavity. When the bladder is empty, it is only 5 to 7.5 centimeters long and its walls are thrown into folds. As urine enters the bladder, it causes the organ to expand. A moderately full bladder is about 12.5 centimeters long and will contain approximately one-half of a liter of urine. A completely full bladder is capable of holding approximately 1 liter of fluid. The kidneys are continually forming urine. Thus, the bladder acts as a temporary storage unit for urine, allowing the individual to empty the bladder when it is convenient.

The urethra is a thin-walled tube that carries urine from the urinary bladder to the exterior of the body. Near where the urethra exits the urinary bladder is a band of smooth muscle which makes up the internal urethral sphincter. This sphincter, which is not under conscious control, acts to keep the urethra shut when urine is not being voided. A second sphincter, the external urethral sphincter, is found further down the length of the urethra and is composed of skeletal muscle. This sphincter is under voluntary control: When it is not convenient to void the urine, it is this sphincter that is used to prevent urination.

The urge to urinate is brought about by the stretching of the bladder. Ordinarily, the urge to urinate occurs when the bladder contains about 200 milliliters of urine. This amount of urine causes a stretching of the bladder which sends impulses to the spinal cord initiating the contraction of the urinary bladder. The contractions of the urinary bladder force urine past the internal urethral sphincter. It is at this time that a person will feel the need to void the urine, a process termed micturition.

DISORDERS AND DISEASES

Renal and urinary disorders can be categorized based on their mechanism of action and the portion of the urinary system that they affect. These disorders include obstructive disorders that interfere with normal urine flow anywhere within the urinary tract, urinary tract infections, and glomerular disorders, which affect the glomeruli in the kidneys.

Obstructive disorders of the urinary system can be caused by many different factors. Obstruction of the passage of the urine will usually cause a backing up of the urine into the kidney or kidneys. The result is a swelling of the kidney termed hydronephrosis.

Perhaps the most common obstruction is that caused by kidney stones, also referred to as renal calculi. Kidney stones consist of crystallized minerals such as calcium, magnesium, or uric acid salts that form hard stones in the distal end of the collecting ducts. If the stones are small, they will pass through the remainder of the urinary tract. Larger stones, however, get caught in the ureters, thus blocking the passage of urine from the kidneys to the urinary bladder. This blockage usually results in intense pain as the ureters rhythmically contract in an effort to dislodge the stone; this condition is sometimes referred to as renal colic. If the stone does not move from its position of blockage, a buildup of urine in the kidney may occur; if this continues, damage may be done to the kidneys.

Damage to the nerves that innervate the bladder, termed neurogenic bladder, can also result in an obstructive disorder. Damage to these nerves results in the loss of normal control over the voiding of urine from the bladder. Consequently, there is a retention of urine in the bladder since there is no signal telling the bladder to contract.

Tumors of the urinary system may also cause obstruction of urine flow. Another cause of obstruction is the loss of the fat surrounding the kidney. When this occurs, one or both kidneys may drop from their normal position, a condition referred to as renal ptosis. When the kidneys drop, there is a chance that the ureters exiting the kidney may become kinked and prevent the normal flow of urine from the kidneys to the urinary bladder.

Urinary tract infections are usually caused by bacteria and can involve the urethra, ureters, urinary bladder, kidneys, or all the above. Urinary infections in the urethra are termed urethritis and result in the inflammation of the urethra. The two most common bacteria involved in urethritis are gonorrhea and chlamydia. Males are more likely than females to have urethritis.

Cystitis refers to any inflammation of the urinary bladder. This condition usually results from bacterial infections, but it may also be caused by tumors or by the presence of stones in the bladder. Cystitis occurs more frequently in women than in men and is characterized by pelvic pain, a frequent urge to urinate, and possibly blood in the urine.

Nephritis is a general term used to describe inflammatory kidney diseases. The inflammation of the nephrons within the kidney is referred to as pyelonephritis. Pyelonephritis is often attributable to bacterial infection but may also be caused by viral infections, tumors, kidney stones, or pregnancy.

Glomerulonephritis is a term that refers to any type of glomerular disorder. It can be further subdivided into two categories: acute glomerulonephritis and chronic glomerulonephritis. Acute glomerulonephritis is the most common form and may be caused by bacterial infection. Chronic glomerulonephritis refers to noninfectious kidney disorders. It commonly occurs when the immune system reacts to and destroys the body's own glomeruli. This type of glomerulonephritis eventually leads to kidney failure. Acute glomerulonephritis, if it is left untreated or it does not respond to treatment, can become chronic glomerulonephritis.

Renal (kidney) failure is simply the inability of the kidneys to form urine. Renal failure can be classified as either acute or chronic. Acute renal failure is the abrupt loss of kidney function, which may result from excessive loss of blood, severe burns, pyelonephritis, glomerulonephritis, or infection or obstruction of the urinary tract. Chronic renal failure is the slow destruction of the nephrons in the kidney. This form of renal failure may result from infections, glomerulonephritis, tumors, obstructive disorders, or autoimmune diseases. Unless the progression of nephron loss is stopped, chronic renal failure will eventually lead to death.

Diabetes insipidus is a disease that does not directly attack the urinary system, but it has a profound effect on the urinary system through its influence on the pituitary gland and the hypothalamus. With diabetes insipidus, the pituitary gland fails to release antidiuretic hormone, as a result of an injury or tumor of the posterior portion of the pituitary gland or hypothalamus. Because of the decreased amount of antidiuretic hormone, large amounts of urine, and thus water, are flushed from the body daily. If left untreated, diabetes insipidus can lead to dehydration and electrolyte imbalances. To offset the loss of water in the urine, individuals with diabetes insipidus must drink large amounts of water.

PERSPECTIVE AND PROSPECTS

The complexity of the human kidney can be characterized by science's inability to build an artificial kidney that is continually functional and can be inserted into the body in the position of the normal kidney. Until the development of tubing that contained miniature holes, dialysis tubing, kidney failure nearly always resulted in death. Dialysis tubing allowed the development of renal dialysis, which cleanses the blood of toxic substances and helps to regulate electrolyte balance. The process of renal dialysis is carried out using a thin membrane that is permeable to only a few select substances. The tubing is immersed in a bathing solution that is very similar to normal blood plasma. As blood circulates through the tubing, toxic substances and some electrolytes move out of the blood and into the bathing solution. This dialysis tubing and the bathing solution are often referred to as an artificial kidney. Dialysis is usually done three times a week, with each session requiring about four to eight hours. Although effective, dialysis is a far cry from the functioning of the human kidney and is no cure for chronic renal failure. When the kidneys are no longer functioning, the only hope is a kidney transplant.

Because the kidneys are so effective at filtering the blood of toxic substances and drugs, the urine formed by the kidney is the principal fluid used for drug testing and drug screening. Furthermore, the kidney also secretes some white blood cells into the urine. As techniques continue to develop, it will be possible to perform genetic tests on these white blood cells to determine genetic traits such as sex and the color of hair and eyes, as well as the possibility of the presence of genetic diseases or personality traits. Such technology could have considerable impact on the future of individual privacy as many companies and employers require a mandatory analysis of urine, primarily for the presence of drugs in the urine, prior to

the possibility of employment. Thus, with a simple urine sample, the company could know not only the possible drug use of prospective employees but also their genetic makeup.

—*David K. Saunders, Ph.D.*

See also Abdomen; Abdominal disorders; Abscess drainage; Abscesses; Adrenalectomy; Bed-wetting; Candidiasis; Catheterization; Circumcision, male; Cystectomy; Cystitis; Cystoscopy; Cysts; Dialysis; *E. coli* infection; Endoscopy; Fistula repair; Fluids and electrolytes; Geriatrics and gerontology; Glomerulonephritis; Host-defense mechanisms; Hypertension; Incontinence; Internal medicine; Kidney disorders; Kidney transplantation; Kidneys; Laparoscopy; Lithotripsy; Nephrectomy; Nephritis; Nephrology; Nephrology, pediatric; Pediatrics; Penile implant surgery; Renal failure; Reye's syndrome; Schistosomiasis; Stone removal; Stones; Systems and organs; Transplantation; Ultrasonography; Urethritis; Urinalysis; Urinary disorders; Urology; Urology, pediatric.

FOR FURTHER INFORMATION:

Carola, Robert, John P. Harley, and Charles R. Noback. *Human Anatomy and Physiology.* 2d ed. New York: McGraw-Hill, 1992. This text provides an easy-to-follow discussion of the urinary system's structure and function. The illustrations are well done, and the book also contains some photographs of parts of the urinary system in cadavers. Uses flowcharts to help explain the physiological functions of the urinary system.

Guyton, Arthur C., and John E. Hall. *Textbook of Medical Physiology.* 9th ed. Philadelphia: W. B. Saunders, 1996. This textbook gives many examples of diseases and pathological conditions of the urinary system. Does an excellent job of describing how the diseases and pathologies affect the normal function of the urinary system.

Hole, John W., Jr. *Essentials of Human Anatomy and Physiology.* 6th ed. Dubuque, Iowa: Wm. C. Brown, 1993. An introductory college anatomy and physiology book that is easily read and understood. Provides a good general overview of the structure and function of the urinary system.

Marieb, Elaine N. *Essentials of Human Anatomy and Physiology.* 6th ed. Redwood City, Calif.: Benjamin/Cummings, 2000. An excellent book to begin the study of the urinary system. This text is easy to read and understand because it uses little technical jargon and explains the jargon that it does use. Provides good descriptions and drawings of most parts of the urinary system.

_____. *Human Anatomy and Physiology*. 5th ed. Redwood City, Calif.: Benjamin/Cummings, 2000. Provides a detailed look at the urinary system and its function. Nevertheless, written in a style that makes the physiology of the urinary system understandable. Also contains illustrations of the urinary system and photographs from described specimens.

Thibodeau, Gary A., and Kevin T. Patton. *Anatomy and Physiology*. 4th ed. St. Louis: Mosby Year Book, 1993. Provides understandable and logical descriptions of the functions of the urinary system. Excellent illustrations aid the reader in understanding the discussion in the text.

UROLOGY

SPECIALTY

ANATOMY OR SYSTEM AFFECTED: Abdomen, bladder, genitals, kidneys, reproductive system, urinary system

SPECIALTIES AND RELATED FIELDS: Family practice, gynecology, microbiology, nephrology, obstetrics, proctology

DEFINITION: The branch of medicine that deals with the physiology and disorders of the urinary system (kidneys, ureters, bladder, and urethra) and the male genital tract.

KEY TERMS:

-otomy: combining form meaning an opening or incision in an organ or structure; for example, a ureterotomy is an opening in the ureter

ureter: either of the two tubes that carry urine from the kidneys to the bladder

urethra: the tube that carries urine from the bladder, voiding the liquid from the body

-uria: combining form meaning the presence of a substance in urine; for example, hematuria refers to blood in the urine

urinalysis: the physical, chemical, and microscopic analysis of urine

urinary system assessment: the evaluation of the complete urinary tract, including kidneys, bladder, ureters, and urethra; also includes an analysis of the patient's personal medical history

urine: fluid collected in the kidneys that contains metabolic wastes, including urea and salts

urogram: the injection of a radiopaque substance, followed by X rays of the urinary tract as the substance passes through it

SCIENCE AND PROFESSION

The urinary system consists of a complex series of structures which includes the kidneys, ureters, urinary bladder, and urethra. Since in males the urinary tract is closely associated with the genital tract, urology properly deals with disorders of the male genitourinary tract and the female urinary tract. Urologists may also study disorders of the adrenal glands, which are closely associated with the kidneys.

Urine production begins in the kidneys, a pair of bean-shaped organs found within the abdomen. Urine is produced through a complex system of units called nephrons; approximately one million nephrons are found within each kidney. Each nephron consists of a ball-shaped capillary network called the glomerulus, which is surrounded by a capsule (Bowman's capsule) through which the actual filtration of blood takes place. Blood enters the glomerulus under high pressure, forcing the liquid and dissolved material through the basement membrane into the renal tubules that extend from the capsule.

The long, convoluted tubule which extends from each capsule follows a circuitous route through the kidney. As it emerges from the capsule, the proximal convoluted tubule is found within the outer region, or cortex, of the kidney. The tubule then passes through the inner portion, or medulla, of the kidney, forming an extended loop called the loop of Henle. The tubule winds its way back to the cortical region as the distal convoluted tubule. Blood circulates completely through the kidneys about twenty times each hour. Approximately 20 percent of the plasma (liquid portion of the blood) is filtered through the Bowman's capsules during this time, the equivalent of some 180 liters of fluid per day. Much of the plasma and nearly all the nutrient material found within the liquid that passes through the tubules are reabsorbed into the capillary network surrounding the tubules. Approximately 80 percent is absorbed within the proximal convoluted tubule, the remainder as it flows through the tubule system. The rest of the fluid, approximately 1 liter per day for the average person, contains nitrogenous material such as urea, salts, and other metabolic wastes, which are voided.

The distal tubules emerge from the cortex of the kidney and again pass into the medulla, where they now merge into increasingly larger collecting ducts. The collecting ducts form clearly visible pyramids, or papillae, within the medulla. The merging of the largest ducts within the renal pelvis, the lowest portion of the kidney, results in the formation of a single tube, the ureter. One ureter emerges from each kidney to empty the urine into the bladder.

The ureters are thick-walled tubes, about 30 centimeters (6 inches) in length, which extend through the pelvic region. They enter the bladder in a slanted manner, which helps prevent backup of the urine from the bladder when it is full. Urine is actually pumped through the ureters by means of peristaltic, or rhythmic, contraction of the smooth muscle that lines the ureters.

The urinary bladder is a membranous organ in the pelvis which serves to store and discharge urine. The bladder is capable of holding approximately one-third to one-half of a liter of liquid in the average individual. When full, it is quite capable of causing the lower abdomen to bulge visibly. Since the structure is adjacent to the uterus in women, conditions such as pregnancy may significantly lower the carrying capacity of the bladder.

The musculature in the lower portion of the bladder is thickened, forming the bladder neck, and serves to retain the liquid within the organ. The muscle, in turn, is continuous with that of the urethra, the tubular structure that drains the urine from the bladder.

In women, the urethra is 3 to 4 centimeters in length and emerges just in front of the vagina. In men, the tube is approximately 20 centimeters long. Emerging from the bladder in the male, it passes through the prostate gland and into the penis, where it serves both for the elimination of urine and as a passage for semen during ejaculation.

Since urine formation begins in the kidney, the branches of medicine that constitute nephrology and urology may overlap each other at times. Strictly speaking, however, nephrology deals with the kidney as a regulatory organ for fluid and salt levels in the body, in addition to its role as an endocrine gland. Urology deals with disorders of the urinary tract, in addition to problems associated with the genitourinary tract in males, since the two systems are so closely associated.

Approximately 20 percent of adult visits to a physician involve problems associated with the genitourinary tract. Urinalysis—the physical, chemical, and microscopic evaluation of collected urine—thus becomes an important diagnostic tool. The process begins with proper collection of urine into a sterile specimen container. The sample initially undergoes a macroscopic examination in which color and appear-

ance are evaluated. Since recent ingestion of food may result in the discoloration of urine or alteration in its pH, it is best to obtain the sample several hours after the patient has eaten. Generally, the odor is unimportant; for example, by-products of asparagus ingestion may produce a rather characteristic odor in urine that is of no medical significance. Nevertheless, a pungent aroma may signify an infection. Metabolic diseases may also produce by-products that have characteristic smells.

Macroscopic examination of urine also involves a determination of the specific gravity, or density, of the solution, and its pH. Densities outside the normal density range for urine may be indicative of diabetes mellitus or renal dysfunction. The pH is a measurement of hydrogen ion concentration in the fluid. A pH of 7.0 is neutral. Normal levels in urine vary considerably, from an acid level of 4.6 to an alkaline pH of 8.0. Generally, urine samples obtained soon after a meal will be slightly alkaline, but a consistently alkaline level may be indicative of a urinary tract infection. Other macromolecules that may be observed in urine as a result of various pathologies include elevated levels of protein or sugar and the presence of blood (hematuria).

Microscopic analysis of urine is a necessary part of a thorough urinalysis. The urine sample is centrifuged, or spun at high speed, to concentrate material in a smaller volume. The pellet from the centrifugation is stained and observed for bacteria or blood cells. Normally, the number of bacteria and white blood cells in urine is low; indeed, some bacterial contamination of the specimen during collection is common. Large numbers of either, however, may be indicative of an infection. The presence of red blood cells in urine is always considered abnormal and may signify inflammation or bleeding within the urinary system.

DIAGNOSTIC AND TREATMENT TECHNIQUES
A thorough urinary system assessment involving the examination of the kidneys, ureters, bladder, and urethra may be necessary for an accurate diagnosis of certain pathologies. In addition to the normal urinalysis, including the use of a catheter for obtaining a urine sample, the patient's medical history and vital signs are included in the study. The diagnosis of urinary problems may include procedures for obtaining images of the urinary tract: X rays of the kidneys or urinary tract, as well as excretory or intravenous urog-

raphy. The latter involves the injection of a radiopaque solution into the system, either of solids containing barium or of gas (such as air), followed by X-ray analysis as the solution passes through the tract. Direct observation through cystoscopy may also be carried out. Methodology developed during the 1980's also includes computed tomography (CT) scanning and magnetic resonance imaging (MRI).

Depending on the problem, treatment may be as simple as the prescription of antibiotics. Urologic surgery becomes necessary if diagnostic procedures reveal a tumor or obstruction. Under these circumstances, direct surgical removal may be necessary. Surgical reconstruction, as well as possible relocations, may be required for certain problems. For example, damage to the urinary system as a result of neurologic or neoplastic (cancerous) conditions may require the diversion of urine through an opening in the abdomen, a ureteroileostomy, instead of through normal channels.

Pathologic conditions of the urinary tract may take a variety of forms, such as obstructions, which interfere with urinary flow, or infections by any of a wide number of bacteria. Either condition may lead to inflammation and subsequent urinary problems. Damage may also result from external forces, such as injuries caused by falling or blunt force.

Urinary obstructions are generally classified on the basis of several characteristics: the etiology or source of the obstruction, the length of time over which the obstruction takes place (acute or chronic), and the site of the obstruction. The source of obstruction may be congenital, often resulting from a stenosis, or narrowing, of the meatus (opening or tunnel) within the urethra. An additional congenital abnormality may result from the inability of the ureterovesical junction, the site at which the ureters enter the bladder, to prevent urine reflux, or backflow, into the ureter. The result of any obstruction is frequently infection, pyelonephritis, within the urinary system. Since any infection may ascend to the kidney, damage can occur at any site in the urinary tract.

Obstructions may result from injury to the urinary tract, from benign or malignant tumors, or from the formation of stones. In addition, in women extension of the uterus during pregnancy may impinge on the ureters, interfering with normal flow.

The obstructions may develop anywhere along the urinary tract. The lower urinary tract consists of the region along the urethra. An obstruction in this region may cause ballooning or dilation of the urethra; in men, this dilation may extend into the prostate gland. The weakening of the urethral wall may result in the formation of diverticula, pouchlike herniations in the muscle wall. If the region becomes infected, a likely possibility, the increased hydrostatic pressure coupled with the weakening of the wall may cause the urethra to rupture.

Midtract obstructions are associated with the bladder. In order to compensate for increased resistance to urine flow, the muscle of the bladder may initially thicken, sometimes increasing its thickness by a factor of two or three. The increased size in the musculature of the bladder may in turn actually decrease the urine flow from the ureter as a result of the downward pull on these tubes. The resulting backflow may cause damage to the ureters or kidneys.

The increased pressure within the bladder may also force the tissue, or mucosa, between bundles of musculature, resulting in pockets called cellules. Continued pressure may result in larger pockets, or diverticula, being formed within the bladder wall. Since these regions tend to retain urine, infections are common, and surgery may be necessary to remove the diverticula.

Obstructions of the upper urinary tract are associated with the ureters and kidneys. In addition, increased pressure from backflow may cause dilation of the ureter wall, with an increase in muscle development as compensation. This stage is generally followed by one of decompensation, in which the ureters lose their ability to contract and maintain urine flow. Likewise, the kidneys may be subjected to increased pressure. Normally, the pressure from within the urinary tract on the kidneys is very low. When the pressure is increased on the kidney pelvis, the regions in which the collecting ducts form, the pelvis becomes subject to pressure, ultimately having an impact on blood flow. The result is ischemia (lack of oxygen to the region). The kidney itself may atrophy, followed by renal failure.

Generally, obstructions can be visualized through a variety of procedures. Calcified stones within the tract, or tumors, will show on X rays. In addition, an excretory urogram, a technique in which the urinary tract is X-rayed following injection of a radiopaque substance, may reveal the precise site of the obstruction. The urogram is preferred for observation of certain forms of urinary tract stones which may not appear on conventional X rays. The urogram can also be used to observe sites of both dilation and stenosis.

Depending on the source of obstruction, urologic surgery may become necessary for its removal. If kidney function is significantly reduced, temporary or permanent dialysis, even transplantation, may be necessary. On the other hand, temporary urinary diversion may provide relief to the system, allowing natural healing to repair dilated tubes once the obstruction has been removed. For example, ureteroileostomy has been used under such circumstances. With this technique, a portion of the ureter is diverted through an opening, or stoma, in the intestine.

Urinary stones remain the most common cause of obstructions. The formation of stones is related to a variety of causes, including the diet and metabolic state of the patient, genetics, and the anatomic features of the urinary tract. The result is increased deposition of salts such as calcium around an initial foreign body in the urine. Eventual crystallization leads to steady increases in the size of the stone and, unless it is passed naturally within the urine, eventual obstruction. Stones may form anywhere in the tract, but they tend to be less common in the urethra. In general, stones are crystals of either calcium salts or, less often, uric acid.

A variety of techniques exists for the elimination of urinary stones. Stone dissolution, including lithotripsy (the breaking up of the stone with a surgical instrument or shock waves), is preferred, since minimal invasiveness and hospitalization are required. Hemiacidrin, a magnesium-containing solution, has been used successfully in dissolving certain stones. Ultrasonographic lithotripsy, which utilizes ultrasonic vibrations to dissolve the stone, has also been proved successful. Some stones, however, particularly those composed of calcium, may not respond adequately to these forms of treatment. If the obstruction is significant, and particularly if an infection is present, surgical removal may become necessary.

Infections of the urinary tract may be primary (a direct result of contamination) or secondary (the result of other pathological conditions, such as obstructions). Infections may be confined to a single site or may spread to other organs or areas. Since the clinical signs of infection may resemble other conditions, recognition of the microbial cause is necessary for proper treatment. In addition, infections that spread to the kidney may cause significant damage or organ failure.

Infections are categorized as being "specific" or "nonspecific." Specific infections are those in which a particular disease is manifested as a result of a particular agent. For example, sexually transmitted diseases (STDs) are specific in the sense that gonorrhea is caused only by *Neisseria gonorrhoeae* and urinary tuberculosis by *Mycobacterium tuberculosis*. Nonspecific infections are diseases in which the pathology or manifestation may be similar but in which the symptoms may be caused by any of a variety of bacteria. For example, common causes of nonspecific urinary infection include *Escherichia coli* (*E. coli*) and members of the genera *Proteus* and *Staphylococcus*.

The most common cause of urinary tract infections is *E. coli*, a natural colon bacillus. Secondary problems may also result from specific agents. For example, members of the genus *Proteus* produce urease, an enzyme capable of splitting urea to form ammonia. The result is a rise in pH, an alkaline condition which may cause precipitation of magnesium or calcium salts and subsequent stone formation.

The specific physical manifestation of the infection is generally related to the site within the urinary tract. Urethritis, accompanied by reduced or painful urination, often results from STDs. Infection may spread as far up as the kidney, with resulting pyelonephritis. Both *E. coli* and STDs are common causes, though other bacteria may also cause similar types of infections. Proper diagnosis of bacterial infections generally requires the isolation and identification of the organism, if possible, and the ruling out of other possible causes of the symptoms (for example, diabetes). The agent may be isolated from pus, from urine, or through the insertion of a needle into the lesion itself. Treatment usually involves antimicrobials (antibiotics) suited to the particular etiological agent. Abscesses, particularly those in the kidney, may require surgical drainage. If the abscess is too large or does not respond to treatment, then nephrectomy (the surgical removal of a kidney) may be necessary.

Damage from external sources may also result in injury to the urinary tract. Depending on the damage, surgical repair or realignment of the urethra, bladder, or ureters may be necessary. Observations through the use of X rays, cystograms, or urethrograms are routinely used for such assessment.

PERSPECTIVE AND PROSPECTS

The understanding of urine formation and excretion had its roots in the work of the Roman physician

Galen during the second century C.E. Though observations had been carried out before this period, it remained unclear whether the source of urine was the kidney or the bladder. Galen settled the issue by tying off the ureters in animals, demonstrating that no urine would be found below the stricture; urine formation began in the kidney.

Urology as a branch of medicine, and indeed clinical interest in urine formation, arguably began in the early decades of the nineteenth century. In 1827, English physician Richard Bright described a form of chronic nephritis, now called Bright's disease, in which progressive kidney failure generally resulted in the death of the individual. Bright demonstrated that as a result of kidney failure, instead of urine being secreted from the body, its constituents are retained in body fluids. It was also in 1827 that German chemist Friedrich Wöhler chemically synthesized urea, the first demonstration of the synthesis of an organic compound from inorganic materials.

Carl Ludwig, beginning in 1844, attempted to explain urine formation on the basis of a purely physical process. Ludwig suggested the hydrostatic pressure of the blood is sufficiently high that a protein-free filtrate is forced through the kidney glomeruli, followed by passage through the tubules, and ultimately into the ureters. The first definitive work on urine secretion was a 1917 monograph *The Secretion of Urine*, by Arthur Robertson Cushny. Cushny believed—and he was subsequently proved to be essentially correct in this portion of his hypothesis—that urine secretion involves both an active and a passive process: mechanical filtration and movement through the urinary tract, and active tubular reabsorption of most nutrients before the liquid leaves the kidney. (The mechanics of Cushny's reabsorption were less than accurate, however, and were later refined by others.)

The development of noninvasive techniques for the elimination of stones and improved surgical methods for urinary diversion marked much of the progress in urology in the 1970's and 1980's. Extracorporeal shock-wave lithotripsy (ESWL), the use of ultrasonic vibration for the disintegration of stones, eliminated the need for the surgical removal of these obstructions in most cases. The use of ureterosigmoidostomy (implantation of the ureter into the intestinal tract) had dated to the nineteenth century. It was replaced with alternate methods of bladder augmentation. The ureter itself could be replaced with segments of intestinal ileum, or it could be joined to the other ureter (ureteroureterostomy).

—*Richard Adler, Ph.D.*

See also Abdomen; Bed-wetting; Catheterization; Chlamydia; Circumcision, male; Cystectomy; Cystitis; Cystoscopy; Dialysis; *E. coli* infection; Endoscopy; Fluids and electrolytes; Genital disorders, female; Genital disorders, male; Geriatrics and gerontology; Gonorrhea; Hydrocelectomy; Hypospadias repair and urethroplasty; Incontinence; Infertility in males; Kidney disorders; Kidney transplantation; Kidneys; Laser use in surgery; Lithotripsy; Nephrectomy; Nephritis; Nephrology; Nephrology, pediatric; Pediatrics; Pelvic inflammatory disease (PID); Penile implant surgery; Prostate cancer; Prostate gland; Prostate gland removal; Reproductive system; Schistosomiasis; Sex change surgery; Sexual differentiation; Sexual dysfunction; Sexually transmitted diseases; Sterilization; Stone removal; Stones; Syphilis; Testicular surgery; Transplantation; Ultrasonography; Urethritis; Urinalysis; Urinary disorders; Urinary system; Urology, pediatric; Vasectomy; Warts.

FOR FURTHER INFORMATION:

Chisholm, Geoffrey D., and William R. Fair, eds. *Scientific Foundations of Urology.* 3d ed. Chicago: Year Book Medical, 1990. A detailed description of urology. Portions of the book are for the specialist, but numerous illustrations make this a useful reference for the layperson.

Stamm, W. E., and T. M. Hooton. "Current Concepts: Management of Urinary Tract Infections in Adults." *New England Journal of Medicine* 329 (October 28, 1993): 1328-1334. This journal article provides a thorough description of the types and management of urinary tract diseases. A clinical review, but much of the material is appropriate for anyone with an interest in the subject.

Tanagho, Emil A., and Jack W. McAninch, eds. *Smith's General Urology.* 15th ed. Norwalk, Conn.: Appleton and Lange, 2000. A text within the Appleton and Lange series of medical publications. An outstanding overview of kidney structure and function.

Wallace, Robert A., Gerald P. Sanders, and Robert J. Ferl. *Biology: The Science of Life.* 4th ed. New York: HarperCollins, 1996. Contains a nice section on the excretory system. Provides clear illustrations and a text which is concise and without clinical details. A good introduction to the subject.

UROLOGY, PEDIATRIC
SPECIALTY

ANATOMY OR SYSTEM AFFECTED: Abdomen, bladder, genitals, kidneys, reproductive system, urinary system

SPECIALTIES AND RELATED FIELDS: Microbiology, neonatology, nephrology, pediatrics, urology

DEFINITION: The treatment and/or surgical correction of disorders of the urinary tract and associated sexual organs in infants and children.

KEY TERMS:

congenital defect: an anatomic defect present at birth; it is not necessarily hereditary

renal: pertaining to the kidneys

SCIENCE AND PROFESSION

The pediatric urologist, who is usually a urologic surgeon, has received extra training in urological procedures on infants and children. The full course of training for this type of surgeon requires a medical degree followed by two years of general surgery training. The physician then undergoes four years of urology residency and two additional years of training on pediatric cases.

The urinary system is the group of organs responsible for filtering waste chemicals from the blood and excreting them in the urine. It begins in the back of the mid-abdomen with the two kidneys, left and right. As blood passes through the kidneys, water and chemicals are filtered, concentrated, and collected in the central portion of each kidney. This urine is then transported through the ureters, long, thin tubes that run from each kidney to the bladder in the pelvis. Urine is then eliminated from the body through the urethra, which opens in the female's vulva or at the tip of the male's penis.

The pediatric urologist is particularly skilled in the repair of congenital deformities of the urinary tract and in the long-term management of the urinary disorders of childhood. Defects of the urinary tract may be present congenitally. Rarely, the bladder may develop in a defect of the abdominal wall, appearing inside-out at birth. External genitalia that are abnormal in function or appearance may require surgical correction. Males may have an abnormally positioned opening of the urethra. The testes may not be properly positioned in the scrotum. The female urethra may open in an abnormal place, such as the vagina. Such congenital defects may be corrected or improved by urologic surgery.

Many of these abnormalities may lead to frequent urinary tract infections or to backward pressure in the urinary system, eventually damaging the sensitive kidneys. The damage may be severe enough to cause renal failure and the need for dialysis or kidney transplantation.

Urologists are often involved in the evaluation and treatment of recurrent urinary tract infections. Although surgery faded in importance for treating these chronic infections by the 1980's, urologists continue to be important participants in the management of these children.

Another pediatric disorder that requires help from the pediatric urologist is neurogenic bladder. The nerves that control bladder sensations and function come from the spinal cord, leaving the spinal canal in its lowest, sacral region. Spinal cord damage anywhere above this level, because of injury or congenital defects, can result in damage to these nerves. Consequently, the child has no sensation of bladder filling or urination. Also, the muscles of the bladder wall and the sphincter, both of which permit and control urination, develop uncoordinated contractions. As a result, the bladder retains urine between urinations. This urine repeatedly becomes infected, with eventual damage to the bladder, the ureters, and, most important, the kidneys. The pediatric urologist uses a variety of medications and surgical procedures to treat this serious disorder, in an attempt to avoid permanent renal damage.

Family practitioners and pediatricians perform routine circumcisions on newborn males. If routine circumcision is not performed in the first month of life, a pediatric urologist is generally consulted to perform the procedure if it is needed later.

DIAGNOSTIC AND TREATMENT TECHNIQUES

Pediatric urologists usually practice in large cities, often at universities or children's hospitals. Their day typically is divided between the operating room and the clinic. In the clinic, urinary tract disorders are evaluated and treated medically. Surgery is scheduled when it is indicated or when medical treatment fails. The surgical procedures are often quite difficult. Sometimes, multiple procedures are required to remedy a complicated abnormality. The goal is to achieve as near to normal appearance and function of the affected organs as possible.

Common laboratory tests used by the pediatric urologist include complete blood counts, chemistry tests of renal function, and examination of the urine. Urine examination, called urinalysis, involves two steps, which are usually performed by a laboratory technician. First, a plastic strip impregnated with chemicals is dipped in the urine to test for acidity, concentration, sugar, protein, and other compounds. Then, after being concentrated in a centrifuge, the urine specimen is examined microscopically to detect clues of urinary tract disease, such as white and red blood cells, bacteria, and crystals of excreted compounds. If there is suspicion of a urinary tract infection, a small volume of urine is placed on a culture medium to allow the growth of any bacteria that might be present. Normal urine should be sterile. A number of imaging studies, such as renal ultrasonography, bladder X rays, and intravenous pyelography, help assess the urinary tract's anatomy and function.

Pediatric urologists also perform cystoscopy, the examination of the bladder interior with a scope passed through the urethra. Stones of the kidney or bladder, although rare in children, may require removal using the cystoscope or a wire basket passed through it into one of the ureters.

PERSPECTIVE AND PROSPECTS

General urologists have always performed urologic surgery on children. With the increasing technical complexity of many of these procedures, however, the Society for Pediatric Urology was formed in the 1960's to advance the specialty. Pediatric urology fellowships were developed in the 1970's.

A major challenge for the specialty has been to correct congenital anomalies in such a way as to result in normal urinary and, as an adult, normal sexual function for the patient. Improved techniques, including microsurgery, point to increasing success.

—*Thomas C. Jefferson, M.D.*

See also Abdomen; Bed-wetting; Catheterization; Circumcision, male; Cystitis; Cystoscopy; Dialysis; *E. coli* infection; Endoscopy; Fluids and electrolytes; Hydrocelectomy; Hypospadias repair and urethroplasty; Incontinence; Kidney disorders; Kidney transplantation; Kidneys; Nephrectomy; Nephritis; Nephrology; Nephrology, pediatric; Pediatrics; Reproductive system; Schistosomiasis; Sexual differentiation; Surgery, pediatric; Testicular surgery; Transplantation; Ultrasonography; Urethritis; Urinalysis; Urinary disorders; Urinary system; Urology.

FOR FURTHER INFORMATION:

Baskin, Laurence S., Barry A. Kogan, and John W. Duckett, eds. *Handbook of Pediatric Urology.* Philadelphia: Lippincott-Raven, 1997. This convenient handbook is an accessible, reliable guide to the diagnosis and treatment of urologic disorders in infants, children, and adolescents. In an outline format that is ideal for quick reference, the book provides complete information on the full range of urologic problems seen in pediatric patients.

Oski, Frank A., ed. *Principles and Practice of Pediatrics.* 3d ed. Philadelphia: J. B. Lippincott, 1999. Contains many good descriptions and illustrations of different stages of development, various disorders common in children, and several treatments for these disorders.

UTERINE CANCER. *See* CERVICAL, OVARIAN, AND UTERINE CANCERS.

Vaccination. *See* **Immunization and vaccination.**

Vagotomy

Procedure

Anatomy or system affected: Gastrointestinal system, nerves, nervous system, stomach

Specialties and related fields: Gastroenterology, general surgery, neurology, nutrition

Definition: The surgical cutting of the vagus nerve or nerves as part of the treatment for gastric ulcers.

Indications and Procedures

The vagus nerves, the longest nerves in the body, pass from the head through the neck, chest, and abdominal regions. They regulate such processes as speech, coughing, swallowing, heart rate and the hunger sensation. Branches of the vagus nerve also stimulate gastric acid secretions and gastric movements.

Vagotomy is generally carried out in conjunction with treatments for gastric (stomach) and duodenal (intestinal) ulcers. Such peptic ulcers are characterized by the loss of mucous membranes in regions exposed to such stomach secretions as hydrochloric acid and the digestive enzyme pepsin. Mild ulcers may heal on their own, but chronic ulceration may result in significant damage or scarring to the stomach or intestinal wall. In addition to the pain and discomfort associated with an ulcer, under some circumstances the ulcer may become cancerous. While the formation of peptic ul-

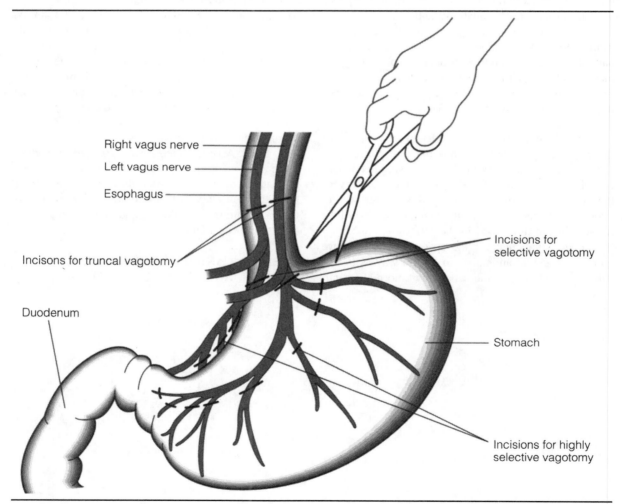

Vagotomy, the severing of the vagus nerve, is a radical treatment for chronic acid reflux, in which gastric juice backs up into the esophagus.

cers is poorly understood, it is known that acid secretion by the stomach can aggravate the condition.

Since the vagus nerve serves to stimulate acid secretions by the parietal cells of the stomach, cutting of the nerve is an effective way to reduce such secretions. Since cutting of the vagus nerve will also reduce or eliminate peristalsis, the rhythmic contraction of muscle which forces food through the stomach, additional procedures are often carried out in combination with vagotomy. For example, an artificial opening between the stomach and small intestine may be created (gastroenterostomy) in order to allow the food to move directly from the stomach to the intestine without the necessity of stomach peristalsis.

The specific region of the vagus nerve on which the vagotomy will be carried out depends on the site of the ulcer. For example, in the case of a duodenal ulcer, the most common form of ulcer, the branch innervating the parietal area of the stomach is severed, reducing the amount of acid produced by the cells in that outer portion of the stomach. Recovery is similar to that for any other general surgical procedure. Medication is provided for pain, and food is reintroduced gradually.

—*Richard Adler, Ph.D.*

See also Digestion; Enzymes; Gastroenterology; Gastrointestinal disorders; Gastrointestinal system; Nervous system; Neurology; Peristalsis; Sympathectomy; Ulcer surgery; Ulcers.

FOR FURTHER INFORMATION:

Carlson, Anton J., Victor Johnson, and H. Mead Cavert. *The Machinery of the Body.* 5th rev. ed. Chicago: University of Chicago Press, 1961.

McMinn, R. M. H., and R. T. Hutchings. *Color Atlas of Human Anatomy.* 4th ed. St. Louis: Mosby Year Book, 1998.

Tortora, Gerard A., and Sandra R. Grabowski. *Principles of Anatomy and Physiology.* 9th ed. New York: John Wiley & Sons, 2000.

VARICOCELE REMOVAL. *See* TESTICULAR SURGERY.

VARICOSE VEIN REMOVAL
PROCEDURE
ANATOMY OR SYSTEM AFFECTED: Blood vessels, circulatory system, legs

SPECIALTIES AND RELATED FIELDS: General surgery, plastic surgery, vascular medicine

DEFINITION: A surgical procedure that is used to rid the body of swollen blood vessels.

INDICATIONS AND PROCEDURES

Varicose veins are caused by an expansion of a superficial vein that is associated with incompetence of the valves within the vein. Conditions such as pregnancy and tumors that increase intra-abdominal pressure contribute to varicose vein formation. Initial treatment involves compression with support stockings.

Sclerotherapy is a more invasive treatment option. In this technique, several injections of a small amount of a solution are injected into the affected vessels over an extended period of time. This solution irritates and destroys the inner lining of the blood vessel. The vein subsequently ceases to carry blood, and circulation is improved by the elimination of this diseased blood vessel. Each vessel usually requires one to six treatments at an interval of three to four weeks. Although the procedure is relatively painless, the fading of vessels is a slow process that can take one to six months.

The traditional method of treating varicose veins is surgery, which is usually performed on an outpatient basis. The most common site of varicose veins is in the lower extremities. The varicose veins are marked out on the surface of the leg. The leg is prepared with iodine and draped from the groin to the toes. A local anesthetic is injected in the skin overlying the ends of the varicose veins. A transverse incision is made over each end. The most distant (distal) end is freed, and a suture is tied around the vein. The surgeon must take care to avoid nearby sensory nerves. The near (proximal) end of the vein is similarly located and tied off. The vein is then cut, and a thin wire is passed from the distal to the proximal incision. A bullet-shaped stripper is tied to the wire; the vein is secured to the stripper. The stripper is slowly pulled out, removing the varicose vein. If a branch prevents the vein from moving, an incision is made, a suture is placed around the branch, and the branch is cut.

After the stripper passes through the entire vein, the varicosity has been removed. The path of the vein is then compressed with warm towels for several minutes to stop small branches from bleeding. Other marked branches are removed. The incisions are closed with sutures or tape. Dressings are placed over the path of the vein, and the leg is wrapped from the toe to groin with rolled, soft gauze and elastic bandages. The patient is instructed to walk but not to sit for prolonged periods of time for at least two days.

Several newer and less invasive techniques for treating varicose veins include radio frequency ablation, ambulatory phlebectomy, laser surgery, and intense pulsed light therapy. Radio frequency ablation or closure is a nonsurgical technique that uses heat in the form of radio frequency energy to collapse and seal varicose veins. The problem vein is essentially shut down, and other, healthy veins take over the blood flow. This procedure is much less invasive than vein stripping. In the closure technique, a thin catheter (flexible tube) is inserted into the vein through a small opening. The catheter delivers the radio frequency energy to the vein wall, causing it to heat up and seal shut. The vein is eliminated by placing the catheter in the lower portion of the vein and then advancing the catheter up the vein using ultrasound guidance. There is no bleeding. After this one-day procedure, patients with little trauma can ambulate more quickly and wear compression dressings for a shorter period of time than in traditional vein stripping.

Ambulatory phlebectomy is a minimally invasive technique in which a varicose vein is removed through small punctures or stab incisions along the path of the vein. Through these tiny holes, the surgeon uses a surgical hook to remove the varicose vein.

In laser surgery, a high intensity laser beam focuses a single wavelength of light at a tiny point on the vein. The light heats the vein but passes through the skin with only minimal surface damage. The underlying vein, however, is damaged by the heat and is then slowly reabsorbed by the body over a period of a few weeks. As opposed to laser surgery, intense pulsed light therapy focuses a broad spectrum of light in a range of wavelengths that are adjustable through the

use of filters and computer-guided parameters of energy delivery. This adjustability allows the physician to customize precisely the characteristics of the light energy according to the needs of each patient, thereby minimizing damage to surrounding tissue and reducing recovery time.

USES AND COMPLICATIONS

Nonabsorbable sutures are removed after a week during a postoperative visit to the surgeon; elastic bandages are used for at least two weeks. Medication for pain may be needed for two to four days. The patient is instructed to walk increasing distances over the next few weeks. Patients who walk rarely experience complications.

PERSPECTIVE AND PROSPECTS

The prevention of varicose veins is preferable to surgical removal. Removing excess weight, exercising, and avoiding articles of clothing that constrict the top of the thighs will help. Varicose veins affect men as well as women, although they are more common among the latter.

—*L. Fleming Fallon, Jr., M.D., Ph.D., M.P.H.;*
updated by Genevieve Slomski, Ph.D.

See also Circulation; Lower extremities; Plastic surgery; Varicose veins; Vascular medicine; Vascular system.

FOR FURTHER INFORMATION:

Cranley, Jack J. *Peripheral Vascular Diseases.* Vol. 11 in *Vascular Surgery.* Hagerstown, Md.: Harper & Row, 1975.

Hobbs, J. T. *The Treatment of Venous Disorders: A Comprehensive Review of Current Practice in the Management of Varicose Veins and the Post-*

The Stripping of Varicose Veins

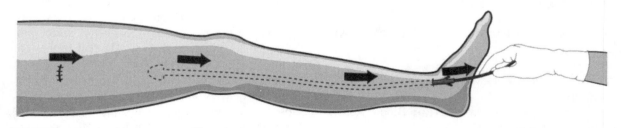

Varicose veins, which are identified by their characteristic swollen appearance, usually occur in the legs; although they are not harmful, many patients wish to have them stripped for cosmetic reasons.

Thrombotic Syndrome. Philadelphia: J. B. Lippincott, 1977.

Sabiston, David C., Jr., ed. *Textbook of Surgery*. 16th ed. Philadelphia: W. B. Saunders, 2001.

VARICOSE VEINS

DISEASE/DISORDER

ANATOMY OR SYSTEM AFFECTED: Blood vessels, circulatory system

SPECIALTIES AND RELATED FIELDS: Cardiology, plastic surgery, vascular medicine

DEFINITION: The distension of superficial veins, usually affecting the legs and causing the appearance of twisted, swollen, blue veins, especially on the backs of the calves.

The main task of normal leg veins is to return blood to the heart and lungs. This is difficult because the blood must be pushed upward, against the constant force of gravity. The force that propels the blood up the leg comes from the contraction of the calf muscles surrounding the deep veins that occurs during the act of walking. This forward momentum is quickly lost as gravity pulls the blood back down; however, one-way valves attached to the inside of the vein wall allow blood to pass up the leg freely, then close before the blood can be pulled back down. With each step taken, the column of blood moves up the leg until it eventually reaches the heart.

The system works well until one of the valves fails. Valves may fail because of congenital defect or because of damage from venous thrombosis (blood clots in the veins of the leg). As one ages, long periods of standing or straining eventually cause even normal veins to become stretched out and dilated, causing the valve leaflets to close improperly. When the vein valves do not close correctly, blood leaks backward, placing extra pressure on the valve beneath it. This increased pressure causes the vein to become dilated and twisted. Such veins are said to be "varicose." If this vein is near the skin, they will bulge out and become visible. These unsightly veins become more pronounced while standing and disappear or become less noticeable when lying down.

Once damaged, the valve cannot repair itself. The increased pressure continues to damage valve after valve until the small bump eventually becomes a large, bluish rope. Varicose veins are frequently accompanied by an aching sensation or a feeling of heaviness in the legs. These symptoms are aggravated by sitting or standing. People who must be on their feet all day usually experience severe discomfort. As the condition worsens, the legs and feet swell. These symptoms, which are often absent upon arising from bed in the morning, usually become more severe as the day progresses.

Although varicose veins are embarrassing and sometimes painful, they are not always a serious condition. Most people experience only minor inconvenience from them. If allowed to progress, however, varicose veins lead to more serious conditions. One of the most common—and most serious—of these complications is a blood clot within the varicose vein. As long as blood is moving quickly in a vessel, it is very difficult for it to clot. When a vein becomes varicose, the dilated portion of the vein allows blood to pool. If blood stagnates, it can become a solid mass of blood called a thrombus, or a blood clot. This blood clot may continue to grow up the vein. It can fill the entire vein from the foot to the groin and enter the deep veins of the leg.

A clot in a deep vein is a potentially life-threatening condition, as it may break loose, pass through the heart, and lodge in the arteries that take blood to the lungs. This condition is referred to as a pulmonary embolism. If this happens, and the blood clot is small, the patient experiences shortness of breath and chest pain. If the clot that breaks loose is big and lodges in a larger lung artery, it can result in sudden death. Blood clots limited to the superficial veins (near the skin) are far less likely to break loose and result in a major pulmonary embolism. The symptoms of clot in the superficial veins are pain and redness directly over the vein involved. The varicose vein may also become hard. This is called a superficial cord. As the clot grows, the redness, pain, and cord move up the leg. This is a serious condition and requires immediate medical attention.

Other complications associated with varicose veins relate to the impact of having increased venous pressure in the legs over a long period of time. When the valves are working, the pressure in the tissue at the ankle is kept at a low level. When varicose veins are severe, the pressure in the tissue becomes so high that blood flow to the skin decreases. If this occurs over a long period of time, the skin becomes discolored and hardens. Ultimately, the skin breaks down, and venous ulcers occur. These open, weeping sores can become infected and become a chronic problem.

TREATMENT AND THERAPY

Minor varicose veins are managed quite effectively—if caught early—with well-fitting elastic compression stockings. These place pressure over the superficial

---

Varicose Veins

Blood flow
Valve

Blood flow
Valve failure

Varicose vein

Backflow creates bulge under valve

In normal veins, the wings of the valves shut completely, preventing backflow of blood; in varicose veins, backflow creates a bulge in the vein that leads to the characteristic appearance of branched blue veins on the legs.

---

veins, giving them support and preventing additional damage to them. This also forces blood into the deep veins. Assuming the deep veins have functioning valves in them, this provides relief and slows progression of the problem. Another popular approach is to surgically remove the damaged vein. This operation, called stripping, removes the veins with damaged valves, forcing blood to go through healthy veins. This can resolve the symptoms of varicose veins altogether. However, other veins may eventually become varicose.

Another intervention to get rid of varicose veins is injection therapy, or sclerotherapy, in which the patient is injected with a material that irritates the varicose vein, causing a clot to form in it. The clot is carefully controlled so that it stays only in the vein being treated. The clot attaches to the vein wall, causing the vein to shrink. This shrinking of the vein makes it seem to disappear. Sclerotherapy is not appropriate in more serious cases of varicose veins.

PERSPECTIVE AND PROSPECTS

Although varicose veins can occur at any time, they are particularly predominant among the elderly; 50 percent of all individuals can expect to develop varicose veins by the age of fifty.

Nothing can be done to change congenital or inherited factors that cause varicose veins. Simple measures, however, can prevent the development of varicose veins before they occur or can slow their progression once they have developed. These preventive measures all have a common theme: avoiding long periods of sitting or standing and keeping the calf muscle active. Doctors advise people who must sit or stand for any length of time to flex and relax their calf muscles by pulling their feet up and pushing them back down. This keeps the blood moving and keeps it from pooling. Other measures include breaking up long periods of inactivity by walking a few minutes every hour, elevating the legs from time to time, and wearing loose clothing that does not restrict blood flow. Some doctors also recommend eating a high-fiber diet since some varicose vein problems result from straining during difficult bowel movements.

—*Steven R. Talbot, R.V.T.*

See also Circulation; Embolism; Lower extremities; Plastic surgery; Thrombosis and thrombus; Varicose vein removal; Vascular medicine; Vascular system; Venous insufficiency.

FOR FURTHER INFORMATION:
Kumar, Vinay, Ramzi S. Cotran, and Stanley L. Robbins, eds. *Basic Pathology*. 6th ed. Philadelphia: W. B. Saunders, 1997.
Sabiston, David C., Jr., ed. *Textbook of Surgery: The Biological Basis of Modern Surgical Practice*. 16th ed. Philadelphia: W. B. Saunders, 2001.
Wyngaarden, James, et al., eds. *Cecil Textbook of Medicine*. 21st ed. Philadelphia: W. B. Saunders, 2000.

VASCULAR MEDICINE
SPECIALTY

ANATOMY OR SYSTEM AFFECTED: Blood vessels, circulatory system, lymphatic system

SPECIALTIES AND RELATED FIELDS: Cardiology, family practice, hematology

DEFINITION: The diagnosis and management of diseases of the arteries, veins, and lymphatic system, exclusive of the heart and lungs.

KEY TERMS:

aneurysm: an abnormal area of an artery (or, less commonly, vein) which enlarges for a variety of reasons and produces a focal ballooning

atherosclerosis: also known as hardening of the arteries; a nonspecific term for the buildup of fatty material in the wall of any artery; over time, this buildup can obstruct the flow of blood through the artery and lead to adverse consequences in the organ it supplies

bypass graft: a surgical procedure that reroutes blood around an obstruction, usually caused by atherosclerosis; the "new" artery can be either plastic or constructed from an expendable, healthy section of vein in another part of the patient's body

embolus: any particle in the arterial or venous system that travels with the flow of blood and eventually lodges in the lungs, brain, or other organ or blood vessel

endarterectomy: a surgical procedure during which an artery is opened and the atherosclerotic material is manually removed, effectively cleaning out the artery and restoring more normal blood flow

ischemia: a state of blood deprivation of any organ in the body; ischemia may occur as a result of atherosclerosis in the main artery which supplies the organ, decreasing the amount of blood that can reach the organ

plaque: the fatty material composed of cholesterol, degenerating cells, and proteinaceous substances that can build up in the wall of any artery

thrombosis: the act of complete clotting of an artery or vein, through which no blood can then flow

SCIENCE AND PROFESSION

Vascular medicine, especially peripheral vascular surgery, has become an important specialty of general surgery. In the past, general surgeons performed surgery on the arteries and veins, but technical advances have led to the creation of vascular surgery as a field of its own.

Western society has produced an older population because of its high level of primary care, but with this older population comes the ravages of atherosclerosis. The modern lifestyle is ideally suited to the formation of atherosclerosis in many arteries as a result of cigarette smoking, stress and high blood pressure, a fatty diet, and a sedentary lifestyle. Peripheral vascular surgeons can contribute in a positive way and help many patients with these diseases. This can be in the form of stroke prevention, the restoration of blood flow to a leg that might otherwise not be saved, and occasionally the saving of a life through repair of a ruptured aortic aneurysm.

One of the most common arteries affected by atherosclerosis is the carotid artery in the neck. This artery branches high in the neck near the jawline. One branch continues up into the brain, supplying a large part of the area that controls motor and sensory function. For some reason, presently unknown, atherosclerosis tends to occur at areas of branching arteries; the carotid bifurcation is no exception. The buildup of material in this location is especially hazardous, because small pieces of the material, called emboli, can break off the arterial wall, travel up the artery, and lodge in the brain. When an embolus lodges in the small arteries of the brain, it blocks the flow of blood to the area of brain tissue supplied by those arteries. This results in ischemia—less blood flow—and the body functions controlled by that part of the brain may be altered. If the ophthalmic artery is involved, then blindness can ensue. If the middle cerebral artery is involved, then symptoms of motor and sensory dysfunction—such as abnormal sensation, numbness, weakness, or paralysis of one side of the body—can occur. Fortunately, very small emboli often do not cause permanent loss of neurological function, and a complete recovery is possible. They are, however, warning signs that atherosclerotic debris resides in the carotid artery, and if treatment is not begun, a permanent stroke might occur if the brain tissue is irreversibly damaged. If a permanent stroke occurs, there is a loss of some neurologic function and patients may be unable to see to their own daily needs. They also may need extensive and expensive rehabilitation. Strokes can be prevented, however, if the warning signs are properly interpreted and acted upon.

Atherosclerosis also results in blockages, or stenoses, in other arteries. Depending on the location of these blockages, a variety of symptoms can result. If the arteries to the intestines are involved, patients can feel abdominal pain which is very difficult to diagnose, given that there are many other causes of abdominal pain (such as ulcer disease, gallbladder problems, and colitis). Intestinal ischemia is somewhat rare and often is not thought of as a cause of abdominal pain. These patients may have to endure this pain for a long period of time and experience severe eating problems, weight loss, and addictions to painkillers. Many patients can be helped with nonsurgical and surgical techniques, however, resulting in the cessation of pain, the regained ability to eat, and thus the maintenance of proper nourishment.

A particularly interesting form of atherosclerotic arterial disease is called renovascular hypertension. In this syndrome, plaque builds up in the renal arteries (kidney arteries). Patients with renovascular hypertension exhibit a type of high blood pressure (hypertension) which is somewhat different from the kind of high blood pressure that effects most of the population. The majority of patients with hypertension have "essential hypertension" for which there is no known cause. For that minority of patients whose hypertension results from pathology in the renal arteries, the blood flow in these arteries is decreased because of atherosclerotic plaques in the arterial walls that severely limit the space through which blood can flow. When this happens, the kidney "senses" this decreased flow and elaborates a variety of chemical hormones that serve to increase the blood flow. These hormones indirectly raise the blood pressure by trying to preserve blood flow to the kidney.

Renovascular hypertension is often difficult to diagnose and to treat medically. Many patients need to take up to five kinds of blood pressure pills to keep their pressure under reasonable control; it is this kind of patient that must be screened for renovascular hypertension. A variety of treatments can be offered to these patients when the diagnosis is made, although the medicines they must take all have significant side effects.

The arteries that supply the muscles and nerves of the extremities also can be affected by atherosclerotic disease. Peculiarly, the upper extremities are usually spared of this disease, whereas the lower extremities are not. The mildest form of lower-extremity disease manifests itself in the form of "claudication" (the term that describes the specific symptoms that develop in an ischemic limb). Most of the time there are no symptoms when a patient is at rest, but when the patient undergoes the physical stress of walking or other exercise, pain develops in the limb in certain areas that correspond to the areas of muscle tissue supplied by the blocked artery. A characteristic pain syndrome develops after a certain amount of exercise and repeats itself regularly. The pain stops after exercise, and this cessation of pain also follows a pattern.

Claudication is the classic example of arterial occlusive disease. If the disease is severe enough, it may cause resting pain. Such patients have profound ischemia of their leg(s), which is limb-threatening and requires intervention. People afflicted with ischemia of the leg have difficulty in healing small scrapes and cuts on the feet, which may turn into large lesions that do not heal. If these lesions become secondarily infected, they can also become limb-threatening and result in amputation. In many patients, however, amputation can be avoided by timely intervention with either surgery or other techniques.

A rather curious phenomenon occurs in some patients whereby there is a focal dilatation of a portion of an artery. The mechanism by which this occurs is largely unknown, but it may be related in some way to the atherosclerotic process. Instead of a buildup of debris in the arterial wall resulting in a blockage in the artery, aneurysms have a thinned-out wall. They enlarge over time and can cause problems. They may clot off entirely or be a source of emboli giving rise to problems further down the arterial tree. The most devastating complication of an aneurysm, however, is acute rupture. Laplace's law of hemodynamics states that wall tension in a tube of fluid is related to the fourth power of the radius. Accordingly, as an aneurysm enlarges, the wall tension increases in exponential fashion. If rupture does occur, it can lead to rapid blood loss if expert medical and surgical care are not readily available.

Aneurysms can form anywhere in the body, but they most commonly occur in the aorta (the main artery coming out from the heart) directly beneath the umbilicus. Because this location is surgically accessible, repair of these aneurysms is a common operation. In this location, most aneurysms will not cause a problem until they measure approximately 5 centimeters in diameter; at that size, the risk of rupture becomes significant. Smaller aneurysms are usually followed with serial examinations over time, and if they do enlarge, then the appropriate therapy can be instituted. Other, less common areas of aneurysm formation include the splenic, renal, iliac, femoral, and popliteal arteries. Similar complications can ensue with these aneurysms.

The majority of peripheral vascular surgery practice deals with the diseases of the arteries, but venous disease is a very common problem that many physicians in many specialties must address. Patients with simple phlebitis of the superficial veins of the leg usually require no more than supportive care until they feel better, but if the clots are in or extend into the deep veins of the leg, much more aggressive treatment is necessary. A clot in this location has a chance of migrating into the lungs (pulmonary embolus) and can be fatal. Therefore, intensive treatment with intravenous and then oral blood thinners (anticoagulants) is mandatory. There are some patients who then have chronic venous problems because the clots in their legs can damage the valves in the veins. This results in severe pain, swelling, and even ulceration of the legs that can be very difficult to treat.

DIAGNOSTIC AND TREATMENT TECHNIQUES

Many patients who suffer from vascular diseases are not treated with surgery right away. They may ultimately need an operation, but often long periods of time elapse before surgery is undertaken. Nonoperative therapy is often all that is needed to control certain aspects of the patient's symptoms, in the form of cessation of cigarette smoking, lowering of serum cholesterol, or an exercise program. Vascular surgeons provide guidelines for patients who need this sort of therapy.

Atherosclerosis may appear in many ways and affect patients differently. For example, a forty-five-year-old postal carrier complains of pain in the thighs of the legs in the same location whenever he walks more than a few hundred feet. He may have been a heavy smoker for many years, his cholesterol levels may be elevated, and there may be many relatives in his family with "hardening of the arteries." Such a person has a classic case of claudication resulting from atherosclerotic occlusive disease of the arteries

that supply the thigh muscles. The patient has several options. Other causes of leg pain must be ruled out, such as nerve problems or back conditions, but when this is accomplished, the field of vascular surgery can help this patient maintain his lifestyle. If the patient would like to investigate options for intervention, an arteriogram is performed next. In this procedure, specially trained radiologists insert a small tube into the arteries and take pictures after dye has been injected. This allows an exact replica of the patient's arterial anatomy to be projected in two dimensions. The arteriogram allows the surgeons and radiologists to determine the best course of action for this patient.

Some atherosclerotic plaques are in particular locations that may allow their treatment with balloon angioplasty rather than open surgery. In this procedure, again performed by trained radiologists or some vascular surgeons, a catheter with a balloon at its end is inserted into the artery and the balloon is inflated in the area of the offending plaque in an effort to open the clogged artery. This procedure is often performed on the arteries of the heart, but it can also be performed on other arteries: those of the kidneys, intestines, and legs. A vascular surgeon usually oversees the care of the patient, as not all the balloon procedures are completely successful and open surgery is sometimes necessary. Open surgery might include a bypass graft with a woven or knitted prosthetic artery or a graft made with an expendable vein in the patient's leg, utilizing the same vein as for heart bypass surgery. The postal worker described above could be a candidate for a balloon procedure or a surgical bypass graft, but in either case he should be restored to almost normal walking capability and be able to return to his job.

Another common scenario might involve a more serious situation. A person may have an open sore on his foot that has been there for more than six months and is getting bigger, perhaps infected. This person may also be a heavy smoker with cholesterol problems and severe diabetes mellitus. He has not walked more than a block in the past few years because his feet hurt when he does. His problem may relate to poor blood flow to his legs and feet, and the diabetes certainly does not help. Before vascular surgery techniques became popular, this patient ultimately would have required an amputation of his leg either below or above the knee. It is physically and emotionally difficult for patients to cope with such a loss: The long, expensive period of rehabilitation includes learning to walk with a prosthetic extremity. This patient would be a good candidate for an arteriogram and would undoubtedly need some surgery. This would most likely be in the form of a bypass graft, which could stretch from the groin all the way to the foot, crossing the knee and the ankle. Ultimately, a successful outcome would be healing of the open sore and control of the infection; the patient would then be able to continue walking with his own leg.

Another situation that might involve vascular surgery is as follows. A patient has a history of deep vein clots following prior major surgery. Treatment consisted of long-term blood thinners, and the patient may have had no major problems since that time. The patient now needs a hip operation, however, and hip operations carry a high risk of blood clot formation in the deep veins of the leg. Because deep-vein thrombosis carries risks of a pulmonary embolus as well as chronic problems in the leg, a vascular surgeon is called upon to help design a program that can prevent these complications from occurring. The usual methods of prophylaxis do not necessarily apply in this patient, and as the patient is labeled "high-risk," it might be most prudent to place a device in the body to catch any pulmonary emboli if they occur. The theory behind this management is that, in the high-risk patient, the formation of blood clots in the legs is almost unavoidable and that the majority of effort should be aimed at preventing the most serious, potentially fatal complication, the pulmonary embolus. In this circumstance, vascular surgeons could place a filter device in the main vein that carries blood to the heart and lungs, which would effectively trap any free-floating emboli that could cause a problem.

PERSPECTIVE AND PROSPECTS

Peripheral vascular surgery has assumed a paramount role in medical practice. By 1900, significant contributions had been made regarding the basic reconstructive techniques needed to sew arteries together. The work of Alexis Carrel in the early twentieth century is considered the most important contribution to the technical art of vascular surgery. He reported the techniques of transplanting organs and sewing arteries together that are still routinely performed. By the 1950's, synthetic materials were introduced as arterial replacements, which became acceptable treatment for many patients.

Nonsurgical techniques for opening blocked arteries and veins to improve blood flow have so far been somewhat disappointing in peripheral vascular surgery, but new techniques are being developed and tested at a rapid pace and may eventually become commonplace. Although technically performing a bypass graft is feasible, the graft cannot approach the durability and performance of a native artery. Research involving the transplantation of human arteries may solve some of these problems and allow more patients to benefit from surgery.

Vascular surgery can benefit large numbers of people simply because of the nature of atherosclerosis. It may be a product of habits, the environment, and/or genetic makeup, but it is widely accepted that as the population ages, more and more people will suffer from diseases that can be helped by vascular surgery, allowing them to maintain lifestyles that are as productive as possible. Basic scientific research of the mechanisms of atherosclerosis may yield important answers and guide new therapies for patients with this disease.

—*Mark Wengrovitz, M.D.*

See also Amputation; Aneurysmectomy; Aneurysms; Angiography; Angioplasty; Arteriosclerosis; Biofeedback; Bleeding; Blood and blood disorders; Bypass surgery; Catheterization; Cholesterol; Circulation; Claudication; Diabetes mellitus; Dialysis; Embolism; Endarterectomy; Exercise physiology; Glands; Healing; Hematology; Hematology, pediatric; Hemorrhoid banding and removal; Hemorrhoids; Histology; Hypercholesterolemia; Hyperlipidemia; Ischemia; Lipids; Lymphatic system; Mitral valve prolapse; Phlebitis; Podiatry; Shunts; Strokes; Systems and organs; Thrombolytic therapy and TPA; Thrombosis and thrombus; Transfusion; Varicose vein removal; Varicose veins; Vascular system; Venous insufficiency.

FOR FURTHER INFORMATION:

Ancowitz, Arthur. *Strokes and Their Prevention: How to Avoid High Blood Pressure and Hardening of the Arteries.* New York: Van Nostrand Reinhold, 1975. Provides useful information on nonpharmacological treatments of vascular disease. Available in most public libraries.

Ernst, Calvin B., and James C. Stanley, eds. *Current Therapy in Vascular Surgery.* 4th ed. St. Louis: Mosby, 2000. This advanced textbook is superbly edited and has contributions by the leaders in the vascular surgical field. Discusses treatments for all vascular disorders.

Krames Communications. *Understanding Carotid Ar-*

tery Problems. Daly City, Calif.: Author, 1988. This pamphlet, often found in doctor's offices, presents an excellent review of carotid artery problems. Written for the general public.

Rutherford, Robert B., ed. *Vascular Surgery.* 5th ed. Philadelphia: W. B. Saunders, 2000. Long considered to be the classic text on vascular surgery by many surgeons, this book provides a wealth of information on all vascular diseases.

VASCULAR SYSTEM

ANATOMY

ANATOMY OR SYSTEM AFFECTED: Blood vessels, circulatory system, legs

SPECIALTIES AND RELATED FIELDS: Cardiology, exercise physiology, hematology, vascular medicine

DEFINITION: The pipeline through which every cell of the body receives oxygen, vitamins, hormones, and the metabolic fuels necessary to sustain life.

KEY TERMS:

arteries: the vessels that carry blood from the heart to all parts of the body

atherosclerosis: the buildup of lipid-containing (fatty) materials beneath or within the inner wall of an artery, which can lead to narrowing or occlusion of the artery

capillaries: minute blood vessels that connect the smallest arteries (arterioles) to the smallest veins (venules); they allow passage of oxygen and nutrients from the arteries into the tissue and passage of waste products from the tissues into the veins

collaterals: small vessels that enlarge to compensate for the obstruction or narrowing of another vessel

heart attack: sudden and permanent damage to a part of the heart muscle as a result of impaired blood flow through the coronary arteries

metabolism: the chemical changes that occur when the body transforms oxygen and nutrients into energy or heat

stroke: permanent damage to part of the brain as a result of impaired blood flow

veins: blood vessels that carry blood from the cells back to the heart

venous thrombosis: the presence of blood clots in the veins, usually in the legs or arms

STRUCTURE AND FUNCTIONS

The vascular system is faced with the enormous task of supplying every cell of the human body with a constant supply of oxygen and nutrients needed to sustain life. This elaborate system circulates more than 2,000 gallons of blood per day through more than 12,000 miles of arteries, veins, and capillaries. Moreover, the job of the vascular system is not done when the nutrients arrive at the cell. After the cell uses the nutrients, waste products that are left over from metabolism must be carried away and disposed of before they damage the cell. For this reason, several kinds of vessels exist within the human body that differ in structure and function. They can be broken into three categories: arteries, veins, and capillaries.

The term "arteries" came from ancient times when arteries were thought to be filled with air. (This misconception evolved because after death much of the blood usually pumped through the arteries had been pumped out, leading scientists of the time to conclude that air, rather than blood, was circulated within them.) Arteries are thick-walled blood vessels that vary in size from about 1 inch in diameter to a fraction of an inch. They carry oxygen-rich blood from the left side of the heart to all parts of the body. The blood circulating within them is usually moving at high velocities and exerts pressure against the artery walls, creating an expansion of the artery during the contraction of the heart. This expansion, called a pulse, can be palpated in areas where the arteries are large and close to the surface of the skin: in the neck (the carotid artery) or in the wrist (the radial artery). The pressure being exerted against the artery varies greatly. A doctor taking a blood pressure reading is measuring this variation in pressure. A blood pressure of 120/80, for example, would mean that the force from the heart is exerting 120 millimeters of mercury pressure against the artery wall while the heart is contracting (the systolic pressure) and 80 millimeters of mercury when the heart is at rest (the diastolic pressure). Clearly, the artery has to be a very strong structure.

Veins, on the other hand, are thin-walled, almost transparent vessels that return blood back to the heart after it has visited the cells. There are far more veins in the body than there are arteries. The blood moving in the veins is under very little pressure and usually is moving quite slowly in comparison to the flow in the arteries. The flow in the veins is slow because most of the force from the contraction of the heart was dissipated when the blood passed through the cell. For this reason, the flow in the veins must be helped along by contraction of the muscles around these blood vessels. For example, with each step, the muscles in the calves of the legs propel the blood in the calf veins upward with great force. For this reason, the calf of the leg is sometimes referred to as the "venous heart." If this pump is not active, blood flow in the veins can stagnate and life-threatening clots can form in the veins.

Another problem for the venous circulation is that its blood is often moving against gravity. If the veins were built like arteries (simple hollow tubes), the blood would flow upward toward the heart with the contraction of the muscles but would fall back down as soon as the contraction stopped. Fortunately, the veins are equipped with one-way valves not found in arteries. These valves open when blood is moving toward the heart and close when blood starts to fall backward. Veins are also different from arteries in that they can expand to several times their normal size. This allows the veins to be used as a storage area for blood. When the body's need for blood is low, such as during a resting state, the veins enlarge and fill with the blood that is not being actively circulated. When the need for blood increases, as during strenuous activity, the stored blood is forced back into active circulation. Because veins have such thin walls and stretch so easily, one might think that they are not as strong as arteries. In reality, veins are strong enough to be used as surgical substitutes for failed arteries and hold up quite well under arterial pressure.

Capillaries are extremely small vessels with very thin walls. These vessels connect the smallest arteries (arterioles) with the smallest veins (venules). Although their size can vary, the average diameter of a capillary is about 8 microns (0.008 millimeter), which is about the size of a single red blood cell. The nutrients carried in the blood pass through tiny pores in the vessel wall directly into the cell, which uses the nutrients to produce energy and heat. During this process, waste products are created that are poisonous to the cell; they must be removed quickly or the cell will die. The waste products then pass from the cell into the capillaries and then into tiny veins that will carry the waste products away.

A trip through the system of arteries, capillaries, and veins—to deliver nutrients to one cell in a calf muscle, for example—would begin in the left ventricle of the heart, where blood is pumped through the aorta (the largest artery) with great force. The aorta has branches that serve the structures of the head and neck (which includes the most important organ—the brain), the upper extremities, the abdomen, and the lower extremities. On this imaginary trip, one passes

through the aortic arch and travels down the main artery in the abdomen called the abdominal aorta. This artery eventually branches into two arteries (at about the level of the navel) that send blood to each leg. This artery continues to branch into smaller and smaller arteries until one reaches the capillaries serving the particular cell of the calf muscle in the leg. Here the nutrients are delivered to the cell. The waste products are dumped back into the capillaries. From the capillaries, one travels into tiny veins called venules. These tiny veins become continually larger until one is finally moving up through a large vein just behind the knee called the popliteal. Soon one is back in the abdomen in the large vein called the vena cava, which enters the heart at the right atrium. The blood then travels through the right ventricle and eventually into another large vessel called the pulmonary artery (the only artery that carries blood that is not oxygenated). This artery leads into the lungs, where the waste products of metabolism are released and exchanged for oxygen. With a new load of oxygen, one travels through the pulmonary veins (the only veins that carry oxygenated blood), into the left atrium of the heart, and into the left ventricle, where the journey began. In a normal person, this entire voyage takes only eighteen to twenty-four seconds.

DISORDERS AND DISEASES

When the vascular system is functioning correctly, all the cells of the body are receiving the right amount of blood at all times. Many problems can arise, however, in the complex functioning of the human organism, and the vasculature must have ways of meeting these challenges. Such problems include the obstruction of vital vessels by plaque formation (a buildup of fatty deposits called atherosclerosis), thrombus (blood clot) formation, and vasospasm (a closing down of a blood vessel in response to cold or trauma). Moreover, some organs in the body cannot survive for more than a few minutes without oxygen before damage occurs. For example, the brain can only survive for a few minutes without oxygen, while the cells in the arms and legs can be deprived of oxygen for a matter of hours without irreversible damage. For this reason, whenever there is a problem the vascular system must be able to set priorities about which systems receive blood flow and which systems do not. When there is a life-threatening problem, the vessels in the arms and legs contract, forcing blood out of the extremities; this allows more flow to reach the brain, where it is most urgently needed. When an artery is narrowed by plaque, the vascular system will compensate by enlarging smaller vessels in the area to help maintain flow. If the artery is totally obstructed, this system of collateral vessels takes over.

While these and other mechanisms work quite well, sudden obstruction or other disease processes involving an artery or vein can result in major problems. The major problems that can result from arterial disease include stroke, myocardial infarction (heart attack), and peripheral artery disease. Problems involving the veins may include deep vein thrombosis, pulmonary embolism, and varicose veins.

A stroke is a condition in which part of the brain is deprived of oxygen long enough to cause permanent damage. The medical term for such an event is a cerebrovascular accident, or CVA. The symptoms may include one-sided weakness or numbness, headache, difficulty in speaking, or transient blindness in one eye. If these symptoms completely resolve within twenty-four hours, the event is referred to as a transient ischemic attack, or TIA. The difference between a TIA and a CVA is that the damage done by the TIA is not permanent. TIAs, however, are often precursors of impending full-blown strokes. Therefore, patients who experience them should see a doctor immediately so that steps can be taken to prevent another, perhaps more severe, episode. The treatment for patients who experience TIA may include surgery to remove plaque buildup from the carotid artery, bypass surgery (in which another vessel is used to bypass a narrowed area), the use of blood-thinning drugs, or the use of antiplatelet drugs (such as aspirin). Rehabilitation, the use of blood-thinning and or antiplatelet drugs, and lifestyle modification are often prescribed for those who have already suffered major strokes.

Myocardial infarction is one of the leading killers in Western societies. A heart attack occurs when blood flow is inadequate to the heart muscle and part of the heart muscle dies. The symptoms include pain in the chest (especially pain that is brought on by exertion), shortness of breath, sweating, nausea, and fatigue. Similar, although usually less severe, symptoms may be present with a condition called angina, in which blood flow to the heart muscle is impaired but there is no permanent damage. Acute treatment for heart attacks can include rest (to reduce additional damage to the heart muscle), treatment with blood-thinning drugs, treatment with drugs that dissolve blood clots,

balloon catheters (to help open narrowed arteries), or coronary bypass surgery.

Peripheral artery disease—the narrowing or blockage of arteries in the arms or legs—is also quite common. Symptoms may include pain in the limb, loss of feeling, coolness, and discoloration; in severe cases, tissue loss may result. This disease process is usually progressive. A patient may first notice pain in the calf of the leg that comes on only with walking and goes away as soon as the exercise stops. This condition, called intermittent claudication, indicates that there is minimal narrowing of the arteries in the leg. As more of the artery narrows, the pain occurs even without exercise. Finally, blood flow to the limb is not sufficient to maintain the cells, and tissue begins to die. Treatment of peripheral artery disease may include medication and exercise (during the early stages) and progress to the surgical bypass of narrowed arteries (in later stages). Sometimes arteries in the extremities become clogged by a thrombus instead of plaque. If this is the case, drugs that dissolve blood clots or surgical operations to remove the clot may be used. If treatment for severe peripheral disease is unsuccessful, amputation may be necessary.

The risk factors for developing arterial disease—of the coronary carotid, or peripheral arteries—include high blood pressure, smoking, diabetes, elevated cholesterol levels, stress, a family history of arterial disease, obesity, and advancing age.

Veins do not develop plaque as do arteries; instead, blood can stagnate and form clots that can obstruct them. When this happens, a condition called venous thrombosis, blood stagnates in the veins behind the clot and a larger clot forms. It is not unusual for clots to fill all the major veins in the leg once this process begins. These clots cause swelling and pain in the leg but do not usually threaten the leg as obstruction of the arteries does. Instead, the danger lies in the possibility of a clot breaking loose and traveling to the lungs. This clot, called a pulmonary embolism, can be fatal. The risk factors for developing venous thrombosis include anything that can slow blood flow in the veins, such as prolonged sitting or standing, a long airplane trip or car trip, a surgical operation, or pregnancy. Injury to the vein can also trigger clots, as can an imbalance of clotting factors in the blood. The best way to prevent venous thrombosis is to keep active.

Another venous problem that strikes as many as one of every four women and one of every five men is a condition most commonly known as varicose veins. The veins become stretched out and elongated to the point where they bulge out when the patient is sitting or standing. Although this is mostly a cosmetic problem, severe cases can lead to blood pooling in the leg and tissue damage.

Perspective and Prospects

The vasculature of the human body has not always been understood, even in recent times. The ancient Egyptians knew about the importance of the heart and the pulse, but this knowledge was not passed on to more modern civilizations. Hippocrates (c. 460- c. 370 B.C.E.) had serious misconceptions about the functions of the circulatory system: He thought that the pulse was caused by movements of the blood vessels. Other great thinkers such as Aristotle and Galen made similar errors in their study of the vascular system, errors that influenced medicine for many years.

In 1628, a doctor in London named William Harvey published a paper introducing his radical theories about how the blood circulates. He changed the way medical people thought about this system by describing it as a closed circuit with blood being forced through it via contractions of the heart. He postulated that blood passed from the arteries into the veins at the cellular level. It was not until the 1660's, when early microscopes were developed, that this theory could be confirmed.

In 1733, a clergyman named Stephen Hales became the first person to measure blood pressure within the arterial system. He inserted a large, hollow glass tube into the neck artery of a horse. To his amazement, the blood rose 9 feet up the tube. This method of measuring blood pressure was not practical, however, and it was not until the late 1800's that the sphygmomanometer was developed to measure blood pressure utilizing blood pressure cuffs and air pressure.

Another pioneer in the understanding of the vascular system was German physician and biologist Rudolf Virchow, who theorized about how blood clots formed in veins. He concluded that clots formed when the blood flow was slowed down, the vein wall was injured, or an imbalance of clotting factors in the blood existed. These observations were astonishingly correct considering that, at this time, many people still thought blood clots in the veins were composed of pus. Understanding of these principles makes possible modern treatments and prevention techniques.

In the late 1800's, modern vascular surgery began with development of techniques to repair blood vessels. By the early 1900's, methods for connecting the ends of vessels with a watertight suture became commonplace. In 1948, a surgeon in Paris took a saphenous vein and used it to bypass a blockage in an artery in the leg. In the 1950's, the technology necessary to support sustained heart surgeries was introduced, and heart surgery has since become routine. Blood vessels can now be surgically repaired, bypassed, or cleaned out. Laser surgery and clot-dissolving drugs are becoming routine.

—*Steven R. Talbot, R.V.T.*

See also Amputation; Aneurysmectomy; Aneurysms; Angiography; Angioplasty; Arteriosclerosis; Biofeedback; Bleeding; Blood and blood disorders; Bypass surgery; Catheterization; Cholesterol; Circulation; Claudication; Diabetes mellitus; Dialysis; Embolism; Endarterectomy; Exercise physiology; Glands; Healing; Hematology; Hematology, pediatric; Hemorrhoid banding and removal; Hemorrhoids; Histology; Hypercholesterolemia; Hyperlipidemia; Ischemia; Lipids; Lymphatic system; Mitral valve prolapse; Phlebitis; Podiatry; Shunts; Strokes; Systems and organs; Thrombolytic therapy and TPA; Thrombosis and thrombus; Transfusion; Varicose vein removal; Varicose veins; Vascular medicine; Venous insufficiency.

For Further Information:

Gray, Henry. *Gray's Anatomy.* Edited by Peter L. Williams et al. 38th ed. New York: Churchill Livingstone, 1999. One of the most complete anatomy reference books available. Contains hundreds of illustrations.

Hershey, Falls B., Robert W. Barnes, and David S. Sumner, eds. *Noninvasive Diagnosis of Vascular Disease.* Pasadena, Calif.: Appleton Davies, 1984. This book, written for medical personnel, may be difficult reading for the layperson. Nevertheless, valuable for its detailed description of the anatomy, physiology, and pathology involved in vascular disease, as well as for its discussion of diagnostic methods.

Kibbe, Constance V. *Standard Textbook of Cosmetology.* Rev. ed. Bronx, N.Y.: Milady, 1989. Although this is a cosmetology textbook, it contains a short and concise chapter on arteries, veins, and capillaries that is very clearly written. Written for a lay audience, this work is an excellent source for gaining a better understanding of the basics of circulation.

VASECTOMY

PROCEDURE

ANATOMY OR SYSTEM AFFECTED: Genitals, reproductive system

SPECIALTIES AND RELATED FIELDS: Family practice, general surgery, urology

DEFINITION: A surgical means of birth control for males which involves the interruption of the tubes that transport sperm to the semen.

KEY TERMS:

ejaculation: the expulsion from a man's erect penis at the time of orgasm of a fluid made up of semen and sperm

elective surgical sterilization: a voluntary operation that is intended to produce permanent birth control

local anesthesia: the injection of medication into the body that renders the immediate area free of pain, allowing surgery in that area to be performed

scrotum: the genital skin sac that holds the testicles and related structures

semen: fluid produced by a man's prostate gland, which makes up 95 percent of the fluid that is ejaculated

sperm: a man's reproductive cells, made in the testicles, they carry the man's genetic traits to a woman's egg, resulting in conception and pregnancy

vas (pl. vasae): the small, muscular tube that carries the sperm from the testicle to the prostate gland

INDICATIONS AND PROCEDURES

The term "vasectomy" describes a minor surgical procedure performed on a man who desires a permanent form of birth control. Vasectomy—which literally means "cutting the tubes"—results in sterilization because it obstructs the passageway through which sperm travel to reach the female ovum. A man's testicles produce both male hormones (that stimulate male characteristics and sex drive) and sperm. A collection of small tubes called the epididymis along each testicle mature and deliver sperm to a single tube called the vas, which is about the width of a spaghetti noodle. Each vas runs through the scrotum, up the groin on each side, and through the wall of the abdomen, ending in a storage area called the seminal vesicle, which is next to the prostate gland near the base of the penis. From there, the sperm mix with semen from the prostate gland and are expelled from the penis during ejaculation.

Vasectomy occludes (closes off) the vas to block the passage of sperm without affecting the important hormonal functions of the testicle. The surgery is done in the first, straight part of the vas, above the testicle and through the skin of the scrotum, making the procedure relatively easy and safe to perform.

Physicians performing vasectomy come from the specialties of urology, family practice, general practice, or general surgery. Since the procedure is relatively simple, in comparison with other surgeries, physicians' expertise usually depends more on specific training and interest in performing vasectomies and following up on the procedure than on their particular specialty training.

Vasectomies are usually done on an outpatient basis, either in a physician's office or in a hospital-based or free-standing ambulatory surgery facility. Local anesthesia of the skin and the vasae is produced by an injection into the scrotum, which can be briefly uncomfortable until the medication has taken its full effect (usually after several seconds). Because of anxiety on the part of many men about having any discomfort in this area, many patients and physicians also choose to use sedation in the form of either tranquilizer pills or an injection for both mental and physical relaxation during vasectomy.

A number of techniques can be used safely and effectively by a physician performing a vasectomy, but the procedure can be thought of in terms of accomplishing three basic goals: The first is anesthesia, or the placement of numbing or freezing medication into the scrotum; the second is to gain access to the vas; and the third is its occlusion to prevent the passage of sperm.

Vasectomy can be made almost completely painless when local anesthesia in the form of medication such as lidocaine is used; this drug is similar to the anesthesia commonly used for dental procedures. By blocking the local nerves that send pain messages to the brain, normally painful procedures can be performed with little or no discomfort. A man having a vasectomy will feel the needle used to inject the medication into the skin and then a brief stinging sensation until it takes effect. The rest of the injection into the vas tubes themselves may or may not cause further discomfort, what some men describe as a pulling sensation.

The standard access procedure that the physician uses can vary with training and experience. It involves making either one incision into the scrotum in the middle of the front side or two incisions, one on either side. The incisions are made after the physician positions the vas directly under the skin, and then the

Vasectomy

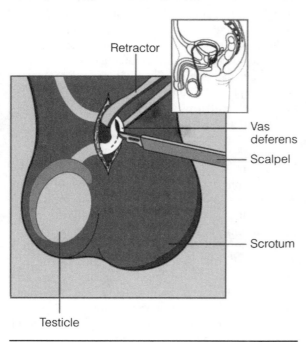

Retractor

Vas deferens

Scalpel

Scrotum

Testicle

The most popular method of sterilization for men is vasectomy, which involves the severing of the vas deferens, the tube that transports sperm from the testes; the inset shows the location of the vas deferens in the male reproductive system.

other layers of tissue are separated to expose the vas itself. After each vas is occluded, the incision, which is between 1 and 1.5 centimeters long, must be closed with stitches, usually the type that dissolve and do not have to be removed.

A refinement of the access procedure, called the "no-scalpel" vasectomy, was introduced into the United States in the late 1980's. It originated in China in 1974, and a study comparing it with a standard technique found a more than 80 percent reduction in postoperative complications. It is being adopted only gradually by United States physicians, however, because performing it requires two simple but specially designed surgical instruments and because some physician retraining is required. Many physicians with experience in the new procedure believe that it should become the new standard for the vasectomy access procedure.

The occlusion of the vas is important because it determines the success of the vasectomy in preventing

pregnancy. The physician can choose to occlude the vas ends by simple tying, folding back and tying, applying small metal clips, or cauterizing (burning with heat or special electrical current). In addition, one of the vas ends can be covered with a layer of the tissue that surrounds it to form a further barrier to sperm. Although all occlusion methods have been effective, cautery of the opening of the vasae may be the most reliable because it depends less on the technical precision of the physician doing the vasectomy than do the other methods, which can fail if applied too loosely or too tightly.

Finally, some physicians perform an open-ended technique, in which the end of the vas coming from the testicle is left open while only the outgoing end is occluded. This is thought to reduce the amount of backed-up sperm that can cause later complications and to make it easier to perform a vasectomy reversal. Some physicians believe, however, that the rate of vasectomy failure is higher with this technique.

Men from all over the world choose to have vasectomy performed, including about half a million Americans every year. Vasectomy has been commonly available in the United States since the 1960's and is the fourth most commonly used birth control method overall, with one in eight women stating that they rely on this contraceptive method.

USES AND COMPLICATIONS

Most physicians make recommendations to the patient about what should be done, or not done, following a vasectomy, including activity restriction, pain control strategies, and follow-up. A period of rest for about forty-eight hours after a vasectomy helps to prevent pain and complications such as postoperative bleeding into the scrotum, which causes swelling. All sexual activity should be avoided for up to a week. Many men find more relief from an ice pack applied to the scrotum for the first few days following the surgery than from any medication, although acetaminophen (such as Tylenol) or mild prescription narcotics are often helpful as well. Aspirin and ibuprofen, although effective for pain, are generally best avoided in the first few days following a vasectomy because they have a blood-thinning effect which may increase the tendency to bleed. Because aspirin has a longer-lasting blood-thinning effect on platelets (the small blood cells that initiate normal blood clotting and stop minor bleeding), it should also not be taken for about ten days prior to the vasectomy.

Follow-up with a physician should be available in case complications occur in the period immediately following the vasectomy. The physician must also check the semen to ensure that no sperm are present. If sperm remain, it may indicate that one or both vasae remain open or have grown back together, meaning that the procedure has failed and the man remains fertile. If there are no sperm in the semen three to six months after the vasectomy, then it is extremely unlikely that a failure can still occur. Most doctors do not recommend any further follow-up unless a problem arises.

Informed consent means that the patient who will undergo a treatment has been given the opportunity to understand the risks and benefits of that treatment. In the case of vasectomy, the risks are pain, complications, the chance that it will fail, and the possibility that there will be a change of heart and that the man will want to father more children. The benefit is having very reliable, safe, and permanent birth control without ongoing costs or effort required.

The complications of vasectomy are best thought of in terms of those occurring early and late. Early complications include infection and hematoma. Infection is fairly uncommon but can include symptoms of pain, swelling, fever, redness, and abnormal drainage from the vasectomy wound. Treatment consists primarily of antibiotic medication. A hematoma is a collection of blood in a localized area such as the scrotum. Blood vessels in the scrotum that are cut or torn during vasectomy and not tied, clipped, or cauterized can ooze a small or large amount of blood. In the worst case, surgery to remove the blood may be considered to relieve pain and pressure. Fortunately, small hematomas resolve without surgery in a few weeks' time, and the more serious ones are rare, probably occurring in far less than 1 percent of vasectomies.

Later complications include problems with the area between the vasectomy incision and the testicles. Because the sperm are blocked from leaving the vas, and therefore the testicle, they can accumulate and cause three possible problems. First, sperm may back up at the site of the vasectomy and form a knot of sperm and inflamed scar tissue known as a sperm granuloma. It can be a painless lump, tender to pressure, or in rare cases it may be painful enough to require surgery to remove it. If swelling occurs because of accumulated sperm along the collecting area between the straight vas and the testicle (called the epididymis), the area can become tender or painful; this is known as congestive epididymitis. If this process extends backward to the testicle, it is known as orchitis. Fortunately, it is also rare for surgical removal of the entire epididymis to be required for relief of pain; sperm production slows in response to the pressure, and the body reabsorbs old sperm, eventually eliminating the pressure. Therefore, it is usually recommended that congestive epididymitis be treated with anti-inflammatory pain relievers such as ibuprofen, as well as with soaking in a warm bath.

Since there are many misconceptions about the risks and complications of vasectomy, it is useful to point out some problems that are not associated with the procedure. The complications of vasectomy are relatively minor and very rarely require hospitalization. Deaths and major surgical complications are largely unheard of. Impotence, loss of sexual drive, and changes in male characteristics such as beard growth, body hair, and voice do not occur. An apparent link between vasectomy and the hardening of the arteries that causes heart attacks has been disproven since the only such study was publicized in the late 1970's. Although a slight statistical association between vasectomy and cancer of the prostate gland was noted in two studies published in 1993, experts do not believe that vasectomy causes or contributes to prostate cancer because there is no reasonable mechanism for it to do so. Many men with milder forms of prostate cancer never die from it, and the statistics can be misleading because men who have seen a doctor for a vasectomy are also more likely to see a doctor for a prostate examination. Therefore, vasectomy may lead not to a greater risk of prostate cancer but to better detection of this disease.

PERSPECTIVE AND PROSPECTS

Vasectomy has been performed to cause sterility since 1925, but its common use for that purpose started in the 1960's. The concepts of birth control and the desirability of limiting family size became increasingly valued in industrialized countries. Some states in the United States removed legal barriers to sterilization around this time, and the oral contraceptive or birth control pill became available to large numbers of women. These developments and the increased openness to discussion of sexual topics helped to form the basis for what was labeled the "sexual revolution." In this environment, vasectomy became quite popular. It exceeded female sterilization by the early 1970's, driven in part by reports of the side effects of birth control pills. Sterilization for women (also called tubal ligation, literally "tying the tubes") is more invasive than vasectomy because the surgeon must enter the woman's abdomen to occlude the tubes that enable eggs to pass into her uterus. Therefore, vasectomy is somewhat safer when seen in the perspective of family planning. The women's movement of the 1960's placed a new emphasis on the control that women have over their bodies, especially in relation to health and medical decisions. Because the man can assume some of the reproductive responsibility and undergo a safer procedure, vasectomy also has a philosophical advantage for many couples.

Technological innovation by the mid-1970's had produced the first laparoscopic instruments, which enabled a gynecologic surgeon to enter a women's abdomen through two pencil-sized openings and identify and occlude her Fallopian tubes. This procedure, safer than the old one, with visibly smaller scars, and performed by obstetrician-gynecologists (the physicians whom women see most often), quickly became more popular than vasectomy, and has remained so ever since. In spite of its high degree of safety, laparoscopic tubal ligation still occasionally results in deaths from general anesthesia and abdominal complications necessitating major surgery. Yet, even though tubal ligation costs three to five times more than vasectomy, it is still done more than twice as often. There are probably several reasons for this discrepancy, one of the most important being that when a woman has to make the sterilization decision alone, only tubal ligation can be chosen. When a woman is single or in a relationship with a lower level of commitment, or when there is a lack of consensus or support for the decision between the two partners, it is often easier for the woman to choose a tubal ligation. When a decision is made by a couple together, however, the risks and benefits give a comparative advantage to the male sterilization procedure.

When a couple makes a well-informed and mutual decision to choose vasectomy, the feelings in the months following the procedure most commonly include an increased sense of relaxation about sex because of lack of fear of unwanted pregnancy and an absence of anxiety and/or side effects related to contraceptive methods. On the other hand, if one of the partners was not ready and feels pressured into acceptance, the vasectomy decision can create irreconcilable conflict in the relationship.

Most doctors and clinics that counsel men about vasectomy emphasize the fact that vasectomy should be regarded as permanent. Every year, thousands of men seek the reversal of their vasectomies. Although the vasae can be surgically "spliced" back together in a safe and minor operation called vasovasostomy, sometimes years after a vasectomy, there are many reasons not to expect a simple reversal of the procedure. Reversal is expensive and often not covered by medical insurance, and the chances of restored fertility (as measured by later pregnancy) are only about 50 percent. The odds of reversal can be improved if the surgeon (usually a urologist) has substantial experience in the procedure, a microsurgical technique is used, and the vasectomy was relatively recent, and perhaps if the open-ended technique was used as well. Reversal certainly offers hope to someone who has undergone a divorce or personal tragedy and wants to start a new family, but an ambivalent couple should not be reassured that after vasectomy they can change their minds and easily reverse the procedure.

The decision process by a man or a couple to pursue a vasectomy for family planning reasons often begins years before the procedure is actually done. First, they must feel that they have completed their family and be aware of vasectomy as a birth control option. Dissatisfaction with other birth control methods because of inconvenience and real or feared side effects often presses the decision. Discussion about vasectomy with one or more patients who have had one is a very common prerequisite to the decision for many men. Finally, a scare that an unwanted pregnancy can occur—such as a late period or a broken condom discovered too late—or even an actual unplanned pregnancy itself may be the last straw for many couples. The high rates of satisfaction with vasectomy may be attributable to strong sense of comfort that follows this long and thorough decision process.

—*John J. Seidl, M.D.*

See also Contraception; Electrocauterization; Pregnancy and gestation; Reproductive system; Sterilization; Testicular surgery.

FOR FURTHER INFORMATION:

Haldar, N., et al. "How Reliable Is a Vasectomy? Long-Term Follow-up of Vasectomised Men." *The Lancet* 356, no. 9223 (July 1, 2000): 43-44. This article discusses the failure rate of vasectomy, which decreases dramatically in the first year following the procedure. The pregnancy rate after vasectomy is about one in two thousand.

Marquette, Catherine M., Lisa M. Koonin, Libby Antarsh, and Paul M. Gargiullo, et al. "Vasectomy in the United States, 1991." *American Journal of Public Health* 85, no. 5 (May, 1995): 644-649. This article examines statistics of men who had vasectomies in the United States in 1991. Illustrated.

Miller, Karl E. "No-Scalpel Technique vs. Standard Incision." *American Family Physician* 61, no. 5 (March 1, 2000): 1464. The major drawbacks to this otherwise safe and effective method of contraception are the adverse effects related to the incision and the delay between the procedure and sterility.

Morse, David. "The Private Club." *Men's Health* 4, no. 2 (Summer, 1989): 52. A personalized and introspective view written by a teacher. Offers well-researched facts, always using the author's own viewpoint to frame a thoughtful, almost soul-searching discussion of his experience with vasectomy.

Paulson, David. "Diary of a Vasectomy." *American Health* 12 (July, 1993): 70-75. Written in a light and humorous style by a radio talk show host, this article addresses both the emotional and the factual aspects of vasectomy accurately and concisely, with up-to-date information.

Shapiro, Howard I. *The New Birth-Control Book: A Complete Guide for Women and Men.* New York: Prentice Hall, 1988. A comprehensive and factual resource on all types of contraception, with a ten-page section on vasectomy which is equally thorough. Perhaps too technical for some readers.

Silber, Sherman J. *How Not to Get Pregnant.* New York: Charles Scribner's Sons, 1987. Contains a long chapter on vasectomy by an expert in vasectomy reversals. Nicely written from a human-interest perspective, it may overstate the effectiveness of vasectomy reversal because the author's own skill in performing the procedure is superior to that of most physicians who do reversals.

VENEREAL DISEASES. *See* SEXUALLY TRANSMITTED DISEASES.

VENOUS INSUFFICIENCY
DISEASE/DISORDER

ANATOMY OR SYSTEM AFFECTED: Blood vessels, circulatory system, legs

SPECIALTIES AND RELATED FIELDS: Cardiology, vascular medicine

DEFINITION: An abnormality characterized by decreased blood return from the legs to the trunk that is caused by inefficient valves in the veins.

CAUSES AND SYMPTOMS

Venous insufficiency can be either reversible (acute) or irreversible (chronic). It is caused by conditions that increase the amount of circulating blood combined with a decrease in venous flow and is most commonly manifested by thrombophlebitis, varicose veins, and leg ulcers. Thrombophlebitis and varicose veins may be reversible in acute insufficiency.

Thrombophlebitis is an inflammation of the vein, commonly occurring in the legs. It may impede blood flow, resulting in pain, tenderness, redness, warmth along the vein, and edema (swelling). Thrombi (clots) may also form, enlarge, break off, and produce an embolus (dislodged clot) obstructing circulation and causing death. Varicose veins are large, protruding, and painful veins unable to return blood adequately to the trunk as a result of inefficient valves. They may be caused by pregnancy, congenital valve or vessel defects, obesity, pressure from prolonged standing, and poor posture. Leg ulcers are open, draining, painful wounds resulting from an inadequate supply of oxygen and other nutrients. They may also develop on skin surrounding varicose veins because of the stasis (slowing or halting) of the blood flow.

TREATMENT AND THERAPY

The treatment for thrombophlebitis includes rest; leg elevation; warm, moist heat to decrease pain and discomfort; and anticoagulant (blood-thinning) therapy to assist with circulation and to impede clot formation. Elastic stockings or ace bandages assist the return of blood to the heart. Drugs may be used to dissolve clots and to dilate vessels, improving circulation.

The conservative treatment of varicose veins includes the use of elastic stockings or ace bandages and rest. Aggressive treatment may include injecting the vein with sclerosing agents to occlude it and stop blood flow, thereby collapsing it. Surgical treatment may include ligating (tying off) the vein and then stripping and removing it.

Leg ulcer treatment include debridement (the chemical or surgical removal of dirt or dead cellular tissue), cleansing and dressing the wound with ointments, pressure bandages, and the application of medicated castlike (unna) boots. Skin grafting may be attempted if other measures are not effective.

—*John A. Bavaro, Ed.D., R.N.*

See also Circulation; Edema; Embolism; Phlebitis; Thrombosis and thrombus; Ulcers; Varicose vein removal; Varicose veins; Vascular medicine; Vascular system.

FOR FURTHER INFORMATION:

Ernst, Calvin B., and James C. Stanley, eds. *Current Therapy in Vascular Surgery.* 4th ed. St. Louis: Mosby, 2000.

Gaudin, Anthony J., and Kenneth C. Jones. *Human Anatomy and Physiology.* New York: Harcourt Brace Jovanovich, 1989.

Hershey, Falls B., Robert W. Barnes, and David S. Sumner, eds. *Noninvasive Diagnosis of Vascular Disease.* Pasadena, Calif.: Appleton Davies, 1984.

Memmler, Ruth L., Barbara J. Cohen, and Dena L. Wood. *The Human Body in Health and Disease.* 7th ed. Philadelphia: J. B. Lippincott, 2000.

VETERINARY MEDICINE

SPECIALTY

ANATOMY OR SYSTEM AFFECTED: All

SPECIALTIES AND RELATED FIELDS: All

DEFINITION: The health care and medical treatment of animals—both domestic (pets and livestock) and wild (native and exotic species)—which includes preventive health care, sanitary and environmental management, and the treatment of diseases and injuries.

KEY TERMS:

clinical examination: the physical examination of an individual animal, including its medical history and an evaluation of its environment

diagnosis: the determination of what is causing a particular medical problem

epidemiological examination: a systematic explanation of patterns of disease among a group of animals and the use of this information in the treatment of the disease found in one or more of these animals

etiology: the cause of a disease, or the study of such cases

laboratory examination: the use of biochemical, biophysical, or hematological tests in the laboratory to assist in the diagnosis of disease

necropsy: a postmortem (after-death) examination of the animal's body, similar to an autopsy performed on a human corpse

physiological parameters: measurable characteristics determined to represent the normal biochemistry or functioning of a body fluid, organ, or system

subclinical disease: a medical problem with symptoms so slight that it is not diagnosed in a clinical examination

zoonoses: diseases communicable between animals and humans

SCIENCE AND PROFESSION

Animals become sick, get injured, or do not perform as well as they should, just as humans do. Humans, however, have developed a much more sophisticated medical expertise about themselves than they have about the wide variety of other animals. The basics of this medical knowledge apply to other animals, but the physiological differences of each of the many kinds of animal species preclude the application of human medical care. Much of veterinary knowledge has traditionally been concerned with a few common species, such as cats, dogs, cattle, sheep, goats, swine, horses, and some birds. Other species are receiving increasing attention, however, and their medical needs are becoming more widely acknowledged and better understood.

Most of the medical fields concerned with human health apply to veterinary health practice, including anatomy, anesthesiology and pharmacology, biochemistry, cardiovascular medicine, cell biology, dental medicine, dermatology, disease pathology, emergency and critical care, endocrinology, epidemiology, gastroenterology, genetics, geriatric medicine, hematology, immunology, internal medicine, microbiology, nephrology and renal medicine, neurology, obstetrics, oncology, ophthalmology, orthopedics, osteopathic medicine, otorhinolaryngology, physiology, psychiatry, surgery, and urology. There has been much progress in the veterinary applications of these medical fields. In addition, there has been considerable progress in the application of the expertise, techniques, and equipment used in these medical fields to an increasingly wider variety of animal species. This development is attributable to both an improved knowledge and interest in these other species and an ethical concern for this wider range of species.

Not only have humans become knowledgeable about how to care for less common domestic and wild animals, but it has also become acceptable to do so. As a result, veterinarians have become involved with a much wider range of employment opportunities in government, business, universities, and zoological parks, although most are still in private practice dealing with farm livestock, horses, cats, and dogs. In addition, veterinarians are also working in a wider range of locations, including in the clinic, in the research laboratory, on the farm, in the field, at zoological parks, and in the wild. There are also more employment opportunities for veterinary technicians, paraprofessionals who assist the veterinarian or who carry out certain veterinary duties when the veterinarian is not available.

Veterinary medicine is both a distinct medical field and an extension of human medical fields. It deals with species quite different from humans, the degree of difference ranging from slight (such as primates) to great (such as birds, reptiles, amphibians, and fish). While the medical doctor deals with only one species, the veterinarian is concerned with a multitude of species. Therefore, the medical doctor tends to specialize in a medical field, while the veterinarian tends to specialize in particular kinds of animals. There are some similarities, and many differences, between human medicine and veterinary medicine, with a common ground in zoonoses, those diseases that can be transmitted between humans and other animals. These degrees of similarity and differences among species is a primary concern for the veterinarian and are one of the things that make veterinary medicine such an interesting subject.

In addition to routine clinical work (both in the office and in the field) dealing with farm livestock, domestic pets, and racing horses and dogs, some veterinarians are involved in other kinds of work. Veterinarians may work with exotic pets, exotic livestock (such as ostrich farms or alligator farms), zoological park and aquarium animals, and laboratory animals. They may maintain healthy game herds and flocks (such as deer and turkeys), translocate wild animals from one area to another, work with teams doing scientific research that involves animals, help with efforts to save endangered species (either in the wild or in captivity), work with beached porpoises and whales, and advise government agencies concerned with animal welfare issues.

In addition to treating sick and injured animals, veterinary medicine involves advising on preventive measures, making routine observations of individual animals or groups of animals, evaluating herd management, examining environmental and housing conditions, assisting with births, and performing necropsies.

Veterinarians working with laboratory animals, zoological park animals, native game species, or endangered species may also provide advice on reducing stress, assisting with propagation strategies (including various artificial propagation techniques), tranquilization, translocation techniques, the gathering of tissue samples, and other animal welfare matters.

The control of epidemic diseases in farm livestock or native wildlife is also carried out by veterinarians. Also of interest are diseases that may be introduced by imported animals, particularly exotic species. For example, parrots imported for the pet trade are capable of transmitting diseases that could affect poultry, as could migrating native bird species. Imported exotic hoofstock can introduce diseases that could affect farm livestock, as could the importation of farm livestock from already infested areas.

For these reasons, species similar to those on farms and ranches (usually birds and hoofstock) are subjected to medical quarantines and other medical restrictions. The transfer of animals or animal products from one country to another by private citizens is also strictly controlled. Diseases that can be passed to humans by animals, particularly those sold as pets, are another situation that is closely monitored. Another problem involving both medical doctors and veterinarians is those diseases that can be passed from native wild animals to humans, either directly or through other host species, such as insects.

Veterinarians working in the field on medical problems involving native wildlife, imported exotic species, or endangered species are often on their own, working at remote sites and often carrying their clinics on their backs. Improvisation, creativeness, and adventure are often a part of their practice.

Thus, the application of veterinary medicine involves the same kinds of medical fields as those used in human medicine, but the methods, techniques, equipment, medicines, and treatments are different. The amount of difference depends on the species and the area of operation, which in turn ranges from the urban clinic, to the rural farm, to the wilds of remote wilderness areas.

DIAGNOSTIC AND TREATMENT TECHNIQUES

Most medical fields are much better developed for use with humans than with animals because humans know so much more about themselves than they do about the other animal species. Humans only constitute one species—a species that has been studied in depth for quite some time. Unlike human medicine, veterinary medicine is concerned with a large number of animal species, each of which has its own physiological parameters. In addition, different categories of animals—mammals, birds, reptiles, amphibians, and fishes—have significantly different body systems. These different categories and species have to be treated differently when determining whether an animal is normal and healthy and when prescribing treatment for a sick animal.

The best understood groups of animals are the ones that have been of concern to the veterinary profession for the longest period of time, particularly farm livestock and pets. More recently, other groups have received attention, including those used in sporting events, those in zoological parks, laboratory animals, native wildlife, and endangered species. As ethical concerns extend out beyond the human race, more concern has been shown for the health of all animal species. There is much to learn, however, about many species that are not dealt with on a regular basis by veterinarians.

The diagnosis and treatment of an illness or injury depends on the kind of animal being examined. Since the animal cannot tell the owner or the veterinarian what is wrong, it is up to the veterinarian to discover this information. The diagnosis is therefore particularly important. First, the veterinarian must analyze the abnormality. On a clinical level, this means a general physical examination, a special examination of the suspect system or organ, a special examination of the problem area, and a medical history; on a subclinical level, it means laboratory tests and a comparison with peer performance standards. Second, one must analyze the pattern of occurrence of the abnormality in the herd (if necessary), which includes an epidemiological examination; an evaluation of general management, environmental factors, and time of season; nutritional status; and genetics. The veterinarian then categorizes and defines the abnormality, prescribes a treatment, follows up on the treatment, and advises the owner on prevention.

The first step in providing care is to know when an animal is sick. An injury is easier to detect, but it may still be difficult to determine the extent of the injury. Lack of performance may, or may not, be a medical problem. Obviously, an animal is not able to relate any information pertaining to its medical problems. It is easier to determine when an illness is present in animals with which humans are very familiar, such as pets, horses, or livestock. It becomes more difficult with other mammals and birds, and especially with fish, reptiles, and amphibians.

The species of the animal must be known, along with the physiological parameters for that species. The medical history of the individual (and, if applicable, the other individuals with which it is associated, such as a herd) is also necessary. A clinical examination is then used to determine the current medical situation, supplemented by a laboratory examination and an epidemiological examination. From this information, a diagnosis is made and a treatment is prescribed.

These examinations include consideration of past diseases and treatments, nutrition, behavior, general appearance, skin condition, voice, eating habits, defecation and urination, posture and gait, the inspection of the specific body regions, a physical examination (for example, temperature and pulse), the consideration of environmental factors (such as housing, source of water supply, sanitation, and chemical contaminations), and the consideration of laboratory tests on specimen samples from the animal and the environment.

A diagnosis based on these examinations should provide information on the disease or injury, the etiology of the disease, and the clinical manifestation of the disease, that is, the severity or extensiveness of the disease. From the diagnosis, a treatment can be prescribed. This treatment may involve additional care, surgery, the use of medication, a change in diet, or a change in the animal's environment.

Follow-up on the treatments may also be necessary. For animals, medicines can have side effects and multiple medicines can have synergistic effects. Another problem is that animals tend to care for themselves by licking, pulling at bandages, and other behaviors that tend to undo what the veterinarian has done. Also, animals are not able to say whether they are feeling better, although this can often be determined by observing the animal's return to normal behavior. Continued monitoring and reexamination by the veterinarian may be necessary.

Preventive health care is as important for animals as it is for humans. This kind of care may include vaccination shots, pills, proper nutrition, dental care, reduction of stress, exercise, sanitation and proper housing, the quarantine of exotic species, or simply the observation of behavior.

Low performance may be a medical problem, but is difficult to detect because the problem tends to be a subclinical disease. Economically efficient performance of livestock, or peak racing performance in horses and dogs, have become important matters requiring the attention of the veterinarian. The efficient performance of livestock is economically important to the farmer. An assessment of a herd's productivity is usually done by comparing its performance with a standard that is based on known performances of peer herds. Productivity can have several meanings: the amount of milk or meat produced per animal or per hectare, reproductive efficiency, calf survival rate, longevity, and acceptability or quality of the milk or meat at market. Low performance might be caused by a number of factors: inadequate nutrition, poor genetic inheritance, improper housing, stress, lack of herd management expertise, subclinical diseases, physiological abnormalities, or anatomical problems.

Although some veterinarians specialize in a particular medical field, for the most part, a veterinarian has to be familiar with all medical fields in order to treat an animal. While these fields of medicine are basically the same whether one is treating a human or an animal, it must be kept in mind that each species has different body structures and different physiological parameters. Also, different equipment and techniques are necessary in applying these medical fields to animals. For example, the principles of anesthesiology are well understood, but applying anesthesia to a human is not the same as applying it to a dog, a horse, or an elephant: The gases used, the equipment needed, and the procedures used must be tailored to the particular kind of animal being treated. Similar examples could be given for the application of each medical field.

Most veterinary work is carried out in the clinic, particularly small-animal practice (usually cats, dogs, and other common pets). Large-animal practice (usually farm livestock and horses) is often done at specially designed on-site areas at a farm or ranch. Veterinary schools also have both small-animal and large-animal clinics. While small animals are easily handled, large animals need pens, squeeze cages, tilting tables (tilting from a vertical position, in which the animal is strapped onto it, to a horizontal position), and other equipment to restrain them during the examination. Large-animal veterinarians working on a farm or ranch also use veterinary vehicles that are stocked with whatever the veterinarian normally needs. In rural areas, the veterinarian is too far away from the clinic to go back continually to the clinic for supplies while making rounds from farm to farm. Therefore, their vehicles are specially adapted (by the veterinarian or by commercial companies) as mobile clinics.

PERSPECTIVE AND PROSPECTS

Animal domestication developed around 8000 B.C.E. With humankind's increasing dependency on domestic animals, it became necessary to care for their medical needs. The Mesopotamian Code of Hammurabi (a legal code from about 2200 B.C.E.) mentions payments to animal doctors if they successfully cared for an animal, and punishment if they were not successful. Papyrus from ancient Egypt contain the oldest known veterinary prescriptions (c. 1900 B.C.E.). The first veterinarian known by name was from India (c. 1800 B.C.E.). It was also in India that the first known animal hospitals were established (c. 250 B.C.E.). The Aztecs of ancient America also had animal doctors for the large royal animal collections. Ancient civilizations treated diseases with herbs and rituals, some surgical procedures were performed, and some injuries were treated. Medical instruments were crude, and care was based on magic and folklore. This, however, was not unusual during a time when medicine, science, and religion were integrated into one limited body of knowledge. The fact that an effort was made to care for animals indicates their importance to these early societies.

While medical knowledge increased in ancient China and Greece, veterinary medicine did not. In the Roman and medieval periods, practitioners simply compiled and transcribed what had already been done. Nevertheless, the advances made in medical knowledge were to affect veterinary medicine—for example, the determination that diseases were derived from natural causes rather than divine causes, and improved knowledge of how the body functioned.

The Renaissance brought about a renewed interest in many areas of study, including in veterinary medicine. In particular, there was concern about farm livestock and horses because of their increasing economic importance to society. In addition, much of the medical research conducted during this time was done with animals. Advances in veterinary medicine coincided with those in medicine in general but were eventually made for their own sake. The first short-lived veterinary schools appeared in Spain (c. 1490), and the first modern ones appeared in Europe during the eighteenth century. It was not until the nineteenth century, however, that methodological observation and examination became the foundation for diagnoses, and veterinary medicine passed from the common practitioner to the academic or professional practitioner.

One significant effect of the growth of veterinary medicine and its acceptance among the general public has been the concept of animal rights, which has increased the provision of medical care to pets, exotic animals exhibited at zoological parks, and native wildlife. At the same time, veterinary knowledge has been extended to amphibians, reptiles, and fish, as well as to a larger array of birds and mammals.

—*Vernon N. Kisling, Jr., Ph.D.*

See also Animal rights vs. research; Education, medical; Ethics; Zoonoses.

FOR FURTHER INFORMATION:

Blood, D. C., O. M. Radostits, and J. A. Henderson. *Veterinary Medicine.* 8th ed. London: Bailliere Tindall, 1994. A textbook on the diseases of cattle, sheep, pigs, goats, and horses. Intended primarily for use by veterinary students.

Fowler, Murray E., ed. *Zoo and Wild Animal Medicine.* 4th ed. Philadelphia: W. B. Saunders, 1999. A text concerning the veterinary care of nondomestic animals. Covers preventive medicine, sanitation, stress, restraint, and the medical care of mammals, birds, reptiles, and amphibians. More specialized books dealing with these animal groups (in the wild, in zoos, or as pets) are also available.

Fraser, C. M., ed. *Merck Veterinary Manual.* 7th ed. Rahway, N. J.: Merck, 1991. A concise and authoritative reference covering the pathology, clinical findings, and treatment of medical problems related to the various biological body systems. Also covers behavior, clinical values, husbandry, nutrition, toxicology, pharmacology, and zoonoses.

Kirk, Robert W., and Stephen I. Bistner, eds. *Kirk and Bistner's Handbook of Veterinary Procedures and Emergency Treatment.* 7th ed. Philadelphia: W. B. Saunders, 2000. A concise and authoritative reference on the procedures used for the emergency treatment of specific conditions, for interpreting signs of disease, and for interpreting laboratory tests.

Wallach, Joel D., and William J. Boever. *Diseases of Exotic Animals.* 19th ed. Philadelphia: W. B. Saunders, 1998. An authoritative text arranged by broad taxonomic groups within the mammals, birds, reptiles, amphibians, and fishes. Covers biological
data, housing, nutrition, restraint, behavior, and medicine for each of these groups.

VIRAL INFECTIONS

DISEASE/DISORDER

ANATOMY OR SYSTEM AFFECTED: All

SPECIALTIES AND RELATED FIELDS: Epidemiology, family practice, internal medicine, virology

DEFINITION: A wide range of diseases, from mild (such as the common cold) to fatal (such as rabies, smallpox, and AIDS), caused by viruses, life forms that function as intracellular parasites.

KEY TERMS:

capsid: the protein coat of a virus, composed of subunits known as capsomeres

envelope: an additional covering found on animal viruses; it is composed of lipids and proteins and surrounds the genome and the protein coat of the virus

genome: the genetic material of a virus; in a virion, the genome consists of deoxyribonucleic acid (DNA) or ribonucleic acid (RNA) and is protected by the capsid

lysogenic (temperate) virus: a virus that integrates its genome into the genome of the host cell; such viruses exist in a latent state and do not produce progeny viruses

lytic virus: a virus that guides the production of progeny viruses and that ultimately causes the death and lysis (disintegration) of the host cell

virion: the form of the virus as it exists outside the host cell

HOW VIRUSES WORK

Viruses are entities that infect the cells of all organisms. Some scientists classify viruses as living organisms based on their ability to reproduce inside an appropriate host cell. Yet, viruses lack cellular structure and have no metabolic capability of their own. They are completely dependent on host cells to reproduce. In addition, some viruses can be crystallized and thus have properties of complex molecules rather than of living organisms.

Viruses can only be visualized with an electron microscope. They are small in size, ranging from approximately 10 to 300 nanometers in either length or diameter. Because viruses cannot easily be seen within the host cells that they infect, studies of viral structure often utilize the extracellular form of the virus, called the viral particle or virion.

Viruses are quite variable with respect to size, shape, and biological properties, but they do have some common features. All viruses contain a genome, which is genetic material in the form of either deoxyribonucleic acid (DNA) or ribonucleic acid (RNA). A protein coat known as a capsid that is composed of protein subunits called capsomeres protects the genome of a virus. The capsid is arranged either into a symmetrical structure with spherical (round) or up to twenty-sided (icosahedral) symmetry. Alternatively, the capsid can assume a helical shape.

Some viruses contain additional protein structures that aid in their attachment and penetration of host cells. Other viruses, especially the ones that infect animal cells, are surrounded by a complex membrane structure known as the envelope. While the lipids in the envelope are derived from host cells, the proteins and glycoproteins contained in the envelope are usually viral-specific structures that are encoded by the genetic material of the virus. In animal viruses, the genetic material and protein coat, together called the nucleocapsid, constitute the core of the virus. In addition to these features, some viruses carry enzymes that are necessary for the virus to infect a host cell or to replicate.

Most viruses can infect only one type of host; that is, they display species specificity. The virus that causes rabies is a notable exception since it can infect a variety of mammalian species. All types of organisms—bacteria, protozoa, fungi, plants, and animals—are known to be hosts to viruses. Viruses that infect bacteria are called bacteriophages, or phages. The elucidation of many of the aspects of viral structure and the stages of viral infection was derived from the study of the mechanism by which phages infect their specific bacterial hosts.

Slow virus diseases are a class of viruses that reproduce very slowly, often over months or years. They are difficult to study. A common result of slow virus infections is a condition called spongiform encephalopathy, which is a degeneration of brain cells that ultimately causes death. Recent research has shown that slow viruses cause such diseases as kuru and Creutzfeldt-Jakob disease in humans and scrapie in sheep.

Several steps have been identified in the process by which viruses infect host cells. Because they lack motility, viruses must come into contact with host cells by chance. They are transmitted from host to host in the same ways as other microorganisms: through air,

water, or food or by physical contact. A common mode of transmission is by aerosols produced when an infected individual coughs, sneezes, or breathes. Virions in the aerosols gain access to the host by means of the respiratory system. Common cold and influenza viruses are transmitted in this manner, as

Types of Viral Infection

Family		Conditions
Adenoviruses		Respiratory and eye infections
Arenaviruses		Lassa fever
Coronaviruses		Common cold
Herpesviruses		Cold sores, genital herpes, chickenpox, herpes zoster (shingles), glandular fever, congenital abnormalities (cytomegalovirus)
Orthomyxoviruses		Influenza
Papovaviruses		Warts
Paramyxoviruses		Mumps, measles, rubella
Picornaviruses		Poliomyelitis, viral hepatitis types A and B, respiratory infections, myocarditis
Poxviruses		Cowpox, smallpox (eradicated), molluscum contagiosum
Retroviruses		AIDS, degenerative brain diseases, possibly various kinds of cancer
Rhabdoviruses		Rabies
Togaviruses		Yellow fever, dengue, encephalitis

are the viruses that cause common childhood diseases such as chickenpox, measles, and mumps. As a result, these viruses are very contagious; they are easily spread from person to person.

Some viruses, such as the poliomyelitis (polio) virus, can be transmitted in contaminated food or water. The virus gains entry to the host through the mouth and digestive system. Other viruses will also gain entry after contact, which may be direct (person to person) or indirect (via an inanimate object). Viruses will also enter a host if they are directly introduced into the bloodstream, which can occur via a cut or wound or through use of a contaminated needle. Hepatitis B virus and the human immunodeficiency virus (HIV), which causes acquired immunodeficiency syndrome (AIDS), can infect individuals in this manner. Transmission of these viruses occurs at a high rate among intravenous drug users who share needles. In addition to the above methods of transmission, mosquitoes may transmit viruses such as the encephalitis virus and the yellow fever virus.

All viruses must first attach themselves to their respective host cells. This phase of viral infection is sometimes referred to as adsorption. The attachment process is very specific and is controlled (mediated) by receptors present on the host cell, most of which are glycoproteins. It is the specific nature of this attachment process that accounts for the fact that a virus will infect host cells of only one species. Some viruses are also specific for the type of host cell to which they will adsorb. For example, poliovirus adsorbs only to cells of the central nervous system and gastrointestinal tract.

Following adsorption, the virus penetrates the host cell. In the case of bacteriophages, only the viral genome reaches the interior of the host cell; the protein coat of the virus remains outside. In contrast, the entire animal virus penetrates its host cell. Once inside, the viral genome is separated from the protein coat and envelope. During this stage of viral infection, the virus cannot be visualized by electron microscopy.

The viral genome is responsible for the next stages of viral infection. Many viruses begin a process that will eventually result in the replication of the viral genome and the production of progeny viruses. These viruses are referred to as lytic viruses because the death and lysis of the host cell accompany infection. The infecting lytic virus uses many of the host cell's biochemical processes to replicate its DNA or RNA. It also causes the host to make proteins that will

constitute the capsids of the newly made viruses. New viral particles assemble spontaneously. In many cases, hundreds of these progeny will be released as the host cell disintegrates. These newly produced viruses are then available to infect other cells. This type of virus causes diseases such as chickenpox and polio. In some cases, progeny viruses are continuously shed from host cells. The host cell remains viable for long periods of time and releases large numbers of viruses.

Some viruses do not produce progeny after they penetrate host cells. Instead of being used to produce new viruses, the genetic material of these viruses becomes part of the host cell genome in a process called integration. These viruses are referred to as lysogenic or temperate viruses. In order for these viruses to integrate into the host cell genome, they must either consist of double-stranded DNA or be capable of forming double-stranded DNA within the host cell. RNA viruses that are capable of lysogeny contain an enzyme known as reverse transcriptase that enables the virus to produce a DNA copy of the viral RNA. These viruses are known as retroviruses. Several medically important viruses, such as some tumor viruses and HIV, belong to this category.

Although integrated into the viral genome, lysogenic viruses do not multiply to produce new viral particles. They remain in an apparently latent state. There is evidence, however, that these viruses can make some types of protein and, in some cases, can alter the properties of their host cells. For example, when a virus called SV40 integrates into the genome of certain host cells, it will cause these cells to divide rapidly and grow in a manner that resembles tumor cells. Not all lysogenic viruses remain latent. Ultraviolet light is known to cause latent herpesvirus to switch to a lytic mode of infection, an effect known as induction. Other factors, such as stress, may also be responsible for viral induction.

DIAGNOSIS AND TREATMENT

The extent of a viral disease can usually be explained by the biological properties of the particular virus involved. Some viral infections may be mild, such as the common cold, or entirely unnoticed. Other viral infections can be more serious, debilitating, or even fatal, such as polio, influenza, and AIDS. In some cases, viral infection is acute; an individual is sick for a short period of time and then fully recovers. Other viral infections are chronic; the virus persists for long periods of time. The disease that it causes periodically erupts and then subsides.

Diagnosis of viral diseases often relies on an analysis of the symptoms associated with each type of viral infection. Some viral illnesses cause typical rashes such as those seen in chickenpox, measles, and rubella. Influenza virus infection results in typical flulike symptoms, including throat pain, fever, and muscle aches. It is much more difficult to diagnose viral infections when the virus is latent or not actively causing damage to the host. Sometimes it is important to detect individuals who are infected with a latent virus or who are not symptomatic. Such individuals may be carriers of the virus and thus have the potential to transmit the disease to others. It is possible to identify such individuals by testing for the presence of viral proteins or by examining their immune response to the virus.

The major host defense against viral infections in higher organisms is the immune system. Cells of the immune system recognize many disease-causing viruses, either as virions circulating within the host or by the presence of virus-specific proteins on infected host cells. In either case, the virus is eliminated, although damage to host cells is sometimes a natural consequence of this type of protection. This active immune response against the virus will often result in lifelong protection from subsequent infections by the same virus. It is extremely rare for a person who has recovered from measles or mumps to have another occurrence of that particular disease.

Some viruses are not completely eliminated when recovery occurs. Varicella-zoster virus is the cause of chickenpox, a common childhood disease. In the United States, more than 90 percent of the population has been infected with this virus by the time they reach adulthood. Chickenpox usually runs its course in about two weeks, and complete clinical recovery is observed. Yet, the virus is not necessarily eliminated. It has been tracked to the nervous system, where it can remain dormant for decades. The virus can be reactivated, usually in older adults or in those individuals whose immune systems are compromised. It will travel via the nerves and cause shingles (herpes zoster). Shingles is a condition characterized by a rash that is described as burning, itching, tingling, and by pain that may be quite severe.

Vaccines. Vaccines protect against viral infections by utilizing the host's own immune system. For use in vaccines, the virus is either inactivated, and thus is no longer capable of causing an infection, or infectious but of a much milder strain. Viruses are commonly inactivated for vaccine preparation by chemical treatments that essentially kill the virus. The virus is then no longer able to infect and multiply within host cells. These types of vaccines must be administered at repeated time intervals (months or years, depending on the vaccine) to ensure a sufficient level of immunity.

Live viruses are used in some vaccines, but the harmful or pathogenic form of the virus is never employed. Instead, a weaker version of the virus is selected. These weaker variants, called attenuated strains, can sometimes be found when the virus is grown under laboratory conditions. The advantage of live viral vaccines is that the virus can multiply within the host and cause a significantly higher stimulation of the host's immune system than is usually seen with inactivated viral vaccines. Attenuated strains of the poliovirus are used to produce the oral polio vaccine that is commonly administered to infants in the United States. In rare cases, serious problems do occur with live vaccines. A few individuals among the millions who have been vaccinated, or their family contacts, have been known to develop polio as a result of exposure to the live polio vaccine.

Another method of vaccine preparation involves the use of parts of the viral envelope, particularly the viral-coded proteins. These proteins can be mass-produced using modern genetic engineering technology and then incorporated into various vaccine preparations. This method has the advantage of reducing the risks involved with live vaccines.

The important result of vaccination is that the immune system is stimulated to recognize the virus and thus eliminate its harmful form when the virus is next encountered. Vaccination programs have been highly effective in decreasing the incidence of viral diseases in countries where they are administered. The most striking success of a major vaccination program was the virtual global elimination of smallpox that occurred by 1976.

For some viral infections, the immune system does not offer adequate protection from the harmful effects of the virus. In still other cases, effective vaccines that offer long-term protection against viral infection have not been developed. With some viral infections, an encounter with the virus does not guarantee immunity from future infections: The virus is able to alter its envelope proteins and thus appears different to the immune system when it is encountered again. This is the case with influenza viruses.

Chemical agents. Chemical antiviral agents have also been developed. These chemical agents have been useful because they limit or inhibit important steps in the viral reproductive cycle. For example, acyclovir inhibits the replication of viral DNA in herpesviruses. Among the problems encountered with the use of these chemical agents, however, are their restricted action (they work only for certain viruses) and their toxic effects on the host.

A naturally produced agent with antiviral activity is interferon. Interferon is actually a group of proteins produced by the host during a viral infection. These proteins are only active in the host species in which they are produced. They have the ability to interfere with viral multiplication and are therefore potentially useful agents in the treatment of viral infection and certain human cancers.

Cancer and viruses. The link between viruses and cancer, induced in experimental animals, was established in the early part of the twentieth century. The role of viruses as causative agents of human cancers has been less conclusive. Many viruses are associated with human cancers. They are often integrated into the genomes of cancer cells. Yet, the presence of a virus and its association with a certain type of cancer do not constitute proof that the virus is actually responsible for the cancerous condition. There is evidence that a type of liver cancer is caused by a virus. Hepatocellular carcinoma is thought to be caused by hepatitis B virus. A specific form of leukemia has been linked to human T-cell leukemia viruses. The Epstein-Barr virus is associated with a rare type of cancer, Burkitt's lymphoma. Viruses may be involved in many other types of human cancer, along with other genetic and environmental factors.

The growing evidence for the involvement of viruses in human cancers, either directly or indirectly, provides further impetus for developing an understanding of the biology of these viruses, as well as methods to protect individuals from infection. Molecular biologists continue to elucidate the strategies by which cancer viruses gain entry into host cells and alter the properties and functions of these cells. Understanding such events will provide important clues that could be utilized to interrupt the processes that cause normal cells to become cancer cells.

Prevention. Very few antiviral agents have proven effective in combating viral illnesses. One of the best

approaches in dealing with viral infection is prevention. This can be accomplished by identifying the mode of transmission of the virus and developing measures to block the transmission whenever possible. The most powerful method of preventing viral diseases, however, is through the use of vaccines to immunize individuals against viral infection. Vaccine programs have been tremendously successful in eliminating smallpox worldwide and greatly reducing the number of new cases of polio and chickenpox throughout the Western Hemisphere and Europe. Continued efforts are needed to produce safe and effective vaccines. These vaccines must also be stable and easily administered so that they can be used in parts of the world where populations need protection from serious viral diseases.

Preventive measures cannot be used in all cases. For example, it is extremely difficult to block the transmission of viruses that are carried in the air. There are also many viral diseases for which safe vaccines may not be available. Furthermore, some viruses are able to evade the immune defenses of the host, thus greatly reducing the usefulness of a vaccine. The influenza virus has a strategy for escaping detection by the host's immune system. This virus is able to alter its envelope proteins so that the newer forms are no longer recognized by the immune system of an individual who has recovered from a previous bout with the flu. Thus, an individual who has had one strain of flu is susceptible to another occurrence of the illness caused by a different strain. Although flu vaccines have been developed, their usefulness is limited by the changing nature of the virus.

PERSPECTIVE AND PROSPECTS

From their discovery as the causative agent of tobacco mosaic disease in the late 1890's by the Dutch microbiologist Martinus Beijernick, viruses have been implicated in numerous plant and animal diseases. Human diseases caused by viruses range from very mild to fatal and are often difficult to treat. Epidemics caused by viruses have plagued humankind for centuries. Outbreaks of smallpox, polio, yellow fever, and other viral diseases were once quite commonplace. Viral illnesses such as influenza still appear yearly in epidemic proportions. A severe worldwide outbreak of influenza was responsible for the deaths of 20 million people between 1918 and 1919.

The virus that causes AIDS has the potential to cause millions of deaths worldwide. It is spread relatively easily, and the time between exposure and apparent disease can be a decade or longer. Unfortunately, AIDS is uniformly fatal. Many experts are working to create a vaccine for AIDS, but they have not yet been successful. The AIDS virus is sending a warning that humans must be careful with viruses.

—*Barbara Brennessel, Ph.D.;
updated by L. Fleming Fallon, Jr.,
M.D., Ph.D., M.P.H.*

See also Acquired immunodeficiency syndrome (AIDS); Arthropod-borne diseases; Cancer; Chickenpox; Childhood infectious diseases; Chlamydia; Chronic fatigue syndrome; Common cold; Creutzfeldt-Jakob disease and mad cow disease; Cytomegalovirus (CMV); Disease; Ebola virus; Encephalitis; Fever; Fifth disease; Glomerulonephritis; Hand-foot-and-mouth disease; Hanta virus; Hepatitis; Herpes; Human immunodeficiency virus (HIV); Infection; Influenza; Measles; Microbiology; Mononucleosis; Mumps; Parasitic diseases; Pelvic inflammatory disease (PID); Pityriasis rosea; Poliomyelitis; Prion diseases; Pulmonary diseases; Rabies; Rheumatic fever; Rhinitis; Roseola; Rubella; Sexually transmitted diseases; Shingles; Smallpox; Tonsillitis; Warts; Yellow fever; Zoonoses.

FOR FURTHER INFORMATION:

Fettner, Ann Giudici. *The Science of Viruses: What They Are, Why They Make Us Sick, How They Will Change the Future.* New York: Quill/William Morrow, 1990. The author of this popular work is a writer who specializes in issues of science and health. In dealing with the topic of viruses and society, she traces the history of viral epidemics through the ages and describes the more recent advances in modern virology.

Fields, Bernard N., David M. Knipe, and Peter M. Howley. *Fields' Virology.* Vols. 1 and 2. Rev. 3d ed. Philadelphia: Lippincott-Raven, 1996. The third edition of this classic reference is thoroughly revised to incorporate recent discoveries about the replication, molecular biology, pathogenesis, and medical aspects of viruses.

Garrett, Laurie. *The Coming Plague: Newly Emerging Diseases in a World Out of Balance.* New York: Farrar, Straus & Giroux, 1994. This book contains an excellent discussion of several viral diseases and the efforts of the World Health Organization to control or eradicate them.

Henig, Robin Marantz. *A Dancing Matrix: Voyages Along the Viral Frontier.* New York: Alfred A. Knopf, 1993. The author provides a description of viruses and their relationship to public health and discusses the global impact of viruses from economic, political, and environmental perspectives.

Liberski, P. P. *The Enigma of Slow Viruses: Facts and Artifacts.* Amsterdam: Springer-Verlag, 1993. This text provides a good summary of slow virus diseases. It is accessible to general readers.

Montagnier, Luc, and Stephen Sartarelli. *Virus: The Co-Discoverer of HIV Tracks Its Rampage and Charts the Future.* London: W. W. Norton, 1999. This work traces the early life of Luc Montagnier, the discoverer of human immunodeficiency virus (HIV), and the events leading up to his famous discovery. Includes a description of the epidemiology and biology of HIV.

Radetsky, Peter. *The Invisible Invaders: The Story of the Emerging Age of Viruses.* Boston: Little, Brown, 1991. The author provides a selected history of virology that highlights important viral diseases such as influenza and hepatitis. The major discoveries in virology are discussed, as are the scientists involved.

Regush, Nicholas. *The Virus Within: A Coming Epidemic.* New York: Dutton, 2000. News journalist Regush introduces readers to a virus called human herpes virus-6 and the debate over whether it might play a role in acquired immunodeficiency syndrome (AIDS), multiple sclerosis, chronic fatigue syndrome, schizophrenia, and several other seemingly unrelated diseases.

Ryan, Frank. *Virus X: Tracking the New Killer Plagues out of the Present and into the Future.* New York: Little, Brown, 1997. The author, a member of both the Royal College of Physicians and the New York Academy of Medicine, painstakingly chronicles numerous outbreaks, including those of hanta virus in the American Southwest in 1993; Ebola virus in Sudan and Zaire in 1976 and in Reston, Virginia, in 1989; and HIV.

VISUAL DISORDERS
DISEASE/DISORDER
ANATOMY OR SYSTEM AFFECTED: Eyes
SPECIALTIES AND RELATED FIELDS: Geriatrics and gerontology, ophthalmology, optometry
DEFINITION: Diseases or abnormalities of the eyes, including poor vision and infections.

KEY TERMS:

aqueous fluid: a clear, watery liquid that fills the region inside the front of the eyeball between the lens and cornea

cataract: a loss of transparency in the lens of the eye, commonly associated with aging

cornea: the transparent, curved front surface of the eyeball, which provides protection and focuses light

glaucoma: an increase in the eye's internal pressure that can damage the optic nerve and eventually lead to blindness

laser: a very intense beam of light; used in eye surgery for glaucoma, a detached retina, or hemorrhaging blood vessels

macular degeneration: a deterioration of vision, primarily among the elderly, caused by small hemorrhages in the most sensitive central region of the retina

retina: a thin membrane, lining the inside back surface of the eyeball, where light is transformed into electrical signals that are transmitted to the brain

trachoma: a contagious eye infection, leading to blindness, which affects millions of people in developing countries

CAUSES AND SYMPTOMS

The most common defects in human vision are nearsightedness (myopia), farsightedness (hyperopia), and astigmatism. All three of these conditions are called refractive errors because the cornea-lens focusing system of the eye bends light rays either too much or too little, so that the image formed on the retina is blurred. Fortunately, refractive errors can be corrected by means of eyeglasses or contact lenses. In the United States, almost 60 percent of the population, or about 150 million people, use some form of vision correction, and more than 27 million of them wear contacts.

Myopia and hyperopia are caused by a mismatch between the focusing power of the cornea-lens combination and the length of the eyeball. For a nearsighted person, the incoming light comes to a focus in front of the retina; a diverging lens is needed to move the image further back. For a farsighted person,

Anatomy of the Eye

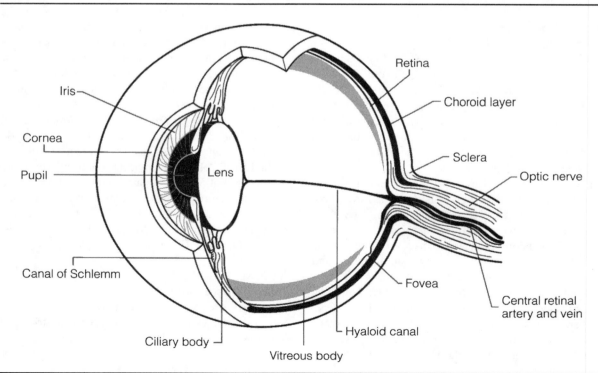

the situation is reversed; a converging lens is prescribed to provide extra focusing power.

The problem of astigmatism is attributable to a difference in the focal length of the eye for two perpendicular directions, which can occur if the eyeball is slightly deformed (like a grape being squeezed between two fingers). The curvature of the corneal surface would be different in two perpendicular planes. An optometrist can correct for astigmatism by prescribing glasses with different focal lengths in the two planes. The prescription must specify the angle at which the deformation of the eyeball is maximized.

A vision problem that is common among older adults is the formation of cataracts, in which the lens of the eye becomes cloudy. Cataracts are a normal part of the aging process, like wrinkled skin or gray hair. In rare cases, however, children have them at birth or after an eye injury. Cataracts form on the inside of the lens capsule, not on the surface of the eye. Once started, their growth is irreversible. The only treatment is surgical removal of the defective eye lens, followed by implantation of an artificial (plastic) replacement. With developments in ophthalmology, such microsurgery has a success rate of better than 95 percent. What causes eye cataracts in the elderly is not yet well understood. One suggested explanation is the Maillard reaction, in which glucose and protein molecules combine when heated to form a brown product. This chemical reaction is responsible for the browning of bread or cookies during baking. The same process is thought to occur even at body temperature, but very slowly over a period of years. It has been suggested that the onset of cataract formation can be delayed by a good diet, regular exercise, and a generally healthy lifestyle.

Glaucoma is a vision problem that afflicts about 2 percent of the adult population, normally after the age of forty. Excessive fluid pressure develops inside the eye, causing damage to the optic nerve. Peripheral vision gradually decreases—a decrease which the patient may not even notice until it is detected by an optometrist during an eye examination. The usual treatments are medicated eyedrops to reduce pressure and laser surgery to improve fluid drainage. Glaucoma has nothing to do with red or watery eyes because these symptoms occur on the exterior of the eyeball.

The retina is a paper-thin membrane at the back of the eye, nourished by a network of tiny blood vessels. A frequent problem encountered by diabetics is the enlargement and possible hemorrhaging of these blood vessels. For older adults, macular degeneration is a condition associated with arteriosclerosis, sometimes leading to retinal bleeding. The most sensitive, central region of the retina deteriorates, causing an irreversible loss in reading ability that cannot be corrected with glasses.

Another retinal problem is its detachment from the back wall of the eye. This is an emergency situation requiring immediate medical attention. A detached retina can be caused by an accumulation of fluid behind the retina resulting from leakage through a small tear in the membrane. It can also come from a blow to the eye, as with a sports injury. Laser surgery has become an effective treatment for the various types of retinal damage.

Conjunctivitis, commonly called pinkeye, is an inflammation of the mucous membrane underneath the eyelids. It is caused by a bacterial infection, a virus, or an allergy. Itchiness and the formation of pus are common symptoms. It is important for patients not to rub their eyes, in spite of the irritation. Frequent eye washing and an antibiotic ointment can usually clear up the infection.

Trachoma is a contagious eye infection, similar to conjunctivitis, that affects more than 400 million people worldwide and has caused an estimated 20 million cases of blindness. It is rarely found in the United States and other Western countries but is common in Africa, South America, and Asia. The World Health Organization and other international relief organizations have set up programs to halt this disabling disease by supplying antibiotics, especially for young children.

TREATMENT AND THERAPY

During an eye examination, the optometrist tries to detect any deviations from normal vision. If the patient is nearsighted or farsighted or has astigmatism, appropriate corrective lenses can be prescribed. If cataracts, glaucoma, or a retinal problem exists, the patient will be referred to an ophthalmologist, who has received specialized medical training in eye surgery.

The history of eyeglasses has been traced back to the thirteenth century, when Roger Bacon, a Catholic scholar, wrote about using convex glass to make writing appear larger. Some medieval paintings show elderly noblemen wearing eyeglasses. No significant innovations were made until Benjamin Franklin invented bifocals in 1780, to aid people whose eyes did not focus properly at either near or far distances. Until

Visual Disorders

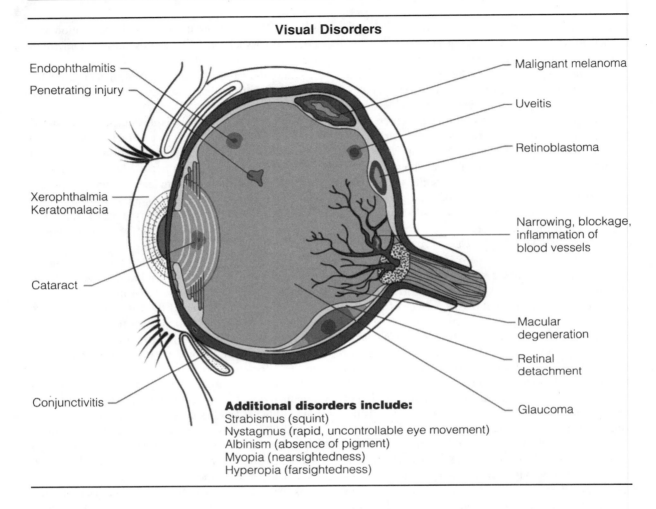

Endophthalmitis

Penetrating injury

Xerophthalmia
Keratomalacia

Cataract

Conjunctivitis

Malignant melanoma

Uveitis

Retinoblastoma

Narrowing, blockage,
inflammation of
blood vessels

Macular
degeneration

Retinal
detachment

Glaucoma

Additional disorders include:
Strabismus (squint)
Nystagmus (rapid, uncontrollable eye movement)
Albinism (absence of pigment)
Myopia (nearsightedness)
Hyperopia (farsightedness)

the late 1940's, prescription eyeglasses were always made out of glass. Then plastic lenses were introduced; they had the advantages of lighter weight and greater resistance to breakage. The main problem with plastic is that it scratches more easily, but coatings have been developed to overcome this drawback. More than 80 percent of the eyeglasses worn in the United States are now made of plastic.

An alternative to eyeglasses came in the 1950's with the development of contact lenses. They were made out of a hard plastic and covered the front of the cornea, floating on a thin layer of tears. They provided good vision but were uncomfortable to insert. Also, hard contacts cannot transmit oxygen and carbon dioxide to nourish the surface of the cornea, causing dryness and irritation for the wearer. Such lenses are now virtually obsolete. Daily-wear soft contact lenses became available in the 1970's. They were much more comfortable than the hard plastic material and were gas-permeable. The soft lenses had an affinity for infection-causing bacteria, however, requiring a tedious, nightly sterilizing procedure with heat or chemicals. The technology of contact lenses continues to evolve. More recent developments are soft contacts for extended wear (up to two weeks without removal), bifocal gas-permeable contacts, and inexpensive, disposable contacts (to be discarded after two or three weeks). Contact lens wearers are cautioned to have regular eye check-ups to make sure that the cornea is not being damaged.

Starting in the 1970's, eye specialists began to investigate the possibility of reshaping the eyeball to do away with eyeglasses completely. The first attempt utilized a hard lens pressing directly against the cornea to flatten it, in much the same way that orthodontic braces are used to straighten teeth. The change induced in the shape of the eye generally was only temporary, so lenses still were needed afterward.

A Soviet physician, Svyatoslav Fyodorov, developed radial keratotomy (RK), a surgical procedure to flatten the cornea permanently. A series of shallow incisions is made in the outer part of the cornea in a radial pattern, like the spokes of a wheel. The center of the cornea is not touched. As the incisions heal, the cornea bulges slightly near the edges, thus reducing its curvature in the middle. In this way, a permanent cure for nearsightedness can be accomplished. In the United States between 1980 and 1993, about 200,000 patients had RK surgery. Nevertheless, the procedure remained controversial. The main problem was that the number of incisions and their depth could overcorrect or undercorrect the original refractive error. Also, some ophthalmologists were concerned about possible long-term aftereffects of scars on the cornea. RK soon decreased in popularity.

Another technique to alter the shape of the cornea is called keratomileusis. The outer half of the patient's cornea is removed and frozen, and then reshaped with a computer-controlled lathe to a predetermined curvature. After thawing, the cornea is sewn back into place, where it acts as a permanent contact lens. Keratomileusis can correct both myopia and hyperopia.

The laser, invented by physicists in the 1960's, is a very intense beam of light that can be adapted particularly well for surgery on the retina of the eye. The light beam passes successively through the transparent cornea, aqueous fluid, and lens without being absorbed. Its energy is then concentrated into a tiny spot on the retina, causing localized vaporization, or "welding," to occur. Laser in-situ keratomileusis (LASIK) became quite popular at the end of the twentieth century. In LASIK surgery, the cornea is reshaped to help patients overcome myopia, hyperopia, or astigmatism. The procedure is done with a cool beam laser that removes thin layers of tissue from selected sites on the cornea to change its curvature. Success rates are high: 90 to 95 percent of the patients get 20/40 vision, and 65 to 75 percent of the patients get 20/20 vision or better. Lasers can also be used to excise leaking blood vessels and to repair or reattach a damaged retina.

Another surgical technique is to use a corneal transplant from an organ donor. The new cornea is shaped to the proper curvature with a lathe and is sewn on top of the patient's own cornea.

The standard treatment for cataracts is surgical removal of the defective lens, followed by implantation of an artificial, plastic lens. Cataract surgery is very

In The News: Improving Reading by Using Only One Eye

In a January, 2000, report in the neurological journal *Brain*, Professors J. F. Stein, A. J. Richardson, and M. S. Fowler of Oxford University reported the results of a study in which 143 children who had been referred to a reading clinic participated. All the children had unstable binocular control at the beginning of the study: A person who has unstable binocular control finds it difficult to maintain eye control and, when reading, finds it difficult to focus on words. Children who have unstable binocular control often report that words and letters jump about on the page.

Of the 143 participants in the study, half were randomly assigned to a group whose members, while reading, wore yellow glasses in which the left eye was covered. The other half of the participants were assigned to a group whose members wore yellow glasses when reading, but their glasses had neither eye covered.

At the end of the nine-month study, of those children who had worn glasses with the left eye covered, 59 percent gained binocular stability whereas of those who did not wear glasses with a covered eye, only 36 percent gained binocular stability. Over the entire nine-month period, children who gained binocular vision nearly doubled their progress in reading compared to those whose binocular stability remained unstable. In follow-up examinations the reading progress of those who used the glasses with the covered left eye was significantly better than that of those students who did not use covered-eye glasses. The research indicated that using the glasses with a covered eye helped children to achieve greater reading progress than did other remedial reading methods.

—*Annita Marie Ward, Ed.D.*

common in the United States, comprising more than 40 percent of all eye operations. Ophthalmologists routinely perform cataract surgery using only local anesthetic, so that the patient can go home without an overnight hospital stay.

Glaucoma, a condition of excess pressure in the eye, affects more than two million Americans and has caused approximately 70,000 cases of blindness. The first line of treatment is the use of the daily medication in the form of eyedrops to reduce the fluid pressure. Eventually, surgery may be necessary. The procedure used enlarges an opening at the edge of the iris to allow for better drainage of the aqueous fluid between the lens and cornea. The incision can be made with either a miniature scalpel or a laser. Glaucoma damage to the optic nerve cannot be repaired, but prompt treatment can prevent further deterioration of vision.

PERSPECTIVE AND PROSPECTS

The human eye is the most important sense organ for individuals to gather information about their environment. An amazingly high 40 percent of all nerve fibers going to the brain come from the retina of the eye. Any defect or deterioration from normal vision is a serious limitation. During the Middle Ages, few people learned to read and write, so the need for seeing at close range was not important. In modern society, however, people with poor eyesight are greatly handicapped. For example, students, computer operators, airplane pilots, and athletes cannot function without good vision.

Society is gradually becoming more sympathetic to people with handicaps, including blindness. Braille printing, guide dogs, and books recorded on audiotape are helpful developments for the blind. The U.S. Congress in 1992 passed the Americans with Disabilities Act, which mandates improved access for the visually impaired in facilities that serve the general public. Nevertheless, retaining good vision and preventing further deterioration will continue to be a vital part of overall health care.

—*Hans G. Graetzer, Ph.D.*

See also Albinos; Astigmatism; Blindness; Blurred vision; Cataract surgery; Cataracts; Chlamydia; Color blindness; Conjunctivitis; Corneal transplantation; Diabetes mellitus; Eye surgery; Eyes; Glaucoma; Gonorrhea; Laser use in surgery; Macular degeneration; Microscopy, slitlamp; Myopia; Ophthalmology; Optometry; Optometry, pediatric; Sense organs; Strabismus; Toxoplasmosis; Transplantation.

FOR FURTHER INFORMATION:

Anshel, Jeffrey. *Healthy Eyes, Better Vision: Everyday Eye Care for the Whole Family.* Los Angeles: Body Press, 1990. A good overview of eye problems typical during childhood, midlife, and old age. The advantages and disadvantages of various types of contact lenses are evaluated. Other topics include eye hazards from work or sports and eye emergencies.

Berns, Michael W. "Laser Surgery." *Scientific American* 264 (June, 1991): 84-90. An excellent article explaining how lasers are used as medical tools. Photographs of blood vessels in the retina of the eye before and after surgery are shown, along with other applications of this technology.

Cassel, Gary H., Michael D. Billig, and Harry G. Randall. *The Eye Book: A Complete Guide to Eye Disorders and Health.* Reprint. Baltimore: The Johns Hopkins University Press, 2001. With particular attention on degeneration of the eye, the combined expertise of three eye care professionals produces a primer on the physiology of the eye and its dysfunctions.

Eden, John. *The Physician's Guide to Cataracts, Glaucoma, and Other Eye Problems.* Yonkers, N.Y.: Consumer Reports Books, 1992. An authoritative guide to all types of eye problems and their treatment, addressed to the general reader. Developments in extended-wear contact lenses and corneal surgery are described, with cautionary remarks about their limitations.

Ross, Linda M. *Ophthalmic Disorders Sourcebook.* Detroit: Omnigraphics, 1997. A popular work that describes such eye diseases as glaucoma, cataracts, macular degeneration, strabismus, and refractive disorders.

VITAMINS AND MINERALS

BIOLOGY

ANATOMY OR SYSTEM AFFECTED: All

SPECIALTIES AND RELATED FIELDS: Endocrinology, family practice, internal medicine, nutrition

DEFINITION: Chemicals that supply the body with the means of metabolizing (extracting and using the energy from) the macronutrients (fats, carbohydrates, and proteins) it ingests; essential ingredients of the diet.

KEY TERMS:

fat-soluble vitamins: vitamins that, because of their structure and solubility, migrate to fatty tissues in the body, where they are stored

macronutrients: materials ingested in large amounts to supply the energy and materials for physical bodies

megadose: ten or more times the recommended daily allowance of a nutrient

micronutrients: substances of which only milligrams are needed in the daily diet, such as vitamins and minerals

mineral: an inorganic salt of particular metals or elements needed for good health

recommended daily (or dietary) allowance (RDA): the intake levels of the essential nutrients that are considered adequate to meet the known nutritional needs of most healthy persons

trace elements: elements needed in the diet at levels of less than 100 milligrams per day

vitamin: an organic compound constituent of food that is consumed in relatively small amounts (less than 0.1 gram per kilogram of body weight per day) and that is essential to the maintenance of life

water-soluble vitamins: vitamins that, because of their structure, show strong solubility in water; they normally pass through the body in a relatively short time

STRUCTURE AND FUNCTIONS

Vitamins are organic compounds (that is, compounds made up of carbon, oxygen, nitrogen, sulfur, or hydrogen) that are constituents of food and that are crucial to the maintenance of life and good health. They make possible the production of energy and the formation of coherent body tissues from the macronutrients normally consumed in a regular diet. They are, among other things, coenzymes that serve as oxidizing, reducing, and transfer chemicals at the active sites of enzymes. Vitamins are part of the one hundred or so organic compounds that are of the proper size and stability to be absorbed from the digestive tract into the bloodstream without digestion or breakdown. Nevertheless, they are not produced in the body in amounts large enough to keep a person healthy—because they have always been available in food, there was probably no need for the human metabolism to produce them. Vitamins are synthesized by plants, and therefore plants constitute the principal natural source of these compounds.

Vitamins are divided into two main groups: the water-soluble and the fat-soluble vitamins. Structural differences account for the two types of solubility. Fat-soluble vitamins (such as vitamins A, D, E, and K) consist mainly of hydrocarbon groupings (nonpolar hydrocarbon chains and rings compatible with nonpolar oil and fat) and are structurally similar to fats, whereas water-soluble vitamins have polar hydroxyl (-OH) and carboxyl (-COOH) groups that are attracted to and form hydrogen bonds with water. One of the most important differences between vitamins is the result of their solubility: Fat-soluble vitamins are stored in the body tissues and organs for relatively long periods of time, while water-soluble vitamins are eliminated from the body in a relatively fast manner, sometimes in a matter of hours.

Vitamin A (retinol) maintains the health of eyes, skin, and mucous membranes and is particularly important for good vision in dim light. There are various physiological equivalents to vitamin A, that is, compounds with closely related structures that can be used as the vitamin itself. Beta carotene is a provitamin (a substance that can be easily converted to a vitamin) of vitamin A found in carrots. The vitamin can also be found in liver and liver oils. Lack of vitamin A can cause night or total blindness.

The B vitamins are often considered as a group, called the B complex, because they work together as coenzymes in biochemical reactions leading to growth and energy production. They are water soluble and easily eliminated from food in the cooking process. Members of this group include pyridoxine (B_6), involved in at least sixty enzyme reactions (mostly in the metabolism and synthesis of proteins); thiamine (B_1), a coenzyme in carbohydrate metabolism and involved in energy production, digestion, and nerve activity; riboflavin (B_2), used in obtaining energy from foods; pantothenic acid (B_3), needed for proper growth; niacin (B_4), needed for the production of healthy tissues; cobalamin (B_{12}), involved in the production and growth of red blood cells; and folic acid (B_9), also involved in the production of red blood cells and in metabolism. They are present in various foods, especially meat and dairy products. Deficiency symptoms include anemia, skin disorders, and nervous system disorders.

Vitamin C, or ascorbic acid, is involved in the destruction of invading bacteria, in the synthesis and activity of interferon (which prevents entry of viruses into cells), decreasing the effect of toxic substances, such as drugs and pollutants), and in the formation of connective tissue. Humans are one of the few species of animals for which ascorbic acid is actually a vitamin, since other species produce it in their metabolic processes. Deficiency symptoms include the degeneration of tissue and scurvy. Vitamin C is found mostly in citrus fruits.

Vitamin D (calciferol) promotes the absorption of calcium and phosphorus through the intestinal wall and into the bloodstream. Its deficiency induces the disease rickets and, in adults, the malformation of bones. Unlike other vitamins, it forms in the body through the action of the sun's ultraviolet light. As with the vitamin B complex, vitamin D has a set of closely related molecular structures, called D_1, D_2, D_3, and so on. All these structures have the same physiological function. Because of limited sun exposure, copious clothing, and indoor living and working conditions, humans need to add vitamin D to their diet, as in fortified milk, cod liver oil, or vitamin supplements.

Vitamin E (alpha tocopherol) is an antioxidant of polyunsaturated fatty acids (fatty acids with numerous double bonds). These fatty acids readily form peroxides, which are particularly damaging because they can lead to runaway oxidation in cells. Vitamin E protects the integrity of cell membranes, which contain considerable amounts of fat. It also helps maintain the integrity of the circulatory and central nervous systems; is involved in the functioning of the kidneys, lungs, liver, and genitalia; and detoxifies poisonous materials absorbed by the body. Since aging, in some theories, is considered to be the cumulative effect of free radicals (reactive atoms) running wild in the body, the antioxidant properties of vitamin E may make it a good candidate for inhibiting aging, or at least preventing premature aging. Its deficiency symptoms in humans are unknown. Vitamin E is present in various foods, especially in grain oils.

Biotin (also called vitamin H) participates in metabolism by acting as a carboxyl carrier for a number of enzymes. Its sources are liver, cereals, and egg yolks. Symptoms of deficiency include alopecia (the loss or absence of hair) and skin rashes.

Vitamin K completes the list of vitamins. It participates in the clotting of blood, and its deficiency can cause hemorrhage and liver damage. This vitamin is commonly found in plants and vegetables.

The term "minerals," when used in a nutritional context, includes all the nutritional chemical elements of foods obtained from macronutrients, except for carbon, hydrogen, nitrogen, oxygen, and sulfur. This term also refers to metal elements combined with others in compounds such as soluble inorganic salts. It is in this combined form that they serve indispensable functions in the body.

Minerals pass slowly through the body and are excreted in the feces, urine, and sweat. Therefore, they must be replaced and an appropriate balance continuously maintained. Because living beings cannot generate minerals in their own bodies, they must obtain them from foods or food supplements. Plants pick up minerals directly from the soil, and animals get them from the plants that they ingest. As opposed to vitamins, which are synthesized by plants, minerals cannot be generated if they are not in the soil. Among their many functions, minerals are components of enzymes, are structural components of body parts such as bones, are involved in maintaining the electrolyte balance in body fluids, and transport materials, as hemoglobin does in blood.

There are seventeen known minerals, although many others may exist. Since most of them are present in the body in relatively small amounts, their functions have been determined through the symptoms of various dietary deficiencies. Minerals can be grouped into two classes. The major elements, among them calcium, phosphorus, and magnesium, are required in amounts of 1 gram or more per day. The trace elements, such as chromium, chlorine, cobalt, copper, fluorine, iodine, iron, manganese, molybdenum, nickel, selenium, sulfur, vanadium, and zinc, are needed in milligram or microgram quantities each day.

Calcium, probably the best known mineral, is present in the body in a greater amount than any other mineral: up to 1.5 or 2.0 percent of total body weight, 99 percent of which is in bones and teeth. In the nervous system, it is used to slow down the heartbeat, and it is metabolized in the body by a hormone synthesized from calciferol (vitamin D). Excess calcium can give rise to kidney stones. Its deficiency is common in postmenopausal women, who produce less estrogen. This decrease encourages bone dissolution, and when bones are dissolved, calcium is lost. Calcium is found in milk and dairy products, fish, and green vegetables. Phosphorus, the second most common mineral, is a structural component of bones and soft tissue. It is found in nearly all foods.

Sodium and potassium cations (positively charged atoms) work in the conservation of electrolytic balance in cell fluids. Potassium governs the activity of many cellular enzymes, while sodium keeps the water content of cellular fluids in a healthy balance. In order for the body to work properly, it needs the appropriate ratio of sodium to potassium. Potassium ions concentrate outside the cell, while sodium ions concentrate inside the cell. Natural unprocessed foods have high sodium-to-potassium ratios. Because sodium and potassium compounds are very soluble in water, however, they dissolve during processing and cooking and are discarded. Sodium is replenished by adding salt to the food, but this is not the case with potassium, which is not added to food. Care must be taken in this matter, either by eating more fresh foods or by using a specialized table salt which contains a mixture of sodium chloride and potassium chloride. The retention of sodium leads to water retention and edema (swollen legs and ankles) and to high blood pressure in some individuals. Sodium is mostly found in table salt, and potassium is found in meat, dairy products, and fruit.

Magnesium and chloride ions are the most common minerals in cell fluids, as they regulate fluid balances and electrical charges. Magnesium controls the formation of proteins inside the cell and the transmission of electrical signals from cell to cell. Chloride is present in the stomach as hydrochloric acid, or stomach acid. Magnesium is found in whole-grain cereals, dried fruits, and leafy green vegetables, and chloride is found in table salt.

Trace elements work in various ways, with most of them incorporated into the structure of enzymes, hormones, and related molecules or acting in conjunction with vitamins. Among the trace elements, one of the more important ones is iron, which is a critical part of the hemoglobin molecule of red blood cells and is involved in oxygen transport. Fluoride, another trace element, helps harden the enamel of teeth to make them resistant to decay; zinc plays an important role in growth, the healing of wounds, and the development of male sex glands; and manganese is needed for healthy bones and a well-functioning nervous system. Iodine is involved in the proper operation of the thyroid gland, chromium is important in the metabolism of glucose, and cobalt aids in cell function. Copper and selenium are other trace elements needed by the body. Most trace elements are found in fish, meat, fruits, and vegetables.

RELATED DISEASES

Vitamin deficiencies are not common in the United States and other Western countries. A well-balanced diet provides ample vitamins of all kinds. Megadoses of vitamins can create harmful effects, however, as a

toxic dose exists for many vitamins. For example, vitamin A, when taken in excess, can cause headache, nausea, vomiting, fatigue, swelling, hemorrhage, pain in the arms and legs, and birth defects. An acute deficiency of the vitamin, however, can impair vision and eventually cause blindness. Consequently, there must be a balance in vitamin intake. This balance can be achieved by following the recommended daily (or dietary) allowances (RDAs).

In the United States, the Food and Nutrition Board of the National Academy of Sciences and the National Research Council determined the daily needs for some vitamins and minerals. The Food and Drug Administration (FDA) made these findings the basis for its list of RDAs. These allowances are presented in units of grams or milligrams, and this amount is determined using international units of biological activity. (Some vitamins come in several forms, all of which are physiologically equivalent.) RDAs do not cover every single vitamin and mineral needed for good health, nor do they cover the more extreme nutritional requirements that result from illness or unusual genetic makeup. They just serve as general guidelines for healthy individuals. For some substances lacking specific RDAs, such as chromium and a handful of other elements, the FDA lists the daily ranges of these micronutrients that it considers to be safe and effective. RDAs depend on gender, age, weight, and other conditions and are normally presented in food labels as percentages of the daily dietary requirement.

The activity of a vitamin or mineral depends only on its molecular structure, not on its source. Therefore, the synthetic vitamins found in food supplements provide the same nutrients as naturally occurring ones. It is crucial to remember, however, that other substances or nutrients are present in the food that is being consumed to obtain the necessary vitamin and mineral requirements. Authentic food often contains additional substances that enhance the absorption and utilization of its nutrients. For example, the calcium that is naturally present in food is more likely to carry with it any vitamin D or phosphorus that the body might need for its optimum use than is the calcium found in an antacid tablet or a food supplement. A balanced diet provides a diversity of nutrients that no pills can match.

The major medical use of the vitamins is in curing the deficiency diseases—that is, those caused by their absence from the diet. Nine vitamins have been judged by an FDA panel to be safe and effective as over-the-counter drugs. Supplementation is commonly thought of as a means of maintaining nutritional equilibrium in the body.

Many different analytical methods—such as ultraviolet-visible and infrared spectroscopy; paper, thin-layer, and gas-liquid chromatography; and mass spectroscopy—as well as biological assays have been used for the detection and identification of vitamins. They have greatly helped to explain the complex structures of these compounds. These methods are also used in the determination of the vitamin content of a particular food item, providing the consumer with valuable nutritional information.

PERSPECTIVE AND PROSPECTS

Vitamin deficiency diseases such as scurvy, beriberi, and pellagra have plagued the world at least since the existence of written records. The concept of a vitamin or "accessory growth factor" was developed in the early part of the twentieth century. In 1912, Casimir Funk, a Polish biochemist, isolated a dietary growth factor from the outer covering of rice grains and found that, when added to the food of those who had beriberi, it cured the disease. The factor was an organic compound called an amine (that is, a compound containing nitrogen combined with carbon and hydrogen). Funk coined the term "vitamine" (meaning "life-giving amine") for the compound, which is now called thiamin or vitamin B_1. In the next five decades, there was an exciting era of the isolation, identification, and synthesis of vitamins. It was soon found that these compounds were not all amines, and the term was changed to "vitamins." As more information on the structure of vitamins was obtained, names changed from general ones (such as vitamin C) to more specific ones (such as ascorbic acid). These discoveries led to the availability of inexpensive synthetic vitamins and to a dramatic reduction in overt vitamin deficiency disease.

The technology has been developed to identify the risk of developing a vitamin deficiency, which in its turn has increased the awareness and concern over the effects of marginal vitamin deficiencies. Small amounts of vitamins are essential for good health, but the benefits of taking megadoses of certain vitamins to prevent or cure certain ailments are often debated. Even so, there is evidence that the use of high levels of vitamins can prevent or alleviate a number of diseases. Improvements in the analytical methods used in the detection and identification of vitamins have led to better and more sensitive detection limits for these compounds. The result has been increased knowledge of vitamins and minerals and their function.

—*Maria Pacheco, Ph.D.;*
updated by Lisa Levin Sobczak, R.N.C.
See also Anorexia nervosa; Antioxidants; Beriberi; Bulimia; Cholesterol; Digestion; Eating disorders; Food biochemistry; Food poisoning; Hyperlipidemia; Kwashiorkor; Lactose intolerance; Lead poisoning; Malnutrition; Nutrition; Obesity; Osteoporosis; Phenylketonuria (PKU); Poisoning; Rickets; Scurvy; Self-medication; Supplements.

FOR FURTHER INFORMATION:

Balch, James F., and Phyllis A. Balch. *Prescription for Nutritional Healing: A Practical A to Z Reference to Drug-Free Remedies Using Vitamins, Minerals, Herbs, and Food Supplements.* 3d ed. Garden City Park, N.Y.: Avery, 2000. A guide to nutritional, herbal, and complementary therapies. Includes the latest research and theories on treatment of aging, HIV, and a host of other subjects.

Clark, Nancy. *Nancy Clark's Sports Nutrition Guidebook.* 2d ed. Brookline, Mass.: Human Kinetics, 1997. A balanced and scientifically sound, practical guide for persons interested in healthy eating and sports medicine. Written by a registered dietitian.

Frank, Robyn C., and Holly Berry Irving, eds. *Directory of Food and Nutrition Information for Professionals and Consumers.* 2d ed. Phoenix, Ariz.: Oryx Press, 1992. A good reference for other information sources that will be useful for consumers interested in nutritional issues.

Hendler, Sheldon Saul. *The Doctors' Vitamin and Mineral Encyclopedia.* New York: Simon & Schuster, 1990. An excellent presentation of the nutritional value of herbs, and a good introduction to micronutrients and other food supplements and their relation to health and diseases.

Herbert, Victor, and Genell J. Subak-Sharpe, eds. *The Mount Sinai School of Medicine Complete Book of Nutrition.* New York: St. Martin's Press, 1990. A series of short essays by numerous authors, presenting a commonsense approach to nutrition. Includes numerous sample menus, calorie information, and useful nutrition tables.

Machlin, Lawrence J., ed. *Handbook of Vitamins: Nutritional, Biochemical, and Clinical Aspects.* 2d ed.

New York: Marcel Dekker, 1991. Although somewhat on the technical side, this book presents a wealth of information on vitamins, including their history, chemistry, synthesis, content in food, methods of analysis, metabolism, transport, biochemical function, deficiency signs, nutritional requirements and assessment, and toxic doses.

Snyder, Carl H. *The Extraordinary Chemistry of Ordinary Things.* New York: John Wiley & Sons, 1992. An excellent, nontechnical presentation of nutrition is found in chapter 16, emphasizing vitamins and minerals. A good reference for those who are in search of a chemistry-oriented introduction to nutrition, but who are more interested in the practical than the theoretical aspects of the topic.

Weil, Andrew. *Eight Weeks to Optimum Health: A Proven Program for Taking Full Advantage of Your Body's Natural Healing Power.* New York: Alfred A. Knopf, 1997. A step-by-step program for enhancing and protecting present and lifelong health, written by a medical researcher. Includes the latest information about personal health and healing.

VOICE AND VOCAL CORD DISORDERS
DISEASE/DISORDER

ANATOMY OR SYSTEM AFFECTED: Respiratory system, throat

SPECIALTIES AND RELATED FIELDS: Otorhinolaryngology, speech pathology

DEFINITION: Physical disorders of the vocal system in the larynx, pharynx, or oral cavity.

CAUSES AND SYMPTOMS

The human vocal apparatus consists of the larynx (voice box), the vocal tract (the pharynx and the nasal and oral cavities), and the nose and mouth (sound radiators). The main sound source is the larynx, containing the vocal cords; the thyroid, forming the projection on the front of the neck known as the Adam's apple; and the arytenoids, which control the size of the glottis (the opening between the vocal cords). The arytenoids are usually well separated to permit breathing; however, they pull together and vibrate during vocalization. Disorders of the vocal system may occur at the larynx or the palate (the roof of the mouth). Such disorders are sometimes caused by nonorganic emotional disturbances.

Laryngitis, or inflammation of the larynx, may be acute or chronic. The acute form may be caused by

bacterial infection, chemical agents (such as chlorine), overuse of the vocal cords, or trauma. During acute laryngitis, the membrane lining the larynx swells and secretes a thick mucous substance which obstructs the vocal cords. Vocal strain following prolonged talking or singing may cause chronic hoarseness or roughening of the voice. Abuse of the voice consists of yelling or screaming, being forced to talk loudly in noisy surroundings, or having a faulty vocal technique.

Chronic laryngitis, produced by excessive smoking, alcoholism, or constant abuse of the vocal cords, dries the mucous membrane and often results in nodular growths on the vocal cords. These growths obstruct the normal functioning of the cords or cause erratic vibration. Hoarseness is symptomatic of a vocal cord problem. Sinusitis or any pulmonary disease that results in a chronic cough is particularly damaging to the voice. Chronic bronchitis may permanently injure the vocal apparatus because coughing is particularly traumatic to the vocal folds, which close tightly just prior to the cough and then open abruptly to permit the explosive air blast.

When the palate is not fused, a congenital deformity termed cleft palate, sound in the mouth cavity leaks into the nasal cavity. The resulting speech sounds have a nasal quality. (For normal speech, nasal sounds are produced when the soft palate at the back of the throat opens to allow sound into the nasal cavity.) The speaker with cleft palate may not be able to develop sufficient pressure in the mouth cavity to enunciate stops and fricatives.

Laryngeal granuloma, or contact ulcer, is a vocal cord lesion resulting from the insertion of a tube into the trachea (as with general anesthesia) or from an inappropriate configuration of the vocal cords during speech. This condition is suspected when a patient complains of pain or hoarseness after prolonged talking. Symptoms are slight hoarseness and a peculiar feeling in the throat.

A papilloma, or vocal nodule, is a small, benign, wartlike growth (polyp) attached to the vocal cords. It most often occurs in singers, announcers, and people who frequently use their voices strenuously. A patient with a vocal nodule may complain of chronic hoarseness or some ill-defined difficulty in speaking.

Laryngeal carcinoma is a malignant tumor caused by chronic irritation or by alcohol and tobacco abuse. Both types of laryngeal carcinoma—intrinsic, which attacks the vocal cords, and extrinsic, which grows in the area above the vocal cords—produce immediate symptoms of hoarseness, discomfort, and coughing. In the intrinsic form, if the symptoms are diagnosed correctly in the early stages of tumor growth, the patient has a good chance of recovery after the tumor is removed.

TREATMENT AND THERAPY

There are two treatments for chronic laryngitis. Surgery, followed by vocal exercises to correct the cause, will restore the contours of a larynx which has developed polyps or become thickened. In some cases, however, the larynx appears entirely normal but the voice tires or roughens with prolonged use. The problem is repeated vocal cord strain from excessive subglottal pressure or the inappropriate application of breath during phonation. Relief must come from a voice teacher or speech therapist.

A cleft palate is surgically corrected by closing the hole in the palate. When the original palate is inadequate for simple closure, plastic surgery may restore it to its intended purpose, or a prosthesis may be fitted to effect an artificial closure.

Laryngeal granuloma is readily corrected by surgically removing the lesion. When the ulcer occurs as a result of prolonged talking, speech therapy or vocal training will prevent a recurrence. After careful diagnosis, a vocal nodule (polyp), is also removed by means of surgical forceps. The patient is ordinarily restored to normal talking or singing within two to six weeks. Since nodules usually result from vocal abuse, the cause must also be identified and corrected.

Carcinoma of the larynx can be successfully removed surgically, or treated by radiotherapy, when detected early. The extent of surgical intervention is directly dependent on the site and extent of the tumor. If the tumor is restricted to the surface of the vocal folds, a laryngofissure may be performed, but more extensive penetration requires a laryngectomy. When the tumor is known to be of low malignancy, a hemilaryngectomy and immediate skin graft preserve the natural airway and leave a functional, although inefficient, voice.

—*George R. Plitnik, Ph.D.*

See also Aphasia and dysphasia; Bronchitis; Cleft lip and palate; Cleft lip and palate repair; Hearing loss; Laryngectomy; Laryngitis; Nasopharyngeal disorders; Otorhinolaryngology; Pharyngitis; Sinusitis; Sore throat; Speech disorders; Stuttering; Tumor removal; Tumors.

FOR FURTHER INFORMATION:

Colton, Raymond H., and Janina K. Casper. *Understanding Voice Problems: A Physiological Perspective for Diagnosis and Treatment.* 2d ed. Baltimore: Williams & Wilkins, 1996. This text, which is illustrated with color photographs, addresses the physiopathology behind voice disorders.

Greene, Margaret C. L. *The Voice and Its Disorders.* 5th ed. London: Whurr, 1989. A detailed compendium of the normal vocal apparatus, vocal disorders and their correction, and vocal therapies.

Ramig, Lorraine Olson, Katherine Verdolini. "Treatment Efficacy: Voice Disorders." *Journal of Speech, Language, and Hearing Research* 41, no. 1 (February, 1998): S101-S116. Ramig and Verdolini review the literature on the efficacy of treatment for voice disorders primarily using studies published in peer-reviewed journals.

Strong, W. J., and G. R. Plitnik. *Music, Speech, Audio.* Provo, Utah: Soundprint, 1992. Comprehensive treatment for the layperson, covering many aspects of human speech, including chapters on vocal sound production, vocal tract effects, speech characteristics, prosodic features, speech defects, degraded speech, machine processing, and singing.

Tucker, Harvey M. *The Larynx.* 2d ed. New York: Thieme Medical, 1993. Includes detailed presentations of the anatomy and physiology of the larynx, as well as of laryngeal pathology and congenital disorders.

VOMITING. *See* NAUSEA AND VOMITING.

WARTS

DISEASE/DISORDER

ANATOMY OR SYSTEM AFFECTED: Feet, genitals, hands, reproductive system, skin

SPECIALTIES AND RELATED FIELDS: Dermatology, gynecology, urology, virology

DEFINITION: A family of generally benign epidermal tumors of the skin and adjacent mucous membranes; genital warts are more serious, sometimes precursors of cervical cancer.

KEY TERMS:

condylomata acuminata: the most common form of genital warts

epidermis: the superficial outer layer of skin, which consists of an outer dead layer and inner living layers of cells

epidermodysplasia verruciformis: the development of numerous small, flat warts that result from a noncontagious, genetic predisposition; they often develop into forms of skin cancer

keratosis: a skin growth that results from the overproduction of keratin, a protein which is the primary component of skin, hair, and nails

myrmeciae: deep plantar warts often found in teenagers; they may occur singly or in small groups

papillomaviruses: small, cuboidal viruses that replicate in the nuclei of epithelial cells

plantar warts: warts that develop on the sole of the foot, usually at points of pressure; consist of a soft core surrounded by a callouslike ring

verruca: a benign, warty skin lesion caused by a member of the papillomaviruses

CAUSES AND SYMPTOMS

More than fifty different types of wart have been characterized on the basis of the type of lesion or its location. Though all warts are associated with infections by members of the papillomavirus genus, certain forms of warts are associated with specific viral strains or types. Regardless, all warts have certain characteristics in common. Their appearance is usually rough, with an irregular surface. A typical wart is an overgrowth or thickening of surface keratin, a condition sometimes referred to as hyperkeratosis. Generally, warts are painless unless they are found in an area subject to irritation or pressure, as in the genital area or on the soles of the feet.

While the association of warts with an infectious agent has been known since the 1890's, the role played by papillomaviruses was only confirmed in the early

1950's. These are small, cuboidal viruses in which the genetic material is deoxyribonucleic acid (DNA). These viruses are widespread in nature, though they are highly species-specific. Thus human papillomaviruses (HPV), as the name implies, are restricted to human infections.

More than seventy subtypes of HPV have been recognized; development of various forms of warts is associated with specific subtypes. For example, plantar warts are mainly associated with infections by HPV types 1 and 4, while anogenital warts are commonly associated with types 6, 11, 16, and 18. Despite the association of various types of HPV with distinct forms of lesions, certain features of infection are held in common. Thus, all types of HPV exhibit tropism for surface epithelial cells of the skin, specifically for the keratinocytes. Replication of the virus is found mainly within these cells. HPV virus particles may be found on the surface of the wart, resulting in their spread to other mucosal surfaces, including those of another person. The wart itself results from hyperkeratosis and thickening of the upper layers of skin following infection, in addition to hypertrophy (overgrowth) of the underlying basal layer of cells.

The most common types of warts are cutaneous warts. In general, these are encountered during childhood. They fall into three major groups: plantar and deep plantar warts, common warts, and plane or flat

Hand Warts

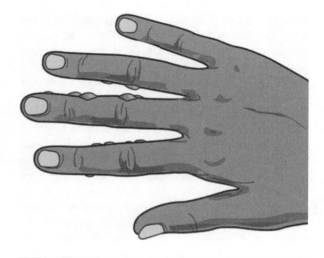

Warts come in more than fifty varieties; a common site is the fingers of the hand.

warts. Each of these forms of warts is most often associated with specific types of papillomaviruses.

Plantar warts (or myrmeciae), particularly types of deep plantar warts, are sometimes referred to as verrucas. They exhibit a rough, raised appearance, with a horny surrounding collar. Often they are found on the sole of the foot, resulting in pain or discomfort when walking. Large numbers of virus particles can be found in the wart tissue, which makes these forms of warts particularly contagious.

Common warts (verruca vulgaris) are generally found on the hands, usually singly or in small groups. Because they contain viruses, scratching of the wart may result in spread to other areas of the body. The wart may become quite large, nearly a half-inch in diameter, with a gray, irregular surface.

A type of common wart is the butcher's wart, so called because it was often seen among members of that profession, though it is also found among those in other professions that utilize cutting utensils (such as fishermen). These warts are typically large and cauliflower-shaped and are associated particularly with HPV 7, the only form of wart generally associated with this strain of virus.

Plane warts (or verrucae planae) are small, flat papules (pimplelike structures) that may have a slight scalelike appearance. They usually develop on the back of the hands or on the face, generally among children. Variations of these warts are often associated with different strains of papillomaviruses. For example, plane warts associated with HPV 3 are usually small and flat, while those associated with HPV 10 are often larger, with some horny appearance. Plane warts are usually found in groups. They may last for several years, but they eventually undergo spontaneous regression.

Condylomata acuminata, or anogenital warts, are the most common form of warts found in this region, occurring in the soft skin or mucous tissue around the vulva, penis, or anal regions. They usually begin as small, verrucous papules, developing and merging into large, cauliflower-like masses. These warts may also spread into the urethra, anus, and vagina, and even into the cervix. Subclinical or latent infections of the genital tract may occur in women who have anogenital warts. During pregnancy, warts may appear in the genital tract, raising the danger of infection of the baby as it passes through the birth canal. Development of anogenital warts is nearly always the result of infection through sexual intercourse. Their oc-

currence in children is so rare that the presence of anogenital warts is reason for suspicion of child abuse. As is true for other types of warts, anogenital lesions are associated with particular strains of HPV.

With rare exceptions, warts do not develop into malignancies. Epidermodysplasia verruciformis is a noncontagious, potentially malignant form of wartlike lesion associated with a recessive genetic trait. It is characterized by the development of large numbers of small, flat papules during childhood. Approximately one-third of these persons will develop skin cancers at the sites of the warts by the second decade of life. Development of skin cancer is exacerbated by sunlight. Many of these patients have depressed immune systems, further supporting claims of the congenital nature of this form of cancer.

Papillomavirus infections are known to result in malignant transformations of infected cells under certain circumstances. Thus certain strains of HPV, particularly types 16, 18, and 31, appear to be associated with the development of cervical cancer. Since these viruses are most commonly transmitted through sexual intercourse, this would imply that cervical cancer can be a form of sexually transmitted disease. (It must be emphasized that cancer of the cervix does appear, although less often, in women who are not sexually active.) The association between sexual activity and cervical cancer has been known since the mid-nineteenth century, when it was noted that the disease is more common among married women than among virgins or nuns. The possible role played by HPV in the development of the disease, however, first became apparent in the 1970's. Since then, the consistent finding of HPV DNA in nearly all forms of cervical cancer tissue, coupled with the finding that the expression of certain genes within HPV DNA may cause the transformation of laboratory cells, has strongly supported the suspicion that these viruses are the cause of this form of cancer.

TREATMENT AND THERAPY

In few other areas of medicine is the use of folk tradition as widespread as it is in the treatment of warts. In great part, this fact is attributable to the significant rate of spontaneous regression; as many as 50 percent of warts regress on their own. This feature has sometimes made it difficult to assess the value of alternative treatments. In addition, multiple rounds of treatment are often required in the elimination of warts, treatments that are sometimes uncomfortable or even painful.

Methods for treating warts date nearly as far back in history as the first medical observations. The Roman medical author Celsus (c. 25 B.C.E.-c. 50 C.E.) recommended the use of ash from wine-lees to burn off warts and a mixture of alum and sandarac resin along with a poultice of lentil meal. The Greek physician Galen (129-c. 199 C.E.) reported seeing a treatment which consisted of biting off and sucking plantar warts for their removal; no record indicates the success of the procedure.

Since warts frequently regress on their own, it is not surprising that large numbers of folk cures developed over time. Mary Bunney has cited a number of reported cures over the centuries. For example, in the sixteenth century Sir Francis Bacon reportedly cured his own warts by rubbing them with pork fat, which was then hung out to dry—as the sun melted the fat, so too did the warts disappear. Other folk methods of treatment included rubbing the warts with a green alder stick or with a potato (subsequently buried) and attending wart shrines, as in Japan. Some modern treatments have applied changes in diet, as in the use of various amino acid supplements.

In some instances, folk treatments may contain a factual basis; the willow bark sometimes rubbed on warts contains salicylic acid, a component similar to that found in aspirin. The modern use of a preparation of 16 percent salicylic acid in collodion, sometimes in combination with lactic acid, has had some success. The preparation is used daily by the patient, either by soaking the area or through maintenance of exposure by covering the preparation with a gel or plaster. The salicylic acid preparation apparently does not kill the virus directly. Rather, by destroying the connection between the upper and underlying layers of cells, the portion of the skin containing the virus is removed. In addition, the procedure promotes vascularization of the dermal tissue, aiding the immune response in removing the virus. With a success rate as high as 80 percent, the use of salicylic acid remains the most common daily treatment of warts.

Modern treatment of warts has the goal of maintaining wart-free remissions for as long as possible. Given the nature of the viral infection of the skin area, warts often reappear. In individuals who are immunocompromised—that is, lacking an effective immune system—the problem of elimination is even more difficult.

The most common treatment, particularly for those on the hands or feet, is the physical removal of the warts. Cryotherapy using liquid nitrogen is the method used most commonly by physicians. Essentially, the wart is burned off using the supercold "liquid." The liquid nitrogen is applied for five-second to fifteen-second periods, usually about twice a month. The process can be painful, and if not carried out properly, may cause localized scarring. If blistering occurs, as on the soles of the feet, the patient may undergo additional inconvenience. The process may also cause depigmentation in dark-skinned individuals.

On occasion, the wart may be surgically excised. Other than rapid removal, little advantage is observed with this method. The process involves the application of a local anesthetic, followed by surgical removal at the base of the wart. The process has a high rate of recidivism (30 percent), may be painful, and often leaves a scar.

Additional preparations used on occasion in the treatment of warts include formalin and glutaraldehyde. Formalin consists of a 40 percent solution of formaldehyde. More commonly known as a tissue fixative, formalin appears to act by dehydrating the outer layers of tissue. Since many persons may find the treatment irritating and some develop contact dermatitis, a localized allergic reaction, patients should be monitored in their use of formalin. On the other hand, evidence exists that the allergic reaction may be a key element in the elimination of the warts following formalin treatment. Since formalin may be destructive to underlying layers of skin, its use is often confined to treatment of plantar warts, as the keratin layer of skin is thicker on the bottom of the foot. Glutaraldehyde treatment appears to be as effective as the use of formalin. This chemical may combine with keratin, however, causing the area of the skin to turn brown.

A variety of other topical treatments is also available. Cantharidin, an extract of Spanish fly, is often used in the treatment of plantar warts. As with other topical treatments, localized blistering may occur, but scarring is usually minimal. Podophyllin resin is used to treat plantar warts and, by some physicians, in the treatment of anogenital warts. The chemical is an antimitotic agent obtained from the roots of podophyllum. The drug can be extremely irritating and can be absorbed within the body. Thus it is not used to treat infants or pregnant women. Dinitrochlorobenzene (DNCB) may be effective in the treatment of warts resistant to removal by other methods. The chemical seems to act through the induction of contact dermatitis. The ensuing immune reaction acts to clear the area of virus-infected cells.

Warts developing in the anogenital region are particularly difficult to treat. They are often small and difficult to find, and the latent, or dormant, virus is difficult to eradicate. Some topical agents are used, including podophyllin and trichloroacetic acid, but neither agent seems to have a cure rate above 50 percent and the warts often recur. Liquid nitrogen cryotherapy is used on occasion, with a cure rate of approximately 70 percent.

Other modern methods for treatment include the use of laser therapy. This procedure utilizes a carbon dioxide laser which vaporizes the tissue. The process can be painful, with a significant period of time required for recovery (from weeks to months). The procedure is more effective in the treatment of plantar warts. Among the drawbacks is the creation of a virus aerosol as the tissue is vaporized.

Immunotherapy as treatment for warts remains disappointing. Some reagents such as DNCB and formalin may act in part through indirect induction of an immune response, but direct stimulation of the immune system has not been particularly successful. Interferon alpha-2a appears to inhibit viruses grown in the laboratory, and use of the chemical in treatment often will cause shrinkage of the lesion. Yet neither the topical use of the chemical in the form of a gel nor the intralesional administration of interferon shows long-term effectiveness.

At best, treatment of warts has a success rate that is anywhere from 50 to 80 percent, depending on the type of wart. The treatment of anogenital warts in particular is often unsatisfactory, with a high rate of recidivism, while treatment of warts on the hands and plantar warts has a greater chance of success. Treatment procedures are often painful; warts often recur. On the other hand, most warts will, with time, disappear on their own. Generally speaking, warts pose no long-term threat to health, with the exception of those caused by oncogenic strains of papillomaviruses. Nevertheless, they can be painful and unsightly. The result is a dilemma with regard to whether, and how, to treat warts.

PERSPECTIVE AND PROSPECTS

Knowledge of warts dates back to the ancient Greeks and Romans; many of the modern terms relating to the nature of warts were first used by medical writers of that period. For example, the Latin word *verruca* re-

ferred to a small hill and was subsequently applied to mean the warts on the skin. The term "wart" itself was derived from the Anglo-Saxon word *wearte*, which referred to a callouslike growth.

As cited by Mary Bunney, the Roman medical writer Celsus recognized three distinct forms of warts: acrochordon, the multiple form of warts often affecting children; thymion, equivalent to the plantar warts and used by that writer to also apply to genital warts; and myrmecia, a deeper form of plantar wart. Celsus also pointed out the spontaneous regression, and reappearance, typical of many forms of warts. He also was aware that some forms of genital warts may be sexually transmitted.

The infectious nature of warts was first noted by Joseph Payne in 1891. Payne, an English physician, reported that he developed warts on his thumb, after it came into contact with an extract from the warts that he had been treating on a patient. In 1894, C. Licht and G. Variot independently demonstrated the transmission of warts by injecting extracts under the skin of volunteers, confirming the infectious nature of material from the wart.

It was during this period, from 1890 to 1910, that the viral nature of many forms of illness was becoming apparent. Though the exact nature of viruses was not understood, and indeed would not be for some decades, it was clear that cell-free filtrates of material from some diseases were still able to transmit the "contagium." Thus, in 1907, the Italian physician G. Ciuffo infected himself with cell-free filtrates of wart extract; the development of warts confirmed their viral nature. In 1950, a team working under Joseph Melnick first visualized the wart virus by using an electron microscope. Though a wide array of warts had been described, once the nature of the virus had been demonstrated it became clear that all warts resulted from infection by similar types of viruses. The wart virus was later grouped with other papillomaviruses.

Papillomaviruses were first described in 1933, when Richard Shope demonstrated that cutaneous papillomatosis in the cottontail rabbit was caused by a papillomavirus. Subsequently, similar viruses were found to cause warts in a variety of animals, and eventually in humans. Difficulty in growing the virus in the laboratory hampered its study for many years. Indeed, it was not until the 1970's, when the virus genome could be cloned in bacteria, that the nature of the viral proteins could be studied in detail.

A possible association between papillomavirus infection and human malignancy dates to as early as 1922, when certain types of infection were found in association with the rare epidermodysplasia verruciformis. It was not until the 1970's, however, that the possibility of papillomaviruses being associated with more common forms of cancer was fully explored. In the 1980's, it became apparent that certain subsets of human papillomaviruses, particularly some associated with genital lesions, may be the etiological agents for some forms of cancers. In particular, cervical carcinoma may result from papillomavirus infection, as viral genetic material is often found in association with these malignant cells. The viral proteins associated directly with malignant transformation continue to be the subject of intense study.

—*Richard Adler, Ph.D.*

See also Cancer; Cervical, ovarian, and uterine cancers; Cryotherapy and cryosurgery; Dermatology; Dermatopathology; Genital disorders, female; Genital disorders, male; Keratoses; Malignancy and metastasis; Sexually transmitted diseases; Skin; Skin cancer; Skin disorders; Skin lesion removal; Tumor removal; Tumors; Viral infections.

FOR FURTHER INFORMATION:

Bunney, Mary H., Claire Benton, and Heather Cubie. *Viral Warts: Biology and Treatment*. 2d ed. New York: Oxford University Press, 1992. A thorough overview on the nature and treatment of warts. The text is written in a concise manner and is profusely illustrated.

Fields, Bernard N., and David M. Knipe, eds. *Fundamental Virology*. 3d ed. Philadelphia: Lippincott-Raven, 1996. Provides thorough coverage of all major groups of viruses. The section on papillomaviruses is extensive and detailed, and it includes a discussion of the role of these viruses in certain types of cancers.

Rosenfeld, Isadore. *The Best Treatment*. New York: Bantam Books, 1992. A collection of short synopses on treatments of common illnesses. Included is a section on types of warts and methods of treatment. Does not contain a large amount of detail, but provides basic facts.

Tierney, Lawrence M., Jr., et al., eds. *Current Medical Diagnosis and Treatment: 2001*. 39th ed. New York: McGraw-Hill, 2000. The text contains summaries of the diagnosis and treatment for most major forms of infectious illness. The section on

papules (warts) is brief, but it contains an adequate overview of the nature of warts and a good summary of modern methods of treatment.

WEANING
PROCEDURE

ANATOMY OR SYSTEM AFFECTED: Gastrointestinal system, stomach

SPECIALTIES AND RELATED FIELDS: Family practice, nutrition, pediatrics

DEFINITION: The training of an infant to accept food other than breast milk.

KEY TERMS:

engorgement: an uncomfortable, often painful condition in which the breasts are overly full with milk

overfeeding: the provision of more milk or formula for an infant than is necessary; may result in regurgitation

INDICATIONS AND PROCEDURES

For a woman who is well-informed about breast-feeding, the appropriate time to wean her infant will become clear if she is sensitive to the child's cues. Other factors affecting a mother's decision to wean her child include family or cultural pressures, pressure from the partner, and personal beliefs about when weaning should occur. Often, weaning takes place between periods of great developmental activity for the child: between eight to nine months, twelve to fourteen months, eighteen months, two years, or three years of age. Most babies are weaned before nine months of age.

Mothers who want to wean their children from breast milk to a bottle before nine months of age need to prepare the child for the process long before by introducing a bottle when the infant is about six to eight weeks old. Infants who are not used to the bottle after that age are more reluctant to accept it later. If the mother decides to wean the baby before one year of age, a commercial formula should be used for supplementation. Cow's milk is not appropriate for infants under one year of age. Honey should never be used to sweeten the formula because of the danger of infant botulism.

When a mother decides to wean her child from breast milk, she should supplement one bottle (or cup) of formula for the least important breast-feeding session of the day. This should be done over a period of two days to a week. If weaning is conducted abruptly, the mother's breasts may become painfully engorged with milk. Breast-feeding sessions associated with meals can be easily forgone, as the child has less desire for milk during those times. Gradually, the mother can substitute more breast-feeding sessions with bottle-feeding. Many mothers continue to breast-feed their infants in the morning and/or in the evenings for many months before weaning is completed. This has many advantages, in that both the baby and the mother will have time to adjust to their new feeding schedule. Weaning mothers should continue to drink plenty of fluids, as restricting fluid intake will not prevent engorgement. Typically, this late form of engorgement passes in one or two days after the weaning process begins.

When bottle-feeding babies, mothers should assume the same position with their infants as they did when breast-feeding. Most women cradle their infants in the crook of their arm for comfort and intimacy. The bottle's nipple should have a hole big enough to allow milk to flow in drops when turned upside down. Too big a hole, however, can lead to overfeeding and regurgitation by the baby. Cleanliness is important when bottle-feeding; appropriate methods of formula preparation and the sterilization of bottles must be followed.

Related to weaning is getting an infant to discontinue the use of a pacifier. Just as in weaning a baby from breast milk, this process has to be gradual and gentle. The best time to wean a baby from a pacifier is when he or she becomes more mobile, in order to prevent the pacifier from becoming a habit. The parent can remove the pacifier after the baby is asleep. Gradually, pacifier use can be restricted to nap time and bedtime. Parents should encourage the baby to stop using the pacifier by offering praise and being patient.

Once a baby starts to use a cup, it is important to make sure that the cup is heavy enough to be stable on a flat surface such as a table or high chair tray. The cup needs to be small enough for the baby to hold properly. Special training cups with spill-proof tops are widely available. Using a floor mat often saves the parent time in cleaning up after a spill.

USES AND COMPLICATIONS

If both the mother and the child are comfortable with the timing of the weaning, it can be accomplished with minimal difficulty. Nevertheless, weaning is a time of emotional separation for mother and child,

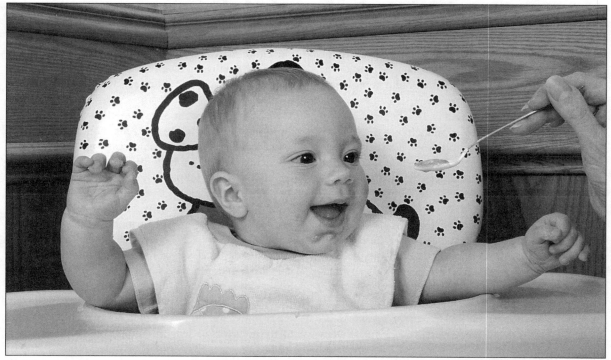

An infant who can sit upright and swallow properly is ready for solid foods, although many more months may pass before complete weaning takes place. (PhotoDisc)

and they may be unwilling to give up the closeness that nursing offers. Hence, it is important to plan comforting, consoling, and play activities to replace breast-feeding. Weaning is best conducted in a gradual manner.

One worry that mothers often express when switching from breast to bottle is uncertainty as to how much milk an infant needs. Parents should avoid overfeeding or feeding infants every time they cry. They should also avoid setting artificial goals such as "the baby must consume 8 ounces," feeding the infant until the goal is reached even though the baby may no longer be hungry. Overfeeding results in obesity.

PERSPECTIVE AND PROSPECTS

In recent years, the American Pediatrics Association has emphasized the importance of breast-feeding through a baby's first year. Physiologically, breast milk helps the infant fight infections by supplying antibodies and by coating the intestines with bacteria-fighting liquids. Developmentally, it has been found that breast-feeding mothers are more likely to engage in frequent interactive behavior with their infants, report that their infants have "easy temperaments," and engage in more flexible caregiving. It has been found that infants who are breast-fed retain an advantage in cognitive ability as measured by intelligence quotient (IQ) tests well into their third year of life.

For a majority of women who terminate breast-feeding prior to one year, inadequate milk supply and employment are the major reasons cited. Whether the result of choice or necessity, weaning is a natural process and a milestone for both mother and child.

—Gowri Parameswaran

See also Bonding; Breast-feeding; Developmental stages; Food poisoning; Malnutrition; Nutrition; Obesity; Pediatrics; Teething; Thumb sucking.

FOR FURTHER INFORMATION:

Bengson, Diane. *How Weaning Happens.* Schaumburg, Ill.: La Leche League International, 1999. This volume, with accounts from the personal experiences of hundreds of La Leche League mothers, informs mothers of the emotional and physical changes they will encounter when weaning their children.

Bumgarner, Norma Jane. *Mothering Your Nursing Toddler.* Schaumburg, Ill.: La Leche League International, 2000. This updated volume offers new research into when and how a baby should be weaned

and urges mothers who want to nurse beyond the typical few weeks or months to feel comfortable doing so.

Markel, Howard, and Frank A. Oski. *The Practical Pediatrician: The A to Z Guide to Your Child's Health, Behavior, and Safety.* New York: W. H. Freeman, 1996. Topics covered run the gamut from ways to determine when abdominal pain demands medical attention to diagnosing zoster (shingles). Other topics include how to select and evaluate day-care options, how to discipline and negotiate with a child, and injuries that can be prevented with simple safety precautions.

Spock, Benjamin, and Steven J. Parker. *Dr. Spock's Baby and Child Care.* 7th ed. New York: Pocket Books, 1998. For more than a half a century, this book has been a virtual bible for parents seeking trustworthy information on child care. Informative, easy to use, and responsive to the changes in society, this revised and updated seventh edition makes a classic work more essential than ever.

WEIGHT LOSS AND GAIN

BIOLOGY

ANATOMY OR SYSTEM AFFECTED: Gastrointestinal system, muscles, muscuoskeletal system, psychic-emotional system, stomach

SPECIALTIES AND RELATED FIELDS: Endocrinology, gastroenterology, nutrition, psychology

DEFINITION: Weight loss occurs when more energy is expended than ingested, while weight gain occurs when more energy is ingested than expended; both conditions may exist as a consequence of physical or psychological disease.

KEY TERMS:

basal metabolism: the energy used to fuel the involuntary activities necessary to sustain life (respiration, circulation, and hormonal activity)

energy balance: the state in which kilocalories from ingested food are equal to kilocalories expended

energy-yielding nutrient: nutrients that supply the body with energy (fat provides 9 kilocalories per gram, while carbohydrates and protein provide 4 kilocalories per gram)

kilocalorie: the amount of heat necessary to raise the temperature of a kilogram of water 1 degree Celsius; the unit of measure for the energy content of foods, also called a Calorie

nutrient density: the amount of nutrients provided per kilocalorie of food *wasting:* severe weight loss characterized by the loss of muscle tissue and body fat deposits

PROCESS AND EFFECTS

Whether a person gains or loses weight is dependent on the balance of energy expended versus energy ingested. Thus, weight is determined by how many kilocalories are in the foods eaten and how many kilocalories of energy are expended. Normal day-to-day fluctuations in weight are typically minor changes attributed to shifts in body fluid and are not related to energy balance (input versus output). Input kilocalories refer to those from fat, protein, carbohydrates, and alcohol. Although alcohol is not considered an energy-yielding nutrient, it provides 7 kilocalories per gram. Output kilocalories are used to maintain the body's basal metabolism; to chew, digest, and process food; to fuel muscular activity for physical exercise; and to help the body adapt to environmental changes. When energy intake exceeds output, a person gains weight. When energy output exceeds intake, a person loses weight.

Body weight is determined by the amounts of body fat, water, lean tissue (muscle), and bones. Ideally, what people want to lose when dieting is body fat, not lean tissue. It takes approximately 3,500 excess kilocalories to store a pound of body fat, whereas approximately 2,000 to 2,500 kilocalories are required to gain one pound of lean tissue. Any excess food kilocalories—whether from fat, carbohydrates, protein, or alcohol—can be converted into body fat. There is no limit to body fat stores.

During periods of caloric deficit (meaning that input is less than output), a person will lose weight. A deficit of 500 kilocalories per day translates into a loss of about one pound per week. Not all the body weight lost is fat. During a deficit or fasting, the body draws on stores to provide energy. During the first four to six hours without eating, either while sleeping during the night or while awake and active during the day, the body draws its energy primarily from liver carbohydrate stores called glycogen. If no food is consumed after these periods, the body begins to break down muscle (also called lean body tissue) as fuel. Although people lose weight under these circumstances, it is the result of muscle loss and fluid shifts, not fat loss. Body fat supplies fuel during fasting but cannot prevent muscle wasting unless a regular supply of carbohydrates is present. The fat used during fasting is not efficiently metabolized and can cause

medical problems if the fast continues for more than a few days. Fat loss can be accomplished by eating balanced regular meals that contain fewer kilocalories than those typically eaten.

Caution should be used before an individual undergoes either a weight loss or a weight gain plan. Starvation diets or very low kilocalorie diets and meal skipping are not wise. These diets promote water and muscle loss, not a steady body fat loss. A reduction in kilocalories of about 500 per day will promote safe, effective fat loss without medical hazards. The central nervous system cannot use stored body fat as fuel, making prolonged fasting a dangerous practice. By consuming a balanced diet which contains all five food groups in moderate portions, exercising, and modifying poor dietary behaviors (such as snacking while watching television), an individual can achieve lasting weight loss. Nutrient-dense foods—those which are low in kilocalories and fat yet still contain ample amounts of vitamins and minerals—should be chosen. Understanding the kilocaloric content of foods is not always necessary if a person uses exchange lists (diabetic exchanges), which are portion-controlled groupings of foods with similar energy contents that can be used to form an adequate diet. Exercise is important because it not only tones the body but also allows for more energy expenditure. Research has shown that regular exercise speeds up the basal metabolic rate, which also helps control weight.

Usually individuals seeking weight gain want to gain muscle, not body fat. Weight gain of this type can be accomplished by physical conditioning and a high kilocalorie diet. The amount of muscle gained is under hormonal control. In healthy individuals, an excess of 700 to 1,000 kilocalories per day is sufficient to add 1 to 2 pounds per week. This excess must be accompanied by exercise training, however, or only body fat deposits will increase.

Healthy individuals desiring weight gain need to exercise and to ingest more kilocalories in order to increase muscle size. Consuming more kilocalories can be problematic, especially for athletes. These individuals must take time to eat perhaps five to six times per day. These individuals should eat more kilocalorically dense foods—the exact foods avoided during weight loss. Emphasis should still be placed on nutrient-wise choices, not simply empty kilocalories. If someone is underweight, increasing fat in the diet is not considered a major heart disease risk because the fat will prevent muscle wastage.

COMPLICATIONS AND DISORDERS

Not all weight gain or loss is voluntary. Weight changes can be warning signs or consequences of disease. Several diseases are frequently accompanied by severe weight loss and wasting, such as acquired immunodeficiency syndrome (AIDS), cancer, colitis, chronic obstructive pulmonary diseases (such as emphysema), cystic fibrosis, and kidney diseases. Wasting is characterized by decreased muscle mass and depleted fat stores. This is a result of inadequacies in both kilocalories and nutrient intake. Lack of appetite, termed anorexia, could be a consequence of disease, drug therapy, or both, complicating a person's desire to eat. Severe weight loss is compounded by other nutrient losses caused by diarrhea, loss of blood, or drug interactions. Individuals with AIDS can experience extreme weight loss, perhaps losing up to 34 percent of ideal body weight.

Thus, with illness a vicious cycle occurs: A lack of adequate food energy promotes the risk of infection; infections require more food energy for healing, further depleting energy reserves; and patients lose more weight, placing them at greater risk for subsequent infections. Extreme weight loss makes AIDS patients prone to other infections, which subsequently compromise weight status because more kilocalories are needed to combat these infections. Similarly, patients with cancer, colitis, and chronic obstructive pulmonary disease who experience weight loss become nutritionally compromised, placing them at risk for infections and delayed wound healing. Extra kilocalories are required to support the labored breathing accompanying chronic obstructive pulmonary disease. People with emphysema, a type of this disease, are often too weak to ingest enough food to prevent weight loss. Diseases of the gastrointestinal tract magnify poor nutritional status because energy-yielding nutrients cannot be absorbed.

Weight loss is also a symptom of cystic fibrosis. Cystic fibrosis is a genetic disorder which affects the pancreas and lungs. Individuals with this disease become malnourished because the normal release of pancreatic digestive enzyme secretions is impaired and because of high nutritional needs to combat lung infections. In an effort to clear congested lungs, individuals with severe cystic fibrosis cough so forcefully that frequently they vomit any food substances that they were able to consume.

Treatment for illness-related weight loss is complex. Individuals do not always want to eat, for both physical and psychological reasons. More frequent meals, higher fat intakes, and even special nutritional supplements are required. In severe cases, intravenous solutions, tube feedings, and hyperalimentation (feeding higher-than-normal amounts of nutrients through tube feeding or veins) may be implemented.

Sudden, dramatic weight loss could be a sign of dehydration. Athletes exercising during hot weather must pay attention to weight loss after practice and replenish fluids immediately. Rapid weight loss in teenagers, especially girls, may be attributable to eating disorders such as anorexia nervosa (self-induced starvation) and bulimia (periods of binge eating followed by intentional vomiting, or purging). Being underweight increases the risk of infections and often causes infertility in women.

Patterns of weight gain or loss are important indicators of childhood growth. Rapid changes may signal illnesses or psychological problems that have manifested themselves as overeating or undereating. Tracking weight gain during pregnancy is also important. Gaining weight too rapidly may be a sign of fluid imbalance forewarning pregnancy complications. Weight gain may precipitate non-insulin-dependent (type 2) diabetes mellitus. Although people with this type of diabetes are overweight, they are hungry because the energy that they ingest cannot enter the body's cells; consequently they continue to overeat, fostering further weight gain. The location of excess weight on the body is also important. Individuals who gain excess weight in the waist area are considered to be at risk for hypertension, type 2 diabetes, and other disorders.

PERSPECTIVE AND PROSPECTS

It is now well known that weight loss, the predominant goal of people with nonmedical weight-related concerns, cannot usually be achieved and sustained by dieting. It is estimated that one-fifth to one-third of the otherwise healthy adult population in the United States is "on a diet" at any given time. Going on a diet is not the way to get control of weight. Diets can produce weight loss; they rarely produce weight control over the long term. Repeated cycles of weight loss through deprivation of favorite high-calorie foods and weight gain when the motivation to tolerate this deprivation wanes, so-called yo-yo dieting, are hazardous. The cycles usually reduce individual metabolic rates, reduce lean tissue, discourage the individual, and make subsequent weight loss extremely difficult.

Weight management is a long-term endeavor resulting from myriad short-term decisions. Success comes with setting and achieving realistic goals. Family or group support, positive and tolerant attitudes, regular meals representative of all food groups, and behavioral modification will sustain healthy weight. Twenty to thirty minutes of exercising the large muscle groups, every other day, can prove a modest, effective way to burn fat and increase one's metabolic rate. It also produces more lean muscle tissue, a goal for both dieters and gainers.

Whether weight gain or loss is the goal, healthful eating habits require one to make wise choices and understand that weight control is a lifestyle, not a quick fix. Individuals experiencing a weight gain or loss who are not voluntarily altering exercise or food intake should have a thorough physical examination to determine the root cause.

—*Wendy L. Stuhldreher, Ph.D., R.D.;*
updated by Paul Moglia, Ph.D.

See also Acquired immunodeficiency syndrome (AIDS); Alcoholism; Anorexia nervosa; Bulimia; Cancer; Cholesterol; Colitis; Cystic fibrosis; Diabetes mellitus; Eating disorders; Emphysema; Growth; Hyperadiposis; Hyperlipidemia; Malnutrition; Metabolism; Nutrition; Obesity; Pregnancy and gestation; Vitamins and minerals; Weight loss medications.

FOR FURTHER INFORMATION:

American Dietetic Association. "Position of the American Dietetic Association: Weight Management." *Journal of the American Dietetic Association* 97 (1997): 71-74. Presents the official position of the association regarding approaches to weight management, including pharmacotherapy. A terse, more technical source.

Brownell, Kelly D. *The LEARN Program for Weight Control.* 7th ed. Dallas: American Health, 1997. A popular workbook, presenting a how-to, step-wise program for weight management utilizing sound principles and user-friendly format. Recommended for those who want to start a realistic program on their own or with others. Contains many behavioral suggestions and much nontechnical nutritional information.

Stransky, Fred W., and R. Todd Haight. *The Good News About Nutrition, Exercise, and Weight Control.* Troy, Mich.: Momentum Books, 2001. This volume offers helpful hints on weight loss, nutrition, and health.

Summerfield, Liane. *Nutrition, Exercise, and Behavior: An Integrated Approach to Weight Management.* Pacific Grove, Calif.: Wadsworth/Thomson Learning, 2000. This text presents the basic principles of weight management and examines the role that nutrition and physical fitness play in weight control.

Wardlaw, George M. *Perspectives in Nutrition.* 4th ed. Boston: WCB/McGraw-Hill, 1999. This easy-to-read introductory nutrition text has chapters on energy balance and weight control.

Whitney, Eleanor Noss, Corinne Balog Cataldo, and Sharon Rady Rolfes. *Understanding Normal and Clinical Nutrition.* 5th ed. Belmont, Calif.: West/Wadsworth, 1998. Offers an introductory normal nutrition section with a chapter on weight control and a section on nutrition during disease which contains information on how illness impairs nutritional status and how proper nutritional support can aid in recovery or improve quality of life.

WEIGHT LOSS MEDICATIONS
TREATMENT

ANATOMY OR SYSTEM AFFECTED: Brain, endocrine system

SPECIALTIES AND RELATED FIELDS: Endocrinology, family practice, internal medicine, nutrition

DEFINITION: The use of drugs to assist in weight loss.

INDICATIONS AND PROCEDURES

By the mid-1990's, several drugs had come onto the market showing promise in helping people achieve weight loss. The most widely sought and prescribed of these were Fen-Phen (combining serotonergic fenfluramine and amphetamine-like phentermine) and Redux (dexfenfluramine, with similar properties and actions to fenfluramine). Fen-Phen inhibits the brain's utilization of the neurochemical serotonin, which acts on the brain's appetite control center in the hypothalamus, and suppresses appetite directly, much as traditional over-the-counter diet pills do. Other drugs, less widely used, included phentermine, mazindol, and fluoxitine.

The hope and early evidence were that these medications would produce improved cardiac function, cholesterol and triglyceride profiles, blood sugar concentrations, and blood pressure; assist in the treatment of bulimia; and reduce weight in the obese and prevent weight gain in those at high risk for it, such as when an individual quits smoking. The drugs were intended to assist those with morbid obesity, obese persons with serious medical conditions, and obese persons who had failed to manage their weight using more conservative nutritional and behavioral methods. At no point did researchers intend the medications as quick fixes for those unwilling to exercise or unwilling to change their eating habits. Nevertheless, many physicians prescribed them to patients who were not significantly obese or who were merely overweight.

USES AND COMPLICATIONS

Multiple studies across many different populations tended to show the same results. Measurable weight loss in those taking the drugs was between 5 and 15 percent, with weight regained one year after patients had stopped taking the drug. While the medications had few initial side effects—dry mouth, constipation, and drowsiness being the most common—and were unlikely to become physically addicting, concerns grew over the drugs' potential to cause neurotoxicity and primary pulmonary hypertension. Health providers across all disciplines were particularly concerned that some patients were coming to rely on these medications to the prohibition of the sustained, hard work of developing lifestyle habits of healthy, proportional eating and exercise. In 1997, the Food and Drug Administration (FDA) withdrew approval of these medicines for treating obesity, and their marketing and distribution were discontinued.

—*Paul Moglia, Ph.D.*

See also Addiction; Anorexia nervosa; Bulimia; Eating disorders; Malnutrition; Nutrition; Obesity; Weight loss and gain.

FOR FURTHER INFORMATION:

American Dietetic Association. "Position of the American Dietetic Association: Weight Management." *Journal of the American Dietetic Association* 97 (1997): 71-74.

Peikin, Steven R. *The Complete Book of Diet Drugs: Everything You Need to Know About Today's Prescription and Over-the-Counter Weight Loss Products.* New York: Kensington Books, 2000.

WELL-BABY EXAMINATIONS

PROCEDURE

ANATOMY OR SYSTEM AFFECTED: All

SPECIALTIES AND RELATED FIELDS: Neonatology, nursing, pediatrics, perinatology

DEFINITION: The art and scientific procedure of the pediatric physical examination.

KEY TERMS:

alopecia: hair loss

dehydration: excessive loss of the body's water content; in infants, manifests as increased pulse, sunken fontanelle, decreased blood pressure, dry mucous membranes, and decreased skin turgor

periodic breathing: rapid breathing followed by several seconds of no breathing; more than ten-second pauses are abnormal

trichotillomania: excessive hair pulling

INDICATIONS AND PROCEDURES

A pediatrician or nurse practitioner usually performs the routine physical examination of an infant. Because the child may be frightened, some steps in the examination may be performed while the baby is being held in the parent's lap. If the baby or child is ill, the health care provider will look for signs of dehydration and possible lethargic mental status. Dehydration is always checked in cases where fever is present. A child's normal oral temperature is similar to an adult's (98.6 degrees Fahrenheit). A rectal temperature will typically be 1 degree higher. It is not uncommon for a young child to have a temperature of 105 degrees with even a minor infection.

Respiration and pulse are measured. Young children and infants breathe with their diaphragm; therefore, the movements of the abdomen can be counted. Periodic breathing is common in infants. Respiratory rates for newborns are 30 to 50 respirations per minute. Toddlers average rates of 20 to 40 respirations per minute. The pulse of a newborn baby is detected best over the brachial artery. The rate is usually in the range of 120 to 160 beats per minute; this figure declines as the child grows older.

Blood pressure, length, weight, and head circumference charts are measured and checked against charts showing norms. Infants are weighed without clothing and are measured on a firm table. The head is measured at the maximum point of the occipital protuberance posteriorly and at the mid forehead anteriorly. The shape of the child's head, such as flatness or swelling, is observed. Hair is checked for quantity, color, texture, and infestations. The presence of a fungus can be indicated by alopecia (hair loss), but this cause must be distinguished from trichotillomania. Hypothyroidism can be indicated by dry, coarse hair.

An eye examination can give information about sys-

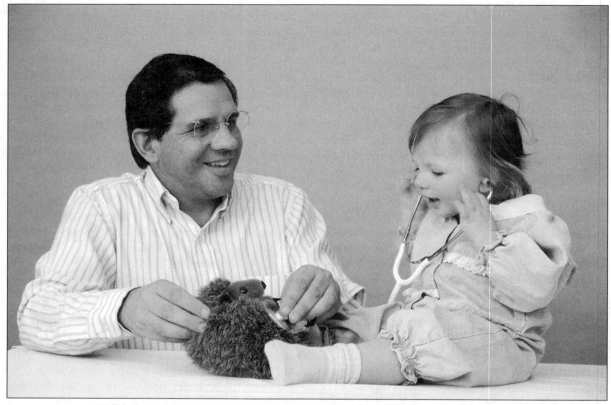

Well-baby examinations assess a young child's health and development. (PhotoDisc)

temic problems and about the eyes themselves. The eyes are observed working together; reaction to light, pupil size, cornea haziness, excess tearing, vision, visual fields, and the distance between the eyes are checked. Observations for nystagmus (involuntary movement of the eyes) and for the abnormal upward outward eye slant and epicanthal folds associated with Down syndrome are also made. Newborns have about 20/400 vision, which improves to 20/40 by six months of age.

During an ear examination, the tympanic membrane is checked for perforations, color, lucency, and bulging (indicating pus and/or fluid) in the middle ear. A rough hearing acuity may be determined by eliciting from the child a startle reflex to sound.

The nose is checked interiorly, and the nasal mucus is checked for watery discharge (indicating allergy) and mucopurulent discharge (indicating infection). The nasal septum and passages are also checked, and any foreign bodies are removed.

The oral cavity examination consists of checking the lips for asymmetry, fissures, clefts, lesions, and color. The tongue is examined for color, size, coating, and dryness. The tonsils are observed for signs of infection and color, while the palate is observed for arch and possible lesions. The throat is examined for signs of inflammation and other problems. The neck is checked for tilt and range of motion. The thyroid gland is palpitated and evaluated for symmetry, consistency, and surface characteristics. Any other swellings are noted and their causes determined.

The neurologic examination is extensive and begins with an assessment of a child's milestones. An infant's primitive reflexes—Moro, asymmetric tonic neck, Babinski, palmar grasp, rooting, and parachute reflexes—are checked. Cranial nerves that can be assessed at the child's stage of development may be assessed. General sensation and response to touch and muscle tone and movement are checked for unusual responses. The musculoskeletal system and extremities are checked for gross deformities and congenital anomalies. Gait and stance are observed, as well as muscle tone and range of motion. Posture in older children may be observed for spinal curvatures.

The lungs are checked to evaluate air movement, to identify breath sounds and chest sounds, and to inspect the shape of the chest. The physician will note any physical deformities and listen to rhythms that could indicate abnormal blood circulation. Indications of circulatory system problems in infants are cyanosis, clubbing of fingers or toes, tachycardia, peripheral edema, and tachypnea. Examining the abdominal contour and auscultation and palpation of the abdomen are done. In newborns, the genitals are checked for ambiguity, and the rectal area is checked for fissures or anal prolapse. Skin is checked for color, pigmentation, rashes, or burns.

Vaccinations—either oral or by injection—and boosters are a part of some well-baby visits. Occasionally, blood or urine samples are taken for analysis.

USES AND COMPLICATIONS
The challenge of keeping the child calm enough for the clinician to perform a valid exam is important in the diagnostic process. Although an older child can usually be examined easily in standard adult order, this does not work well for pediatric patients. The younger the patient, the more important it is that crucially affected areas be examined first, before the child becomes upset or cries. Physicians and parents should work together to minimize a child's fears during the examination.

—*Patricia A. Ainsa, M.P.H., Ph.D.*

See also Bones and the skeleton; Cardiology, pediatric; Childhood infectious diseases; Cognitive development; Colic; Cradle cap; Dermatology, pediatric; Developmental stages; Diaper rash; Endocrine system; Endocrinology, pediatric; Failure to thrive; Gastroenterology, pediatric; Gastrointestinal system; Growth; Immune system; Immunization and vaccination; Motor skill development; Neonatology; Nervous system; Neurology, pediatric; Physical examination; Pulmonary medicine, pediatric; Reflexes, primitive; Reproductive system; Respiration; Screening; Umbilical cord; Urinary system; Urology, pediatric.

FOR FURTHER INFORMATION:
Albright, Elizabeth K. *Pediatric History and Physical Examination.* 4th ed. Laguna Hills, Calif.: Current Clinical Strategies, 2000. This handbook teaches the fine art of history and physical examination of children. It is organized by disease and symptom, featuring a complete review of history, physical examination, and differential diagnosis for each disease.

Barness, Lewis A. *Manual of Pediatric Physical Diagnosis.* 6th ed. St. Louis: Mosby Medical, 1991. Topics discussed include diagnosing pediatric disease through physical examination. Includes an index and illustrations.

Schwartz, M. William, ed. *Clinical Handbook of Pediatrics.* 2d ed. Baltimore: Williams & Wilkins, 1999. A guide to assessing and managing seventy-four common problems in children. Each chapter has information on presenting symptoms, differential diagnosis, laboratory assessment, and treatments, plus suggested readings and tables of normal lab values.

Zitelli, Basil J., and Holly W. Davis, eds. *Atlas of Pediatric Physical Diagnosis.* 3d ed. St. Louis: Mosby-Wolfe, 1997. This is an excellent book, and although it is not quite as comprehensive as a major textbook of medicine, it is very concise and readable.

WHOOPING COUGH
DISEASE/DISORDER
ALSO KNOWN AS: Pertussis

ANATOMY OR SYSTEM AFFECTED: Chest, heart, neck, respiratory system, throat

SPECIALTIES AND RELATED FIELDS: Bacteriology, critical care, family practice, otorhinolaryngology, pediatrics

DEFINITION: A highly contagious respiratory disease characterized by uncontrollable coughing that ends in a loud whoop as the patient attempts to inhale.

KEY TERMS:
catarrhal stage: the early stage of pertussis, characterized by sneezing and dry cough

DPT vaccine: a trivalent vaccine that provides immunization against diphtheria, pertussis, and tetanus

dyspnea: difficulty in breathing

epiglottis: tissue that lies over the larynx to prevent food from entering the windpipe

paroxysmal stage: the second stage of pertussis, characterized by deep, rapid coughing accompanied by sharp intakes of breath with sound of "whooping"

CAUSES AND SYMPTOMS
The etiological agent of whooping cough is *Bordetella pertussis*, a small, gram-negative, rod-shaped bacterium. A similar organism, *Bordetella parapertussis*, causes a less severe form of the disease. Symptoms

and tissue damage are the result of a toxin secreted by the organism.

The diagnosis of pertussis is primarily clinical, based on the characteristic whoop that accompanies the paroxysmal stage. The most definitive diagnosis involves the actual isolation of the organism. Most pathogenic strains of *Bordetella* are fastidious in their requirements. Nasal swabs from the patient are obtained, with the organism grown on a special Bordet-Gengou medium.

The clinical manifestation of whooping cough is arbitrarily divided into the catarrhal, paroxysmal, and convalescent stages. The average incubation period following exposure is about seven days. During this period, the patient develops a dry cough, often accompanied by sneezing. A mild fever may be present. Early symptoms resemble bronchitis or influenza.

The severity of the cough gradually increases over the next ten to fourteen days; it may be triggered by exercise or even eating. As the patient enters the paroxysmal stage, the cough becomes deeper and more pronounced. It is often characterized as a series of short bursts, followed by a whooping sound as the patient attempts to inhale; the sound itself is caused by possible spasm of the epiglottis.

Large quantities of mucus may be expelled during the coughing spells, which in severe cases may occur forty to fifty times a day. The patient may exhibit dyspnea and become cyanotic from lack of air. In infants, choking is common during this stage and can prove fatal. The severity of the cough has also been known to result in hemorrhaging from the throat.

The paroxysmal stage of the disease lasts from four to six weeks. Gradually, the cough disappears as the patient enters the convalescent stage. The entire period of illness may last six to eight weeks, with the cough persisting for months afterward.

The disease is highly contagious, with the agent passing from person to person by means of respiratory droplets. The patient is most infectious during both the catarrhal stage and the early portion of the paroxysmal stage, a period lasting two to three weeks.

TREATMENT AND THERAPY

Routine treatment of whooping cough consists of bed rest and the provision of adequate food and water. Infants are most at risk and are generally hospitalized. The administration of oxygen may be helpful in the relief of dyspnea and cyanosis. If there is prolonged vomiting, intravenous therapy may be necessary. Ad-

ministration of corticosteroids has also been shown to ameliorate the severity of the cough.

Because paroxysmal symptoms are associated with production of a toxin secondary to the initial infection, antibiotics are of little help. An antibiotic such as erythromycin, however, may be administered to reduce secondary infections or to limit transmission to other persons. If erythromycin is administered early during the development of the disease, during the incubation period, or even during the first week of the catarrhal stage, it may prevent the disease or limit its severity. Persons coming into contact with the patient should also receive a course of antibiotic treatment.

Immunoglobulin is available, but its actual effectiveness is in dispute. Active immunization with pertussis vaccine is recommended to protect against the initial infection. Usually, this is a portion of the DPT vaccine administered in a series of injections beginning at about two months of age.

PERSPECTIVE AND PROSPECTS

The earliest known description of whooping cough was that by G. Baillou in 1578. It was Robert Watt, an English physician, who in 1813 provided the first complete clinical description of the disease. Watt also described the results of autopsies that he had performed on children who had died of the disease during his thirty years of observations; two of these children were his own. Watt also noted the highly contagious nature of whooping cough.

In 1906, Jules Bordet and his brother-in-law, Octave Gengou, isolated the infectious agent from the sputum of Bordet's son, who had contracted the disease. Known initially as *Haemophilus pertussis*, the organism was eventually renamed *Bordetella pertussis* after its discoverer. Bordet also determined that the virulent nature of the disease resulted from the production of a toxin. The special substance needed to grow the organism in the laboratory became known as Bordet-Gengou medium.

Initial attempts to develop a pertussis vaccine by Bordet and Gengou using inactivated toxin were largely unsuccessful. In the 1940's, however, an inactivated whole cell suspension was introduced and proved effective in immunizing children against the disease. In the United States, the pertussis vaccine was combined with inactivated diphtheria and tetanus preparations into a trivalent vaccine, DPT, which proved effective in immunizing children against all three diseases simultaneously.

Because of rare side effects in some children receiving the pertussis preparation, questions developed as to the safety of the vaccine. The development of alternative vaccines using either inactivated toxin or purified extracts from the organisms themselves may eliminate such concerns. Since human beings represent the only reservoir of whooping cough, the disease may eventually face eradication.

—*Richard Adler, Ph.D.*

See also Antibiotics; Bacterial infections; Childhood infectious diseases; Coughing; Immunization and vaccination; Lungs; Pulmonary diseases; Pulmonary medicine; Pulmonary medicine, pediatric; Respiration.

FOR FURTHER INFORMATION:

Armstrong, Donald, and Jonathan Cohen, eds. *Infectious Diseases*. London: Mosby, 1999. This book discusses syndromes by body system, special problems, HIV and AIDS, anti-infective therapy, and clinical microbiology. Includes helpful illustrations, bibliographical references and an index.

Kiple, Kenneth F., ed. *The Cambridge World History of Human Disease*. New York: Cambridge University Press, 1993. In addition to being an encyclopedia describing human diseases, this book provides an epidemiological history of disease and discusses possible origins and treatments.

Ryan, Kenneth, and Stanley Falkow. "Haemophilus and Bordetella." In *Sherris Medical Microbiology*, edited by Ryan. 3d ed. Norwalk, Conn.: Appleton and Lange, 1994. A chapter in an introductory text focusing on infectious diseases. Aimed at the medical professional.

WISDOM TEETH

ANATOMY

ALSO KNOWN AS: Third molars

ANATOMY OR SYSTEM AFFECTED: Gums, mouth, teeth

SPECIALTIES AND RELATED FIELDS: Dentistry, orthodontics

DEFINITION: The common term used to refer to the permanent third molars, which usually emerge into the mouth in the late teenage years.

STRUCTURE AND FUNCTIONS

The four wisdom teeth, two upper and two lower, are normally the last of the thirty-two permanent teeth to emerge into the mouth, usually between the ages of seventeen and twenty-one. They show considerable variation in size and shape between individuals, as well as in the timing of their emergence.

One or more of the wisdom teeth may not be able to fit completely into the mouth because of lack of space in the jaws. These impacted teeth may be completely covered by gum tissue or partly erupted. In some individuals, one or more of the wisdom teeth may not develop at all.

DISORDERS AND DISEASES

Impacted wisdom teeth may need to be extracted as a result of dental decay or recurrent inflammation of the surrounding gum tissue (referred to as pericoronitis). Occasionally, there may be other associated problems, such as cyst formation. Infection of the gums around an impacted wisdom tooth can cause pain and swelling, as well as bad breath and an unpleasant taste in the mouth.

Dentists obtain X-ray films of the jaws before extraction of wisdom teeth so that they can examine the roots of the teeth and their relationship to surrounding structures. If extraction is necessary, it is usually preferable to perform the procedure at a younger age, before the roots of the wisdom teeth have fully formed and while the surrounding bone is relatively elastic. When extraction is likely to be difficult, a dentist may refer a patient to an oral and maxillofacial surgeon, who may remove the teeth under general anesthesia.

PERSPECTIVE AND PROSPECTS

From an evolutionary standpoint, it seems that a lack of tough abrasive foods in modern diets has been associated with a disproportionate reduction in jaw size compared with tooth size, leading to a high incidence of impacted wisdom teeth in industrialized populations.

—*Grant Townsend, Ph.D., D.D.Sc.*

See also Dental diseases; Dentistry; Dentistry, pediatric; Orthodontics; Teeth; Tooth extraction; Toothache.

FOR FURTHER INFORMATION:

Christensen, Gordon J. "When It Is Best to Remove a Tooth." *Journal of the American Dental Association* 128, no. 5 (May, 1997): 635-636.

Klatell, Jack, Andrew Kaplan, and Gray Williams, Jr., eds. *The Mount Sinai Medical Center Family Guide to Dental Health*. New York: Macmillan, 1991.

Smith, Rebecca W. *The Columbia University School of Dental and Oral Surgery's Guide to Family Dental Care.* New York: W. W. Norton, 1997.

WORLD HEALTH ORGANIZATION

ORGANIZATION

DEFINITION: A specialized agency of the United Nations that fights illness and disease all over the globe.

KEY TERMS:

ecology: a branch of science concerned with the relationships of organisms and their environments

ecosystem: an ecological community considered together with the nonliving factors of its environment

epidemic: an unarrested spread of something, as of a disease

epidemiology: a science that deals with the incidence, distribution, and control of disease in a population

etiology: the investigation of the causes of any disease

meningitis: inflammation of a membrane which envelopes the brain or spine, caused by bacteria

pandemic: pertaining to a high proportion of a population

vaccine: any substance for preventive inoculation to build immunity

FUNCTIONS AND RESPONSIBILITIES

The World Health Organization (WHO) is a specialized agency of the United Nations. With its headquarters in Geneva, Switzerland, the organization has grown from 26 member countries in 1948 to more than 140, improving health conditions on every continent of the earth. It functions under the aegis of the United Nations' Economic and Social Council. The governing body of WHO is the World Health Assembly, which is composed of delegations from all member states. The assembly decides the policies, programs, and budget of the organization. It selects the countries that will place one member each on its twenty-four-member executive board, which oversees the programs and budget for the coming year. These plans are presented for approval by the director general, who, with a staff of two thousand, is responsible for conducting investigations and surveys.

The World Health Organization is divided into six regional subdivisions working in Europe, the Americas, Africa, the middle eastern Mediterranean, south-eastern Asia, and the western Pacific. These regional organizations have headquarters in Copenhagen, Denmark; Washington, D.C.; Brazzaville, Congo; Alexandria, Egypt; New Delhi, India; and Manila, the Philippines, respectively.

The regular budget is contributed directly to WHO by its member states. The United Nations also devotes many resources to the Fund for Technical Assistance to Underdeveloped Countries, of which a substantial part is for health work. Other financial sources are individual donations for promoting good health practices and eradicating malaria. Despite these incomes, there is a continual drain on funds because many underdeveloped countries cannot afford to pay for the drugs, vaccines, or technical medical assistance that they receive.

One of WHO's enduring achievements has been to communicate to the world an understanding and acceptance of the idea of a common, basic list of drugs. The model Essential Drug List has been a powerful tool in providing scientific justification for the improvement of health standards and practices through publicity, workshops, and training in the Third World. The first list of essential drugs was published in 1977 and included 205 drugs; the list published in 1990 contained 268 preparations. Drugs are included based on recommendations of expert committees from both developing and developed countries. The committees consist of clinical pharmacologists, health officials, and university professors. The drugs are chosen for efficacy, safety, quality, and stability. By emphasizing generic agents, the list has stimulated international competition among drug suppliers and brought down prices—an important consideration since some countries spend 40 percent of their slim health budgets on drugs.

WHO concerns itself with the needs of those billions of people in the world who are still without regular access to the most basic drugs at the primary health care level. It seeks to establish equitable access to essential drugs for people. The organization has helped more than 90 percent of its member nations to develop a partly or fully developed essential drugs policy. The Essential Drug List is a valuable resource for countries trying to develop their own national lists. Changes have been made in the list for several reasons, including oversight or omission, accumulation of more conclusive evidence of the therapeutic advantages of various drugs, and changes in the perceived role of the list itself.

WHO attacks communicable diseases in every country through prevention, control, and treatment. The cornerstone of prevention and control is education. Public information is of crucial importance in controlling epidemics. Also vital to many populations is information on nutrition, breast-feeding, personal hygiene, cleanliness, and the use of safe water. Stress is placed on the public's ability to play an important role in prevention and early detection. With full and accurate information, symptoms may be correctly interpreted and conditions correctly diagnosed, thus preventing the spread of disease.

Various WHO commissions continue working on projects to improve health standards. Efforts continue for increasing the number of trained medical personnel in many countries. Systems for selecting, procuring, storing, and distributing drugs and supplies more efficiently are continually being refined. WHO is cognizant of a global range of concerns, from promoting a healthy environment to revising guidelines for ethical conduct in research on an international level.

THE EFFORTS OF WHO AROUND THE WORLD

The World Health Organization monitors the spread or decline of disease all over the world. An example of how beneficial such knowledge can be when applied internationally is the organization's work on inoculation in Egypt and Brazil. Public information services led to the success. In 1973, a study supported by WHO to test the effectiveness of a newly perfected meningitis vaccine was conducted in Egypt, with 250,000 schoolchildren participating. After the first year, it was clear that the vaccine was extremely effective.

Then a major meningitis epidemic broke out in Brazil. King Faisal of Saudi Arabia, aware of the successful results in Alexandria, Egypt, donated 4 million U.S. dollars to send the vaccine to Brazil in order to reduce international concern. Immunization against meningitis was later carried out in Sudan, with the population of Khartoum and surrounding areas receiving vaccinations in 1987 when the disease began to break out across the country.

In Saudi Arabia, vaccination against meningitis is particularly important in preventing disease at the time of the annual pilgrimage to the holy city of Mecca. The health authorities insist that all pilgrims be vaccinated against meningitis before they arrive in Saudi Arabia, and, if they have not, they are offered vaccina-

tion on arrival. People living in the pilgrimage area—in the cities of Jeddah, Mecca, and Medina—who come into contact with the pilgrims are also vaccinated against meningitis regularly. Thus no cases are expected among them.

The exchange of information has also led to spectacular success in Egypt in the control of diarrheal diseases. Authorities have used a proven method: After recognizing the seriousness of the problem, they have developed a simple preventive message and have used public personalities to deliver it. Egypt has also made effective use of all information channels, employing various methods to give the same message. Egypt's national program to control diarrheal diseases is recognized as one of the best in the world. It has demonstrated the value of using the media for advocating health. The country is no longer concentrating only on curing these diseases but instead is giving equal emphasis to prevention. These practices are also used to educate mothers about nutrition, breast-feeding, personal hygiene, cleanliness, and the use of safe water for drinking, cooking, and bathing.

Vaccinating newborns against the hepatitis B virus, a contagious infection of the liver, is another successful campaign by WHO. Immunizing poor children is an ongoing, worldwide program. Medical experts are also looking ahead at trying to take care of the orphaned children of the victims of acquired immunodeficiency syndrome (AIDS).

Prenatal care and safe childbirth practices are also global concerns of WHO, which contends that there is no need to die in giving birth. Every time a woman in Africa becomes pregnant, her risk of dying as a result is more than one hundred times greater than for a woman in the industrialized world. Conferences are held regularly in order to try to stop this waste of life. Involved in the exchanges and preparations are public health officials, midwives, doctors, and the representatives of nongovernmental agencies.

It is estimated that south of the Sahara 150,000 women die every year as the result of becoming pregnant. Epidemiological studies have brought together twenty-two French-speaking governments in Africa to act to reduce maternal mortality. Apart from such specific causes as excessive blood clots, difficult confinements, infections, and other complications, additional factors in maternal mortality include anemia, malnutrition, malaria, or simply overwork—many African women toil twelve to fourteen hours a day.

WHO contends that the heavy price that African

women pay for maternity is not inevitable. There are inexpensive methods that can put a stop to such tragedy. Some of the most important are family planning, prenatal and postnatal care, supervision of the confinement, and recourse to well-equipped and well-staffed primary health care centers. To achieve these goals, WHO coordinates the mobilization of resources with the help of both national commitment and international cooperation.

Heavy publicity and effort attend the multifaceted WHO campaign to cope with the dramatic rise in the global AIDS toll. Statistics show that human immunodeficiency virus (HIV) infection has spread rapidly among women and children in sub-Saharan Africa and in Asia. An estimated 3 million women were developing AIDS by the 1990's, at least 80 percent of which are in Africa south of the Sahara. Millions of HIV-infected babies are being born to these women. AIDS is the leading cause of death of women aged twenty to forty in some central African cities. Infant mortality is also on the rise, with an increase of as much as 30 percent.

Experts working in the field of AIDS have noted that one of the greatest obstacles to prevention is the general lack of basic health care in the developing world, as well as among the poor in urban cities. A lack of resources and medicine compounds the seriousness of AIDS in countries such as Zaire and Tanzania. At times, there is not the money to buy medicine, even if the supply of medicine existed.

Without a cure for AIDS in sight, common treatments are the drugs zidovudine (formerly known as azidothymidine, or AZT) and standard sulfa drugs for *Pneumocystis carinii*, a type of pneumonia seen in immunocompromised patients. Unfortunately, access to these medications is severely limited for people with AIDS in Africa and Asia. Even elsewhere in the world, zidovudine is an expensive option. WHO continues to promote better distribution and use of sulfa drugs in the developing world. It is also financing drug development studies for promising agents in these countries.

The fight against communicable diseases continues to be fought and won on various fronts. Oral rehydration tablets to cope with diarrhea among children, for example, have proven effective, reducing infant mortality in many countries by 50 percent. Early in the 1950's, Professor Samir Najjar of Lebanon produced a formula for oral rehydration which differed only slightly from the present oral rehydration formula. Then in 1962, a hospital training course in oral rehydration was organized in Alexandria, Egypt, another pioneering effort. Eventually, oral rehydration salts became the standard worldwide treatment of diarrhea in the 1970's.

PERSPECTIVE AND PROSPECTS

The World Health Organization's efforts to fight diseases of all kinds and to improve health are so impressive that international successes in all fields seem almost inevitable. Yet the world's health problems also have a larger cause, one that is more difficult to solve. It is now increasingly evident that many diseases stem from the degradation to the environment caused by humans. The harmful effects of industrial development on the global ecosystem are now better known. Some of these ecological wounds are depletion of the ozone layer, acid rain, changes in climate, deforestation, and chemical pollution.

In Europe, thirty-two member nations of WHO have agreed to a single health policy, including environmental issues. It contains measurable objectives to which each nation has agreed to be publicly accountable on an annual basis. The program is called Health for All, and it is based on four sweeping policy goals. The goals have thirty-eight targets supported by more than one hundred measurable indicators, all of which are aimed at achieving a symbolic health standard and improving the environment of Europe.

Communicable diseases are a continual problem. Susceptible populations have to be monitored for their appearance, and the latest medical information and practices need to be made accessible. Like environmental problems, the spread of diseases must be prevented, controlled, treated, and, wherever possible, eradicated completely.

The polio vaccine has been so effective that the illness has been eradicated in the United States, but in tropical areas such as Central and South America, the disease remains. The rate of effectiveness for the vaccine is 60 to 80 percent in the tropics, compared with 90 percent in the United States. Since 1985, however, the Pan American Health Organization (PAHO) has carried out an extensive four-year vaccination program, immunizing 40 million children in forty-seven countries and territories in the Americas. The number of new cases plummeted from 930 in 1986, to 130 in 1989, to only 11 in 1990, causing PAHO to believe firmly that it will be able to eradicate polio in the tropics.

The World Health Organization plans to use the same type of intensive immunization program for polio in other areas of the world, including areas where the incidence is high: Africa, China, and India. Millions more children have also been immunized against diphtheria, pertussis (whooping cough), measles, and tetanus. Using advanced biotechnology, scientists are working on keeping vaccines cool in transit to recipients in the tropics.

Still other endeavors by WHO are "no tobacco" days, vaccination programs against hepatitis B virus, laws to facilitate the distribution of drugs and medical supplies, the reduction of prices charged by manufacturers, the provision of more X-ray machines, the elimination of iron deficiency among the destitute, and advanced research on amino acids. For example, WHO predicts that 500 million people will die because of tobacco-related disease, based on current long-term trends. Smoking could reduce the lives of persons aged thirty-five to sixty-nine by fifteen to twenty years, the *NCI Cancer Weekly* reported in 1990, when 3 million were expected to die annually. Furthermore, children's health is at risk from adult smoking. If women stopped smoking, it is estimated that fetal and infant deaths would drop by 10 percent.

In the area of nutrition, WHO is helping to publicize the fact that requirements for each amino acid may be higher than professionally recommended. Amino acids are the molecular units that combine to make proteins. Adult humans need eight amino acids in the diet. Other amino acids required for protein synthesis are manufactured in the body and do not need to be consumed in food. If new, higher levels are accepted, as WHO recommends, better protein nutrition could be achieved and food aid programs could be improved.

—*Walter Appleton*

See also Acquired immunodeficiency syndrome (AIDS); Centers for Disease Control and Prevention (CDC); Childbirth; Childbirth complications; Childhood infectious diseases; Diarrhea and dysentery; Environmental diseases; Environmental health; Epidemiology; Ethics; Hepatitis; Immunization and vaccination; Malnutrition; Meningitis; National Institutes of Health (NIH); Nutrition; Poliomyelitis; Preventive medicine; Tropical medicine.

FOR FURTHER INFORMATION:

Beigbeder, Yves. *The World Health Organization.* Boston: M. Nijhoff, 1998. This work, written by a former World Health Organization official, presents a broad outline of the activities and evolution of WHO. Research was based on the official documentation of WHO, both open and restricted.

Bier, Dennis M., Peter L. Pellett, and Vernon R. Young. "A Theoretical Basis for Increasing Current Estimates of the Amino Acid Requirements in Adult Man, with Experimental Support." *American Journal of Clinical Nutrition* 50 (July, 1989): 80-92. A concise, up-to-date report on ongoing research in the field of amino acids and their effect on nutrition.

D'Adesky, Anne-Christine. "WHO Predicts Dramatic Rise in Global AIDS Toll." *UN Chronicle* 27 (December, 1990): 66-68. Grim predictions of the devastating spread of AIDS in Africa and how it is seeking a hold in India, Thailand, and other Asian countries.

Dickman, Steven. "Vaccine Research: WHO Calls the Shots." *Nature* 347 (September 20, 1990): 218. A clear depiction of the Children's Vaccine Initiative and its tremendous successes in underdeveloped countries.

Gibbons, Anna. "Saying 'So Long' to Polio." *Science* 251 (March 1, 1991): 1020. The story of how effective the polio vaccine was in northern climates and the need to devise ways of transporting cool vaccines to tropical areas.

Goldbeck, Willis. "The European Business Council for Health." *Business and Health* 8 (January, 1990): 48. A formal report on a number of remarkable health programs and the valuable lessons they portend for the United States and other countries.

Howard, N. J., and R. O. Laing. "Changes in the Essential Drug Lists of the World Health Organization." *The Lancet* 338 (September 21, 1991): 743-745. A history of how the list was developed and how it has evolved. The value and importance of the list is stressed.

Nakajima, Hiroshi. "A Wounded Planet." *World Health*, January/February, 1990, 3. A dire warning that the environment is deteriorating rapidly and that the nations of the earth must undertake to halt further deterioration.

WORMS

DISEASE/DISORDER

ANATOMY OR SYSTEM AFFECTED: Abdomen, gastrointestinal system, intestines, respiratory system

SPECIALTIES AND RELATED FIELDS: Gastroenterology, internal medicine, pediatrics, public health

DEFINITION: Invertebrates, usually flatworms or roundworms, that act as human parasites.

In common usage, the term "worm" includes many other wormlike organisms, a few with medical importance: Some fly larvae (or maggots) can cause human infections, some caterpillars are covered with irritating hairs, and leeches have had a place in medical history (of misuse to "bleed" victims and, more recently, of help with swelling or the reattachment of limbs). To control many parasitic worms, a society must be affluent enough to provide water treatment, plumbing, and sewage treatment; fuel to cook fish and meat thoroughly; and regular medical care for the general population.

Flatworms. Flatworms are primitive organisms in the phylum Platyhelminthes. The class Turbellaria are mostly free-living, planaria-like worms, although some are in intermediate stages of becoming parasitic. Tapeworms in the class Cestoda and flukes in the class Trematoda are the most serious parasitic worms, particularly in tropical and subtropical regions. Flukes that are medically important to humans are in the order Digenea. Schistosomes are flukes that live in the blood system; other adult flukes live in bile ducts, in the lungs, or along the digestive tract. A few are known to infect the body cavity, urogenital system, or eyes of victims. Control requires understanding not only the effect that the adults have on a human host but also the complex life cycle that flukes have developed to ensure a continuous chain of offspring in successive hosts.

Blood flukes affect more than 200 million people and are second only to malaria as a world health problem. The human blood fluke, *Schistosoma mansoni*, has both male and female individuals and is long and hairlike. This blood fluke feeds on blood and clings to the walls of small veins in the large intestine. The strategy of all parasitic worms is to produce vast numbers of eggs. Some of these breach the intestinal wall and pass out with human wastes into the environment. Modern plumbing and sewage treatment can stop the fluke life cycle at this point. In poorer tropical countries, however, the fluke eggs are soon washed into ponds, ditches, or rice paddies, where they immediately hatch. The larvae, coated with cilia, swim about in search of a snail. Boring into the flesh of the snail, the larva sheds its cilia and develops into

a sporocyst. This sporocyst absorbs nutrients and asexually subdivides; eventually, as many as 200,000 tadpolelike cercarias will develop from the one larva. Erupting through the surface of the snail, the cercarias swarm near the water surface. People working in rice paddies or wading or swimming in streams are infected when the cercaria bores through the skin to reach a blood vessel and complete its life cycle.

The Chinese liver fluke, *Clonorchis sinensis*, represents a life history involving two intermediate hosts. In this more representative fluke, the adults are hermaphroditic—possessing both male and female organs. Large numbers of eggs are released from the host's liver into the bile duct, where they pass through the digestive tract and are shed in the feces. When the eggs are washed into the bottoms of ponds, streams, and paddies, many are eaten by snails. This releases the larva, which burrows into the snail's tissues and becomes a sporocyst. The sporocyst subdivides into redia, an active feeding stage that eventually develops many cercariae. The cercariae erupt from the snail and swim through the water to infect native fish. The cercariae encyst in the meat of the fish and wait until the fish is eaten by a human or other mammal. If the fish is not thoroughly cooked, the cyst coating will be digested in the intestine and the young fluke will emerge. From there, it will eventually move to the smaller bile passages of the liver. Using its suckers to anchor, the fluke feeds on blood, causing both anemia and liver blockage.

Tapeworms are unique parasitic flatworms where adults are specialized for living in the digestive tract of vertebrates. By relying on the host's digestive system, tapeworms have lost all evidence of an alimentary canal in both larval and adult stages. A tapeworm possesses a head with hooks and suckers by which it hangs on the gut lining. Beyond a short growing region are bags called proglottids which are constantly budded off, younger ones nearer the neck show developing testes and ovaries, while the most distant proglottids are large sacs of maturing eggs. One common large tapeworm of humans is the beef tapeworm. When eggs are shed with human feces, some eggs may find their way to vegetation and be eaten by cattle. The tapeworm egg coating is digested, and the larval tapeworm migrates across the intestinal wall and flows with the blood to the muscle. There it grows into a tapeworm bladder, which can be seen as measly beef by meat inspectors. When such meat is not thoroughly cooked, digestion releases the enclosed tapeworm, which begins to grow in the intestine of the new host. Mature beef tapeworms can grow to 10 meters in length and release thousands of egg-laden proglottids.

Roundworms. Most roundworms, of the phylum Nematoda, are free-living. They are widely distributed across the land, streams, and oceans. The large *Ascaris lumbricoides* is a roundworm parasite that invades the human intestine. A mature female worm can produce 200,000 eggs a day, which are expelled with the host's feces. These minute eggs are easily washed through the soil and ingested by a new host. Hatching in the small intestine, the baby worms burrow into the body and are soon in the bloodstream or lymph. Fine capillaries of the lungs eventually filter them out; the worms bore across into the bronchial tubes, where they are coughed up and then swallowed, returning the roundworms to the intestine to mature. Damage occurs when the worms migrate through the body or when infestations are very large and cause blockage, especially in small children. Among the more serious diseases caused by roundworms are elephantiasis and trichinosis.

—*John Richard Schrock, Ph.D.*

See also Arthropod-borne diseases; Elephantiasis; Parasitic diseases; Pinworm; Roundworm; Schistosomiasis; Tapeworm; Trichinosis; Tropical medicine; Zoonoses.

FOR FURTHER INFORMATION:

Desowitz, Robert S. *New Guinea Tapeworms and Jewish Grandmothers*. New York: W. W. Norton, 1987. This collection of essays by a distinguished professor of tropical medicine focuses on parasitic diseases. These profiles of schistosomes, tapeworms, and filarial worms are readable true stories.

Schmidt, Gerald D., Larry S. Roberts, and John Janovy. *Foundations of Parasitology*. 5th ed. Boston: Wm. C. Brown, 1996. This book, designed for upper division courses in general parasitology, includes sections on the biology, physiology, morphology, and ecology of human and domestic animal parasites.

Zeibig, Elizabeth A. *Clinical Parasitology: A Practical Approach*. Philadelphia: W. B. Saunders, 1997. Presents all the guidelines needed to perform, read, and interpret parasitology tests. Each chapter contains thorough descriptions of parasitic forms, drawings with structures labeled, typical characteristics, and look-alike parasites.

WOUNDS

DISEASE/DISORDER

ANATOMY OR SYSTEM AFFECTED: All

SPECIALTIES AND RELATED FIELDS: Critical care, emergency medicine, family practice, internal medicine

DEFINITION: Disruptions or breaks in the continuity of any body tissue.

Wounds might arise because of violence, accident, or intentional procedure, such as surgery. They may be classified according to the instrument responsible, such as a knife, bullet, or shrapnel, or according to the way in which they occurred, such as a burn or a crushing wound.

Surgeons describe wounds according to their general appearance. A wound may be described as incised, when a sharp cutting instrument is involved; lacerated, when damage is due to a jagged instrument; contused, when the edges are cut; avulsed, when part of the tissue is torn apart; punctured, when the outer opening is rather small; penetrating; and nonpenetrating, when the external tissue remains intact. Fractures are also classified in several terms, such as spiral, impacted, and comminuted. The depth of the tissue injury classifies burns as first, second, or third degree.

Generally, wounds may be classified as open or closed. Closed wounds involve no external hemorrhage, and their degree of seriousness is related to the force of the blow and its direction, the age of the victim, and other physiological and anatomical factors. Normally, internal hemorrhage stops abruptly, with the blood and fluid absorbed within a few days. More bleeding occurs when larger internal vessels are damaged, with subsequent collection of the blood in the tissues forming a hematoma that may take several weeks to be absorbed. The impact on a body part may result in damage to a part that is not directly involved at the time of impact. Thus, a fall on an outstretched hand may injure not only the flesh and bones of the hand itself but also the scaphoid part of the wrist, or even the elbow or shoulder. During a car accident, a stationary body part may be heavily affected by the transmission of impact from a relatively mobile part; when occurring in the neck, this type of injury is commonly known as whiplash. First aid procedures for fractures, sprains, and strains include ice packs, crutches, elevation, and splinting.

Infections resulting from wounds. Open wounds take place when the skin and/or the mucous membranes are broken, thus allowing the invasion of hazardous foreign material, such as bacteria or dirt, into the tissues. This invasion may lead to infection, which is particularly serious when the disruption of the skin is considerable. Generally, injuries from sharp instruments (such as a needle, knife, or bullet) cause little tissue damage, except to the part that they penetrate. The great danger lies in the injury of a vital organ and from the foreign objects that are on the surface of the instrument. Injuries from irregular objects (such as bomb fragments or a jagged knife) create much more damage which leads to longer recuperation periods. Skin is elastic and well supplied with blood, which means that superficial cuts heal easily. The subcutaneous fatty tissues and muscles are not as rich in blood supply, and their damage is more serious and long-lasting, especially because it is easier for infection to occur. Fragmentation of bone in an open wound is particularly troublesome, since the fragments cannot survive without blood and will act as foreign substances, thus creating a serious infection. Injuries to joints, nerves, or major capillaries (such as arteries) will complicate the state of the open wound.

The contamination of the wound may start immediately after the causative incident. Nonbacterial contamination is more serious when organic substances are involved. In bacterial contamination, the most serious results are seen with virulent bacteria that are nourished by dead tissue and organic foreign material, sometimes leading to gas gangrene. Such infection generally spreads unchecked and can be stopped only by surgical removal or amputation, in order to avoid death. Other infections are caused by streptococcal and staphylococcal bacteria and are characterized by the local production of pus. Finally, tetanus is another type of wound infection. It starts with serious muscle spasms a few days after the injury and, left untreated, often leads to death.

The healing process. When an open wound occurs, the tissues are cut and the edges of the wound separate, pulled apart by the elasticity of the skin. Blood flowing from the wound fills the resulting cavity, fibrin is produced, and the blood clots, creating a scab. During the first twenty-four hours after the injury, the scab shrinks, drawing the edges of the skin together. Special cells called histiocytes and macrophages digest the debris in the wound, such as blood seepage, dead cells, and other foreign bodies. Connective tissue cells called fibroblasts grow inward from the margins of the wound to close the cavity. The fibroblasts produce a protein called collagen that provides strength to the new skin.

The red-colored capillaries slowly disappear and are replaced by white collagen. Thus, upon removal of the scab a layer of reddish granulation tissue appears, which covers the subcutaneous tissue. A thin, gray membrane extends outward from the skin edges and covers the whole surface. Contraction brings the epithelial sheets from the two sides together, and eventually the skin around the wound is reproduced. Wounds that cross normal skin creases become depressed below the level of the surrounding skin. The resulting scars, which are very low in capillaries, do not become tanned with sunlight exposure, and they produce neither hair nor sweat, which is indicative of skin that is less than fully functional. They are much whiter than the surrounding skin.

Treatment. Medical treatment of wounds requires first the control of bleeding, bandaging. Dead tissue is removed surgically through amputation. Sutured wounds heal faster because stitches bring the skin edges together. Foreign material in a wound may be absorbed by the tissues, which is exactly what happens when catgut is used to close the wounded tissue. Disinfection is particularly helpful in the healing process. In the case of small cuts, methods of disinfection include the external use of oxidizing agents (such as hydrogen peroxide) and of nonpolar ointments (such as petroleum jelly) to combat the invading polar bacteria. Body factors are also crucial in the overall healing; these include age, the concurrent presence of diseases, and nutrition that includes adequate quantities of protein and antioxidants, such as vitamin C. Hospitals take elaborate precautions to prevent infections through sterilization, good air filtration, the use of ultraviolet light to kill bacteria in the operating room, and the administration of antibiotics. The skin in the area of any surgery is treated with antiseptics and is carefully protected with sterilized cloth.

—*Soraya Ghayourmanesh, Ph.D.*

See also Amputation; Bites and stings; Bleeding; Burns and scalds; Concussion; Fracture and dislocation; Fracture repair; Frostbite; Gangrene; Grafts and grafting; Healing; Infection; Laceration repair; Necrotizing fasciitis; Plastic surgery; Shock; Tetanus; Transfusion.

FOR FURTHER INFORMATION:

Browner, Bruce D., Lenworth M. Jacobs, and Andrew N. Pollak, eds. *Emergency Care and Transportation of the Sick and Injured.* 7th ed. Boston: Jones and Bartlett, 1999. Includes new and expanded coverage of patient assessment, anatomy and physiology, stroke and seizure, trauma injuries, and special chapters on pediatrics and geriatrics.

Handal, Kathleen A. *The American Red Cross First Aid and Safety Handbook.* Boston: Little, Brown, 1992. A comprehensive, fully illustrated guide outlining basic first aid and emergency care steps to be taken until medical assistance can be obtained. Updated materials can also be obtained directly from local Red Cross Association chapters listed in telephone books.

Leikin, Jerrold B. *American Medical Association Handbook of First Aid and Emergency Care.* Edited by Bernard J. Feldman. New York: Random House, 2000. Covering urgent emergency situations as well as the common injuries and ailments that occur in every family, this AMA guide takes the reader step-by-step through basic first-aid techniques.

Thygerson, Alton L. *First Aid and Emergency Care Workbook.* Boston: Jones and Bartlett, 1987. Concise information packed into a workbook format, produced in cooperation with the National Safety Council. Charts, drawings, photographs, and tables outline common emergency care, covering a wide range of topics for the general public.

WRINKLES

DISEASE/DISORDER

ANATOMY OR SYSTEM AFFECTED: Skin
SPECIALTIES AND RELATED FIELDS: Dermatology, plastic surgery
DEFINITION: Lines in the skin caused by structural changes over time.

CAUSES AND SYMPTOMS

All human body fibers are formed by specialized cells in the tissues and can be classified as inelastic or elastic. Inelastic fibers are rigid and provide support to the surrounding tissue, while elastic fibers are more malleable. With the passage of time, inelastic fibers tend to become even tougher because of structural changes that occur in collagen, the major protein found in skin, bones, and ligaments. The dermis, the inner layer of the skin, contains large amounts of collagen, which is responsible for the skin's mechanical characteristics, such as strength and texture. The skin cells that make and reproduce damaged collagen are called fibroblasts.

As a person ages, collagen tends to form cross-links between different parts of the molecule or between similar molecules that are near each other, thus creating a rigidity that leads to skin sagging and wrinkling. Moreover, the recoiling ability of elastic fibers appears to be reduced, a condition that is often enhanced by calcification. Skin wrinkling is much more pronounced with prolonged exposure to wind and ultraviolet light. The effect appears to be cumulative along with collagen degeneration and epidermis thinning, as seen with people of outdoor professions. Other studies suggest that heavy cigarette smoking contributes to the risk of wrinkling.

TREATMENT AND THERAPY

Application of collagen-containing creams does not seem to create a desired change because the applied collagen molecules are too large to penetrate the dermis. Such applications only temporarily cover wrinkles. Injecting collagen under the wrinkles in a way that pushes the groove up, causing it to become smooth, has some positive cosmetic effect but also serious drawbacks. The main problem comes from the animal source of the collagen, which may lead to serious allergic reactions by the immune system and may, in rare cases, trigger a long-lasting autoimmune disease. Moreover, the smoothing effect of the injections appears to be brief because of the inability of the animal collagen to integrate itself into the skin's collagen mesh. Better results are observed when biotechnology-synthesized collagen is used or when the patient's own fibroblasts are removed, grown in a laboratory, and reinjected into the body. The careful administration of vitamin C, collagen amino acids, or very small quantities of copper peptides appears to stimulate the skin to produce more collagen. In addition, the topical application of growth factors and hormones that enhance the collagen-forming process of cells seems to give favorable results.

Chemical peels have been used to correct facial wrinkling in face lift or eyelid surgeries. A mixture of chemicals is applied to the skin, leading to extreme swelling and consequent peeling of the old skin, thus providing a fresh skin in two weeks. Carbon dioxide lasers were first developed in 1964, but experiments that combined them with computer technology did not begin until the 1990's. This resurfacing technique, which affects an area of skin no more than one hair in thickness for no more than one thousandth of a second, works in a way similar to chemical peel. It is considered best for patients of fair to medium complexion who have good healing qualities and who have not used acutane in the previous year.

—*Soraya Ghayourmanesh, Ph.D.*

See also Aging; Dermatology; Face lift and blepharoplasty; Plastic surgery; Skin; Skin disorders.

FOR FURTHER INFORMATION:

Bonner, Joseph, and William Harris. *Healthy Aging: New Directions in Health, Biology, and Medicine.* Claremont, Calif.: Hunter House, 1988.

Carper, Jean. *Stop Aging Now!* New York: Harper-Collins, 1995.

Fries, James F. *Aging Well.* Reading, Mass.: Addison-Wesley, 1989.

Rossman, Isadore. *Looking Forward: The Complete Medical Guide to Successful Aging.* New York: E. P. Dutton, 1989.

X RAYS. *See* **IMAGING AND RADIOLOGY.**

YEAST INFECTIONS. *See* **CANDIDIASIS.**

YELLOW FEVER
DISEASE/DISORDER
ANATOMY OR SYSTEM AFFECTED: Blood, brain, heart, liver, muscles, musculoskeletal system, nervous system

SPECIALTIES AND RELATED FIELDS: Epidemiology, public health, virology

DEFINITION: Yellow fever is an acute viral infection of the liver, kidneys, and heart muscle which is transmitted by *Aedes aegypti* mosquitoes. About three to fourteen days after being infected, a patient develops headache, fever, and muscle pain. In more advanced cases, fever is high and the person may become disoriented. With severe infection also comes delirium, slow and weak pulse, the vomiting of blood, and the presence of protein in the urine; the person may also become yellow from jaundice. Treatment of yellow fever involves bed rest, fluid maintenance, anticoagulant therapy, and blood transfusions. Up to 20 percent of those infected will die. Travelers to areas where yellow fever is known to exist should be immunized at least ten days prior to the trip.

—*Jason Georges and Tracy Irons-Georges*
See also Arthropod-borne diseases; Bites and stings; Epidemiology; Jaundice; Tropical medicine; Viral infections.

FOR FURTHER INFORMATION:
Busvine, James R. *Disease Transmission by Insects: Its Discovery and Ninety Years of Effort to Prevent It.* New York: Springer-Verlag, 1993.

_____. *Insects, Hygiene, and History.* 3d ed. London: Athlone Press, 1983.

Learmonth, Andrew. *Disease Ecology: An Introduction to Ecological Medical Geography.* Oxford, England: Basil Blackwell, 1988.

Snow, Keith R. *Insects and Disease.* New York: John Wiley & Sons, 1974.

YOGA
PROCEDURE
ANATOMY OR SYSTEM AFFECTED: All

SPECIALTIES AND RELATED FIELDS: Alternative medicine, preventive medicine, psychology

DEFINITION: A mental discipline, originating in India, designed to master consciousness, to offer spiritual insight, and to induce tranquillity.

INDICATIONS AND PROCEDURES
The word "yoga" is related to the English term "yoke." Of Sanskrit origin, yoga has a double implication. One meaning of the word is "union," the joining (or "yoking") of the individual to the ultimate reality behind the universe. A second inference is the concept of discipline, the training or subjugation of the self, as the mind prevails over both matter and itself, to bring consciousness into perfect harmony with the power behind the cosmos.

Common in the major Eastern religions of Hinduism, Buddhism, and Jainism, yoga originated in ancient India as a spiritual technique to help the individual obtain release (*moksha*) from *karma*, or the endless cycle of birth-death-rebirth, and attain *nirvana* (the bliss of self-transcendence). The Hindu classic the *Bhagavad Gītā* (the song of the Blessed Lord), dating from the second century B.C.E., envisioned three types of release: the way of knowledge (*jnana marga*), the way of action (*karma marga*), and the way of devotion (*bhakti marga*). Building on the philosophy of release, yoga facilitated techniques for the person to transcend the physical, mental, and spiritual bonds to the "world of illusion."

Of the many forms of yoga, *Hatha Yoga* (or "physical yoga"), involving bodily discipline, has been extremely popular in the West. In the East, *Raja Yoga* (or "royal yoga"), pioneered by the Indian philosopher Patanjali, who lived in the second century B.C.E., has been popular. *Raja Yoga* moves through eight steps: vows of nonviolence and restraint (*yama*), an attempt at internal control and tranquillity (*niyama*), the perfection of particular bodily postures (*asana*), a mastery of breath control (*pranayama*), discipline of the senses to exclude the external world (*pratyahara*), concentration on a single object (*dharana*), meditation (*dhyana*), and the trance-state (*samadhi*), accomplished through a union with Brahman (ultimate reality).

USES AND COMPLICATIONS
Until relatively recently, yoga has been neglected by Western medicine because it operates from a different set of premises. Yoga is based on the belief that a "subtle body" exists within the body (paralleling the physiological system) that has seven major centers (*chakras*), each with its own particular energy and

Typical Positions in Yoga

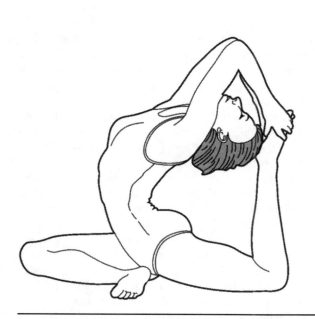 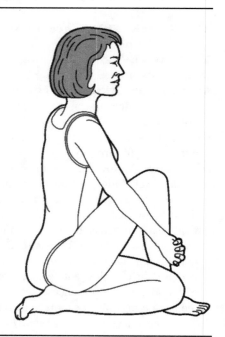

The movements and body positions employed in yoga are now recognized in medicine for their promotion of flexibility and their use in stress reduction.

functions. Yoga is designed to tap into the power contained in each of these centers. Recent studies suggest that the various yoga techniques do, in fact, produce the effects that their teachers predict, including reduction of tension, heart rate, blood pressure, and anxiety. The more remarkable powers claimed by yoga masters—such as levitation, total immunity to pain, and mental projection—have yet to be demonstrated in parapsychology laboratories.

—*C. George Fry, Ph.D.*

See also Alternative medicine; Meditation; Stress; Stress reduction.

FOR FURTHER INFORMATION:

Goldberg, Burton, comp. *Alternative Medicine: The Definitive Guide.* Puyallup, Wash.: Future Medicine, 1993.

Jacobs, Jennifer, ed. *The Encyclopedia of Alternative Medicine: A Complete Family Guide to Complementary Therapies.* Rev. ed. Boston: Journey Edition, 1997.

Kastner, Mark, and Hugh Burroughs. *Alternative Healing: The Complete A-Z Guide to over 160 Different Alternative Therapies.* New York: Henry Holt, 1996.

Mills, Simon, and Steven J. Finando. *Alternatives in Healing.* London: Grange Books, 1995.

Zoonoses

Disease/disorder

Anatomy or system affected: All

Specialties and related fields: Bacteriology, epidemiology, public health, virology

Definition: Diseases that can be transferred to humans from their primary animal hosts, including farm animals, laboratory research animals, tropical insects and animals, and common housepets, and including poliomyelitis, malaria, rabies, and toxoplasmosis.

Key terms:

inoculate: to introduce immunologically active material in order to treat or prevent a disease

malaise: a feeling of lack of health or debility, often indicating or accompanying the onset of illness

mycobacterium: any of a genus of nonmotile aerobic bacteria that are difficult to stain and include numerous saprophytes and the organisms causing tuberculosis and leprosy

organism: a complex structure of interdependent and subordinate elements whose relations and properties are largely determined by their function as a whole

pathogen: a specific causative agent (as a bacterium or virus) of disease

rabies: an acute virus disease of the nervous system of warm-blooded animals, usually transmitted through the bite of a rabid animal

toxoplasma: any of a genus of parasitic microorganisms that are typically serious pathogens of vertebrates

toxoplasmosis: the infection of humans, other mammals, or birds with disease caused by toxoplasmas that invade the tissues and may seriously damage the central nervous system, especially that of an infant

tuberculosis: a highly variable, communicable disease of humans and some other vertebrates caused by the tubercle bacillus; characterized by toxic symptoms of allergic manifestations that in humans primarily affect the lungs

vaccinate: to administer a vaccine, usually by injection

vaccine: a preparation of killed microorganisms or living, virulent organisms that is administered to produce or increase immunity to a particular disease

Causes and Symptoms

There are many types of contact between humans and animals. Some produce pleasure, such as stroking a kitten's fur; some have strictly utilitarian considerations, such as farming or meat processing; and some are to help animals themselves, such as the veterinary sciences. Unfortunately, some also result in the transmission of infectious diseases to humans, which are called zoonoses. The most common symptoms of zoonoses are headache, fevers, general malaise, diarrhea or bloody stool, and sometimes skin rashes, eruptions, or inflammation (in the event of a bite or sting).

Approximately 150 types of zoonoses can be transmitted either directly or indirectly to human beings. Direct exposure results from coming in contact with an infected animal or its excrement, blood, or saliva. Indirect exposure results from being bitten by an insect carrying an infected animal's blood. In either case, a disease may or may not develop.

Although many diseases transmissible to humans from animals now can be cured, it is important to avoid the methods of transmittal, especially the handling of infected animals. Humans must wash their hands after handling animals, especially after cleaning cages or litter boxes. Small children should be discouraged from kissing and cuddling pets. In rural or mountainous areas, humans should be discouraged from handling wild animals. In some communities, especially rural areas, keeping wild animals such as wolves or raccoons as pets is popular. Unfortunately, wild animals can carry many serious diseases that can be passed to humans, notably rabies.

Incubation periods for zoonoses can range from a few days to several years. If it is suspected that a human has contracted a disease from an animal, it is important to seek medical attention. Most zoonoses can be diagnosed and treated. In most cases, treatment will clear up the disease with no lasting aftereffects. If the infected person waits too long for treatment, however, therapy may take longer, and problems may persist. In rare cases, surgery is necessary, and in even rarer cases, death can occur.

Zoonoses vary greatly in their symptoms and sources. Among the most important of these diseases are anthrax, brucellosis, cat-scratch fever, encephalitis, Lyme disease, malaria, cattle tuberculosis, plague, rabies, ringworm, Rocky Mountain spotted fever, roundworm, salmonella poisoning, sporotrichosis, and toxoplasmosis.

Anthrax is an infectious disease of warm-blooded animals such as cattle or sheep, caused by the bacterium *Bacillus anthracis*. The disease can be transmitted to humans by the handling of infected products, such as the animals' hair. The disease is characterized by lesions in the lungs and by external ulcerating nodules.

Brucellosis is characterized by repeated fevers accompanied by weakness and joint pain. It is contracted from the amniotic and fetal membranes of pregnant and newborn animals. More typical in farm animals, it can also be present in dogs that are bred. While it is not fatal, it does cause severe flulike symptoms. It can be difficult to treat and cure completely.

Not as serious as toxoplasmosis, which can also be transmitted through a bite or scratch from a cat, cat-scratch fever is a bacterial infection which can result when a human is bitten, nipped, or scratched by a feline. Symptoms include a blistery inflammation at the site of the infection, fever, malaise, and sometimes swelling of the lymph nodes. Such symptoms appear two to thirty days after the skin is broken and generally last about a month. The infection will generally clear up on its own, but, after washing the affected area with soap and water, a consultation with a physician is recommended. Approximately twenty thousand people are infected annually with cat-scratch fever, mostly children. It is important for parents to instruct children not to play roughly with cats.

The bite of mosquitoes infected with encephalitis can cause this disease in humans. The illness is an infection of the lining of the brain; symptoms include a high fever, general malaise, and usually a very strong headache. Another disease transmitted by the bite of mosquitoes is malaria, which is caused by sporozoan parasites. Symptoms include intermittent chills and fever. Malaria may persist for years, and once the disease has been contracted, those affected are discouraged from donating blood, to avoid passing it on to others.

Lyme disease is an insect-related disease that is usually caused by the bite of a deerfly or tick. The disease was named for an area of Connecticut where it was first discovered. A doctor treating patients with flulike symptoms and skin inflammations realized that patients complaining of the symptoms had all been walking in woody areas and had been in contact with brush, weeds, and flowers where the tiny ticks and deerflies could have been harbored. The insects preyed on deer and other animals in the area, then probably jumped off or were brushed off the host animal into the grass. (Bitten animals may become infected with the disease as well.) Cases of Lyme disease have been found in almost every state, with the highest percentage being reported in the Midwest and on the East Coast. Although humans can develop the disease from a tick or deerfly bite, there is no evidence yet that a bite or scratch from an infected animal can transmit the disease.

The bacterium *Borrelia burgdorferi* is responsible for Lyme disease. Its symptoms include inflammation, skin lesions and redness, joint inflammation, fever, fatigue, general malaise, and headaches or a stiff neck. These symptoms may last for weeks after the bite. Nerve-related disorders and heart ailments may follow the preliminary symptoms. Early treatment is a fourteen-day regimen of antibiotics, which can then be followed by treatment with antimicrobial agents until symptoms cease. Later stages of Lyme disease, such as arthritis and heart disorders, can be treated with penicillin-type antibiotics. Nevertheless, joint and muscle pain may persist for several weeks.

Rocky Mountain spotted fever is another disease caused by tick bites. The disease is found in all areas of the United States, not only in the Rocky Mountains. Symptoms include headache, fever, and skin rash. Early diagnosis and antibiotic treatment are very important in order to prevent more serious complications.

An infection that often strikes herded animals such as cows, deer, or elk is a subspecies of tuberculosis caused by *Mycobacterium bovis*. Individuals who come in contact with such animals, such as veterinarians, farmers, and slaughterhouse workers, are most susceptible to this disease because they breathe in the tiny droplets of bacteria. In addition to lung infections, other diseases are reported to be associated with the *M. bovis* bacterium. Treatment for infected individuals is with antibiotics.

Plague is an infectious disease transmitted by the bite of a rodent flea infected with the bacillus *Yersinia pestis*. Two forms of plague affected millions of humans in Asia and Europe during the Middle Ages and continue to occur today, although not in epidemic form. Bubonic plague results in the formation of buboes, or swellings of the lymph glands. The Black Death was caused by the same bacterium and was probably pneumonic plague; this form is transmissible between people and is characterized by black patches appearing on the skin of its victims. Both types cause fevers and heavy coughing. Before the discovery of antibiotics, most victims died from this very contagious disease.

Rabies is an acute viral disease of the nervous system of warm-blooded animals, usually transmitted through the bite of the infected animal. Rabies can be found in a small number of animal species across the world. There are two main types: urban rabies, carried mainly by domesticated animals such as dogs; and sylvatic rabies, carried by wild animals such as bats. Symptoms of the disease include fever, nausea, vomiting, shortness of breath, abdominal pain, and a cough. If left untreated, the muscles become paralyzed and breathing and heartbeats stop, causing death. There are three methods of treating the disease: vaccination of people at risk of exposure before any exposure has occurred; animal control and immunization, especially preexposure immunization; and postinfection treatment, usually a series of expensive, painful shots.

Generally, the incubation period for rabies in humans is three weeks to three months. There have been cases, however, in which the victim was bitten by a rabid animal a year before the onset of the disease. Two documented cases showed that the victims were bitten by infected dogs while traveling in Asia six or seven years prior to the onset of the illness. Worldwide, approximately eighteen thousand people per year are treated for possible rabies infection. While domesticated animals, such as dogs and cats, can be treated against the development of rabies, it is difficult to inoculate wild animals, mostly because vaccines are not licensed for use on them. One method to attempt to control rabies in wild animals is the use of edible bait laced with vaccine.

Ringworm is a skin disease caused by a fungus, not a worm. The fungus usually occurs on exposed skin, especially the scalp, and looks inflamed and scaly. Diagnosis in animals is made by exposing the hair or fur to an ultraviolet lamp (the infected area will appear greenish in color). In humans, antifungal soaps or drugs will cure the disease.

Salmonella bacteria in food cause gastroenteritis, inflammation of the mucous membrane of the stomach and intestine. Symptoms of the disease are severe, bloody diarrhea and sometimes dehydration. The illness is very contagious and often spread rapidly in day care or home settings. While usually found in uncooked meat, it has been discovered that the salmonella bacteria can be present on pet turtles raised on farms. Thus parents buying pet turtles for their children may unknowingly bring the disease into their homes. Many of these strains of salmonella are quite resistant to commonly used antibiotics, thus making treatment difficult and allowing the disease to spread.

When this information came to the attention of the United States government, the shipping of live turtles from their farms was banned and various laws were enacted to restrict the interstate and international trade of the reptiles. Shipment of turtle eggs is still allowed, however, and as many as 20 percent of these eggs may carry the bacteria.

Most spider bites result in redness and itchiness or soreness at the site. They usually heal by themselves in a few days. The bites of some venomous spiders, however, such as the brown recluse, or violin, spider (*Loxosceles reclusa*), can cause serious complications in humans. Symptoms of the bite of a brown recluse spider include an eruption which turns black in the center, surrounded with a characteristic bull's-eye pattern of red, white, and blue circles. The sore is accompanied by flulike symptoms, weight loss, and extreme fatigue. If treatment is not sought, the flesh at the site becomes gangrenous, and surgery is necessary.

Almost all newborn puppies carry roundworms, and because children love to cuddle puppies, the children often pick up the worms without knowing it. Symptoms in humans are a cough, fever, headache, and poor appetite. Treatment for both humans and puppies is with anthelmintic (worm-destroying) drugs. It is important that all puppies be seen by a veterinarian when very young.

Sporotrichosis is a fungal infection transmitted by cats. The fungus is found as mold on decaying vegetation, soil, and timber, usually found along southern U.S. waterways and in places with similar climates. Left untreated, the fungus can spread throughout the human body. The organism enters the body through a cut or abrasion in the skin or through inhalation of the fungus. Therefore, it is a good idea to wash one's hands after handling cats.

Protozoan toxoplasmas are found in undercooked meat, unwashed raw fruits, and in the feces of cats, and cause a condition called toxoplasmosis. The toxoplasmas may enter the human body through the skin or by respiration. Extreme care should be taken, especially by pregnant women, when disposing of used cat litter. In pregnant women, the disease invades fetal tissues, causing damage to the baby's central nervous system. The antibiotic spiramycin is effective in combating the disease's effects. Toxoplasmosis also poses a threat to AIDS patients as a major cause of encephalitis (inflammation of the brain or brain's lining). Experiments have been conducted with the drug clindamycin in treating toxoplasmic encephalitis in AIDS or HIV-positive patients; however, such side effects as diarrhea and rashes have resulted.

TREATMENT AND THERAPY

Zoonoses are transmitted either directly from an animal (by handling it or coming in contact with its feces or saliva) or indirectly (by being bitten or stung by an insect which is carrying tainted blood from an infected animal). Symptoms of infection in humans usually consist of headache, fevers, general malaise, nausea, diarrhea, and skin eruptions or inflammation. If any of these symptoms is present after receiving an animal bite or scratch, or even after handling an animal, a visit to medical personnel is necessary.

Prevention plays the largest part in avoiding transmission of these diseases. People should wash their hands after touching or being in contact with animals, even if they do not appear to be sick or infected. Parents should instruct children to be careful when playing with pets. Humans should not care for wild animals as housepets. Hunters and hikers should take care when traveling through wooded areas so as not to pick up ticks or other insects; wearing clothing that covers the body, with socks rolled over pantlegs and gloves fitting over long sleeves, can help in these instances. Finally, pregnant women should avoid contact with animal feces (someone else, for example, should change the cat's litterbox) in order to avoid contracting toxoplasmosis.

PERSPECTIVE AND PROSPECTS

Zoonoses have been in existence ever since humans and other animals have been together. There is probably no way to completely eliminate such diseases from the human world. Since zoonoses can be transmitted in any environment in which animals and humans live, work, or play together, such eradication would be impossible. It is, therefore, extremely important for people to take precautions when handling animals or animal by-products (such as meat).

Although there are approximately 150 known zoonoses, new diseases that are transmissible between humans and animals are being identified. Most zoonoses are relatively rare and can be treated once a proper diagnosis is made by medical personnel. With common sense and precautionary measures, the contraction of such diseases can be controlled.

—*Carol A. Holloway*

See also Anthrax; Arthropod-borne diseases; Bacterial infections; Bites and stings; Encephalitis; Fungal infections; Lice, mites, and ticks; Lyme disease; Malaria; Parasitic diseases; Plague; Poliomyelitis; Protozoan diseases; Rabies; Roundworm; Salmonella infection; Tapeworm; Toxoplasmosis; Tuberculosis; Viral infections; Worms.

FOR FURTHER INFORMATION:

"AAP Issues Policy on Treatment of Lyme Disease in Children." *American Family Physician* 44, no. 1 (July, 1991): 308. While there is much information written about Lyme disease in general, this clinical article focuses on treatment for infected children. The symptoms are listed, and the detection of antibodies and antibiotic regimens for early treatment are discussed.

Biddle, Wayne. *Field Guide to Germs.* New York: Henry Holt, 1995. This comprehensive book is easily accessible to the nonspecialist and includes a discussion of nearly every virus, bacterium, and fungus known to cause human and nonhuman animal disease.

Folkenberg, Judy. "Pet Ownership: Risky Business?" *FDA Consumer* 24 (April, 1990): 28-30. This three-page article focuses on a list of the most common zoonoses transmitted from domesticated animals, such as housepets. The targeted audience consists of adults who are contemplating becoming pet owners.

Hugh-Jones, Martin E., William T. Hubbert, and Harry V. Hagstad. *Zoonoses: Recognition, Control, and Prevention.* Ames: Iowa State University Press, 2000. Preceding synopses of parasitic, fungal, and viral agents are sections on the principles and history of zoonoses recognition, new disease agents, and advances in control and prevention.

"Human Rabies: Strain Identification Reveals Lengthy Incubation." *The Lancet* 337, no. 8745 (April 6, 1991): 822. In this clinical article, virus-typing techniques are presented to show the many strains of rabies. Case histories of victims who did not demonstrate any symptoms for several years after infection are cited.

Palmer, S. R., Lord Soulsby, and D. I. H. Simpson, eds. *Zoonoses: Biology, Clinical Practice, and Public Health Control.* New York: Oxford University Press, 1998. This volume covers the history, scientific basis for control, microbiology of the causative agent, pathogenesis, clinical features, symptoms and signs, diagnosis, treatment, and prognosis for each disease.

"Salmonella and Pet Turtles." *Child Health Newsletter* 8 (April, 1991): 21. This article highlights the dangers lurking in pet turtles and their eggs, with a warning to adults seeking to buy such pets for their children. A list of symptoms is presented, along with contagion issues.

Schlossberg, David, ed. *Infections of Leisure.* Washington, D.C.: ASM Press, 1999. This volume brings together a collection of essays, each addressing a different setting for the transmission of disease. Chapter titles include "At the Shore," "Freshwater: From Lakes to Hot Tubs," "The Camper's Uninvited Guests," and "Perils of the Garden."

Swabe, Joanna. *Animals, Disease, and Human Society: Human-Animal Relations and the Rise of Veterinary Medicine.* New York: Routledge, 1999. This book takes a historical perspective on zoonoses, discussing such things as the intensification of livestock production and the domestication of animals and how these trends have effected disease transmission.

Woodruff, Bradley A., Thomas R. Eng, and Jeffrey L. Jones. "Human Exposure to Rabies from Pet Wild Raccoons in South Carolina and West Virginia, 1987 Through 1988." *The American Journal of Public Health* 81, no. 10 (October, 1991): 1328. This clinical article focuses on the risk of transmission of rabies to humans as a result of attempts to domesticate wild animals.

"Zoonoses: Unseen Dangers." *Current Health* 17 (March 2, 1991): 11-13. This three-page article is written for the general reader and highlights the basic manners in which zoonoses can be transmitted—through family pets, hunting, hiking, and wildlife. Prevention tips are given in an inset box.

GLOSSARY

Abandonment: The failure of a health care provider to continue emergency medical treatment.

Abdomen: The part of the body between the thorax (chest) and the pelvis.

Abortion: Termination of a pregnancy before the stage of viability (about twenty weeks); may occur from natural causes (spontaneous abortion) or may be induced by medical intervention.

Abscess: A pocket of infection or inflammation.

Absorption: A process transporting digested food from the small intestine into blood vessels, blood, and body cells.

Acid-base chemistry: The interaction between acids and bases in the cells of the body, the proper functioning of which is crucial in digestive metabolism, respiration, and the buffering capacity of body fluids.

Acidosis: A condition of high blood carbon dioxide levels and low pH that results from such diseases as emphysema and pneumonia.

Acne: A group of skin disorders; acne vulgaris usually affects teenagers, while acne rosacea usually afflicts older people.

Acquired immunodeficiency syndrome (AIDS): A progressive loss of immune function and susceptibility to secondary infections that arises from chronic infection with the human immunodeficiency virus (HIV).

Action potential: An electrochemical event in which nerve cells send signals along their cellular extensions in the nervous system.

Active euthanasia: The administration of a drug or some other means that directly causes death.

Active immunity: Immunity resulting from antibody production following exposure to an antigen.

Acupressure: An ancient Chinese mode of therapy performed by applying pressure to specific points on the body.

Acupuncture: Insertion of long, fine needles at particular points on the body located along one of fourteen major meridian lines, thought to be the major channels of life force. Developed by the Chinese.

Acute: Referring to a disease process of sudden onset and short duration.

Acute confusion: A transient condition caused by social and/or biological stressors, which may include inattention, disorganized thinking, other mental impairments, and emotional problems.

Acute rejection: The rejection of a transplanted organ by cells of the immune system; acute rejection is common days to weeks after cadaveric organ transplants and can usually be treated successfully with antilymphocytic drugs.

Adaptation: A decreased sensitivity to a stimulus, even though the stimulus may still be present, resulting in slowing of nerve impulses until the impulses stabilize or stop entirely.

Addiction: A psychological and sometimes physiological process whereby an organism comes to depend on a substance; characterized by a persistent need to use the substance, increases in the dosage used in order to counteract tolerance, and withdrawal symptoms when the substance is withheld or the dosage is reduced.

Addison's disease: A chronic condition in which the adrenal glands do not produce adequate amounts of corticosteroid hormones.

Adenoids: A group of lymph nodes located above the tonsils, at the back of the nasal passage; usually disappear after childhood but are sometimes surgically removed (adenoidectomy) if they become swollen and cause blockage or infection.

Adenosine triphosphate (ATP): A high-energy compound found in the cell that provides energy for all bodily functions.

Adhesion: The "gluing" together by scar tissue of internal organs and tissues, often caused by endometriosis or infections; a common cause of pelvic pain.

Adipose tissue: Fat, a soft tissue of the body composed of cells (adipocytes) that contain triglyceride, a compound consisting of glycerol and fatty acids.

Adjustment (chiropractic): A thrust delivered into the spine or its articulations in order to reestablish normal joint and nerve function.

Adjuvant therapy: Therapy used in addition to surgery in order to control the growth of remaining cancer cells.

Adrenal glands: Small organs near the kidneys that are responsible for the production of certain sex hormones, including testosterone and small amounts of estrogen, and of hormones involved in metabolism and stress responses.

Adrenalectomy: Surgical removal of one or both of the adrenal glands.

Advanced life support (ALS): Procedures to sustain life such as intravenous therapy, pharmacology, cardiac monitoring, and electrical defibrillation.

Aerobic exercise: Exercise that requires oxygen for energy production and that can be sustained for prolonged periods of time; involves large muscle groups, increases the heart rate and/or breathing rate, and is rhythmic and continuous.

Aerobic respiration: The chemical reactions that use oxygen to produce energy.

Aerospace medicine: The medical specialty concerned for the health of the operating crews and passengers of air and space vehicles.

Affective disorders: Mental conditions characterized by a primary disturbance of mood as distinct from thinking or behavior.

Ageism: Discrimination against individuals based on their age; the overlooking of individuals' abilities to make positive contributions to society because of their age.

Agglutination: A clumping of blood cells caused by antibodies joining with antigens on the cell surfaces.

Aging: The process of growing older, which begins at conception and eventually leads to death; the gradual effects of aging include changes in every organ and body system.

Agnosia: Inability to recognize persons or various objects despite being able to see them clearly.

Agonist: A drug which acts in a similar fashion to a hormone or neurotransmitter normally found in the body.

AIDS. *See* Acquired immunodeficiency syndrome (AIDS).

Albinos: Individuals who have an inherited defect in the production of melanin characterized by a lack of pigmentation.

Alcohol: An organic compound containing a hydroxyl group attached to a carbon atom; ethyl alcohol is the compound found in alcoholic beverages.

Alcoholism: The compulsive drinking of and dependency on alcoholic beverages; viewed as psychological in origin, it can be arrested but not cured.

Alkalosis: A condition of abnormally low carbon dioxide levels that results from hyperventilation (rapid breathing).

Alkylating agents: Drugs that introduce alkyl groups to biologically important cell constituents, whose function is then impaired.

Alleles: Alternate forms of a gene; an individual has two alleles of each gene (one from each parent), which may be the same or different.

Allergen: A substance (such as pollen, dust, or animal dander) that causes an allergic reaction.

Allergies: Exaggerated immune reactions to materials that are intrinsically harmless; the body's release of pharmacologically active chemicals during allergic reactions may result in discomfort, tissue damage, or, in severe responses, death.

Allied health: A designation used to describe the services and personnel that support the providers of direct patient care within the larger health care system.

Allogeneic: Of the same species.

Allograft: A graft of tissue from one individual to another individual, usually between close relatives.

Alloimmunization: Immunization by means of antibodies from another person.

Allopathic medicine: The traditional course of study leading to a doctorate in medicine; most practicing physicians are allopathic physicians.

Alternative medicine: Any of a variety of nontraditional therapies and treatments (such as acupuncture, herbal medicine, and homeopathy) which are not practiced by the established medical community. These alternative treatments range in the degree to which their efficacy and legitimacy have been accepted, from highly experimental and non-science-based to well established.

Altitude sickness: A condition resulting from altitude-related hypoxia (low oxygen levels).

Alveolar cell: Also known as an acinar cell; the fundamental secretory unit of the mammary glandular tissue.

Alveoli: Tiny air sacs deep within the lungs.

Alzheimer's disease: A progressive disease characterized by a loss of brain cells; it causes increasing memory impairment and cognitive deficits.

Ambulatory care: Health care provided outside the hospital, usually in a clinic, office, or home.

Amenorrhea: A lack of menstruation in girls by the age of eighteen or its suppression, often as a result of overly strenuous exercise, rapid weight loss or gain, or emotional trauma.

American Medical Association: The largest voluntary association of physicians in the United States, with most of its members engaging directly in the practice of medicine.

Amino acid: The fundamental building block of proteins; there are twenty amino acids.

Amnesia: An impairment of memory, which may be total or limited, sudden or gradual.

Amniocentesis: A procedure in which a small amount of fluid is removed from the amniotic sac of a pregnant woman to detect abnormalities that may be present in the fetus.

Amniotic fluid: Fluid within the amniotic cavity produced by the amnion during the early embryonic period (two to eight weeks) and later by the lungs and kidneys; it protects the fetus from injury and helps to maintain a stable temperature.

Amniotic sac: A thin, tough, membranous sac that contains amniotic fluid and the embryo or fetus of mammals, birds, and reptiles.

Amputation: Surgical removal of all or part of a limb or digit (finger or toe), often as a last resort to prevent fatal infection from gangrene.

Amylase: The enzyme responsible for breaking down carbohydrates in the small intestine; amylase enters the intestinal tract from the salivary glands and the pancreas.

Amyloidosis: A condition characterized by the deposit of waxy substances in animal organs.

Amyotrophic lateral sclerosis: Also called Lou Gehrig's disease; the most common form of motor neuron disease, in which the nerves that control muscle movement degenerate in the brain and spinal cord.

Anabolic steroids: A class of steroids that stimulate body reactions to build up more complex molecules and structures from simpler molecules; most are synthetic derivatives of testosterone.

Anaerobic: Occurring in the absence of oxygen.

Anal incontinence: The inability to control defecation.

Analgesic: A medication (such as aspirin) that reduces or eliminates pain.

Analyte: Any chemical substance undergoing measurement; includes charged electrolytes found in the blood, such as sodium or potassium.

Anastomosis: The surgical connection of one tubular organ to another.

Anatomy: The structure of the human body—its parts, systems, and organs.

Andrology: The study of the physiological functions relating to male reproductive capacity.

Anemia: A condition characterized by a deficiency of red blood cells or hemoglobin; anemia is sometimes caused by a decrease in hemoglobin production, an increase in cell destruction, or blood loss.

Anesthesia: A state characterized by the loss of sensation, caused by or resulting from drugs that induce pharmacological depression of normal nerve function.

Anesthesiology: The branch of medicine specializing in the application of anesthetics.

Anesthetic: Any of a variety of drugs used to cause a patient to become unconscious and amnesic for a brief period of time.

Anesthetist: A health care specialist who administers anesthetics.

Aneurysm: A localized enlargement of a vessel, usually an artery, caused by the stretching of a weak place in the vessel wall.

Aneurysmectomy: Surgical removal of an aneurysm.

Angina: Chest pain often caused by coronary artery disease.

Angiography: A radiological technique for visualizing the interior of the arteries. Involves the placement of a catheter in an artery and the injection of dye.

Angioplasty: Compression of arterial plaque by insertion of a catheter into the artery and inflation of a balloon at the end of the catheter.

Anomia: An inability to remember the names of persons or objects even though the patient sees and recognizes the persons or objects.

Anorectal: Associated with the anal portion of the large intestine.

Anorexia nervosa: An eating disorder characterized by a compulsive aversion to food, caused by a fear of obesity and a distorted body image, that may result in severe malnutrition.

Anosmia: A loss of the ability to detect aromas.

Antagonist: A drug that acts to block the effects of a hormone or neurotransmitter normally found in the body.

Anterior: Toward the front of the body.

Anthropology: The study of human culture.

Antibiotic: Any substance that destroys or inhibits the growth of microorganisms, such as bacteria.

Antibody: A protein produced in the body by the immune system that recognizes and binds selectively to foreign material (antigens) to facilitate their elimination; antibodies combat bacterial, viral, chemical, and other invasive agents in the body.

Anticholinergic: Referring to drugs that oppose the action of acetylcholine in nerve-impulse transmission.

Anticoagulant: A drug that reduces the clotting of the blood.

Anticonvulsant: A drug that prevents or diminishes convulsions.

Antidote: Anything that counteracts the effect of a substance.

Antiemetic: A drug that prevents or relieves the symptoms of nausea and/or vomiting.

Antifungal agent: A drug that kills or inhibits the growth of fungi.

Antigen: A molecule that induces the production of antibodies; antigens are generally proteins.

Anti-inflammatory drugs: Drugs that counter the effects of inflammation, either locally or throughout the body; the three classes of these drugs are steroidal, immunosuppressant, and nonsteroidal.

Antimetabolites: Chemotherapeutic agents that act by inhibiting enzymes in the DNA synthetic pathway or by incorporating in DNA itself.

Antiserum: The fluid portion of blood that contains specific antibodies.

Anxiety: A condition characterized by nervousness or agitation.

Anxiety disorders: Problems in which physical and emotional uneasiness, apprehension, and fear are the dominant symptoms.

Aphasia: The total absence of such language skills as speaking, reading, writing, and comprehension.

Apheresis: The removal of whole blood from a donor, followed by its separation into components, the retention of the desired component, and the return of the recombined remaining elements.

Apothecary: A pharmacist or druggist.

Appendectomy: The surgical removal of the vermiform appendix.

Appendicitis: Inflammation of the vermiform appendix, which may require its removal.

Aqueous humor: A clear, watery liquid that fills the region inside the front of the eyeball between the lens and cornea; also called the vitreous humor.

Arch bar: A pliable piece of metal that is fitted along the teeth to prevent jaw movement.

Areola: The pigmented tissue immediately surrounding the nipple.

Aromatherapy: The use of scents to facilitate physical, mental, and emotional well-being.

Arrhythmia: An abnormal heart rhythm, either in speed or force.

Arteries: Vessels that take blood away from the heart and toward the tissues.

Arteriosclerosis *or* **Atherosclerosis:** Hardening and thickening of the walls of the arteries caused by a buildup of fatty deposits or plaques.

Arthritis: Joint inflammation.

Arthroplasty: Replacement or repair of a joint using metal or plastic parts.

Arthropods: Small animals including mites, ticks, insects, and related organisms that may be vectors to animal or human hosts.

Arthroscopy: The use of an endoscope to examine the interior of a joint.

Articulation: A joint between two bones of the skeleton; also called an arthrosis.

Aseptic techniques: Sterilization and other procedures that allow surgeons to operate in a germ-free environment.

Asphyxiation: An impaired exchange of oxygen and carbon dioxide in the lungs; if prolonged, this condition leads to death.

Aspiration: The removal of a substance using suction; a cyst can be aspirated using a needle and syringe to withdraw its contents.

Assessment: The systematic process of collecting, validating, and communicating patient data; these data will include information gathered from the patient's history and the results of the physical examination and laboratory tests.

Asthma: A disorder of the lungs, experienced as wheezing and mucus blockage of the bronchi.

Astigmatism: A visual disorder in which either the cornea of the eye or the lens is not symmetrical.

Asymptomatic: Lacking or without any symptoms.

Ataxia: An inability to coordinate the muscles in voluntary movement.

Athlete's foot: A contagious fungal infection of the skin on the feet.

Atom: The smallest chemically and biologically active unit of matter; composed of electrons enclosing an atomic nucleus containing protons and neutrons.

ATP. *See* Adenosine triphosphate (ATP).

Atrioventricular (A-V) node: A small region of specialized heart muscle cells that receives the electrical impulse from the atria and begins its transmission to the ventricles.

Atrium (*pl.*** atria):** One of the two upper chambers

of the heart; the right atrium receives blood returning through the veins, while the left atrium receives oxygenated blood from the lungs.

Atrophy: The wasting of tissue, an organ, or an entire body as the result of a decrease in the size and/or number of the cells within that tissue, organ, or body.

Attenuation: The weakening or elimination of the pathogenic properties of a microorganism; ideally, the organism is rendered harmless.

Audiology: The study of hearing disorders and hearing loss.

Audiometer: A calibrated electronic device for the purpose of measuring human hearing to determine the magnitude of loss and the probable rehabilitative course.

Auditory nerve: The nerve that conducts impulses originating in hair cells of the cochlea to the brain for processing as the sensation of sound.

Auditory system: The human hearing mechanism, including the pinna, the external ear canal, the middle-ear structures, the cochlea, and the ascending neural pathway that terminates in the auditory cortex of the brain.

Aural rehabilitation: A program for hearing-impaired individuals which may include auditory prosthesis, auditory training, and speech reading training.

Auscultation: Active listening, usually with the aid of a stethoscope, to sounds generated by the body.

Autism: An emotional disturbance found in children in which communication, social interactions, and language skills are severely impaired.

Autoantibody: An antibody produced against tissue antigens within a host; self-antigens.

Autograft: A graft of tissue transferred from one part of an individual's body to another.

Autoimmune disorders: Disorders in which the immune system starts to attack the body's cells as foreign matter.

Autologous: Self-derived.

Autonomic nervous system: The division of the nervous system that regulates involuntary actions, such as vital functions; comprises the sympathetic and parasympathetic systems.

Autopsy: Examination of a dead body to determine cause of death.

Autosomal: Refers to all chromosomes except the X and Y chromosomes (sex chromosomes) that determine body traits.

Autosomal recessive gene: A gene (other than the X

or Y chromosome) that must be on both chromosomes in order to be expressed.

Autotransplantation: The transplantation of tissue or organs in which the recipient serves as his or her own donor (such as a skin graft); may also refer to transplantation between genetically identical individuals (identical twins).

Axon: The cellular extension of the neuron that conducts electrical information, transmitting it to the dendrite of the next neuron through the synaptic gap between them.

AZT. *See* Zidovudine.

B lymphocyte: A blood and lymphatic cell that plays a role in the secretion of antibodies.

Bacillus Calmette-Guérin (BCG): A weakened version of *Mycobacterium bovis*, which is used in vaccines to protect against tuberculosis; also, the vaccine itself.

Bacteremia: A condition in which bacteria enter the bloodstream and thus can be disseminated throughout the body.

Bacteria: Single-celled microorganisms that exist throughout the environment.

Bacterial endocarditis: Bacterial infection of the heart, which may scar or destroy a valve.

Bacteriology: The study of bacteria.

Balloon catheterization: The use of a balloonlike device on the tip of a catheter to widen blood vessels, as in angioplasty.

Barrier method: The use of a contraceptive that physically prevents sperm from meeting the ovum, including the male condom, female condom, diaphragm, cervical cap, and vaginal sponge.

Basal cell carcinoma: The most common type of skin cancer; it grows slowly and seldom spreads beneath the skin.

Basal cells: Cells at the base of the epidermis that migrate upward and become the principal source of epidermal tissue.

Basic life support (BLS): A variety of life-support procedures, including rescue breathing and chest compressions, often given to a heart attack victim by the first person responding to the patient; public training in such procedures is available from the Red Cross and the American Heart Association.

BCG. *See* Bacillus Calmette-Guérin (BCG).

Becquerel: The international unit of radioactivity, defined as a radioactive sample that is decaying at the rate of one disintegration per second.

Bed-wetting: A condition characterized by an inability of the bladder to contain the urine during sleep, often a developmental condition in children.

Bell's palsy: A sudden paralysis of one side of the face, including muscles of the eyelid.

Beneficence: A principle of medical ethics which requires that actions be taken for the patient's good.

Benign: Referring to a tumor made of a mass of cells which do not leave the site where they develop.

Benign senescent forgetfulness: A common source of frustration in old age, associated with memory impairment; unlike dementia, it does not interfere with the individual's social and professional activities.

Bereavement: The general, overall process of mourning and grieving; considered to have progressive stages which include anticipation, grieving, mourning, postmourning, depression, loneliness, and reentry into society.

Beriberi: A serious vitamin deficiency caused by an inadequate intake of thiamine (B_1).

Bile: Fluid produced by the liver and stored in the gallbladder to be secreted into the intestine; contains salts, bile pigments (bilirubin), cholesterol, and other waste products.

Biliary colic: A distinct pain syndrome characterized by severe intermittent waves of right-sided, upper abdominal pain, often brought on by the ingestion of fatty foods; pain occurs when a gallstone obstructs the outflow of bile and usually resolves when the gallstone moves away from the outflow area.

Bilirubin: A major component of bile, derived from the breakdown products of red blood cells.

Bioengineering: The combination of biological principles and engineering concepts and/or methodology to improve knowledge in both areas.

Biofeedback: Receiving information about involuntary bodily responses in an effort to modify these responses to some extent, thus learning how to reduce stress and induce or maintain other positive behavior.

Biomedicine: The branch of medical science concerned with the capacity of human beings to survive and function in abnormally stressful environments, as well as with the protective modification of such environments.

Bionics: The medical application of biological and engineering knowledge to the design of artificial systems that act in the place of natural systems.

Biophysics: The application of the theories and laws of physics to the study of biological processes.

Biopsy: The removal of tissue from a suspected site of disease, such as cancer, in order to identify abnormal cells under microscopic examination.

Biopsychosocial model: A model that examines the effects of illness on all spheres in which the patient functions—the biological sphere, the psychological sphere, and the social sphere.

Biostatistics: The application of statistical analyses to the study of biological data.

Biotechnology: The medical application of biological and engineering knowledge at the molecular and genetic levels of these natural systems in order to diagnose, treat, cure, or learn more about diseases.

Bipolar disorder: A syndrome characterized by alternating periods of mania and depression; formerly called manic-depressive disorder.

Birth defect: A genetic abnormality in the tissue development of a certain body part of the fetus; in some cases the defect is minor, but in others it may be medically dangerous to the fetus and/or the mother.

Blackout: Memory loss, usually as a result of taking substances known to disrupt memory, in which the affected person may function as if aware of what is happening, despite having no memory of activities.

Bladder: The organ that stores urine until it is discharged from the body.

Blastocyst: A small, hollow ball of cells which typifies one of the early embryonic stages in humans.

Blepharoplasty: The removal of excess tissue around the eyelids.

Blood: The fluid that circulates in the veins and arteries, carrying oxygen and nutrients through the body, transporting waste materials to excretory channels, and participating in the body's defense against infection.

Blood bank: A temporary storehouse of blood, kept at reduced temperatures, for transfusions into persons needing an additional supply; such transfers are vital in surgery and in unexpected emergency procedures.

Blood group system: A classification of individuals into groups on the basis of their possession or nonpossession of specific blood substances.

Blood pressure: A measure of how much the fluid in the blood vessels pushes against the walls of the vessels.

Blood testing: The withdrawal of blood from an individual and its analysis for one of many purposes, including blood typing and a search for acquired or genetic disease indicators.

Blood type: A blood classification group based on the presence or absence of certain antigens on red blood cells.

Blood typing: The identification of the blood-group substances of individuals so as to classify them in specific blood groups; individuals may have blood types A, B, or O and be Rh negative or Rh positive.

Body mass index (BMI): Weight in kilograms divided by height in meters, squared (kg/m^2).

Bolus: Food that has been mixed with saliva and formed into a ball; the bolus passes from the mouth to the stomach through a process called swallowing, or deglutition.

Bone grafting: The transplantation of a section of bone from one part of the body to another, or from one individual to another.

Bone marrow: The soft substance that fills the cavities within bones and that is the site of blood cell production.

Bone marrow transplantation: The removal of bone marrow from an immunologically matched individual for infusion into a patient whose bone marrow has been destroyed.

Bone scan: A diagnostic technique using a radioactive tracer which is strongly absorbed by a tumor, whose location then can be detected by radiation counters.

Bones: Hard tissues that form the skeleton, providing support while allowing flexibility.

Botulism: Food poisoning caused by bacteria which produce a toxin that is absorbed by the digestive tract and spread to the central nervous system.

Bowman's capsule: The group of cells in the kidneys that forms the cup of a nephron; fluids that seep from glomerular capillaries into the hollow wall of the capsule will be transformed into urine during their passage through the renal tubule leading from the capsule.

Bowman's glands: One of three sources in the nasal cavity of the mucus that moisten the membranes of the olfactory center, thereby allowing odoriferous molecules to adhere to the olfactory hairs; glands that are located between olfactory supporting cells.

Bradycardia: Slowness of the heartbeat.

Brain: The most complex organ in the body, which is used for thinking, learning, remembering, seeing, hearing, and many other conscious and subconscious functions.

Brain death: Irreversible brain damage so extensive that the organ enjoys no potential for recovery and can no longer maintain the body's internal functions.

Brain stem: The medulla oblongata, pons, and mesencephalon portions of the brain, which perform motor, sensory, and reflex functions (such as respiration) and which contain the corticospinal and reticulospinal tracts.

Breast: The mammary gland, along with the nipple in front of it and the surrounding fatty tissue.

Breast biopsy: The surgical removal of a lump or tissue from the breast to determine whether it is malignant.

Breast cancer: Malignancy occurring in breast tissue and possibly involving the associated lymph nodes.

Breech position: A commonly encountered abnormal fetal presentation in which the buttocks is first delivered, rather than the head; may require a cesarean section.

Bronchi: The airways conducting air from the mouth to the depths of the lungs.

Bronchitis: An inflammation of the bronchial tree of the lungs.

Bronchoscopy: The visual examination of the respiratory system using a flexible tube composed of optic fibers.

Buffer: A solution which contains components that enable a solution to resist large changes in pH when small quantities of acids and bases are added.

Bulbourethral gland: The bulbous portion of the male urethra adjacent to the prostate gland.

Bulimia: A compulsive eating disorder characterized by food binges and purges (either through self-induced vomiting or the use of laxatives).

Bunion: A swelling of the big toe caused by an inflamed bursa, often a complication of footwear.

Bursa: A connective tissue sac filled with fluid that reduces friction at joints.

Bursitis: An inflammation of a bursa, one of the membranes that surround joints.

Bypass graft: A surgical procedure that reroutes blood around an obstruction, usually caused by atherosclerosis; the "new" artery can be either plastic or constructed from an expendable, healthy section of vein in another part of the patient's body.

Bypass surgery: Heart surgery to bypass a clogged

artery by use of an unclogged vein, usually taken from the leg.

Calcification: The deposit of lime salts in organic tissue, leading to the buildup of calcium in the arterial wall.

Calcitonin: A hormone made and released by the thyroid gland that lowers the level of calcium in the blood by stimulating the formation of bone.

Calculi (*sing.* calculus): Any of a variety of stones formed by calcium deposits, cholesterol, and other materials which may accumulate in the kidneys, gallbladder, or elsewhere in the urinary or digestive tract.

Calorie: The basic unit of energy; the amount of heat needed to change the temperature of 1 liter of water from 14.5 degrees Celsius to 15.5 degrees Celsius.

Cancer: Inappropriate and uncontrollable cell growth within specialized tissues, which threatens normal cell and organ function.

Candidiasis: An overgrowth of the fungus *Candida albicans*, which may affect the vagina, mouth, or skin; commonly called a yeast infection.

Cannula: A tube used to drain body fluids or to administer medications.

Capacitation: A change in sperm when in the female reproductive tract that causes them to swim more vigorously.

Capillaries: Minute blood vessels that connect the smallest arteries (arterioles) to the smallest veins (venules); they allow passage of oxygen and nutrients from the arteries into the tissue and passage of waste products from the tissues into the veins.

Carbohydrates: A group of organic compounds that includes the sugars and the starches; one of three classes of nutrients and a basic source of energy.

Carbon dioxide: The gas produced by the body from the use of oxygen; carbon dioxide and the hydrogen ions that it can create may become toxic if not excreted by the body.

Carcinogen: A chemical or radiation mutagen that causes changes in genes, leading to the cancerous state in a cell.

Carcinoma: A malignant neoplasm arising from the epithelial cells that make up the surface layers of skin or other membranes.

Cardiac catheterization: The guidance of a catheter into the heart or great blood vessels to measure function, assess problems, and identify treatment options.

Cardiac muscle: A type of muscle, found only in the heart, that makes up the major portion of the heart; involved in the movement of blood through the body.

Cardiac rehabilitation: The activities that ensure the physical, mental, and social conditions necessary for returning cardiac patients to good health.

Cardiology: The branch of medicine specializing in the diagnosis and treatment of heart disease.

Cardiomyopathy: A serious acute or chronic disease in which the heart becomes inflamed; it may result from multiple causes, including viral infection, and may involve obstructive damage.

Cardiopulmonary resuscitation (CPR): A method of restoring normal breathing to a patient in cardiac arrest using chest compressions and artificial ventilation.

Cardiovascular: Relating to or involving the heart and blood vessels.

Cardiovascular disease: Any of a group of diseases that affect the heart, including coronary artery disease, hypertension, congestive heart failure, congenital heart defects, and valvular heart disease.

Carpal tunnel syndrome: Tingling and pain in the thumb, index, and middle fingers caused by pressure on a nerve that passes through an area in the hand called the carpal tunnel.

Carpus: The wrist.

Cartilage: White, fibrous connective tissue attached to the articular surfaces of bones.

Case management: An interdisciplinary approach to medical care characterized by the inclusion of physical, psychological, social, emotional, familial, financial, and historical data in patient treatment.

Casuistry: A form of moral reasoning whereby specific cases about which there is moral uncertainty are compared to other cases about which there is moral certainty.

Catalysis: An increase in the speed of a chemical reaction.

Cataract: A dark region in the lens of the eye that causes gradual loss of vision.

Cataract surgery: The removal of an eye lens with cataracts and the implantation of a plastic replacement using microsurgery.

Catheter: A flexible tube inserted into a body cavity to distend it or maintain an opening.

Catheterization: The insertion of a tube into a cavity of the body to withdraw fluids from or introduce fluids into that cavity.

Cathode-ray tube (CRT): A display device used for the presentation of nuclear medicine data; it displays images in real time.

Cauterization: A means of sealing blood vessels with heat used to prevent bleeding.

Cavities: Disintegrations in tooth enamel; also called tooth decay or dental caries.

Cecum: The dividing passageway between the small intestine and the large intestine (or colon).

Cell: The basic functional unit of the body, which contains a set of genes and all the other materials necessary for carrying out the processes of life.

Cell therapy: The injection of fetal lamb cells for the purpose of rejuvenation.

Cellular biology: The study of the processes that take place within a cell.

Cellular respiration: The chemical reactions that produce energy in the cell; these reactions can be aerobic or anaerobic.

Cellular transformation: The process in which a cell becomes cancerous, which begins with abnormal changes in gene expression and cell differentiation.

Cementum: The outer covering of the root of a tooth.

Centers for Disease Control and Prevention (CDC): The government agency charged with monitoring the spread of infectious diseases in the United States.

Central nervous system: The brain and spinal cord.

Centrifugation: The spinning of blood or another fluid to separate out certain components for laboratory analysis.

Cerebral palsy: A group of nonprogressive disorders of the upper neurologic system resulting in abnormal muscle tone and lack of muscular control.

Cerebrospinal fluid (CSF): The extracellular fluid of the central nervous system; it flows through the ventricles of the brain and the central canal of the spinal cord, circulating nutrients and providing a cushion for the brain.

Cerebrum: The largest and uppermost section of the brain, which integrates memory, speech, writing, and emotional responses.

Certification: The formal notice of certain privileges and abilities after completion of certain training and testing.

Cervical vertebrae: The first seven bones of the spinal column, located in the neck.

Cervix: The entrance to the uterus from the vagina; it secretes mucus, which appears as vaginal discharge.

Cesarean section: Delivery of a baby through the lower abdomen by means of surgery.

Charge: The quantity of electricity responsible for attraction and repulsion among atoms and molecules.

Chemical energy: The energy locked up in the chemical bonds that hold the atoms of a molecule together; food molecules, such as glucose, contain considerable energy in their bonds.

Chemoreception: Sensitivity to chemical stimuli.

Chemoreceptors: Specific structures that respond to chemical stimuli, producing such sensations as taste and odor.

Chemotherapeutic index: For antibiotics, the ratio of the maximum dose that can be administered without causing serious damage to a person to the minimum dose that will cause serious damage to the infecting microorganism; a measure of selective toxicity.

Chemotherapy: The use of chemicals to kill or inhibit the growth of cancer cells.

Chest: The region of the body from the diaphragm to the neck, both within the rib cage (heart and lungs) and in front of it (breasts and muscles).

Ch'i: The Chinese concept of the vital essence; when Ch'i is unbalanced, disease results.

Chickenpox: A very contagious but mild disease caused by the herpes zoster virus whose symptoms include fever, abdominal pain, and skin eruptions.

Chiropractic: Manipulation of the musculoskeletal and nervous structures (often the spine) to allow the body to use its natural recuperative systems to restore or maintain health.

Chlamydia: A sexually transmitted disease characterized by discharge, pain, and swelling of the genitals; if a pregnant woman is infected, the disease chlamydia can infect her infant's eyes during childbirth.

Choking: A condition in which the breathing passage (windpipe) is obstructed.

Cholecystectomy: The surgical procedure that results in the removal of the gallbladder in its entirety. The two main techniques are the traditional open method and the laparoscopically aided method.

Cholecystitis: Inflammation or bacterial infection of the gallbladder, usually caused by the presence of gallstones.

Cholelithiasis: The formation of gallstones in the gallbladder or the ducts that connect the gallbladder to the liver or small intestine.

Cholera: An infection of the small intestine caused by *Vibrio cholerae*, a comma-shaped bacterium.

Cholesterol: A lipid substance that is a structural component of cell membranes and which makes up the surface of lipoproteins.

Chordee: The downward curvature of the penis, most apparent on erection, caused by the shortness of the skin on the downward side of the penile shaft.

Chorionic villi: The fingerlike projections of the placenta that function in oxygen, nutrient, and waste transportation between a fetus and its mother.

Chromosomal abnormality: Any change to the number, shape, or appearance of the forty-six chromosomes in each human cell; the presence of many such abnormalities will prevent the normal development of an individual and lead to miscarriage.

Chromosomes: The parts of a cell's nucleus that contain genetic information, made of DNA covered with protein; each human cell has twenty-three pairs of chromosomes.

Chronic: Referring to a lingering or long-term disease process.

Chronic fatigue syndrome: Chronic fatigue syndrome is a multifaceted disease state characterized by debilitating fatigue.

Chronic rejection: The rejection of a transplanted organ months or years after transplantation.

Chronobiology: The study of the timing of biological processes (such as growth, development, aging, and accompanying cycles) within an individual.

Chyle: The product that results from the emulsification of fat by pancreatic juice during the digestive process.

Chyme: The semiliquid state of food as it is found in the stomach and first part of the small intestine.

Cilia: Hairlike structures on cells that sweep mucus, containing bacteria and foreign particles, out of the airways.

Ciliary body: A ring of tissue that surrounds the eye; the uveal portion of this tissue contains the ciliary muscle that adjusts the degree of curvature of the lens.

Circadian rhythm: A cyclical variation in a biological process or behavior that has a duration of slightly greater than twenty-four hours.

Circulation: The flow of blood throughout the body; the circulatory system consists of the heart, lungs, arteries, and veins.

Circulator: The worker in the operating room whose responsibility is to keep records and to open sterile supplies for the team members wearing gowns and gloves.

Circumcision: Surgical removal of an area surrounding a body part, most often used to denote removal of the male foreskin (prepuce).

Cirrhosis: A condition of the liver in which injured or dead cells are replaced with scar tissue.

Claudication: Muscle cramps that occur when arterial blood flow does not meet the muscles' demand for oxygen.

Cleavage: The process by which the fertilized egg undergoes a series of rapid cell divisions, which results in the formation of a blastocyst.

Cleft lip: Incomplete fusion of the two sides of the lips during embryonic development; often associated with cleft palate.

Cleft palate: Incomplete fusion of the two sides of the palate in the mouth during embryonic development.

Clinical examination: The physical examination of an individual animal, including its medical history and an evaluation of its environment.

Clinical laboratory: A general term for those areas of a medical facility where analyses of body fluids are performed.

Clinical trial: A research study to compare standard treatment against potentially better treatment.

Cloning: The making of many identical copies; the techniques that genetic engineers use to recombine DNA from different sources and to reproduce those fragments in bacteria or other organisms.

Clot: A clumping of platelets, blood, fibrin, and clotting factors that normally accumulates in damaged tissue as part of the body's healing process; also called a thrombus.

Clotting factors: Chemicals circulating in the blood that are necessary for the process of blood clotting.

Cluster headaches: Headaches characterized by intense pain behind one eye.

Coagulation: The process of blood clotting.

Cochlea: A structure in the inner ear that receives sound vibrations from the ossicles and transmits them to the auditory nerve.

Cognitive: Relating to the mental process by which knowledge is acquired.

Cognitive functioning: A general term describing mental processes such as awareness, knowing, reasoning, problem-solving, judging, and imagining.

Colitis: Inflammation of the mucous membranes of the colon.

Collagen: A protein found in bone and other connective tissues; collagen fibers are well suited for support and protection because they are sturdy, flexible, and resist stretch.

Collaterals: Small vessels that enlarge to compensate for the obstruction or narrowing of another vessel.

Collimator: A device used for restricting and directing gamma rays by passing them through a grid made of metal, which absorbs the rays.

Colon: The large intestine, divided from the small intestine by the cecum (a controlled passageway) and ending at the sigmoid, which leads food waste into the rectum.

Colon therapy: The irrigation of the colon with water in order to detoxify it.

Colonoscopy: Use of an endoscope to examine the interior of the colon visually.

Color blindness: A genetic condition of the eye in which the patient is unable to distinguish between some colors.

Colostomy: The surgical creation of an artificial opening for the colon.

Colostrum: Thin, yellow milky secretions of the mammary gland just a few days before and after childbirth; it contains more proteins and less fat and carbohydrates than does milk.

Coma: A loss of consciousness from which a person cannot be aroused; a symptom signifying a variety of causes.

Commissurotomy: The severing of corpus callosum, the fiber tract joining the two cerebral hemispheres.

Common cold: A class of respiratory infections that can be caused by one of hundreds of different viruses; also called rhinitis.

Communicative skills: Those skills required to express thoughts, desires, and feelings effectively through verbal and nonverbal communication.

Complement: A series of about twenty serum proteins that, when sequentially activated by immune complexes, may trigger cell damage.

Compound: To mix or combine; to make by combining parts of elements.

Compulsion: A persistent, irresistible urge to perform a stereotyped behavior or irrational act, often accompanied by repetitious thoughts (obsessions) about the behavior.

Computed tomography (CT) scanning: A method of displaying the outline of a tumor, utilizing a computer to combine information from multiple X-ray beams.

Conception: A process encompassing all the events

from fertilization of an egg to its first cell divisions.

Concordance: The inheritance of the same trait by both twins.

Concussion: Temporary neural dysfunction, causing confusion, dizziness, nausea, headache, lethargy, and short-term amnesia; often results when the head is struck by a hard blow or shaken violently.

Conductive loss: A hearing loss caused by an outer-ear or middle-ear problem which results in reduced transmission of sound.

Confidential: A situation distinguished by the willing disclosure of intimate information because of assurances that the information will be protected from general distribution or unauthorized disclosure; information which, if disclosed, has the potential to be damaging or dangerous to the person providing the information, their reputation, status, or their associates.

Congenital: Referring to a condition present at birth; it may result from an inherited trait or damage before birth.

Congenital disorders: Abnormalities present at birth that occurred during fetal development as a result of genetic errors, exposure to toxins and microorganisms, illness, or unknown causes.

Congenital heart disease: Conditions resulting from malformations of the heart that occur during embryonic and fetal development.

Congestive heart failure: Abnormal heart function characterized by circulatory congestion caused by cardiac disorders, especially myocardial infarction of the ventricles.

Conjunctivitis: An inflammation of the white part of the eye, the conjunctiva.

Connective tissues: Tissues containing large amounts of matrix outside the cells, such as tendons and ligaments.

Conscious: Having an awareness of one's existence, behavior, and surroundings.

Constipation: The slow passage of feces through the bowels or the presence of hard feces.

Contact dermatitis: A common skin allergy characterized by inflamed skin; it occurs when skin comes in contact with substances such as poison ivy or allergenic cosmetics.

Contact lens: A small, shell-like glass or plastic lens that rests directly on the external surface of the eye; used to correct refractive error as an alternative to spectacles, to protect the eye, or to serve as a prosthetic device promoting a more normal appearance of a disfigured eye.

Continuing medical education (CME): Medical lectures given by hospitals, medical societies, and conferences.

Contraception: Avoidance of conception by either natural means (such as abstinence) or artificial means (use of condoms, spermicides, diaphragms, intrauterine devices, or chemical hormone regulators such as birth control pills). No method of contraception except abstinence is completely effective.

Contraction: A squeezing action of the muscles, such as the squeezing of the uterus that results in birth.

Control group: A group of patients receiving either a standard treatment or a placebo, allowing comparison with the experimental treatment.

Contusion: A bruise; injury to tissue without breaking the skin.

Convulsion: An instance of high-frequency and amplitude-random electrical activity in the brain.

Cooper's ligament: Projections of breast parenchyma covered by fibrous connective tissue that extend from the skin to the deep layer of superficial fascia.

Cornea: The curved, transparent front surface of the eyeball, which provides protection and partial light focusing.

Coronary arteries: The arteries that supply blood to the heart muscle.

Coronary artery bypass graft (CABG): A surgical procedure in which a blocked coronary artery is bypassed using a vein or artery; this intervention provides a blood supply to areas beyond the distal attachment of the graft.

Coronary artery disease: A disease that results in a narrowing of the coronary arteries and a concomitant reduction of oxygen supply to the heart muscle.

Coronavirus: A microorganism causing respiratory illness; one of the most prevalent causes of the common cold.

Coroner: An officer, often a layperson, who holds inquests in regard to violent, sudden, or unexplained deaths.

Corpora cavernosa: Two parallel erectile cylinders on the upper side of penis that are filled with blood during a natural erection.

Corpus luteum: A yellow cell mass produced from a graafian follicle after the release of an egg.

Corpus spongiosum: A third cylinder in the penis below the corpora cavernosa; the urethra passes through it, and the glans penis forms the front end of the cylinder.

Corpuscle: A minute particle; a protoplasmic cell floating free in the blood.

Correlation: A number between −1 and +1 that describes the strength and direction of the relationship between two variables.

Corrosives: Having a burning (caustic) and locally destructive effect.

Corticosteroid: A fatlike molecule (or steroid), produced by the adrenal gland or made synthetically, that can be used to treat inflammation.

Cosmetic surgery: The application of plastic surgical techniques to alter the patient's appearance.

CPR. *See* Cardiopulmonary resuscitation (CPR).

Craniotomy: Any surgical incision into the cranium.

Creatine phosphate: An energy-containing molecule present in significant quantities in muscle tissue; energy is stored in a high-energy bond similar to that of ATP.

Creatinine: A nitrogen-containing by-product of metabolism; levels of creatinine may be indicative of kidney function.

Cretinism: A severe hypothyroidism in which infants are born with insufficiently developed thyroid tissue.

Critical care: Care, in a hospital or other clinical setting, for a patient who is termed "in critical condition," or in imminent danger of death.

Crohn's disease: A chronic inflammation of the bowel, often as a result of an autoimmune disease.

Crown: That portion of the tooth, normally covered with enamel, which is exposed in the oral cavity above the gingiva (gum).

Cryogenic agent: One of various mediums used to achieve the low temperatures needed to produce therapeutic effects.

Cryoprobe: An instrument used by physicians to apply cryogenic agents to diseased tissue; cryoprobes have differently shaped tips that affect the size and depth of the freezing.

Cryosurgery: The destruction of tissue by the application of extreme cold.

Cryotherapy: Use of cold temperatures to treat disease.

Crypt: A pit or cavity in the surface of a body organ (such as a tonsil).

CSF. *See* Cerebrospinal fluid (CSF).

CT scanning. *See* Computed tomography (CT) scanning.

Culdocentesis: Retrieval of a small amount of fluid,

by means of needle aspiration, from the recto-vaginal pouch for diagnostic purposes.

Current: The flow of electrical charges through space or a material.

Cusp: The conical projection of the chewing surface of the tooth.

Cuspid: The longest anterior tooth; also called the canine tooth or the eyetooth.

Cutaneous: Pertaining to the skin.

Cuticle: Cutaneous or skin tissue that surrounds the nail plate on its proximal sides and provides a protective barrier to the nail bed; it is attached to the proximal nail fold and to the nail plate.

Cybernetics: A field of study, closely associated with bionics, which is concerned with communication and control in living systems and their application to artificial systems.

Cyst: A swelling or nodule containing fluid or soft material, resulting from a blocked duct or abnormal growth in fluid-producing tissue.

Cystectomy: Surgical removal of the urinary bladder or the gallbladder; also, surgical removal of a cyst.

Cystic fibrosis: A genetic disease that affects the exocrine glands and most physical systems of the body, resulting in death usually between the ages of sixteen and thirty.

Cystitis: Inflammation of the bladder, primarily caused by bacterial infection and resulting in pain, urgency in urination, and sometimes hematuria (blood in the urine).

Cystoscopy: Use of an endoscope to examine the urinary bladder.

Cytokines: Proteins which are used by white blood cells to communicate with similar cells.

Cytopathology: The study of disease states as they manifest themselves within cells.

Cytoskeleton: A network of filaments (including microtubules, microfilaments, and intermediate filaments) that supports the cytoplasm and extensions of the cell surface.

D & C. *See* Dilation and curettage.

Debridement: The removal of all foreign material and contaminated and devitalized tissues from or adjacent to a traumatic or infected lesion until surrounding tissue is exposed.

Decubitus ulcer: Ulceration of the skin and subcutaneous tissues resulting from protein deficiency and prolonged, unrelieved pressure on bony prominences.

Defibrillation: The application of electrical energy through the chest in order to correct abnormal heart function and restore a normal heart rhythm.

Delayed primary closure: A procedure in which the wound is left open four to six days and then sewn closed; used for infected or contaminated wounds.

Dementias: Disorders characterized by a general deterioration of intellectual and emotional functioning, involving problems with memory, judgment, emotional responses, and personality changes.

Dendrite: The extension of the neuron that receives electrical information from neurotransmitters.

Dental arch: The arched bony part of the upper and lower jaws in which the teeth are found.

Dentin: The substance that comprises the major portion of the tooth internally.

Dentistry: The study, diagnosis, treatment, and maintenance of the teeth, gums, and other parts of the oral anatomy. Also known as odontology.

Deoxyribonucleic acid (DNA): A long, spiral-shaped molecule in chromosomes; the sequence of DNA subunits contains the genetic information of the cell and organism.

Department of Health and Human Services: A federal organization, headed by a member of the U.S. president's cabinet, concerned with the health of the nation's citizens.

Dependence: A condition related to maladaptive substance use and characterized by tolerance, withdrawal, and contrived use despite psychosocial or physical impairment because of use of the substance or efforts to acquire it.

Depression: A condition characterized by persistent feelings of despair, weight change, sleep problems, thoughts of death, thinking difficulties, diminished interest or pleasure in activities, and agitation or listlessness.

Dermatitis: A general term for nonspecific skin irritations that may be caused by bacteria, viruses, or fungi.

Dermatology: The study of the skin: its chemistry, physiology, histopathology, cutaneous lesions, and the relationships of these lesions to systemic disease.

Dermatopathology: The study of diseased skin tissue.

Dermatoses: Disorders of the skin.

Dermis: The second layer of skin, immediately below the epidermis; it contains blood and lymphatic vessels, nerves, glands, and (usually) hair follicles.

Detector: A device or substance that can sense ionizing radiation and produce an indication of its presence for visual display; examples are photographic film, certain phosphors such as calcium tungstate, and crystals such as sodium iodide.

Detoxification: The process by which toxic substances are removed from the body, often as a function of the body's natural responses over time; in alternative medicine, such methods as juice therapy or colon therapy may be used to aid this process.

Development: The process of progressive change that takes place as one matures from birth to death; development can be gradual (as on a continuum) or ordered (as in distinctly different stages).

Diabetes mellitus: A hormonal disorder in which the pancreas is unable to produce sufficient insulin to process and maintain a proper level of sugar in the blood; if left untreated, may lead to circulatory problems, heart disease, blindness, dementia, kidney failure, and death.

Diagnosis: The determination of what is causing a particular medical problem.

Diagnostic: Relating to the determination of the nature of a disease.

Dialysis: The filtration of crystalloid from colloid substances. Most commonly used to refer to the medical procedure performed periodically on individuals whose kidneys have failed to remove waste products and other toxic substances that build up in the blood.

Diaphragm: The muscular partition that separates the abdominal and thoracic cavities; also, a contraceptive device that covers the cervix.

Diarrhea: Loose, watery, and copious bowel movements.

Diastole: The period of relaxation of the heart between beats.

Diastolic blood pressure: The pressure of the blood within the artery while the heart is at rest.

Diathermy: The heating of body tissues because of the resistance to the passage of high-frequency electromagnetic radiation, electric current, or ultrasonic waves; also known as electrocoagulation.

Differentiation: The process of gradual change of tissues in the embryo or fetus.

Diffusion: The process in which substances move from an area of high concentration to an area of low concentration; if given enough time, the concentration of the substance will be the same everywhere.

Digestion: The chemical breakdown of food materials in the stomach and small intestine and the ab-

sorption into the bloodstream of essential nutrients through the intestinal walls.

Dilation: The opening of the cervix to allow passage of the fetus through the birth canal.

Dilation and curettage (D & C): Dilation of the cervix to allow scraping of tissue from the endometrium (lining of the uterus), used both to diagnose and treat disease.

Diminished capacity: Partial insanity; a legal determination that a defendant does not have the ability to achieve the state of mind required to commit a crime.

Diopter: A unit of power of a lens equal to the reciprocal of the focal length of the lens in meters.

Diphtheria: A highly contagious bacterial infection that usually affects the respiratory system.

Diploid: Containing a double set of chromosomes.

Dipstick: A chemically treated paper strip used for the chemical analysis of urine or saliva.

Disarticulation: The amputation of a limb through a joint, without cutting the bone.

Disease: An abnormal condition of the body, with characteristic symptoms associated with it.

Disk: A soft, cushionlike structure that lies between bony vertebrae from the base of the skull to the sacrum of the pelvis; it has a soft liquid in the center and is surrounded by a thickened ligament.

Disk prolapse: The protrusion (herniation) of intervertebral disk material, which may press on spinal nerves.

Dislocation: The forceful separation of bones in a joint.

Disorder: A persistent or repetitive maladaptive pattern in thinking, behaving, or feeling that necessitates treatment.

Distal: Away from the point of origin.

Diuretic: A drug that stimulates the kidneys to eliminate more salt and water from the body.

Diverticulitis: The painful inflammation of diverticula.

Diverticulosis: A disease involving multiple outpouchings, or diverticuli, of the wall of the colon.

Diverticulum: A pouchlike, weakened region of the colon wall, which can cause pain and bleeding.

Dizygotes: Fraternal twins; born from two ova separately fertilized by two sperms.

DNA. *See* Deoxyribonucleic acid (DNA).

DNA testing: A technique for identifying a person based on matching unique gene-bearing proteins from an organic sample taken from that person (such as hair, blood, or tissue) with another organic sample retrieved from the scene of a crime.

Domestic violence: Assaultive behavior intended to punish, dominate, or control another in an intimate family relationship; physicians are often best able to identify situations of domestic violence and assist victims to implement preventive interventions.

Dominant allele: The version of a gene that produces a recognizable trait in offspring when present in only one of the two chromosomes of a pair.

Dominant genetic disease: A disease caused by a mutation in a gene that need be inherited from only one parent in order to exert its effect.

Doppler shift: The increase in frequency of sound waves as the source of the waves approaches the observer or instrument; Doppler techniques are often used to assess blood flow in body channels such as veins.

Down syndrome: An inherited disease caused by a defect in chromosome 21 that produces moderate to severe mental retardation.

Drug: Any chemical substance that can be ingested into the body to modify bodily functions and responses.

Drug interactions: The chemical effects of taking drugs in combination, where the effects will reduce, magnify, or alter the desired effects of the drug.

Duodenum: The initial part of the small intestine, where most of the digestion of food occurs.

Duplex scan: An ultrasound representation of echo images of tissues and blood vessels combined with a Doppler representation of blood-flow patterns.

Durable power of attorney: Designation of a person who will have legal authority to make health care decisions if the patient becomes incapable of making decisions for himself or herself.

Dwarfism: Underdevelopment of the body, most often caused by a variety of genetic or endocrinological dysfunctions and resulting in either proportionate or disproportionate development, sometimes accompanied by other physical abnormalities and/or mental deficiencies.

Dys-: A prefix denoting wrong, painful, or difficult.

Dysfunction: The disordered or impaired function of a body system, organ, or tissue.

Dyskinesia: A neurologic disorder causing difficulty in the performance of voluntary movements.

Dyslexia: Severe reading disability in children with average to above-average intelligence.

Dysmenorrhea: Painful menstruation; primary dysmenorrhea is generally harmless and occurs in young women, while secondary dysmenorrhea may be caused by endometriosis, pelvic inflammatory disease, or tumors.

Dyspareunia: Painful sexual intercourse.

Dyspepsia: A general term applied to several forms of indigestion.

Dysphasia: A disturbance of such language skills as speaking, reading, writing, and comprehension.

Dysplasia: Any form of abnormal tissue development.

Dystrophy: A progressive condition that occurs when required nutrients do not reach tissues or organs, causing an inability of these structures to carry out their proper functions.

Dysuria: Painful or difficult urination, often the result of urinary tract infection or obstruction.

E. coli. See *Escherichia coli.*

Eardrum: The membrane separating the outer ear canal from the middle ear that changes sound waves into movements of ossicles; also called the tympanic membrane.

Ears: The organs responsible for both hearing and balance.

Eating disorder: An emotional disorder centering on body image that leads to a misuse of food, such as overeating, overeating and purging (bulimia), or undereating (anorexia nervosa).

ECG waves: The repeated deflections of an electrocardiogram; one complete wave consists of a P wave, followed by a QRS complex, and then a T wave and represents one complete cardiac cycle, or heartbeat.

Echocardiogram: A graph of cardiac motion and heart valve closure produced by sending sound waves to the heart and recording their deflections.

Echocardiography: The use of sound waves to record activities within the heart and great arteries and to examine heart structures.

Eclampsia: Hypertension induced by pregnancy, in its convulsive form.

Ecology: A branch of science concerned with the relationships between organisms and their environments.

Ecosystem: An ecological community considered together with the nonliving factors of its environment.

-ectomy: A suffix denoting surgical removal; for example, an appendectomy is the removal of the appendix.

Ectopic pregnancy: The development of a fertilized egg in a Fallopian tube instead of the uterus; can be fatal to the mother unless it is corrected surgically.

Eczema: A skin disorder characterized by reddening, swelling, blistering, crusting, and scabbing; also called dermatitis.

Edema: The abnormal accumulation of fluid in tissues or cavities of the body.

Effector: A general term referring to skeletal, smooth, and cardiac muscles or glands that respond to impulses produced by the nervous system.

Efficacy: The extent to which a drug or procedure works as expected under ideal conditions, such as in the laboratory; efficacy must be proven before a drug or procedure may be applied in a clinical environment.

Ejaculation: The release of sperm from the male's body during sexual activity.

Elbow: The joint between the upper arm and the forearm.

Electric anesthesia: The use of pulses of electricity to deaden nerve cells or cause unconsciousness.

Electrical shock: The physical effect of an electrical current entering the body and the resulting damage.

Electrocardiography (ECG or EKG): The recording of heartbeat activity using electrodes attached to the chest.

Electrocauterization: The use of a high-frequency electrical current or electrically heated metal to sear tissue.

Electroconvulsive therapy: The use of electric shocks to induce seizure in depressed patients as a form of treatment.

Electrodermal response biofeedback: The monitoring and displaying of information about the conductivity of the skin; used for anxiety reduction, asthma treatment, and the treatment of sleep disorders.

Electroencephalography (EEG): The recording of brain-wave activity using electrodes attached to the scalp.

Electrolytes: Chemicals that, when dissolved in water, dissociate to form positive and negative ions so that the resulting solution is an electrical conductor.

Electromyograph: An instrument that is capable of monitoring and displaying information about electrochemical activity in a group of muscle fibers.

Electromyography (EMG): An electrodiagnostic technique for recording the extracellular activity (action and evoked potentials) of skeletal muscles at rest, during voluntary contractions, and during electrical stimulation.

Electron: A tiny particle with an electronic charge; a component of an atom.

Electron volt: A unit of energy defined as the energy acquired by an electron traveling through a potential difference of 1 volt.

Elephantiasis: A grossly disfiguring disease caused by a roundworm parasite; it is the advanced stage of the disease Bancroft's filariasis, contracted through roundworms.

Embolism: The blockage of an artery by matter (such as a blood clot) that has broken off from another area.

Embolus: Any particle in the arterial or venous system that travels with the flow of blood and eventually lodges in the lungs, brain, or other organ or blood vessel.

Embryo: In humans, the cells growing from conception until the eighth week of pregnancy.

Embryology: The study of the development of the (human) organism from conception to birth.

Emergency medical services: The complete chain of human and physical resources that provides patient care in cases of sudden illness or injury.

Emergency medicine: The branch of medicine that addresses conditions (such as cardiac arrest, severe wounds, poisoning, seizures) requiring immediate medical treatment.

Emergency room: A health care facility where rapid evaluation and treatment of sudden illnesses, accidents, and traumas occurs.

Emetic: Something that causes vomiting (emesis).

Emphysema: A disease characterized by an increase in the size of air spaces at the terminal ends of bronchioles in the lungs, which reduces the ability of the lungs to exchange oxygen and carbon dioxide.

Enamel: The tissue that covers the crown of the tooth; the hardest tissue in the body.

Encephalitis: A family of diseases resulting from viral infection or complications from another disease; inflammation of the brain resulting in a variety of usually serious symptoms and sometimes death.

Encephalopathy: Any abnormality in the structure or function of the brain.

End-stage renal disease: The final phase of long-standing kidney disease, characterized by a nearly complete loss of kidney function.

Endarterectomy: A surgical technique for excising atherosclerotic plaque or the diseased endothelial lining of an artery.

Endemic disease: A disease that is usually present in a specific population such that the frequency of disease occurrence does not fluctuate greatly.

Endocarditis: Inflammation of the lining of the heart and its valves.

Endocrine: Referring to a process in which cells from an organ or gland secrete substances into the blood, which in turn act on cells elsewhere in the body.

Endocrine glands: Ductless glands that secrete hormones directly into the bloodstream.

Endocrine pancreas: Specialized secretory tissue dispersed within the pancreas called islets of Langerhans, which are responsible for the secretion of glucagon and insulin.

Endocrine system: The system of glands located throughout the body that produces hormones and secretes them directly into the blood for delivery by the circulatory system.

Endocrinology: The study of the endocrine system, the glands that produce hormones and the functioning of those hormones.

Endodontic disease: Diseases of the dental pulp found within teeth and diseases of the surrounding tissues, the gums.

Endodontics: The dental specialty that treats diseases of infected pulp tissue.

Endogenous: Something occurring or naturally found within the body.

Endometrial biopsy: A procedure designed to obtain a sample of the uterine lining (endometrium) for diagnostic analysis.

Endometriosis: A female reproductive disease in which cells from the uterine lining (the endometrium) grow outside the uterus, causing severe pain and sometimes infertility or the need for hysterectomy.

Endoplasmic reticulum: A system of cytoplasmic membrane-bound sacs that, with attached ribosomes, synthesize proteins destined to enter membranes or to be stored or secreted.

Endoscope: A lighted, flexible, hollow instrument used for examination and the placement of surgical instruments.

Endoscopic retrograde cholangiopancreatography: An endoscopic procedure in which dye is injected into the common bile duct and pancreatic ducts for visualization with X rays.

Endoscopy: The process of passing a fiber-optic instrument into the gastrointestinal tract for visualization.

Endospore: A modified bacterial cell that is extraordinarily resistant to heat, desiccation, and other environmental extremes.

Endothelium: The inner surface of the cornea, which is separated from the rest of the eye by a layer of transparent fluid.

Endotracheal tube: A flexible tube inserted through the mouth or nose into the trachea (windpipe) to carry anesthetic gas and oxygen directly to the lungs.

Enema: Any one of a variety of procedures for cleaning out the lower colon or injecting food or diagnostic substances.

Energy: A measure of a system's capacity to do work.

Enuresis: Bed-wetting.

Environment: The biological, physical, cultural, and mental factors that influence health; anything external to an individual.

Environmental diseases: Conditions and diseases resulting from largely human-mediated hazards in both the natural and artificial environments.

Environmental health: The control of all factors in the physical environment that exercise, or may exercise, a deleterious effect on human physical development, health, and survival.

Environmental medicine: The branch of medical science that addresses the impact of chemical and physical stressors and biological hazards on the individual or group in a community.

Environmental toxicology: The study of the impact of chemical pollutants on biological organisms; human health is the primary consideration, but the specialty also examines the effects of toxins on nonhuman organisms.

Enzyme: A protein secreted by a cell that acts as a catalyst to induce chemical changes in other substances, remaining apparently unchanged itself in the process.

Enzyme therapy: The administration of enzymes to aid digestive problems.

Epidemic: A marked increase in the frequency of a disease in a population, compared to historical experience.

Epidemiology: The study of the spread of disease in large groups of people.

Epidermis: The outer layer of the skin, consisting of a dead superficial layer and an underlying cellular section.

Epididymis: An organ attached to the testis in which newly formed sperm reach maturity (that is, become capable of fertilizing an egg).

Epidural anesthesia: Anesthesia produced by injecting a local anesthetic between the vertebral spines and beneath the ligamentum flavum into the extradural space; also known as extradural anesthesia.

Epilepsy: Uncontrollable excessive activity in either all or part of the central nervous system.

Episiotomy: Surgical incision into the area between the anus and the vagina to enlarge the vaginal opening during childbirth.

Epithelia: Tissues that originate in broad, flat surfaces.

Erection: A complex phenomenon involving nerves, blood vessels, and the mind that leads to the entrapment of blood in the penis, making it rigid.

Erythematous: Related to or marked by reddening.

Erythrocyte: The nonnucleated, disk-shaped blood cell that contains hemoglobin; also called a red blood cell.

Escherichia coli: A common bacterium which inhabits the human intestinal tract; used by genetic engineers to carry and propagate cloned DNA fragments and to produce proteins from the cloned genes.

Esophagectomy: Surgical removal of all or part of the esophagus.

Esophagus: The muscular tube through which food passes from throat to the stomach.

Essential nutrient: A substance that must be included in the diet because it cannot be synthesized by the body.

Ester: The relatively non-water-soluble compound formed when an alcohol reacts with a carboxylic acid.

Estrogen: The female sex hormone produced by the ovaries and the adrenal gland that is responsible for the development of female secondary sex characteristics; the three types naturally produced by the body are estradiol, estrone, and estriol.

Ether: A volatile liquid that causes unconsciousness when inhaled.

Ethics: A philosophical discipline that attempts to analyze systematically the way in which moral decisions are made; in medicine, ethics involves defining appropriate patient care, humane biological research, an equitable distribution of scarce medical resources, and a just health care delivery system.

Etiology: The investigation of the causes of any disease.

Eustachian tube: The tube connecting the middle ear to the back of the throat; air exchange through this tube equalizes air pressure in the middle ear with the outside air pressure.

Euthanasia: The medical inducement of death to relieve suffering. Though performed routinely on non-human animals, euthanasia on humans is against the law in most, but not all, societies.

Evolution: A theory that explains the development of all organisms from simple ancestor organisms.

Excision: The surgical removal of an organ or tissue.

Excisional biopsy: Biopsy by incision to excise and completely remove an entire lesion, including adjacent portions of normal tissue.

Exercise physiology: The science that studies the effects on the body of various intensities and types of physical activity, including cellular metabolism, cardiovascular responses, respiratory responses, neural and hormonal adaptations, and muscular adaptations to exercise.

Exocrine glands: Glands that excrete their products into tubes or ducts that empty onto the skin's surface.

Exogenous: Originating outside the body.

Expiration: The act of breathing out, which partly collapses the lungs.

Extended care: Long-term, ongoing medical care for individuals with serious, chronic, or terminal conditions; may be performed in a medical or hospice facility or at the individual's home.

Extended care facility: A facility that can be found in several settings, outside the home, where specialized medical care can be rendered under a physician's orders.

Extension: Movement that increases the angle between the bones, causing them to move further apart; straightening or extension of the ankle occurs when the toes point away from the shin.

Exteroreceptors: Sensory receptors generally located on the skin or body surfaces that supply the brain with information about the external environment in which the body is located.

Extracellular fluid: The internal environment of the human body that surrounds the cells; the fluid contains ions, gases, and the nutrients needed by cells for proper functioning and is constantly circulated throughout the body by the blood and into tissues by diffusion.

Extracellular respiration: The process of oxygen transport from the lungs to the cells and carbon dioxide transport from cells back to the lungs.

Eyes: The body structures that receive and transform information about objects into neural impulses that can be translated by the brain into visual images.

Face lift: The separation of the skin of the face from the underlying fascia and its tightening until the desired degree of wrinkle elimination is achieved; also called rhytidectomy.

Facial nerve: The seventh cranial nerve pair, which relays signals from the face and the front region of the tongue up to the pons of the brain stem; conducts impulses related to taste, salivation, and facial expression.

Fallopian tube: One of the two tubes through which egg cells travel from the ovaries, in which they originate, to the uterus.

Family practice: The branch of medical practice concerned with treating individuals comprehensively on a long-term basis, often along with, or in the context of, all members of that person's immediate family.

Farsightedness: The inability of the eye to focus on close objects; also called hyperopia.

Fascia: Connective tissues such as tendons and ligaments.

Fasciculation: A brief, spontaneous contraction of muscle fibers associated with disorders of the lower motor neurons.

Fasciectomy: Surgical removal of any part of the fascia.

Fatigue: A general symptom of tiredness, malaise, depression, and sometimes anxiety associated with many diseases and disorders; in some cases, no specific cause can be found.

Fats: A group of organic compounds, also called lipids, that store energy; one of three classes of nutrients.

Fatty acid: An organic compound that is composed of a long hydrocarbon chain with a carboxyl group at one end.

Fecalith: A hardened piece of fecal matter that often begins the events leading to appendectomy by blocking the appendix.

Fee-for-service: The traditional way of paying for medical care by billing patients when services are rendered (in contrast to a health maintenance organization).

Feedback: A system in which two parts of the body communicate and control each other, often through hormones; through such a system, hormones trigger other hormones' production (stimulatory feedback) or inhibition (inhibitory feedback).

Femur: The thigh bone.

Fenestration: The surgical opening of a passage in a closed or narrowing ear canal in order to allow sound to pass.

Fermentation: A chemical reaction that splits complex organic compounds into relatively simple substances.

Fertilization: The process in which the sperm head penetrates the ovum, resulting in the formation of an embryo.

Fetal alcohol syndrome: Growth retardation and mental or physical abnormalities in a child resulting from alcohol consumption by the mother during pregnancy.

Fetal tissue transplantation: The controversial use of tissue from aborted human fetuses to replace damaged tissue in patients with diseases in which the patient's own tissue has been destroyed (such as Parkinson's disease or diabetes mellitus).

Fetus: The unborn child from the eighth week after fertilization until birth.

Fever: A symptom associated with a variety of diseases and disorders, characterized by body temperature above normal.

Fiber: Food material derived from plant substances that retain the full structure of their cell walls despite the chemical effects of the digestive process.

Fiber optics: The transmission of light through thin, flexible tubes.

Fibrillation: Rapid and chaotic contractions of the heart muscle.

Fibrinolysis: The breakdown of fibrin, a major component of blood clots, that occurs after the broken vessel wall has healed; fibrinolytic agents are used to dissolve unwanted clots.

Fibula: The smaller of the two bones in the lower leg, on the lateral side.

Fight-or-flight response: A stressful biochemical reaction in animals, usually involving the adrenal hormone epinephrine, that prepares the animal for confrontation with predators or competitors.

Filiform papillae: The small, rounded projections that form the tough, yet velvetlike, texture of the tongue surface; lacking any chemoreceptors, these papillae do not function in the process of taste.

Fistula: Any of a variety of abnormal openings from an internal organ to the body's surface.

Flagellum: A long, whiplike structure at the base of the sperm that propels it forward.

Flexion: A bending movement that decreases the angle of the joint and brings two bones closer together; for example, flexion of the ankle pulls the foot closer to the shin.

Flora: The microorganisms that are commonly found on or in the human body; also called microflora.

Fluid: An intracellular or extracellular solution of water and other substances, the concentrations of which must be regulated to achieve proper physiological functioning.

Fluoroscopy: Examination of the deep structures of the body by means of a fluoroscope, which renders visible X-ray shadows by projecting them on a screen.

Foliate papillae: The folded papillae found on the soft edges of the tongue and just ahead of the V shape formed by the vallate papillae; although found in the regions that detect bitter or sour tastes, foliate papillae are not specific receptors for bitter or sour tastes.

Follicle: A small, saclike cavity for secretion or excretion, such as a hair follicle; also, spherical structures in the ovary that contain the maturing ova (eggs).

Food biochemistry: The breakdown of food by cells, a process in which nutrients are converted to energy and other components needed by the body.

Food poisoning: Food-borne illness caused by bacteria, viruses, or parasites consumed in food and resulting in acute gastrointestinal disturbance that may include diarrhea, nausea, vomiting, and abdominal discomfort.

Forearm: The region from the elbow joint to the wrist; also called the antebrachium.

Foremilk: The milk released early in a nursing session, which is low in fat and rich in nutrients.

Forensic: Having to do with a court of justice; forensic medicine and its various subspecialties apply medical science to the purposes of the law.

Forensic autopsy: A systematic investigation to determine the cause of death, providing the pathologist with information to state an informed opinion about the manner and mechanism of death in cases that are of public interest.

Forensic pathology: The branch of medicine that applies medical knowledge to legal situations, particularly crimes. Forensic specialists, for example, gather data to determine the causes and circumstances surrounding a death when the death is believed to be a homicide.

Forensic toxicology: The branch of toxicology that interacts regularly with the legal community and law enforcement.

Fourier-transform: A mathematical method which allows MRI to utilize one radiofrequency pulse and thereby examine all wavelengths, as opposed to examining each wavelength individually with a continuous wave.

Fracture: A break in a bone, which may be partial or complete.

Free radical theory: The idea that aging may be brought about by the production within the body of very reactive chemicals (free radicals) that damage chromosomes and other cell parts.

Frequency: The number of complete events per period of time; for example, sound is measured in cycles per second, and one cycle per second is equal to 1 hertz.

Frostbite: Localized freezing of tissue, usually of extremities exposed to low temperatures.

Frozen section: An extremely thin tissue section cut by a specially designed instrument called a microtome from tissue that has been rapidly frozen, for the purpose of microscopic evaluation and rendering a diagnosis.

Full-term: Referring to a gestation period of nine months.

Functional disease: A derangement in the way that normal anatomy operates; also, a disorder without any known organic basis (sometimes suggesting that the basis may be psychological).

Fungal infections: Infections caused by fungi, ranging from minor skin disease to serious, disseminated disease of the lungs and other organs.

Fungiform papillae: The papillae scattered about the tongue surface, in no specific array, that are responsive to tastant molecules; they do not exhibit specificity for a particular type of taste.

Fungus (*pl.* fungi): A plantlike organism that does not produce its own food through photosynthesis, instead living as a heterotroph that absorbs complex carbon compounds from other living or dead organisms.

Gallstones: Particles of cholesterol and other substances that form in the gallbladder when the solubility of bile components is altered.

Gametes: The reproductive cells in either sex (the sperm and the ova).

Gamma camera: A type of radiation-detection instrument that detects gamma rays external to the body and makes an image of the radionuclide distribution in body organs; also known as a scintillation camera.

Gamma ray: A type of electromagnetic radiation that has the same physical properties as X rays but is emitted by unstable nuclei in their decay process; gamma rays are capable of penetrating soft tissue, thereby allowing their detection outside the body to produce images of organs.

Ganglion: A benign swelling or nodule surrounding a tendon, usually in the wrists, fingers, or feet.

Gangrene: Necrosis (tissue death) caused by obstruction of the blood supply; it may be localized to a small area or involve an entire extremity.

Gas exchange: The movement of oxygen and carbon dioxide across the membrane of the lungs; other gases, such as nitrogen, may also cross the membrane.

Gastrectomy: Surgical removal of all or part of the stomach.

Gastric: Pertaining to the stomach.

Gastritis: Any inflammation of the stomach.

Gastroenteritis: Inflammation of the mucous membrane of the stomach and/or the small intestine.

Gastroenterology: The medical specialty devoted to care of the digestive tract and related organs.

Gastrointestinal: Referring to the stomach and to the small and large intestines.

Gastrointestinal system: A compartmentalized tube that reduces food, mechanically and chemically, to a state in which it is absorbed by the body; includes the mouth, esophagus, stomach, small intestine, and colon, as well as the salivary glands, pancreas, liver, and gallbladder.

Gastrointestinal tract: The digestive tract; a tube-like series of organs that includes the mouth, pharynx, esophagus, stomach, small intestine, large intestine, and anus.

Gastrostomy: Surgical incision into the stomach.

Gender: Strictly speaking, the behavioral and social aspects of being one sex versus the other; loosely used to refer to the biological and physical aspects of being male or female as well.

Gender identity: The mental view of oneself as male or female.

Gender role: Behaviors and self-presentations that are associated with being male or female and that one uses to identify or recognize others as male or female; also implies societal and/or cultural expectations.

Gene: The basic unit of inheritance; at the molecular level, a gene consists of a segment of DNA that codes for a particular protein.

Gene regulation: The control of whether a gene is active (that is, encoding messenger RNA and protein) or inactive (that is, not encoding RNA or protein), a process often affected by hormones.

General anesthesia: Anesthesia that induces unconsciousness.

General practice: A primary care field in which health care is provided by physicians who usually have completed less than three years of residency training.

Generic drugs: Copycat versions of brand-name originals that are no longer protected by patents.

Genetic: Imparted at conception and incorporated into every cell of an organism.

Genetic counseling: Physician-provided advice to a couple who plan to have a child who might inherit a condition or disorder.

Genetic disease: A disease state that exists because of a decrease in or the absence of normal protein activity as the result of an alteration in the information carried in DNA.

Genetic engineering: A group of scientific techniques that allow scientists to alter genes. Also called recombinant DNA research.

Genetic screening: A program designed to determine whether individuals are carriers of or are affected by a particular genetic disease.

Genome: The total complement of genes inherited by an organism.

Genotype: The genetic makeup of an individual; it is usually expressed as a list of alleles.

Geriatrics: The branch of medicine that treats the conditions and diseases associated with aging and old age.

German measles. *See* Rubella.

Gerontology: The branch of medicine focused on the process of aging and the conditions and diseases that affect the elderly.

Gestation: The period from conception to birth in which the fetus reaches full development in order to survive outside the mother's body.

Gigantism: A rare endocrine disorder characterized by an overgrowth of all bones and body tissues.

Gingiva: The gum tissue surrounding the neck of the tooth.

Gingivitis: A superficial inflammation of the gums associated with the destructive buildup of dental plaque; if left untreated, it can result in periodontitis.

Gland: An organ or area of the body that produces, stores, and secretes fluids, exerting a profound effect on growth, energy production, chemical balance, reproduction, and health.

Glans penis: The head of the penis; also called the glans.

Glaucoma: An eye disease characterized by increased intraocular pressure, which can lead to degeneration of the optic nerve and ultimately blindness if left untreated.

Glial cells: Nonexcitable cells of the nervous system; they include astrocytes, microglial cells, oligodendrocytes, and Schwann cells.

Glomerular filtration: The first step in urine formation; passive filtration in which fluids and solids dissolved in the fluid (solutes) are forced through a membrane, resulting in filtration of the blood.

Glomerulonephritis: Inflammation of the glomeruli, the clusters of blood vessels and nerves found throughout the kidney.

Glomerulus (*pl.* glomeruli): One of the very small units in the kidney, in which blood is filtered through a membrane.

Glossopharyngeal nerve: The ninth cranial nerve, which relays signals pertaining to or controlling salivation; it sends neurological information to and from the posterior region of the tongue to the medulla oblongata of the brain stem.

Glucagon: A pancreatic hormone which signals an elevated concentration of glucose circulating in the blood.

Glucocorticoids: Steroid hormones that regulate the metabolism of glucose and other organic molecules.

Glucosuria: A condition in which the concentration of blood glucose exceeds the ability of the kidney to reabsorb it; as a result, glucose spills into the urine, taking with it body water and electrolytes.

Glycerol: A three-carbon alcohol that has one hydroxyl compound on each carbon atom.

Glycogen: The form that glucose takes when it is stored in the muscles and liver.

Glycolysis: The chemical process of splitting a molecule of glucose in order to obtain energy for other cellular processes; at times of intense activity, glycolysis produces most of the energy used by muscles.

Goiter: Enlargement of the thyroid gland in the neck.

Golgi complex: A system of membrane sacs in which proteins are chemically modified, sorted, and routed to various cellular destinations.

Gonad: The male or female organ (testis or ovary, respectively) in which the essential gametes are formed for reproduction.

Goniometry: The measurement of angles, particularly those for the range of motion of a joint.

Gonorrhea: An infection of the urogenital tract that is a common sexually transmitted disease.

Gout: Painful arthritis of the peripheral joints, often in the big toe.

Graafian follicle: Any of the ovarian follicles that produce eggs.

Graft-versus-host disease: A genetic incompatibility between tissues in which immune system cells from the grafted tissue attack host tissue.

Grafting: A surgical graft of skin from one part of the body to another or from one individual to another.

Gram staining: The use of a stain to classify bacteria as either gram-positive (they retain the primary stain of crystal violet when subjected to treatment with a decolorizer) or gram-negative (no coloration).

Grand mal: A type of epileptic seizure characterized by severe convulsions, body stiffening, and loss of consciousness during which victims fall down.

Granulocyte: A white blood cell characterized by large numbers of cytoplasmic granules, including neutrophils, eosinophils, and basophils.

Granuloma: A nodular, inflammatory lesion that is usually small, firm, and persistent and contains proliferated macrophages.

Graves' disease: A common type of hyperthyroidism in which the thyroid gland produces an oversupply of hormone.

Gross pathology: The study of that which is visible to the naked eye (macroscopic) during inspection.

Growth: The development of the human body from conception to adulthood.

Guillain-Barré syndrome: An acute degeneration of peripheral motor and sensory nerves, known to physicians as acute inflammatory demyelinating polyneuropathy, a common cause of acute generalized paralysis.

Gustation: The ability to taste, which is independent of smell (olfaction) or textural and temperature enhancements; ageusia, or apogeusia, is the loss of taste sensation.

Gynecology: The branch of medicine that focuses on the conditions and disorders affecting the female reproductive system.

Hair transplantation: The surgical relocation of healthy hair follicles to a part of the scalp where shrunken follicles are producing short, thin hair or no hair.

Half-life: The time required for half of the nuclei in a radioactive sample to decay.

Halitosis: Bad breath, usually the result of drinking alcohol, smoking, and eating pungent foods.

Hallucinations: The perception of sensations without relevant external stimuli.

Hallucis: A term referring to the big toe; the flexor hallucis longus is a muscle that flexes the big toe.

Hammertoe: An abnormality of the tendon in a toe which causes the main joint to curve upward and can be painful as a result of shoe pressure.

Haploid: Containing only a single set of chromosomes; mature gametes are haploid.

Hard palate: The bony portion of the roof of the mouth, contiguous with the soft palate.

Hare lip. *See* Cleft lip.

Hashimoto's disease: Thyroiditis; among the earliest characterized autoimmune diseases.

HDLs. *See* High-density lipoproteins.

Headaches: Pain localized in the head or neck, often caused by tension but also the result of a range of disorders.

Healing: The process of mending damaged tissue by which an organism restores itself to health.

Health: A condition in which all functions of the body, mind, and spirit are normally active.

Health maintenance: The practice of anticipating, finding, preventing, and/or dealing with potential or established medical problems at the earliest possible stage to minimize adverse effects on the patient.

Health maintenance organization (HMO): A group of general practitioners, specialists, and allied health professionals who provide medical services to subscribers paying a regular maintenance fee.

Hearing loss: Loss of sensitivity to sound pressure changes as a result of congenital factors, disease, traumatic injury, noise exposure, or aging.

Heart: The muscle that pumps blood through the body by means of rhythmic contractions.

Heart attack: Sudden and permanent damage to a part of the heart muscle as a result of impaired blood flow through the coronary arteries; the common term for myocardial infarction.

Heart block: A delay or blockage of the electrical signal traveling through the heart muscle, which upsets the synchronization between contractions of the upper and lower chambers.

Heart failure: A condition in which the heart pumps inefficiently, allowing fluid to back up into the lungs or body tissue.

Heart rate: The number of times the heart contracts, or beats, per minute.

Heart transplantation: The removal of a diseased heart and its replacement with a healthy donor heart.

Heart valve replacement: A surgical procedure involving the removal of a defective heart valve and its replacement with another tissue valve or with a mechanical valve.

Heartburn: The presence of a burning sensation in the chest and throat caused by the reflux of stomach acids.

Heat: The transfer of energy across a boundary because of a temperature difference.

Heat exhaustion: Mild shock caused by a decrease in the amount of fluid in the blood.

Heat stroke: A medical emergency in which high body temperatures result in organ damage.

Heel spur: A bony outgrowth on the heel of the foot.

Helminths: A general term for roundworms (nematodes) and flatworms (platyhelminths), many of which are parasites of humans and animals.

Hematology: The study of the blood, including its normal constituents and such blood disorders as anemia, leukemia, and hemophilia.

Hematoma: A localized collection of clotted blood in an organ or tissue as a result of internal bleeding.

Hematopoiesis: The production of red and white cells and platelets, which occurs mainly in bone marrow.

Hematosis: The formation of blood.

Hematuria: The abnormal presence of blood in the urine.

Hemiplegia: Paralysis or weakness on one side of the body.

Hemodialysis: The removal of toxins from blood through the process of dialysis.

Hemodynamics: The study of blood circulation.

Hemoglobin: The oxygen-carrying iron-containing pigment present in red blood cells that is responsible for oxygen exchange in cells and tissues.

Hemolytic anemia: Anemia resulting from hemolysis, the excessive destruction of red blood cells.

Hemophilia: A hereditary blood defect (occurring almost exclusively in males) characterized by delayed clotting of the blood and consequent difficulty in controlling bleeding even after minor injuries.

Hemorrhage: The loss of a large amount of blood in a short period of time.

Hemorrhoids: Dilated blood vessels in the anus or rectum that are itchy and painful.

Hemostasis: The control of bleeding.

Hepatic: Of or referring to the liver.

Hepatitis: Inflammation of the liver.

Hepatitis A virus: The virus associated with certain forms of hepatitis; generally contracted through fecal contamination of food and water.

Hepatitis B virus: The agent associated with severe forms of viral hepatitis; contracted through contaminated blood or hypodermic needles or through contaminated body fluids.

Hepatitis C virus: Formerly referred to as the etiological agent for non-A, non-B viral hepatitis; most often passed in contaminated blood.

Hepato-: A prefix denoting an association with the liver; for example, a hepatocyte is a liver cell.

Hepatocyte: The functional cell of the liver.

Herbal medicine: A nontraditional form of medicine that uses different types of herbs for therapy and health maintenance.

Hernia: A pouch of intestines and/or vital organs of the abdomen that protrudes through the abdominal wall.

Herpes: A family of viruses that cause several diseases, including infectious mononucleosis, cold sores, genital herpes, and chickenpox.

Heterosexual: Being principally attracted to and aroused by opposite-gender persons.

Heterozygous: Having two different alleles for a particular gene.

Heuristics: Methods used to aid and guide in the discovery of a disease process when incomplete knowledge exists.

High-density lipoproteins (HDLs): A form of cholesterol in the blood that appears to be associated with a lower risk of arterial and heart disease.

Hindmilk: The milk released late in a nursing session, which is higher in fat content.

Hippocratic oath: A document written in the fifth century B.C.E. to offer guidelines for the emerging medical profession.

Histamine: A compound released during allergic reactions which causes many of the symptoms of allergies.

Histamine II blockers: Various drugs that combat the chemical action of ulcers by reducing the secretion of gastric juices, or "stomach acids."

Histocompatibility: Tissue compatibility, as determined by histocompatibility protein antigens present on the cell membranes of all tissue cells.

Histology: The branch of medicine that focuses on the study of cells and tissues as they relate to their function.

Histopathology: The histologic or microscopic description of abnormal pathologic tissue changes; these changes can be seen under the microscope.

HIV. *See* Human immunodeficiency virus (HIV).

Hodgkin's disease: A neoplastic disorder originating in the tissues of the lymphatic system, recognized by distinctive histologic changes and defined by the presence of Reed-Sternberg cells.

Holistic: The philosophy that individuals function as complete units or integrated systems and are not understood merely through their parts.

Holistic medicine: An approach to the practice of medicine based on the philosophy that treatment must occur taking into consideration the entire organism, both physiological and psychological.

Home care: The provision of outside services to a patient living in a home setting.

Homeopathy: A nontraditional approach to treatment which is based on a theory of Samuel Hahnemann, the "law of similars." The theory posits that substances which provoke disease may be used in small doses to treat the disease.

Homeostasis: The maintenance of a constant internal environment; the systems of the body work together to maintain a constant temperature, pH, oxygen availability, water content, ion concentrations, and so on.

Homosexual: Being principally attracted to and aroused by persons of one's own gender; two synonymous terms are "gay," which can refer to all homosexuals or to homosexual males exclusively, and "lesbian," which refers only to homosexual females.

Homozygous: Having two identical alleles of a particular gene.

Hormone: A substance which creates a specific effect in an organ distant from its site of production.

Hormone receptor: A molecule contained in or on a cell that allows it to respond to a hormone; if receptors are not present, the hormone will have no effect.

Hormone replacement therapy: Treatment protocols using estrogens, with or without progesterone, to reduce the rate of bone mineral loss which occurs after the menopause.

Hospice: A program designed to ease the suffering and grief for terminally ill patients and their families; care can be rendered in the home or in a special hospice setting with special emphasis on the relief of pain.

Hospital: An institution focused on the management, prevention, and treatment of illness, utilizing a staff of medical and allied health professionals to provide medical, surgical, and psychiatric treatments, along with emergency care and evaluation.

Host: The body of the person or animal infected with a pathogen, especially a parasite.

Host-defense mechanisms: Immunological methods that the body uses to protect against external infectious agents and to maintain internal homeostasis, such as skin, sweat, urine, tears, phagocytes, and "helpful" bacteria.

Host-versus-graft disease: A tissue rejection in which the immune system cells of the graft recipient attack the grafted tissue from a donor individual.

Human immunodeficiency virus (HIV): The virus that causes acquired immunodeficiency syndrome (AIDS); it may be transmitted through blood or semen.

Human leukocyte antigens (HLAs): Structures located on the surface of each cell that are unique to an individual; also called transplantation antigens.

Humerus: The bone that forms the structural beam of the upper arm.

Hydro-: A prefix denoting water or fluid.

Hydrocarbon: An organic compound composed of only hydrogen and carbon atoms that does not dissolve in water (water-insoluble).

Hydrocele: A fluid-filled area around the testis often caused by infection or inflammation.

Hydrocelectomy: Surgical removal of a hydrocele.

Hydrocephalus: An excessive collection of cerebrospinal fluid in the brain.

Hydrophilic: "Water-loving" or water-attracting; a term given to molecules or regions of molecules that interact favorably with water.

Hydrophobic: "Water-hating" or "water-repelling"; a term given to molecules or regions of molecules that do not interact favorably with water.

Hydrotherapy: A form of treatment which uses water, externally, to aid in recovery or ease pain.

Hygiene: The science of health and the prevention of disease.

Hyper-: A prefix denoting "high" or more than normal.

Hyperlipidemia: The presence of abnormally large amounts of lipids in the blood.

Hypernatremia: A high salt concentration in the blood that can result in seizure and coma.

Hyperopia: The inability of the eye to focus on close objects; also called farsightedness.

Hyperparathyroidism: The excessive, uncontrolled secretion of parathyroid hormone.

Hyperplasia: A state of hormonal stimulation causing an increase in the number of cells in a tissue, resulting in an oversized organ.

Hypersensitivity: An overreaction by the immune system to the presence of certain antigens; this overreaction often results in some damage to the person as well as the antigen.

Hypertension: A condition in which the blood pressure is higher than what is considered to be normal.

Hyperthermia: The elevation of the body core temperature of an organism above a normal range.

Hypertrophy: The growth of a tissue or organ as a result of an increase in the size of existing cells.

Hypnosis: The induction of an altered state of consciousness.

Hypo-: A prefix denoting "low" or less than normal.

Hypochondriasis: A condition in which the patients believe strongly that they are suffering from one or more serious illnesses, even when this belief is unsupported by medical evidence.

Hypodermis: The layer of fat under the dermis that contains carotene.

Hypoglycemia: A condition in which the concentration of glucose in the blood is too low to meet the needs of key organs, especially the brain.

Hypoparathyroidism: The reduced secretion of parathyroid hormone.

Hypospadias: An abnormal urethral opening in the penis, either on the underside or on the perineum.

Hypotension: Decrease in blood pressure to the point that insufficient blood flow causes symptoms.

Hypothalamus: The region of the brain called the diencephalon, forming the floor of the third ventricle, including neighboring, associated nuclei.

Hypothermia: A subnormal body temperature; clinically, it is a sustained cooling of the body to lower-than-normal temperatures.

Hypothyroidism: A condition in which the thyroid gland produces an insufficient supply of hormone.

Hypoxia: A deficiency in the amount of oxygen reaching the body tissues.

Hysterectomy: The surgical removal of the uterus. In a total hysterectomy, the uterus, ovaries, and Fallopian tubes are removed.

Iatrogenic: Referring to a complication or negative reaction resulting from physician intervention or contracted as a result of actions taken in a clinical setting.

Idiopathic: Referring to a medical condition with no known cause.

IgE. *See* Immunoglobulin E (IgE).

Ileostomy: The surgical creation of a fistula through which the lower part of the small intestine (ileum) passes to create an artificial bowel.

Ileum: The lower third of the small intestine, which joins with the colon.

Illicit drugs: Drugs that are illegal to possess, have addiction potential, and lack approved medical uses.

Imaging: Any one of a wide variety of technologies for creating visual depictions of the internal structures of the body, including (among others) X radiation, magnetic resonance imaging (MRI), CT scanning, PET scanning, ultrasonography, and radionuclide scanning.

Immune response: The reaction of an intricate system of cells, which identify, attack, immobilize, and remove foreign tissue from the body through chemical signals.

Immune system: The body system that is responsible for fighting off infectious disease.

Immunity: Resistance to infection by a particular disease-causing microorganism, often acquired by vaccination.

Immunization: The process of creating an immunity to a disease through the introduction of vaccines or other agents designed to produce the immunity.

Immunoassay: The use of antibody-antigen recognition as the basis of a medically useful method of detecting and measuring a substance in body fluids.

Immunocompromised: Referring to a condition in which the immune system is impaired in some way, such as being not fully developed, deficient, or suppressed.

Immunodeficiency disorders: Genetic or acquired disorders in which the normal functioning of the immune system is disturbed.

Immunoglobulin: The globulin fraction of serum protein.

Immunoglobulin E (IgE): A type of antibody associated with the release of granules from basophils and mast cells; ordinarily, a relatively rare antibody, but in patients with atopic dermatitis, levels can be significantly higher than in the general population.

Immunology: The branch of medicine that studies the immune system: its function and processes and agents that affect its function either positively or negatively, including allergies.

Immunopathology: The study of conditions or diseases that impair the immune system.

Immunosuppression: A decrease in the effectiveness of the immune system; drugs are sometimes used to depress the immune system in order to lower the probability of rejection in organ transplantation.

Implant: A section of endometrial tissue found outside the uterus; also, an artificial part or device inserted surgically in a part of the body (such as a breast).

Implantation: The process in which the embryo attaches to the uterine lining; also, the surgical process of adding an artificial body part, such as a pacemaker.

Impotence: The inability to achieve an erection.

In utero: A Latin term meaning "in the womb."

In vitro fertilization: Fertilization of an ovum outside the female body, in an artificial culture in a test tube or dish.

In vivo fertilization: Fertilization of an ovum naturally, within the female body.

Incidence: The number of new illnesses or events occurring over a specified period of time among a specific population.

Incision: A cut made with a scalpel.

Incisional biopsy: The biopsy of a selected sample of lesion.

Incisor: One of the front teeth, used primarily to cut or shear food with a scissoring motion.

Incontinence: The inability to retain urine.

Incubator: In the nursery, a plexiglass unit that encloses the premature or sick infant to allow strict temperature regulation.

Indigestion: A digestive disorder characterized by a burning sensation in the chest and throat, sometimes by abdominal pain, bloating, nausea, vomiting, and diarrhea; also called dyspepsia.

Infant: A young child from birth to twelve months of age.

Infarction: Damage resulting from insufficient blood supply to a tissue or organ.

Infection: The invasion of healthy tissue by a pathogenic microorganism, resulting in the production of toxins and subsequent injury of tissue.

Infectious disease: An illness caused by a microorganism or its products, in contrast to diseases caused by factors such as heredity or poor nutrition.

Infectivity: The ability of an organism to enter and reproduce within a host.

Inferior: Situated below another part; for example, the ankle bones are inferior to the bones of the lower leg.

Inflammation: Irritation caused by such things as infection, injury, allergy, or toxins; symptoms include redness, swelling, warmth, pain, and drainage.

Influenza: Any one of a group of serious respiratory diseases caused by viruses; different strains of the "flu" have been responsible for worldwide epidemics.

Informed consent: The process of educating a patient fully about the purpose, benefits, and risks of a clinical trial.

Inguinal hernia: The most common form of hernia, in which the hernial sac protrudes into the lower groin area.

Inhalant: Medication that is inhaled into the lungs.

Inheritance: The passage of traits from parents to offspring in discrete units called genes.

Inner ear: An organ that includes the cochlea (for detection of sound) and the labyrinth (for detection of movement).

Inoculate: To introduce immunologically active material in order to treat or prevent a disease.

Inotropic agent: A drug that improves the ability of the heart muscle to contract.

Inpatient care: Evaluation and treatment services requiring an overnight stay in a medical facility.

Insane: A legal term referring to a state wherein a person is said to be incapable of appreciating the wrongfulness of certain acts or of conforming to the requirements of the law.

Insemination: The placement of semen in the female reproductive tract, which may occur naturally as a result of sexual intercourse or artificially as a result of a medical procedure.

Insomnia: Disturbed sleep; insomnia can be caused by many factors, such as dysfunctional sleep cycle, breathing problems, leg jerking, underlying medical and psychiatric disorders, and the side effects of medication.

Inspiration: The act of breathing in, which expands the lungs.

Instinctual drives: Libido (the seeking of gratification of sexual impulses) and aggression (the seeking of gratification of destructive impulses).

Insulin: A hormone secreted by the pancreas that is essential in regulating blood glucose, as well as in assimilating carbohydrates for growth and energy.

Intensive care: Continuous medical treatment involving vigilant monitoring of the vital signs of patients with grave physical conditions.

Interferons: A family of proteins; some induce an antiviral state within a cell, while others serve to regulate aspects of the immune response.

Internal medicine: The branch of medicine that focuses on the diagnosis and treatment of diseases, particularly of the internal organs, in adults. Practitioners of internal medicine, called internists, often act as primary care physicians.

Internship: A synonym for the first year of residency training for a variety of masters' and doctoral-level practitioners in diverse fields.

Interstitial: Referring to the spaces within the tissues or other structures of the body, but not the large body cavities.

Interstitial pulmonary fibrosis (IPF): A disease characterized by scarring and thickening of lung tissue, which causes breathing difficulty.

Intervertebral disks: Flattened disks of fibrocartilage that separate the vertebrae and allow cushioned flexibility of the spinal column.

Intervertebral foramina: Openings between two adjacent vertebrae to permit the exit of nerve structures from the spinal cord.

Intestines: The section of the gut between the anus and the stomach, consisting of the rectum, colon, and small bowel (subdivided into the ileus, jejunum, and duodenum).

Intoxication: Poisoning of the body by toxins, such as drugs; also, alcohol intoxication (drunkenness).

Intracellular fluid: The fluid within cells.

Intraocular pressure: The degree of firmness of the eyeball, as controlled by the proper secretion and drainage of the aqueous humor.

Intravascular fluid: The fluid carried within the blood vessels; it is in a constant state of motion because of the pumping action of the heart.

Intravenous (IV) therapy: The introduction of medication into a vein with a special needle.

Intubation: The introduction of a tube into a body cavity, as into the larynx.

Invasive: Referring to any process (such as disease) that spreads throughout an area of the body or any procedure (such as diagnostic or therapeutic surgery) that requires entry into the body through the skin.

Involuntary muscle contractions: Muscle contractions that occur unconsciously, such as those of the intestines.

Ionization: A process in which a neutral atom loses one or more of its orbital electrons because of light, heat, or electrical collisions.

Ions: Small chemical substances that have a positive or negative charge; the most important ions with a positive charge are sodium, potassium, hydrogen, and calcium, while the most important negative ion is chloride.

Ipecac: A plant extract that will induce vomiting when orally administered; the syrup can be used to induce vomiting after ingestion of a poisonous substance.

IPF. *See* Interstitial pulmonary fibrosis (IPF).

Iris: The circular pigmented membrane behind the cornea, perforated by the pupil; the most anterior portion of the vascular tunic of the eye.

Iron-deficiency anemia: Anemia characterized by low serum iron concentration.

Ischemia: A local anemia or area of diminished or insufficient blood supply caused by mechanical obstruction of the blood supply (commonly, the narrowing of an artery).

Islets of Langerhans: Clusters of cells scattered throughout the pancreas; they produce three hormones involved in sugar metabolism: insulin, glucagon, and somatostatin.

Itching: An irritating skin sensation that provokes a desire to scratch the affected area; also called pruritus.

-itis: A suffix denoting inflammation; for example, laryngitis is an inflammation of the larynx.

Jaundice: A yellowish coloration of the skin and mucous membranes caused by high levels of bilirubin in the blood; the result of liver malfunction.

Jejunum: A region of the small intestine located below the duodenum.

Jet lag: The malaise, headache, fatigue, gastrointestinal disorders, and other symptoms that may result from traveling across several time zones within a few hours.

Joint: The conjunction of two or more bones.

Joint replacement. *See* Arthroplasty.

Karyotype: A photograph of the chromosomes taken from the cells of an individual; a karyotype can beused to predict the chromosomal set of a fetus or the presence of a large chromosomal abnormality.

Keratin: An extremely tough protein that is the chief constituent of the epidermis, hair, nails, and tooth enamel.

Keratinocytes: Matrix basal epithelial cells that differentiate, fill with keratin, and form the dead horny substance making up the nail plate.

Keratitis: A state of inflammation of the cornea that may cause partial or total opacity, leading to loss of vision.

Keratoses: Wartlike growths caused by the excessive production of the skin protein keratin, usually occurring in elderly people.

Keratotomy: Surgical incision into the cornea of the eye to correct myopia (nearsightedness) or astigmatism.

Ketones: The by-products of fat metabolism; their presence may be indicative of diabetes mellitus.

Kidney transplantation: A surgical procedure that replaces the recipient's diseased, nonfunctioning kidney with a donated one.

Kidneys: The organs that control the amount and composition of body water by separating the blood into waste products (which leave the body as urine) and nutrients (which are returned to the blood).

Kilocalorie: The unit measurement of food energy defined as the amount of heat needed to raise the temperature of 1 kilogram of water 1 degree Celsius; also known as a Calorie.

Kinase: An enzyme that catalyzes the transfer of phosphate from adenosine triphosphate (ATP) to another molecule.

Kinesiology: The study of the body's movement and the function of structures involved in that movement.

Kluver-Bucy syndrome: A series of symptoms following temporal-lobe removal, such as psychic blindness, abnormal oral tendencies, and changes in sexuality.

Knee: The joint between the thigh and the lower leg.

Knockout mouse: A mouse in which a specific gene has been inactivated or "knocked out."

Kupffer cells: Specialized cells in the liver that perform the function of removing bacterial debris from the blood that has circulated throughout the body.

Kwashiorkor: A protein-deficiency disease that usually affects young children in developing countries.

L-dopa (L-dihydroxyphenylalanine or levodopa): An amino acid that is the parent compound for dopamine; used to treat parkinsonism.

Labia: The folds of tissue along the external portion of a woman's vagina and urethra.

Labor: The physiological process by which the fetus and placenta are expelled from the uterus; labor involves strong uterine contractions.

Laboratory tests: The collection and analysis of body fluids such as blood and urine in order to establish a diagnosis or to monitor a treatment regimen.

Labyrinth: A structure consisting of three fluid-filled, semicircular canals at right angles to one another in the inner ear; they monitor the position and movement of the head.

Laceration: A torn, jagged wound, or an unintentional cut (as opposed to an incision).

Lacteals: Lymphatic capillaries in the villi of the small intestine that absorb fat, producing a milky substance called chyle.

Lactiferous duct: A single excretory duct from each lobe of mammary glandular tissue that converges yet opens separately at the tip of the nipple; the mammary gland has fifteen to twenty lactiferous ducts.

Lamellar keratoplasty: The partial removal or transplantation of a portion of the cornea; usually possible in younger patients or those with less advanced disorders.

Lamina (*pl.* laminae): An arch of the vertebral bones.

Laminaria: A type of seaweed that absorbs water and swells; it can be used to dilate the cervix.

Laminectomy: Surgical removal of part or all of a lamina to relieve pressure on the spinal cord. Sometimes called fusion surgery.

Laparoscopy: A surgical procedure in which an instrument is inserted into the abdominal cavity through tiny incisions in the abdomen. Usually performed without hospitalization.

Laparotomy: A surgical procedure, often exploratory in nature, carried out through the abdominal wall; it may be used to correct endometriosis.

Laryngectomy: Surgical removal of all or part of the larynx.

Laryngitis: Inflammation of the larynx, characterized by hoarseness in the voice and sometimes the inability to speak.

Larynx: The voice organ, lying between the pharynx and the trachea; commonly called the voice box.

Laser: An acronym for "*l*ight *a*mplification by *s*timulated *e*mission of *r*adiation"; a laser produces a high-intensity light beam at a single wavelength.

Latent: Lying hidden or undeveloped within a person; unrevealed.

Lateral: On the outer side; for example, toward the little toe when in reference to the leg.

LDLs. *See* Low-density lipoproteins.

Lead poisoning: Poisoning as the result of ingestion or inhalation of abnormally high levels of lead, which disrupts kidney function and damages the nervous system.

Learning disabilities: A variety of disorders involving the failure to learn an academic skill despite normal levels of intelligence.

Leg: The lower extremity, excluding the foot; the upper leg runs from the hip to the knee, and the lower leg runs from the knee to the ankle.

Legionnaires' disease: Acute bacterial pneumonia that resembles influenza and that may prove fatal to older persons or those individuals with previous lung damage.

Leishmaniasis: One of several diseases associated with the single-celled protozoan species *Leishmania*, transmitted by the bite of a sandfly, which cause ulcers in the skin or internal organs.

Lens: A transparent, flexible structure, convex on both surfaces and lying directly behind the iris of the eye; it focuses light rays onto the retina.

Leprosy: A bacterial infection that affects the skin and nerves, causing symptoms ranging from numbness to disfigurement.

Lesion: A visible local tissue abnormality such as a wound, sore, rash, or boil, which can be benign, cancerous, gross, occult, or primary.

Leukemia: A condition characterized by the presence of an increased number of leukocytes in the blood, with the specific disorder classified according to the predominant proliferating cells, the clinical course, and the duration of the disease.

Leukocyte: A white or colorless blood corpuscle.

Leukopenia: An abnormal decrease in white blood cells.

Liability: Responsibility for wrongdoing.

Ligament: A tough, rubber band-like structure that connects one bone to another and prevents the abnormal motion of these bones in relationship to each other.

Light therapy: A nontraditional form of therapy that employs light to alleviate symptoms such as depression.

Lingual: Related to the tongue; in dentistry, the inner sides or faces of the teeth.

Lipases: Enzymes secreted by the pancreas into the small intestine that break down fatty materials (triglycerides) in the first intestinal stage of digestion.

Lipids: Any of a group of fatty substances including triglycerides, phospholipids, and sterols (such as cholesterol).

Lipopolysaccharide (LPS): A major component of the cell walls of gram-negative bacteria; the toxicity of LPS is associated with illnesses caused by gram-negative organisms.

Lipoproteins: Lipid aggregates that transport fat and cholesteryl esters in the circulation; associated apolipoproteins determine how rapidly they are taken up by the liver or other tissues.

Liposuction: A cosmetic method for removing body fat by a surgical vacuuming procedure.

Lithium: A drug used in the treatment of bipolar disorder.

Lithotripsy: Pulverization of stones (calculi) located in the kidneys, bladder, or urethra by means of high-frequency sound waves.

Liver: A vital organ that controls blood sugar levels; metabolizes carbohydrates, lipids, and proteins; stores blood, iron, and some vitamins; degrades steroid hormones; and inactivates and/or excretes certain drugs and toxins.

Liver transplantation: Surgery performed to replace a diseased, nonfunctional liver with one that is healthy and capable of carrying out normal liver functions.

Living will: A legally binding document instructing a physician not to prolong life by externally administered life-support systems if the patient is unable to express his or her decision concerning physician-recommended forms of medical treatment.

Lobectomy: The removal of a lobe of the brain, or a major part of a lobe.

Lobotomy: The separation of either an entire lobe or a major part of a lobe from the rest of the brain.

Local anesthesia: The injection of medication into the body that renders the immediate area free of pain, allowing surgery in that area to be performed.

Lockjaw. *See* Tetanus.

Loss-of-control syndrome: A pattern of behavior characterized by violent and emotional outbursts, occasionally associated with temporal-lobe seizures.

Lou Gehrig's disease. *See* Amyotrophic lateral sclerosis.

Low-density lipoproteins (LDLs): A form of cholesterol in the blood that appears to be associated with a higher risk of arterial and heart disease.

Lower extremities: The legs (thighs, lower legs, and feet), which are attached to the pelvis at the hip joint and which consist of muscles, bones, blood vessels, lymph vessels, nerves, skin, and toenails.

Lumbar puncture: A procedure to extract cerebrospinal fluid from the lumbar region of the spine (between the ribs and the pelvis), usually to diagnose disease (such as meningitis) or to administer therapeutic drugs (in leukemia treatment, for example).

Lumbar vertebrae: The five bones of the spinal column in the lower back, which experience the greatest stress in the spine.

Lumen: The space within an artery, vein, or other tube.

Lumpectomy: Surgical removal of a lump, often in the female breast.

Lungs: Vital organs that allow gas exchange between an organism and its environment.

Lunula: A whitish, crescent-shaped area at the end of the proximal nail fold that marks the end of the nail matrix and is the site of mitosis and nail growth.

Lupus: Systemic lupus erythematosus; a chronic inflammatory disease characterized by an arthritic condition and a rash.

Lyme disease: Lyme disease involves a mild-to-serious infection caused by the bacteria *Borrelia burgdorferi*, which is spread by the bite of infected ticks.

Lymph: The straw-colored fluid of the lymphatic system; as much as 1 to 2 liters is collected from tissue each day and returned to the bloodstream.

Lymph node: A small, oval structure that filters tissue fluids; lymph nodes are found in areas such as the armpits, groin, mouth, and neck, and serve as sites of immune response.

Lymphadenopathy: Enlarged lymph nodes, which may be caused by any disorder related to the lymphatic vessels or lymph nodes.

Lymphatic system: A bodily system, consisting of lymphatic vessels and lymph nodes, that transports lymph (the fluid containing infection-fighting lymphocytes) through tissues and organs and drains it back into the bloodstream. A major part of the body's immune system.

Lymphocyte: A small white blood cell constituting about 25 percent of all blood cells; two basic types are B cells (antibody production) and T cells (cellular immunity).

Lymphoma: A group of cancers that affect lymphatic tissue.

Macrophage: Any of several forms of either circulating or fixed phagocytic cells of the immune system.

Macular degeneration: The progressive breakdown of the macula, the part of the eye that allows for detailed sight in the center of the field of vision, with a dense concentration of rods and cones.

Magnetic field therapy: A practical and inexpensive modality that uses magnets to relieve chronic and acute pain incurred through overuse or trauma.

Magnetic resonance imaging (MRI): A diagnostic technique used to see the outline of an internal organ or a tumor without using X rays.

Malaise: A feeling of lack of health or debility, often indicating or accompanying the onset of illness.

Malaria: A serious parasitic infection spread by mosquitoes and characterized by fever, chills, sweating, vomiting, and damage to the kidneys, brain, and liver.

Malignancy: Any condition that becomes progressively worse, especially the growth of a cancerous tumor.

Malignant melanoma: A fast-growing, highly dangerous form of skin cancer.

Malnutrition: A physical state characterized by an imbalance of dietary proteins, carbohydrates, fats, vitamins, and minerals, given an individual's physical activity and health needs.

Malocclusion: An incorrect fit of the upper and lower teeth when they are brought together.

Malpractice: The failure to care for patients in accordance with professional standards, for which injured patients are allowed to sue for compensation.

Malpractice insurance: Insurance policies held by physicians in order to protect them financially in the event of a patient-initiated lawsuit alleging incidents of improper medical decisions or incompetence.

Mammography: The use of X rays to image the female breast, primarily in the detection and diagnosis of malignant breast tumors before they can be felt.

Mandible: The lower jawbone.

Manic-depressive disorder. *See* Bipolar disorder.

Marasmus: The condition that results from consuming a diet that is deficient in both energy and protein.

Mast cells: Cells in connective tissue capable of releasing chemicals that cause allergic reactions.

Mastectomy: Surgical removal of the female breast.

Mastication: The act of chewing food.

Mastitis: Infection of the breast, which results in inflammation, tenderness, swelling, and pain.

Mastoidectomy: The surgical removal of the temporal or mastoid bone, which is located behind the ear.

Materia Medica: The homeopathic pharmacopoeia, a list of remedies with their associated symptoms and uses.

Matrix: Organic or inorganic material occurring in connective tissues but located outside the cells.

Maxilla: The upper jawbone.

Maxillofacial surgery: Surgery of the face and neck, a form of cosmetic and reconstructive surgery.

Maximal oxygen uptake: The maximum rate of oxygen consumption during exercise.

Measles: A childhood infectious disease, also known as rubeola, characterized by a rash and fever; it can be controlled through immunization.

Mechanoreceptors: Sensory receptors that, when mechanically deformed (such as being pressed on), send nerve impulses causing sensations of pressure and touch.

Medial: Closer to an imaginary midline dividing the body into equal right and left halves than another part.

Medical College Admission Test (MCAT): A test of problem-solving skills taken by all candidates to medical school in the United States; used to predict which students will be successful.

Medicare: A U.S. federal program that covers many of the hospital costs and doctor bills for elderly and disabled persons and those with end-stage renal (kidney) disease.

Medicine: The science and art of diagnosing, treating, curing, and preventing disease; relieving pain; and improving and preserving health. Also, any drug or other substance used in treating disease, healing, or relieving pain.

Meditation: A mental exercise to enhance personal understanding of the self and the universe.

Megadose: Ten or more times the recommended daily allowance of a nutrient, such as a vitamin.

Megaloblastic anemia: Anemia caused by the failure of red blood cells to mature; also known as pernicious anemia, Addisonian anemia, or maturation failure.

Meiosis: A special kind of cell division whereby four cells are produced; each cell has only half of the original number of chromosomes; meiosis produces the sex cells (eggs and sperm).

Meissner's corpuscles: Receptors at which the sense of a light touch or low-frequency vibrations are detected; also called corpuscles of touch.

Melanin: A polymer made up of several compounds (including the amino acid tyrosine) that causes pigmentation in the skin, hair, and eyes.

Melanoma: Cancer of the melanocytes, the cells that produce melanin.

Melatonin: A hormone produced by the pineal gland within the epithalamus of the forebrain; it is usually released into the blood during the night phase of the light-dark cycle.

Membrane: A thin layer of lipid and protein molecules that controls transport of molecules and ions between the cell and its exterior and between membrane-bound compartments within the cell.

Menarche: The first menstrual cycle in a woman.

Ménière's disease: Progressive dysfunction of the inner ear that causes vertigo and eventually results in total hearing loss.

Meningitis: Inflammation of the membrane that envelopes the brain or spine; caused by bacteria.

Menopause: The permanent cessation of the menstrual cycle, signifying the conclusion of a woman's reproductive life.

Menorrhagia: Excessive or prolonged bleeding during menstruation.

Menstruation: The cyclic bleeding that normally occurs, usually in the absence of pregnancy, during the reproductive period of the human female; typically occurs at twenty-eight day intervals.

Mental retardation: A condition characterized by a below-average intelligence quotient (IQ) and deficits in adaptive functioning before the age of eighteen years; the degree of retardation ranges from mild to severe.

Meridians: Designated points in the body that react to acupuncture or acupressure stimulation.

Merkel's disks: Sensory receptors in the skin located in deeper layers of the epidermis; also called tactile disks.

Messenger ribonucleic acid (mRNA): A single-stranded ribonucleic acid that arises from and is complementary to double-stranded deoxyribonucleic acid (DNA); it passes from the nucleus to the cytoplasm, where its information is translated into proteins.

Metabolic equivalent (MET): A unit used to estimate the metabolic cost of physical activity; 1 MET is equal to 3.5 milliliters of oxygen consumed per kilogram of body weight per minute.

Metabolic rate: A measurement of the Calories (kilocalories) that are converted into heat energy in order to maintain body temperature and/or for physical exertion.

Metabolism: The chemical and physical processes involved in the interconversion of foods and the maintenance of life.

Metastasis: The transfer of disease-producing cells to other parts of the body.

Metastasize: To spread by means of the bloodstream to other parts of the body.

Methotrexate: A powerful drug, originally developed to treat cancer, that is used to treat patients with severe cases of psoriasis.

Microbiology: The study of organisms too small to be seen by the unaided human eye, especially the identification, transmission, and control of microorganisms that cause disease.

Microorganism: An organism that is too small to be seen without a magnifying lens; also known as a microbe.

Microscopy: The use of a microscope to enlarge extremely small objects to make them visible.

Microsurgery: Surgery done with the aid of a microscope.

Micturition: The act of urinating.

Middle ear: The air-filled cavity in which vibrations are transmitted from the eardrum to the inner ear via the ossicles.

Migraine headaches: Severe, incapacitating headaches that may be preceded by nausea and vomiting or by visual, sensory, and motor disturbances.

Milk line: A line that originates as a primitive milk streak on each front side of the fetus; it extends from axilla to vulva, where rudimentary breast tissues or nipples could be located.

Mineralocorticoids: Steroid hormones that regulate the body levels of sodium and potassium.

Minerals: Inorganic compounds that are essential for human life; seventeen are required in the diet.

Miscarriage: The expulsion of the embryo or fetus before it is viable outside the uterus; also called spontaneous abortion.

Mitochondrion: A membrane-bound cytoplasmic organelle that constitutes the primary location of oxidative reactions providing energy for cellular activities.

Mitosis: The type of cell division that occurs in nonsex cells, which conserves chromosome number by equal allocation to each of the newly formed cells.

Mitral valve: The valve between the heart's left auricle and ventricle.

Mitral valve prolapse: The inability of the mitral valve in the heart to close properly; also called mitral insufficiency.

Modality: The ability to distinguish one sensation from another; the ability to discriminate light or heavy touch, pain, pressure, vibratory, or hot and cold sensations from one another.

Molars: The back teeth, which are used to grind food into smaller portions prior to swallowing.

Molecular biology: The study of the interactions that occur among the molecules making up living organisms.

Molecule: A collection of atoms bonded together; normally neutral because it has an equal number of protons and electrons.

Momentum: The product of mass and velocity for a particle; inverse with wavelength (the distance between peaks of a wave).

Monoclonal antibodies: Antibodies (proteins that protect the body against disease-causing foreign bodies such as bacteria and viruses) produced in large quantities from cloned cells.

Mononucleosis: An infectious respiratory illness caused by the Epstein-Barr virus.

Monozygotes: Identical twins; born of a single ovum that divides after a single sperm fertilizes it.

Morbid obesity: Excessive accumulation of fat (more than 100 pounds overweight or 100 percent overweight).

Morbidity: In medical statistics, the occurrence of clinical disease, in contrast to mortality (death) and occurrence (which includes subclinical infections).

Mordant: A chemical that acts to fix a stain within a physical structure; the role played by iodine in Gram staining.

Morgue: A place, usually cooled, where dead bodies are temporarily kept, pending proper identification, autopsy, or burial.

Motility: Spontaneous motion, such as of the gastrointestinal tract or of sperm.

Motion sickness: A feeling of nausea brought on by motion.

Motor: Referring to parts of the nervous system having to do with movement production.

Motor neuron: A nerve that functions either directly or indirectly to control movement in a target organ.

Motor neuron diseases: Progressive, debilitating, and eventually fatal diseases affecting nerve cells in muscles.

Motor weakness: Muscle weakness resulting from the failure of motor nerves.

MRI. *See* Magnetic resonance imaging (MRI).

Mucosa: The tissue lining the interior of the gastrointestinal tract, through which nutrients pass into the bloodstream.

Mucous membrane: The soft, pink layer of cells that produce mucus to keep body structures lubricated; found in eyelids, respiratory, and urinary tracts.

Mucus: A fluid excreted by many body membranes as a lubricant.

Müllerian ducts: The pair of tubes in the early embryo that will develop into the internal female organs (uterus, oviducts, and upper vagina).

Multiple sclerosis: An incurable, debilitating disease of the nervous system.

Multipotent: Referring to stem cells derived from adults that may develop into one specific type of tissue.

Mumps: An infectious, viral childhood disease characterized by swelling of the salivary glands in front of and below the ears.

Murmur: The sound made by blood flowing backward through a heart valve.

Muscle: A bundle of contractile cells that is responsible for the movement of organs and body parts.

Muscle contraction: The shortening of a muscle that results in movement of a particular body part.

Muscle fibers: Elongated muscle cells that make up skeletal, cardiac, and smooth muscles.

Muscle relaxant: Any of a number of medications used to paralyze the muscles of the patient temporarily before delivering an electrical stimulus; the main medication used for this purpose is succinylcholine.

Muscular dystrophy: A group of progressive genetic diseases that attack the muscles.

Musculature: The arrangement of skeletal muscles in the body.

Musculoskeletal: Pertaining to or comprising the skeleton and the muscles.

Mutagen: A chemical or an ionizing radiation that causes a change in the nucleotide sequence of the DNA of a gene, possibly affecting the gene's normal expression.

Mutation: Damage to a gene that changes how it works.

Myco-: A prefix denoting fungus.

Mycobacterium: Any of a genus of nonmotile aerobic bacteria that are difficult to stain and include numerous saprophytes and the organisms causing tuberculosis and leprosy.

Mycosis: Any disease of humans, plants, or animals caused by a fungus.

Myocardial infarction. *See* Heart attack.

Myocardium: The muscle tissue that forms the walls of the heart, varying in thickness in the upper and lower regions.

Myoclonus: Involuntary twitching or spasm of muscle.

Myomectomy: Surgical removal of a noncancerous muscle tumor (myoma).

Myopia: The inability of the eye to focus on distant objects; also called nearsightedness.

Myringotomy: Incision of the tympanic membrane, used to drain fluid and reduce middle-ear pressure.

Narcolepsy: An apparently inherited disorder of the nervous system characterized by brief, numerous, and overwhelming attacks of sleepiness throughout the day.

Narcotics: A group of potent painkilling drugs characterized by their ability to cause the user to develop tolerance and therefore dependency (physical addiction); such drugs include morphine, codeine, heroin, and other opium-like compounds.

Nasopharyngeal: Referring to the nose and pharynx (the upper part of the throat that leads from the mouth to the esophagus).

Nausea: An unpleasant sensation followed by stomach and intestinal discomfort, which may lead to vomiting.

Nearsightedness: The inability of the eye to focus on distant objects; also called myopia.

Necropsy: A postmortem (after-death) examination of an animal's body, similar to an autopsy performed on a human corpse.

Necrosis: The death of one or more cells or a portion of a tissue or organ, resulting from irreversible damage.

Needle biopsy: The obtaining of tissue fragments by the puncture of a tumor, through a large-caliber needle, syringe, and plunger; the tissue within the lumen of the needle is obtained through the rotation and withdrawal of the needle.

Negative feedback: A homeostatic control system designed to respond to a stress by returning body conditions to normal physiologic levels.

Negligence: Failure to perform an important or necessary medical technique, or the performance of such a technique in a careless or unskilled manner so as to cause further injury.

Neonatal intensive care unit: A hospital nursery with advanced equipment and specially trained staff to maintain the vital functions of sick newborns and to monitor their progress closely.

Neonatal period: The first month of life; derived from the Greek *neo* (meaning "new") and the Latin *natum* (meaning "birth").

Neonate: A newborn infant.

Neonatology: The study of diseases, conditions, and treatments of newborns (infants between the time of birth and approximately one month old).

Neoplasm: An uncontrolled growth of cells, which can develop into a tumor; may be malignant (cancerous) or benign.

Nephrectomy: Kidney removal.

Nephritis: Any disease or pathology of the kidney that results in inflammation.

Nephrology: The study of kidney diseases.

Nephron: A tiny blood-processing unit located in the kidneys (composed of the renal corpuscle, the loop of Henle, and renal tubules) that carries out the processes that form urine; each kidney contains approximately one million nephrons.

Nephrotic syndrome: An abnormal condition of the kidneys characterized by a variety of conditions, including edema and proteinuria; often accompanies glomerular dysfunction and diabetes.

Nephroureterectomy: A procedure similar to a radical nephrectomy, with the additional removal of the ureter and a cuff of the bladder; performed to treat transitional cell carcinomas of the ureters and the pelvis of the kidneys.

Nerve: A bundle of sensory and motor neurons held together by layers of connective tissue.

Nervous system: The bodily system that receives and interprets stimuli and transmits impulses to and from the brain and other organs.

Neural tube: The embryonic structure that gives rise to the central nervous system.

Neuralgia: Pain associated with a nerve, often caused by inflammation or injury.

Neuritis: An inflammatory or degenerative lesion of a nerve, marked by pain and the loss of normal reflexes.

Neurofibrillary tangles: A hallmark lesion of Alzheimer's disease and several other disorders consisting of intracellular aggregates of the structural protein tau.

Neuroglial cell: A supportive cell for neurons within the central nervous system of animals.

Neurologic: Dealing with the nervous system and its disorders.

Neurology: The study of the central nervous system, which is composed of the brain and spinal cord.

Neuromusculoskeletal: Pertaining to the interrelationship between the body's nerves, muscles, and skeleton.

Neuron: The principal nervous system cell that conducts electrical information from its dendritic extensions, through its cell body, to its axonal extensions, and on to other cells and is capable of releasing neurotransmitters.

Neuropathy: Any disorder of the nerves.

Neuroscience: The scientific specialization that seeks to understand mental processes, occurrences, and disturbances in terms of underlying mechanisms in the brain and the nervous system.

Neurosis: A psychic disturbance and defect from childhood that develops into a particular pattern of emotional illness and dysfunctional behavior.

Neurosurgery: Surgery to correct disorders of the nervous system, including the brain.

Neurotransmitter: A chemical substance released by one nerve cell to stimulate or inhibit the function of an adjacent nerve cell; a chemical message released by a neuron.

Neutrophil: A circulating white blood cell that serves as one of the principal phagocytes for the immune system.

Nicotinamide adenine dinucleotide (NAD): A molecule used to hold pairs of electrons when they have been removed from a molecule by some biological process; the empty molecule is denoted by NAD+, while it is denoted as NADH when it is carrying electrons.

Nitrous oxide: An anesthetic; sometimes called "laughing gas" because people appear to become intoxicated after inhaling it.

Nocturia: Involuntary nighttime urination.

Noninvasive: Referring to a procedure that does not require entering the body.

Nonmaleficence: A principle of medical ethics which requires that the actions taken not harm the patient.

Nonsteroidal anti-inflammatory drugs (NSAIDs): A drug such as ibuprofen that is used to reduce swelling and pain.

Normal: A term of reference that can mean average (as in statistically normal), functional (as in adaptive), or socially appropriate (as in within cultural bounds of acceptability).

Novocaine: A local anesthetic, commonly used in dentistry, whose chemical structure is similar to cocaine.

NSAIDs. *See* Nonsteroidal anti-inflammatory drugs (NSAIDs).

Nuclear medicine: The branch of medicine that employs radioactive substances to diagnose or treat disease.

Nucleic acids: Very large molecules, located on DNA molecules, that control the synthesis of proteins and carry basic information determining heredity.

Nucleolus: A nuclear structure formed through the activity of chromosome segments in the production of ribosomal RNA and the assembly of ribosomal subunits.

Nucleotide: A chemical subunit of DNA; different sequences of linked nucleotides spell out instructions for the assembly of proteins.

Nucleus: A large spherical mass occupying up to one-third of the volume of a typical plant or animal cell; also, the dense, positively charged, central core of an atom, containing its massive protons and neutrons.

Null hypothesis: A statement about a population that can be tested statistically which presupposes that there are no differences between what is being compared.

Nulliparity: Having never given birth to a viable infant.

Numbness: A reduction or loss of feeling in an area of skin.

Nursing: The profession of providing health care that assists a patient to recover from an illness, injury, or surgical or other procedure, performed in a variety of settings. Also, the act of breast-feeding.

Nursing home: A type of extended care facility that can be classified as either skilled or intermediate, depending on the type of care; physicians oversee medical care that is rendered around the clock by a nursing staff.

Nutrients: Substances needed by the body for maintenance, growth, and repair; the six classes of nutrients are carbohydrates, fats, proteins, vitamins, minerals, and water.

Nutrition: The study of those substances found in foods that are needed by the body for maintenance, growth, and repair, as well as those substances that increase the risk of disease.

Obesity: A medical condition defined as being in excess of 20 percent above ideal weight.

Obsession: A recurrent, unwelcome, and intrusive thought.

Obsessive-compulsive disorder: An anxiety disorder characterized by intrusive and unwanted thoughts and/or the need to perform ritualized behaviors.

Obstetrics: The branch of medicine specializing in the problems and needs of pregnant women and their fetuses from conception through delivery and postnatal care.

Obstruction: Partial or complete blockage of the gastrointestinal tract.

Occlusion: The fit of the upper and lower teeth when they are brought together; also, the blockage of any vessel in the body, which may be caused by a thrombus or other embolus.

Occult blood: Fecal blood, as detected by microscopic or chemical testing.

Occupational health: Those health disciplines collectively concerned with the conditions, diseases, and injuries that occur within or as a result of the work setting.

Occupational medicine: A medical specialty focused on providing all levels of preventive medical services to working men and women in order to preserve, maintain, or restore health and well-being.

Occupational toxicology: A subspecialty of environmental toxicology that focuses on the effects of chemicals on the health of a workplace population.

Odontology: The study of teeth.

Oedipus complex: The experience of having sexual feelings toward the parent of the opposite sex that can occur in young children.

Olfaction: The sense of smell; a process in which nerve impulses caused by chemicals interacting with chemoreceptors in the nose arrive in the olfactory center of the brain and are classified as certain kinds of odor.

Olfactory adaptation: The relatively quick response to and subsequent fatigue of the sense of smell that allows the presence of odoriferous chemicals to be recognized quickly and then become less and less noticed until they are soon ignored.

Olfactory bulb: An extension of the brain located below the frontal lobes of the cerebrum and above the ethmoid bone (extending back from nose); one of a pair of gray masses into which the olfactory nerves terminate, thus serving as the first synaptic sites in olfactory neural pathways.

Olfactory knobs: Unmyelinated, tiny, rounded nerve endings of the sensory cells found at the mucus-coated olfactory membrane; each knob has five to eight extensions, called olfactory hairs, that branch out into the nasal cavity and monitor the environment.

Oncogene: A gene within the chromosomes of all the cells of an individual organism that triggers cancerous cellular transformation when it is expressed incorrectly.

Oncology: The branch of medicine specializing in the study of tumors, especially malignant tumors, and their treatment.

Onychomycosis: Common nail disorder in which fungal organisms invade the nail bed causing progressive changes in the color, texture, and structure of the nail.

Oophorectomy: Removal of the ovaries, which is often necessary in cases of severe endometriosis.

Oophoritis: Inflammation of the ovary.

Operating room: A room in which surgical procedures are performed.

Operator: A person who induces a hypnotic state; synonymous with "hypnotist" and "suggestor."

Ophthalmology: The branch of medicine concerned with the study of the eye and its structures, disorders, conditions, and treatments.

Opioids: Drugs derived from opium; also known as narcotics or opiates.

Opportunistic infection: Any infection caused by pathogens that take advantage of a dysfunctional immune system; much of the morbidity and mortality of AIDS results from opportunistic infections.

Optic disc: The portion of the optic nerve at its point of entrance into the rear of the eye.

Optical fiber: A very thin thread made of high-purity glass, plastic, or quartz; used to transmit light from a laser into the body.

Optometry: The practice of diagnosing visual problems and diagnosing correctional devices such as eyeglasses and contact lenses.

Oral hygiene: Care of the teeth and mouth.

Oral surgery: The dental specialty that surgically removes diseased teeth and oral tissues and treats bone fractures of the jaws.

Orchiectomy: Surgical removal of the testicle for benign or malignant conditions.

Orchiopexy: Fixation of the testicle to the internal lining of the scrotum to eliminate the possibility of testicular torsion.

Orchitis: Inflammation of the testis.

Organelles: Specialized parts of cells.

Organic: Pertaining to, arising from, or affecting a body organ.

Organic brain syndromes: Clusters of behavioral and psychological symptoms involving impaired brain function, where etiology is unknown; includes delirium, delusions, amnesia, intoxication, and dementias.

Organic disease: A disease caused or accompanied by an alteration in the structure of the tissues or organs.

Organic mental disorders: Mental and emotional disturbances from transient or permanent brain dysfunction, with known organic etiology; includes drug or alcohol ingestion, infection, trauma, and cardiovascular disease.

Organism: A complex structure of interdependent and subordinate elements whose relations and properties are largely determined by their function as a whole.

Organs. *See* Systems and organs.

Orthodontics: The branch of dentistry that diagnoses and treats malformed teeth.

Orthognathic surgery: Jaw reconstruction.

Orthopedics: The branch of medicine that specializes in the surgical repair or correction of injured or malformed bones and joints and the structures (such as muscles) associated with them.

Orthotic device: A podiatric appliance or prosthesis that is used to correct a foot deformity.

Orthotopic: Referring to the placement of a transplanted organ in the position occupied by the original organ.

Oscilloscope: An instrument that displays a visual representation of electrical variations on the fluorescent screen of a cathode-ray tube.

Osmosis: The diffusion of molecules through a semipermeable membrane until there is an equal concentration on either side of the membrane.

Ossicles: Three small bones in the middle ear that transmit vibrations from the eardrum to the fluid of the inner ear.

Ossification: The formation of bone tissue.

Osteoarthritis: A degenerative disease of the joints and surrounding tissues.

Osteoblast: A bone cell that can produce and form bone matrix; osteoblasts are responsible for new bone formation.

Osteoclast: A large bone cell that can destroy bone matrix by dissolving the mineral crystals.

Osteocyte: The primary living cell of mature bone tissue.

Osteopathic medicine: A form of medicine, founded by Andrew Taylor Still in 1874, that emphasizes the health of the musculoskeletal system as well as a holistic approach to the functioning of the body.

Osteoporosis: A loss of bone mass accompanied by increasing fragility and brittleness.

Ostomy: A popular term for any operation that results in a stoma.

Otitis: Any inflammation of the outer or middle ear.

Otologist: A medical doctor who specializes in diseases and disorders of the ear.

-otomy: A suffix meaning an opening or incision in an organ or structure; for example, a ureterotomy is an opening in the ureter.

Otorhinolaryngology: The branch of medicine concerned with the diseases, conditions, and treatment of the ear, nose, and throat.

Otosclerosis: A condition in which the stapes becomes progressively more rigid and hearing loss results.

Otoscope: An instrument for viewing the ear canal and the eardrum.

Outer ear: The visible, fleshy part of the ear and the ear canal; it transmits sound waves to the eardrum.

Outpatient care: Evaluation and treatment services not requiring an overnight stay in a medical facility.

Ovarian cysts: Benign growths in the ovaries, which may cause pain.

Ovariectomy: The removal of the ovaries.

Ovaries: The pair of structures in the female that produce ova (eggs) and hormones.

Over-the-counter drugs: Pharmaceutical products, vitamins, herbal remedies, and other medicines that can be purchased by anyone, without a doctor's prescription.

Oviducts: The pair of tubes leading from the top of the uterus upward toward the ovaries; also called the Fallopian tubes.

Ovulation: The release of an ovum from its follicle in the ovary.

Ovum (*pl.* ova): The female gamete; a large round cell that carries the female's chromosomes that is released from the ovaries during ovulation.

Oxygen therapy: Application of pure or high-oxygen gas to assist in recovery from oxygen deprivation (as in respiratory diseases).

Oxytocin: The maternal pituitary hormone that regulates milk production and uterine contraction.

Pacemaker: A device surgically implanted in a patient suffering from heart disease in order to maintain a healthy heartbeat; also, a region of the heart called the sinoatrial (S-A) node, which maintains the regular heartbeat.

Pacinian corpuscles: Receptors at which the sensations of heavy touch or deep pressure originate; also called lamellated corpuscles.

Paget's disease: A disorder characterized by a progressive thickening and weakening of the bones.

Pain: Physical distress that is often associated with disorder and injury.

Pain management: The alleviation of pain, either completely or to a point of tolerance, by means of a variety of therapies, both chemical (as with drugs) and physical (as with exercise therapy).

Palliative treatments: Therapies that reduce symptoms without completely eradicating a disorder.

Palpation: Application of the hands, or touching, to determine the size, texture, consistency, and location of body structures.

Palpitation: The sensation of being aware of one's own heartbeat, usually because the heart is beating rapidly or more forcefully than normal.

Palsy: Partial or complete paralysis of a nerve followed by muscle weakness and wasting.

Pancreas: A secretory organ behind the stomach and connected to the duodenum. It produces enzymes to digest food and insulin to metabolize sugar.

Pancreatitis: Inflammation of the pancreas.

Pandemic: Pertaining to a high proportion of a population.

Panic attack: A sudden feeling of intense apprehension, fear, doom, and/or terror that can cause shortness of breath, palpitations, chest pain, chills, nausea, and light-headedness.

Pap smear: A simple diagnostic test for the presence of cervical cancer involving the removal of cervical tissue cells and the subsequent biopsy of these cells.

Papillomaviruses: Small, cuboidal viruses that replicate in the nuclei of epithelial cells.

Paralysis: The loss of muscle function or sensation as a result of trauma or disease.

Paramedic: A person who is not generally a physician but is trained to provide emergency treatment in critical situations, such as resuscitation after a heart attack or seizure, arrest of bleeding, dressing wounds, and setting broken bones.

Paramedical: Related to the science or practice of medicine.

Paranoia: Pervasive distrust and suspiciousness of others and a tendency to interpret others' motives as malevolent.

Paraplegia: Partial or complete paralysis of both legs caused by damage to the spinal cord.

Parasite: An organism whose principal food source is another living organism; in medicine, the term refers to both unicellular and multicellular animals.

Parasympathetic nervous system: The part of the autonomic nervous system that stimulates digestion, slows the heart, and dilates blood vessels, acting in opposition to sympathetic nerves.

Parathyroid gland: One of four small endocrine glands, situated underneath the thyroid gland, whose main product is parathyroid hormone; this hormone is responsible for the regulation of serum calcium levels.

Parathyroidectomy: Removal of part or all of one or both of the parathyroid glands.

Parkinson's disease: A disease in which the dopamine-secreting cells of the midbrain degenerate, resulting in uncontrolled movement and rigidity.

Paroxysm: An uncontrolled spasm or convulsion which may sometimes be violent.

Partial pressure of a gas in a gas: The measure of the contribution of one gas of a mixture of gases to the total pressure pushing on the walls containing it; it is the pressure that would be exerted if all the other gases were removed from the container, leaving only the gas of interest.

Parturition: The process or action of giving birth.

Passive euthanasia: Ending life by refusing or withdrawing life-sustaining medical treatment.

Passive immunity: Immunity resulting from the introduction of preformed antibodies.

Pathogen: Any disease-causing organism, including a virus, bacterium, protozoan, mold or yeast, or other parasite.

Pathogenicity: The ability of an organism to cause disease.

Pathologic: Pertaining to the study of disease and the development of abnormal conditions.

Pathology: The study of the nature and consequences of disease.

Pathophysiology: An alteration in function as seen in disease.

Patient advocacy: The representation of the patient's interest in medical diagnosis and treatment decisions, in which the physician acts as an information source and counselor for the patient.

Patient assessment: The systematic gathering of information in order to determine the nature of a patient's illness.

Pediatric: Pertaining to neonates, infants, and children up to the age of twelve.

Pediatrics: The branch of medicine specializing in the conditions, diseases, and development of infants and children.

Pedodontics: The dental specialty that treats children.

Pelvic inflammatory disease (PID): An infection of the female reproductive organs that may be caused by a sexually transmitted disease.

Penis: The male genital organ containing the urethra, through which both urine and semen pass; sufficient erection of the penis is required for intercourse.

Pepsin: A substance in the stomach that breaks down most proteins.

Peptic ulcer: Open sores that develop in the lining of the stomach as a result of excessive secretion of gastric juices.

Peptidoglycans: Repeating units of sugar derivatives that make up a rigid layer of bacterial cell walls; found in both gram-positive and gram-negative cells.

Percussion: Gentle tapping by the medical examiner's finger, which has been positioned on the patient; a hollow sound is heard over air-filled structures, while a dull thud is heard over solid areas or liquid-filled structures.

Percutaneous transluminal coronary angioplasty (PTCA): A procedure undertaken to increase the internal diameter of a coronary artery by inflating a small balloonlike device at the site or sites where the artery has narrowed because of plaque buildup.

Perforation: An abnormal opening, such as a hole in the wall of the colon.

Perfusion: The flow of blood through the lungs or other vessels in the body.

Perfusionist: A health care specialist who operates extracorporeal circulation equipment when it is necessary to support or replace a patient's circulatory or respiratory function.

Peri-: A prefix denoting "around," either in a literal sense (as in "pericarditis") or in a figurative sense (as in "perinatal").

Pericarditis: A disease of the membrane that surrounds the heart, caused by an inflammation that can lead to constriction of the heart muscle.

Perinatology: The branch of medicine that treats the mother and child during the late stages of pregnancy and the first month or so following birth.

Perineum: The short bridge of flesh between the anus and vagina in women and the anus and base of the penis in men.

Period: The length of one complete cycle of a rhythm; ultradian rhythms are about twenty-four hours (twenty to twenty-eight hours), and infradian rhythms are longer than twenty-eight hours.

Periodontics: The dental specialty that treats the diseases of the supporting tissues of the teeth.

Periodontitis: The inflammation and infection of the gums, which may cause loss of the supporting bone and eventually tooth loss.

Periodontium: Those tissues supporting the tooth in the jaws, including the gingiva, the jawbone, and the periodontal ligament that attaches the root of the tooth into the jaw.

Periosteum: The thick, fibrous membrane that covers the entire surface of a bone except for the cartilage within joints.

Peripheral: Referring to a part of the body away from the center.

Peripheral nervous system: A system consisting of the nerves not located in the central nervous system (brain and spinal cord); these nerves carry impulses from the central nervous system to the target muscles and relay sensory impulses from the rest of the body to the central nervous system.

Peripheral vision: Side vision, or the visual perception to all sides of the central object being viewed.

Peristalsis: The wavelike muscular contractions that move food and waste products through the intestines. Problems with peristalsis are called motility disorders.

Peritoneal cavity: The abdominal cavity, that contains the visceral organs.

Peritoneal dialysis: The removal of toxins from blood by dialysis in the peritoneal cavity.

Peritoneum: The membrane lining the walls of the abdominal cavity and enclosing the viscera.

Peritonitis: Infection of the abdominal (peritoneal) cavity in which the visceral organs are found.

Peroxisome: A membrane-bound organelle that contains reaction systems linking biochemical pathways taking place elsewhere in the cell; also called a microbody.

Personality disorders: Pervasive, inflexible patterns of perceiving, thinking, and behaving that cause long-term distress or impairment, beginning in adolescence and persisting into adulthood.

Pertussis: A serious bacterial infection of the respiratory tract that usually strikes very young children; commonly known as whooping cough.

PET scanning. *See* Positron emission tomography (PET) scanning.

Petechiae (*sing.* petechia): Minute, pinhead-sized spots caused by hemorrhage or bleeding into the skin.

Petit mal: A mild type of epileptic seizure characterized by a very short lapse of consciousness, usually without convulsions or falling.

Peyer's patches: Lymphatic nodules in the ileum of the intestine; Peyer's patches are one kind of mucosal associated lymphoid tissue (MALT), which, unlike lymph nodes, is not enclosed by tissue capsules.

pH: A value that represents the relative acidity or alkalinity of a solution; values below pH 7 are acidic, while values above pH 7 are basic.

Phagocyte: Any cell capable of surrounding, ingesting, and digesting microbes or cell debris; in a certain sense, phagocytes function as scavengers.

Phagocytosis: The ingestion and destruction of a pathogen or abnormal tissue by specialized white blood cells known as phagocytes.

Pharmaceutical: Of or relating to pharmacy; a medicinal drug.

Pharmaceutical care: The responsible provision of drug therapy to improve a patient's quality of life.

Pharmacist: A person with a license to dispense or sell drugs prescribed by a medical practitioner, such as a dentist, physician, or veterinarian.

Pharmacodynamics: Changes in tissue sensitivity or physiologic systems in response to pharmacological substances.

Pharmacognosy: The preparation of medicinal agents from natural sources.

Pharmacokinetics: The action of pharmacological substances within a biological system; pharmacologic substance absorption, distribution, metabolism, and elimination by an organism.

Pharmacology: The science that deals with the chemistry, effects, and therapeutic use of drugs.

Pharmacy: The art or profession of preparing and dispensing drugs and medicine.

Pharyngitis: Inflammation of the pharynx.

Pharynx: The throat; the part of the respiratory-digestive passage that extends from the nasal cavity to the larynx (voice box).

Phenylketonuria (PKU): A genetic disease characterized by the absence of the enzyme that breaks down the amino acid phenylalanine; the resulting buildup can lead to brain damage.

Phimosis: The narrowing of the opening of the skin covering the head of the penis sufficient to prevent retraction of the skin back over the glans.

Phlebitis: The inflammation of a vein, often in the legs; may be accompanied by blood clots.

Phlebotomy: The act or practice of opening a vein for letting blood.

Phobia: Any abnormal or exaggerated fear of a particular object or situation.

Photocoagulation: The condensation of protein material by the controlled use of an intense beam of light (such as a xenon arc light or argon laser).

Photon: A particle of light whose energy depends on its wavelength (that is, its color); many billions of individual photons make up a light beam.

Photophobia: Dread or avoidance of light.

Photoreception: Sensitivity to light.

Photoreceptor: A light-responsive nerve cell or receptor that is located in the retina of the eye.

Phrenic: Of or relating to the diaphragm.

Physiatry: The branch of medicine dealing with the prevention, diagnosis, and treatment of disease or injury and the rehabilitation from resultant impairments and disabilities; it uses physical agents such as light, heat, cold, water, electricity, therapeutic exercise, mechanical apparatus, and pharmaceutical agents.

Physical deconditioning: A condition that results when a person who has previously been exercising (has become conditioned) stops exercising for a significant period of time.

Physical examination: A step in the diagnostic process in which the physician makes general observations about the patient and examines structures of the patient's body through touching (palpation), tapping (percussion), and listening, usually with the aid of a stethoscope (auscultation).

Physical modalities: The physical means of addressing a disease, which include heat, cold, electricity, exercises, braces, assistive devices, and biofeedback.

Physical rehabilitation: The discipline devoted to the restoration of normal bodily function, primarily of the muscles and skeleton.

Physician assistant: A health care provider who works under the supervision of a licensed physician and who is trained to perform physical examinations, diagnose illnesses, interpret laboratory tests, set fractures, and assist in surgeries.

Physiological: Characteristic of or appropriate to an organism's healthy or normal functioning.

Physiology: The study of how the body functions, both at the cellular level and at the anatomical level.

PID. *See* Pelvic inflammatory disease (PID).

Pigmentation: The color of the skin, hair, and eyes, caused by the degree and distribution of melanin in the skin.

Piles: A common term for hemorrhoids.

Pilosebaceous: Referring to hair follicles and the sebaceous glands.

Pimple: The common term for a papule (a solid elevation in the skin) or a pustule (a papule containing pus).

Pituitary gland: A very small gland at the base of the brain that is referred to as the master gland; with the hypothalamus, it regulates most of the endocrine systems.

PKU. *See* Phenylketonuria (PKU).

Placebo: An inactive substance resembling the experimental drug that might be given to a control group, especially when no standard treatment exists.

Placenta: The oval, spongy tissue containing blood vessels that provides the fetus with nutrients and oxygen from the mother via the umbilicus.

Plague: A serious, and sometimes fatal, bacterial infection transmitted by fleas.

Plaintiff: A person or corporation that brings legal action against another person or corporation.

Plantar: Having to do with the sole of the foot.

Plantar warts: Warts that develop on the soles of the feet, usually at points of pressure; the wart consists of a soft core surrounded by a callous-like ring.

Plaque: The fatty material composed of cholesterol, degenerating cells, and proteinaceous substances that can build up in the wall of any artery; also, an accumulation of decomposing matter on the teeth which promotes tooth decay.

Plasma: The fluid portion of blood, in which white and red blood cells are suspended and which contains water, proteins, minerals, nutrients, hormones, and wastes.

Plasma proteins: Any proteins found in the plasma of blood, which include those proteins necessary for blood clotting and some necessary for the transport of other molecules; most are produced by the liver.

Plasmin: An enzyme present in the blood that can dissolve clots; plasmin is normally found in its inactive form, plasminogen, until needed.

Plastic surgery: Surgery performed to repair defects of the skin and underlying tissues caused by injury or malformations.

Plasticity: A phenomenon of many animal nervous systems, particularly those in higher vertebrates, in which central nervous system neurons grow in patterns based on input information.

Platelets: Specialized blood-clotting particles that travel in the blood and become sticky when they come in contact with a damaged blood vessel.

Pleurisy: The inflammation and swelling of the pleurae, the membranes that enclose the lungs and line the chest cavity.

Pluripotent: Referring to stem cells that have the capacity to develop into most of the specialized tissues of the body, but not an entire individual.

PMS. *See* Premenstrual syndrome (PMS).

Pneumocystis pneumonia: A form of pneumonia caused by the single-celled parasite *Pneumocystis carinii*; dangerous mainly to persons with impaired immune systems, particularly patients with AIDS.

Pneumonia: An inflammation of the lungs or bronchial passageways caused by viral or bacterial infection.

Podiatry: The branch of medicine that treats diseases and conditions of the foot.

Poisoning: Exposure to any substance in a quantity sufficient to cause health problems.

Poisonous plants: Plants that cause gastrointestinal or dermatological reactions in humans.

Poliomyelitis: A viral illness that may cause meningitis and permanent paralysis; it can be prevented through immunization.

Polycythemia: An abnormal increase in red blood cells.

Polydactyly: A congenital anomaly characterized by excess fingers or toes.

Polymethylmethacrylate: A material used in the fixation of bones.

Polyp: A tumorlike growth, such as of the colorectal mucous lining.

Polypharmacy: The prescription of many drugs at one time, often resulting in excessive use of medications and adverse drug interactions.

Polyspermy: Entry of more than one sperm into an egg, resulting in too many sets of chromosomes.

Population: All the people, research animals, or other items of interest in a particular study.

Porphyria: One of several rare, genetic disorders caused by the accumulation of substances called porphyrins.

Portacaval: Referring to a type of shunt used to carry blood from the portal vein to the inferior vena cava, allowing blood to bypass the liver.

Portal system: A system of veins, unique to the liver, that carry nutrient-rich blood from the digestive organs to the liver.

Positive feedback: When a stimulus causes more of the same to occur; can be useful in some instances, such as with blood clotting and uterine contractions during childbirth.

Positron emission tomography (PET) scanning: A technique for creating three-dimensional images of tissues in the body by tracking radioisotopes injected into the body, allowing for diagnosis of tumors or metabolic diseases and conditions, especially of the brain.

Positrons: A type of radiation, similar to electrons but with positive charge, emitted by radioactive atoms.

Posterior: Toward the back or rear of the body or any structure.

Postpartum depression: Depression following childbirth brought on by hormonal changes and sometimes by underlying social or emotional problems.

Potency: The effectiveness of a drug.

Preeclampsia: Hypertension induced by pregnancy, in its nonconvulsive form.

Pregnancy: The development of an embryo or fetus within the uterus, which begins with conception.

Premature: Referring to a birth that is less than full term.

Premenstrual syndrome (PMS): A common condition involving tension, irritability, headaches, depression, and bloating in the week prior to menstruation.

Premolars: The teeth between the cuspids and the molars, used in crushing and grinding food; also called bicuspids.

Prep: A short form of the word "prepare"; to prep means to wash and shave the surgical area and to clean the skin surface immediately before a surgical procedure.

Prescription drugs: Medicines that can only be obtained with the prescription of a doctor.

Presenilins: Proteins linked to several forms of inherited Alzheimer's disease, which are believed to play a role in the production of Aβ.

Pressure: The measure of how much a gas or a liquid pushes on the walls of its container.

Prevalence: The number of individuals at a particular time who have a disease or a given characteristic.

Preventive medicine: An approach to health care that emphasizes behaviors and therapies (such as exercise and proper diet) designed to minimize contraction of disease before it happens.

Prima facie: The concept that one ethical principle is morally binding unless the action it requires violates another equal or greater principle.

Primary care: General medical services provided in family practice, internal medicine, pediatrics, geriatrics, obstetrics, and emergency care (in contrast to specialties, such as urology or cardiac surgery).

Primary infection: A person's first infection with a particular agent such as a virus.

Privacy: The state of being free from unwanted or unauthorized observation, company, or other intrusion.

Probability: A number varying between 0 (for an impossible event) to 1 (for an absolutely certain event).

Procedure: Any medical treatment that involves physical manipulation or invasion of the body.

Proctology: The study and treatment of diseases of the rectum.

Professional licensing: State-granted privileges to health care and other professionals allowing them to deliver services or to participate in certain activities; a privilege that is revokable and subject to censure; a privilege usually only granted after thorough examination of the skill and practice of a person seeking licensure.

Progesterone or progestin: A hormone produced in the ovaries, adrenal gland, and placenta (of pregnant women) that prepares for and sustains pregnancy.

Prognosis: The outlook for a patient with a disease condition.

Prolactin: A hormone secreted from the anterior pituitary gland that signals the breast to start and sustain milk production.

Prone: The position of the body when lying face downward, on the abdomen.

Prophylactic treatment: A treatment focusing on preventing disease, illness, or their symptoms from occurring.

Prostaglandins: Chemical messengers that are not carried in the blood and that function only locally; they cause pain, contractions, and a variety of other effects.

Prostate gland: An accessory reproductive gland whose main function is to secrete into semen vital additive components that increase the fertilizing potential of sperm.

Prosthesis: A fabricated, artificial substitute for a missing part of the body, such as a limb.

Prosthetist: An individual skilled in constructing and fitting prostheses.

Prosthodontics: The dental specialty that restores missing teeth with fixed or removable dentures.

Prostoglandular carcinoma: The general pathological nomenclature for cancers located in the prostate gland.

Protein: Large molecules made up of amino acids connected by peptide bonds; the sequence of amino acids in a protein determines its three-dimensional structure.

Protein kinase: An enzyme type that often is encoded by oncogenes; this enzyme attaches phosphate molecules to certain amino acids on specifically targeted proteins.

Protozoan (*pl.* protozoa): A single-celled organism that is more closely related to animals than are bacteria and is often a vector of disease; only a few drugs are available that will kill protozoa without harming their animal hosts.

Proving: The testing of a substance or remedy on healthy volunteers (provers), who take repeated doses and record in detail any symptoms produced by it.

Proximal: Toward the origin.

Psoriasis: A chronic skin disease characterized by red, scaly patches overlaid with thick, silvery gray scales.

Psyche: The human mind, which according to Sigmund Freud is divided into id, ego, and superego; the id contains instincts and repressed feelings, the ego directs everyday behavior, and the superego guides the ego.

Psychedelic drugs: Substances that cause alterations in perception and thinking, such as changes in awareness, sense of self, or hallucinations.

Psychiatry: The branch of medicine, practiced by physicians, that treats emotional and behavioral problems through both medication and non-drug therapies such as counseling.

Psychoanalysis: A form of treatment for mental illness that employs interviews designed to elicit information from the patient, which the analyst then interprets in the light of theories developed by Sigmund Freud.

Psychoanalyst: A person, usually a psychiatrist, who has received several years of postgraduate training and supervised practice in using psychoanalysis to diagnose and treat clients. Psychoanalysts are often, but not always, medical doctors.

Psychogenic: Psychological (rather than physical) in origin; set off by psychologically stressful events.

Psychosis: A condition occurring where a person is severely out of touch with reality and unable to function in an adaptive manner.

Psychosomatic: Referring to physical symptoms caused by psychological problems.

Psychosurgery: The surgical removal or destruction of part of the brain of depressed patients as a form of treatment.

Psychotherapy: Treatment using the mind, body, and behavior to remedy problems related to disordered behavior or thinking, emotional problems, or disease.

Psychotic: Referred to a disabling mental state characterized by poor reality testing (inaccurate perceptions, confusion, disorientation) and disorganized speech, behavior, and emotional experience.

Psychotropic drugs: Substances primarily affecting behavior, perception, and other psychological functions.

Ptosis: Downward drooping or sagging of tissue, caused by the influence of gravity or the loss of muscular or other support.

Puberty: The physiological sequence of events by which a child is transformed into an adult; the growth of secondary sexual characteristics occurs, reproductive functions begin, and the differences between males and females are accentuated.

Public health: The well-being of humankind, both as a community and as individuals, accomplished by using scientific skills and beliefs that assist in health maintenance and health improvement.

Pulmonary: Referring to the lungs, both the lung tissue and the bronchial tree.

Pulmonary edema: Accumulation of fluid in the lungs, which may lead to death.

Pulmonary medicine: The field of medicine concerned with all the diseases that may afflict the lungs or in which the lungs may be involved.

Pulp: The internal, living tissue of the tooth, consisting of nerves, blood vessels, and dental cells.

Pulse: The rhythmical dilation of an artery, produced by the increased volume of blood forced into the vessel by the contraction of the heart; the frequency of the pulse corresponds to the heart rate.

Pulsed laser: A laser technique used to deliver a light beam of high power for a very short time in order to localize the heating effect without damaging surrounding tissue.

Pupil: The opening at the center of the iris through which light passes.

Pyloric stenosis: A narrowing of the passageway between the stomach and the duodenum.

Pyorrhea: The second stage of gingivitis.

Pyridostigmine bromide: A chemical that prevents damage from possible nerve gas exposure.

Pyrogens: Protein substances that appear at the outset of the process that leads to a fever reaction.

Qi gong: A Chinese meditative exercise that improves cardiovascular circulation, restores deep breathing, and relieves stress.

Quadriplegia: Partial or complete paralysis of the arms, legs, and trunk caused by damage to the spinal cord in the neck.

Quantum theory: The theory that energy, momentum, and other physical quantities appear in indivisible units of finite quantity.

Quickening: The stage during a pregnancy when the mother begins to feel the movements of the fetus, usually in the second trimester.

Rabies: A viral infection, usually transmitted through the bite of a rabid animal, that attacks the nervous system; it can be cured through immediate immunization but is nearly always fatal once symptoms occur.

Radial: Toward the edge of the forearm and hand containing the radius and thumb.

Radiation dose: The amount of radiation absorbed, depending on the intensity of the source and the time of exposure; measured in units of rads or grays.

Radiation sickness: Acute, sometimes fatal illness that occurs with exposure to a sudden, large dose of radiation.

Radiation therapy: The use of radiation to kill cancer cells or shrink cancerous growth. When high and full doses of radiation (measured in units called rads) are used, the patient is said to be given a "megavoltage."

Radical surgery: Any surgery that removes all of the organ or tissue affected by a disease, as well as tissue surrounding the area, in an attempt to eradicate the disease.

Radioimmunoassay: The quantitative measurement of a hormone using an unlabeled hormone to inhibit the binding of a radiolabeled hormone to an antibody.

Radioimmunotherapy: A cancer therapy using radionuclides; the radionuclides attach themselves to antibodies that tend to target cancer cells in the body, thus eradicating the cancer cells through selective irradiation.

Radioisotope: A radioactive atom.

Radiology: The branch of medicine that focuses on imaging technologies such as X rays, magnetic resonance imaging (MRI), scanning techniques, and ultrasonography.

Radionucleotide scanning: A technique that develops an image of an internal bodily structure by detecting radiation emitted from a substance injected into the body to see how the bodily structure reacts to it.

Radionuclide: An unstable atomic nucleus that, in the process of decay, emits radiation; also referred to as a radioisotope.

Radiopharmaceutical: A sterile, radioactively tagged compound that is administered to a patient for diagnostic or therapeutic purposes.

Radius: The shorter of the two forearm bones, on the thumb side.

Random sample: A sample in which every member of the population has the same probability of being included.

Rash: A skin disorder, usually temporary, characterized by red, inflamed areas or spots; generally a symptom of an underlying condition, such as a skin disease, autoimmune disorder, infectious disease, or bleeding disorder.

RDA. *See* Recommended daily (or dietary) allowance (RDA).

Receptor: A molecular structure at the cell surface or inside the cell that is capable of combining with hormones or neurotransmitters and causing a change in cell metabolism.

Recessive allele: A version of a gene that must be present on both chromosomes of a pair in order to produce a recognizable trait in offspring.

Recessive genetic disease: A disease caused by a mutation in a gene that must be inherited from both parents in order for an individual to show the symptoms of the disease; such a disease may show up only occasionally in a family history, especially if the mutation is rare.

Recombinant DNA technology: Manipulation of genetic material or DNA whereby pieces of DNA are separated and interchanged in order to obtain a desired result.

Recombination: The reciprocal exchange of segments between the two chromosomes of a pair, producing new combinations of alleles.

Recommended daily (or dietary) allowance (RDA): The amount of nutrients needed daily by a healthy person to maintain health; age and gender affect the listed RDAs.

Reconstructive surgery: Surgery designed to rebuild or replace a body part malformed at birth, damaged as a result of injury, or surgically removed for therapeutic reasons.

Recovery room: The room where a patient returns to full consciousness after a surgical procedure; in an outpatient facility, patients can change clothes in the recovery room, which may serve double duty as the preoperative waiting room.

Rectal prolapse: The protrusion of the rectum through the anus.

Rectum: The intestinal storage area for feces between the colon and anus.

Recurrence: The appearance of an infection or disease after initial treatment has been completed.

Red blood cells: Blood cells that contain hemoglobin; their role is to transport oxygen.

Reduction: The restoration of a fractured bone to its normal position; also a decrease in the total volume or mass of breast tissue, usually to correct undesirable ptosis.

Reed-Sternberg cell: A large, atypical macrophage with multiple nuclei; found in patients with Hodgkin's disease.

Referred pain: Pain that is not felt at the site of injury or disease, as a result of neural pathways.

Reflux: The abnormal backward flow of a fluid which normally flows in the opposite direction (such as bile or urine).

Refraction: The bending of light rays by the cornea and lens to form an image on the retina.

Regeneration: The renewal, regrowth, or restoration of destroyed or missing tissue; the production of new tissue.

Regional anesthesia: Insensibility caused by the interruption of nerve conduction in a region of the body.

Regurgitation: The leakage of blood backward through a valve; also vomiting.

Rehabilitation: The restoration of normal form and function after injury or illness; the restoration of the ill or injured patient to optimal functional level in the home and community in relation to physical, psychosocial, vocational, and recreational activity.

Rejection: A cellular and chemical attack by the immune system on transplanted tissues or organs, which are recognized as foreign to the body.

Reliability: The concept that repeated tests will produce the same result.

Renal: Referring to the kidneys.

Renal cell carcinoma: Cancer of the small tubules of the kidney; generally known as kidney cancer.

Renal failure: The inability of the kidneys to process waste products in the blood and excrete them through the urine.

Renal pelvis: The central pocket or sac of each kidney, which collects urine from all nephrons and channels it into the ureter.

Renal tubule: The tubular portion of a nephron that allows renal fluid to flow from the Bowman's capsule to the renal pelvis; these tubules, shaped like hairpins, are crucially important in the production of urine.

Repertory: In homeopathy, a published index of symptoms, with each heading listing the drugs known to cause the symptom.

Replication: The process by which the DNA of a cell is duplicated so that the information stored there can be passed on to new cells after cell division.

Reproductive system: The organs of the female (the vagina, uterus, Fallopian tubes, ovaries, and mammary glands) and the male (the penis, testes, vas deferens, and prostate gland) that are necessary for the production of offspring.

Reservoir: An animal population that is infected with a disease which can be transmitted either to other animals or to humans; also called an alternate host.

Residency: A course of clinical medical education undertaken after receiving an M.D. or D.O. degree and leading to certification in a generalist or specialist branch of medicine.

Resorption: The process in which bones dissolve and return their components to the body fluids.

Respect for autonomy: A principle of medical ethics which requires that the autonomous decisions of patients be honored.

Respiration: A process which includes both air conduction (the act of breathing) and gas exchange (oxygen and carbon dioxide transfer between the air and blood).

Respirator: A machine that inflates and deflates the lungs, imitating normal breathing; connected to patient through a tube placed into the windpipe.

Respiratory diseases: Any of a wide variety of diseases which affect the lungs and/or the process of respiration, including emphysema, lung cancer, and pneumonia.

Respiratory distress syndrome: A life-threatening illness primarily of premature infants; immature lungs lack a vital substance that keeps the tiny air sacs (alveoli) from collapsing upon exhalation.

Rest pain: Pain noted in the most distal portion of the extremity at rest, relieved by analgesics.

Restriction endonuclease: An enzyme that responds to a specific, short sequence of nucleotides within a DNA molecule by binding to that sequence and breaking the DNA strands near the sequence.

Resuscitation: The return of a person to consciousness or the restoration of a person's vital signs after an injury, seizure, or heart attack by means of artificial respiration, CPR (cardiopulmonary resuscitation), electrical shock treatment, chemical, or other means.

Retina: A thin membrane at the back of the eyeball where light is converted into nerve impulses that travel to the brain.

Retrocochlear hearing loss: Any disruption of neural information processing beyond the cochlea.

Retrovirus: Any of a family of RNA viruses to which HIV belongs, characterized by a multiplication cycle that includes reverse transcription.

Revascularization: Procedures to reestablish the circulation to a diseased portion of the body.

Reverse transcriptase: An enzyme, encoded by an HIV gene, that causes a DNA copy of the HIV genes to be inserted into the chromosomes of the target cell; drugs directed against HIV target reverse transcriptase.

Reye's syndrome: A somewhat rare, noncontagious disease of the liver and central nervous system that strikes individuals under the age of eighteen.

Rh factor: Any one of several "factors," or elements present in the blood, according to one system of blood-type classification. The presence of one of these factors, the D factor, is an important cause of Rh incompatibility between sexual partners, which may lead to diseases of a child of the coupling.

Rh$_0$(D) immune globulin (human): A type of gamma globulin protein injected into Rh-negative mothers who may have an Rh-positive fetus in order to protect the fetus from an immune reaction.

Rheumatic fever: A complication of untreated streptococcal infections characterized by swollen joints, rashes, fever, and sometimes heart disorders; evidence of heart valve damage may emerge later in life.

Rheumatoid arthritis: A disease affecting the muscles, cartilage, and joints characterized by stiffness, pain, and swelling.

Rheumatology: The study and treatment of rheumatoid arthritis and related diseases.

Rhinitis: Inflammation of the mucous membrane that lines the nose, resulting from an allergic reaction or a common cold virus.

Rhinoplasty: Surgical alteration of the structure of

the nose, performed for both therapeutic and cosmetic reasons.

Rhinovirus: A microorganism causing respiratory illness; one of the most prevalent causes of the common cold.

Ribonucleic acid (RNA): The material contained in the core of many viruses that is responsible for directing the replication of the virus inside the host cell.

Ribosome: A cytoplasmic particle assembled from ribosomal RNA and ribosomal proteins that uses messenger RNA molecules as directions for synthesizing proteins.

Ribs: The bones that support the chest and define its outline.

Rickets: A deficiency in vitamin D, calcium, and phosphorus that results in soft bones.

Risk assessment: The process that establishes whether a health risk exists for a population exposed to a toxic substance.

Risk factors: The situations, circumstances, or conditions that increase the probability of the occurrence of disease or accident.

RNA. *See* Ribonucleic acid (RNA).

Root: That portion of the tooth which is below the crown and is embedded in a bony socket of the jaw.

Root canal treatment: Surgery to save a tooth whose pulp has become diseased or has died.

Root hair plexus: A network of sensory receptors located at hair roots that generates an impulse when hairs are moved.

Rosacea: The chronic inflammation of facial skin; also known as acne rosacea or adult acne.

Roseola: A common and contagious childhood disease characterized by high fever and a skin rash.

Roundworm: Intestinal parasites in humans which thrive in the gastrointestinal tract.

Rubella: A mild, contagious viral illness that is dangerous only when contracted by women during the early months of pregnancy, when it is likely to cause birth defects; also called German measles.

Rubeola. *See* Measles.

Ruffini endings: Sensory receptors that respond to heavy and continuous touch and pressure; also called type II cutaneous mechanoreceptors or the end organs of Ruffini.

Rule of nines: A system used to designate areas of the body, represented by various body parts. Used in determining the extent of a burn.

Salicylates: A group of drugs that includes aspirin and related compounds used to relieve pain, reduce inflammation, and lower fever.

Salivary glands: The glands that produce saliva.

Salmonella: Bacteria that cause a general infection of the gastrointestinal tract and lymphatic system when ingested.

Sample: The members of a population that are actually studied or whose characteristics are measured.

Sanatorium: An institution designed for the treatment of chronic illnesses, such as tuberculosis.

Sanitation: The application of measures designed to protect public health.

Saponification: A reaction in which a strong basic solution splits a molecule into a carboxylic acid unit and an alcohol unit.

Sarcoma: A malignant tumor originating in connective tissue, including bone and muscle.

Sarin: A nerve gas that can cause convulsions and death.

Scabies: Skin infestation by mites, causing a rash and severe itching.

Scarlet fever: An acute, contagious childhood disease caused by bacterial infection.

Schistosomiasis: A chronic illness caused by parasitic worms that live in the blood vessels around the liver and bladder.

Schizophrenia: A mental disturbance characterized by psychotic features during the active phase and deteriorated functioning in occupational, social, or self-care abilities.

Schwann cell: A supportive cell for neurons in the peripheral nervous system of vertebrate animals that wraps around and insulates axons using the protein myelin.

Sciatica: Painful inflammation of one of the sciatic nerves.

Scientific method: A method of scientific investigation of a problem through observation, the formation of a hypothesis (a possible explanation to a problem), experimentation, and the reevaluation of data.

Scintillation: The production of flashes emitted by luminescent substances when excited by high-energy radiation.

Sclera: The opaque portion of the outer layer of the eye; commonly referred to as the "white of the eye."

Scoliosis: Abnormal curvature of the spine, which is often progressive.

Screening: A strategy used by physicians and public health professionals to diagnose disease or the potential for disease at an early stage, when it may be treatable or preventable; may be a mandatory procedure for a specific population or a voluntary activity requested by individuals.

Scrotum: The genital skin sac that holds the testicles and related structures.

Scrub: To wash one's hands and forearms in preparation for donning gown and gloves, which protect the patient from the surgeon and staff and protect the surgeon and staff from the patient.

Scurvy: A disease caused by a prolonged inadequate intake of vitamin C.

Seasonal affective disorder (SAD): A depression that undergoes a seasonal fluctuation as a result of various factors, both unknown and known.

Sebaceous glands: Glands in the skin that usually open into the hair follicles.

Sebum: A semifluid, fatty substance secreted by the sebaceous glands into the hair follicles.

Secondary infection: A bacterial, viral, or other infection that results from or follows another disease.

Seizure: A sudden, violent, and involuntary contraction of a group of muscles; may be paroxysmal and episodic, also called a convulsion.

Semen: Fluid produced by a man's prostate gland, which makes up 95 percent of the fluid that is ejaculated.

Semipermeable membrane: A barrier that allows some materials to pass but blocks others.

Semisynthetic: Referring to natural products, such as antibiotics, that have been chemically modified to be more useful for a particular application.

Senile plaques: A hallmark lesion of Alzheimer's disease, composed of Aβ amyloid.

Senility: An outmoded term for dementia often applied to the elderly.

Sense organs: Specialized structures anatomically suited to a particular sense—the eyes for vision, the nose for smell (olfaction), the taste buds for taste, the ears for hearing and balance, and the skin for such cutaneous sensations as warmth, cold, light touch, deep pressure, and pain.

Sensitivity: The ability of a screening technique to identify correctly people who have a disease.

Sensorineural hearing loss: The loss of sensory or neural tissue of the auditory system as a result of disease, age, and acquired or congenital factors.

Sensory: Referring to perception by the senses: touch, sight, hearing, smell, and other senses such as hunger.

Sepsis: An infection in the circulating blood.

Septic pyelophlebitis: Inflammation of the veins that carry blood away from the kidneys.

Septic shock: A dangerous condition in which there is tissue damage and a dramatic drop in blood pressure as a result of septicemia.

Septicemia: Serious, systemic infection of the blood with pathogens that have spread from an infection in a part of the body, characteristically causing fever, chills, prostration, pain, headache, nausea, and/or diarrhea.

Septum: A membrane which serves as a wall of separation; in the heart, the interatrial septum divides the two atria, and the interventricular septum divides the two ventricles.

Serology: The branch of medicine specializing in the clear portion of the blood called the serum, often focused on analysis of the serum as a means of diagnosing disease.

Seronegative: The test result seen when blood does not contain the specific antibody or antigen being sought and the particular antigen-antibody reaction is not present.

Seropositive: The test result seen when blood contains the specific antibody or antigen being sought and the particular antigen-antibody reaction is present.

Serotonin: An abundant chemical nerve signal in the brain which is involved in modulating aggression.

Serotype: A subgroup member within a larger species; similar, but not identical, to other members of the species.

Serum: The fluid part of blood, without red blood cells and clotting factors.

Set point: A mechanism, thought to be formed by a series of feedback systems, for maintaining such characteristics as temperature and body weight.

Sex change surgery: A set of procedures designed to convert the secondary sexual characteristics of an anatomic male to a female or an anatomic female to a male.

Sex glands: The ovaries in the female and the testes in the male, which secrete hormones involved in reproduction.

Sex steroids: Steroid hormones such as androgens and estrogens that influence the activity of sexual organs and activity.

Sexual differentiation: The process by which an embryo becomes male or female under the influence of genetic and hormonal factors.

Sexually transmitted disease: Any disease that can be acquired through sexual contact or passed from a pregnant woman to her fetus, including syphilis, gonorrhea, chlamydia, herpes, and acquired immunodeficiency syndrome (AIDS).

Shigellosis: An intestinal infection caused by *Shigella* bacteria.

Shingles: A disease of the central nervous system characterized by painful red blisters that join together and rapidly rupture and become crusted.

Shock: A life-threatening condition in which the heart is unable to pump enough blood to the vital organs; symptoms include rapid and shallow breathing, clammy skin, low blood pressure, and dizziness.

Shock wave: A miniature explosion caused by intense local heating with a laser beam; used to fragment stones in the kidney or gallbladder.

Shunt: An opening established by surgery to maintain easy access to an internal area of the body for various purposes, such as application of medication or drainage of excess body fluids.

Sickle-cell disease: An inherited blood disorder in which abnormally high amounts of hemoglobin cause red blood cells to become sickle-shaped and block capillaries.

Side effect: A secondary and usually adverse effect (as of a drug); also known as an adverse effect or reaction.

SIDS. *See* Sudden infant death syndrome (SIDS).

Sigmoidoscopy: Endoscopy performed on the lower section of the colon.

Sign: Objective evidence of disease; a finding noted by the physician during the course of the physical examination.

Signal-averaged electrocardiogram: A sophisticated ECG that detects subtle and potentially lethal cardiac conduction defects.

Silicone: A plastic made primarily of silicon polymer.

Sinoatrial (S-A) node: A cluster of cells above the right atrium that emit electrical signals that initiate contractions of the heart; also called natural pacemaker cells.

Sinusitis: The inflammation of the lining of the nasal sinuses.

Skeletal muscle: A type of muscle that attaches to bone and causes movement of body parts; the only type that is under conscious, voluntary control.

Skeleton: The bony framework of the body.

Skin: The largest organ of the body, which is vital to the survival of an organism for its protection against dehydration and abrasion, regulation of body temperature, and sensory reception.

Sleep disorder: Any abnormal pattern of sleep which threatens normal function, including conditions that cause too much as well as too little sleep, and which may be both organic and nonorganic in origin.

Sleeping sickness: An infectious protozoan disease transmitted through the bite of a tsetse fly.

Slipped disk: A supportive ligament surrounding a vertebra in the neck or back that has broken through the spinal column and into the spinal canal; also called a herniated disk or a ruptured disk.

Small intestine: The region of gut between the stomach and the colon that comprises the duodenum, jejunum, and ileum; also called the small bowel.

Smallpox: A contagious, often-fatal viral infection that has been eradicated through vaccination.

Smegma: A pasty accumulation of shed skin cells and secretions of the sweat glands, which collects in the moist areas of the foreskin-covered base of the glans (in men) and around the clitoris and labia minora (in women).

Smell: A special sense in which chemicals interact with receptor sites in specialized structures of the nasal cavity and the resulting nerve impulses are classified as certain kinds of odor.

Smooth muscle: Muscle that, when viewed under a microscope, does not have striations, which are stripes seen in skeletal muscle cells; smooth muscle contracts involuntarily and is related to the functioning of the stomach, intestines, and urinary bladder; involved in the movement of food through the digestive tract.

Sodium pentothal: A fast-acting anesthetic that is injected into the vein; first developed for military hospitals during World War II.

Soft palate: A structure of mucous membrane, muscle fibers, and mucous glands suspended from the posterior border of the hard palate in the mouth.

Soma: The body of a cell, where the cell's genetic material and other vital structures are located.

Sonography: The use of sound waves deflected from internal body organs to find growing masses (including fetuses) and abnormal lesions; also called ultrasound.

Sore throat: Discomfort and/or pain experienced in the throat, which sometimes indicates the presence of a more serious disorder.

Spastic: Characterized by uncontrollable spasms.

Spasticity: A rigidity or resistance to passive limb movement, usually occuring in limbs that are weak, respond in an impaired way to voluntary control, and whose weakness is thought to be due to observed lesions in the upper motor neurons.

Specialist: Any physician who practices in a specialty other than the generalist areas of family practice, general internal medicine, general pediatrics, or obstetrics and gynecology.

Specific gravity: The density of a solution relative to that of water; abnormal values can be indicative of elevated sugar or protein levels in urine.

Specificity: The ability of a screening technique to identify correctly people who do not have a disease.

Spectacles: A pair of ophthalmic lenses held together with a frame or mounting; also called glasses.

Spectrum of activity: The range of microbial species that can be inhibited by an antibiotic; broad-spectrum antibiotics can control more than one kind of infection, but narrow-spectrum antibiotics avoid unintentional damage to the normal microbiota.

Speech disorder: A dysfunction in the brain-coordinated use of speech organs, such as problems with language, vocal quality, articulation, fluency, and dementia.

Sperm: The male gamete; the mature sperm has an oval head that contains the male's chromosomes and a long tail that allows it to swim in fluid.

Spermicide: A chemical that kills sperm after they are ejaculated.

Sphincter: A ringlike muscle that acts as a one-way valve to control the flow of fluids and waste.

Sphincterectomy: Surgical removal of the sphincter.

Sphygmomanometer: A device that uses a column of mercury to measure blood pressure.

Spina bifida: A genetic abnormality in which the spine has failed to fuse, sometimes exposing the spinal cord and nerves.

Spinal anesthesia: The injection of an anesthetic at the base of the spine to produce loss of feeling in the lower part of the body and legs; also known as a subarachnoid block.

Spinal cord: A cord in the trunk containing nerve cells that transmit impulses to and from the brain.

Spinal tap. *See* Lumbar puncture.

Spine: The combined spinal cord and the vertebral (spinal) column.

Spinous processes: Bony projections from vertebrae (horizontally in the neck, tilting downward in the thoracic area, and horizontally in the lumbar area) that are connected to one another by the interspinous and supraspinous ligaments and that control extremes of trunk motion.

Spleen: A lymphatic organ, found between the stomach and the diaphragm, that destroys old blood cells and filters foreign material from the blood.

Splenectomy: Surgical removal of the spleen.

Spondylitis: Inflammation and stiffening of the joints between the vertebrae of the spine.

Spondylosis: A condition characterized by restriction of movement of the vertebral bones; occurs naturally as a child grows.

Sports medicine: A medical subspecialty concerned with the care and prevention of athletic injuries, primarily those related to the musculoskeletal system.

Sprain: An injury in which ligaments are stretched or torn.

Squamous cell carcinoma: A form of skin cancer starting as a small, painless lump and often resembling a wart; common in fair-skinned individuals, especially in later life.

Staging: A numerical classification system used by physicians to describe how far a cancerous growth has advanced.

Staining: The artificial coloring of tissue sections and cells to facilitate their microscopic study.

Stapedectomy: The surgical removal of all or part of the stapes or innermost ossicle of the ear.

Stapes: The ossicle that makes contact with the cochlea.

Staphylococcal infections: A variety of infections caused by staphylococcus bacteria, including boils, abscesses, pneumonia, bone infections, and toxic shock syndrome.

Stem cell: A master cell from which other blood cells develop; these cells are primarily located in the bone marrow.

Stenosis: The narrowing of heart valves or blood vessels.

Stereotaxic computed tomography: A method of imaging using a series of X rays that are compiled by a computer to give a three-dimensional image of internal structures.

Sterile field: An area in which only sterile supplies may be placed and which only those wearing sterile gowns and gloves may touch; includes the surgical wound, the surgical drapes, and the extra tables.

Sterilization: Any procedure that makes it impossible for a person to reproduce, whether chemical or surgical.

Sternum: The breastbone, which is found in the midline of the chest cavity and lying over the heart.

Steroids: A group of drugs that work like hormones. The two main types of steroids are the corticosteroids (adrenal in nature) and the anabolic steroids (similar to male reproductive hormones).

Sterol: A steroid that has long side chains of carbone compounds attached to it and contains at least one hydroxyl group; cholesterol is one type of sterol.

Stethoscope: An instrument for listening to sounds in the body, such as the heartbeat.

Stillbirth: A condition in which a fetus has died within the uterus and is born after the twenty-eighth week of pregnancy.

Stimulus: Anything capable of producing a response.

Stoma: A surgically created passage between the intestines and the outer skin.

Stone: A deposit of cholesterol and calcium that may form in the gallbladder, kidneys, ureters, bladder, or urethra; also called a calculus (*pl.* calculi).

Stool: The waste matter of digestion excreted from the body through the anus or a stoma.

Strain: An injury in which muscles or tendons are stretched or torn.

Stratum corneum: The outermost layer of the epidermis; its cells are normally dead, hard, and constantly removed by normal bathing.

Strep throat: A contagious bacterial infection by streptococcal bacteria that causes inflammation of the pharynx.

Streptococcal infections: A variety of infections caused by streptococcus bacteria, including tonsillitis, strep throat, pneumonia, endocarditis, urinary tract infections, and otitis media.

Stress: Physical, environmental, or psychological strain experienced by an individual that requires adjustment.

Stress reduction: A set of procedures with the goal of decreasing bodily and mental tension by increasing rest and coping skills.

Stricture: The narrowing of a passageway.

Stroke: Permanent damage to part of the brain as a result of impaired blood flow.

Stroke volume: The blood volume leaving either the right or the left side of the heart with each beat; each side usually ejects the same volume per beat.

Stuttering: The repetition of sounds or syllables or the inability to formulate words in a spoken sentence.

Subclinical: Referring to a medical problem in which the patient has no symptoms of disease or symptoms so slight that the disease is not diagnosed.

Subcutaneous: Under the skin.

Subluxation: An incomplete or partial dislocation of a joint, which creates abnormal neurological and physiological symptoms in neuromusculoskeletal structures and/or other body systems via interference with nerve impulse transmission.

Substance abuse: Ongoing, chronic ingestion of a substance (usually drugs such as alcohol, nicotine, or narcotics), which threatens health and may cause death if not arrested.

Substantia nigra: A clump of cells located near the base of the cerebral hemispheres that secrete the neurotransmitter dopamine.

Substrates: Reactants that enzymes convert into products; every enzyme is specific for one specific substrate.

Succussion: Violent shaking at each stage of dilution in the preparation of a homeopathic remedy.

Sudden infant death syndrome (SIDS): The abrupt death of any infant or young child in which postmortem examination fails to demonstrate an adequate cause.

Suggestion: A communication that evokes a nonvoluntary response reflecting the ideational content of the communication.

Superinfection: An infection caused by destruction of the normal microbiota by antibiotic therapy, which allows for proliferation of a pathogen other than the one targeted by the antibiotic.

Superior: Above another part or closer to the head; the ankle bones are superior to the bones of the feet.

Supine: Lying face-upward.

Suppressor T cell: A type of T lymphocyte that is believed to modulate the immune response.

Suprachiasmatic nuclei: Two clusters of nerve cell bodies located in the hypothalamus of the forebrain; these structures display circadian rhythms and seem to be the source of rhythmicity for many of the body's other cycles.

Surgery: The treatment of diseases or disorders by physical intervention, which usually involves cutting into the skin and other tissues.

Surgical pathology: The branch of pathology that deals with the interpretation of biopsies.

Surgical team: The people working together in the operating room during a surgical procedure, including the surgeon, first assistant, surgical technologist, anesthesiologist and/or anesthetist, and circulator.

Surgical technologist: A surgical team member whose primary functions are to prepare surgical instruments and hand them to the surgeon as needed and to prevent infection by maintaining a sterile field in the operating room.

Suspiciousness: A range of symptoms from increasing distrust of others to paranoid delusions of conspiracies.

Suture: A thread used to unite parts of the body.

Sympathectomy: The surgical process of removing or destroying nerves that may be afflicted by frostbite or other injury.

Sympathetic nervous system: The division of the autonomic nervous system concerned primarily with preparing the individual to expend energy.

Symptom: Subjective evidence of disease, provided by the patient.

Symptomatic treatment: A treatment focusing on aborting disease, illness, or their symptoms once they have occurred.

Synapse: An area of close contact between nerve cells that is the functional junction where one cell communicates with another.

Syndactyly: A congenital anomaly characterized by the fusion of the fingers or toes.

Syndrome: A collection of complaints (symptoms) and signs (abnormal findings on clinical examination) which do not match any specific disease.

Synergistic effects: The combined effects of drugs interacting with one another, such that the effects of the drugs together have a compounded effect, greater than that of any one alone.

Synovial: Referring to the lubricating fluid in the joints or the membrane surrounding the joints.

Synovium: The cellular lining of a joint, having a blood supply and a nerve supply; the synovium secretes fluid for lubrication and protects against injury and injurious agents.

Syphilis: A serious sexually transmitted disease that can be fatal if left untreated.

Systems and organs: Groups of tissues and organs dedicated to particular functions, all of which must work together to perform efficiently.

Systole: The period of contraction of the heart when blood moves out of the heart chambers and into the arteries.

Systolic blood pressure: The pressure of the blood within the artery while the heart is contracting.

T lymphocyte: A type of immune cell which kills host cells infected by bacteria or viruses or produces a chemical compound which mediates the host cells' destruction.

Tachycardia: Rapid beating of the heart.

Tai Chi Chuan: A Chinese physical and mental discipline which consists of set routines of deliberate, slow movements designed to increase energy "flow."

Tapeworm: An intestinal parasite in humans transmitted through eating improperly cooked or raw pork, beef, or fish or by being bitten by a larva-carrying flea.

Target heart rate range: A heart rate range that is to be maintained during exercise training.

Tarsus: The ankle.

Taste: A special sense in which chemicals interact with receptor sites in specialized structures of the tongue, and the resulting nerve impulses are classified as certain kinds of taste.

Taste bud: A special sensing structure for taste found on taste-responsive papillae; taste buds are made of three cell types—gustatory or taste cells, supporting cells, and basal cells.

Taste cell: The cellular compartment of a taste bud that contains chemoreceptors; taste hairs, one type of chemoreceptor, are found at the taste pore (or entry point) of a taste cell.

Teeth: Structures that aid animals in processing food prior to swallowing, bringing food into the mouth and grinding; may also be used for defense, the killing of prey, and displays of either hostility or pleasure.

Tendinitis: Inflammation of a tendon or a tough band of tissue that connects muscle to the bone.

Tendon: A structure of tough connective tissue that attaches a muscle to a bone.

Tensile strength: The greatest stress that can be placed on a tissue without tearing it apart; it is relative to the strength of a tissue.

Teratogens: Substances that induce congenital malformations when embryonic tissues and organs are exposed to them.

Teratology: The study of congenital malformations.

Testes (*sing.* testis): The male reproductive organs, a pair of gonads that are suspended in the scrotum and produce sperm; also known as the testicles.

Testicular torsion: Twisting of the testicle in the scrotum, with compromise of the blood supply to the testicle, as a result of spermatic cord rotation.

Testosterone: The male sex hormone that gives rise to male fertility and secondary sexual characteristics, such as body hair and musculature.

Tetanus: An often fatal nervous system disease characterized by painful, sustained, and violent muscle spasms; it can be prevented through vaccination.

Thalassemia: An inherited form of anemia in which red blood cells contain less hemoglobin than normal.

Thalidomide: A sedative and sleep-inducing drug that was found to produce phocomelia (a birth defect in which hands or feet are attached to the body by short, flipperlike stumps) in developing fetuses.

Thanatology: The study and investigation of life-threatening actions, terminal illness, suicide, homicide, death, dying, grief, and bereavement.

Therapeutics: The use of chemicals in the diagnosis, prevention, or treatment of disease.

Thermogenesis: The combustion of fuels to provide energy in excess of that required to perform biological work in order to maintain body temperature.

Thermoregulatory set point: The ultimate neural control that maintains the human internal body temperature at 37 degrees Celsius and can either raise or lower it as a defense mechanism against disease.

Thigh: The upper segment of the leg, from the hip joint to the knee.

Thoracic: Pertaining to the chest.

Thoracic duct: The largest lymphatic vessel, which collects lymphatic fluid and returns it to the bloodstream at the left subclavian vein in the region of the neck.

Thorax: The part of the trunk above the diaphragm, containing the ribs; also called the chest.

Thrombocytes: Small, irregularly shaped cells in the blood that participate in blood clotting; also called platelets.

Thromboembolism: The blockage of a blood vessel by a fragment that has broken off from a thrombus in another blood vessel.

Thrombolytic drugs: A group of drugs that dissolve blood clots by increasing the level of plasmin in the blood.

Thrombosis: The act of complete clotting of an artery or vein, through which no blood can then flow.

Thrombus: A blood clot that has formed inside an intact blood vessel; a thrombus can be life-threat-

ening if it occludes a vessel which supplies the heart or brain.

Thymus: The lymphatic gland in which T lymphocytes mature; located in humans just below the thyroid.

Thyroid gland: A gland found in the neck that secretes the hormones responsible for the synthesis and breakdown of proteins and the metabolism of carbohydrates.

Thyroidectomy: Surgical removal of the thyroid gland.

Thyroxine: The chief hormone of the thyroid gland, an iodine-containing derivative of the amino acid tyrosine.

TIA: *See* Transient ischemic attack.

Tibia: The larger of the two bones in the lower leg, on the medial side.

Tincture: A homeopathic remedy in liquid form, normally with alcohol and water as a solvent; the most concentrated form is called the mother tincture, from which all dilutions are made.

Tissue: A specialized region of cells that forms organs within the body; the four principal types are epithelial, connective, nervous, and muscular; tissues have specific functions.

Tissue plasminogen activator (TPA or tPA): A substance produced by the body to prevent abnormal blood clots by stimulating the formation of plasmin from plasminogen; can also be administered to dissolve blood clots.

Tissue typing: The process of identifying a person's transplantation antigens.

Tolerance: With repeated substance abuse, the need for increasing amounts of a substance to achieve the same effect.

Tomography: All types of body-section imaging techniques; that is, a visual representation restricted to a specified section or "cut" of tissue within an organ.

Tonometer: An instrument used to measure the eye's intraocular pressure, thus checking for the presence of glaucoma.

Tonsillectomy: Surgical removal of one or both tonsils.

Tonsillitis: Infection and inflammation of the tonsils; if severe or chronic, it may require removal of the tonsils.

Tonsils: Masses of lymphatic tissue lying on either side of the entrance to the throat near the back of the tongue.

Tooth decay: The common term for dental caries.

Tooth extraction: The surgical removal of a tooth because it is damaged by decay, disease, or trauma; threatening the health of other teeth; or near the site of significant disease.

Tooth pulp: The tissue at the center of teeth, surrounded by dentin.

Toothache: Pain in the teeth or gums ranging from a dull, throbbing sensation to intense, sharp pains.

Tophus (*pl.* tophi): A lump in the cartilage or joints of chronic gout suffers, caused by crystals of uric acid.

Tort: A wrongful act for which civil courts, rather than criminal courts, are empowered to render justice.

Totipotence: The capacity for cells of a given tissue type to regenerate and replace killed or damaged cells within a given body region.

Touch: A special sense in which nerve endings and specialized structures in the skin and other tissues send the brain data about the organism's environment, both internal and external.

Toxemia: The presence of toxins in the blood produced by bacteria, which may be ingested or caused by an infection in the body; also called blood poisoning or septicemia.

Toxicokinetics: The study of the time course of chemical absorption, distribution, metabolism, and elimination of toxic chemicals in the body; when the chemicals considered are therapeutic drugs, the correct term is "pharmacokinetics."

Toxicology: The science devoted to the study of poisons.

Toxin: A poisonous substance that is a product of the chemical processes of a living organism.

Toxoid: A toxin that has been chemically treated to eliminate its toxic properties but that retains the same antigens as the original.

Toxoplasmosis: An infection caused by parasitic microorganisms that invade tissues and that may cause damage to the central nervous system, especially in fetuses.

TPA: *See* Tissue plasminogen activator.

Trace elements: Elements needed in the diet at levels of less than 100 milligrams per day.

Trace evidence: Minute, often microscopic, signs or indications of an event or a presence.

Tracer: A radioactive substance introduced into the body, the progress of which may be followed by means of an external radioactive detector; it must not affect the process that it is used to measure.

Trachea: The tube that leads from the throat to the lungs; commonly called the windpipe.

Tracheostomy: Surgical creation of an opening in the trachea.

Trachoma: A contagious eye infection, leading to blindness, which affects millions of people in developing countries.

Tract: A collection of nerve fibers (axons) in the brain or spinal cord that all have the same place of origin and the same place of termination.

Transcription: The process by which the information stored in DNA is copied into the structure of RNA for transport to the cytoplasm.

Transducer (probe): A device designed to transfer ultrasound waves into the body noninvasively, receive the returning echoes, and transform those echoes into electrical voltages.

Transference: The unconscious tendency of a person to re-create preexisting nonfunctional relationship patterns with others; psychoanalytic treatment depends on the development of transference between client and analyst.

Transfusion: Injection directly into the bloodstream of a large amount of blood or blood components, usually to correct loss of blood as a result of injury or during surgery.

Transient ischemic attack (TIA): A brief loss of blood to the brain, accompanied by temporary impairment of vision and numbness.

Transitional cell carcinoma: Cancer arising from the lining of the urine collection system of the kidneys, ureters, and bladder.

Translation: The process by which the copied information in RNA is utilized in the production of a protein.

Transplantation: The movement of one part of the body (such as an organ) or one area of tissue to another, either within the same individual or from one individual to another.

Transsexuals: Individuals who genuinely believe that they exist in the body of the wrong sex, despite the fact that they are anatomically normal.

Transverse processes: Projections from the sides of vertebrae, to which are attached muscles and ligaments, that assist in motor function by enhancing leverage and limiting extremes of motion.

Trauma: Physical injury to bodily tissue.

Treatment: Any specific procedure used for the cure or improvement of a disease or pathological condition.

Trephination: The opening of a hole in the skull.

Trephine: A specialized surgical instrument which is used to cut a perfectly vertical incision in bone or corneal tissue.

Triage: A process in which patient needs are evaluated and prioritized by a health care team and preliminary treatment plans are made.

Tricyclics: Medications used to relieve the symptoms of depression.

Trimester: An arbitrary division of a human pregnancy into three-month divisions based on development changes in the fetus over time.

Tropical medicine: The area of medicine concerned particularly with diseases, often arthropod-borne (such as malaria, yellow fever, schistosomiasis), that thrive in tropical latitudes.

Trunk: The central part of the body, to which the extremities are attached.

Tubal ligation: A procedure for rendering a woman sterile by cutting, constricting, or otherwise blocking the Fallopian tubes so that sperm cannot reach the ovum.

Tuberculosis: A chronic, highly infectious lung disease.

Tubular reabsorption: The process of returning important solutes that were filtered out of the blood back into the blood; these important solutes include glucose, amino acids, vitamins, and most ions.

Tubular secretion: The process of tubular reabsorption in reverse; important solutes moved from the filtrate to the urine include hydrogen and potassium ions, organic acids, ammonia, and creatine.

Tumor: An abnormal mass of tissue which may be malignant (growing larger) or benign (not spreading).

Turgor: Fullness and firmness; the quality of normal skin in a healthy young person.

Twins: The presence of two fetuses in the womb.

Tympanic membrane: The eardrum, which separates the external ear canal from the middle ear and ossicles and which transmits sound vibration to the ossicles.

Tympanoplasty: A surgical procedure to repair the tympanic membrane.

Typhoid fever and typhus: Acute infectious diseases caused by bacteria or rickettsiae.

Ulcer: A lesion that destroys tissue.

Ulcerative colitis: An inflammatory disease that causes ulcers in the large intestine.

Ulna: The larger of the two forearm bones, forming the principal part of the elbow joint with the humerus.

Ulnar: Toward the edge of the forearm and hand containing the ulna and little finger.

Ultrasonic: Referring to any frequency of sound that is higher than the audible range—that is, higher than 20,000 cycles per second (20 kilohertz).

Ultrasonography: An imaging technique that employs sound waves to form an image, still or moving, of internal organs.

Ultraviolet radiation: Radiation that is potentially damaging to the skin; it is not visible to humans.

Umbilicus: The cord that contains the blood vessels connecting the fetus to the placenta.

Unconsciousness: A state in which an individual is unaware of either surroundings or self and lacks response to stimuli; includes sleep, fainting, and coma.

Upper arm: The region from the shoulder joint to the elbow joint; also called the brachium.

Upper extremities: The arms (upper arms, forearms, and hands), which are attached to the shoulder blade at the shoulder joint and which consist of muscles, bones, blood vessels, lymph vessels, nerves, skin, and fingernails.

Urea: A waste product of protein metabolism, which represents the form in which nitrogen is eliminated from the body.

Uremia: The presence of excessive amounts of urea and other nitrogenous waste products in the blood.

Ureter: Either of the two tubes that carry urine from the kidneys to the bladder.

Ureterolithotomy: The surgical removal of a stone in the ureter.

Urethra: The tube that drains from the bladder to outside the body; in the male, the urethra passes through the penis and carries sperm during ejaculation, while in the female, the urethra opens in front of the vagina but does not have a reproductive function.

Urethritis: Inflammation or infection of the urethra as a result of bacterial infection.

Urethroplasty: Surgical repair of the urethra.

-uria: A suffix meaning the presence of a substance in urine; for example, hematuria refers to blood in the urine.

Urinalysis: Laboratory analysis of urine to determine presence, absence, or quantity of compounds that may point to disease.

2496 • Glossary

Urinary bladder: A stretchable, muscular sac that functions to store urine.

Urinary system: A system, composed of the kidneys, ureters, urinary bladder, and urethra, that removes body waste, maintains the proper amount of body water, and regulates the acid-base balance of the blood.

Urinary tract infections: Infections of the bladder, kidneys, the urethra, and the ureters (which connect the bladder to the kidneys); infection may be limited to one area of these organs or spread throughout the urinary tract.

Urine: Fluid collected in the kidneys that contains metabolic wastes, including urea and salts.

Urolithiasis: The formation of stones in the urinary tract.

Urology: The branch of medicine specializing in the urinary tracts of both sexes, and the genitourinary tract of the male.

Uterus: The organ that supports the embryo during its development.

Uvea: The iris and ciliary body of the eye.

Uveitis: Inflammation of the uvea of the eye.

Vaccine: Any substance used for preventive inoculation to build immunity.

Vaccinia: A virus that causes a poxlike illness in cattle (cowpox); it serves as a smallpox vaccine in humans because of its similarity to the smallpox virus.

Vagina: The tube-shaped cavity of the female into which the male's penis is inserted during intercourse and through which a baby is delivered; the diaphragm, cervical cap, vaginal sponge, or spermicide can be inserted into the vagina as contraceptives.

Vagotomy: Surgical incision into the vagus nerve.

Vagus nerve: The tenth cranial nerve, which carries taste messages from the limited number of taste buds located in obscure sites such as the palate, epiglottis, uvula, and other structures at the entrance of the esophagus; also sends important information from the thoracic and abdominal viscera to the brain.

Valgus: A musculoskeletal deformity in which a limb is twisted outward from the body.

Validity, selective: A preliminary indication of a screening technique's capability to identify persons with preclinical disease as test-positive and those without preclinical disease as test-negative.

Vallate papillae: The seven to ten papillae mounds arranged in a V shape that can be seen when the tongue is fully extended; these taste sensors lack taste specificity.

Valves: Structures that close periodically to allow the passage of blood, such as those that connect heart chambers to each other and to the great arteries.

Variable: Any quantity which varies, such as height or cholesterol level.

Varicocele: An enlarged vein surrounding the testicle as a result of incompetent venous valves; most commonly found surrounding the left testicle.

Varicosis: The distension of superficial veins, often in the legs; also known as varicose veins.

Varus: A musculoskeletal deformity in which a limb is twisted toward the body.

Vas deferens: The duct that carries the male seminal fluid.

Vascular: Relating to or containing blood vessels.

Vascular medicine: The diagnosis and management of diseases of the arteries, veins, and lymphatic system, exclusive of the heart and lungs.

Vascular system: The pipeline through which every cell of the body receives oxygen, vitamins, hormones, and the metabolic fuels necessary to sustain life.

Vascularized transplant: Transplanted tissue or organs that must have blood vessels reattached in the recipient in order to function (such as a kidney); corneal or bone marrow transplants are examples of nonvascularized transplants.

Vasculature: All the blood vessels, including the arteries (blood vessels carrying oxygenated blood away from the heart), the capillaries (the smallest blood vessels, where fluid and nutrients are exchanged between arteries and veins), and the veins (blood vessels that return deoxygenated blood to the heart).

Vasectomy: A surgical procedure to render a male sterile by cutting the two vas deferens, the ducts carrying sperm from the testes to the seminal vesicles.

Vasoconstriction: A decrease in the diameter of vessels transporting blood throughout the body, reducing blood flow and oxygen transport.

Vasodilation: An increase in the diameter of arteries, which decreases the amount of work required for the heart to move blood.

Vector: An organism, usually an insect or other arthropod, which transmits a disease from one host to another; the vector may itself be a host in which the pathogen multiplies, or it may merely transmit the pathogen mechanically.

Veins: Blood vessels that carry blood from the cells back to the heart.

Venereal disease: *See* Sexually transmitted disease.

Venipuncture: A method of obtaining blood from a vein using a tourniquet, needle, and syringe.

Venous insufficiency: An abnormality characterized by decreased blood return from the legs to the trunk that is caused by inefficient valves in the veins.

Venous thrombosis: The presence of blood clots in the veins, usually in the legs or arms.

Ventricles: The two lower chambers of the heart; the right ventricle pumps blood to the lungs, and the left ventricle pumps oxygenated blood to the body.

Ventriculoperitoneal: Referring to a type of shunt used to carry cerebrospinal fluid from the brain to the abdominal cavity.

Vertebra: A bony structure in the back with a central spinal canal surrounded by an arch; the back part of the arch (the lamina) and the front part of the arch (the pedicle) are joined together by muscles, ligaments, and cartilage for motion, stability, and posture.

Vestibular: Referring to the parts of the ear concerned with balance.

Veterinary medicine: The health care and medical treatment of animals, both domestic (pets and livestock) and wild (native and exotic species); includes preventive health care, sanitary and environmental management, and the treatment of diseases and injuries.

Villi: Fingerlike projections on the intestinal lining that absorb essential body nutrients after enzymes break down chyme.

Virus: A subcellular particle that enters cells and causes cellular damage; it uses cellular mechanisms to reproduce itself.

Visual acuity: Clarity or clearness in vision.

Vital organs: Organs of the body essential to life, usually considered to be the brain, the heart, the lungs, the liver, and sometimes the kidneys.

Vitamins: Organic compounds, essential for life but required in very minute quantities, that participate in biochemical reactions and help to release energy from the three classes of nutrients.

Vitiligo: A skin disorder in which patches of skin are lacking pigment, resulting in white areas contrasting with darker areas.

Vitrectomy: Surgical removal of the vitreous humor.

Vitreous humor: The clear, jelly-like substance that fills the eyeball; also called the aqueous humor.

Voltage: Energy per unit charge; typical biological voltages range from hundredths to tenths of a volt.

Voluntary euthanasia: A patient's consent to a decision that results in the shortening of his or her life.

Vomiting: The regurgitation of the contents of the stomach.

Von Neumann machine: A cellular automaton or machine which can think and self-replicate; based on the attempts of the physicist John von Neumann to duplicate the human nervous system in computers.

Wart: A generally benign tumor of the skin and mucous membranes caused by a Papillomavirus.

Wasting: Severe weight loss characterized by the loss of both muscle tissue and body-fat deposits.

Wavelength: A property used to measure colors in the spectrum of light from infrared to ultraviolet; usually expressed in units of microns (1 micron is equal to one-millionth of a meter).

Wedge argument: A logically contrived argument supporting a morally acceptable action which subsequently leads to other actions that are considered morally unacceptable.

Whiplash: Injury to the ligaments, joints, and soft tissues of the neck region of the spine due to a sudden, violent jerking motion.

White blood cells: Colorless, large blood cells that work together to combat infections.

Whole blood: Blood from which none of the elements has been removed.

Withdrawal: A physical and mental condition following decreased intake of an abusable substance, with symptoms ranging from anxiety to convulsions.

Wolffian ducts: The pair of tubes in the early embryo that will develop into the internal male organs (the epididymis, the vas deferens, and the seminal vesicles).

Work: A form of energy transfer; it may take the form of mechanical work (force multiplied by distance), electrical work (moving an electric charge against a voltage gradient), or chemical work (chemical synthesis or maintaining a difference in concentration across a membrane).

World Health Organization: A specialized agency of the United Nations that fights illness and disease all over the globe.

2498 • Glossary

Worms: Invertebrates, usually flatworms or round-worms, that act as human parasites.

Wounds: Injuries classified as open or closed depending on whether the skin is broken; types of open wounds include abrasions, lacerations, avulsions, punctures, and incisions.

X and Y chromosomes: The chromosomes that determine genetic sex; males carry an XY pair and females carry an XX pair.

X radiology: The use of ionizing radiation of short wavelength to detect abnormalities in primarily dense portions of the body.

X-ray tube: A high-voltage electronic device used to produce X rays; X-ray tubes are used in X-ray machines, fluoroscopes, and CT scanners.

X rays: Penetrating radiation produced by means of a high-voltage machine; useful for both the diagnosis and the treatment of cancerous tissue.

Xanthomatosis: A condition in which fatty deposits appear anywhere in the body, including various areas of the skin, internal organs, eyes, and tendons.

Xenobiotics: Drugs and chemical compounds foreign to the body; the terms "xenobiotic," "toxin," "drug," and "chemical" are used interchangeably when discussing toxicology, since all substances are poisonous at some concentration.

Xenotransplantation: The transplantation of tissue or organs between different species (such as baboon to human).

Yang: The Chinese concept of the positive, male element of the universe.

Yeast infection: Candidiasis, an infection caused by the fungus *Candida albicans*; commonly infects the vaginal area and causes intense itching.

Yellow fever: An acute viral infection of the liver, kidneys, and heart muscle transmitted by *Aedes aegypti* mosquitoes.

Yin: The Chinese concept of the negative, female element of the universe.

Yoga: A mental discipline, originating in India, designed to master consciousness, to offer spiritual insight, and to induce tranquillity.

Zeugmatography: A name applied to MRI characterizing the close relationship of nuclear magnetic forces and electromagnetic waves (from the Greek *zeugma*, meaning "to yoke together").

Zidovudine: A drug, formerly known as azidothymidine (AZT), used to treat HIV infection; it interferes with the functioning of the virus' reverse transcriptase enzyme.

Zona pellucida: A translucent layer surrounding the mammalian egg; it promotes fertilization by causing the acrosome reaction in the sperm and also prevents polyspermy.

Zoonoses: Diseases communicable between animals and humans.

Zygoma: The cheekbone.

Zygote: A fertilized ovum before multicelluar development begins.

MEDICAL JOURNALS

AACN Clinical Issues: Advanced Practice in Acute and Critical Care

AARC Times (American Association for Respiratory Care)

Academic Medicine

Academic Psychiatry

Acta Diabetologica

Acta Medica Scandinavica (to 1988). Continued by *Journal of Internal Medicine*

Acta Medica Scandinavica. Supplement (to 1988)

Acta Neurologica Scandinavica

Acta Neurologica Scandinavica. Supplement

Acta Obstetrica et Gynecologica. Supplement (to 1997)

Acta Obstetrica et Gynecologica Scandinavica

Acta Ophthalmologica

Acta Ophthalmologica. Supplement

Acta Paediatrica

Acta Paediatrica. Supplement

Acta Paediatrica Scandinavica (to 1991). Continued by *Acta Paediatrica*

Acta Paediatrica Scandinavica. Supplement (to 1992)

Acta Psychiatrica Scandinavica

Acta Psychiatrica Scandinavica. Supplement

Addiction

Addictive Behaviors

Advances in Mind-Body Medicine

Advances in Nursing Science

Age and Aging

Aggression and Violent Behavior

AIDS

AIDS Care

AIDS Research and Human Retroviruses

Alcohol

Alcohol Health and Research World

Alcoholism Treatment Quarterly

Alternative Health Practitioner

Alternative Therapies in Health and Medicine

Ambulatory Surgery

American Annals of the Deaf

American Family Physician

American Fitness

American Heart Journal

American Industrial Hygiene Association Journal

American Journal of Audiology

American Journal of Cardiology

American Journal of Clinical Nutrition

American Journal of Clinical Pathology

American Journal of Diseases of Children (to 1993). Continued by *Archives of Pediatrics and Adolescent Medicine*

American Journal of Electroneurodiagnostic Technology

American Journal of Epidemiology

American Journal of Family Therapy

American Journal of Gastroenterology

American Journal of Health Promotion: AJHP

American Journal of Health Studies

American Journal of Hematology

American Journal of Human Genetics

American Journal of Hypertension

American Journal of Infection Control

American Journal of Medicine

American Journal of Nursing

American Journal of Obstetrics and Gynecology

American Journal of Occupational Therapy

American Journal of Ophthalmology

American Journal of Orthopsychiatry (to 1990)

American Journal of Pathology

American Journal of Physical Medicine (to 1987). Continued by *American Journal of Physical Medicine and Rehabilitation*

American Journal of Physical Medicine and Rehabilitation

American Journal of Physiology-Cell Physiology

American Journal of Physiology-Endocrinology and Metabolism

American Journal of Physiology-Gastrointestinal and Liver Physiology

American Journal of Physiology-Heart and Circulatory Physiology

American Journal of Physiology-Lung Cellular and Molecular Physiology

American Journal of Physiology-Regulatory, Integrative, and Comparative Physiology

American Journal of Physiology-Renal Physiology

American Journal of Preventive Medicine

American Journal of Psychiatry, The

American Journal of Psychoanalysis, The

American Journal of Psychology

American Journal of Psychotherapy

American Journal of Public Health
American Journal of Respiratory and Critical Care
    Medicine
American Journal of Roentgenology
American Journal of Science
American Journal of Speech-Language Pathology
American Journal of Sports Medicine
American Journal of Surgery, The
American Journal on Addictions
American Laboratory
American Medical News
American Nursing Research
American Review of Respiratory Disease (to 1993).
    Continued by American Journal of Respiratory
    and Critical Care Medicine
American Surgeon
Analytical Biochemistry
Anatomy and Embryology
Annals of Biomedical Engineering
Annals of Clinical Psychiatry
Annals of Diagnostic Paediatric Pathology
Annals of Emergency Medicine
Annals of Epidemiology
Annals of Hematology
Annals of Human Genetics
Annals of Internal Medicine
Annals of Nutrition and Metabolism
Annals of Occupational Hygiene, The
Annals of Otology, Rhinology, and Laryngology
Annals of Science
Annals of Surgery
Annals of Thoracic Surgery, The
Annual Review of Biochemistry
Annual Review of Biomedical Engineering
Annual Review of Genetics
Annual Review of Immunology
Annual Review of Medicine
Annual Review of Microbiology
Annual Review of Neuroscience
Annual Review of Nutrition
Annual Review of Pharmacology and Toxicology
Annual Review of Psychology
Annual Review of Public Health
ANS, Advances in Nursing Science
Antimicrobial Agents and Chemotherapy
Aphasiology
Apoptosis
Appetite
Applied and Environmental Microbiology
Applied Microbiology and Biotechnology

Applied Nursing Research
Applied Psychophysiology and Biofeedback
Applied Radiation and Isotopes
Applied Radiology
Archives of Biochemistry and Biophysics
Archives of Clinical Neuropsychology
Archives of Disease in Childhood
Archives of Environmental Contamination and
    Toxicology
Archives of Environmental Health
Archives of General Psychiatry
Archives of Gerontology and Geriatrics
Archives of Gynecology and Obstetrics
Archives of Internal Medicine
Archives of Medical Research
Archives of Microbiology
Archives of Neurology
Archives of Ophthalmology
Archives of Otolaryngology (to 1985). Continued
    by Archives of Otolaryngology—Head and Neck
    Surgery
Archives of Otolaryngology—Head and Neck
    Surgery
Archives of Pathology and Laboratory Medicine
Archives of Pediatrics and Adolescent Medicine
Archives of Physical Medicine and Rehabilitation
Archives of Surgery
Archives of Virology
Archives of Women's Mental Health
Arteriosclerosis, Thrombosis, and Vascular Biology
Asia Pacific Journal of Clinical Nutrition
Atherosclerosis
Auris Nasus Larynx
Australasian Psychiatry
Australian and New Zealand Journal of Mental
    Health Nursing
Australian and New Zealand Journal of Psychiatry
Australian Journal of Rural Health
Australian Occupational Therapy Journal
Autonomic Neuroscience

Behavioral and Brain Sciences
Behavioural Brain Research
Biochemical Education
Biochemical Genetics
Biochemical Journal
Biochemical Medicine and Metabolic Biology
Biochemical Pharmacology
Biochemistry
Biological Psychiatry

Biological Psychology
Biology of Reproduction
Biology of the Cell
Biomedicine & Pharmacotherapy
Biomedical Instrumentation and Technology
Biotechnic & Histochemistry
Biotechnology and Applied Biochemistry
Blood
Blood Cells, Molecules, and Diseases
BMJ
Bone
Brain: A Journal of Neurology
Brain and Mind
Brain, Behavior, and Evolution
Brain, Behavior, and Immunity
Brain Injury
Brain Research
Brain Research Bulletin
British Journal of Clinical Psychology
British Journal of Educational Psychology
British Journal of Medical Psychology
British Journal of Nutrition
British Journal of Occupational Therapy
British Journal of Psychology
British Medical Journal (to 1988). Continued by
  BMJ
Bulletin de l'Institut Pasteur (Bulletin of the
  Pasteur Institute)
Bulletin of Environmental Contamination and
  Toxicology
Bulletin of the History of Medicine
Bulletin of the Medical Library Association
Bulletin of the World Health Organization/Bulletin
  de l'Organisation Mondiale de la Santé
Burns

Cambridge Quarterly of Healthcare Ethics
Canadian Journal of Medical Laboratory Science
Canadian Journal of Medical Radiation
  Technology
Canadian Journal of Occupational Therapy
Canadian Journal of Public Health/Revue
  Canadienne de Sant Publique
Canadian Medical Association Journal
Canadian Nurse/L'infirmière Canadienne
Cancer
Cancer Causes & Control
Cancer Cytopathology
Cancer Detection and Prevention
Cancer Genetics and Cytogenetics

Cancer Nursing
Cancer Research
Carcinogenesis
Cardiovascular Pathology
Cardiovascular Radiation Medicine
Cardiovascular Research
Cardiovascular Surgery
Cell
Cell and Tissue Research
Cell Biology and Toxicology
Cell Biology International
Cell Proliferation
Cell Transplantation
Cellular Immunology
Cellular Microbiology
Cellular Physiology and Biochemistry
Chemical Research in Toxicology
Chest
Child Psychiatry and Human Development
Circulation
Circulation Research
Clinical and Diagnostic Laboratory Immunology
Clinical and Diagnostic Virology
Clinical and Experimental Immunology
Clinical Biochemistry
Clinical Chemistry
Clinical Child and Family Psychology Review
Clinical Electroencephalography
Clinical Eye and Vision Care
Clinical Immunology
Clinical Immunology and Immunopathology
Clinical Immunology Newsletter
Clinical Kinesiology: Journal of the American
  Kinesiotherapy Association
Clinical Laboratory Science
Clinical Medicine & Health Research
Clinical Microbiology Newsletter
Clinical Microbiology Reviews
Clinical Neurology and Neurosurgery
Clinical Neurophysiology
Clinical Nurse Specialist
Clinical Nursing Research
Clinical Psychology Review
Clinical Psychology: Science and Review
Clinics in Dermatology
Community Mental Health Journal
Comparative Biochemistry and Physiology, Part C:
  Pharmacology, Toxicology, and Endocrinology
Comparative Hematology International
Computerized Medical Imaging and Graphics

Computers and Biomedical Research
Computers in Biology and Medicine
Computers in Human Behavior
Computers in Nursing
Conn's Current Therapy
Consciousness and Cognition
Contemporary Family Therapy
Contraception
Critical Reviews in Oncology/Hematology
Culture, Medicine, and Psychiatry
Cumulative Index to Nursing & Allied Health
  Literature
Current Genetics
Current Microbiology
Current Opinion in Biotechnology
Current Opinion in Cell Biology
Current Opinion in Genetics & Development
Current Opinion in Immunology
Current Opinion in Microbiology
Current Opinion in Neurobiology
Current Opinion in Oncology
Current Therapy (to 1983). Continued by Conn's
  Current Therapy
Cytogenetics and Cell Genetics
Cytokine

Dental Assistant
Dental Materials
Dermatology Nursing
Developmental and Comparative Immunology
Developmental Neuroscience
Diabetes, Obesity & Metabolism
Diabetes Research and Clinical Practice
Diabetologia
Diagnostic Microbiology and Infectious Disease
Digestive Disease and Sciences
Disability and Rehabilitation
Disease Management and Clinical Outcomes
Diseases of the Colon and Rectum
Drug and Alcohol Review
Drug Metabolism and Disposition
Drug Topics
Drugs
Dysphagia

Ear and Hearing
Ecotoxicology and Environmental Safety
Educational Gerontology
Electroencephalography and Clinical
  Neurophysiology

Emergency Medical Services
Emergency Medicine
Environmental Microbiology
Environmental Nutrition
Environmental Pollution
Environmental Toxicology and Pharmacology
Epidemiology and Infection
Epilepsy Research
European Addiction Research
European Archives of Psychiatry and Clinical
  Neuroscience
European Child & Adolescent Psychiatry
European Heart Journal
European Journal of Biochemistry
European Journal of Cancer
European Journal of Cancer Care
European Journal of Cardio-Thoracic Surgery
European Journal of Clinical Nutrition
European Journal of Epidemiology
European Journal of Heart Failure
European Journal of Internal Medicine
European Journal of Neuroscience
European Journal of Nutrition
European Journal of Obstetrics & Gynecology and
  Reproductive Biology
European Journal of Pain
European Journal of Pediatrics
European Journal of Pharmaceutical Sciences
European Journal of Pharmaceutics and
  Biopharmaceutics
European Journal of Pharmacology
European Journal of Radiology
European Neuropsychopharmacology
European Psychiatry
Evidence-based Healthcare

FASEB Journal
Federation Proceedings (to 1987). Continued by
  FASEB Journal
FEMS Immunology and Medical Microbiology
FEMS Microbiology Ecology
Fertility and Sterility
Food and Chemical Toxicology
Food Microbiology
Forensic Science International
Foundations of Science
Free Radical Biology and Medicine
Frontiers in Neuroendocrinology
Fundamental and Applied Toxicology
Fungal Genetics and Biology

Gait and Posture
Gastroenterology
Gene
General and Comparative Endocrinology
General Hospital Psychiatry
General Pharmacology
Genesis: The Journal of Genetics and Development
Genetica
Genetical Research
Genetics
Geriatric Nursing
Geriatrics
Gerontologist
Gerontology
Gynecologic Oncology

Health
Health Affairs
Health & Place
Health Care for Women International
Health Care Management Review
Health Education and Behavior
Health Progress
Hearing Research
Heart and Lung
Hematology and Cell Therapy
Hepatology Research
Heredity
HIV Medicine
Holistic Nursing Practice
Home Healthcare Nurse
Hormones and Behavior
Hospital Practice
Hospitals
Hospitals and Health Networks
Human Gene Therapy
Human Genetics
Human Immunology
Human Molecular Genetics
Hypertension

Immunity
Immunogenetics
Immunology
Immunology and Cell Biology
Immunology Today
ImmunoMethods
Immunopharmacology
Immunotechnology
Infection and Immunity

Injury
Integrative Medicine
Intensive & Critical Care Nursing
Intensive Care Medicine
International Archives of Occupational and
    Environmental Health
International Immunology
International Journal for Parasitology
International Journal for Quality in Health Care
International Journal of Biochemistry and Cell
    Biology, The
International Journal of Cardiology
International Journal of Developmental
    Neuroscience
International Journal of Eating Disorders
International Journal of Epidemiology
International Journal of Fatigue
International Journal of Food Microbiology
International Journal of Gynecology and Obstetrics
International Journal of Hematology
International Journal of Immunopharmacology
International Journal of Medical Infomatics
International Journal of Nursing Practice
International Journal of Nursing Studies
International Journal of Palliative Nursing
International Journal of Pediatric
    Otorhinolaryngology
International Journal of Pharmaceutics
International Journal of Psycho-Analysis
International Journal of Psychophysiology
International Journal of Radiation Oncology,
    Biology, Physics
International Journal of Stress Management
International Nursing Review
Interventional Cardiology Newsletter
Investigative Ophthalmology & Visual Science
Issues in Comprehensive Pediatric Nursing
Issues in Mental Health Nursing

JAAPA/Journal of the American Academy of
    Physician Assistants
JAMA: Journal of the American Medical Association
JEMS: Journal of Emergency Medical Services
JONA: The Journal of Nursing Administration
Journal for Nurses in Staff Development
Journal of Abnormal Child Psychology
Journal of Adolescent Health
Journal of Advanced Nursing
Journal of Affective Disorders
Journal of Allergy and Clinical Immunology

Journal of Allied Health

Journal of Anxiety Disorders

Journal of Applied Developmental Psychology

Journal of Applied Psychoanalytic Studies

Journal of Athletic Training

Journal of Autism and Developmental Disorders

Journal of Autoimmunity

Journal of Back and Musculoskeletal Rehabilitation

Journal of Bacteriology

Journal of Behavior Therapy and Experimental
    Psychiatry

Journal of Behavioral Medicine

Journal of Biochemistry

Journal of Biotechnology

Journal of Bone and Joint Surgery

Journal of Burn Care and Rehabilitation

Journal of Cancer Research and Clinical Oncology

Journal of Cardiopulmonary Rehabilitation

Journal of Cataract & Refractive Surgery

Journal of Cell Biology

Journal of Cellular Biochemistry

Journal of Child and Adolescent Group Therapy

Journal of Child Language

Journal of Child Psychology and Psychiatry

Journal of Chronic Diseases (to 1987). Continued
    by Journal of Clinical Epidemiology

Journal of Clinical Anesthesia

Journal of Clinical Endocrinology and Metabolism

Journal of Clinical Epidemiology

Journal of Clinical Investigation

Journal of Clinical Microbiology

Journal of Clinical Neuroscience

Journal of Clinical Nursing

Journal of Clinical Psychiatry

Journal of Clinical Virology

Journal of Communication Disorders

Journal of Comparative Neurology

Journal of Contemporary Psychotherapy

Journal of Deaf Studies and Deaf Education

Journal of Dental Hygiene

Journal of Dentistry

Journal of Dermatological Science

Journal of Developmental and Physical Disabilities

Journal of Diabetes and Its Complications

Journal of Diagnostic Medical Sonography

Journal of Emergency Medicine

Journal of Emergency Nursing: JEN

Journal of Environmental Psychology

Journal of Epilepsy

Journal of Ethnopharmacology

Journal of Experimental Child Psychology

Journal of Experimental Medicine

Journal of Extra-Corporeal Technology

Journal of Family Nursing

Journal of Fluency Disorders

Journal of General Physiology

Journal of General Virology

Journal of Hand Surgery (B&E)

Journal of Head Trauma Rehabilitation

Journal of Health and Social Behavior

Journal of Healthcare Management

Journal of Heart and Lung Transplantation, The

Journal of Hematotherapy & Stem Cell Research

Journal of Holistic Nursing: Official Journal of the
    American Holistic Nurses' Association

Journal of Human Genetics

Journal of Human Nutrition & Dietetics

Journal of Immunological Methods

Journal of Immunology

Journal of Infectious Diseases

Journal of Intellectual Disability Research

Journal of Interferon & Cytokine Research

Journal of Internal Medicine

Journal of Intravenous Nursing

Journal of Investigative Dermatology

Journal of Laboratory and Clinical Medicine

Journal of Laryngology and Otology

Journal of Lipid Research

Journal of Medical Education

Journal of Medical Ethics

Journal of Medical Humanities

Journal of Memory and Language

Journal of Molecular and Cellular Cardiology

Journal of Natural Products

Journal of Nervous and Mental Disease

Journal of Neuroimmunology

Journal of Neurology, Neurosurgery & Psychiatry

Journal of Neuroscience

Journal of Neuroscience: The Official Journal of
    the Society for Neuroscience

Journal of Nuclear Medicine Technology

Journal of Nurse-Midwifery

Journal of Nutrition

Journal of Nutrition Education

Journal of Nutrition for the Elderly

Journal of Nutritional Biochemistry

Journal of Obstetric, Gynecologic, and Neonatal
    Nursing: JOGNN

Journal of Orthopaedic and Sports Physical
    Therapy

Journal of Paediatrics and Child Health
Journal of Pain and Symptom Management
Journal of Pediatric Psychology
Journal of Pediatrics, The
Journal of Pharmaceutical Sciences
Journal of Pharmacology and Experimental
  Therapeutics
Journal of Professional Nursing
Journal of Psychiatric & Mental Health Nursing
Journal of Psychiatric Research
Journal of Psychosomatic Research
Journal of Rehabilitation
Journal of Speech, Language and Hearing
  Research
Journal of Studies on Alcohol
Journal of Substance Abuse Treatment
Journal of the American Academy of Audiology
Journal of the American Academy of Child
  Psychiatry
Journal of the American Association of Audiology
Journal of the American College of Cardiology
Journal of the American College of Surgeons
Journal of the American Dental Association
Journal of the American Dietetic Association
Journal of the American Geriatrics Society
Journal of the American Medical Association (see
  JAMA)
Journal of the American Society of
  Echocardiography
Journal of the American Society of Nephrology
Journal of the Canadian Dietetic Association
Journal of the European Academy of Dermatology
  and Venereology
Journal of the National Cancer Institute
Journal of the Neurological Sciences
Journal of the Royal Society of Medicine
Journal of Toxicology—Clinical Toxicology
Journal of Urology
Journal of Virology
Journal of X-Ray Science and Technology
JPO: Journal of Prosthetics and Orthotics

Laboratory Medicine
Lancet
Lippincott's Primary Care Practice
Lung Cancer

Magnetic Resonance Imaging
Marketing Health Services
Maternal and Child Health Journal

MCN, American Journal of Maternal Child
  Nursing
Medical Education
Medical Journal of Australia
Medicine
Medicine and Science in Sports
Methods: A Companion to Methods in
  Enzymology
Microbiology
Midwifery
MLO: Medical Laboratory Observer
Modern Healthcare
Molecular Aspects of Medicine
Molecular Medicine Today
Molecular Microbiology
Molecular Pharmacology

Nature
Nature Biotechnology
Nature Genetics
Nature Medicine
Nature Neuroscience
Neurobiology of Aging
Neurobiology of Disease
Neurobiology of Learning and Memory
Neurogenetics
Neurology
Neuromuscular Disorders
Neuropharmacology
Neuropsychopharmacology
Neurorehabilitation
Neuroscience
Neurosurgery
Neurotoxicology and Teratology
New England Journal of Medicine
Nuclear Medicine and Biology
Nurse Educator
Nurse Practitioner, The
Nurse Practitioner Forum
Nursing and Health Sciences
Nursing and Healthcare Perspectives
Nursing Case Management
Nursing Forum
Nursing Outlook
Nursing Research
Nursing Science Quarterly
Nursing Times
Nursing 2000
Nutrition
Nutrition in Clinical Care

Obstetrical and Gynecological Survey
Obstetrics and Gynecology
Occupational and Environmental Medicine
Occupational Therapy in Health Care
Occupational Therapy in Mental Health
Occupational Therapy Journal of Research
Oncologist, The
Oncology Nursing Forum
Ophthalmic and Physiological Optics
Oral Oncology
Oral Surgery, Oral Medicine, and Oral Pathology
  (to 1994). Continued by Oral Surgery, Oral
  Medicine, Oral Pathology, Oral Radiology, and
  Endodontics
Oral Surgery, Oral Medicine, Oral Pathology, Oral
  Radiology, and Endodontics
OT Week (American Occupational Therapy
  Association)

Pain
Palliative Care Letter
Pathophysiology
Patient Education and Counseling
Pediatric Neurology
Pediatric Physical Therapy
Pediatrics
Pediatrics International
Perfusion
Pharmaceutical Science & Technology Today
Pharmacology and Therapeutics
Physical and Occupational Therapy in Geriatrics
Physical and Occupational Therapy in Pediatrics
Physical Therapy
Physician and Sportsmedicine, The
Physician Assistant
Physiotherapy
Physiotherapy Canada
Plastic and Reconstructive Surgery
PMA: Professional Medical Assistant
Postgraduate Medical Journal
Postgraduate Medicine
Practitioner
Preventive Medicine
Primary Care Update for OB/GYNS
Proceedings of the National Academy of Sciences
Progress in Retinal and Eye Research
Psychiatric Quarterly
Psychiatric Services
Psychiatry
Psychiatry in Practice

Psychiatry in Progress
Psychiatry Research
Psychoneuroendocrinology
Psychopharmacology
Psychosomatics
Psychotherapy and Psychosomatics
PT: Magazine of Physical Therapy
Public Health Nursing
Public Health Nutrition
Pulmonary Pharmacology
Pulmonary Pharmacology & Therapeutics

Radiologic Technology
Radiology
Radiotherapy and Oncology
Reproductive Toxicology
Research in Nursing and Health
Respiratory Care
Resuscitation
RN
RRT: The Canadian Journal of Respiratory
  Therapy

Scandinavian Audiology
Scandinavian Journal of Clinical and Laboratory
  Investigation
Scandinavian Journal of Clinical and Laboratory
  Investigation. Supplement
Scandinavian Journal of Public Health
Science
Sexual Dysfunction
Social Psychiatry and Psychiatric Epidemiology
South African Medical Journal
Speech Communication
Steroids
Stroke
Studies in History and Philosophy of Science
  Part C: Studies in History and Philosophy of
  Biological and Biomedical Sciences
Surgery
Surgery, Gynecology and Obstetrics (to 1993).
  Continued by Journal of the American College
  of Surgeons
Surgical Neurology
Surgical Oncology
Surgical Technologist
Survey of Ophthalmology

Theoretical Medicine & Bioethics
Topics in Emergency Medicine

Topics in Geriatric Rehabilitation
Topics in Health Information Management
Toxicological Sciences
Toxicology
Toxicology and Applied Pharmacology
Transfusion
Transplantation Proceedings
Trends in Biotechnology
Trends in Cardiovascular Medicine
Trends in Cell Biology
Trends in Endocrinology and Metabolism
Trends in Genetics
Trends in Microbiology
Trends in Neurosciences

Trends in Pharmacological Sciences
Tropical Medicine and International Health

Ultrasonic Imaging
Ultrasound in Medicine and Biology
Urologic Oncology
Urology

Vaccine
Virology

Women's Health Issues
World Journal of Microbiology and Biotechnology

—Compiled by Peter B. Heller, Ph.D.

Types of Health Care Providers

Biotechnologists

Training and Degrees: Undergraduate degree program; graduate degree recommended
—Bachelor of Science (B.S.), Master of Science (M.S.)
Duties: The performance of research or application studies in the field of biology
Specializations: All medical fields

Chiropodists

Training and Degrees: Two years of premedical studies (minimum), followed by four years of podiatry school; state license
—Doctor of Surgical Chiropody (D.S.C.) or Doctor of Podiatry (Pod.D.)
Duties: The treatment of foot disorders
Specialization: Doctor of Podiatric Medicine (the recipient of a postgraduate degree awarded for further studies)

Chiropractors

Training and Degrees: Two years of premedical studies (minimum), followed by four years of chiropractic school
—Doctor of Chiropractic (D.C.)
Duties: The mechanical manipulation of the spinal column for the maintenance of health
Specializations: The use of radiology or physiotherapy to supplement manipulation

Counselors

Training and Degrees: Varies; may range from personal experience to specialized training
—Bachelor of Arts (B.A.) or Bachelor of Science (B.S.), with possible advanced degree
Duties: One-on-one work with a patient to deal with specific emotional problems
Specializations: All areas of health care

Cytologists

Training and Degrees: Undergraduate degree program, followed by graduate program and postgraduate training
—Doctor of Philosophy (Ph.D.) or Doctor of Medicine (M.D.)
Duties: The microscopic study of cells or tissue
Specializations:
Hematology (the observation and study of blood cells or tissues associated with blood cell formation)
Histology (the observation and study of tissue)

Dentists

Training and Degrees: Two years of undergraduate studies (minimum), followed by three to four years of dental college
—Doctor of Dental Surgery (D.D.S.) or Doctor of Dental Medicine (D.M.D.)
Duties: The repair, restoration, and cleaning of teeth
Specializations:
Endodontics (the diagnosis and treatment of diseases of dental pulp and tissue)
Oral pathology or surgery (the diagnosis and surgical repair of oral disorders)
Orthodontics (the diagnosis and treatment of tooth irregularities)
Pedodontics (the diagnosis and treatment of the dental problems of children)
Periodontics (the diagnosis and treatment of disorders in tissue surrounding teeth)
Prosthodontics (the production of artificial devices for tooth replacement)

Dietetic Technicians

Training and Degrees: A two-year dietetic program
—Associate degree in a program approved by the American Dietetic Association
Duties: The assessment, design, and implementation of nutritional programs
Specializations:
Dietitian (a person trained in nutritional care)
Geriatric dietician (a person trained in the nutritional care of the elderly)
Pediatric dietician (a person trained in the nutritional care of children)

Immunologists

Training and Degrees: Undergraduate degree program; graduate or professional program
—Master of Science (M.S.); Doctor of Philosophy (Ph.D.)

Duties: The observation and study of the body's immune system
Specializations: None

Interns
Training and Degrees: The completion of a postgraduate program in the field of health care
—Master of Science (M.S.) or doctoral degree
Duties: The learning of medical procedures under the supervision of residents or other physicians
Specializations: All areas of health care

Laboratory Technicians
Training and Degrees: A two-year or four-year school
—Associate degree, Bachelor of Science (B.S.) or Master of Science (M.S.)
Duties: The collection, preparation, and testing of tissues or fluids for diagnostic purposes; the carrying out of medical procedures under the direction of physicians
Specializations: Many medical fields

Medical Doctors
Training and Degrees: Undergraduate degree program followed by medical school; specializations are generally based on training that begins during the years as a resident
—Doctor of Medicine (M.D.)
Duties: The assessment and diagnosis of medical problems; the administration of procedures or drugs for treatment
Specializations:
Anesthesiology (the administration of anesthetics for the relief or prevention of pain)
Cardiology (the diagnosis and treatment of disorders of the heart)
Dermatology (the diagnosis and treatment of skin disorders)
Family practice (the diagnosis and treatment of disorders among all individuals, rather than specialization based on age or sex)
Gastroenterology (the study of disorders of the stomach and intestinal tract)
Geriatrics (the treatment of disorders of the elderly)
Gynecology (the diagnosis and treatment of disorders of the female reproductive system)
Internal medicine (the diagnosis and treatment of disorders affecting internal organs)

Nephrology (the diagnosis and treatment of disorders associated with the kidneys)
Obstetrics (the diagnosis and treatment of disorders dealing with pregnancy and childbirth)
Oncology (the diagnosis and treatment of tumors)
Ophthalmology (the diagnosis and treatment of disorders associated with the eyes)
Pediatrics (the diagnosis and treatment of disorders of children)
Plastic surgery (the surgical repair or restoration of visible areas of the body)
Proctology (the diagnosis and treatment of disorders affecting the anus, colon, or rectum)
Psychiatry (the diagnosis and treatment of mental disorders)
Pulmonology (the diagnosis and treatment of disorders of the lungs or respiratory system)
Rheumatology (the diagnosis and treatment of disorders affecting connective tissue)
Urology (the diagnosis and treatment of disorders affecting the urinary tract)
Vascular medicine (the diagnosis and treatment of disorders associated with the circulatory system)

Microbiologists
Training and Degrees: Undergraduate degree program; graduate degree recommended
—Bachelor of Science (B.S.), Master of Science (M.S.)
Duties: The research, maintenance, or identification of microorganisms
Specializations:
Bacteriology (the identification and study of bacteria)
Mycology (the identification and study of molds)
Virology (the identification and study of viruses)

Midwives
Training and Degrees: Program in midwifery; registration and license to practice
Duties: The supervision of pregnancy, labor, delivery, and the postpartum period, in addition to counseling and family planning
Specialization: Certified nurse midwife (a person who is certified as both a nurse and a midwife)

Nurses
Training and Degrees: Undergraduate degree program, followed by study at an approved school of nursing; passage of the National Council

Licensure Examination (NCLEX-RN) is required to become a Registered Nurse

—Associate Degree in Nursing (A.D.N.), Bachelor of Science in Nursing (B.S.N.) (four-year program), Master of Science in Nursing (M.S.N.), Registered Nurse (R.N.)

Duties: The administration of medical treatments recommended by physicians; the monitoring and facilitation of medical care

Specializations:

Clinical nurse specialist (R.N. with experience in dealing with overall health care; requires M.S.N.)

Nurse educator (R.N. trained in the teaching of nurses)

Nurse practitioner (R.N. with advanced training and experience in a particular branch of nursing)

Obstetric nurse (R.N. specializing in pregnancy and childbirth)

Pediatric nurse (R.N. trained in the nursing care of children)

Surgical nurse (R.N. trained to assist during surgical procedures)

Optometrists

Training and Degrees: Two years of undergraduate studies (minimum), followed by four years of optometry college; state license

—Doctor of Optometry (D.O.)

Duties: Testing of the eyes for visual acuity; the prescription of corrective lenses

Specialization: Optician (a person who makes or sells corrective lenses)

Osteopaths

Training and Degrees: Undergraduate degree program, followed by medical school and an internship, or graduation from a college of osteopathy

—Doctor of Medicine (M.D.), Doctor of Osteopathy (D.O.)

Duties: The manipulation of body structures as supplemental treatment for disease

Specialization: Doctor of Medicine (M.D.)

Pathologists

Training and Degrees: Undergraduate degree program, followed by medical school

—Doctor of Medicine (M.D.)

Duties: The observation of the effects of disease on the body

Specializations:

Autopsy (the determination of the cause of death)

Clinical pathology (the assessment of disease states as reflected in changes within the body)

Pharmacists

Training and Degrees: A two-year undergraduate program, followed by a two-year to three-year program in an approved school of pharmacy; state license

—Doctor of Pharmacology (Pharm.D.)

Duties: The formulation and dispensation of medications

Specializations: None

Pharmacologists

Training and Degrees: Undergraduate degree program; graduate program

—Master of Science (M.S.); Doctor of Philosophy (Ph.D.)

Duties: The study of the properties and use of drugs or other pharmacologic agents

Specializations: None

Physical Therapists

Training and Degrees: Undergraduate program in physical therapy, or a one-year certified course in conjunction with a degree program in a related field

Duties: The testing and treatment of persons who are physically handicapped, either temporarily or permanently

Specializations: None

Physician Assistants

Training and Degrees: A two-year program for national certification by the American Association of Physician Assistants (AAPA)

Duties: The provision of assistance as requested by supervising physicians

Specializations:

Radiology (providing aid during X-ray and related procedures)

Surgery (assisting surgeons during operations)

Psychological Assistants

Training and Degrees: Undergraduate degree program, graduate degree, and an internship

—Master's degree or higher

Duties: The administration of psychological tests or

their assessment under the supervision of psychologists

Specializations:

Child psychology (the assessment of children)

Clinical psychology (the assessment of behavioral disorders)

Educational psychology (the preparation and administration of tests)

Psychologists

Training and Degrees: Undergraduate degree program, graduate degree, an internship, and postdoctoral experience

—Doctor of Philosophy (Ph.D.), Doctor of Psychology (Psy.D.), Doctor of Education (Ed.D.)

Duties: The assessment diagnosis, and administration of psychological tests and treatments for mental disorders and physical conditions that are affected by mental conditions

Specializations:

Child psychology (the diagnosis and treatment of emotional disorders in children)

Clinical psychology (the diagnosis and treatment of personality or behavioral disorders)

Educational psychology (the application of psychology to education or testing procedures)

Radiologists

Training and Degrees: Undergraduate degree program, followed by medical school and generally a residency in radiology

—Doctor of Medicine (M.D.)

Duties: The use of radioactive materials for the diagnosis and treatment of disease

Specializations:

Diagnostic radiology (the use of radioactive materials for imaging)

Nuclear medicine (the performance of diagnostic procedures and imaging involving the internal use of radiochemicals)

Therapeutic radiology (the use of radiochemicals for the treatment of disorders)

Residents

Training and Degrees: Undergraduate degree program, followed by medical school and one year of internship

—Doctor of Medicine (M.D.)

Duties: Clinical duties in hospitals in any of several specialties

Specializations: All medical fields

Respiratory Therapists

Training and Degrees: Undergraduate degree from a school approved by American Medical Association, with training appropriate for passing the registry examination

—Associate degree or Bachelor of Science (B.S.)

Duties: The carrying out of treatments designed to improve or correct functions of the respiratory tract, under the direction of physicians

Specialization: Registered respiratory therapist (the graduate of an advanced program from the National Board of Respiratory Care)

Toxicologists

Training and Degrees: Undergraduate degree program; graduate program

—Master of Science (M.S.), Doctor of Philosophy (Ph.D.)

Duties: The study of poisonous compounds

Specializations: None

GENERAL BIBLIOGRAPHY

ACQUIRED IMMUNODEFICIENCY SYNDROME (AIDS). *See also* SEXUALLY TRANSMITTED DISEASES

Bartlett, John G. *The Johns Hopkins Hospital 1998 Guide to Medical Care of Patients with HIV Infection.* 8th ed. Philadelphia: Lippincott Williams & Wilkins, 1998.

Cotton, Deborah, and Heather D. Watts, eds. *The Medical Management of AIDS in Women.* New York: Wiley-Liss, 1997.

DeVita, Vincent T., Jr., et al., eds. *AIDS: Etiology, Diagnosis, Treatment, and Prevention.* 4th ed. Philadelphia: Lippincott Williams & Wilkins, 1997.

Fahey, John L., and Diana Shin Flemmig, eds. *AIDS/HIV Reference Guide for Medical Professionals.* 4th ed. Philadelphia: Lippincott Williams & Wilkins, 1997.

Libman, Howard, and Robert A. Witzburg, eds. *HIV Infection: A Primary Care Manual.* 3d ed. Philadelphia: Lippincott Williams & Wilkins, 1996.

Masci, Joseph R. *Outpatient Management of HIV Infection.* 2d ed. St. Louis: C. V. Mosby, 1996.

Merigan, Thomas C., Jr., et al. *Textbook of AIDS Medicine.* 2d ed. Philadelphia: Lippincott Williams & Wilkins, 1999.

Pizzo, Philip A., and Catherine M. Wilfert, eds. *Pediatric AIDS: The Challenge of HIV Infection in Infants, Children, and Adolescents.* 3d ed. Philadelphia: Lippincott Williams & Wilkins, 1998.

Sande, Merle A., and Paul A. Volberding, eds. *The Medical Management of AIDS.* 6th ed. Philadelphia: W. B. Saunders, 1999.

Scharer, Lawrence L., and John M. McAdam. *Tuberculosis and AIDS.* New York: Springer, 1996.

ALLERGY

Bierman, C. Warren, et al., eds. *Allergy, Asthma, and Immunology from Infancy to Adulthood.* 3d ed. Philadelphia: W. B. Saunders, 1996.

Kaplan, Allen P., ed. *Allergy.* 2d ed. Philadelphia: W. B. Saunders, 1997.

Lieberman, Phil, and John A. Anderson, eds. *Allergic Diseases: Diagnosis and Treatment.* Totowa, N.J.: Humana Press, 1997.

Metcalfe, Dean D., et al., eds. *Food Allergy: Adverse Reactions to Foods and Food Additives.* 2d ed. Boston: Blackwell Science, 1997.

Middleton, Elliott, Jr., et al., eds. *Allergy: Principles and Practice.* 5th ed. St. Louis: C. V. Mosby, 1998.

Patterson, Roy, ed. *Allergic Diseases: Diagnosis and Management.* 5th ed. Philadelphia: Lippincott Williams & Wilkins, 1997.

ALTERNATIVE/COMPLEMENTARY MEDICINE

Blumenthal, Mark, ed. *Therapeutic Guide to Herbal Medicines.* Boston: Integrative Medicine Communication, 1998.

Cohen, Michael H. *Complementary and Alternative Medicine: Legal Boundaries and Regulatory Perspectives.* Baltimore: The Johns Hopkins University Press, 1998.

Gordon, Rena J., et al. *Alternative Therapies: Expanding Options in Health Care.* New York: Springer, 1998.

Mitchell, Annie, and Maggie Cormack. *The Therapeutic Relationship in Complementary Health Care.* Philadelphia: W. B. Saunders, 1998.

AMBULATORY CARE

Barker, L. Randol, et al., eds. *Principles of Ambulatory Medicine.* 5th ed. Philadelphia: Lippincott Williams & Wilkins, 1999.

Dershewitz, Robert A., ed. *Ambulatory Pediatric Care.* 3d ed. Philadelphia: Lippincott Williams & Wilkins, 1999.

Dornbrand, Laurie, et al., eds. *Manual of Clinical Problems in Adult Ambulatory Care with Annotated Key References.* 3d ed. Philadelphia: Lippincott Williams & Wilkins, 1997.

Mengel, Mark B., and L. Peter Scwiebert, eds. *Ambulatory Medicine: The Primary Care of Families.* 3d ed. Stamford, Conn.: Appleton & Lange, 1999.

Rucker, Lisa M., ed. *Essentials of Adult Ambulatory Care.* Philadelphia: Lippincott Williams & Wilkins, 1997.

ANATOMY

Bo, Walter J., et al. *Basic Atlas of Sectional Anatomy with Correlated Imaging.* 3d ed. Philadelphia: W. B. Saunders, 1998.

Eroschenko, Victor P. *Di Fiorés Atlas of Histology with Functional Correlations.* 8th ed. Philadelphia: Lippincott Williams & Wilkins, 1996.

Junqueira, Luis C., et al. *Basic Histology.* 9th ed. Stamford, Conn.: Appleton & Lange, 1998.

McMinn, Robert M. H., et al. *McMinn's Functional and Clinical Anatomy.* St. Louis: C. V. Mosby, 1995.

Moore, Keith L. *Clinically Oriented Anatomy.* 4th ed. Philadelphia: Lippincott Williams & Wilkins, 1999.

Moore, Keith L., and T. V. N. Persaud. *The Developing Human: Clinically Oriented Embryology.* 6th ed. Philadelphia: W. B. Saunders, 1998.

Snell, Richard S. *Clinical Neuroanatomy for Medical Students.* 4th ed. Philadelphia: Lippincott Williams & Wilkins, 1997.

Williams, Peter L., ed. *Gray's Anatomy: The Anatomical Basis of Medicine and Surgery.* 38th ed. Philadelphia: W. B. Saunders, 1995.

Woelfel, Julian B., and Rickne C. Scheid. *Dental Anatomy: Its Relevance to Dentistry.* 5th ed. Philadelphia: Lippincott Williams & Wilkins, 1997.

ANESTHESIOLOGY

Ashburn, Michael A., and Linda J. Rice, eds. *The Management of Pain.* Philadelphia: W. B. Saunders, 1998.

Benumof, Jonathan L., ed. *Anesthesia and Uncommon Diseases.* 4th ed. Philadelphia: W. B. Saunders, 1998.

Brown, David L., ed. *Regional Anesthesia and Analgesia.* Philadelphia: W. B. Saunders, 1996.

Collins, Vincent J., ed. *Physiologic and Pharmacologic Bases of Anesthesia.* Philadelphia: Lippincott Williams & Wilkins, 1996.

DiNardo, James A. *Anesthesia for Cardiac Surgery.* 2d ed. Stamford, Conn.: Appleton & Lange, 1998.

Gambling, David R., and M. Joanne Douglas, eds. *Obstetric Anesthesia and Uncommon Disorders.* Philadelphia: W. B. Saunders, 1998.

Hurford, William E., et al., eds. *Clinical Anesthesia Procedures of the Massachusetts General Hospital.* 5th ed. Philadelphia: Lippincott Williams & Wilkins, 1998.

Kaplan, Joel A., ed. *Cardiac Anesthesia.* 4th ed. Philadelphia: W. B. Saunders, 1999.

Lake, Carol L. *Pediatric Cardiac Anesthesia.* 3d ed. Stamford, Conn.: Appleton & Lange, 1998.

Longnecker, David E., et al., eds. *Principles and Practice of Anesthesiology.* 2d ed. St. Louis: C. V. Mosby, 1998.

Longnecker, David E., and Frank L. Murphy, eds. *Dripps/Eckenhoff/Vandam Introduction to Anesthesia.* 9th ed. Philadelphia: W. B. Saunders, 1997.

Miller, Ronald D., ed. *Anesthesia.* 5th ed. Philadelphia: W. B. Saunders, 1999.

Morell, Robert C., and John H. Eichhorn, eds. *Patient Safety in Anesthetic Practice.* Philadelphia: W. B. Saunders, 1997.

Motoyama, Etsuro K., and Peter J. Davis, eds. *Smith's Anesthesia for Infants and Children.* 6th ed. St. Louis: C. V. Mosby, 1996.

Sosis, Mitchel B., ed. *Anesthesia Equipment Manual.* Philadelphia: Lippincott Williams & Wilkins, 1997.

White, Paul F., ed. *Ambulatory Anesthesia and Surgery.* Philadelphia: W. B. Saunders, 1997.

_____. *Textbook of Intravenous Anesthesia.* Philadelphia: Lippincott Williams & Wilkins, 1997.

Yao, Fun-Sun F., ed. *Yao and Artusio's Anesthesiology: Problem-Oriented Patient Management.* 4th ed. Philadelphia: Lippincott Williams & Wilkins, 1998.

BIOCHEMISTRY

Cohn, Robert M., and Karl S. Roth. *Biochemistry and Disease: Bridging Basic Science and Clinical Practice.* Philadelphia: Lippincott Williams & Wilkins, 1996.

Devlin, Thomas M., ed. *Textbook of Biochemistry with Clinical Correlations.* 4th ed. New York: Wiley-Liss, 1997.

Murray, Robert K., et al. *Harper's Biochemistry.* 25th ed. Stamford, Conn.: Appleton & Lange, 1999.

Stryer, Lubert. *Biochemistry.* 4th ed. New York: Freeman, 1995.

CARDIOVASCULAR SYSTEM

Alexander, Wayne, et al., eds. *Hurst's The Heart: Arteries and Veins.* 9th ed. New York: McGraw-Hill, 1998.

Baim, Donald S., and William Grossman, eds. *Cardiac Catheterization, Angiography, and Intervention.* 5th ed. Philadelphia: Lippincott Williams & Wilkins, 1996.

Braunwald, Eugene, ed. *Heart Disease: A Textbook of Cardiovascular Medicine.* 5th ed. Philadelphia: W. B. Saunders, 1997.

Cheitlin, Melvin D., et al. *Clinical Cardiology.* 7th ed. Stamford, Conn.: Appleton & Lange, 1999.

Crawford, Michael H. *Current Diagnosis and Treat-*

ment in Cardiology. Stamford, Conn.: Appleton & Lange, 1995.

Dolgin, Martin, et al., eds. *Nomenclature and Criteria for Diagnosis of Diseases of the Heart and Great Vessels*. 9th ed. Philadelphia: Lippincott Williams & Wilkins, 1994.

Ellestad, Myrvin H. *Stress Testing: Principles and Practice*. 4th ed. Philadelphia: Davis, 1996.

Fuster, Valentin, et al., eds. *Atherosclerosis and Coronary Artery Disease*. Philadelphia: Lippincott Williams & Wilkins, 1996.

Garson, Arthur, Jr., et al., eds. *The Science and Practice of Pediatric Cardiology*. 2d ed. Philadelphia: Lippincott Williams & Wilkins, 1998.

Goldberger, Ary L. *Clinical Electrocardiography: A Simplified Approach*. 6th ed. St. Louis: C. V. Mosby, 1999.

Goldman, Lee, and Eugene Braunwald. *Primary Cardiology*. Philadelphia: W. B. Saunders, 1998.

Julian, Desmond G., and Nanette K. Wenger, eds. *Women and Heart Disease*. St. Louis: C. V. Mosby, 1997.

Kaplan, Norman M. *Clinical Hypertension*. 7th ed. Philadelphia: Lippincott Williams & Wilkins, 1998.

Kvetan, Vladimir, and David R. Dantzker, eds. *The Critically Ill Cardiac Patient: Multisystem Dysfunction and Management*. *Philadelphia:* Lippincott Williams & Wilkins, 1996.

Mandel, William J., ed. *Cardiac Arrhythmias: Their Mechanisms, Diagnosis, and Management*. 3d ed. Philadelphia: Lippincott Williams & Wilkins, 1995.

Mills, Roger M., Jr., and James B. Young. *Practical Approaches to the Treatment of Heart Failure*. Philadelphia: Lippincott Williams & Wilkins, 1998.

Otto, Catherine M. *The Practice of Clinical Endocardiography*. Philadelphia: W. B. Saunders, 1997.

Paradis, Norman A., et al., eds. *Cardiac Arrest: The Science and Practice of Resuscitation Medicine*. Philadelphia: Lippincott Williams & Wilkins, 1996.

Pepine, Carl J., ed. *Diagnostic and Therapeutic Cardiac Catheterization*. 3d ed. Philadelphia: Lippincott Williams & Wilkins, 1998.

Perloff, Joseph K., and John S. Child. *Congenital Heart Disease in Adults*. 2d ed. Philadelphia: W. B. Saunders, 1998.

Snider, A. Rebecca, et al. *Echocardiography in Pediatric Heart Disease*. 2d ed. St. Louis: C. V. Mosby, 1997.

Talley, J. David, ed. *Cardiovascular Involvement in Systemic Diseases*. New York: Igaku-Shoin, 1997.

Young, Jess R., et al., eds. *Peripheral Vascular Diseases*. 2d ed. St. Louis: C. V. Mosby, 1996.

CRITICAL CARE

Civetta, Joseph M., et al., eds. *Critical Care*. 3d ed. Philadelphia: Lippincott Williams & Wilkins, 1997.

Fuhrman, Bradley P., and Jerry J. Zimmerman. *Pediatric Critical Care*. 2d ed. St. Louis: C. V. Mosby, 1998.

Hall, Jesse B., et al., eds. *Principles of Critical Care*. 2d ed. New York: McGraw-Hill, 1998.

Irwin, Richard S., et al., eds. *Irwin and Rippe's Intensive Care Medicine*. 4th ed. Philadelphia: Lippincott Williams & Wilkins, 1999.

Marini, John J., and Arthur P. Wheeler. *Critical Care Medicine: The Essentials*. 2d ed. Philadelphia: Lippincott Williams & Wilkins, 1997.

Marino, Paul L. *The ICU Book*. 2nd ed. Philadelphia: Lippincott Williams & Wilkins, 1998.

Matthay, Michel A., and David E. Schwartz, eds. *Complications in the Intensive Care Unit: Recognition, Prevention, and Management*. New York: Chapman & Hall, 1997.

Murray, Michael J., et al., eds. *Critical Care Medicine: Perioperative Management*. Philadelphia: Lippincott Williams & Wilkins, 1997.

Shoemaker, William C., et al., eds. *Textbook of Critical Care*. 4th ed. Philadelphia: W. B. Saunders, 1999.

Tobin, Martin J., ed. *Principles and Practice of Intensive Care Monitoring*. New York: McGraw-Hill, 1998.

DENTISTRY

Cohen, Stephen, and Richard C. Burns, eds. *Pathways of the Pulp*. 7th ed. St. Louis: C. V. Mosby, 1998.

Donoff, R. Bruce. *Massachusetts General Hospital Manual of Oral and Maxillofacial Surgery*. 3d ed. St. Louis: C. V. Mosby, 1997.

Eisen, Drore, and Denis P. Lynch. *The Mouth: Diagnosis and Treatment*. St. Louis: C. V. Mosby, 1998.

Graber, Thomas M., et al. *Dentofacial Orthopedics with Functional Appliances*. 2d ed. St. Louis: C. V. Mosby, 1997.

Little, James W., and Donald A. Falace. *Dental Management of the Medically Compromised Patient*. 5th ed. St. Louis: C. V. Mosby, 1997.

Misch, Carl E. *Contemporary Implant Dentistry.* 2d ed. St. Louis: C. V. Mosby, 1999.

Peterson, Larry J., ed. *Contemporary Oral and Maxillofacial Surgery.* 3d ed. St. Louis: C. V. Mosby, 1998.

Wood, Norman K., and Paul W. Goaz. *Differential Diagnosis of Oral and Maxillofacial Lesions.* 5th ed. St. Louis: C. V. Mosby, 1997.

Zambito, Raymond E., et al. *Hospital Dentistry: Practice and Education.* St. Louis: C. V. Mosby, 1997.

DERMATOLOGY

Arndt, Kenneth A., et al., eds. *Lasers in Cutaneous and Aesthetic Surgery.* Philadelphia: Lippincott Williams & Wilkins, 1997.

Arndt, Kenneth A., et al. *Primary Care Dermatology.* Philadelphia: W. B. Saunders, 1997.

Braverman, Irwin M. *Skin Signs of Systemic Disease.* 3d ed. Philadelphia: W. B. Saunders, 1998.

Elder, David, ed. *Lever's Histopathology of the Skin.* 8th ed. Philadelphia: Lippincott Williams & Wilkins, 1997.

Fitzpatrick, Thomas B., et al. *Color Atlas and Synopsis of Clinical Dermatology: Common and Serious Diseases.* 3d ed. New York: McGraw-Hill, 1997.

Freedberg, Irwin M., et al., eds. *Fitzpatrick's Dermatology in General Medicine.* 5th ed. New York: McGraw-Hill, 1999.

Goldstein, Beth G., and Adam O. Goldstein. *Practical Dermatology.* 2d ed. St. Louis: C. V. Mosby, 1997.

Habif, Thomas P. *Clinical Dermatology: A Color Guide to Diagnosis and Therapy.* 3d ed. St. Louis: C. V. Mosby, 1996.

Helm, Klaus F., and James G. Marks, Jr. *Atlas of Differential Diagnosis in Dermatology.* Philadelphia: W. B. Saunders, 1998.

Litt, Jerome Z. *Drug Eruption Reference Manual.* New York: Parthenon, 1998.

Marks, James G., Jr., and Vincent A. DeLeo. *Contact and Occupational Dermatology.* 2d ed. St. Louis: C. V. Mosby, 1997.

Sauer, Gordon C., and John C. Hall. *Manual of Skin Diseases.* 8th ed. Philadelphia: Lippincott Williams & Wilkins, 1999.

Sontheimer, Richard D., and Thomas T. Provost, eds. *Cutaneous Manifestations of Rheumatic Diseases.* Philadelphia: Lippincott Williams & Wilkins, 1996.

Sybert, Virginia P. *Genetic Skin Disorders.* New York: Oxford University Press, 1997.

Usatine, Richard P., et al. *Skin Surgery: A Practical Guide.* St. Louis: C. V. Mosby, 1998.

Weston, William L., et al. *Color Textbook of Pediatric Dermatology.* 2d ed. St. Louis: C. V. Mosby, 1996.

DIAGNOSIS

Berkow, Robert, ed. *The Merck Manual of Diagnosis and Therapy.* 17th ed. Rahway, N.J.: Merck, 1999.

Bickley, Lynn, and Robert A. Hoekelman. *Bates' Guide to Physical Examination and History Taking.* 7th ed. Philadelphia: Lippincott Williams & Wilkins, 1999.

Bouchier, I. A. D., et al., eds. *French's Index of Differential Diagnosis.* 13th ed. Boston: Butterworth-Heinemann, 1996.

Conn, Rex B., at al. *Current Diagnosis 9.* Philadelphia: W. B. Saunders, 1997.

DeGowin, Richard. *DeGowin and DeGowin's Diagnostic Examination.* 7th ed. New York: McGraw-Hill, 1999.

Friedman, H. Harold, ed. *Problem-Oriented Medical Diagnosis.* 6th ed. Philadelphia: Lippincott Williams & Wilkins, 1996.

Seidel, Henry M., et al. *Mosby's Guide to Physical Examination.* 4th ed. St. Louis: C. V. Mosby, 1999.

Seller, Robert H. *Differential Diagnosis of Common Complaints.* 3d ed. Philadelphia: W. B. Saunders, 1996.

Silen, William. *Cope's Early Diagnosis of the Acute Abdomen.* 19th ed. New York: Oxford University Press, 1996.

Swartz, Mark H. *Textbook of Physical Diagnosis: History and Examination.* 3d ed. Philadelphia: W. B. Saunders, 1998.

DICTIONARIES AND DIRECTORIES

Anderson, Kenneth N., et al., eds. *Mosby's Medical, Nursing, and Allied Health Dictionary.* 5th ed. St. Louis: C. V. Mosby, 1998.

Armitage, Peter, and Theodore Colton, eds. *Encyclopedia of Biostatistics.* New York: Wiley, 1998.

Aspen Reference Group, ed. *Infectious Disease Resource Manual.* Gaithersburg, Md.: Aspen, 1999.

Dorland, W. A. Newman, ed. *Dorland's Illustrated Medical Dictionary.* 29th ed. Philadelphia: W. B. Saunders, 2000.

Izenberg, Neil, ed. *Human Diseases and Conditions.* New York: Charles Scribner's Sons, 2000.

Lynn, Stephan G., and Pamela Weintraub, eds. *Medi-*

cal Emergency: The St. Luke's-Roosevelt Hospital Center Book of Emergency Medicine. New York: Hearst Books, 1996.

McGraw-Hill Encyclopedia of Science and Technology. 8th ed. New York: McGraw-Hill, 1997.

Magalini, Sergio, et al. Dictionary of Medical Syndromes. 4th ed. Philadelphia: Lippincott Williams & Wilkins, 1997.

Miller, Benjamin F., ed. Miller-Keane Encyclopedia and Dictionary of Medicine, Nursing, and Allied Health. 6th ed. Philadelphia: W. B. Saunders, 1997.

The PDR Family Guide: Encyclopedia of Medical Care. New York: Three Rivers Press, 1997.

Professional Guide to Diseases. 7th ed. Springhouse, Pa.: Lippincott Williams & Wilkins, 2001.

Stedman, Thomas Lathrop, ed. Stedman's Medical Dictionary. 27th ed. Philadelphia: Lippincott Williams & Wilkins, 2000.

Thomas, Clayton L., et al., eds. Taber's Cyclopedic Medical Dictionary. 19th ed. Philadelphia: Davis, 2001.

Wagman, Richard J., et al., eds. The New Complete Medical and Health Encyclopedia. Chicago: Ferguson, 2000.

EMERGENCY MEDICINE

Barkin, Roger M., et al., eds. Pediatric Emergency Medicine: Concepts and Clinical Practice. 2d ed. St. Louis: C. V. Mosby, 1997.

Brillman, Judith C., and Ronald W. Quenzer, eds. Infectious Disease in Emergency Medicine. 3d ed. Philadelphia: Lippincott Williams & Wilkins, 1998.

Edwards, Libby. Dermatology in Emergency Care. Philadelphia: W. B. Saunders, 1997.

Howell, John M., ed. Emergency Medicine. Philadelphia: W. B. Saunders, 1998.

Knoop, Kevin J., et al. Atlas of Emergency Medicine. New York: McGraw-Hill, 1997.

Mengert, Terry J., et al., eds. Emergency Medical Therapy. 4th ed. Philadelphia: W. B. Saunders, 1996.

Pearlman, Mark D., and Judith E. Tintinalli, eds. Emergency Care of the Woman. New York: McGraw-Hill, 1998.

Roberts, James R., and Jerris R. Hedges, eds. Clinical Procedures in Emergency Medicine. 3d ed. Philadelphia: W. B. Saunders, 1998.

Rosen, Peter, and Roger M. Barkin, eds. Emergency Medicine: Concepts and Clinical Practice. 4th ed. St. Louis: C. V. Mosby, 1998.

Salluzzo, Richard F., et al., eds. Emergency Department Management: Principles and Applications. St. Louis: C. V. Mosby, 1997.

Scaletta, Thomas A., and Jeffrey J. Schaider. Emergent Management of Trauma. New York: McGraw-Hill, 1996.

Schwartz, George R., et al., eds. Principles and Practice of Emergency Medicine. 4th ed. Philadelphia: Lippincott Williams & Wilkins, 1999.

Wolfson, Allan B., and Paul M. Paris, eds. Diagnostic Testing in Emergency Medicine. Philadelphia: W. B. Saunders, 1996.

ENDOCRINOLOGY AND METABOLISM

Abelow, Benjamin. Understanding Acid-Base. Philadelphia: Lippincott Williams & Wilkins, 1998.

Avioli, Louis V., and Stephen M. Krane, eds. Metabolic Bone Disease and Clinically Related Disorders. 3d ed. San Diego, Calif.: Academic Press, 1998.

Braverman, Lewis E., and Robert D. Utiger, eds. Werner and Ingbar's the Thyroid: A Fundamental and Clinical Text. 7th ed. Philadelphia: Lippincott Williams & Wilkins, 1996.

DeGroot, Leslie J., et al., eds. Endocrinology. 3d ed. Philadelphia: W. B. Saunders, 1995.

Falk, Stephen A., ed. Thyroid Disease: Endocrinology, Surgery, Nuclear Medicine, and Radiotherapy. 2d ed. Philadelphia: Lippincott Williams & Wilkins, 1997.

Felig, Philip, et al., eds. Endocrinology and Metabolism. 3d ed. New York: McGraw-Hill, 1995.

Greenspan, Francis S., and Gordon Strewler, eds. Basic and Clinical Endocrinology. 5th ed. Stamford, Conn.: Appleton & Lange, 1997.

Moore, W. Tabb, and Richard C. Eastman, eds. Diagnostic Endocrinology. 2d ed. St. Louis: C. V. Mosby, 1996.

Porte, Daniel, Jr., and Robert S. Sherwin, eds. Ellenberg and Rifkin's Diabetes Mellitus. 5th ed. Stamford, Conn.: Appleton & Lange, 1997.

Sperling, Mark A., ed. Pediatric Endocrinology. Philadelphia: W. B. Saunders, 1996.

Wilson, Jean D., et al., eds. Williams' Textbook of Endocrinology. 9th ed. Philadelphia: W. B. Saunders, 1998.

ETHICS

American Medical Association. Council on Ethical and Judicial Affairs. Code of Medical Ethics: Cur-

rent Opinions with Annotations. Chicago: Author, 1998.

Beauchamp, Tom L., and James F. Childress. *Principles of Biomedical Ethics.* 4th ed. New York: Oxford University Press, 1994.

Brody, Baruch A. *The Ethics of Biomedical Research: An International Perspective.* New York: Oxford University Press, 1998.

Jamison, Stephen. *Assisted Suicide: A Decision-Making Guide for Health Professionals.* San Francisco: Jossey-Bass, 1997.

Jonsen, Albert R., et al. *Clinical Ethics: A Practical Approach to Ethical Decisions in Clinical Medicine.* 4th ed. New York: McGraw-Hill, 1998.

Lo, Bernard. *Resolving Ethical Dilemmas: A Guide for Clinicians.* Philadelphia: Lippincott Williams & Wilkins, 1995.

Mappes, Thomas A., and Jane S. Zembaty, eds. *Biomedical Ethics.* 4th ed. New York: McGraw-Hill, 1996.

Monagle, John F., and David C. Thomasma. *Health Care Ethics: Critical Issues for the Twenty-first Century.* 2d ed. Gaithersburg, Md.: Aspen, 1998.

Schneider, Carl E. *The Practice of Autonomy: Patients, Doctors, and Medical Decisions.* New York: Oxford University Press, 1998.

Vaetch, Robert M., ed. *Medical Ethics.* 2d ed. Sudbury, Mass.: Jones and Bartlett, 1997.

EVIDENCE-BASED MEDICINE

Friedland, Daniel J., ed. *Evidence-Based Medicine: A Framework for Clinical Practice.* Stamford, Conn.: Appleton & Lange, 1998.

Greenhalgh, Trisha. *How to Read a Paper: The Basics of Evidence-Based Medicine.* London: BMA, 1997.

Lee, Burton W., et al., eds. *Quick Consult Manual of Evidence-Based Medicine.* Philadelphia: Lippincott Williams & Wilkins, 1997.

Mulrow, Cynthia, and Deborah Cook, eds. *Systematic Reviews: Synthesis of Best Evidence for Health Care Decisions.* Philadelphia: American College of Physicians, 1998.

Sackett, David L., et al. *Evidence-Based Medicine: How to Practice and Teach EBM.* Philadelphia: W. B. Saunders, 1997.

FAMILY MEDICINE

Goroll, Allan H., et al., eds. *Primary Care Medicine: Office Evaluation and Management of the Adult Patient.* 3d ed. Philadelphia: Lippincott Williams & Wilkins, 1995.

Graber, Mark A., et al., eds. *The Family Practice Handbook: University of Iowa.* 3d ed. St. Louis: C. V. Mosby, 1997.

Rakel, Robert E. *Textbook of Family Practice.* 5th ed. Philadelphia: W. B. Saunders, 1995.

_____, ed. *Essentials of Family Practice.* 2d ed. Philadelphia: W. B. Saunders, 1998.

Rudy, David R., and Kurt Kurbowski. *Family Medicine.* Philadelphia: Lippincott Williams & Wilkins, 1997.

Taylor, Robert B., et al., eds. *Family Medicine: Principles and Practice.* 5th ed. New York: Springer, 1998.

_____. *Manual of Family Practice.* Philadelphia: Lippincott Williams & Wilkins, 1997.

GASTROENTEROLOGY

Altschuler, Steven M., and Chris A. Liacouras. *Clinical Pediatric Gastroenterology.* Philadelphia: W. B. Saunders, 1998.

Castell, Donald O., ed. *The Esophagus.* 3d. ed. Philadelphia: Lippincott Williams & Wilkins, 1999.

Feldman, Mark, et al., eds. *Sleisenger and Fordtran's Gastrointestinal and Liver Disease: Pathophysiology/Diagnosis/Management.* 6th ed. Philadelphia: W. B. Saunders, 1998.

Friedman, Gerald, et al., eds. *Gastrointestinal Pharmacology and Therapeutics.* Philadelphia: Lippincott Williams & Wilkins, 1997.

Grendell, James H., et al., eds. *Current Diagnosis and Treatment in Gastroenterology.* Stamford, Conn.: Appleton & Lange, 1996.

Groher, Michael E., ed. *Dysphagia: Diagnosis and Management.* 3d ed. Boston: Butterworth-Heinemann, 1997.

Haubrich, William S., et al., eds. *Bockus Gastroenterology.* 5th ed. Philadelphia: W. B. Saunders, 1995.

Johanson, John F., ed. *Gastrointestinal Diseases: Risk Factors and Prevention.* Philadelphia: Lippincott Williams & Wilkins, 1997.

Kirsner, Joseph B., and Roy G. Shorter, eds. *Inflammatory Bowel Disease.* 4th ed. Philadelphia: Lippincott Williams & Wilkins, 1995.

Longo, Walter E., et al., eds. *Intestinal Ischemia Disorders: Pathophysiology and Management.* St. Louis: Quality Medical, 1999.

Lott, John A., ed. *Clinical Pathology of Pancreatic Disorders.* Totowa, N.J.: Humana Press, 1997.

Ming, Si-Chun, and Harvey Goldman, eds. *Pathology of the Gastrointestinal Tract*. 2d ed. Philadelphia: Lippincott Williams & Wilkins, 1998.

Schiff, Eugene R., et al., eds. *Schiff's Diseases of the Liver*. 8th ed. Philadelphia: Lippincott Williams & Wilkins, 1999.

Sherlock, Sheila, and James Dooley. *Diseases of the Liver and Biliary System*. 10th ed. Boston: Blackwell Science, 1997.

Silverstein, Fred E., and Guido N. J. Tytgat. *Gastrointestinal Endoscopy*. 3d ed. Boston: Blackwell Science, 1997.

Taylor, Mark B., ed. *Gastrointestinal Emergencies*. 2d ed. Philadelphia: Lippincott Williams & Wilkins, 1997.

Welch, John P., et al., eds. *Diverticular Disease: Management of the Difficult Surgical Case*. Philadelphia: Lippincott Williams & Wilkins, 1998.

Zakim, David, and Thomas D. Boyer, eds. *Hepatology: A Textbook of Liver Disease*. 3d ed. Philadelphia: W. B. Saunders, 1996.

GENETICS AND HEREDITY

Gelehrter, Thomas D., et al. *Principles of Medical Genetics*. 2d ed. Philadelphia: Lippincott Williams & Wilkins, 1998.

Jameson, J. Larry, ed. *Principles of Molecular Medicine*. Totowa, N.J.: Humana Press, 1998.

Jorde, Lynn B., et al. *Medical Genetics*. 2d ed. St. Louis: C. V. Mosby, 1999.

Korf, Bruce R. *Human Genetics: A Problem-Based Approach*. Boston: Blackwell Science, 1996.

McKusick, Victor A., et al. *Mendelian Inheritance in Man: A Catalog of Human Genes and Genetic Disorders*. 12th ed. Baltimore: The Johns Hopkins University Press, 1998.

Rimoin, David L., et al., eds. *Emery and Rimoin's Principles and Practice of Medical Genetics*. 3d ed. Philadelphia: W. B. Saunders, 1997.

Scriver, Charles R., et al., eds. *The Metabolic and Molecular Bases of Inherited Disease*. 7th ed. New York: McGraw-Hill, 1995.

Semenza, Gregg L. *Transcription Factors and Human Disease*. New York: Oxford University Press, 1998.

GERIATRICS

Cassel, Christine K., et al., eds. *Geriatric Medicine*. 3d ed. New York: Springer, 1997.

Duthie, Edmund H., Jr., and Paul R. Katz, eds. *Practice of Geriatrics*. 3d ed. Philadelphia: W. B. Saunders, 1998.

Gauthier, Serge, ed. *Clinical Diagnosis and Management of Alzheimer's Disease*. 2d ed. Boston: Butterworth-Heinemann, 1998.

Hazzard, William R., et al., eds. *Principles of Geriatric Medicine and Gerontology*. 4th ed. New York: McGraw-Hill, 1999.

Kaiser, Fran E., et al., eds. *Cardiovascular Disease in Older People*. New York: Springer, 1997.

Ouslander, Joseph G., et al. *Medical Care in the Nursing Home*. 2d ed. New York: McGraw-Hill, 1997.

Reichel, William, et al., eds. *Care of the Elderly: Clinical Aspects of Aging*. 4th ed. Philadelphia: Lippincott Williams & Wilkins, 1995.

Tallis, Raymond, et al., eds. *Brocklehurst's Textbook of Geriatric Medicine and Gerontology*. 5th ed. Philadelphia: W. B. Saunders, 1998.

Yoshikawa, Thomas T., et al., eds. *A Practical Ambulatory Geriatrics*. 2d ed. St. Louis: C. V. Mosby, 1998.

GYNECOLOGY AND OBSTETRICS

Altchek, Albert, and Liane Deligdisch, eds. *Diagnosis and Management of Ovarian Disorders*. New York: Igaku-Shoin, 1996.

Berek, Jonathan S., ed. *Novak's Gynecology*. 12th ed. Philadelphia: Lippincott Williams & Wilkins, 1996.

Bland, Kirby L., et al., eds. *The Breast: Comprehensive Management of Benign and Malignant Diseases*. 2d ed. Philadelphia: W. B. Saunders, 1998.

Briggs, Gerald G., et al. *Drugs in Pregnancy and Lactation: A Reference Guide to Fetal and Neonatal Risk*. 5th ed. Philadelphia: Lippincott Williams & Wilkins, 1998.

Burrow, Gerard N., and Thomas F. Ferris, eds. *Medical Complications During Pregnancy*. 5th ed. Philadelphia: W. B. Saunders, 1999.

Creasy, Robert K., and Robert Resnik. *Maternal-Fetal Medicine*. 4th ed. Philadelphia: W. B. Saunders, 1999.

Cunningham, F. Gary, et al. *Williams Obstetrics*. 20th ed. Stamford, Conn.: Appleton & Lange, 1997.

Curtis, Michele G., and Michael P. Hopkins, eds. *Glass's Office Gynecology*. 5th ed. Philadelphia: Lippincott Williams & Wilkins, 1999.

DeCherney, Alan H., and Martin L. Pernoll, eds. *Current Obstetric and Gynecologic Diagnosis and*

Treatment. 9th ed. Stamford, Conn.: Appleton & Lange, 1999.

DiSaia, Philip J., and William T. Creasman. *Clinical Gynecologic Oncology.* 5th ed. St. Louis: C. V. Mosby, 1997.

Emans, S., Jean Herriot, et al., eds. *Pediatric and Adolescent Gynecology.* 4th ed. Philadelphia: Lippincott Williams & Wilkins, 1998.

Foley, Michael R., and Thomas H. Strong, Jr., eds. *Obstetric Intensive Care: A Practical Manual.* Philadelphia: W. B. Saunders, 1997.

Gleicher, Norbert, ed. *Principles and Practice of Medical Therapy in Pregnancy.* 3d ed. Stamford, Conn.: Appleton & Lange, 1998.

Hacker, Neville F., and J. George Moore, eds. *Essentials of Obstetrics and Gynecology.* 3d ed. Philadelphia: W. B. Saunders, 1998.

Hulka, Jaroslav F., and Harry Reich. *Textbook of Laparoscopy.* 3d ed. Philadelphia: W. B. Saunders, 1998.

Lindsay, Robert, et al., eds. *Estrogens and Antiestrogens: Basic and Clinical Aspects.* Philadelphia: Lippincott Williams & Wilkins, 1997.

Mishell, Daniel R., Jr., et al. *Comprehensive Gynecology.* 3d ed. St. Louis: C. V. Mosby, 1997.

Niswander, Kenneth R., and Arthur T. Evans, eds. *Manual of Obstetrics.* 5th ed. Philadelphia: Lippincott Williams & Wilkins, 1996.

Rock, John A., and John D. Thompson, eds. *Te Linde's Operative Gynecology.* 8th ed. Philadelphia: Lippincott Williams & Wilkins, 1997.

Scott, James R., et al., eds. *Danforth's Obstetrics and Gynecology.* 8th ed. Philadelphia: Lippincott Williams & Wilkins, 1999.

Seibel, Machelle M., ed. *Infertility: A Comprehensive Text.* 2d ed. Stamford, Conn.: Appleton & Lange, 1997.

Speroff, Leon, et al. *Clinical Gynecologic Endocrinology and Infertility.* 6th ed. Philadelphia: Lippincott Williams & Wilkins, 1999.

Steege, John F., et al., eds. *Chronic Pelvic Pain: An Integrated Approach.* Philadelphia: W. B. Saunders, 1998.

Sweet, Richard L., and Ronald S. Gibbs. *Infectious Diseases of the Female Genital Tract.* 3d ed. Philadelphia: Lippincott Williams & Wilkins, 1995.

Wallis, Lila A., ed. *Textbook of Women's Health.* Philadelphia: Lippincott Williams & Wilkins, 1998.

Warren, Michelle P., and Mona M. Shangold. *Sports Gynecology: Problems and Care of the Athletic Female.* Boston: Blackwell Science, 1997.

HEMATOLOGY

Beutler, Ernest, et al., eds. *Williams Hematology.* 5th ed. New York: McGraw-Hill, 1995.

Embury, Stephen H., et al., eds. *Sickle Cell Disease: Basic Principles and Clinical Practice.* Philadelphia: Lippincott Williams & Wilkins, 1994.

Hillman, Robert S., and Kenneth A. Ault. *Hematology in Clinical Practice: A Guide to Diagnosis and Management.* 2d ed. New York: McGraw-Hill, 1998.

Hoffman, Ronald, et al., eds. *Hematology: Basic Principles and Practice.* 3d ed. Philadelphia: W. B. Saunders, 1999.

Jandl, James H. *Blood: Textbook of Hematology.* 2d ed. Philadelphia: Lippincott Williams & Wilkins, 1996.

Lee, G. Richard, et al., eds. *Wintrobe's Clinical Hematology.* 10th ed. Philadelphia: Lippincott Williams & Wilkins, 1999.

Miller, Denis R., et al., eds. *Blood Diseases of Infancy and Childhood: In the Tradition of C. H. Smith.* 7th ed. St. Louis: C. V. Mosby, 1995.

Nathan, David G., and Stuart H. Orkin, eds. *Nathan and Oski's Hematology of Infancy and Childhood.* 5th ed. Philadelphia: W. B. Saunders, 1998.

Spiess, Bruce D., et al., eds. *Perioperative Transfusion Medicine.* Philadelphia: Lippincott Williams & Wilkins, 1998.

Winslow, Robert M., et al., eds. *Blood Substitutes: New Challenges.* Boston: Birkhauser, 1996.

HOSPITALS AND ADMINISTRATION

American Hospital Association. *Hospital Statistics: The Source for Aggregate Data and Trend Analysis for U.S. Community Hospitals—Nonfederal, Short-Term General, and Other Special Hospitals.* Chicago: Author, 1999.

Binstock, Robert H., et al., eds. *The Future of Long-Term Care: Social and Policy Issues.* Baltimore: The Johns Hopkins University Press, 1996.

Bodenheimer, Thomas S., and Kevin Grumbach. *Understanding Health Policy: A Clinical Approach.* 2d ed. Stamford, Conn.: Appleton & Lange, 1998.

Cleverley, William O. *Essentials of Health Care Finance.* 4th ed. Gaithersburg, Md.: Aspen, 1997.

Joint Commission on Accreditation of Healthcare Organizations. *Comprehensive Accreditation Manual for Hospitals: The Official Handbook: Accreditation Policies, Standards, Scoring, Aggregation Rules, Decision Rules.* Oakbrook Terrace, Ill.: Author, 1999.

Kavaler, Florence, and Allen D. Spiegel. *Risk Management in Health Care Institutions: A Strategic Approach.* Boston: Jones and Bartlett, 1997.

Kovner, Anthony R., ed. *Jonas and Kovner's Health Care Delivery in the United States.* 6th ed. New York: Springer, 1999.

Langlais, K. J. *Managing with Integrity for Long Term Care: The Key to Success for Building Stability in Staffing.* New York: McGraw-Hill, 1997.

Longest, Beaufort B., Jr. *Health Professionals in Management.* Stamford, Conn.: Appleton & Lange, 1996.

McConnell, Charles R. *The Effective Health Care Supervisor.* 4th ed. Gaithersburg, Md.: Aspen, 1997.

Shi, Leiyu, and Douglas A. Singh. *Delivering Health Care in America: A Systems Approach.* Gaithersburg, Md.: Aspen, 1998.

Sultz, Harry A., and Kristina M. Young. *Health Care USA: Understanding Its Organization and Delivery.* Gaithersburg, Md.: Aspen, 1997.

Wolper, Lawrence F., ed. *Health Care Administration: Planning, Implementing, and Managing Organized Delivery Systems.* 3d ed. Gaithersburg, Md.: Aspen, 1999.

IMMUNOLOGY

Frank, Michael M., et al., eds. *Samter's Immunologic Diseases.* 5th ed. Philadelphia: Lippincott Williams & Wilkins, 1995.

Paul, William E. ed. *Fundamental Immunology.* 4th ed. Philadelphia: Lippincott Williams & Wilkins, 1999.

Roitt, Ivan M. *Roitt's Essential Immunology.* 9th ed. Boston: Blackwell Science, 1997.

Roitt, Ivan M., et al., eds. *Immunology.* 5th ed. St. Louis: C. V. Mosby: 1998.

Rose, Noel R., et al., eds. *Manual of Clinical Laboratory Immunology.* 5th ed. Washington, D.C.: American Society for Microbiology, 1997.

Stiehm, E. Richard. *Immunologic Disorders in Infants and Children.* 4th ed. Philadelphia: W. B. Saunders, 1996.

Stites, Daniel P., et al., eds. *Medical Immunology.* 9th ed. Stamford, Conn.: Appleton & Lange, 1997.

INFECTIOUS DISEASES

Benenson, Abram S., ed. *Control of Communicable Diseases Manual: An Official Report of the American Public Health Association.* 16th ed. Washington, D.C.: American Public Health Association, 1995.

Bennett, John V., and Philip S. Brachman, eds. *Hospital Infections.* 4th ed. Philadelphia: Lippincott Williams & Wilkins, 1998.

Connor, Daniel H., et al., eds. *Pathology of Infectious Diseases.* Stamford, Conn.: Appleton & Lange, 1997.

Feigin, Ralph D., and James D. Cherry, eds. *Textbook of Pediatric Infectious Diseases.* 4th ed. Philadelphia: W. B. Saunders, 1998.

Fein, Alan M., et al., eds. *Sepsis and Multiorgan Failure.* Philadelphia: Lippincott Williams & Wilkins, 1997.

Gorbach, Sherwood L., et al., eds. *Infectious Diseases.* 2d ed. Philadelphia: W. B. Saunders, 1998.

Horsburgh, C. Robert, Jr., and Ann Marie Nelson, eds. *Pathology of Emerging Infections.* Washington, D.C.: American Society for Microbiology, 1997.

Katz, Samuel L., et al., eds. *Krugman's Infectious Diseases of Children.* 10th ed. St. Louis: C. V. Mosby, 1998.

Mandell, Gerald L., et al., eds. *Mandell, Douglas, and Bennett's Principles and Practice of Infectious Diseases.* 4th ed. Philadelphia: W. B. Saunders, 1995.

Plotkin, Stanley A., and Edward A. Mortimer, Jr. *Vaccines.* 3d ed. Philadelphia: W. B. Saunders, 1999.

Reese, Richard E., and Robert F. Betts, eds. *A Practical Approach to Infectious Diseases.* 4th ed. Philadelphia: Lippincott Williams & Wilkins, 1996.

Remington, Jack S., and Jerome O. Klein, eds. *Infectious Diseases of the Fetus and Newborn Infant.* 4th ed. Philadelphia: W. B. Saunders, 1995.

Schlager, Seymour I. *Clinical Management of Infectious Diseases: A Guide to Diagnosis and Therapy.* Philadelphia: Lippincott Williams & Wilkins, 1998.

Shulman, Stanford T., et al., eds. *The Biologic and Clinical Basis of Infectious Diseases.* 5th ed. Philadelphia: W. B. Saunders, 1997.

INTERNAL MEDICINE

Andreoli, Thomas E., et al. *Cecil Essentials of Medicine.* 4th ed. Philadelphia: W. B. Saunders, 1997.

Bennett, J. Claude, and Fred Plum, eds. *Cecil Textbook of Medicine.* 20th ed. Philadelphia: W. B. Saunders, 1996.

Fauci, Anthony S., et al., eds. *Harrison's Principles of Internal Medicine.* 14th ed. New York: McGraw-Hill, 1998.

Ferri, Fred F. *Practical Guide to the Care of the Medical Patient.* 4th ed. St. Louis: C. V. Mosby, 1998.

Fihn, Stephan D., and Dawn E. DeWitt, eds. *Outpatient Medicine.* 2d ed. Philadelphia: W. B. Saunders, 1998.

Fishman, Mark C., et al. *Medicine.* 4th ed. Philadelphia: Lippincott Williams & Wilkins, 1996.

Gross, Richard J., and Gregory M. Caputo, eds. *Kammerer and Gross' Medical Consultation: The Internist on Surgical, Obstetric, and Psychiatric Services.* 3d ed. Philadelphia: Lippincott Williams & Wilkins, 1998.

Harrington, John T. *Consultation in Internal Medicine.* 2d ed. St. Louis: C. V. Mosby, 1997.

Hurst, John Willis, et al., eds. *Medicine for the Practicing Physician.* 4th ed. Stamford, Conn.: Appleton & Lange, 1996.

Kelley, William N., et al., eds. *Textbook of Internal Medicine.* 3d ed. Philadelphia: Lippincott Williams & Wilkins, 1997.

Rubenstein, Edward, and Daniel D. Federman, eds. *Scientific American Medicine.* New York: Scientific American, 1999.

Stein, Jay H., ed. *Internal Medicine.* 5th ed. St. Louis: C. V. Mosby, 1998.

Stobo, John D., et al., eds. *The Principles and Practice of Medicine.* 23d ed. Stamford, Conn.: Appleton & Lange, 1996.

Tierney, Lawrence M., et al., eds. *Current Medical Diagnosis and Treatment 2000.* 39th ed. Stamford, Conn.: Appleton & Lange, 2000.

Washington University School of Medicine, Department of Medicine. *The Washington Manual of Medical Therapeutics.* 29th ed. Philadelphia: Lippincott Williams & Wilkins, 1998.

LABORATORY METHODS

Dufour, D. Robert. *Clinical Use of Laboratory Data: A Practical Guide.* Philadelphia: Lippincott Williams & Wilkins, 1998.

Fenton, John. *The Laboratory and the Poisoned Patient: A Guidebook for Interpreting Laboratory Data.* Washington, D.C.: AACC Press, 1998.

Henry, John Bernard, ed. *Clinical Diagnosis and Management by Laboratory Methods.* 19th ed. Philadelphia: W. B. Saunders, 1996.

Ravel, Richard. *Clinical Laboratory Medicine: Clinical Application of Laboratory Data.* 6th ed. St. Louis: C. V. Mosby, 1995.

Sacher, Ronald A. *Widmann's Clinical Interpretation of Laboratory Tests.* 11th ed. Philadelphia: Davis, 1999.

Wallach, Jacques. *Interpretation of Diagnostic Tests.* 6th ed. Philadelphia: Lippincott Williams & Wilkins, 1996.

LEGAL MEDICINE

American College of Legal Medicine. *Legal Medicine.* 4th ed. St. Louis: C. V. Mosby, 1998.

Miller, Robert D. *Problems in Health Care Law.* 7th ed. Gaithersburg, Md.: Aspen, 1996.

Pozgar, George D., and Nina Santucci Pozgar. *Legal Aspects of Health Care Administration.* 7th ed. Gaithersburg, Md.: Aspen, 1999.

Tsushima, William T., and Kenneth K. Nakano. *Effective Medical Testifying: A Handbook for Physicians.* Boston: Butterworth-Heinemann, 1998.

MANAGED CARE

Halverson, Paul K., et al., eds. *Managed Care and Public Health.* Gaithersburg, Md.: Aspen, 1998.

Herzlinger, Regina E. *Market-Driven Health Care: Who Wins, Who Loses in the Transformation of America's Largest Service Industry.* Reading, Mass.: Addison-Wesley, 1997.

Knight, Wendy. *Managed Care: What It Is and How It Works.* Gaithersburg, Md.: Aspen, 1998.

Kongstvedt, Peter R., ed. *Essentials of Managed Health Care.* 2d ed. Gaithersburg, Md.: Aspen, 1997

Patterson, Dennis J. *Indexing Managed Care: Benchmarking Strategies for Assessing Managed Care Penetration in Your Market.* New York: McGraw-Hill, 1997.

Saxton, James W., and Thomas L. Leaman. *Managed Care Success: Reducing Risk While Increasing Patient Satisfaction.* Gaithersburg, Md.: Aspen, 1998.

MEDICAL INFORMATICS

Berner, Eta S., ed. *Clinical Decision Support Systems: Theory and Practice.* New York: Springer, 1999.

Friedman, Charles P., and Jeremy C. Wyatt. *Evaluation Methods in Medical Informatics.* New York: Springer, 1997.

Goodman, Kenneth W. *Ethics, Computing, and Medicine: Informatics and the Transformation of Health Care.* New York: Cambridge University Press, 1998.

Smith, Roger P., and Margaret J. A. Edwards. *The Internet for Physicians*. 2d ed. New York: Springer, 1999.

MICROBIOLOGY

Baron, Samuel, ed. *Medical Microbiology*. 4th ed. Galveston: University of Texas Medical Branch, 1996.

Brooks, George F., et al. *Jawetz, Melnick, and Adelberg's Medical Microbiology*. 21st ed. Stamford, Conn.: Appleton & Lange, 1998.

Evans, Alfred S., and Richard A. Kaslow, eds. *Viral Infections of Humans: Epidemiology and Control*. 4th ed. New York: Plenum, 1997.

Garcia, Lynne Shore, and David A. Bruckner. *Diagnostic Medical Parasitology*. 3d ed. Washington, D.C.: ASM Press, 1997.

Isenberg, Henry D., ed. *Essential Procedures for Clinical Microbiology*. Washington, D.C.: ASM Press, 1998.

Koneman, Elmer W., et al. *Color Atlas and Textbook of Diagnostic Microbiology*. 5th ed. Philadelphia: Lippincott Williams & Wilkins, 1997.

Murray, Patrick R., et al. *Medical Microbiology*. 3d ed. St. Louis: C. V. Mosby, 1998.

Murray, Patrick R., et al., eds. *Manual of Clinical Microbiology*. 7th ed. Washington, D.C.: ASM Press, 1999.

NEUROLOGY

Adams, Raymond D., et al. *Principles of Neurology*. 6th ed. New York: McGraw-Hill, 1997.

Barnett, Gene H., et al., eds. *Image-Guided Neurosurgery: Clinical Applications of Surgical Navigation*. St. Louis: Quality Medical, 1998.

Biller, José, ed. *Iatrogenic Neurology*. Boston: Butterworth-Heinemann, 1998.

Castillo, Mauricio. *Neuroradiology Companion: Methods, Guidelines, and Imaging Fundamentals*. 2d ed. Philadelphia: Lippincott Williams & Wilkins, 1999.

Engel, Jerome, Jr., and Timothy A. Pedley, eds. *Epilepsy: A Comprehensive Textbook*. Philadelphia: Lippincott Williams & Wilkins, 1998.

Feldman, Robert G. *Occupational and Environmental Neurotoxicology*. Philadelphia: Lippincott Williams & Wilkins, 1999.

Gilman, Sid, and Sarah Winans Newman. *Manter and Gatz's Essentials of Clinical Neroanatomy and Neurophysiology*. 9th ed. Philadelphia: Davis, 1996.

Jankovic, Joseph, and Eduardo Tolosa, eds. *Parkinson's Disease and Movement Disorders*. 3d ed. Philadelphia: Lippincott Williams & Wilkins, 1998.

Keane, Robert W., and William F. Hickey, eds. *Immunology of the Nervous System*. New York: Oxford University Press, 1997.

Low, Phillip A., ed. *Clinical Autonomic Disorders: Evaluation and Management*. 2d ed. Philadelphia: Lippincott Williams & Wilkins, 1997.

Menkes, John H. *Textbook of Child Neurology*. 5th ed. Philadelphia: Lippincott Williams & Wilkins, 1995.

Niedermeyer, Ernst, and Fernando Lopes da Silva, eds. *Electroencephalography: Basic Principles, Clinical Applications and Related Fields*. 4th ed. Philadelphia: Lippincott Williams & Wilkins, 1999.

Rowland, Lewis P., ed. *Merritt's Textbook of Neurology*. 9th ed. Philadelphia: Lippincott Williams & Wilkins, 1995.

Scheld, W. Michael, et al., eds. *Infections of the Central Nervous System*. 2d ed. Philadelphia: Lippincott Williams & Wilkins, 1997.

Siegel, George J., et al., eds. *Basic Neurochemistry: Molecular, Cellular, and Medical Aspects*. 6th ed. Philadelphia: Lippincott Williams & Wilkins, 1998.

Waxman, Stephen G. *Correlative Neuroanatomy*. 24th ed. Stamford, Conn.: Appleton & Lange, 1999.

Young, G. Bryan, et al., eds. *Coma and Impaired Consciousness: A Clinical Perspective*. New York: McGraw-Hill, 1998.

NURSING

Hill, Dorothy R., and Henry N. Stickell, "Brandon/Hill Selected List of Print Nursing Books and Journals," Nursing Outlook 48, no. 1 (January/February, 2000): 10-22.

NUTRITION

Bendich, Adrianne, and Richard J. Deckelbaum. *Preventive Nutrition: The Comprehensive Guide for Health Professionals*. Totowa, N.J.: Humana Press, 1997.

Buchman, Alan. *Handbook of Nutritional Support*. Philadelphia: Lippincott Williams & Wilkins, 1997.

Heimburger, Douglas C., and Roland L. Weinster. *Handbook of Clinical Nutrition*. 3d ed. St. Louis: C. V. Mosby, 1997.

National Research Council. *Recommended Dietary*

Allowances. 10th ed. Washington, D.C.: National Academy Press, 1989.

Pennington, Jean A. T. *Bowes and Church's Food Values of Portions Commonly Used.* 17th ed. Philadelphia: Lippincott Williams & Wilkins, 1998.

Rombeau, John L., and Rolando Rolandelli. *Clinical Nutrition: Enteral and Tube Feeding.* 3d ed. Philadelphia: W. B. Saunders, 1997.

Shils, Maurice E., et al., eds. *Modern Nutrition in Health and Disease.* 9th ed. Philadelphia: Lippincott Williams & Wilkins, 1998.

ONCOLOGY

American Joint Committee on Cancer. *AJCC Cancer Staging Manual.* 5th ed. Philadelphia: Lippincott Williams & Wilkins, 1997.

Andrassy, Richard J. *Pediatric Surgical Oncology.* Philadelphia: W. B. Saunders, 1998.

Balch, Charles M., et al., eds. *Cutaneous Melanoma.* 3d ed. St. Louis: Quality Medical, 1998.

DeVita, Vincent T., Jr., et al., eds. *Cancer: Principles and Practice of Oncology.* 5th ed. Philadelphia: Lippincott Williams & Wilkins, 1997.

Donegan, William L., and John S. Spratt, eds. *Cancer of the Breast.* 4th ed. Philadelphia: W. B. Saunders, 1995.

Fischer, David S., et al. *The Cancer Chemotherapy Handbook.* 5th ed. St. Louis: C. V. Mosby, 1997.

Henderson, Edward S., et al., eds. *Leukemia.* 6th ed. Philadelphia: W. B. Saunders, 1996.

Holland, James F., et al., eds. *Cancer Medicine.* 4th ed. Philadelphia: Lippincott Williams & Wilkins, 1997.

Hoskins, William J., et al., eds. *Principles and Practice of Gynecologic Oncology.* 2d ed. Philadelphia: Lippincott Williams & Wilkins, 1997.

Isaacs, Hart, Jr. *Tumors of the Fetus and Newborn.* Philadelphia: W. B. Saunders, 1997.

Johnson, Frank E., et al. *Cancer Patient Follow-up.* St. Louis: C. V. Mosby, 1997.

Levesque, Jerome, et al. *A Clinical Guide to Primary Bone Tumors.* Philadelphia: Lippincott Williams & Wilkins, 1998.

Meyers, Morton A., ed. *Neoplasms of the Digestive Tract: Imaging, Staging, and Management.* Philadelphia: Lippincott Williams & Wilkins, 1998.

Myers, Eugene N., and James Y. Suen, eds. *Cancer of the Head and Neck.* 3d ed. Philadelphia: W. B. Saunders, 1996.

Oesterling, Joseph E., and Jerome P. Richie, eds.

Urologic Oncology. Philadelphia: W. B. Saunders, 1997.

Pizzo, Philip A., and David G. Poplack, eds. *Principles and Practice of Pediatric Oncology.* 3d ed. Philadelphia: Lippincott Williams & Wilkins, 1997.

Schottenfeld, David, and Joseph F. Fraumeni, Jr., eds. *Cancer Epidemiology and Prevention.* 2d ed. New York: Oxford University Press, 1996.

OPHTHALMOLOGY

Apple, David, and Maurice F. Rabb. *Ocular Pathology: Clinical Applications and Self-Assessment.* 5th ed. St. Louis: C. V. Mosby, 1998.

Elander, Richard, et al. *Principles and Practice of Refractive Surgery.* Philadelphia: W. B. Saunders, 1997.

Epstein, David, ed. *Chandler and Grant's Glaucoma.* 4th ed. Philadelphia: Lippincott Williams & Wilkins, 1997.

Jaffe, Norman S., et al. *Cataract Surgery and Its Complications.* 6th ed. St. Louis: C. V. Mosby, 1997.

Kaufman, Herbert E., et al., eds. *The Cornea.* 2d ed. Boston: Butterworth-Heinemann, 1998.

MacCumber, Mathew W., ed. *Management of Ocular Injuries and Emergencies.* Philadelphia: Lippincott Williams & Wilkins, 1998.

Nelson, Leonard B., ed. *Harley's Pediatric Ophthalmology.* 4th ed. Philadelphia: W. B. Saunders, 1998.

Newell, Frank W. *Ophthalmology: Principles and Concepts.* 8th ed. St. Louis: C. V. Mosby, 1996.

Regillo, Carl D., and William E. Benson. *Retinal Detachment: Diagnosis and Management.* 3d ed. Philadelphia: Lippincott Williams & Wilkins, 1998.

Roy, Frederick Hampton. *Ocular Differential Diagnosis.* 6th ed. Philadelphia: Lippincott Williams & Wilkins, 1997.

Sassani, Joseph W., ed. *Ophthalmic Pathology with Clinical Correlations.* Philadelphia: Lippincott Williams & Wilkins, 1997.

Shields, M. Bruce. *Textbook of Glaucoma.* 4th ed. Philadelphia: Lippincott Williams & Wilkins, 1998.

Varma, Rohit. *Essentials of Eye Care: The Johns Hopkins Wilmer Handbook.* Philadelphia: Lippincott Williams & Wilkins, 1997.

Vaughan, Daniel, et al. *General Ophthalmology.* 15th ed. Stamford, Conn.: Appleton & Lange, 1998.

Walsh, Thomas J., ed. *Walsh and Hoyt's Clinical Neuro-Ophthalmology: The Essentials.* 5th ed. Philadelphia: Lippincott Williams & Wilkins, 1999.

Zimmerman, Thom J., et al., eds. *Textbook of Ocular*

Pharmacology. Philadelphia: Lippincott Williams & Wilkins, 1997.

ORIENTAL MEDICINE
Alphen, Jan Val, and Anthony Aris, eds. *Oriental Medicine: An Illustrated Guide to the Asian Arts of Healing.* Boston: Shambhala, 1996.

ORTHOPEDICS
Borenstein, David G., et al. *Low Back Pain: Medical Diagnosis and Comprehensive Management.* 2d ed. Philadelphia: W. B. Saunders, 1995.

Bradford, David S., ed. *The Spine.* Philadelphia: Lippincott Williams & Wilkins, 1997.

Callaghan, John J., et al., eds. *The Adult Hip.* Philadelphia: Lippincott Williams & Wilkins, 1998.

Canale, S. Terry, ed. *Campbell's Operative Orthopaedics.* 9th ed. St. Louis: C. V. Mosby, 1998.

Cooney, William P., et al., eds. *The Wrist: Diagnosis and Operative Treatment.* St. Louis: C. V. Mosby, 1998.

Dee, Roger, et al. *Principles of Orthopaedic Practice.* 2d ed. New York: McGraw-Hill, 1997.

Greenspan, Adam, and Wolfgang Remagen. *Differential Diagnosis of Tumors and Tumor-Like Lesions of Bones and Joints.* Philadelphia: Lippincott Williams & Wilkins, 1998.

Koval, Kenneth J., and Joseph D. Zuckerman, eds. *Fractures in the Elderly.* Philadelphia: Lippincott Williams & Wilkins, 1998.

Lonstein, John E., et al. *Moe's Textbook of Scoliosis and Other Spinal Deformities.* 3d ed. Philadelphia: Lippincott Williams & Wilkins, 1995.

McCarthy, Edward F., and Frank J. Frassica. *Pathology of Bone and Joint Disorders with Clinical and Radiographic Correlation.* Philadelphia: W. B. Saunders, 1998.

Morrissy, Raymond T., and Stuart L. Weinstein, eds. *Lovell and Winter's Pediatric Orthopaedics.* 4th ed. Philadelphia: Lippincott Williams & Wilkins, 1996.

Riggs, B. Lawrence, and L. Joseph Melton III, eds. *Osteoporosis: Etiology, Diagnosis, and Management.* 2d ed. Philadelphia: Lippincott Williams & Wilkins, 1995.

Rockwood, Charles A., Jr., et al., eds. *Rockwood and Green's Fractures in Adults.* 4th ed. Philadelphia: Lippincott Williams & Wilkins, 1996.

Rockwood, Charles A., Jr., and Frederick Matsen III. *The Shoulder.* 2d ed. Philadelphia: W. B. Saunders, 1998.

OTORHINOLARYNGOLOGY
Ballenger, John Jacob, and James B. Snow, Jr., eds. *Otorhinolaryngology: Head and Neck Surgery.* 5th ed. Philadelphia: Lippincott Williams & Wilkins, 1996.

Baloh, Robert W. *Dizziness, Hearing Loss, and Tinnitus.* Philadelphia: Davis, 1998.

Bluestone, Charles D., et al., eds. *Pediatric Otolaryngology.* 3d ed. Philadelphia: W. B. Saunders, 1996.

Donald, Paul J., et al., eds. *The Sinuses.* Philadelphia: Lippincott Williams & Wilkins, 1995.

Fried, Marvin P., ed. *The Larynx: A Multidisciplinary Approach.* 2d ed. St. Louis: C. V. Mosby, 1996.

Hughes, Gordon B., et al., eds. *Clinical Otology.* 2d ed. New York: Thieme, 1997.

Johnson, Jonas T., and Victor L. Yu, eds. *Infectious Diseases and Antimicrobial Therapy of the Ears, Nose, and Throat.* Philadelphia: W. B. Saunders, 1997.

Lucente, Frank E., and Steven M. Sobol, eds. *Essentials of Otolaryngology.* 4th ed. Philadelphia: Lippincott Williams & Wilkins, 1999.

McCaffrey, Thomas V. *Rhinologic Diagnosis and Treatment.* New York: Thieme, 1997.

Myers, Eugene N., ed. *Operative Otolaryngology: Head and Neck Surgery.* Philadelphia: W. B. Saunders, 1997.

PALLIATIVE CARE
Doyle, Derek, et al., eds. *Oxford Textbook of Palliative Medicine.* 2d ed. New York: Oxford University Press, 1998.

Dunlop, Robert. *Cancer: Palliative Care.* New York: Springer, 1998.

Faull, Christina, et al., eds. *Handbook of Palliative Care.* Boston: Blackwell Science, 1998.

MacDonald, Neil, et al., eds. *Palliative Medicine: A Case-Based Manual.* New York: Oxford University Press, 1998.

Randall, Fiona, and R. S. Downie. *Palliative Care Ethics: A Good Companion.* New York: Oxford University Press, 1996.

PATHOLOGY
Atkinson, Barbara F., and Jan F. Silverman. *Atlas of Difficult Diagnoses in Cytopathology.* Philadelphia: W. B. Saunders, 1998.

Bibbo, Marluce, ed. *Comprehensive Cytopathology.* 2d ed. Philadelphia: W. B. Saunders, 1997.

Cotran, Ramzi S., et al., eds. *Robbins Pathologic Basis of Diseases.* 6th ed. Philadelphia: W. B. Saunders, 1999.

Damjanov, Ivan, and James Linder, eds. *Anderson's Pathology.* 10th ed. St. Louis: C. V. Mosby, 1996.

Hasleton, Philip Simon. *Spencer's Pathology of the Lung.* 5th ed. New York: McGraw-Hill, 1996.

Jennette, J. Charles, et al., eds. *Heptinstall's Pathology of the Kidney.* 5th ed. Philadelphia: Lippincott Williams & Wilkins, 1998.

Majno, Guido, and Isabelle Joris. *Cells, Tissues, and Disease: Principles of General Pathology.* Boston: Blackwell Science, 1996.

Milikowski, Clara, and Irwin Berman. *Color Atlas of Basic Histopathology.* Stamford, Conn.: Appleton & Lange, 1997.

Rosal, Juan. *Ackerman's Surgical Pathology.* 8th ed. St. Louis: C. V. Mosby, 1996.

Sternberg, Stephen S., et al., eds. *Diagnostic Surgical Pathology.* 3d ed. Philadelphia: Lippincott Williams & Wilkins, 1999.

Stocker, J. Thomas, and Louis P. Dehner, eds. *Pediatric Pathology.* 2d ed. Philadelphia: Lippincott Williams & Wilkins, 1998.

Wick, Mark R., et al., eds. *Pathology of Pseudoneoplastic Lesions.* Philadelphia: Lippincott Williams & Wilkins, 1997.

Zaino, Richard J. *Interpretation of Endometrial Biopsies and Curettings.* Philadelphia: Lippincott Williams & Wilkins, 1996.

PATIENT EDUCATION

Bartlett, John G., and Ann K. Finkbeiner. *The Guide to Living with HIV Infection: Developed at the Johns Hopkins AIDS Clinic.* 4th ed. Baltimore: The Johns Hopkins University Press, 1998.

Berkow, Robert, ed. *The Merck Manual of Medical Information.* Whitehouse Station, N.J.: Merck, 1997.

Blaivas, Jerry G. *Conquering Bladder and Prostate Problems: The Authoritative Guide for Men and Women.* New York: Plenum, 1998.

Buckman, Robert. *What You Really Need to Know About Cancer: A Comprehensive Guide for Patients and Their Families.* Baltimore: The Johns Hopkins University Press, 1997.

Duvoisin, Roger C., and Jacob Sage. *Parkinson's Disease: A Guide for Patient and Family.* 4th ed. Philadelphia: Lippincott Williams & Wilkins, 1996.

Moore, Stephen W. *Griffith's Instructions for Patients.* 6th ed. Philadelphia: W. B. Saunders, 1998.

Muma, Richard D., et al., eds. *Patient Education: A Practical Approach.* Stamford, Conn.: Appleton & Lange, 1996.

Saudek, Christopher D., et al. *The Johns Hopkins Guide to Diabetes: For Today and Tomorrow.* Baltimore: The Johns Hopkins University Press, 1997.

PEDIATRICS

Barness, Lewis A. *Handbook of Pediatric Physical Diagnosis.* Philadelphia: Lippincott Williams & Wilkins, 1998.

Barone, Michael A., ed. *The Harriet Lane Handbook: A Manual for Pediatric House Officers.* 14th ed. St. Louis: C. V. Mosby, 1996.

Baskin, Laurence S., et al., eds. *Handbook of Pediatric Urology.* Philadelphia: Lippincott Williams & Wilkins, 1997.

Behrman, Richard E., et al., eds. *Nelson Textbook of Pediatrics.* 15th ed. Philadelphia: W. B. Saunders, 1996.

Burg, Fredric D., et al. *Gellis and Kagan's Current Pediatric Therapy 16.* Philadelphia: W. B. Saunders, 1999.

Cloherty, John P., and Ann R. Stark, eds. *Manual of Neonatal Care.* 4th ed. Philadelphia: Lippincott Williams & Wilkins, 1998.

Fanaroff, Avroy A., and Richard J. Martin, eds. *Neonatal-Perinatal Medicine: Diseases of the Fetus and Infant.* 6th ed. St. Louis: C. V. Mosby, 1997.

Feld, Leonard G. *Hypertension in Children: A Practical Approach.* Boston: Butterworth-Heinemann, 1997.

Finberg, Laurence. *Saunders Manual of Pediatric Practice.* Philadelphia: W. B. Saunders, 1998.

Fletcher, Mary Ann. *Physical Diagnosis in Neonatology.* Philadelphia: Lippincott Williams & Wilkins, 1998.

Friedman, Stanford B., et al., eds. *Comprehensive Adolescent Health Care.* 2d ed. St. Louis: C. V. Mosby, 1998.

Gomella, Tricia Lacy, et al., eds. *Neonatology: Management, Procedures, On-Call Problems, Diseases, and Drugs.* 4th ed. Stamford, Conn.: Appleton & Lange, 1999.

Hay, William W., Jr., et al., eds. *Current Pediatric Diagnosis and Treatment.* 14th ed. Stamford, Conn.: Appleton & Lange, 1999.

Hoekelman, Robert A., et al., eds. *Primary Pediatric Care.* 3d ed. St. Louis: C. V. Mosby, 1997.

Jones, Kenneth Lyons. *Smith's Recognizable Patterns*

of Human Malformation. 5th ed. Philadelphia: W. B. Saunders, 1997.

Kemper, Kathi. *The Holistic Pediatrician: A Parent's Comprehensive Guide to Safe and Effective Therapies for the Twenty-five Most Common Childhood Ailments.* New York: Harper Perennial, 1996.

Long, Sarah S., et al., eds. *Principles and Practice of Pediatric Infectious Diseases.* Philadelphia: W. B. Saunders, 1997.

Merenstein, Gerald B., et al. *Handbook of Pediatrics.* 18th ed. Stamford, Conn.: Appleton & Lange, 1997.

Monteleone, James A., ed. *Child Maltreatment.* 2d ed. St. Louis: G. W. Medical, 1998.

Rudolph, Abraham M., et al., eds. *Rudolph's Pediatrics.* 20th ed. Stamford, Conn.: Appleton & Lange, 1996.

Taeusch, H. William, and Roberta A. Ballard, eds. *Avery's Diseases of the Newborn.* 7th ed. Philadelphia: W. B. Saunders, 1998.

Wyllie, Robert, et al., eds. *Pediatric Gastrointestinal Disease.* Philadelphia: W. B. Saunders, 1999.

Yaster, Myron, et al., eds. *Pediatric Pain Management and Sedation Handbook.* St. Louis: C. V. Mosby, 1997.

PHARMACOLOGY AND THERAPEUTICS

Bressler, Rubin, and Michael D. Katz, eds. *Geriatric Pharmacology.* New York: McGraw-Hill, 2000.

Brody, Theodore M., et al., eds. *Human Pharmacology: Molecular to Clinical.* 3d ed. St. Louis: C. V. Mosby, 1998.

Brust, John C. M. *Neurotoxic Side Effects to Prescription Drugs.* Boston: Butterworth-Heinemann, 1996.

Craig, Charles R., and Robert E. Stitzel, eds. *Modern Pharmacology: With Clinical Applications.* 5th ed. Philadelphia: Lippincott Williams & Wilkins, 1997.

Drug Facts and Comparisons. St. Louis: Facts and Comparisons, 2000.

Hansten, Philip D., and John R. Horn. *Hansten and Horn's Drug Interactions, Analysis, and Management.* Vancouver, Wash.: Applied Therapeutics, 2001.

Hardman, Joel Griffith, et al., eds. *Goodman and Gilman's The Pharmacological Basis of Therapeutics.* 9th ed. New York: McGraw-Hill, 1996.

Katzung, Bertram G., ed. *Basic and Clinical Pharmacology.* 7th ed. Stamford, Conn.: Appleton & Lange, 1998.

Keltner, Norman L., and David G. Folks. *Psycho-tropic Drugs.* 2d ed. St. Louis: C. V. Mosby, 1997.

McCormack, James, et al., eds. *Drug Therapy: Decision Making Guide.* Philadelphia: W. B. Saunders, 1996.

Mosby's GenRx 1999: The Complete Reference for Generic and Brand Drugs. 9th ed. St. Louis: C. V. Mosby, 1999.

PDR: Physicians' Desk Reference. 54th ed. Montvale, N.J.: Medical Economics Data, 2000.

Physicians Desk Reference for Nonprescription Drugs and Dietary Supplements. 21st ed. Montvale, N.J.: Medical Economics Data, 2000.

Rakel, Robert E., ed. *Conn's Current Therapy 2000: Latest Approved Methods of Treatment for the Practicing Physician.* Philadelphia: W. B. Saunders, 2000.

United States Pharmacopeial Convention. *USP DI 2000.* 20th ed. Rockville, Md.: Author, 2000.

Youngkin, Ellis Quinn, et al., eds. *Pharmacotherapeutics: A Primary Care Clinical Guide.* Stamford, Conn.: Appleton & Lange, 1999.

Zucchero, Frederic J., et al., eds. *Evaluations of Drug Interactions.* St. Louis: First Data Bank, 2000.

PHYSICAL MEDICINE AND REHABILITATION

Basmajian, John V., and Sikhar N. Banerjee, eds. *Clinical Decision Making in Rehabilitation: Efficacy and Outcomes.* Philadelphia: W. B. Saunders, 1996.

Cassvan, Arminus, et al. *Cumulative Trauma Disorders.* Boston: Butterworth-Heinemann, 1997.

DeLisa, Joel A., et al., eds. *Rehabilitation Medicine: Principles and Practice.* 3d ed. Philadelphia: Lippincott Williams & Wilkins, 1998.

Johnson, Ernest W., and William S. Pease. *Practical Electromyography.* 3d ed. Philadelphia: Lippincott Williams & Wilkins, 1997.

Lazar, Richard B., ed. *Principles of Neurologic Rehabilitation.* New York: McGraw-Hill, 1998.

Tan, Jackson C. *Practical Manual of Physical Medicine and Rehabilitation: Diagnostics, Therapeutics, and Basic Problems.* St. Louis: C. V. Mosby, 1998.

PHYSIOLOGY

Berne, Robert M., and Matthew N. Levy, eds. *Physiology.* 4th ed. St. Louis: C. V. Mosby, 1998.

Ganong, William F. *Review of Medical Physiology.* 19th ed. Stamford, Conn.: Appleton & Lange, 1999.

Guyton, Arthur C., and John E. Hall. *Textbook of*

Medical Physiology. 9th ed. Philadelphia: W. B. Saunders, 1996.

Johnson, Leonard R., ed. *Essential Medical Physiology.* 2d ed. Philadelphia: Lippincott Williams & Wilkins, 1998.

PREVENTIVE MEDICINE AND PUBLIC HEALTH

Last, John M. *Public Health and Human Ecology.* 2d ed. Stamford, Conn.: Appleton & Lange, 1998.

Lee, Philip R., and Carroll L. Estes, eds. *The Nation's Health.* 5th ed. Boston: Jones and Bartlett, 1997.

Loue, Sana, ed. *Handbook of Immigrant Health.* New York: Plenum, 1998.

Newcomer, Robert J., and A. E. Benjamin, eds. *Indicators of Chronic Health Conditions: Monitoring Community-Level Delivery Systems.* Baltimore: The Johns Hopkins University Press, 1997.

Rom, William N. *Environmental and Occupational Medicine.* 3d ed. Philadelphia: Lippincott Williams & Wilkins, 1998.

Wagner, Kathryn D., ed. *Environmental Management in Healthcare Facilities.* Philadelphia: W. B. Saunders, 1998.

Wallace, Robert B., ed. *Maxcy-Rosenau-Last Public Health and Preventive Medicine.* Stamford, Conn.: Appleton & Lange, 1998.

PRIMARY HEALTH CARE. *See* FAMILY MEDICINE; INTERNAL MEDICINE

PSYCHIATRY

American Psychiatric Association. *Diagnostic and Statistical Manual of Mental Disorders: DSM-IV-TR.* Rev. 4th ed. Washington, D.C.: American Psychiatric Press, 2000.

Busse, Ewald W., and Dan G. Blazer, eds. *The American Psychiatric Press Textbook of Geriatric Psychiatry.* 2d ed. Washington, D.C.: American Psychiatric Press, 1996.

Cassem, Ned H., ed. *Massachusetts General Hospital Handbook of General Hospital Psychiatry.* 4th ed. St. Louis: C. V. Mosby, 1997.

Goldman, Howard H., ed. *Review of General Psychiatry.* 5th ed. Stamford, Conn.: Appleton & Lange, 1999.

Hubbard, John R., and Delmar Short, eds. *Primary Care Medicine for Psychiatrists: A Practitioner's Guide.* New York: Plenum, 1997.

Kaplan, Harold I., and Benjamin J. Sadock. *Kaplan and Sadock's Synopsis of Psychiatry: Behavior Sciences/Clinical Psychiatry.* 8th ed. Philadelphia: Lippincott Williams & Wilkins, 1998.

_____, eds. *Comprehensive Textbook of Psychiatry/VI.* 6th ed. Philadelphia: Lippincott Williams & Wilkins, 1995.

Klykylo, William M., et al., eds. *Clinical Child Psychiatry.* Philadelphia: W. B. Saunders, 1998.

Lyons, John S., et al. *The Measurement and Management of Clinical Outcomes in Mental Health.* New York: Wiley-Liss, 1997.

Okpaku, Samuel O., ed. *Clinical Methods in Transcultural Psychiatry.* Washington, D.C.: American Psychiatric Press, 1998.

Rundell, James R., and Michael G. Wise, eds. *The American Psychiatric Press Textbook of Consultation-Liaison Psychiatry.* Washington, D.C.: American Psychiatric Press, 1996.

Sederer, Lloyd I., and Barbara Dickey, eds. *Outcomes Assessment in Clinical Practice.* Philadelphia: Lippincott Williams & Wilkins, 1996.

Sederer, Lloyd I., and Anthony J. Rothschild, eds. *Acute Care Psychiatry: Diagnosis and Treatment.* Philadelphia: Lippincott Williams & Wilkins, 1997.

Shea, Shawn Christopher. *Psychiatric Interviewing, the Art of Understanding: A Practical Guide for Psychiatrists, Psychologists, Counselors, Social Workers, Nurses, and Other Mental Health Professionals.* 2d ed. Philadelphia: W. B. Saunders, 1998.

Wiener, Jerry M., ed. *Textbook of Child and Adolescent Psychiatry.* 2d ed. Washington, D.C.: American Psychiatric Press, 1997.

Yudofsky, Stuart C., and Robert E. Hales, eds. *The American Psychiatric Press Textbook of Neuropsychiatry.* 3d ed. Washington, D.C.: American Psychiatric Press, 1997.

RADIOLOGY AND IMAGING

Bassett, Lawrence W., et al. *Diagnosis of Diseases of the Breast.* Philadelphia: W. B. Saunders, 1997.

Berman, Claudia G., et al., eds. *Oncologic Imaging: A Clinical Perspective.* New York: McGraw-Hill, 1998.

Brower, Anne C., and Donald J. Flemming. *Arthritis in Black and White.* 2d ed. Philadelphia: W. B. Saunders, 1997.

Eisenberg, Ronald L. *Clinical Imaging: An Atlas of Differential Diagnosis.* 3d ed. Philadelphia: Lippincott Williams & Wilkins, 1997.

_____. *Gastrointestinal Radiology: A Pattern Approach*. 3d ed. Philadelphia: Lippincott Williams & Wilkins, 1996.

Fishman, Elliot K., and R. Brooke Jeffrey, Jr., eds. *Spiral CT: Principles, Techniques, and Clinical Applications*. 2d ed. Philadelphia: Lippincott Williams & Wilkins, 1998.

Fleckenstein, James L., et al., eds. *Muscle Imaging in Health and Disease*. New York: Springer, 1996.

Fleischer, Arthur C., et al., eds. *Clinical Gynecologic Imaging*. Philadelphia: Lippincott Williams & Wilkins, 1997.

Gerson, Myron C., ed. *Cardiac Nuclear Medicine*. 3d ed. New York: McGraw-Hill, 1997.

Goaz, Paul W., and Stuart C. White. *Oral Radiology: Principles and Interpretation*. 4th ed. St. Louis: C. V. Mosby, 1999.

Halperin, Edward C., et al. *Pediatric Radiation Oncology*. 3d ed. Philadelphia: Lippincott Williams & Wilkins, 1999.

Kopans, Daniel B. *Breast Imaging*. 2d ed. Philadelphia: Lippincott Williams & Wilkins, 1998.

Lee, Joseph K. T., et al., eds. *Computed Body Tomography with MRI Correlation*. 3d ed. Philadelphia: Lippincott Williams & Wilkins, 1998.

Mettler, Fred A., Jr., and Milton J. Guiberteau. *Essentials of Nuclear Medicine Imaging*. 4th ed. Philadelphia: W. B. Saunders, 1998.

Mirowitz, Scott A. *Pitfalls, Variants, and Artifacts in Body MR Imaging*. St. Louis: C. V. Mosby, 1996.

Novelline, Robert A. *Squire's Fundamentals of Radiology*. 5th ed. Cambridge, Mass.: Harvard University Press, 1997.

Perez, Carlos A., and Luther W. Brady, eds. *Principles and Practice of Radiation Oncology*. 3d ed. Philadelphia: Lippincott Williams & Wilkins, 1998.

Reed, James C. *Chest Radiology: Plain Film Patterns and Differential Diagnoses*. 4th ed. St. Louis: C. V. Mosby, 1997.

Resnick, Donald. *Bone and Joint Imaging*. 2d ed. Philadelphia: W. B. Saunders, 1996.

Rumack, Carol M., et al., eds. *Diagnostic Ultrasound*. 2d ed. St. Louis: C. V. Mosby, 1998.

Silverman, Paul M., ed. *Helical (Spiral) Computed Tomography: A Practical Approach to Clinical Protocols*. Philadelphia: Lippincott Williams & Wilkins, 1998.

Som, Peter M., and Hugh D. Curtin, eds. *Head and Neck Imaging*. 3d ed. St. Louis: C. V. Mosby, 1996.

Stoller, David W. *Magnetic Resonance Imaging in Orthopaedic and Sports Medicine*. 2d ed. Philadelphia: Lippincott Williams & Wilkins, 1997.

Wilson, Michael A., ed. *Textbook of Nuclear Medicine*. Philadelphia: Lippincott Williams & Wilkins, 1998.

RESPIRATORY SYSTEM

Barnes, Peter J., et al., eds. *Asthma*. Philadelphia: Lippincott Williams & Wilkins, 1997.

Baum, Gerald L., and Emanuel Wolinsky, eds. *Textbook of Pulmonary Diseases*. 6th ed. Philadelphia: Lippincott Williams & Wilkins, 1997.

Benumof, Jonathan L., ed. *Airway Management: Principles and Practice*. St. Louis: C. V. Mosby, 1996.

Bordow, Richard A., and Kenneth M. Moser, eds. *Manual of Clinical Problems in Pulmonary Medicine*. 4th ed. Philadelphia: Lippincott Williams & Wilkins, 1996.

Chernick, Victor, and Thomas F. Boat, eds. *Kendig's Disorders of the Respiratory Tract in Children*. 6th ed. Philadelphia: W. B. Saunders, 1998.

Fishman, Alfred P., ed. *Fishman's Pulmonary Diseases and Disorders*. 3d ed. New York: McGraw-Hill, 1998.

Goldstein, Donald H., et al., eds. *A Practical Approach to Pulmonary Medicine*. Philadelphia: Lippincott Williams & Wilkins, 1997.

Hyatt, Robert E., et al. *Interpretation of Pulmonary Function Tests: A Practical Guide*. Philadelphia: Lippincott Williams & Wilkins, 1997.

Irwin, Richard S., et al., eds. *Diagnosis and Treatment of Symptoms of the Respiratory Tract*. Armonk, N.Y.: Futura, 1997.

Kradin, Richard L., and Bruce W. S. Robinson, eds. *Immunopathology of Lung Disease*. Boston: Butterworth-Heinemann, 1996.

RHEUMATOLOGY

Clements, Philip J., and Daniel E. Furst, eds. *Systemic Sclerosis*. Philadelphia: Lippincott Williams & Wilkins, 1996.

Harris, Edward D., Jr. *Rheumatoid Arthritis*. Philadelphia: W. B. Saunders, 1997.

Kelley, William N., et al., eds. *Textbook of Rheumatology*. 5th ed. Philadelphia: W. B. Saunders, 1997.

Klippel, John H., and Paul A. Dieppe. *Rheumatology*. 2d ed. St. Louis: C. V. Mosby, 1998.

Koopman, William J., ed. *Arthritis and Allied Conditions: A Textbook of Rheumatology*. 13th ed. Philadelphia: Lippincott Williams & Wilkins, 1997.

Rosenbaum, Richard B., et al. *Clinical Neurology of Rheumatic Diseases.* Boston: Butterworth-Heinemann, 1996.

Sontheimer, Richard D., and Thomas T. Provost, eds. *Cutaneous Manifestations of Rheumatic Diseases.* Philadelphia: Lippincott Williams & Wilkins, 1996.

Wallace, Daniel J., and Bevra Hannahs Hahn, eds. *Dubois' Lupus Erythematosus.* 5th ed. Philadelphia: Lippincott Williams & Wilkins, 1997.

SEXUALLY TRANSMITTED DISEASES. *See also* ACQUIRED IMMUNODEFICIENCY SYNDROME (AIDS)

Borchardt, Kenneth A., and Michael A. Noble, eds. *Sexually Transmitted Diseases: Epidemiology, Pathology, Diagnosis, and Treatment.* Boca Raton, Fla.: CRC Press, 1997.

Eng, Thomas R., and William T. Butler, eds. *The Hidden Epidemic: Confronting Sexually Transmitted Diseases.* Washington, D.C.: National Academy Press, 1997.

Holmes, King K., et al., eds. *Sexually Transmitted Diseases.* 3d ed. New York: McGraw-Hill, 1998.

Morse, Stephen A., et al., eds. *Atlas of Sexually Transmitted Diseases and AIDS.* 2d ed. St. Louis: C. V. Mosby, 1996.

SPORTS MEDICINE

American College of Sports Medicine. *ASCM's Guidelines for Exercise Testing and Prescription.* 5th ed. Philadelphia: Lippincott Williams & Wilkins, 1995.

Andrews, James R., et al. *On-Field Evaluation and Treatment of Common Athletic Injuries.* St. Louis: C. V. Mosby, 1997.

Foss, Merle L., and Steven J. Keteyian. *Fox's Physiological Basis for Exercise and Sport.* 6th ed. New York: McGraw-Hill, 1998.

Guten, Gary N., ed. *Running Injuries.* Philadelphia: W. B. Saunders, 1997.

Jordan, Barry D., et al., eds. *Sports Neurology.* 2d ed. Philadelphia: Lippincott Williams & Wilkins, 1998.

Lillegard, Wade A., et al., eds. *Handbook of Sports Medicine: A Symptom-Oriented Approach.* 2d ed. Boston: Butterworth-Heinemann, 1999.

Marder, Richard A., and George J. Lian. *Sports Injuries of the Ankle and Foot.* New York: Springer, 1997.

Mellion, Morris B., et al., eds. *The Team Physician's Handbook.* 2d ed. St. Louis: C. V. Mosby, 1997.

Sallis, Robert E., and Ferdy Massimino, eds. *Essentials of Sports Medicine.* St. Louis: C. V. Mosby, 1997.

Scuderi, Giles R., et al., eds. *Sports Medicine: Principles of Primary Care.* St. Louis: C. V. Mosby, 1997.

Zachazewski, James E., et al., eds. *Athletic Injuries and Rehabilitation.* Philadelphia: W. B. Saunders, 1996.

STATISTICS

Garb, Jane L. *Understanding Medical Research: A Practitioner's Guide.* Philadelphia: Lippincott Williams & Wilkins, 1996.

Glantz, Stanton A. *Primer of Biostatistics.* 4th ed. New York: McGraw-Hill, 1997.

Ingelfinger, Joseph A., et al. *Biostatistics in Clinical Medicine.* 3d ed. New York: McGraw-Hill, 1994.

SUBSTANCE ABUSE

Bukstein, Oscar Gary. *Adolescent Substance Abuse: Assessment, Prevention, and Treatment.* New York: Wiley-Liss, 1995.

Galanter, Marc, and Herbert D. Kleber, eds. *The American Psychiatric Press Textbook of Substance Abuse Treatment.* Washington, D.C.: American Psychiatric Press, 1994.

Lowinson, Joyce H., et al., eds. *Substance Abuse: A Comprehensive Textbook.* 3d ed. Philadelphia: Lippincott Williams & Wilkins, 1997.

Miller, Norman S., et al., eds. *Manual of Therapeutics for Addictions.* New York: Wiley-Liss, 1997.

Miller, Norman S., ed. *The Principles and Practice of Addictions in Psychiatry.* Philadelphia: W. B. Saunders, 1997.

Stoil, Michael J., and Gary Hill. *Preventing Substance Abuse: Interventions That Work.* New York: Plenum, 1996.

SURGERY

Adkins, R. Benton, Jr., and H. William Scott, Jr. *Surgical Care for the Elderly.* 2d ed. Philadelphia: Lippincott Williams & Wilkins, 1998.

Ashcraft, Keith W., and Thomas M. Holder, eds. *Pediatric Surgery.* 3d ed. Philadelphia: W. B. Saunders, 1999.

Aston, Sherrell J., et al., eds. *Grabb and Smith's Plastic Surgery.* 5th ed. Philadelphia: Lippincott Williams & Wilkins, 1997.

Baue, Arthur E., et al., eds. *Glenn's Thoracic and Cardiovascular Surgery.* 6th ed. Stamford, Conn.: Appleton & Lange, 1996.

Corman, Marvin L. *Colon and Rectal Surgery*. 4th ed. Philadelphia: Lippincott Williams & Wilkins, 1998.

Edmunds, L. Henry, Jr., ed. *Cardiac Surgery in the Adult*. New York: McGraw-Hill, 1997.

Feliciano, David V., et al., eds. *Trauma*. 3d ed. Stamford, Conn.: Appleton & Lange, 1996.

Georgiade, Nicholas G., et al., eds. *Georgiade Plastic, Maxillofacial, and Reconstructive Surgery*. 3d ed. Philadelphia: Lippincott Williams & Wilkins, 1997.

Graham, Sam D., ed. *Glenn's Urologic Surgery*. 5th ed. Philadelphia: Lippincott Williams & Wilkins, 1998.

Greenfield, Lazar J., et al., eds. *Surgery: Scientific Principles and Practice*. 2d ed. Philadelphia: Lippincott Williams & Wilkins, 1997.

Harvey, James C., and Edward J. Beattie, eds. *Cancer Surgery*. Philadelphia: W. B. Saunders, 1996.

Khonsari, Siavosh. *Cardiac Surgery: Safeguards and Pitfalls in Operative Technique*. 2d ed. Philadelphia: Lippincott Williams & Wilkins, 1997.

Lanzafame, Raymond J. *Prevention and Management of Complications in Minimally Invasive Surgery*. New York: Igaku-Shoin, 1996.

McQuarrie, Donald G., et al., eds. *Reoperative General Surgery*. 2d ed. St. Louis: C. V. Mosby, 1997.

Merli, Geno J., and Howard H. Weitz. *Medical Management of the Surgical Patient*. 2d ed. Philadelphia: W. B. Saunders, 1998.

Montgomery, William W. *Surgery of the Upper Respiratory System*. 3d ed. Philadelphia: Lippincott Williams & Wilkins, 1996.

Nyhus, Lloyd M., et al., eds. *Mastery of Surgery*. 3d ed. Philadelphia: Lippincott Williams & Wilkins, 1997.

Nyhus, Lloyd M., and Robert E. Condon, eds. *Hernia*. 4th ed. Philadelphia: Lippincott Williams & Wilkins, 1995.

Oldham, Keith T., et al., eds. *Surgery of Infants and Children: Scientific Principles and Practice*. Philadelphia: Lippincott Williams & Wilkins, 1997.

Sabiston, David C., Jr., ed. *Textbook of Surgery: The Biological Basis of Modern Surgical Practice*. 15th ed. Philadelphia: W. B. Saunders, 1997.

Sabiston, David C., Jr., and Frank C. Spencer, eds. *Surgery of the Chest*. 6th ed. Philadelphia: W. B. Saunders, 1995.

Schirmer, Bruce David, and David William Rattner, eds. *Ambulatory Surgery*. Philadelphia: W. B. Saunders, 1998.

Schwartz, Seymour I., et al., eds. *Principles of Surgery*. 7th ed. New York: McGraw-Hill, 1999.

Stoney, Ronald J., and David J. Effeney. *Comprehensive Vascular Exposures*. Philadelphia: Lippincott Williams & Wilkins, 1998.

Wanebo, Harold J., ed. *Surgery for Gastrointestinal Cancer*. Philadelphia: Lippincott Williams & Wilkins, 1997.

Way, Lawrence W., ed. *Current Surgical Diagnosis and Treatment*. 11th ed. Stamford, Conn.: Appleton & Lange, 1999.

Zinner, Michael J., et al., eds. *Maingot's Abdominal Operations*. 10th ed. Stamford, Conn.: Appleton & Lange, 1997.

TOXICOLOGY

Ellenhorn, Matthew J., ed. *Ellenhorn's Medical Toxicology: Diagnosis and Treatment of Human Poisoning*. 2d ed. Philadelphia: Lippincott Williams & Wilkins, 1997.

Goldfrank, Lewis R., et al. *Goldfrank's Toxicologic Emergencies*. 6th ed. Stamford, Conn.: Appleton & Lange, 1998.

Greenberg, Michael I., ed. *Occupational, Industrial, and Environmental Toxicology*. St. Louis: C. V. Mosby, 1997.

Haddad, Lester M., et al., eds. *Clinical Management of Poisoning and Drug Overdose*. 3d ed. Philadelphia: W. B. Saunders, 1998.

Klaassen, Curtis D., ed. *Casarett and Doull's Toxicology: The Basic Science of Poisons*. 5th ed. New York: McGraw-Hill, 1996.

Viccellio, Peter, ed. *Emergency Toxicology*. 2d ed. Philadelphia: Lippincott Williams & Wilkins, 1998.

TROPICAL MEDICINE

Cook, Gordon C., ed. *Manson's Tropical Diseases*. 20th ed. Philadelphia: W. B. Saunders, 1996.

Jong, Elaine C., and Russell McMullen, eds. *The Travel and Tropical Medicine Manual*. 2d ed. Philadelphia: W. B. Saunders, 1995.

Strickland, G. Thomas, ed. *Hunter's Tropical Medicine*. 8th ed. Philadelphia: W. B. Saunders, 1999.

UROLOGY

Brenner, Barry M., ed. *Brenner and Rector's The Kidney*. 5th ed. Philadelphia: W. B. Saunders, 1996.

Coe, Fredric L., et al., eds. *Kidney Stones: Medical and Surgical Management*. Philadelphia: Lippincott Williams & Wilkins, 1996.

Gillenwater, Jay Y., et al., eds. *Adult and Pediatric Urology.* 3d ed. St. Louis: C. V. Mosby, 1996.

Hellstrom, Wayne J. G., ed. *Male Infertility and Sexual Dysfunction.* New York: Springer, 1997.

Koss, Leopold G. *Diagnostic Cytology of the Urinary Tract: With Histopathologic and Clinical Correlations.* Philadelphia: Lippincott Williams & Wilkins, 1996.

Massry, Shaul G., and Richard J. Glassock, eds. *Massry and Glassock's Textbook of Nephrology.* 3d ed. Philadelphia: Lippincott Williams & Wilkins, 1995.

Mitch, William E., and Saulo Klahr, eds. *Handbook of Nutrition and the Kidney.* 3d ed. Philadelphia: Lippincott Williams & Wilkins, 1998.

Murphy, William M., ed. *Urological Pathology.* 2d ed. Philadelphia: W. B. Saunders, 1997.

Nissenson, Allen R., et al. *Clinical Dialysis.* 3d ed. Stamford, Conn.: Appleton & Lange, 1995.

Raz, Shlom, ed. *Female Urology.* 2d ed. Philadelphia: W. B. Saunders, 1996.

Sant, Grannum R., ed. *Interstitial Cystitis.* Philadelphia: Lippincott Williams & Wilkins, 1997.

Schrier, Robert W., ed. *Renal and Electrolyte Disorders.* 5th ed. Philadelphia: Lippincott Williams & Wilkins, 1997.

Schrier, Robert W., and Carl W. Gottschalk, eds. *Diseases of the Kidney.* 6th ed. Philadelphia: Lippincott Williams & Wilkins, 1997.

Tanagho, Emil A., and Jack W. McAninch, eds. *Smith's General Urology.* 15th ed. Stamford, Conn.: Appleton & Lange, 1999.

Walsh, Patrick C., et al., eds. *Campbell's Urology.* 7th ed. Philadelphia: W. B. Saunders, 1998.

—Peter B. Heller, Ph.D.

Web Site Directory

ABORTION

National Abortion Rights Action League
http://www.naral.org

Site offers information about reproductive health issues, including daily news items, publications, organized links, and Act Now opportunities.

National Right to Life Organization
http://www.nrlc.org

Site offers sources of information on pro-life issues in relation to abortion, RU-486, organization support, euthanasia, and federal legislation.

ACCIDENTS

National Center for Emergency Medicine Informatics
http://ncemi.org

Site provides Web links, frequently asked questions, automatic e-mail list subscriber, bibliographies, and articles.

ACQUIRED IMMUNODEFICIENCY SYNDROME (AIDS)

HIV/AIDS Information Index
http://www.arens.com/hiv

Site offers links to information on patient care, clinical trials, advocacy organizations, journals and publications, medical search sites, alternative medicine and treatments, drug company Web sites, government agencies, research centers, and physicians.

ALZHEIMER'S DISEASE

Alzheimer's Association
http://www.alz.org

Site of a voluntary organization dedicated to researching the prevention, cures, and treatments of Alzheimer's disease. The Benjamin B. Green-Field Library and Resource Center collects a wide range of materials related to Alzheimer's disease and related disorders and provides service to family members, educators and students, health professionals, social service agencies and the general public.

AMPUTATION

Amputation Prevention Global Resource Center
http://www.diabetesresource.com

Site offers clinical, educational, and research information on amputation.

AMYOTROPHIC LATERAL SCLEROSIS

ALS Association
http://www.alsa.org

Site describes the mission and service of this national not-for-profit voluntary health organization dedicated solely to the fight against amyotrophic lateral sclerosis, also known as Lou Gehrig's disease.

ANTHRAX

Centers for Disease Control, Division of Bacterial and Mycotic Diseases
http://www.cdc.gov/ncidod/dbmd/diseaseinfo/anthrax_g.htm

Site provides answers to frequently asked questions about anthrax.

ANTIBIOTICS

Medscape DrugInfo
http://promini.medscape.com/drugdb/search.asp

A searchable database that provides information on uses, adverse effects, precautions, drug interactions, overdose and toxicity, pharmacology and chemistry, preparations, and patient handouts for a wide variety of drugs.

ANTI-INFLAMMATORY DRUGS

Medscape DrugInfo
http://promini.medscape.com/drugdb/search.asp

A searchable database that provides information on uses, adverse effects, precautions, drug interactions, overdose and toxicity, pharmacology and chemistry, preparations, and patient handouts for a wide variety of drugs.

ARTHRITIS

Arthritis Foundation
http://www.arthritis.org

The site of the Arthritis Foundation, whose mission is to support research to find the cure for and prevention of arthritis and to improve the quality of life for those affected by arthritis.

ASTHMA
Asthma and Allergy Foundation of America
http://www.aafa.org
Site describes the mission of this not-for-profit organization dedicated to finding a cure for and controlling asthma and allergic diseases.

ATTENTION-DEFICIT DISORDER
Children and Adults with Attention Deficit/Hyperactivity Disorder
http://www.chadd.org
Site describes this parent-based organization formed to better the lives of individuals with attention-deficit disorders and their families.

AURAS
National Institute of Neurological Disorders and Stroke
http://www.ninds.nih.gov/health_and_medical/pubs/seizures_and_epilepsy_htr.htm
Site describes warning signs of an impending seizure.

AUTISM
Autism Society of America
http://www.autism-society.org
Site provides information for parents with newly diagnosed children, general information about the society, and information about local society chapters.

BIONICS AND BIOTECHNOLOGY
National Biotechnology Information Facility
http://www.nbif.org
Site provides access to biotechnology research tools and databases, software, legal and regulatory links, educational resources, images, career resources, conferences and workshops, journals, and news.

BITES AND STINGS
Spiders and Other Arachnids
http://spiders.ucr.edu
Site provides links to information about the spider, scorpion, bee, wasp, and ant species worldwide whose bites cause morbidity and mortality.

BLINDNESS
American Foundation for the Blind
http://www.afb.org
Site of the American Foundation for the Blind (AFB), which publishes materials about blindness for professionals and consumers through AFB Press, and maintains and preserves the Helen Keller Archives, housed at the M.C. Migel Memorial Library, one of the world's largest collections of print materials on blindness. AFB also maintains the Careers Technology Information Bank (CTIB), a network of individuals who are blind from all fifty states and Canada.

National Federation of the Blind
http://www.nfb.org
The site of the National Federation of the Blind (NFB), which provides public education about blindness, information and referral services, scholarships, literature and publications about blindness, aids and appliances and other adaptive equipment for the blind, advocacy services and protection of civil rights, job opportunities for the blind, development and evaluation of technology, and support for blind persons and their families.

BLISTERS AND BOILS
STDs
http://www.safersex.co.za/std_s.html
Site graphically illustrates and describes common blisters and boils associated with sexually transmitted diseases.

BLURRED VISION
National Eye Research Foundation
http://www.nerf.org
Site provides consumers and professionals with access to developing technology for treating impaired vision.

BREAST CANCER
National Alliance of Breast Cancer Organizations
http://www.nabco.org
Site describes this nonprofit resource for information about breast cancer, providing current research information, treatment options, support referrals, and links.

BREAST SURGERY
Women in Health
http://womnhlth.home.mindspring.com
Site provides educational information about silicone and saline breast implants.

BURPING
National Digestive Disease Information Clearinghouse
http://www.niddk.nih.gov/health/digest/pubs/gas/gas.htm

Site titled "Gas in the Digestive System" provides information on burping and the possible signs and symptoms it represents.

CANCER

American Cancer Society
http://www.cancer.org
Site describes the mission of this organization dedicated to helping everyone who faces cancer, through research, patient services, early detection, treatment, and education.

Cancer Care
http://www.cancercare.org
Site provides information, including links and resources, to help people who have cancer, and their families and friends, better cope with the disease.

Centers for Disease Control and Prevention:
  Cancer
http://www.cdc.gov/health/cancer.htm
Site provides information and links covering a wide range of cancers.

Combined Health Information Database
http://chid.nih.gov/simple/simple.html
Site provides a searchable database of titles, abstracts, and citations for health information and health education resources related to cancer prevention and control.

CEREBRAL PALSY

United Cerebral Palsy Association
http://www.ucpa.org/index.cfm
Site provides information on the mission and services of this organization, dedicated to research on cerebral palsy and support for those who suffer from it.

CERVICAL, OVARIAN, AND UTERINE CANCERS

National Cervical Cancer Coalition
http://www.nccc-online.org/index.asp
Site describes this grassroots advocacy coalition for issues concerning cervical cancer screening and the traditional pap smear.

CHILDBIRTH COMPLICATIONS

When Pregnancy Isn't Perfect: A Layperson's Guide to Complications in Pregnancy

http://www.larata.com/index1.htm
Site for a book on pregnancy complications includes a list of links.

CHOLESTEROL

Heart Information Network
http://www.heartinfo.com/reviews/hchol.htm
Site provides information on lowering cholesterol levels, cholesterol and the heart, and the opportunity to join a cholesterol discussion group.

CLINICAL TRIALS

CenterWatch Clinical Trials Listing Service
http://www.centerwatch.com
Site provides national and international listings of clinical trials in all therapeutic areas.

Clinical Research Investigator Registry
http://www.criregistry.com
Site contains vital information about physicians and clinics across the United States who conduct clinical research.

Clinical Trials and Noteworthy Treatments for Brain Tumors
http://virtualtrials.com
Site provides patients, family members, health care professionals, and members of the public access to information on clinical trials for brain tumors.

Clinical Trials Center: Gulf War Syndrome
http://pc176.nhrc.navy.mil/disease/clinical.htm
Site provides information on Veterans Administration and Department of Defense sponsored clinical trials conducted in San Diego by the Naval Health Research Center.

ClinicalTrials.gov
http://www.clinicaltrials.gov
Site sponsored by the National Institutes of Health provides patients, family members, health care professionals, and members of the public access to information on clinical trials for a wide range of diseases and conditions.

Rare Diseases Clinical Research Database
http://rarediseases.info.nih.gov/ord/wwwprot/index
  .shtml
Site provides information on all available rare disease clinical studies.

COLON CANCER
Cancer Care
http://www.cancercare.org/campaigns/colon1.htm
Site provides information, including links and resources, to help people who have colon cancer, and their families and friends, better cope with the disease.

CONTRACEPTION
National Abortion Rights Action League
http://www.naral.org/issues/issues_ru486.html
Site offers an update on RU-486 (mifepristone), as well as information about reproductive health issues, including daily news items, publications, organized links, and Act Now opportunities.

Planned Parenthood Federation of America
http://www.plannedparenthood.org
Site describes the philosophy of Planned Parenthood: that knowledge empowers people to make better choices about their health and sexuality. It offers a wide range of information resources including pamphlets, books, newsletters, videotapes, and Web sites.

CORNEAL TRANSPLANTATION
Tissue Banks International
http://www.tbionline.org
Site describes an international network of eye and tissue banks that recovers and provides ocular and other human tissue for use in transplants and other surgeries.

CREUTZFELDT-JAKOB DISEASE (CJD)
Creutzfeldt-Jakob Disease Foundation, Inc.
http://cjdfoundation.org
Site describes resources to promote the research, education, and awareness of the disease, as well as to provide support services for persons affected by CJD.

DELUSIONS
American Psychiatric Association
http://www.psych.org/clin_res/index.cfm
Site describes selected aspects of the DSM-IV, the diagnostic and statistical manual of the American Psychiatric Association, and provides a search engine to get listings of the APA's current coverage of the topic.

DIABETES MELLITUS
Centers for Disease Control: Diabetes

http://www.cdc.gov/diabetes
Site features state contacts, articles, a diabetes fact sheet, and the opportunity to ask questions about diabetes.

Children with Diabetes
http://www.childrenwithdiabetes.com/index_cwd.htm
Site provides information that helps children with diabetes and their families learn about diabetes, meet people with diabetes, and help others with diabetes.

The Diabetes Mall
http://www.diabetesnet.com
Site identifies books, information, insulin pumps, newsletters, and tapes on diabetes.

Diabetes Monitor
http://www.diabetesmonitor.com
Site monitors diabetes happenings everywhere in cyberspace.

Diabetes.com
http://www.diabetes.com
Site provides an information resource and online community for diabetics. Includes sections on diet and exercise, intimacy, risk factors and prevention, and information on symptoms.

DRUG RESISTANCE
Alliance for the Prudent Use of Antibiotics
http://www.healthsci.tufts.edu/apua/apua.html
Site describes the mission and services of this organization, dedicated to curbing the problem of antibiotic resistance worldwide, and preserving antibiotic effectiveness and public health through the education of health care workers and the general public.

DYSLEXIA
Dyslexia Information.com
http://www.dyslexia-information.com
Site offers basic information, educational support, and homework links to help people with dyslexia.

EMPHYSEMA
National Emphysema Foundation
http://www.emphysemafoundation.org/nefheader.htm
Site offers tips on exercises, inhaler uses, and other helpful items for those with emphysema.

ENCEPHALITIS
National Center for Infectious Diseases: Mosquito-
borne Diseases
http://www.cdc.gov/ncidod/diseases/list_mosquitoborne
.htm
Site offers general questions and answers, local outbreak information, control issues, and more.

ENVIRONMENTAL HEALTH
AT&T's Environmental, Health and Safety Site
http://www.att.com/ehs
Site offers an educational, fun-filled site based on
environmental health and safety tips.

Centers for Disease Control: Environmental Health
http://www.cdc.gov/health/environm.htm
Site provides information and links about a variety of environmental health issues, including air
pollution, carbon monoxide poisoning, and lead poisoning.

Environmental Defense Scorecard
http://www.scorecard.org
Site provides a database allowing users to see chemical pollution on local street maps of their own communities.

Environmental Diseases from A to Z
http://www.niehs.nih.gov/external/a2z/home.htm
Site provides information from the U.S. National
Institute of Environmental Health Sciences, National
Institutes of Health.

EXtension TOXicology NETwork
http://ace.orst.edu/info/extoxnet
Site provides information on pesticide toxicology
and environmental chemistry information for the general public.

HazDat: Hazardous Substance Release/Health Effects
Database
http://www.atsdr.cdc.gov/hazdat.html
Site provides information on hazardous environmental substances.

EYE SURGERY
Beyond Discovery, Preserving the Miracle of Sight:
Lasers and Eye Surgery
http://www4.nationalacademies.org/beyond/
beyonddiscovery.nsf/web/sight?OpenDocument

Site provides information on the use of lasers for
eye surgery.

FOOD POISONING
Food and Drug Administration Center for Food Safety
and Applied Nutrition
http://vm.cfsan.fda.gov/list.html
Site provides information on food safety, nutrition,
and wholesomeness, as well as the regulation of cosmetics safety.

U.S. Department of Agriculture/Food and Drug Administration Foodborne Illness Education Information Center
http://www.nalusda.gov/fnic/foodborne/foodborn.htm
Site provides information on foodborne illnesses.

GENETIC DISEASES
Alliance of Genetic Support Groups
http://www.geneticalliance.org
Site provides information on an international coalition of individuals, professionals, and genetic support
organizations working together to enhance the lives
of everyone impacted by genetic conditions.

Blazing a Genetic Trail
http://www.hhmi.org/genetictrail
Site provides a series of articles, with graphics and
photographs, profiling research on mutant genes and
hereditary diseases, from the Howard Hughes Medical Institute.

Cancer Genome Anatomy Project
http://www.ncbi.nlm.nih.gov/ncicgap
Site provides information on an interdisciplinary
program sponsored by the National Cancer Institute
to establish the information and technological tools
needed to decipher the molecular anatomy of a cancer cell.

Center for Inherited Disease Research at Johns Hopkins University
http://www.cidr.jhmi.edu
Site offers information on genotyping and statistical genetics services to investigators seeking to identify genes contributing to human disease.

Centers for Disease Control: Office of Genetics and
Disease Prevention
http://www.cdc.gov/genetics

Site provides information and global resources on human genetic research, the Human Genome Project, epidemiology, public health, disease prevention, and health promotion.

CFC Family Network
http://www.concentric.net/~Jskd/cfcsyndrome
Site designed for parents and professionals looking for support and information on cardio-facio-cutaneous syndrome.

GeneCards
http://bioinformatics.weizmann.ac.il/cards
Site provides a quick overview of the vast amount of knowledge about human genes, their products, and diseases in which they are involved.

GeneClinics
http://www.geneclinics.org/home.html
Site contains genetics disease database and information relating genetic testing to diagnosis, management, and counseling of individuals and families with inherited disorders.

Genes and Disease
http://www.ncbi.nlm.nih.gov/disease
Site provides an opportunity to learn about the known genetic causes of cancer and immune system, metabolic, muscle and bone, nervous system, and other diseases. Includes chromosome maps showing the locations of disease genes.

Hereditary Disease Foundation
http://www.hdfoundation.org
Site describes the mission of this nonprofit, basic science organization dedicated to the cure of genetic disease.

Human Gene Mutation Database
http://archive.uwcm.ac.uk/uwcm/mg/hgmd0.html
Site attempts to collate known (published) gene lesions responsible for human inherited disease.

National Society of Genetic Counselors
http://www.nsgc.org
Site provides voice, authority, and advocate for the genetic counseling profession.

OMIM: Online Mendelian Inheritance in Man
http://www3.ncbi.nlm.nih.gov/omim
Site sponsored by the National Center for Biotechnology Information offers a catalog of human genes and genetic disorders.

Public Health Genetics Society
http://www.umich.edu/~phgs
Site promotes awareness of the role of genetics in public health and disease and the implications of genetic technology on public health.

A Question of Genes: Inherited Risks
http://www.pbs.org/gene
Site for a 1997 PBS special exploring questions and ethical issues raised by genetic research and testing.

Rare Genetic Diseases in Children
http://mcrcr2.med.nyu.edu/murphp01/homenew.htm
Site serves as a resource directory with links for rare childhood genetic diseases with message boards and parent-matching.

GENETIC ENGINEERING
CropGen
http://www.cropgen.org/databases/cropgen.nsf/
    homepage?OpenForm
Site attempts to make the case for genetically modified crops by helping to achieve a greater measure of realism and better balance in the public debate in the United Kingdom about crop biotechnology.

GULF WAR SYNDROME
Clinical Trials Gulf War Syndrome
http://pc176.nhrc.navy.mil/disease/clinical.htm
Site provides information on two Veterans Administration and Department of Defense sponsored clinical trials conducted in San Diego by the Naval Health Research Center.

HAIR
Regrowth.com
http://www.hairloss.org
Site dedicated to researching treatments for hair loss and verifying product claims for hair growth.

HEARING LOSS
Symphonix
http://www.shareholder.com/symphonix/news/
    20000829-22812.cfm
A commercial site that offers a news release about

the Food and Drug Administration (FDA) approval of the implant Vibrant Soundbridge.

HEART ATTACK

American Heart Association
http://www.americanheart.org/
   Heart_and_Stroke_A_Z_Guide
   Site provides a variety of information on heart health and stroke.

HERBAL MEDICINE

American Botanical Council
http://www.herbalgram.org
   Site provides education for the public on the use of herbs and phytomedicinals.

Herbal Encyclopedia
http://www.wic.net/waltzark/herbenc.htm
   Site provides information on the properties and uses of the various healing herbs. Includes sections on pet care, and how to gather and store herbs properly.

Herbal Hall
http://www.herb.com/opus.htm
   Site offers a discussion list for professional herbalists and a database for medicinal herbalism.

National Center for the Preservation of Medicinal
   Herbs
http://www.ncpmh.org/intro.html
   Site describes issues associated with the preservation of natural remedies native to North America.

National Institute of Medical Herbalists
http://www.btinternet.com/~nimh
   Site describes this British organization, established in 1864, with information and research on medicinal herbs and their uses.

HORMONE REPLACEMENT THERAPY

Menopause Online
http://www.menopause-online.com/treatments.htm
   Site offers dicussions of traditional and alternative treatments for menopause.

HOSPICE

Hospice Association of America
http://www.nahc.org/HAA
   Site describes the mission and services of the Hos-

pice Association of America, a national organization representing more than 2,800 hospices and thousands of caregivers and volunteers who serve terminally ill patients and their families.

IATROGENIC DISORDERS

The Wrong Medicine
http://www.catalase.com/wrongmed.htm
   Site describes issues associated with iatrogenic disorders.

IMMUNE SYSTEM

The Immune Articles Pages
http://www.immuneweb.org/articles
   Site provides information and support for people with chronic fatigue syndrome, multiple chemical sensitivities, lupus, allergies, environmental illness, fibromyalgia, candida, and other immune system disorders.

IMMUNIZATION AND VACCINATION

The Vaccine Page
http://www.vaccines.com
   Site provides access to current news about vaccines and an annotated database of vaccine resources on the Internet.

IMMUNODEFIENCY DISORDERS

National Organization for Rare Disorders
http://www.rarediseases.org
   Site describes the mission and services offered by this organization and provides information on Di George syndrome.

INFLUENZA

Medscape DrugInfo
http://promini.medscape.com/drugdb/search.asp
   A searchable database that provides information on uses, adverse effects, precautions, drug interactions, overdose and toxicity, pharmacology and chemistry, preparations, and patient handouts for a wide variety of drugs. Contains information on the influenza drugs Relenza and Tamiflu.

INSULIN RESISTANCE SYNDROME

The Wound Care Institute, Inc., for the Advancement
   of Wound Healing and Diabetic Foot Pathology
http://www.woundcare.org
   Search this site for a variety of articles on insulin resistance syndrome.

IRRITABLE BOWEL SYNDROME (IBS)

National Digestive Diseases Information Clearing-house

http://www.niddk.nih.gov/health/digest/pubs/irrbowel/irrbowel.htm

Site offers an overview of irritable bowel syndrome, its causes, effects, treatments, and suggestions for further reading.

KIDNEY DISORDERS

Healthlink USA: Kidney Diseases

http://www.healthlinkusa.com/173ent.htm

Site offers excellent information concerning treatment, prevention, personal stories, research, support, and e-mail groups.

LASER USE IN SURGERY

American Society for Laser Surgery and Medicine, Inc.

http://www.aslms.org/

Site offers a database for referral to a laser practitioner, and links to the *Lasers in Surgery and Medicine Journal.*

LEPTIN

Leptin, the Fat Feedback Hormone

http://www.loop.com/~bkrentzman/obesity/leptin.html

Site provided by a medical doctor contains information on this hormone.

MACULAR DEGENERATION

The Macular Degeneration Foundation

http://www.eyesight.org/index.html

Site describes this charitable educational and research foundation dedicated to discovering the cause of and developing cures for macular degeneration.

MAD COW DISEASE

The Official Mad Cow Disease Home Page

http://www.mad-cow.org

Site offers links to over seven thousand articles on mad cow disease, frequently updated.

MAMMOGRAPHY

National Alliance of Breast Cancer Organizations

http://www.nabco.org

Site describes this nonprofit resource for information about breast cancer, providing current research information, treatment options, support referrals, and links.

MASSAGE

American Massage Therapy Association

http://www.amtamassage.org/infocenter/home.html

Site provides information and references about massage, methods and techniques, alternative and holistic care, and general information related to massage therapy.

MASTURBATION

SexEdOnline: Masturbation

http://www.sexedonline.com/nonmembers/masturbation.htm

Site offers information about masturbation resources on the Internet.

MENINGITIS

Healthlink USA: Meningitis

http://www.healthlinkusa.com/203ent.htm

Site offers excellent information concerning treatment, prevention, personal stories, research, support, and e-mail groups.

Medscape DrugInfo

http://promini.medscape.com/drugdb/search.asp

A searchable database that provides information on uses, adverse effects, precautions, drug interactions, overdose and toxicity, pharmacology and chemistry, preparations, and patient handouts for a wide variety of drugs. Contains information on the meningitis drug Prevnar.

MOLD AND MILDEW

The Enviro Village Library

http://www.envirovillage.com/library/papers

Links to articles on toxic molds and how to eliminate them.

MULTIPLE SCLEROSIS

Healthlink USA: Multiple Sclerosis

http://www.healthlinkusa.com/212ent.htm

Site offers excellent information concerning treatment, prevention, personal stories, research, support, and e-mail groups.

Medscape DrugInfo

http://promini.medscape.com/drugdb/search.asp

A searchable database that provides information on uses, adverse effects, precautions, drug interactions, overdose and toxicity, pharmacology and chemistry, preparations, and patient handouts for a wide variety of drugs. Contains information on the MS drug Novanltrone.

NARCOLEPSY

Center for Narcolepsy

http://www-med.stanford.edu/school/Psychiatry/
narcolepsy

Site describes the Stanford University center, providing an outline of the disorder, details of current research, and publications.

OBESITY

Healthlink USA: Obesity

http://www.healthlinkusa.com/623ent.htm

Site offers excellent information concerning treatment, prevention, personal stories, research, support, and e-mail groups.

PARALYSIS

Christopher Reeve Paralysis Foundation

http://www.apacure.com

Site describes this advocacy organization that supports research into spinal cord injuries and nervous system disorders that cause paralysis.

Cure Paralysis Now

http://www.cureparalysis.org

Site offers information for professionals and patients on aims to advance progress to cure for spinal cord paralysis.

PARKINSON'S DISEASE

National Parkinson Foundation, Inc.

http://www.parkinson.org

Site provides the latest news and developments in Parkinson's disease research and includes a list of publications and events.

PHARMACY

Medscape

http://internalmedicine.medscape.com

Site offers a search engine that leads to discussion of several issues that the primary care physician must consider when prescribing multiple medications.

POST-TRAUMATIC STRESS DISORDER

WebMD

http://www.searchwebmd.com

Site offers comprehensive online resource for health information and support needs.

PREMATURE BIRTH

Healthlink USA: Premature Birth

http://www.healthlinkusa.com/533ent.htm

Site offers excellent information concerning treatment, prevention, personal stories, research, support, and e-mail groups.

PROSTATE CANCER

Cancerfacts.net

http://www.cancerfacts.net

Site provides information on prostate cancer treatment options.

RESUSCITATION

American Heart Association Emergency Cardiovascular Care Programs

http://www.cpr-ecc.org

Site offers new cardiopulmonary resuscitation (CPR) guidelines.

SEXUAL DYSFUNCTION

Medscape DrugInfo

http://promini.medscape.com/drugdb/
search.asp

A searchable database that provides information on uses, adverse effects, precautions, drug interactions, overdose and toxicity, pharmacology and chemistry, preparations, and patient handouts for a wide variety of drugs. Contains information on the erectile dysfunction drug Viagra.

SHOCK THERAPY

Mental Health Net

http://mentalhelp.net/guide/ect.htm

Site provides a comprehensive listing of electroconvulsive therapy information and self-help resources online.

SLEEP DISORDERS

National Sleep Foundation

http://www.sleepfoundation.org

Site provides information and resources for sleep disorders, including sleep deprivation.

SPINA BIFIDA

WebMD

http://www.searchwebmd.com

Site offers comprehensive online resource for health information and support needs.

SUDDEN INFANT DEATH SYNDROME (SIDS)
WebMD
http://www.searchwebmd.com
Site offers comprehensive online resource for health information and support needs.

SUPPLEMENTS
American Heart Association
http://www.americanheart.org
Site offers a search engine for information on phytochemicals and cardiovacular disease.

THALIDOMIDE
WebMD
http://www.searchwebmd.com
Site offers comprehensive online resource for health information and support.

TRACHOMA
Healthlink USA: Trachoma
http://www.healthlinkusa.com/314ent.htm
Site offers excellent information concerning treat-ment, prevention, personal stories, research, support, and e-mail groups.

TRANSPLANTATION
Organ Donation
http://www.organdonor.gov
Site provides advice on how to become an organ and tissue donor and answers questions about the many myths and facts surrounding donation.

VARICOSE VEIN REMOVAL
WebMD
http://www.searchwebmd.com
Site offers comprehensive online resource for health information and support.

WEIGHT LOSS MEDICATIONS
Food and Drug Administration
http://www.fda.gov
Site provides Fen-Phen information from the Food and Drug Administration (FDA), Center for Drug Evaluation and Research. A search engine provides Fen-Phen information and Fen-Phen safety update information.

—*Mary Allen Carey, Ph.D.*

RESOURCES

ABORTION. *See* REPRODUCTIVE ISSUES

ACQUIRED IMMUNODEFICIENCY SYNDROME (AIDS) AND HUMAN IMMUNODEFICIENCY VIRUS (HIV)

AIDS Clinical Trials Information Service
800-TRIALS-A
TDD/TTY: 800-243-7012

This federal Public Health Service project maintains a database on AIDS clinical trials. Provides information on the location of AIDS trials, criteria for inclusion or exclusion, and related assistance.

Athletes and Entertainers for Kids
3337 Colorado Street
Long Beach, CA 90814
800-933-KIDS

For children with AIDS and other catastrophic illnesses, this group provides information, educational materials, and a referral service relating to AIDS and the teenage population. Offers counseling services and community outings for affected children and their families.

Centers for Disease Control
AIDS and Diseases Fax Information Service
Health Fax Line
Fax: 888-232-3299

A number of documents related to diseases and other health issues are available from the Centers for Disease Control and Prevention (CDC) Fax Information Service as well as from its Web site. Both nontechnical information for patients and technical information for health care providers can be obtained.

Centers for Disease Control
National AIDS Hotline
800-342-AIDS
800-344-SIDA (Spanish)
TDD/TTY: 800-243-7889

This federal program offers information on AIDS and AIDS-related issues. Provides referrals to physicians, support groups, self-help groups, legal organizations, housing agencies, hospices, and home care services.

Gay Men's Health Crisis
119 W. 24th Street
New York, NY 10011
800-AIDS-NYC
212-807-6655
212-807-6664
TDD: 212-645-7470

Provides support and therapy groups for persons with AIDS and their families. Offers volunteer crisis counselors, a buddy program for assistance with tasks, and an AIDS prevention program.

Project Inform
205 13th Street
Suite 2001
San Francisco, CA 94103
800-822-7422
415-558-8669
E-mail: *web@projinf.org*
Web site: *http://www.projinf.org*

This clearinghouse and hotline provides AIDS and HIV treatment information and advocacy and information on current drugs and where they can be obtained.

Teens Teaching AIDS Prevention (TEENS T.A.P.)
3030 Walnut
Kansas City, MO 64108
800-234-TEEN
816-561-8784

This program is founded and run by teens for teens. Offers a toll-free hotline staffed by trained teens. Provides peer education, peer support and counseling, and a teen buddy program that offers friendship and understanding to teens who have HIV or AIDS or who have family members or other loved ones with HIV or AIDS.

Women Organized to Respond to Life-Threatening Diseases (WORLD)
414 13th Street
2d Floor
Oakland, CA 94612
510-986-0340

Offers support and information for women infected

with or affected by AIDS or HIV. Sponsors retreats and classes.

ADDICTION—ALCOHOL, DRUGS, AND SMOKING

AL-ANON Family Group
1600 Corporate Landing Parkway
Virginia Beach, VA 23454
888-4AL-ANON
757-563-1600
E-mail: *wso@al-anon.org*
Web site: *http://www.al-anon.alateen.org*

Provides a free self-help program of recovery from the family disease of alcoholism, based on the Twelve Steps and Twelve Traditions of Alcoholics Anonymous.

Alateen
1600 Corporate Landing Parkway
Virginia Beach, VA 23454
888-4AL-ANON
757-563-1600
E-mail: *wso@al-anon.org*
Web site: *http://www.alateen.org*

Offers a free self-help program based on the twelve steps and Twelve Traditions of Alcoholics Anonymous for younger family members affected by someone else's drinking. Gives referrals to local meetings and will send free information.

Alcoholics Anonymous World Services
P.O. Box 459
Grand Central Station
New York, NY 10163
212-870-3400
Web site: *http://www.aa.org*

This is a free self-help program for recovery from alcoholism. Members work to recover from alcoholism and help others to achieve sobriety through a twelve-step program, in which members share experiences, strength, and hope with one another.

Centers for Disease Control
Office on Smoking and Health
4770 Buford Highway NE
Atlanta, GA 30341
800-CDC-1311
770-488-5705

Provides information on smoking cessation, smoking and teens, smoking during pregnancy, and passive smoking.

Centers for Disease Control
Smoking Fax Line
Fax: 888-232-3299

A number of documents concerning smoking and related health information are available from the Centers for Disease Control and Prevention (CDC) Fax Information Service as well as from its Web site.

Children of Alcoholics Foundation
164 W. 74th Street
New York, NY 10023
800-359-COAF
212-595-5810
E-mail: *coaf@phoenixhouse.org*
Web site: *http://www.coaf.org*

Provides information on the effects of parental abuse of alcohol and other substances on children. Looks for solutions to the problems of children of alcoholics.

Cocaine Anonymous World Services
P.O. Box 2000
Los Angeles, CA 90049
800-347-8998
310-559-5833
E-mail: *cawso@ca.org*
Web site: *http://www.ca.org*

Refers callers to local self-help twelve-step groups for persons addicted to cocaine and other mind-altering drugs.

Dual Disorders Anonymous
P.O. Box 681264
Schaumburg, IL 60168
847-781-1553

This self-help support group is based on the twelve-steps program; for persons who have alcohol or drug addictions along with mental or emotional disorders.

Families Anonymous
P.O. Box 3475
Culver City, CA 90231
800-736-9805
310-815-8018
E-mail: *fananon@familiesanonymous.org*
Web site: *http://www.familiesanonymous.org*

This twelve-step support group is for persons dealing with drug abuse or related behavior problems of a family member or friend. Refers callers to the nearest meetings, which are held throughout the world. Also provides referrals to other twelve-step programs and other resources and organizations.

Jewish Alcoholics, Chemically Dependent Persons, and Significant Others (JACS)
426 W. 58th Street
Suite 555
New York, NY 10019
212-397-4197
E-mail: *jacs@jacsweb.org*
Web site: *http://www.jacsweb.org*
Promotes and assists recovery from chemical dependency for Jewish alcoholics and addicts, their families, and their friends.

National Clearinghouse for Alcohol and Drug Information
P.O. Box 2345
Rockville, MD 20847
800-729-6686
Provides information on alcohol and other drug abuse and offers referrals to local programs.

National Drug and Alcohol Treatment Referral Hotline
800-662-HELP
800-662-9832 (Spanish)
This government agency provides referrals for substance abuse treatment throughout the country and information on alcohol and drugs. Callers can speak with information specialists on adolescent use of alcohol or drugs or family problems caused by alcohol or drug abuse. Information will be mailed on request.

National Institute on Drug Abuse Infofax
888-644-6432 (English and Spanish)
Sixty-two two- to three-page fact sheets on illegal drug abuse and the health effects, treatment, and prevention of drug abuse.

Pride Institute for Lesbian and Gay Mental Health
168 5th Avenue
Suite 4 South
New York, NY 10010
800-54-PRIDE
Web site: *http://www.pride-institute.com*
Helps lesbian, gay, and bisexual individuals with chemical dependency and mental health problems.

Rapha
5500 Interstate North Parkway
Suite 515
Atlanta, GA 30328
800-383-HOPE
E-mail: *rebecca@intelsys.com*
Web site: *http://www.raphacare.com*
Assists callers in locating Christian psychiatric and substance abuse treatment programs.

Rational Recovery
P.O. Box 800
Lotus, CA 95651
800-303-CURE
530-621-2667
E-mail: *rr@rational.org*
Web site: *http://www.rational.org/recovery*
Nonspiritual self-help program for recovery from substance addictions and overeating.

Secular Organizations for Sobriety
5521 Grosvenor Boulevard
Los Angeles, CA 90066
310-821-8430
This is a nonspiritual, nonreligious recovery program for alcoholics and addicts. Encourages self-reliance and stresses personal responsibility.

Women for Sobriety
P.O. Box 618
Quakertown, PA 18951
800-333-1606
215-536-8026
E-mail: *newlife@nni.com*
Web site: *http://www.womenforsobriety.org*
Self-help group specifically for female alcoholics based on the Thirteen Acceptance Statements.

AGENT ORANGE
National Veterans Service Fund
P.O. Box 2465
Darien, CT 06820
800-521-0198
203-656-0003
E-mail: *natvetsvc@aol.com*
Web site: *http://www.vvnw.org/natvetsvc/index.htm*
Provides information on Agent Orange and works to see that affected veterans receive proper treatment. Helps veterans' children with birth defects.

AGING AND ELDER CARE
Children of Aging Parents
1609 Woodbourne Road
Suite 302A
Levittown, PA 19057
800-227-7294
215-945-6900
Web site: *http://www.careguide.net*
This national information and referral service is for caregivers of elderly persons. Organizes and promotes caregivers' support groups, workshops, seminars, and conferences.

Eldercare Locator
927 15th Street NW
6th Floor
Washington, DC 20036
800-677-1116
202-296-8130
Web site: *http://www.aoa.dhhs.gov/elderpage/locator.html*
A federal service that provides information on state and local resources for community-based elderly services.

Little Brothers—Friends of the Elderly
355 N. Ashland
Chicago, IL 60607
312-455-1000
E-mail: *general.chi@littlebrothers.org*
Web site: *http://www.littlebrothers.org*
Provides friendship and assistance to persons over seventy years of age who live alone and do not have emotional and physical help from families. Sponsors visitation programs and provides transportation, information, and referrals.

National Council on the Aging
409 3d Street SW
Suite 200
Washington, DC 20024
800-424-9046
202-479-1200
TDD/TTY: 202-479-6674
E-mail: *info@ncoa.org*
Web site: *http://www.ncoa.org*
Answers questions on services available to seniors. Sponsors groups relating to such topics as employment for seniors, rural aging, adult day care, senior housing, and volunteer programs for seniors.

ALBINOS
Albinism World Alliance
1530 Locust Street
Suite 29
Philadelphia, PA 19102
800-473-2310
E-mail: *awa@albinism.org*
Provides information on albinism and coordinates and promotes support groups for persons with albinism.

ALLERGIES. *See also* LUNG DISORDERS
American Allergy Association
3104 E. Camelback
Suite 459
Phoenix, AZ 85016
408-368-1238
E-mail: *allergyaid@aol.com*
Provides publications on allergies, diets, recipes, pollen data, and other information.

ALZHEIMER'S DISEASE
Alzheimer's Association
919 N. Michigan Avenue
Suite 1000
Chicago, IL 60611
800-272-3900
312-335-8700
E-mail: *info@alz.org*
Promotes family support systems for relatives of victims of Alzheimer's disease.

Alzheimer's Disease Education and Referral Center
P.O. Box 8250
Silver Spring, MD 20907
800-438-4380
301-495-3311
E-mail: *adear@alzheimers.org*
Web site: *http://www.alzheimers.org*
Federal service that provides information on Alzheimer's disease, including symptoms and current research, and makes referrals to other organizations.

Alzheimer's Family Relief Program
15825 Shady Grove Road
Suite 140
Rockville, MD 20850
800-437-2423
301-948-3244

E-mail: *sbarnard@ahaf.org*
Web site: *http://www.ahaf.org*

Provides emergency financial help for treatment of Alzheimer's patients and offers support to caregivers.

AMPUTATION
National Amputation Foundation
38-40 Church Street
Malverne, NY 11565
516-887-3600
E-mail: *amps76@aol.com*

Assists veterans and other amputees in employment and social and mental rehabilitation. Sponsors a program in which amputees who have returned to normal life visit new amputees.

AMYOTROPHIC LATERAL SCLEROSIS (ALS)
Amyotrophic Lateral Sclerosis Association (ALSA)
27001 Agoura Road
Suite 150
Calabasas Hills, CA 91301
800-782-4747
818-880-9007
E-mail: *alsinfo@alsa-national.org*
Web site: *http://www.alsa.org*

Provides research and information on ALS and patient care.

ANOREXIA NERVOSA AND BULIMIA
American Anorexia Bulimia Association
2165 W. 46th Street
Suite 1108
New York, NY 10036
212-575-5200
E-mail: *amanbu@aol.com*
Web site: *http://www.aabainc.org*

Organizes self-help groups. Provides information, referral, and outreach services.

National Association of Anorexia Nervosa and Associated Disorders
P.O. Box 7
Highland Park, IL 60035
847-831-3438
E-mail: *anad20@aol.com*
Web site: *http://www.anad.org*

This is a resource center and advocacy agency. Provides referral services and early detection programs. Organizes self-help groups and supports local and regional meetings.

National Eating Disorders Organization
6655 S. Yale Avenue
Tulsa, OK 74136
918-481-4044
Web site: *http://www.laureate.com*

Offers a referral service, support group packet, prevention video, and general information on eating disorders.

APNEA
American Sleep Apnea Association
1424 K Street NW
Suite 302
Washington, DC 20005
202-293-3650
E-mail: *asaa@sleepapnea.org*
Web site: *http://www.sleepapnea.org*

Offers educational programs and support groups through the Awake Network.

ARTHRITIS
Arthritis Foundation
1330 W. Peachtree Street
Atlanta, GA 30309
800-283-7800
404-872-7100
Web site: *http://www.arthritis.org*

Provides information on arthritis support groups, exercise classes, and other resources for persons with arthritis. Also offers information, education, and publications specific to juvenile arthritis.

ASTHMA. *See* LUNG DISORDERS

ATAXIA
National Ataxia Foundation
2600 Fernbrook Land N
Suite 119
Minneapolis, MN 55447
612-553-0020
E-mail: *naf@mr.net*
Web site: *http://www.ataxia.org*

Provides services and information to victims of ataxia and their families.

ATTENTION-DEFICIT DISORDER (ADD)
Children and Adults with Attention Deficit Disorder
8181 Professional Place
Landover, MD 20785

800-233-4050
301-306-7070
E-mail: *national@chadd.org*
Web site: *http://www.chadd.org*

Local groups provide information and support for families affected by ADD.

National Attention Deficit Disorder Association

1788 Second Street
Suite 200
Highland Park, IL 60035
847-432-ADDA
E-mail: *mail@add.org*
Web site: *http://www.add.org*

Offers support to persons with attention-deficit disorder and their families. Maintains a database of support groups.

AUTISM
Autism Society of America

7910 Woodmont Avenue
Suite 300
Bethesda, MD 20814
800-AUTISM
301-657-0881
Web site: *http://www.autism-society.org*

Provides information, education, and publications about autism, as well as on-line services and referrals.

AUTOIMMUNE DISORDERS
American Autoimmune and Related Diseases Association

22100 Gratiot Avenue
East Pointe, MI 48021
810-776-3900
E-mail: *aarda@aol.com*
Web site: *http://www.aarda.org*

Provides education and information on autoimmunity, which causes several serious chronic diseases.

National Sjogren's Syndrome Association

5815 N. Black Canyon Highway
Suite 103
Phoenix, AZ 85015
800-395-6772
602-433-9844
Fax: 602-433-9838
E-mail: *nssa@aol.com*

This is a clearinghouse for information about Sjogren's syndrome.

Scleroderma Research Foundation

P.O. Box 200
Columbus, NJ 08022
800-637-4005
609-261-2200

Provides support for parents and families and offers doctor referrals on scleroderma, a rare autoimmune disorder in which the body's immune system attacks its own tissues.

Sjogren's Syndrome Foundation

366 N. Broadway
Jericho, NY 11753
800-475-6473
516-933-6365
E-mail: *ssf@idt.net*
Web site: *http://www.sjogrens.com*

Provides information on Sjogren's syndrome, xerostomia (dry mouth), and keratoconjunctivitis sicca (dry eyes) for patients and families. Sponsors support groups and facilitates patients' sharing their experiences.

United Scleroderma Foundation

89 Newbury Street
Suite 201
Danvers, MA 01923
800-722-HOPE
978-750-4499
E-mail: *sclerofed@aol.com*

Provides education and emotional support for persons and families affected by scleroderma.

Wegener's Granulomatosis Support Group International

P.O. Box 28660
Kansas City, MO 64188
800-277-9474
816-436-8211
E-mail: *wgsg@wgsg.org*
Web site: *http://www.wgsg.org*

Provides information, publications, and support for persons and families affected by Wegener's granulomatosis.

BATTEN'S DISEASE
Batten Disease Support and Research Association

2600 Parsons Avenue
Columbus, OH 43207
800-448-4570

614-927-4298
E-mail: *bdsra1@bdsra.org*
Web site: *http://www.bdsra.org*
Provides support group activities, referrals, and information for families of children with Batten's disease.

BED-WETTING. *See* **INCONTINENCE**

BEHCET'S DISEASE
American Behcet's Disease Association
P.O. Box 280240
Memphis, TN 38168
800-723-4238
E-mail: *nyyy49c@prodigy.com*
Web site: *http://www.netcom.com/~mharting/*
behcet.html
Support and information for persons with Behcet's disease and their families.

BIRTH DEFECTS. *See also* **SPECIFIC TYPES OF DEFECT**
Association of Birth Defect Children
930 Woodcock Road
Suite 225
Orlando, FL 32803
800-313-ABDC
407-245-7035
E-mail: *abdc@marketweb.org*
Web site: *http://www.birthdefects.org*
Provides support and publications for persons with birth defects and places parents of children with similar birth defects in touch with one another. Offers help in dealing with problems that come with deformities.

National Veterans Service Fund
P.O. Box 2465
Darien, CT 06820
800-521-0198
203-656-0003
E-mail: *natvetsvc@aol.com*
Web site: *http://www.vvnw.org/natvetsvc/index.htm*
Helps veterans' children with birth defects.

BLINDNESS. *See* **VISUAL DISORDERS**

BRAIN DISORDERS
American Brain Tumor Association
2720 River Road

Suite 146
Des Plaines, IL 60018
800-886-2282
847-827-9910
E-mail: *info@abta.org*
Web site: *http://www.abta.org*
Provides educational materials and resource information to patients, families, and medical professionals. Mentors support group leaders and offers a database of support groups and a pen-pal program.

Brain Injury Association
105 N. Alfred Street
Alexandria, VA 22314
800-444-6443
703-236-6000
Web site: *http://www.biausa.org*
Provides services to persons with brain injuries and their families as well as information about traumatic brain injury. Links callers with support groups and local resources.

Brain Tumor Society
124 Watertown Street
Suite 3-H
Watertown, MA 02472
800-770-TBTS
617-924-9997
E-mail: *info@tbts.org*
Web site: *http://www.tbts.org*
Support for brain tumor patients and their families.

BULEMIA. *See* **ANOREXIA NERVOSA AND BULIMIA**

BURNS
Phoenix Society for Burn Survivors
2153 Wealthy Street SE
Suite 215
East Grand Rapids, MI 49506
800-888-BURN
616-458-2773
E-mail: *amy@phoenix-society.org*
Web site: *http://www.phoenix-society.org*
This is a self-help service organization for burn survivors and their families. Offers seminars and school and job reentry programs.

Shriner's Hospital Referral Line
2900 Rocky Point Drive

Tampa, FL 33607
800-237-5055
813-281-0300, ext. 3088
800-361-7256 (in Canada)

Gives referrals for free medical care at Shriner's Hospitals for children less than eighteen years of age who have orthopedic problems or burns.

CANCER

American Cancer Society
1599 Clifton Road NE
Atlanta, GA 30329
800-ACS-2345
404-320-3333
Web site: *http://www.cancer.org*

Provides general information on cancer and information on the group's programs and services.

Cancer Hotline
800-433-0464
816-932-8453
E-mail: *hotline@hrbloch.com*
Web site: *http://www.blochcancer.org*

Matches patients with volunteers who have had the same type of cancer. Provides resources, information, and free "Fighting Cancer" booklet.

Cancer Information Service
Office of Cancer Communication
800-4-CANCER

A federal government service that offers information on cancer treatment and diagnosis, clinical trials, rehabilitation, home care, financial aid, palliative care, supportive care for the side effects of treatment, quitting smoking, and cancer prevention. Free publications can be ordered for mail delivery, or callers can talk to trained, nonmedical information specialists. Gives referrals to certified mammography facilities.

Candlelighters Childhood Cancer Foundation
3910 Warner Street
Kensington, MD 20895
800-366-2223
301-962-3520
E-mail: *info@candlelighters.org*
Web site: *http://www.candlelighters.org*

Provides information, support, and advocacy to families of children and adolescents with cancer, survivors of childhood cancer, and professionals who work with them.

Look Good, Feel Better
American Cancer Society
1599 Clifton Road NE
Altanta, GA 30329
800-395-LOOK
Web site: *http://www.cancer.org*

A free, nonmedical program to help women overcome the appearance-related side effects of radiation and chemotherapy treatment. Programs are offered throughout the country. Provides a twenty-four-hour hotline.

National Cancer Institute
Cancer Fax Line
Fax: 301-402-5874

Provides information in English and Spanish on cancer, available by fax. More than one hundred fact sheets about cancer cover information sources, risk factors and possible causes, prevention, detection and diagnosis, cancer sites and types, types of therapies, rehabilitation, and unconventional treatment methods. Treatment statements are arranged by diagnosis, and many are available in two versions, one for patients and one for health care professionals. For technical assistance in using this fax line, call (301) 496-7403.

National Coalition for Cancer Survivorship
1010 Wayne Avenue
Suite 500
Silver Spring, MD 20910
301-650-8868
E-mail: *info@cansearch.org*
Web site: *http://www.cansearch.org*

Provides support to cancer survivors and their families and friends. Facilitates peer support and maintains a list of organizations that are concerned with survivorship.

Susan G. Komen Breast Cancer
Foundation
5005 LBJ
Suite 250
Dallas, TX 75244
800-IM-AWARE
972-855-1600
Web site: *http://www.breastcancerinfo.com*

Trained volunteers provide information and resources to individuals concerned about breast health or breast cancer.

Y-ME Breast Cancer Organization
212 W. Van Buren
5th Floor
Chicago, IL 60607
800-221-2141
312-986-8338
E-mail: *ymeone@aol.com*
Web site: *http://www.y-me.org*

Provides information, referrals, and emotional support to women concerned about or diagnosed with breast cancer. National toll-free hotline is staffed by trained personnel and volunteers who have experienced breast cancer. Publications include information tailored for single women with breast cancer, teens, and partners of women with breast cancer.

CAREGIVERS. *See* **AGING AND ELDER CARE; CHRONIC ILLNESSES**

CELIAC SPRUE. *See also* **DIGESTIVE DISORDERS**
Celiac Sprue Association, U.S.A.
P.O. Box 31700
Omaha, NE 68131
402-558-0600
E-mail: *celiacs@csaceliacs.org*
Web site: *http://www.csaceliacs.org*

Support and information on maintaining a gluten-free diet for persons affected by celiac sprue. Publications include a cookbook for gluten-free cooking.

CEREBRAL PALSY
United Cerebral Palsy Associations, Inc.
1660 L Street NW
Suite 700
Washington, DC 20036
800-872-5827
202-776-0406
TDD: 202-973-7197
Web site: *http://www.ucpa.org*

Provides information and referrals. Local affiliates provide family and individual support, early intervention programs, personal assistance and assistive technology services, and community-integrated living arrangements.

CHILDBIRTH. *See* **REPRODUCTIVE ISSUES**

CHRONIC FATIGUE SYNDROME AND FIBROMYALGIA
National Chronic Fatigue Syndrome and Fibromyalgia Association
P.O. Box 18426
Kansas City, MO 64133
816-313-2000
E-mail: *ncfsfa@aol.com*

Provides information, support, and local groups for sufferers of chronic fatigue and fibromyalgia.

CHRONIC ILLNESSES
Make Today Count
1235 E. Cherokee Street
Springfield, MO 65804
800-432-2273
417-885-3324
417-885-2584

This is a mutual support organization for persons affected by a life-threatening illnesses.

MUMS National Parent-to-Parent Network
150 Custer Court
Green Bay, WI 54301
877-336-5333
920-336-5333
E-mail: *mums@netnet.net*
Web site: *http://www.netnet.net/mums*

For parents or caregivers of a child with a disability, rare disorder, chromosomal abnormality, or serious health condition. Matches parents whose children have similar conditions so they can offer support for one another.

National Family Caregivers' Association
10400 Connecticut Avenue
Suite 500
Kensington, MD 20895
800-896-3650
301-942-6430
E-mail: *info@nfcacares.org*
Web site: *http://www.nfcacares.org*

This association for individual caregivers and others working for the needs of family caregivers offers educational material, a hotline, networking, and other resources.

Parents Helping Parents
3041 Olcott Street
Santa Clara, CA 95054

408-727-5775
E-mail: *maryellen@php.com*
Web site: *http://www.php.com*

Offer support for parents of children with special needs, including chronic or terminal illnesses. Assists new and ongoing parent support groups and resource centers.

Well Spouse Foundation
30 E. 40th Street
Suite PH
New York, NY 10018
800-838-0879
212-685-8815
E-mail: *wellspouse@aol.com*

Provides emotional support network for the spouse or partner of a chronically ill patient. Establishes local groups and provides information and materials.

CLEFT LIP AND PALATE. *See*
  CRANIOFACIAL CONDITIONS

COLITIS. *See* **CROHN'S DISEASE**

COLOSTOMY. *See* **ILEOSTOMY AND**
  COLOSTOMY

COOLEY'S ANEMIA
Cooley's Anemia Foundation
129-09 26th Avenue
Flushing, NY 11354
800-522-7222
718-321-2873
E-mail: *ncaf@aol.com*
Web site: *http://www.thalassemia.org*

Provides patient services, therapy materials, referrals to local medical sources, medical research, and public awareness and education on Cooley's anemia (also known as thalassemia).

CORNELIA DE LANGE SYNDROME
Cornelia de Lange Syndrome Foundation
302 W. Main Street
Suite 100
Avon, CT 06001
800-223-8355
860-676-8166
E-mail: *cdlsintl@iconn.net*
Web site: *http://www.cdlsoutreach.org*

Provides information and support for families,

friends, and professionals dealing with Cornelia de Lange syndrome.

CRANIOFACIAL CONDITIONS
Children's Craniofacial Association
P.O. Box 280297
Dallas, TX 75228
800-535-3643
972-994-9902

Refers callers to network support groups for persons and families affected by craniofacial anomalies. Provides referrals to doctors and explains how to get financial assistance for food, travel, and lodging related to these conditions.

Cleft Palate Foundation
104 South Estes Drive
Suite 204
Chapel Hill, NC 27514
800-242-5338

Provides general information on cleft lip, cleft palate, and craniofacial anomalies to affected persons and their families as well as information about health care teams and support groups for these conditions.

FACES: The National Craniofacial Association
P.O. Box 11082
Chattanooga, TN 37401
800-332-2373
423-266-1632
E-mail: *faces@faces-cranio.org*
Web site: *http://www.faces-cranio.org*

Provides information on related support groups and financial assistance for expenses while traveling for reconstructive surgery, based on financial and medical need. Provides referrals to other resources and organizations, support networks, and a speakers' bureau.

National Foundation for Facial Reconstruction
317 E. 34th Street
New York, NY 10016
212-263-6656
E-mail: *info@nffr.org*
Web site: *http://www.nffr.org*

Works to help children and others with craniofacial conditions to lead productive lives.

CROHN'S DISEASE
Crohn's and Colitis Foundation of America
386 Park Avenue South

17th Floor
New York, NY 10016
800-932-2423
212-685-3440
E-mail: *info@ccfa.org*
Web site: *http://www.ccfa.org*
 Provides support groups, educational publications, and programs on Crohn's disease and ulcerative colitis.

CYSTIC FIBROSIS
Cystic Fibrosis Foundation
6931 Arlington Road
Bethesda, MD 20814
800-344-4823
301-951-4422
E-mail: *info@cff.org*
Web site: *http://www.cff.org*
 Supports more than one hundred specialized care centers for people with cystic fibrosis.

DEATH AND DYING
American Association of Retired Persons
Grief and Loss Program
601 E. Street NW
Washington, DC 20049
202-434-2260
E-mail: *jgibala@aarp.org*
 This national outreach group consists of widowed volunteers who visit, support, and offer referrals to new widows and widowers.

Bereavement Services
Gunderson Lutheran Medical Center
1910 South Avenue
LaCrosse, WI 54601
800-362-9567
608-791-4747
E-mail: *berservs@gundluth.org*
Web site: *http://www.gundluth.org*
 Provides support, information, and referrals for parents who have suffered miscarriage, stillbirth, or infant death. Also offers information on fathers', children's, and grandparents' grief.

Center for Loss in Multiple Birth (CLIMB)
P.O. Box 91377
Anchorage, AK 99509
907-222-5321
907-274-7029
E-mail: *climb@pobox.alaska.net*

Web site: *http://www.climb-support.org*
 Provides peer support for parents who have lost a multiple-birth child during pregnancy or after birth. Newsletter includes resources for dealing with multiple-birth loss and names of parents willing to share experiences.

Children's Hospice International
2202 Mount Vernon Avenue
Suite 3C
Alexandria, VA 32301
800-24-CHILD
703-684-0330
 Provides information on children's hospices, referrals to local hospices, and education for affected children and their families.

The Compassionate Friends
P.O. Box 3696
Oak Brook, IL 60522
630-990-0010
E-mail: *nationaloffice@compassionatefriends.org*
Web site: *http://www.compassionatefriends.com*
 This is a self-help organization for parents and siblings of a child who has died, with chapters throughout the United States.

Heartbeat
2015 Devon Street
Colorado Springs, CO 80909
719-596-2575
719-573-7447
E-mail: *archlj@aol.com*
 Offers support to persons who have lost a loved one to suicide from persons who have resolved their own grief. Includes education aimed at preventing suicide among survivors.

Helping Other Parents in Normal Grieving (HOPING)
P.O. Box 30480
Lansing, MI 48909
517-483-3873
 Provides support for parents who have lost an infant to miscarriage, stillbirth, or infant death from trained parents who have had a similar experience.

Hospice Link
190 Westbrook Road
Essex, CT 06426

800-331-1620
203-767-1620

Provides information on hospices and palliative care. Makes referrals to local hospices, palliative care units, and bereavement support services.

National Hospice Organization
1700 Diagonal Road
Suite 300
Alexandria, VA 22314
800-658-8898
703-243-5900
E-mail: *drsnho@cais.com*
Web site: *http://www.nho.org*

Provides information on caring for terminally ill patients and their families. Gives referrals to hospices throughout the United States.

National Institute for Jewish Hospice
8723 Alden Drive
Suite 5107
Los Angeles, CA 90048
800-446-4448
323-467-7423

Provides terminal patients and their families with information on traditional Jewish views on death, dying, and the management of the loss of a loved one.

Parents of Murdered Children
100 E. 8th Street
Suite B-41
Cincinnati, OH 45202
513-721-5683
888-818-POMC
E-mail: *natlpomc@aol.com*
Web site: *http://www.pomc.com*

This self-help organization offers support for anyone who has had a family member or friend murdered. Provides information about grief and the criminal justice system. Establishes self-help groups that meet regularly. Works on violence prevention programs.

Pen-Parents
P.O. Box 8738
Reno, NV 89507
702-826-7332
E-mail: *penparents@penparents.org*
Web site: *http://www.penparents.org*

Provides support to parents dealing with the death of a child (including during pregnancy) or a teen. Offers support through correspondence for parents who do not have access to regular support groups, who are not comfortable in face-to-face groups, or who prefer written correspondence.

Pregnancy and Infant Loss Center
1421 East Wayzata Boulevard
Suite 70
Wayzata, MN 55391
612-473-9372

Offers referrals to support groups, counseling, or other parents, for parents who have suffered miscarriage, stillbirth, or infant death. Provides information on funerals, high-risk pregnancy, and the problems of surviving siblings.

Ray of Hope
P.O. Box 2323
Iowa City, IA 52244
319-337-9890

This self-help organization for persons coping with suicide, loss, and grief organizes suicide survivor support groups. Gives training and consultation on suicide prevention.

Share: Pregnancy and Infant Loss Support
300 1st Capitol Drive
St. Charles, MO 63301
800-821-6819
636-947-6164
E-mail: *share@nationalshareoffice.com*
Web site: *http://www.nationalshareoffice.com*

Provides support, information, and referrals for parents who have suffered miscarriage, stillbirth, or infant death. Assists local groups in organizing.

THEOS Foundation
322 Boulevard of the Allies
Suite 105
Pittsburgh, PA 15222
412-471-7779

Assists in planning and developing programs for widows and widowers in the United States and Canada.

DEPRESSION. *See* **MENTAL HEALTH**

DIABETES
American Diabetes Association
1701 N. Beauregard Street

Alexandria, VA 22311
800-DIABETES
703-549-1500
E-mail: *customerservice@diabetes.org*
Web site: *http://www.diabetes.org*
Provides training, guidance, and education on diabetes.

Juvenile Diabetes Foundation International
120 Wall Street
New York, NY 10005
800-JDF-CURE
212-785-9500
E-mail: *info@jdfcure.org*
Web site: *http://www.jdfcure.org*
Regional groups offer support and activities for families affected by diabetes. Provides information on specific diabetes needs.

National Diabetes Information Clearinghouse
1 Information Way
Bethesda, MS 20892
301-654-3327
This clearinghouse offers information and publications on diabetes. Gives referrals to support groups and other relevant organizations.

DIGESTIVE DISORDERS. *See also* **CELIAC SPRUE**
National Digestive Diseases Information Clearinghouse
2 Information Way
Bethesda, MD 20892
301-654-3810
E-mail: *nddic@info.niddk.nih.gov*
Web site: *http://www.niddk.nih.gov*
Provides information on the prevention and management of digestive diseases and referrals to relevant support groups and other organizations. Offers publications on many digestive disorders.

DISABILITIES, GENERAL
American Network for Community Options and Resources
4200 Evergreen Lane
Suite 315
Annandale, VA 22003
703-642-6614
E-mail: *ancor@radix.net*
Web site: *http://www.ancor.org*

This umbrella group for several hundred agencies provides services and support to persons with disabilities.

Americans with Disabilities Act Information Line
800-514-0301
TDD: 800-514-0383
Web site: *http://www.usdoj.gov/crt/adahom1.htm*
This government service provides information on Titles II and III of the Americans with Disabilities Act. Information is available over the phone from specialists, or documents may be ordered by fax or mail.

Association for the Help of Retarded Children
200 Park Avenue S
4th Floor
New York, NY 10003
212-780-2500
Web site: *http://www.ahrcnyc.org*
Provides support, training, clinics, and residential facilities for the developmentally disabled and their families.

Federation for Children with Special Needs
1135 Tremont Street
Suite 420
Boston, MA 02120
800-331-0688
617-236-7210
E-mail: *fcsninfo@fcsn.org*
Web site: *http://www.fcsn.org*
Coalition of groups concerned with children and adults with disabilities. Provides information on resources, basic rights, and obtaining services. Works for parent involvement in the care of children with disabilities and chronic illnesses and supports parent training and information.

HEATH Resource Center
American Council on Education
1 Dupont Circle NW
Suite 800
Washington, DC 20036
800-544-3284
202-939-9320
Web site: *http://www.acenet.edu*
This national clearinghouse for people with disabilities who are seeking education or training after high school provides information about access, ac-

commodations, program modifications, and national organizations. Gives referrals to local resources.

Lekotek Toy Resource Helpline
2100 Ridge Avenue
Evanston, IL 60201
800-366-PLAY
708-328-0001
Provides information on choosing appropriate toys and other play materials and creative play ideas, for children with disabilities.

National Information Center for Children and Youth with Disabilities
P.O. Box 1492
Washington, DC 20013
800-333-6293
703-893-6061
E-mail: *nichcy@aed.org*
Web site: *http://www.nichcy.org*
Provides information packets and resources regarding special-education and disability-related issues. Offers technical assistance to parents and groups.

Pilot Parents
1941 42d Street
Suite 122
Omaha, NE 68105
402-346-5220
Provides peer support for parents of children with special needs through a parent-matching program. Provides information on developmental disabilities, medical services, and local support agencies.

DISEASES, RARE. *See* **RARE DISEASES**

DONORS, MARROW AND ORGANS
Center for Organ Recovery and Education
204 Sigma Drive
Pittsburgh, PA 15238
800-366-6777
Web site: *http://www.core.org*
Provides general information on becoming an organ donor. Accepts referrals for potential donors.

The Living Bank
P.O. Box 6725
Houston, TX 77265
800-528-2971
713-961-9431

E-mail: *info@livingbank.org*
Web site: *http://www.livingbank.org*
Maintains a registry of organ donors. Provides educational materials and registration forms for organ donation.

National Marrow Donor Program
3433 Broadway NE
Suite 500
Minneapolis, MN 55413
800-MARROW-2
612-627-5800
E-mail: *chowe@NMDP.org*
Web site: *http://www.marrow.org*
This central registry of unrelated potential volunteer marrow donors provides transplant information for patients with leukemia, aplastic anemia, and other life-threatening diseases.

DOWN SYNDROME
Association for Children with Down Syndrome
4 Fern Place
Plainview, NY 11803
516-933-4700
E-mail: *info@acds.org*
Web site: *http://www.acds.org*
This is a resource and information source for parents of children with Down syndrome. Provides referrals and offers programs in New York State for preschool-age children and their siblings and recreational programs and support groups for older children.

National Down Syndrome Congress
7000 Peachtree Dunwoody Road
Building 5
Suite 100
Atlanta, GA 30328
800-232-NDSC
E-mail: *ndsccenter@aol.com*
Web site: *http://www.ndsccenter.org*
Assists parents in finding solutions to children's needs, coordinates local parents' groups, and provides a clearinghouse for information on Down syndrome.

National Down Syndrome Society
666 Broadway
New York, NY 10012
800-221-4602
212-460-9330

E-mail: *info@ndss.org*
Web site: *http://www.ndss.org*
   Provides information and referral services to families, local support groups, and community programs.

Parents of Children with Down Syndrome
c/o The ARC of Montgomery County
11600 Nebel Street
Rockville, MD 20852
301-984-5777
E-mail: *asachs@arcmontmd.org*
Web site: *http://members.aol.com/podsmc*
   Sponsors meetings, provides referrals and support, and facilitates parent-to-parent counseling for parents of children with Down syndrome.

DWARFISM
Little People of America
P.O. Box 745
Lubbock, TX 79408
888-LPA-2001
E-mail: *lpadatabase@juno.com*
Web site: *http://www.lpaonline.org*
   Provides support, publications, and information for dwarfs and other persons of short stature.

DYSLEXIA
International Dyslexia Association
8600 LaSalle Road
Baltimore, MD 21286
800-ABCD-123
E-mail: *info@interdys.org*
Web site: *http://www.interdys.org*
   Provides information, publications, and a computer database on dyslexia. Makes referrals for diagnosis and treatment.

DYSTROPHY
Reflex Sympathetic Dystrophy Association of
   America
116 Haddone Avenue
Suite D
Haddonfield, NJ 08033
609-795-8845
   Helps in forming groups for people with RSDS. Maintains a national database of research and treatment information.

ELDER CARE. *See* **AGING AND ELDER**
   CARE

EPILEPSY
Epilepsy Foundation
4351 Garden City Drive
Landover, MD 20785
800-332-1000
301-459-3700
E-mail: *info@efa.org*
Web site: *http://www.efa.org*
   Provides referrals and basic information on epilepsy for patients, families, physicians, and others.

FATTY OXIDATION DISORDER
Fatty Oxidation Disorder Family Support
805 Montrose Drive
Greensboro, NC 27410
336-547-8682
336-547-0196
E-mail: *goulddan@aol.com*
   Provides information to families affected by Fatty Oxidation disorder.

FIBROMYALGIA. *See* **CHRONIC FATIGUE**
   SYNDROME AND FIBROMYALGIA

FRAGILE X SYNDROME
National Fragile X Foundation
P.O. Box 190488
San Francisco, CA 94119
510-763-6030
E-mail: *natlfx@sprintmail.com*
Web site: *http://www.fragilex.org*
   Provides information about Fragile X syndrome and gives referrals to specialists and support groups.

GALACTOSEMIA
Parents of Galactosemic Children
885 Del Sol Street
Sparks, NV 89436
Web site: *http://www.galactosemia.org*
   Provides support and information for parents of children with galactosemia.

GAUCHER'S DISEASE
National Gaucher Foundation
11140 Rockville Pike
Suite 350
Rockville, MD 20852
800-GAUCHER
301-816-1515
E-mail: *ngf@gaucherdisease.org*

Web site: *http://www.gaucherdisease.org*

Provides support and information for persons with Gaucher's disease.

GENERAL
AirLifeLine
50 Fullerton Court
Suite 200
Sacramento, CA 95825
800-446-1231
916-641-7800
E-mail: *staff@airlifeline.org*
Web site: *http://www.airlifeline.org*

Offers free air transportation to ambulatory patients who are traveling to and from specialized medical treatment and are in financial need.

Centers for Disease Control
AIDS and Diseases Fax Information Service
Health Fax Line
Fax: 888-232-3299

A number of documents related to diseases and other health issues are available from the Centers for Disease Control and Prevention (CDC) Fax Information Service as well as from its Web site. Diseases covered include AIDS, cholera, Epstein-Barr virus, hepatitis, influenza, Lyme disease, plague, rabies, and tuberculosis. Both nontechnical information for patients and technical information for health care providers can be obtained.

Centers for Disease Control
Injury Prevention and Control Fax Information
  Service
Fax: 888-232-3299

A number of documents related to injury prevention and control are available from the Centers for Disease Control and Prevention (CDC) Fax Information Service as well as from its Web site. Both nontechnical information for patients and technical information for health care providers can be obtained.

MedicAlert Foundation United States
2323 Colorado Avenue
Turlock, CA 95382
800-ID-ALERT
E-mail: *inquiries@medicalert.org*
Web site: *http://www.medicalert.org*

Provides medical facts pertaining to the MedicAlert emblem worn on bracelets or neck chains, with an

emergency hotline number for medical professionals to call for further details. Operators available in many languages. Also gives information on obtaining a MedicAlert emblem.

National Health Information Center
800-336-4797

This is a government-sponsored referral service for individuals with health questions.

National Patient Travel Center
4620 Haygood Road
Suite 1
Virginia Beach, VA 23455
800-296-1217
E-mail: *mercymedical@erols.com*
Web site: *http://www.patienttravel.org*

Provides information on and referral to airline, charitable, and commercial service options for patients needing transport to specialized treatment facilities or places of continuing care.

National Rehabilitation Information Center
1010 Wayne Avenue
Suite 800
Silver Spring, MD 20910
800-34-NARIC
E-mail: *naricinfo@kra.com*
Web site: *http://www.naric.com*

This is a national disability and rehabilitation library and information center. Provides information on assistive devices and products. Also does document searches and takes orders for publications.

Research! America
908 King Street
Suite 400E
Alexandria, VA 22314
800-366-CURE
E-mail: *researcham.@aol.com*
Web site: *http://www.researchamerica.org*

Offers resource referrals, data, and contact names for organizations nationwide that offer support and information on a wide range of diseases and disorders.

St. Jude Children's Research Hospital
501 St. Jude Place
Memphis, TN 38173
800-877-5833
901-522-9733

Provides information on referrals to St. Jude Children's Research Hospital, which serves children who have not received extensive treatment for a disease being studied.

U.S. Office of Minority Health Resource Center
P.O. Box 37337
Washington, DC 20013
800-444-6472
TDD: 301-589-0951

This government agency is primarily for health professionals but gives information and referrals on minority health-related topics to the general public. Also offers resource lists and publications. Provides information to Hispanics and Asians in their native languages.

Visiting Nurse Associations of America
11 Beacon Street
Suite 910
Boston, MA 02108
800-426-2547
617-523-4042
Web site: *http://www.vnaa.org*

Gives referrals to callers' nearest Visiting Nurse Association. Services include general nursing; physical, occupational, and speech therapy; medical social services; case management; personal care; advanced therapies; adult day care; parent aid; care for the dying; nutritional counseling; friendly visit services; AIDS education and treatment; Meals on Wheels; and specialized nursing services.

GENETIC DISEASES. *See also* **SPECIFIC TYPES OF DISEASE**
Alliance of Genetic Support Groups
4301 Connecticut Avenue
Washington, DC 20008
800-336-GENE
202-966-5557
E-mail: *info@geneticalliance.org*
Web site: *http://www.geneticalliance.org*

Provides information and support to persons and families affected by genetic disorders. Offers referrals to appropriate genetic support groups and professionals.

National Neimann-Pick Disease Foundation
3734 E. Olive Avenue
Gilbert, AZ 85234

480-497-6638
Fax: 480-497-6346
E-mail: *stevekenyon@netwrx.net*
Web site: *http://www.nnpdf.org*

Support and phone referrals for parents of children with Neimann-Pick disease. Provides information and aids parents in getting genetic counseling.

GLYCOGEN STORAGE DISEASE
Association for Glycogen Storage Diseases
P.O. Box 896
Durant, IA 52747
319-785-6038

Facilitates communication between patients and families of patients with glycogen storage diseases and provides information to families, patients, and health care professionals. Provides referrals for treatment and helps members get equipment needed to care for GSD patients.

GRIEF. *See* **DEATH AND DYING**

GROWTH DISORDERS
Human Growth Foundation
7777 Leesburg Pike
Suite 202 South
Falls Church, VA 22043
800-451-6434
703-883-1773
E-mail: *hgfound@erols.com*

Provides information and support for individuals suffering from physical growth problems and their families.

GUILLAIN-BARRÉ SYNDROME
Guillain-Barré Syndrome Foundation International
P.O. Box 262
Wynnewood, PA 19096
610-667-0131
E-mail: *gbint@ix.netcom.com*
Web site: *http://www.webmast.com/gbs*

Develops support groups for persons suffering Guillain-Barré syndrome and their families.

HANSEN'S DISEASE. *See* **LEPROSY**

HAY FEVER. *See* **ALLERGIES**

HEADACHE
National Headache Foundation
428 W. St. James Place
2d Floor
Chicago, IL 60614
888-NHF-5552
773-388-6399
Web site: *http://www.headaches.org*
Operates local support groups and provides information for headache sufferers, their families, and physicians.

HEARING LOSS
AT&T Accessible Center
800-233-1222
Sells service and telephone equipment to persons with impaired hearing, speech, motion, or vision.

Dial-a-Hearing Screening Test
P.O. Box 18880
Media, PA 19063
800-222-EARS
800-345-EARS (in PA)
Web site: *http://www.dialatest.com*
Provides numbers for self-help groups, interpreters for the deaf, and other services for the hearing-impaired. Offers information on hearing problems, including tinnitus. Gives local referrals for free, over-the-phone hearing screening tests.

Hear Now
4248 Park Glen Road
Minneapolis, MN 55416
800-648-HEAR
303-695-7797
TDD: 800-648-HEAR
E-mail: *jostelter@aol.com*
Web site: *http://www.leisurlan.com/~hearnow/*
Offers financial assistance programs to people who need cochlear implants or hearing aids.

International Hearing Dog
5901 E. 89th Avenue
Henderson, CO 80640
303-287-3277
Fax: 303-287-3425
E-mail: *ihdi@aol.com*
Trains and places hearing dogs, who alert their hearing-impaired owners to doorbells, crying children, smoke alarms, ringing telephones, and other sounds that require attention or could indicate danger.

Ménière's Network
2000 Church Street
P.O. Box 111
Nashville, TN 37236
800-545-HEAR
615-329-7807
Administers a network of support groups, including peer support pen pals and phone friends, for sufferers of Ménière's disease in the United States. Provides scholarships to hearing-impaired students.

HEART ATTACK/DISEASE/FAILURE
Mended Hearts
7272 Greenville Avenue
Dallas, TX 75231
800-242-8721
214-706-1442
E-mail: *dbonham@heart.org*
Local groups offer advice, encouragement, and support for persons and families affected by heart disease.

HEMOCHROMATOSIS
Hemochromatosis Foundation
P.O. Box 8569
Albany, NY 12208
518-489-0972
Web site: *http://www.hemochromatosis.org*
Helps families and patients dealing with hereditary hemochromatosis by offering treatment and genetic counseling and forming support networks. Provides mailing lists and phone referrals to doctors and research centers who deal with this disease.

HEMOPHILIA
National Hemophilia Foundation
116 West 32d Street
11th Floor
New York NY 10001
212-328-3700
E-mail: *info@hemophelia.org*
Web site: *http://www.hemophelia.org*
Support, education, and information for families affected by hemophilia.

HEPATITIS
Hepatitis Foundation International
30 Sunrise Terrace
Cedar Grove, NJ 07009
800-891-0707
973-239-1035

E-mail: *mail@hepfi.org*
Web site: *http://www.hepfi.org*

Provides education and information about viral hepatitis. Maintains a database of support groups.

HERPES
Herpes Resource Center
P.O. Box 13827
Research Triangle Park, NC 27709
Hotline: 800-227-8922
919-361-8488
Web site: *http://www.ashastd.org*

Provides support and information for persons with recurring genital herpes infections and referrals to self-help groups in the United States and Canada.

HIRSCHSPRUNG'S DISEASE
American Pseudo-Obstruction and Hirschsprung's Disease Society (APHS)
158 Pleasant Street
North Andover, MA 01845
800-394-APHS
918-685-4477
E-mail: *aphs@tiac.net*
Web site: *http://www.tiac.net/users/aphs*

Provides information and support for families affected by these disorders.

HISTIOCYTOSIS
Histiocytosis Association of America
302 N. Broadway
Pitman, NJ 08071
800-548-2758
856-589-6606

Provides peer counseling, information, physician referrals, and parent/patient networking.

HIV. *See* ACQUIRED IMMUNODEFICIENCY SYNDROME (AIDS) AND HUMAN IMMUNODEFICIENCY VIRUS (HIV)

HOSPICE. *See* DEATH AND DYING

HOSPITALS AND HOSPITAL CARE
Hill-Burton Hospital Free Care
800-638-0742
800-492-0359 (in MD)
301-443-8225

This government service for low-income persons provides referrals to and information on free or below-cost hospital care.

National Association of Hospital Hospitality Houses
P.O. Box 18087
Asheville, NC 28814
800-542-9730
E-mail: *hopehouses@aol.com*

Provides information about lodging facilities available in the city to which referral has been made for medical care.

HUNTINGTON'S DISEASE
Huntington's Disease Society of America
158 W. 29th Street
7th Floor
New York, NY 10001
800-345-HDSA
212-242-1968
E-mail: *hdsainfo@hdsa.org*
Web site: *http://www.hdsa.org*

Provides information and referrals to local support groups, chapter social workers, physicians, nursing homes, and other resources. Crisis intervention and other support available.

HYDROCEPHALUS
Guardians of Hydrocephalus Research Foundation
2618 Avenue Z
Brooklyn, NY 11235
800-458-8655
718-743-GHRF

Provides information on hydrocephalus.

Hydrocephalus Association
870 Market Street
Suite 705
San Francisco, CA 94102
888-598-3789
415-732-7040
E-mail: *hydroassoc@aol.com*
Web site: *http://www.hydroassoc.org*

Facilitates networking among families affected by hydrocephalus, creates training for families, and sponsors social gatherings. Provides information in English and Spanish.

ILEOSTOMY AND COLOSTOMY
United Ostomy Association
19772 MacArthur Boulevard
Suite 200
Irvine, CA 92612
800-826-0826
714-660-8624
E-mail: *uoa@deltanet.com*
Web site: *http://www.uoa.org*
Provides information and referrals to support groups for persons who have had a colostomy, ileostomy, or similar surgical operation.

ILLNESSES, CHRONIC. *See* **CHRONIC ILLNESSES**

IMMUNIZATION
Centers for Disease Control
Immunization Fax Information Service
Fax: 888-232-3299
A number of documents related to immunization are available from the Centers for Disease Control and Prevention (CDC) Fax Information Service, as well as from its Web site. Topics include information on immunization schedules and general information on vaccines, information on specific vaccines, and how to report adverse reactions to vaccines. Provides nontechnical information for patients and technical information for health care providers.

IMMUNODEFICIENCY DISORDERS
Immune Deficiency Foundation
25 W. Chesapeake Avenue
Towson, MD 21204
800-296-4433
410-321-6647
E-mail: *idf@clark.net*
Web site: *http://www.primaryimmune.org*
Provides information for patients with inherited immunodeficiency diseases, their families, and medical professionals.

IN VITRO FERTILIZATION. *See* **REPRODUCTIVE ISSUES**

INCONTINENCE
National Association for Continence
P.O. Box 8310
Spartanburg, SC 29305
800-BLADDER

864-579-7900
Web site: *http://www.nafc.org*
This is a clearinghouse for information and services related to incontinence and assistive devices. Provides education, advocacy, and support on the causes, prevention, diagnosis, treatment, and management alternatives for persons with incontinence.

Simon Foundation for Continence
P.O. Box 815
Wilmette, IL 60091
800-23-SIMON
847-864-3913
Fax: 847-864-9758
Provides peer support and a speaker's bureau. Manages educational and self-help support groups on urinary and bowel incontinence and organizes self-help groups.

INFERTILITY. *See* **REPRODUCTIVE ISSUES**

INTRAVENTRICULAR HEMORRHAGE
IVH Parents
P.O. Box 56-1111
Miami, FL 33256-1111
305-232-0381
Provides support and information for parents of children with intraventricular hemorrhage.

IRON OVERLOAD DISEASES
Iron Overload Diseases Association
433 Westwind Drive
North Palm Beach, FL 33408
415-840-8512
415-840-8513
E-mail: *iod@ironoverload.org*
Web site: *http://www.ironoverload.org*
Works with patients, families, and doctors. Offers patient referrals by phone.

JUVENILE ARTHRITIS. *See* **ARTHRITIS**

KIDNEY DISORDERS
American Association of Kidney Patients
100 S. Asley Drive
Suite 280
Tampa, FL 33602
800-749-2257
813-223-7099

E-mail: *aakpnat@aol.com*
Web site: *http://www.aakp.org*

This is an advocacy organization for kidney patients, persons on dialysis, and those with kidney transplants.

American Kidney Fund
6110 Executive Boulevard
Suite 1010
Rockville, MD 20852
800-638-8299
301-881-3052
E-mail: *helpline@akfinc.org*
Web site: *http://www.akfinc.org*

Provides financial assistance for individuals with chronic kidney failure.

Cystinosis Foundation
2516 Stockbridge Drive
Oakland, CA 94611
800-392-8458
E-mail: *achavez@ucsd.edu*

Provides support for families affected by cystinosis.

National Kidney Foundation
30 East 33d Street
Suite 1100
New York, NY 10016
800-622-9010
212-889-2210
Web site: *http://www.kidney.org*

Makes referrals to local agencies. Supports patient services such as transportation, drug banks, and educational projects.

KLINEFELTER SYNDROME
Klinefelter Syndrome Association
P.O. Box 119
Roseville, CA 95678
916-773-2999
E-mail: *ks47xxy@ix.netcom.com*
Web site: *http://www.genetic.org*

Offers support and information for persons and families affected by Klinefelter syndrome. Facilitates networking and the exchange of information.

KLIPPEL-TRENAUNAY SYNDROME. *See also*
    STURGE-WEBER SYNDROME
Klippel-Trenaunay Support Group
5404 Dundee Road

Edina, MN 55436
612-925-2596
E-mail: *jvessey@uswest.net*
Web site: *http://www.k-t.org*

Support and information for persons with Klippel-Trenaunay syndrome and their families. Puts parents in touch with one another.

LEAD POISONING
National Lead Information Center
1019 19th Street NW
Suite 401
Washington, DC 20036
800-424-LEAD

This is a government program providing information about lead poisoning and its prevention.

LEARNING DISABILITIES
Learning Disabilities Association of America
4156 Library Road
Pittsburgh, PA 15234
888-300-6710
412-341-1515
E-mail: *ldanatl@usaor.net*
Web site: *http://www.ldanatl.org*

Information, publications, and referral service concerning learning disabilities. State and local groups provide services to families, including camps and recreation programs.

LEPROSY
American Leprosy Missions (ALM)
1 ALM Way
Greenville, SC 29601
800-543-3131
864-271-7040

Provides medical, rehabilitation, and social care, as well as information about leprosy. Refers callers to treatment centers.

LEUKEMIA
Leukemia Society of America
600 3d Avenue
New York, NY 10016
800-955-4LSA
212-573-8884
E-mail: *infocenter@leukemia.org*
Web site: *http://www.leukemia.org*

Provides callers with referrals in their area and offers educational materials and financial aid.

LEUKODYSTROPHY
United Leukodystrophy Foundation
2304 Highland Drive
Sycamore, IL 60178
800-728-5483
815-895-3211
E-mail: *ulf@tbcnet.com*
Web site: *http://www.ulf.org*

Offers information and support to persons suffering from leukodystrophy and their families. Coordinates communication among families.

LIVER DISORDERS
American Liver Foundation
75 Maiden Lane
Suite 603
New York, NY 10038
800-GO-LIVER
212-668-1000
Web site: *http://www.liverfoundation.org*

Provides physician referrals and information on support groups for persons with liver disease and their families.

LUNG DISORDERS
Lung Facts Automated Information System
800-552-LUNG

Provides free twenty-four-hour recorded messages on more than seventy topics related to the lungs and immunological diseases, including asthma, allergies, chronic bronchitis, emphysema, respiratory infections, tuberculosis, and smoking. Written information is also available.

Lung Line
800-222-LUNG

Registered nurses provide information on the detection, treatment, and prevention of lung and immunological diseases and allergies, and give referrals to local doctors.

LUPUS
L.E. Support Club
8039 Nova Court
North Charleston, SC 29420
803-764-1769
E-mail: *hmesic@awod.com*
Web site: *http://www.galaxymall.com/commerce/lupus*

Provides emotional support and self-help information for patients and families through personal correspondence and newsletter; information on nutrition and medication.

Lupus Foundation of America
1300 Picard Drive
Suite 200
Rockville, MD 20850
800-558-0121
301-670-9292
Web site: *http://www.lupus.org*

Provides information on lupus. Refers callers to local chapters, which provide support group details and physician referrals.

LYME DISEASE
American Lyme Disease Foundation
Mill Pond Offices
293 Route 100
Somers, NY 10589
800-876-LYME
914-277-6970
E-mail: *inquire@aldf.com*
Web site: *http://www.aldf.com*

Provides educational materials and information regarding Lyme disease and maintains a physician referral service.

MAPLE SYRUP URINE DISEASE (MSUD)
MSUD Family Support Group
1106 Old Line Road
Manheim, PA 17545
717- 665-5961
Web site: *http://www.msud-support.org*

Provides information on MSUD. Works for better communication between affected families and health care professionals.

MARFAN SYNDROME
National Marfan Foundation
382 Main Street
Port Washington, NY 11050
800-8-MARFAN
516-883-8721
E-mail: *staff@marfan.org*
Web site: *http://www.margan.org*

Provides information on Marfan syndrome and a support network for patients and families.

MARROW DONORS. *See* **DONORS, MARROW AND ORGANS**

MÉNIÈRE'S DISEASE. *See* **HEARING LOSS**

MENKES' DISEASE. *See* **WILSON'S DISEASE**

MENOPAUSE. *See* **WOMEN'S HEALTH ISSUES**

MENTAL HEALTH
Best Buddies International
100 SE Second Street
Suite 1990
Miami, FL 33131
305-374-2233
E-mail: *bestbuddies@juno.com*
Web site: *http://www.bestbuddies.org*
Facilitates friendships among people with mental retardation and others in the community.

Emotions Anonymous
P.O. Box 4245
St. Paul, MN 55104
651-647-9712
E-mail: *eaisc@emtn.org*
Web site: *http://www.emotionsanonymous.org*
This is a self-help group using the twelve-steps program for recovery from emotional illnesses. Provides publications, information, and referrals to local groups.

Mental Health FAX4U
National Institute of Mental Health
301-443-5158
Fax-on-demand service with four hundred documents on mental illness, Alzheimer's disease, bipolar disorders, depression, seasonal affective disorders, and other topics.

National Alliance for the Mentally Ill
2107 Wilson Boulevard
Suite 300
Arlington, VA 22201
800-950-6264
703-524-7600
Web site: *http://www.NAMI.ORG*
Provides emotional support and practical guidance for the mentally ill and their families. Offers referrals to local groups.

National Depressive and Manic Depressive Association
730 N. Franklin

Suite 501
Chicago, IL 60610
800-826-3632
312-642-0049
Web site: *http://www.ndmda.org*
Provides information on depressive and manic-depressive illnesses as medical diseases and promotes self-help for affected persons and their families.

National Foundation for Depressive Illness
800-239-1297
212-268-4260
Provides referrals to doctors who specialize in treating depression and a list of local support groups.

National Institute of Mental Health Information Service
800-64-PANIC
800-64-PANICO (Spanish)
800-421-4211 (for depression)
A government program which offers information on panic disorders and available treatments, as well information on depression, anxiety, and other conditions.

National Mental Health Association
10121 Prince Street
Alexandria, VA 22314
800-969-NMHA
703-684-7722
Web site: *http://www.nmha.org*
Offers regional support groups, information and referral programs, and other patient advocacy services.

National Mental Health Consumers Self-Help Clearinghouse
1211 Chestnut Street
Philadelphia, PA 19170
800-553-4539
215-751-1810
E-mail: *info@mhselfhelp.org*
Web site: *http://www.mhselfhelp.org*
Provides technical assistance in the development of self-help projects, information referrals, publications, and consulting services.

National Resource Center on Homelessness and Mental Illness
c/o Policy Research Associates
262 Delaware Avenue

Delmar, NY 12054
800-444-7415
518-439-7415

Provides technical assistance and comprehensive information on the treatment, services, and housing needs of homeless persons with severe mental illnesses.

Pride Institute for Lesbian and Gay Mental Health
168 5th Avenue
Suite 4 South
New York, NY 10010
800-54-PRIDE
Web site: *http://www.pride-institute.com*

Helps lesbian, gay, and bisexual individuals with chemical dependency and mental health problems.

Rapha
5500 Interstate North Parkway
Suite 515
Atlanta, GA 30328
800-383-HOPE
E-mail: *rebecca@intelsys.com*
Web site: *http://www.raphacare.com*

Assists callers in locating Christian psychiatric and substance abuse treatment.

TERRAP Programs
932 Evelyn Street
Menlo Park, CA 94025
800-2-PHOBIA

Provides self-help videos, publications, and referral information to phobia centers by mail.

METAL METABOLISM DISEASES. *See*
WILSON'S DISEASE

MISCARRIAGE. *See* **DEATH AND DYING;**
REPRODUCTIVE ISSUES

MUCOPOLYSACCHARIDOSIS (MPS)
National MPS Society
102 Aspen Drive
Downingtown, PA 19335
610-942-7188
E-mail: *presmps@aol.com*
Web site: *http://www.mpssociety.org*

Refers parents whose children have been diagnosed with MPS or mucolipidosis (ML) to other families dealing with these diseases.

MULTIPLE BIRTHS. *See also*
REPRODUCTIVE ISSUES
Center for Loss in Multiple Birth (CLIMB)
P.O. Box 91377
Anchorage, AK 99509
907-222-5321
907-274-7029
E-mail: *climb@pobox.alaska.net*
Web site: *http://www.climb-support.org*

Provides peer support for parents who have lost a multiple-birth child during pregnancy or after birth. A newsletter includes resources for dealing with multiple-birth loss and names of parents willing to share their experiences.

National Organization of Mothers of Twins Clubs
P.O. Box 23188
Albuquerque, NM 87192
800-243-2276
505-275-0955
Web site: *http://www.nomotc.org*

Local groups provide information on twins and twin care.

Triplet Connection
P.O. Box 99571
Stockton, CA 95209
209-474-0885
E-mail: *tc@tripletconnection.org*
Web site: *http://www.tripletconnection.org*

Helps parents of triplets and larger multiple births prepare for and deal with high-risk multiple births. Provides supports and facilitates networking. Offers information on such topics as breast-feeding, medical services, preventing premature births, and clothing and equipment exchanges. Also provides support for mothers who have lost one or more babies of a multiple birth.

Twinless Twins Support Group International
11220 St. Joe Road
Fort Wayne, IN 46835
219-627-5414
E-mail: *twinworld1@aol.com*
Web site: *http://www.fwi.com/twinless/*

Provides support to persons who have lost a multiple-birth sibling through death or disappearance and others dealing with multiple-birth losses. Also works to reunite multiple-birth siblings who were separated through adoption or for other reasons.

MULTIPLE SCLEROSIS
National Multiple Sclerosis Society
733 3d Avenue
New York, NY 10017
800-FIGHTMS
212-986-3240
Fax: 212-986-7981
E-mail: *info@nmss.org*
Web site: *http://www.nmss.org*
   Provides services to persons with multiple sclerosis through local chapters.

MUSCULAR DYSTROPHY
Easter Seals National Headquarters
230 W. Monroe
Suite 1800
Chicago, IL 60606
800-221-6827
312-726-6200
E-mail: *info@easterseals.org*
   Provides information and referrals for people with muscular dystrophy and related conditions.

Muscular Dystrophy Association
   Lifeline
3300 E. Sunrise Drive
Tucson, AZ 85718
800-572-1717
520-529-2000
   Provides referrals to local groups for information about muscular dystrophy support groups, clinics, and summer camps.

MYASTHENIA GRAVIS
Myasthenia Gravis Foundation
123 W. Madison
Suite 800
Chicago, IL 60602
800-541-5454
312-853-0522
E-mail: *myastheniagravis@msn.com*
Web site: *http://www.myasthenia.org*
   Provides publications and information on myasthenia gravis.

NARCOLEPSY
Narcolepsy Network
10921 Reed Hartman Highway
Cincinnati, OH 45242
513-891-3522

E-mail: *narnet@aol.com*
Web site: *http://www.webscience.org/narnet*
   Provides referral service, support group meetings, and communication among members.

NARCOTICS. *See* ADDICTION—ALCOHOL, DRUGS, AND SMOKING

NEPHRITIS. *See* KIDNEY DISORDERS

NEUROFIBROMATOSIS
National Neurofibromatosis Foundation
95 Pine Street
16th Floor
New York, NY 10005
800-323-7938
212-344-6633
Fax: 212-747-0004
E-mail: *nnff@nf.org*
Web site: *http://www.nf.org*
   Provides information, peer counseling, and referral services.

Neurofibromatosis
8855 Annapolis Road
Suite 110
Lanham, MD 20706
800-942-6825
301-577-8984
E-mail: *nfinc1@aol.com*
Web site: *http://www.nfinc.org*
   Offers support, peer counseling, and information for patients and families affected by neurofibromatosis. Provides referrals to medical resources.

NEUROSIS. *See* MENTAL HEALTH

NUTRITION
Consumer Nutrition Hotline
800-366-1655
   Provides referrals to local registered dieticians and answers questions on food and nutrition.

OBESITY AND WEIGHT LOSS
O-Anon General Service Office
P.O. Box 1314
North Fork, CA 96343
559-877-3615
   This is a twelve-step support group for families and friends of compulsive overeaters.

Overeaters Anonymous
6075 Zenith Court NE
Rio Rancho, NM 87124
505-891-2664
E-mail: *overeatr@technet.nm.org*
Web site: *http://www.overeatersanonymous.org*
This is a twelve-step support group for persons who want to stop compulsively overeating.

Take Off Pounds Sensibly (TOPS)
  Club
4575 South 5th Street
P.O. Box 07060
Milwaukee, WI 53207
800-932-8677
414-482-4620
Web site: *http://www.tops.org*
This is a self-help weight loss support group using group dynamics, competition, and recognition. Participants are required to consult with a doctor about weight loss goals and diets.

OBSESSIVE-COMPULSIVE DISORDERS. *See* **MENTAL HEALTH**

ORGAN DONORS. *See* **DONORS, MARROW AND ORGANS**

OSTEOPOROSIS
National Osteoporosis Foundation
1232 22d Street NW
Washington, DC 20037
202-223-2226
E-mail: *nofmail@nof.org*
Web site: *http://www.nof.org*
Provides information about osteoporosis.

PAGET'S DISEASE
Paget Foundation for Paget's Disease of Bone and Related Disorders
120 Wall Street
Suite 1602
New York, NY 10005
800-23-PAGET
212-509-5335
E-mail: *pagetfdn@aol.com*
Provides information, patient assistance, and referrals to medical specialists for persons with Paget's disease, primary hyperparathyroidism, or fibrous dysplasia.

PAIN MANAGEMENT
American Chronic Pain Association
P.O. Box 850
Rocklin, CA 95677
916-632-0922
E-mail: *acpa@pacbell.net*
Web site: *http://www.theacpa.org*
Offers mutual support groups for sufferers of pain lasting more than six months. Provides information on pain management.

National Chronic Pain Outreach
  Association
7979 Old Georgetown Road
Suite 100
Bethesda, MD 20814
301-652-4948
This is an information clearinghouse for pain sufferers, family members, and caregivers. Helps form local support groups for chronic pain sufferers. Provides referrals to health care providers and facilities for chronic pain.

PANIC ATTACKS. *See* **MENTAL HEALTH**

PARALYSIS
National Spinal Cord Injury Association
8701 Georgia Avenue
Suite 500
Silver Spring, MD 20910
800-962-9629
Web site: *http://www.spinalcord.org*
Assists persons with spinal cord injuries or diseases. Facilitates networking for parents of children with spinal cord injuries or related diseases.

PARANOIA. *See* **MENTAL HEALTH**

PARKINSON'S DISEASE
American Parkinson's Disease Association
1250 Hylan Boulevard
Suite 4B
Staten Island, NY 10305
800-223-2732
718-981-8001
E-mail: *apda@admin.con2.com*
Web site: *http://www.apdaparkinson.com*
Maintains information and referral centers and more than eight hundred support groups for patients and families.

National Parkinson Foundation
1501 NW 9th Avenue
Miami, FL 33136
800-327-4545
305-547-6666
Fax: 305-548-4403
E-mail: *mailbox@npf.med.miami.edu*
Web site: *http://www.parkinson.org*
Provides information and referrals to local medical facilities. Offers evaluations at the National Parkinson Foundation Center and sponsors regional support groups.

Parkinson's Disease Foundation
833 W. Washington Boulevard
Chicago, IL 60607
800-457-6676
312-733-1893
Fax: 312-733-1896
E-mail: *pdfchgo@enteract.com*
Web site: *http://www.pdf.org*
Provides information about Parkinson's disease and referrals to physicians and hospitals.

PHENYLKETONURIA (PKU)
Children's PKU Network
1520 State Street
Suite 111
San Diego, CA 92101
800-377-6677
619-233-3202
E-mail: *pkunetwork@aol.com*
Provides support groups, crisis intervention, financial assistance, and discount dietary aids for families affected by PKU.

PKU Parents
P.O. Box 950232
Mission Hills, CA 91395
Provides support and education for parents of children with PKU and gives parents a place in which to exchange information and get services and assistance. Uses a telephone network and conferences to provide specialized information.

PHOBIAS. *See* **MENTAL HEALTH**

POLIOMYELITIS
International Polio Network
4207 Lindell Boulevard

Suite 110
St. Louis, MO 63108
314-534-0475
E-mail: *gini_intl@msn.com*
Facilitates networking among persons who have had polio. Provides information and encourages research into the long-term effects of polio.

PORPHYRIA
American Porphyria Foundation
P.O. Box 22712
Houston, TX 77227
713-266-9617
Web site: *http://www.enterprise.net/apf*
Provides information on porphyria to affected persons, parents, and physicians.

POSTPARTUM DEPRESSION. *See* **REPRODUCTIVE ISSUES**

POST-TRAUMATIC STRESS DISORDER. *See* **MENTAL HEALTH**

PRADER-WILLI SYNDROME
Prader-Willi Syndrome Association, U.S.A.
5700 Midnight Pass Road
Suite 6
Sarasota, FL 34242
800-926-4797
941-312-0400
E-mail: *pwsausa@aol.com*
Web site: *http://www.pwsausa.org*
Provides information, referrals, and publications on Prader-Willi syndrome

PREGNANCY AND GESTATION. *See* **REPRODUCTIVE ISSUES**

PREMATURE BIRTH. *See* **REPRODUCTIVE ISSUES**

PREMENSTRUAL SYNDROME (PMS). *See* **WOMEN'S HEALTH ISSUES**

PSYCHOSIS. *See* **MENTAL HEALTH**

PURINE METABOLIC DISORDERS
Purine Research Society
5424 Beech Avenue
Bethesda, MD 20814

301-530-0354
E-mail: *purine@erols.com*
Web site: *http://www2.dgsys.com/~purine/*
Provides information on purine metabolic disorders, including gout, purine autism, Lesch-Nyban syndrome, and ADA deficiency.

QUADRIPLEGIA. *See* PARALYSIS

RARE DISEASES
National Organization for Rare Disorders
P.O. Box 8923
New Fairfield, CT 06812
800-999-6673
203-746-6518
E-mail: *orphan@rarediseases.org*
Web site: *http://www.nord-rdb.com/~orphan*
Gathers and disseminates information on more than three thousand rare diseases. Facilitates networking between patients with the same disorder.

REPRODUCTIVE ISSUES. *See also*
SURROGATE PARENTING
American Academy of Husband-Coached Childbirth
P.O. Box 5224
Sherman Oaks, CA 91413
800-4-A-BIRTH
818-788-6662
Web site: *http://www.bradleybirth.com*
Refers callers to local teachers of the Bradley method of natural childbirth.

Couple to Couple League
P.O. Box 111184
Cincinnati, OH 45211-1184
513-471-2000
E-mail: *ccli@ccli.org*
Web site: *http://www.ccli.org*
Sponsors local groups for couples who wish to space pregnancies by timing intercourse in accordance with a woman's natural cycle of fertility, rather than by using contraceptives. Educational publications available in English, French, Czech, Hungarian, Polish, Russian, and Spanish.

Depression After Delivery
91 E. Somerset Street
Raritan, NJ 08869
800-944-4773

Clearinghouse for information on postpartum depression, providing referrals, educational materials, and support for affected women and their families.

La Leche League International
1400 Meacham
Schaumburg, IL 60173
800-LA-LECHE
847-519-7730
Provides help, education, and encouragement for mothers who want to or are breast-feeding. Offers informal discussion groups, telephone support, and publications.

Lamaze International
1200 19th Street NW
Suite 300
Washington, DC 20036
800-368-4404
202-857-1128
E-mail: *lamaze@dc.sba.com*
Web site: *http://www.lamaze-childbirth.com*
Provides information about the Lamaze method of prepared childbirth and how to locate a local certified childbirth educator.

National Abortion Federation
1755 Massachusetts Avenue NW
Suite 600
Washington, DC 20036
Hotline: 800-772-9100
202-667-5881
E-mail: *naf@prochoice.org*
Web site: *http://www.prochoice.org*
Provides information and referrals to local abortion providers and information on pregnancy and abortion procedures.

National Infertility Network Exchange
P.O. Box 204
East Meadow, NY 11554
516-794-5772
E-mail: *nine204@aol.com*
Web site: *http://www.nine-infertility.org*
Provides peer support group, education, and referrals for persons who are infertile.

Planned Parenthood National Toll-Free Appointment Line
800-230-PLAN

Automatically connects callers to the local Planned Parenthood health center. Offers information on human sexuality and reproductive health.

Pregnancy Helpline Services
800-542-4453

Twenty-four-hour helpline sponsored by a Christian maternity home that provides housing, education, medical care, and counseling for single, pregnant young women who wish to keep their child or place their child up for adoption.

Pregnancy Hotline
c/o National Life Center
686 N. Broad Street
Woodbury, NJ 08096
800-848-LOVE

Provides guidance on pregnancy; free pregnancy tests; and medical, legal, and professional counseling referrals. Shelter, adoption, maternity care, and baby clothing available through local 1st Way affiliates. Directs callers to nearest pro-life pregnancy service.

REYE'S SYNDROME
National Reye's Syndrome Foundation
P.O. Box 829
Bryan, OH 43506
800-233-7393
419-636-2679
E-mail: *reyessyn@mail.bright.net*
Web site: *http://www.bright.net/~reyessyn*

Provides a resource clearinghouse and support groups for patients with Reye's syndrome and their families. Gives referrals to treatment centers across the United States.

RUBINSTEIN-TAYBI SYNDROME
Rubinstein-Taybi Parent Group
P.O. Box 146
Smith Cendter, KS 66967
888-447-2989
785-697-2984
E-mail: *lbaxter@ruraltel.net*
Web site: *http://www.tucson.com/rts/*

Provides support and information for parents of children with Rubinstein-Taybi syndrome.

SCHIZOPHRENIA. *See* **MENTAL HEALTH**

SCOLIOSIS
Scoliosis Association
P.O. Box 811705
Boca Raton, FL 33481
800-800-0669
561-994-4435
E-mail: *scolioassn@aol.com*
Web site: *http://www.scoliosis-assoc.org*

Provides support for persons suffering from curvature of the spine and related problems.

SELF-HELP ORGANIZATIONS, GENERAL
American Self-Help Clearinghouse
Saint Clares Health Services
25 Pocono Road
Denville, NJ 07834
973-625-3037
973-625-9565
Fax: 973-625-8848
TDD: 973-625-9053
Web site: *http://www.selfhelpgroups.org*

Publishes *The Self-Help Sourcebook*, which lists several hundred state and local self-help groups andself-help clearinghouses and gives information on how to start a self-help group. The publication is inexpensive and updated every other year.

National Mental Health Consumers Self-Help Clearinghouse
1211 Chestnut Street
Philadelphia, PA 19170
800-553-4539
215-751-1810
E-mail: *info@mhselfhelp.org*
Web site: *http://www.mhselfhelp.org*

Provides technical assistance in the development of self-help projects, information referrals, publications, and consulting services.

National Self-Help Clearinghouse
365 5th Avenue
Suite 3300
New York, NY 10016
212-817-1822
Web site: *http://www.selfhelpweb.org*

This clearinghouse offers referrals regarding self-help groups throughout the United States.

SEX CHANGE SURGERY
Renaissance Transgender Association
987 Old Eagle School Road
Suite 719
Wayne, PA 19087
610-975-9119
E-mail: *info@ren.org*
Web site: *http://www.ren.org*

Offers support for transvestites, transsexuals, and their spouses and partners.

SEXUAL DISORDERS AND DYSFUNCTION
Impotence Hotline
800-433-4215

Provides information on the diagnosis and treatment of impotence. Offers physician referrals, seminars, and free information.

Incest Survivors Anonymous
P.O. Box 17245
Long Beach, CA 90807
562-428-5599
E-mail: *bb239@lafn.org*

This program for adult and teenage victims of incest and other sexual abuse is based on the Twelve Steps and Twelve Traditions of Alcoholics Anonymous.

Sex Addicts Anonymous
P.O. Box 70949
Houston, TX 77270
713-869-4902
E-mail: *info@saa-recovery.org*
Web site: *http://www.saa-recovery.org*

This is a twelve-step support group for persons who compulsively repeat sexual behavior that is detrimental to their lives.

Sexaholics Anonymous
P.O. Box 111910
Nashville, TN 37222
615-331-6230
E-mail: *saico@sa.org*
Web site: *http://www.sa.org*

This twelve-step self-help group is for persons who want to stop self-destructive thinking and behavior, such as the use of pornography, adultery, incest, or criminal sexual activity.

SEXUALLY TRANSMITTED DISEASES. *See also* ACQUIRED IMMUNODEFICIENCY SYNDROME (AIDS) AND HUMAN IMMUNODEFICIENCY VIRUS (HIV); HERPES
Centers for Disease Control
Sexually Transmitted Disease and AIDS Hotline
800-227-8922
TDD: 800-243-7889

Provides information on sexually transmitted diseases and gives local and national referrals.

SICKLE-CELL DISEASE
Sickle Cell Disease Association of America
200 Corporate Pointe
Suite 495
Culver City, CA 90230
800-421-8453
310-216-6363

Provides referrals to local chapters for educational materials and medical help.

SLEEP DISORDERS. *See* APNEA

SMOKING. *See* ADDICTION—ALCOHOL, DRUGS, AND SMOKING

SPINA BIFIDA
Spina Bifida Association of America
4590 MacArthur Blvd NW
Suite 250
Washington, DC 20007
800-621-3141
202-944-3285

Provides support and information for families affected by spina bifida. Refers callers to local chapters.

SPONDYLITIS
Spondylitis Association
P.O. Box 5872
Sherman Oaks, CA 91413
800-777-8189
818-981-1616
E-mail: *info@spondylitis.org*
Web site: *http://www.spondylitis.org*

Provides information and support for persons and families of persons suffering from Aknylosing Spondylitis, psoriatic arthritis, and Reiter's syndrome.

STILLBIRTH. *See* **REPRODUCTIVE ISSUES**

STRESS. *See* **MENTAL HEALTH**

STROKES
National Institute of Neurological Disorders and Stroke
800-352-9424
This is a government agency offering information on headaches and other neurological disorders, their causes, and treatment.

Stroke Clubs, International
805 12th Street
Galveston, TX 77550
409-762-1022
E-mail: *strokeclub@aol.com*
Support and information for stroke victims, families, and caregivers. Has a list of more than nine hundred clubs in the United States.

STURGE-WEBER SYNDROME. *See also* **KLIPPEL-TRENAUNAY SYNDROME**
Sturge-Weber Foundation
P.O. Box 418
Mount Freedom, NJ 07970
800-627-5482
973-895-4445
E-mail: *swf@sturge-weber.com*
Web site: *http://www.sturge-weber.com*
Provides information and support for persons suffering from Sturge-Weber syndrome, Klippel-Trenaunay, and port-wine stains, their families, and other concerned persons.

STUTTERING
Stuttering Foundation of America
P.O. Box 1179
Memphis, TN 38111
800-992-9392
901-452-7343
E-mail: *stuttersfa@aol.com*
Web site: *http://www.stutterSFA.org*
Provides referrals to speech pathologists, a nationwide resource list, and free brochures.

SUDDEN INFANT DEATH SYNDROME (SIDS)
SIDS Alliance
1314 Bedford Avenue

Suite 210
Baltimore, MD 21208
800-221-SIDS
410-653-8226
Offers support and information for families affected by SIDS.

SIDS Center of New Jersey
800-996-5002
Provides support services, research, awareness, and education for those affected by the loss of a baby to Sudden Infant Death syndrome.

SUICIDE. *See* **DEATH AND DYING**

SURROGATE PARENTING. *See also* **REPRODUCTIVE ISSUES**
Donors' Offspring
P.O. Box 37
Sarcoxie, MO 64862
417-763-1906
E-mail: *candace1@usa.net*
Web site: *http://www.cubirthparents.org*
This is a self-help support group for donors, recipients, surrogate parents, offspring, and others affected by artificial fertilization. Provides children's services and peer counseling, a referral service, and help in locating medical histories.

National Association of Surrogate Mothers
8383 Wilshire Blvd
Suite 750
Beverly Hills, CA 90211
323-655-2015
E-mail: *centersp@aol.com*
Web site: *http://www.creatingfamilies.com*
Provides support for surrogate mothers, enabling them to share experiences and information.

Organization of Parents Through Surrogacy
P.O. Box 611
Gurnee, IL 60031
847-782-0224
E-mail: *opts@voyager.net*
Web site: *http://www.opts.com*
Provides support for families created through surrogate parenting, including phone and e-mail support for members. Also provides information and referrals to infertile couples.

TAY-SACHS DISEASE
National Tay-Sachs and Allied Diseases Association
2001 Beacon Street
Suite 204
Boston, MA 02135
800-906-8723
617-277-4463
E-mail: *ntsad-boston@worldnet.att.net*
Web site: *http://www.ntsad.org*
Offers support groups for parents of children with Tay-Sachs and related diseases. Also acts as a clearinghouse of information for families and professionals.

TERMINALLY ILL CHILDREN, WISHES FOR
Brass Ring Society
213 N. Washington Street
Snow Hill, MD 21863
800-666-WISH
410-339-6188
E-mail: *brassring@brassring.org*
Web site: *http://www.worldramp.net/brassring*
Seeks to fulfill the wishes of children with life-threatening illnesses.

Children's Wish Foundation International
8615 Roswell Road
Altanta, GA 30350
800-323-9474
770-393-9474
Seeks to fulfill the wishes of terminally ill children.

Dream Factory
1218 S. 3d Street
Louisville, KY 40203
800-456-7556
505-637-8700
E-mail: *dfngtrs@aol.com*
Web site: *http://www.dreamfactoryinc.org*
Seeks to fulfill the wishes of chronically or critically ill children and works to promote a more positive family atmosphere in the face of a prolonged illness.

Make-a-Wish Foundation of America
100 W. Clarendon Street
Suite 2200
Phoenix, AZ 85013

800-722-WISH
602-279-9474
E-mail: *mawfa@wish.org*
Web site: *http://www.wish.org*
Seeks to fulfill the wishes of children with terminal illnesses or other life-threatening conditions.

TERMINALLY ILL: EXTENDED CARE. *See* AGING AND ELDER CARE; DEATH AND DYING

THALASSEMIA. *See* COOLEY'S ANEMIA

TORTICOLLIS
National Spasmodic Torticollis Association
9920 Talbert Avenue
Suite 233
Fountain Valley, CA 92708
800-HURTFUL
714-378-7837
Fax: 714-378-7830
E-mail: *nstamail@aol.com*
Web site: *http://www.torticollis.org*
Provides support for persons with spasmodic torticollis.

TOURETTE'S SYNDROME
Tourette's Syndrome Association
42-40 Bell Boulevard
Bayside, NY 11361
888-486-8738
718-224-2999
E-mail: *tourette@ix.netcom.com*
Web site: *http://tsa.mgh.harard.edu*
Offers physician referrals and provides access to support groups and other services for persons with Tourette's syndrome and their families. Helps people identify and understand Tourette's syndrome.

TUBERCULOSIS. *See* LUNG DISORDERS

TUBEROUS SCLEROSIS
National Tuberous Sclerosis Association
8181 Professional Place
Suite 110
Landover, MD 20785
800-225-NTSA
301-459-9888
Fax: 301-459-0394
E-mail: *nts@ntsa.org*

Web site: *http://www.ntsa.org*

Coordinates a national network of volunteers and provides referrals to state groups and information on tuberous sclerosis.

TURNER SYNDROME
Turner's Syndrome Society of the United States
1313 SE 5th Street
Suite 327
Minneapolis, MN 55414
800-365-9944
612-379-3607
E-mail: *tesch005@tc.umn.edu*
Web site: *http://www.turner-syndrome-us.org*

Provides support and information for families affected by Turner syndrome.

URINARY DISORDERS. *See* INCONTINENCE; KIDNEY DISORDERS

VISUAL DISORDERS
American Council of the Blind
1155 15th Street NW
Suite 1004
Washington, DC 20005
800-424-8666
202-467-5081
E-mail: *info@acb.org*
Web site: *http://www.abc.org*

Promotes the independence and dignity of blind and visually impaired persons. Works for civil rights, employment, rehabilitation services, safe and expanded transportation, travel and recreation, Social Security benefits, and accessibility.

American Foundation for the Blind
11 Pen Plaza
Suite 300
New York, NY 10001
800-AFB-LINE
212-502-7600
E-mail: *afbinfo@afb.net*
Web site: *http://www.afb.org*

This is an information and referral service for organizations for the blind. Includes a reference directory of services in the United States.

Blind Children's Fund
4740 Okemos Road
Okemos, MI 48864

517-347-1357
E-mail: *blindchfnd@aol.com*
Web site: *http://www.blindchildrensfund.org*

Promotes the health, education, and welfare of blind and visually impaired infants and preschoolers.

Blinded Veterans Association Hotline
477 H Street NW
Washington, DC 20001
800-669-7079
202-371-8880
E-mail: *bva@bva.org*
Web site: *http://www.bva.org*

Provides information on benefits and services for blinded veterans.

Council of Citizens with Low Vision
1155 15th Street NW
Suite 720
Washington, DC 20005
800-733-2258
202-467-5081
E-mail: *info@acb.org*
Web site: *http://www.ccivi.org*

Offers outreach programs, advocacy, and educational services for partially sighted and low-vision persons.

Foundation Fighting Blindness
Executive Plaza 1
Suite 800
11350 McCormick Road
Hunt Valley, MD 21031
888-394-3937
410-785-1414
TDD: 410-785-9687 or 800-683-5551

Provides information and referral services and support networks for persons with retinal degeneration, such as retinitis pigmentosa, Usher's syndrome, and macular degeneration.

Guide Dog Foundation for the Blind, Inc.
371 E. Jericho Turnpike
Smithtown, NY 11787
800-548-4337
631-265-2121
E-mail: *wjones@guidedog.org*
Web site: *http://www.guidedog.org*

Provides trained guide dogs to the visually impaired. Provides a training program, a dog, all necessary equipment, and airfare within the United States at no charge to students accepted by the program.

Lighthouse
111 E. 59th Street
New York, NY 10022
800-334-5497
212-821-9713
212-821-9200
E-mail: *info@lighthouse.org*
Web site: *http://www.lighthouse.org*
Provides educational material on vision and childhood development, vision and aging, and low vision. Gives referrals to vision rehabilitation agencies, low-vision resources, and support groups nationwide.

National Association for Parents of the Visually Impaired
P.O. Box 317
Watertown, MA 02272
800-562-6265
617-972-7441
E-mail: *napvi@perkins.pvt.k12.ma.us*
Web site: *http://www.spedex.com/napvi*
Database provides support group of parents of visually impaired persons.

National Eye Care Project
P.O. Box 429098
San Francisco, CA 94142
800-222-EYES
Web site: *http://www.eyenet.org*
Assists disadvantaged elderly persons who cannot afford proper eye care. Participating doctors provide medical eye exams and treat vision conditions or diseases.

National Library Service for the Blind and Physically Handicapped
Library of Congress
1291 Taylor Street NW
Washington, DC 20542
800-424-8567
800-424-9100
202-707-5100
Administers a national library service that provides Braille and audio-recorded books and free loans to persons with vision problems or other physical disabilities that prevent the person from reading. Makes referrals to state and local libraries.

Xavier Society for the Blind
154 E. 23d Street
New York, NY 10010
800-637-9193
212-473-7800
Provides spiritual reading material in the Catholic tradition, periodicals, and a lending library. Publications are available in Braille, in large print, and on cassette tape.

WIDOWHOOD. *See* **DEATH AND DYING**

WILSON'S DISEASE
National Center for the Study of Wilson's Disease
432 W. 58th Street
Suite 614
New York, NY 10019
888-638-6928
212-523-8717
Web site: *http://www.wilsondiseasecenter.org*
Research and information on hereditary diseases of metal metabolism, particularly Wilson's disease and Menkes' disease.

Wilson's Disease Association
4 Navaho Drive
Brookfield, CT 06810
800-399-0266
203-775-9666
E-mail: *hasellner@worldnet.att.net*
Web site: *http://www.wilsonsdisease.org*
Provides support and financial aid to needy families, information, and coordination among members and related organizations.

WOMEN'S HEALTH ISSUES
Endometriosis Association
8585 N. 76th Place
Milwaukee, WI 53223
800-992-3636
414-355-2200
E-mail: *endo@endometriosisassn.org*
Web site: *http://www.endometriosisassn.org*
Sponsors self-help support and informational meetings. Provides brochures in twenty-three languages and publications specifically for teens.

North American Menopause Society
P.O. Box 94527
Cleveland, OH 44101

440-442-7550
E-mail: *info@menopause.org*
Web site: *http://www.menopause.org*

Provides information on midlife medical issues. Maintains a database of menopause care providers and support groups.

Older Women's League (OWL)
666 11th St. NW
Suite 700

Washington, DC 20001
202-783-6686
Web site: *http://www.owl-national.org*

Information on and support for issues affecting middle-aged and older women, such as health care and insurance, maintaining independence, and support for family caregivers.

—Irene Rush

MAGILL'S

MEDICAL GUIDE

ALPHABETICAL LIST OF CONTENTS

Cholesterol
Chorionic villus sampling
Chronic fatigue syndrome
Chronobiology
Circulation
Circumcision, female, and genital mutilation
Circumcision, male
Cirrhosis
Claudication
Cleft lip and palate
Cleft lip and palate repair
Clinical trials
Cloning
Club drugs
Cluster headaches
Cognitive development
Colic
Colitis
Colon and rectal polyp removal
Colon and rectal surgery
Colon cancer
Colon therapy
Colonoscopy
Color blindness
Coma
Common cold
Computed tomography (CT) scanning
Conception
Concussion
Congenital heart disease
Conjunctivitis
Constipation
Contraception
Corneal transplantation
Corns and calluses
Coughing
Cradle cap
Craniosynostosis
Craniotomy
Cretinism
Creutzfeldt-Jakob disease and mad cow disease
Critical care
Critical care, pediatric
Crohn's disease
Croup
Crowns and bridges
Cryotherapy and cryosurgery
Culdocentesis
Cushing's syndrome
Cyst removal
Cystectomy

Cystic fibrosis
Cystitis
Cystoscopy
Cysts
Cytology
Cytomegalovirus (CMV)
Cytopathology

Death and dying
Dehydration
Delusions
Dementias
Dental diseases
Dentistry
Dentistry, pediatric
Dentures
Depression
Dermatitis
Dermatology
Dermatology, pediatric
Dermatopathology
Developmental stages
Diabetes mellitus
Dialysis
Diaper rash
Diarrhea and dysentery
Digestion
Diphtheria
Disease
Disk removal
Diverticulitis and diverticulosis
Dizziness and fainting
DNA and RNA
Domestic violence
Down syndrome
Drug resistance
Dwarfism
Dyslexia
Dysmenorrhea
Dystrophy

E. coli infection
Ear infections and disorders
Ear surgery
Ears
Eating disorders
Ebola virus
Eclampsia
Ectopic pregnancy
Eczema
Edema
Education, medical
Electrical shock
Electrocardiography (ECG or EKG)

Electrocauterization
Electroencephalography (EEG)
Elephantiasis
Embolism
Embryology
Emergency medicine
Emergency medicine, pediatric
Emotions: Biomedical causes and effects
Emphysema
Encephalitis
Endarterectomy
Endocarditis
Endocrine disorders
Endocrinology
Endocrinology, pediatric
Endodontic disease
Endometrial biopsy
Endometriosis
Endoscopy
Enemas
Enterocolitis
Environmental diseases
Environmental health
Enzyme therapy
Enzymes
Epidemiology
Epiglottitis
Epilepsy
Episiotomy
Estrogen replacement therapy
Ethics
Euthanasia
Ewing's sarcoma
Exercise physiology
Eye surgery
Eyes

Face lift and blepharoplasty
Factitious disorders
Failure to thrive
Family practice
Fatigue
Feet
Fetal alcohol syndrome
Fetal tissue transplantation
Fever
Fifth disease
Fistula repair
Flat feet
Fluids and electrolytes
Fluoride treatments
Food and Drug Administration (FDA)

Kinesiology
Klinefelter syndrome
Kneecap removal
Knock-knees
Kwashiorkor
Kyphosis

Laboratory tests
Laceration repair
Lactose intolerance
Laminectomy and spinal fusion
Laparoscopy
Laryngectomy
Laryngitis
Laser use in surgery
Law and medicine
Lead poisoning
Learning disabilities
Legionnaires' disease
Leishmaniasis
Leprosy
Leptin
Leukemia
Lice, mites, and ticks
Light therapy
Lipids
Liposuction
Lisping
Lithotripsy
Liver
Liver cancer
Liver disorders
Liver transplantation
Lower extremities
Lumbar puncture
Lung cancer
Lung surgery
Lungs
Lupus erythematosus
Lyme disease
Lymphadenopathy and lymphoma
Lymphatic system

Macular degeneration
Magnetic field therapy
Magnetic resonance imaging
  (MRI)
Malabsorption
Malaria
Malignancy and metastasis
Malignant melanoma removal
Malnutrition
Malpractice
Mammography

Marfan syndrome
Massage
Mastectomy and lumpectomy
Mastitis
Masturbation
Measles
Medicare
Meditation
Melatonin
Memory loss
Ménière's disease
Meningitis
Menopause
Menorrhagia
Menstruation
Mental retardation
Metabolism
Microbiology
Microscopy
Microscopy, slitlamp
Midlife crisis
Migraine headaches
Miscarriage
Mitral valve prolapse
Mold and mildew
Moles
Mononucleosis
Motion sickness
Motor neuron diseases
Motor skill development
Multiple births
Multiple chemical sensitivity
  syndrome
Multiple sclerosis
Mumps
Münchausen syndrome by proxy
Muscle sprains, spasms, and
  disorders
Muscles
Muscular dystrophy
Mutation
Myomectomy
Myopia
Myringotomy

Nail removal
Nails
Narcolepsy
Narcotics
Nasal polyp removal
Nasopharyngeal disorders
National Cancer Institute (NCI)
National Institutes of Health (NIH)
Nausea and vomiting

Necrotizing fasciitis
Neonatology
Nephrectomy
Nephritis
Nephrology
Nephrology, pediatric
Nervous system
Neuralgia, neuritis, and neuropathy
Neurofibromatosis
Neurology
Neurology, pediatric
Neurosis
Neurosurgery
Nightmares
Noninvasive tests
Nosebleeds
Nuclear medicine
Nuclear radiology
Numbness and tingling
Nursing
Nutrition

Obesity
Obsessive-compulsive disorder
Obstetrics
Obstruction
Occupational health
Oncology
Ophthalmology
Optometry
Optometry, pediatric
Orchitis
Orthodontics
Orthopedic surgery
Orthopedics
Orthopedics, pediatric
Osgood-Schlatter disease
Osteoarthritis
Osteochondritis juvenilis
Osteogenesis imperfecta
Osteomyelitis
Osteopathic medicine
Osteoporosis
Otoplasty
Otorhinolaryngology
Ovarian cysts
Oxygen therapy

Pacemaker implantation
Paget's disease
Pain
Pain management
Palpitations
Palsy

ENTRIES BY ANATOMY OR SYSTEM AFFECTED

Colitis
Colon and rectal polyp removal
Colon and rectal surgery
Colon cancer
Colon therapy
Colonoscopy
Computed tomography (CT) scanning
Constipation
Crohn's disease
Cystectomy
Diabetes mellitus
Dialysis
Diarrhea and dysentery
Digestion
Diverticulitis and diverticulosis
Endoscopy
Enemas
Enterocolitis
Fistula repair
Gallbladder diseases
Gastrectomy
Gastroenterology
Gastroenterology, pediatric
Gastrointestinal disorders
Gastrointestinal system
Gastrostomy
Giardiasis
Hernia
Hernia repair
Hirschsprung's disease
Ileostomy and colostomy
Incontinence
Indigestion
Internal medicine
Intestinal disorders
Intestines
Irritable bowel syndrome (IBS)
Kidney transplantation
Kidneys
Laparoscopy
Liposuction
Lithotripsy
Liver
Liver transplantation
Malabsorption
Nephrectomy
Nephritis
Nephrology
Nephrology, pediatric
Obstruction
Pancreas
Pancreatitis
Peristalsis

Peritonitis
Pregnancy and gestation
Prostate cancer
Pyloric stenosis
Reproductive system
Roundworm
Shunts
Splenectomy
Sterilization
Stomach, intestinal, and pancreatic cancers
Stone removal
Stones
Syphilis
Tubal ligation
Ultrasonography
Urethritis
Urinary disorders
Urinary system
Urology
Urology, pediatric
Worms

ANUS
Colon and rectal polyp removal
Colon and rectal surgery
Colon cancer
Colon therapy
Colonoscopy
Diaper rash
Endoscopy
Enemas
Episiotomy
Fistula repair
Hemorrhoid banding and removal
Hemorrhoids
Hirschsprung's disease
Intestinal disorders
Intestines
Irritable bowel syndrome (IBS)
Soiling
Sphincterectomy

ARMS
Amputation
Bones and the skeleton
Carpal tunnel syndrome
Fracture and dislocation
Fracture repair
Liposuction
Muscles
Pityriasis rosea
Skin lesion removal
Tendon disorders

Tendon repair
Thalidomide
Upper extremities

BACK
Arthritis, juvenile rheumatoid
Bone disorders
Bone marrow transplantation
Bones and the skeleton
Cerebral palsy
Chiropractic
Disk removal
Dwarfism
Gigantism
Kyphosis
Laminectomy and spinal fusion
Lumbar puncture
Muscle sprains, spasms, and disorders
Muscles
Osteoporosis
Pityriasis rosea
Sciatica
Scoliosis
Slipped disk
Spinal cord disorders
Spine, vertebrae, and disks
Spondylitis
Sympathectomy
Tendon disorders

BLADDER
Abdomen
Bed-wetting
Candidiasis
Catheterization
Cystectomy
Cystitis
Cystoscopy
Endoscopy
Fistula repair
Incontinence
Internal medicine
Lithotripsy
Schistosomiasis
Sphincterectomy
Stone removal
Stones
Toilet training
Ultrasonography
Urethritis
Urinalysis
Urinary disorders
Urinary system

Podiatry
Rheumatology
Rickets
Sarcoma
Sarcopenia
Scoliosis
Slipped disk
Spinal cord disorders
Spine, vertebrae, and disks
Sports medicine
Teeth
Temporomandibular joint (TMJ)
    syndrome
Tendon disorders
Tendon repair
Upper extremities

BRAIN
Abscess drainage
Abscesses
Addiction
Alcoholism
Altitude sickness
Alzheimer's disease
Amnesia
Anesthesia
Anesthesiology
Aneurysmectomy
Aneurysms
Angiography
Aphasia and dysphasia
Aromatherapy
Attention-deficit disorder (ADD)
Auras
Biofeedback
Brain
Brain disorders
Cluster headaches
Cognitive development
Coma
Computed tomography (CT) scanning
Concussion
Craniotomy
Creutzfeldt-Jakob disease and mad
    cow disease
Cytomegalovirus (CMV)
Dehydration
Dementias
Developmental stages
Dizziness and fainting
Down syndrome
Dyslexia
Electroencephalography (EEG)
Embolism

Emotions: Biomedical causes and
    effects
Encephalitis
Endocrinology
Endocrinology, pediatric
Epilepsy
Failure to thrive
Fetal alcohol syndrome
Fetal tissue transplantation
Fragile X syndrome
Galactosemia
Gigantism
Gulf War syndrome
Hallucinations
Head and neck disorders
Headaches
Hydrocephalus
Hypertension
Hypnosis
Jaundice
Kinesiology
Lead poisoning
Learning disabilities
Light therapy
Malaria
Melatonin
Memory loss
Meningitis
Mental retardation
Migraine headaches
Narcolepsy
Narcotics
Nausea and vomiting
Neurology
Neurology, pediatric
Neurosurgery
Nuclear radiology
Parkinson's disease
Pharmacology
Pharmacy
Phenylketonuria (PKU)
Poliomyelitis
Positron emission tomography (PET)
    scanning
Prion diseases
Psychiatric disorders
Psychiatry
Psychiatry, child and adolescent
Psychiatry, geriatric
Rabies
Reye's syndrome
Schizophrenia
Seizures
Shock therapy

Shunts
Sleep disorders
Sleeping sickness
Sleepwalking
Stammering
Strokes
Syphilis
Tetanus
Thrombolytic therapy and TPA
Thrombosis and thrombus
Tics
Tourette's syndrome
Toxicology
Toxoplasmosis
Trembling and shaking
Tumor removal
Tumors
Unconsciousness
Weight loss medications
Yellow fever

BREASTS
Abscess drainage
Abscesses
Breast biopsy
Breast cancer
Breast disorders
Breast-feeding
Breast surgery
Breasts, female
Cyst removal
Cysts
Estrogen replacement therapy
Glands
Gynecology
Gynecomastia
Klinefelter syndrome
Mammography
Mastectomy and lumpectomy
Mastitis
Sex change surgery
Tumor removal
Tumors

CELLS
Acid-base chemistry
Bacteriology
Biopsy
Cell therapy
Cells
Cholesterol
Conception
Cytology
Cytomegalovirus (CMV)

Cytopathology
Dehydration
DNA and RNA
E. coli infection
Enzymes
Fluids and electrolytes
Food biochemistry
Genetic counseling
Genetic engineering
Glycolysis
Gram staining
Gulf War syndrome
Host-defense mechanisms
Immunization and vaccination
Immunology
In vitro fertilization
Kinesiology
Laboratory tests
Lipids
Magnetic field therapy
Microbiology
Microscopy
Mutation
Pharmacology
Pharmacy
Toxicology

CHEST
Anatomy
Asthma
Bones and the skeleton
Breasts, female
Bronchiolitis
Bronchitis
Bypass surgery
Cardiac rehabilitation
Cardiology
Cardiology, pediatric
Chest
Choking
Common cold
Congenital heart disease
Coughing
Croup
Cystic fibrosis
Electrocardiography (ECG or EKG)
Embolism
Emphysema
Gulf War syndrome
Heart
Heart transplantation
Heart valve replacement
Heartburn
Hiccups

Interstitial pulmonary fibrosis (IPF)
Legionnaires' disease
Lung cancer
Lungs
Pacemaker implantation
Pityriasis rosea
Pleurisy
Pneumonia
Pulmonary diseases
Pulmonary medicine
Pulmonary medicine, pediatric
Respiration
Respiratory distress syndrome
Resuscitation
Sneezing
Thoracic surgery
Tuberculosis
Whooping cough

CIRCULATORY SYSTEM
Aneurysmectomy
Aneurysms
Angina
Angiography
Angioplasty
Apgar score
Arrhythmias
Arteriosclerosis
Arthritis, juvenile rheumatoid
Biofeedback
Bleeding
Blood and blood disorders
Blood testing
Blue baby syndrome
Bypass surgery
Cardiac rehabilitation
Cardiology
Cardiology, pediatric
Catheterization
Chest
Cholesterol
Circulation
Claudication
Congenital heart disease
Dehydration
Diabetes mellitus
Dialysis
Dizziness and fainting
Ebola virus
Eclampsia
Edema
Electrocardiography (ECG or EKG)
Electrocauterization
Embolism

Endarterectomy
Endocarditis
Exercise physiology
Heart
Heart attack
Heart disease
Heart failure
Heart transplantation
Heart valve replacement
Heat exhaustion and heat stroke
Hematology
Hematology, pediatric
Hemorrhoid banding and removal
Hemorrhoids
Hormones
Hypercholesterolemia
Hypertension
Ischemia
Kidneys
Kinesiology
Liver
Lymphatic system
Mitral valve prolapse
Motor skill development
Nosebleeds
Osteochondritis juvenilis
Pacemaker implantation
Palpitations
Phlebitis
Resuscitation
Reye's syndrome
Rheumatic fever
Septicemia
Shock
Shunts
Smoking
Sports medicine
Steroid abuse
Strokes
Systems and organs
Testicular torsion
Thrombolytic therapy and TPA
Thrombosis and thrombus
Transfusion
Transplantation
Varicose vein removal
Varicose veins
Vascular medicine
Vascular system
Venous insufficiency

EARS
Altitude sickness
Audiology

Auras
Biophysics
Cytomegalovirus (CMV)
Dyslexia
Ear infections and disorders
Ear surgery
Ears
Fragile X syndrome
Hearing aids
Hearing loss
Hearing tests
Ménière's disease
Motion sickness
Myringotomy
Nervous system
Neurology
Neurology, pediatric
Osteogenesis imperfecta
Otoplasty
Otorhinolaryngology
Plastic surgery
Quinsy
Sense organs
Speech disorders

ENDOCRINE SYSTEM
Addison's disease
Adrenalectomy
Biofeedback
Breasts, female
Contraception
Cretinism
Diabetes mellitus
Dwarfism
Eating disorders
Emotions: Biomedical causes and
   effects
Endocrine disorders
Endocrinology
Endocrinology, pediatric
Estrogen replacement therapy
Failure to thrive
Gigantism
Glands
Goiter
Hormone replacement therapy
Hormones
Hyperparathyroidism and
   hypoparathyroidism
Hypoglycemia
Klinefelter syndrome
Liver
Melatonin
Obesity

Pancreas
Pancreatitis
Parathyroidectomy
Postpartum depression
Prostate gland
Prostate gland removal
Sex change surgery
Sexual differentiation
Steroid abuse
Steroids
Systems and organs
Testicular surgery
Thyroid disorders
Thyroid gland
Thyroidectomy
Turner syndrome
Weight loss medications

EYES
Albinos
Arthritis, juvenile rheumatoid
Astigmatism
Auras
Blindness
Blurred vision
Cataract surgery
Cataracts
Chlamydia
Color blindness
Conjunctivitis
Corneal transplantation
Cytomegalovirus (CMV)
Diabetes mellitus
Dyslexia
Eye surgery
Eyes
Face lift and blepharoplasty
Galactosemia
Glaucoma
Gonorrhea
Gulf War syndrome
Jaundice
Laser use in surgery
Macular degeneration
Marfan syndrome
Microscopy, slitlamp
Motor skill development
Multiple chemical sensitivity
   syndrome
Myopia
Ophthalmology
Optometry
Optometry, pediatric
Pigmentation

Ptosis
Sense organs
Strabismus
Styes
Toxoplasmosis
Trachoma
Transplantation
Visual disorders

FEET
Athlete's foot
Bones and the skeleton
Bunions
Corns and calluses
Cysts
Feet
Flat feet
Foot disorders
Fragile X syndrome
Frostbite
Ganglion removal
Gout
Hammertoe correction
Hammertoes
Heel spur removal
Lower extremities
Nail removal
Nails
Orthopedic surgery
Orthopedics
Orthopedics, pediatric
Osteoarthritis
Pigeon toes
Podiatry
Sports medicine
Tendon repair
Thalidomide
Warts

GALLBLADDER
Abscess drainage
Abscesses
Cholecystectomy
Cholecystitis
Fistula repair
Gallbladder diseases
Gastroenterology
Gastroenterology, pediatric
Gastrointestinal disorders
Gastrointestinal system
Internal medicine
Laparoscopy
Liver transplantation
Malabsorption

Nuclear medicine
Stone removal
Stones
Ultrasonography

GASTROINTESTINAL SYSTEM
Abdomen
Abdominal disorders
Allergies
Anthrax
Appendectomy
Appendicitis
Bacterial infections
Botulism
Bulimia
Burping
Bypass surgery
Candidiasis
Celiac sprue
Childhood infectious diseases
Cholera
Cholesterol
Colic
Colitis
Colon and rectal polyp removal
Colon and rectal surgery
Colon cancer
Colon therapy
Colonoscopy
Constipation
Crohn's disease
Cytomegalovirus (CMV)
Diabetes mellitus
Diarrhea and dysentery
Digestion
Diverticulitis and diverticulosis
E. coli infection
Eating disorders
Ebola virus
Emotions: Biomedical causes and
  effects
Endoscopy
Enemas
Enterocolitis
Fistula repair
Food biochemistry
Food poisoning
Gallbladder diseases
Gastrectomy
Gastroenterology
Gastroenterology, pediatric
Gastrointestinal disorders
Gastrointestinal system
Gastrostomy

Giardiasis
Glands
Gulf War syndrome
Halitosis
Heartburn
Hemorrhoid banding and removal
Hemorrhoids
Hernia
Hernia repair
Hirschsprung's disease
Host-defense mechanisms
Ileostomy and colostomy
Incontinence
Indigestion
Internal medicine
Intestinal disorders
Intestines
Irritable bowel syndrome (IBS)
Kwashiorkor
Lactose intolerance
Laparoscopy
Lipids
Liver
Malabsorption
Malnutrition
Metabolism
Motion sickness
Muscles
Nausea and vomiting
Nutrition
Obesity
Obstruction
Pancreas
Pancreatitis
Peristalsis
Pinworm
Poisoning
Poisonous plants
Premenstrual syndrome (PMS)
Proctology
Protozoan diseases
Pyloric stenosis
Radiation sickness
Roundworm
Salmonella infection
Sense organs
Shigellosis
Shunts
Soiling
Stomach, intestinal, and pancreatic
  cancers
Systems and organs
Tapeworm
Taste

Teeth
Toilet training
Trichinosis
Tumor removal
Tumors
Typhoid fever and typhus
Ulcer surgery
Ulcers
Vagotomy
Vitamins and minerals
Weaning
Weight loss and gain
Worms

GENITALS
Candidiasis
Catheterization
Cervical, ovarian, and uterine
  cancers
Cervical procedures
Chlamydia
Circumcision, female, and genital
  mutilation
Circumcision, male
Contraception
Culdocentesis
Cyst removal
Cysts
Electrocauterization
Endometrial biopsy
Episiotomy
Fragile X syndrome
Genital disorders, female
Genital disorders, male
Glands
Gonorrhea
Gynecology
Hermaphroditism and
  pseudohermaphroditism
Herpes
Hydrocelectomy
Hypospadias repair and
  urethroplasty
Infertility in females
Infertility in males
Klinefelter syndrome
Masturbation
Orchitis
Pelvic inflammatory disease (PID)
Penile implant surgery
Reproductive system
Sex change surgery
Sexual differentiation
Sexual dysfunction

Sexuality
Sexually transmitted diseases
Sperm banks
Sterilization
Syphilis
Testicles, undescended
Testicular surgery
Testicular torsion
Toilet training
Urology
Urology, pediatric
Vasectomy
Warts

GLANDS
Abscess drainage
Abscesses
Addison's disease
Adrenalectomy
Biofeedback
Breasts, female
Contraception
Cyst removal
Cysts
Diabetes mellitus
Dwarfism
Eating disorders
Endocrine disorders
Endocrinology
Endocrinology, pediatric
Gigantism
Glands
Goiter
Gynecomastia
Hormone replacement therapy
Hormones
Hyperparathyroidism and
    hypoparathyroidism
Hypoglycemia
Internal medicine
Liver
Mastectomy and lumpectomy
Melatonin
Metabolism
Mumps
Neurosurgery
Nuclear medicine
Nuclear radiology
Obesity
Pancreas
Parathyroidectomy
Prostate gland
Prostate gland removal
Sex change surgery

Sexual differentiation
Steroids
Styes
Testicular surgery
Thyroid disorders
Thyroid gland
Thyroidectomy

GUMS
Abscess drainage
Abscesses
Cavities
Cleft lip and palate
Cleft lip and palate repair
Crowns and bridges
Dental diseases
Dentistry
Dentistry, pediatric
Dentures
Endodontic disease
Fluoride treatments
Gingivitis
Gulf War syndrome
Jaw wiring
Nutrition
Orthodontics
Periodontal surgery
Periodontitis
Root canal treatment
Scurvy
Teeth
Teething
Tooth extraction
Toothache
Wisdom teeth

HAIR
Albinos
Dermatitis
Dermatology
Eczema
Gray hair
Hair loss and baldness
Hair transplantation
Klinefelter syndrome
Lice, mites, and ticks
Nutrition
Pigmentation
Radiation sickness
Radiation therapy

HANDS
Amputation
Arthritis

Bones and the skeleton
Bursitis
Carpal tunnel syndrome
Cerebral palsy
Corns and calluses
Cysts
Fracture and dislocation
Fracture repair
Fragile X syndrome
Frostbite
Ganglion removal
Nail removal
Nails
Neurology
Neurology, pediatric
Orthopedic surgery
Orthopedics
Orthopedics, pediatric
Osteoarthritis
Rheumatoid arthritis
Rheumatology
Skin lesion removal
Sports medicine
Tendon disorders
Tendon repair
Thalidomide
Upper extremities
Warts

HEAD
Altitude sickness
Aneurysmectomy
Aneurysms
Angiography
Brain
Brain disorders
Cluster headaches
Coma
Computed tomography (CT)
    scanning
Concussion
Cradle cap
Craniosynostosis
Craniotomy
Dizziness and fainting
Electroencephalography (EEG)
Embolism
Epilepsy
Fetal tissue transplantation
Hair loss and baldness
Hair transplantation
Head and neck disorders
Headaches
Hydrocephalus

Lice, mites, and ticks
Meningitis
Migraine headaches
Nasal polyp removal
Nasopharyngeal disorders
Neurology
Neurology, pediatric
Neurosurgery
Rhinoplasty and submucous
resection
Seizures
Shunts
Sports medicine
Strokes
Temporomandibular joint (TMJ)
syndrome
Thrombosis and thrombus
Unconsciousness

HEART
Aneurysmectomy
Aneurysms
Angina
Angiography
Angioplasty
Anxiety
Apgar score
Arrhythmias
Arteriosclerosis
Arthritis, juvenile rheumatoid
Biofeedback
Bites and stings
Blue baby syndrome
Bypass surgery
Cardiac rehabilitation
Cardiology
Cardiology, pediatric
Catheterization
Circulation
Congenital heart disease
Electrical shock
Electrocardiography (ECG or EKG)
Embolism
Endocarditis
Exercise physiology
Heart
Heart attack
Heart disease
Heart failure
Heart transplantation
Heart valve replacement
Hypertension
Internal medicine
Kinesiology

Lyme disease
Marfan syndrome
Mitral valve prolapse
Pacemaker implantation
Palpitations
Respiratory distress syndrome
Resuscitation
Reye's syndrome
Rheumatic fever
Shock
Sports medicine
Steroid abuse
Strokes
Thoracic surgery
Thrombolytic therapy and TPA
Thrombosis and thrombus
Toxoplasmosis
Transplantation
Ultrasonography
Yellow fever

HIPS
Aging
Arthritis
Arthroplasty
Arthroscopy
Bone disorders
Bones and the skeleton
Chiropractic
Dwarfism
Fracture and dislocation
Fracture repair
Hip fracture repair
Hip replacement
Liposuction
Lower extremities
Orthopedic surgery
Orthopedics
Orthopedics, pediatric
Osteoarthritis
Osteochondritis juvenilis
Osteoporosis
Physical rehabilitation
Pityriasis rosea
Rheumatoid arthritis
Rheumatology
Sciatica

IMMUNE SYSTEM
Acquired immunodeficiency
syndrome (AIDS)
Allergies
Antibiotics
Arthritis

Arthritis, juvenile rheumatoid
Asthma
Autoimmune disorders
Bacterial infections
Bacteriology
Bites and stings
Blood and blood disorders
Bone grafting
Bone marrow transplantation
Candidiasis
Cell therapy
Cells
Childhood infectious diseases
Chronic fatigue syndrome
Cytology
Cytomegalovirus (CMV)
Cytopathology
Dermatology
Dermatopathology
E. coli infection
Emotions: Biomedical causes and
effects
Endocrinology
Endocrinology, pediatric
Enzyme therapy
Enzymes
Fungal infections
Grafts and grafting
Gram staining
Guillain-Barré syndrome
Gulf War syndrome
Healing
Hematology
Hematology, pediatric
Hives
Homeopathy
Host-defense mechanisms
Human immunodeficiency virus
(HIV)
Immune system
Immunization and vaccination
Immunodeficiency disorders
Immunology
Immunopathology
Leprosy
Lupus erythematosus
Lymphatic system
Magnetic field therapy
Measles
Microbiology
Multiple chemical sensitivity
syndrome
Mumps
Mutation

Oncology
Pancreas
Pharmacology
Poisoning
Poisonous plants
Pulmonary diseases
Pulmonary medicine
Pulmonary medicine, pediatric
Rh factor
Rheumatology
Rubella
Sarcoma
Sarcopenia
Scarlet fever
Serology
Smallpox
Sneezing
Stress
Stress reduction
Systems and organs
Thalidomide
Toxicology
Transfusion
Transplantation

INTESTINES
Abdomen
Abdominal disorders
Appendectomy
Appendicitis
Bacterial infections
Bypass surgery
Celiac sprue
Colic
Colitis
Colon and rectal polyp removal
Colon and rectal surgery
Colon cancer
Colon therapy
Colonoscopy
Constipation
Crohn's disease
Diarrhea and dysentery
Digestion
Diverticulitis and diverticulosis
E. coli infection
Eating disorders
Endoscopy
Enemas
Enterocolitis
Fistula repair
Food poisoning
Gastroenterology
Gastroenterology, pediatric

Gastrointestinal disorders
Gastrointestinal system
Hemorrhoid banding and removal
Hemorrhoids
Hernia
Hernia repair
Hirschsprung's disease
Ileostomy and colostomy
Indigestion
Internal medicine
Intestinal disorders
Intestines
Irritable bowel syndrome (IBS)
Kaposi's sarcoma
Kwashiorkor
Lactose intolerance
Laparoscopy
Malabsorption
Malnutrition
Metabolism
Nutrition
Obesity
Obstruction
Peristalsis
Pinworm
Proctology
Roundworm
Salmonella infection
Soiling
Sphincterectomy
Stomach, intestinal, and pancreatic
    cancers
Tapeworm
Toilet training
Trichinosis
Tumor removal
Tumors
Ulcer surgery
Ulcers
Worms

JOINTS
Amputation
Arthritis
Arthritis, juvenile rheumatoid
Arthroplasty
Arthroscopy
Bursitis
Carpal tunnel syndrome
Cell therapy
Chlamydia
Cyst removal
Cysts
Endoscopy

Exercise physiology
Fracture and dislocation
Fragile X syndrome
Gout
Gulf War syndrome
Hammertoe correction
Hammertoes
Hip fracture repair
Kneecap removal
Lupus erythematosus
Lyme disease
Motor skill development
Orthopedic surgery
Orthopedics
Orthopedics, pediatric
Osteoarthritis
Osteochondritis juvenilis
Osteomyelitis
Physical rehabilitation
Rheumatoid arthritis
Rheumatology
Spondylitis
Sports medicine
Temporomandibular joint (TMJ)
    syndrome
Tendon disorders
Tendon repair

KIDNEYS
Abdomen
Abscess drainage
Abscesses
Adrenalectomy
Cysts
Dialysis
Galactosemia
Glomerulonephritis
Hanta virus
Hypertension
Internal medicine
Kidney disorders
Kidney transplantation
Kidneys
Laparoscopy
Lithotripsy
Metabolism
Nephrectomy
Nephritis
Nephrology
Nephrology, pediatric
Nuclear medicine
Nuclear radiology
Renal failure
Reye's syndrome

Edema
Embolism
Emphysema
Endoscopy
Exercise physiology
Hanta virus
Heart transplantation
Hiccups
Influenza
Internal medicine
Interstitial pulmonary fibrosis (IPF)
Kaposi's sarcoma
Kinesiology
Legionnaires' disease
Lung cancer
Lung surgery
Lungs
Measles
Multiple chemical sensitivity
    syndrome
Oxygen therapy
Plague
Pleurisy
Pneumonia
Pulmonary diseases
Pulmonary medicine
Pulmonary medicine, pediatric
Respiration
Respiratory distress syndrome
Resuscitation
Smoking
Sneezing
Thoracic surgery
Thrombolytic therapy and TPA
Thrombosis and thrombus
Toxoplasmosis
Transplantation
Tuberculosis
Tumor removal
Tumors
Whooping cough

LYMPHATIC SYSTEM
Angiography
Bacterial infections
Blood and blood disorders
Breast cancer
Breast disorders
Cancer
Cervical, ovarian, and uterine
    cancers
Chemotherapy
Circulation
Colon cancer

Edema
Elephantiasis
Histology
Hodgkin's disease
Immune system
Immunology
Immunopathology
Liver cancer
Lower extremities
Lung cancer
Lymphadenopathy and lymphoma
Lymphatic system
Malignancy and metastasis
Mononucleosis
Oncology
Prostate cancer
Skin cancer
Sleeping sickness
Splenectomy
Stomach, intestinal, and pancreatic
    cancers
Systems and organs
Tonsillectomy and adenoid removal
Tonsillitis
Tumor removal
Tumors
Upper extremities
Vascular medicine
Vascular system

MOUTH
Candidiasis
Cavities
Cleft lip and palate
Cleft lip and palate repair
Crowns and bridges
Dental diseases
Dentistry
Dentistry, pediatric
Dentures
Endodontic disease
Fluoride treatments
Gingivitis
Halitosis
Hand-foot-and-mouth disease
Herpes
Jaw wiring
Lisping
Nutrition
Orthodontics
Periodontal surgery
Periodontitis
Root canal treatment
Sense organs

Taste
Teeth
Teething
Temporomandibular joint (TMJ)
    syndrome
Thumb sucking
Tooth extraction
Toothache
Ulcers
Wisdom teeth

MUSCLES
Acupressure
Amputation
Amyotrophic lateral sclerosis
Anesthesia
Anesthesiology
Apgar score
Ataxia
Bed-wetting
Bell's palsy
Beriberi
Biofeedback
Botulism
Breasts, female
Cerebral palsy
Chest
Childhood infectious diseases
Chronic fatigue syndrome
Claudication
Creutzfeldt-Jakob disease and mad
    cow disease
Cysts
Ebola virus
Emotions: Biomedical causes and
    effects
Exercise physiology
Feet
Flat feet
Foot disorders
Glycolysis
Guillain-Barré syndrome
Gulf War syndrome
Head and neck disorders
Hemiplegia
Hiccups
Kinesiology
Lower extremities
Mastectomy and lumpectomy
Motor neuron diseases
Motor skill development
Multiple chemical sensitivity
    syndrome
Multiple sclerosis

Spine, vertebrae, and disks
Sports medicine
Systems and organs
Teeth
Tendon disorders
Tendon repair
Tetanus
Tics
Tourette's syndrome
Trembling and shaking
Trichinosis
Upper extremities
Weight loss and gain
Yellow fever

NAILS
Anemia
Dermatology
Fungal infections
Malnutrition
Nail removal
Nails
Nutrition
Podiatry

NECK
Asphyxiation
Choking
Cradle cap
Cretinism
Endarterectomy
Goiter
Head and neck disorders
Hyperparathyroidism and
   hypoparathyroidism
Laryngectomy
Laryngitis
Otorhinolaryngology
Paralysis
Parathyroidectomy
Quadriplegia
Spine, vertebrae, and disks
Sympathectomy
Thyroid disorders
Thyroid gland
Thyroidectomy
Tonsillectomy and adenoid removal
Tonsillitis
Torticollis
Tracheostomy

NERVES
Anesthesia
Anesthesiology

Bell's palsy
Biofeedback
Brain
Carpal tunnel syndrome
Cells
Creutzfeldt-Jakob disease and
   mad cow disease
Cysts
Emotions: Biomedical causes and
   effects
Epilepsy
Guillain-Barré syndrome
Hemiplegia
Leprosy
Lower extremities
Motor neuron diseases
Motor skill development
Multiple chemical sensitivity
   syndrome
Multiple sclerosis
Nervous system
Neuralgia, neuritis, and
   neuropathy
Neurology
Neurology, pediatric
Neurosurgery
Numbness and tingling
Palsy
Paralysis
Paraplegia
Parkinson's disease
Physical rehabilitation
Poliomyelitis
Ptosis
Quadriplegia
Sciatica
Seizures
Sense organs
Shock therapy
Skin
Spina bifida
Spinal cord disorders
Spine, vertebrae, and disks
Sympathectomy
Tics
Touch
Tourette's syndrome
Upper extremities
Vagotomy

NERVOUS SYSTEM
Abscess drainage
Abscesses
Acupressure

Addiction
Alcoholism
Altitude sickness
Alzheimer's disease
Amnesia
Amputation
Amyotrophic lateral sclerosis
Anesthesia
Anesthesiology
Aneurysmectomy
Aneurysms
Anxiety
Apgar score
Aphasia and dysphasia
Apnea
Aromatherapy
Arthropod-borne diseases
Ataxia
Attention-deficit disorder (ADD)
Auras
Autism
Balance disorders
Bell's palsy
Beriberi
Biofeedback
Botulism
Brain
Brain disorders
Carpal tunnel syndrome
Cells
Cerebral palsy
Chiropractic
Claudication
Cluster headaches
Cognitive development
Coma
Computed tomography (CT)
   scanning
Concussion
Craniotomy
Cretinism
Creutzfeldt-Jakob disease and mad
   cow disease
Cysts
Dementias
Developmental stages
Diabetes mellitus
Diphtheria
Disk removal
Dizziness and fainting
Down syndrome
Dwarfism
Dyslexia
E. coli infection

Ear surgery
Ears
Eclampsia
Electrical shock
Electroencephalography (EEG)
Emotions: Biomedical causes and effects
Encephalitis
Endocrinology
Endocrinology, pediatric
Epilepsy
Eyes
Fetal alcohol syndrome
Fetal tissue transplantation
Gigantism
Glands
Guillain-Barré syndrome
Hallucinations
Hammertoe correction
Head and neck disorders
Headaches
Hearing aids
Hearing loss
Hearing tests
Heart transplantation
Hemiplegia
Hydrocephalus
Hypnosis
Irritable bowel syndrome (IBS)
Kinesiology
Lead poisoning
Learning disabilities
Leprosy
Light therapy
Lower extremities
Lyme disease
Malaria
Memory loss
Meningitis
Mental retardation
Migraine headaches
Motor neuron diseases
Motor skill development
Multiple chemical sensitivity syndrome
Multiple sclerosis
Narcolepsy
Narcotics
Nausea and vomiting
Nervous system
Neuralgia, neuritis, and neuropathy
Neurofibromatosis
Neurology
Neurology, pediatric

Neurosurgery
Nuclear radiology
Numbness and tingling
Orthopedic surgery
Orthopedics
Orthopedics, pediatric
Paget's disease
Palsy
Paralysis
Paraplegia
Parkinson's disease
Pharmacology
Pharmacy
Phenylketonuria (PKU)
Physical rehabilitation
Poisoning
Poliomyelitis
Porphyria
Precocious puberty
Premenstrual syndrome (PMS)
Prion diseases
Quadriplegia
Rabies
Reye's syndrome
Sciatica
Seizures
Sense organs
Shingles
Shock therapy
Shunts
Skin
Sleep disorders
Sleeping sickness
Sleepwalking
Smell
Snakebites
Spina bifida
Spinal cord disorders
Spine, vertebrae, and disks
Sports medicine
Stammering
Strokes
Stuttering
Sympathectomy
Syphilis
Systems and organs
Taste
Tay-Sachs disease
Teeth
Tetanus
Thrombolytic therapy and TPA
Tics
Touch
Tourette's syndrome

Toxicology
Toxoplasmosis
Trembling and shaking
Unconsciousness
Upper extremities
Vagotomy
Yellow fever

NOSE
Allergies
Aromatherapy
Auras
Childhood infectious diseases
Common cold
Fifth disease
Halitosis
Nasal polyp removal
Nasopharyngeal disorders
Nosebleeds
Otorhinolaryngology
Plastic surgery
Pulmonary medicine
Pulmonary medicine, pediatric
Respiration
Rhinitis
Rhinoplasty and submucous resection
Rosacea
Sense organs
Sinusitis
Skin lesion removal
Smell
Sneezing
Sore throat
Taste
Viral infections

PANCREAS
Abscess drainage
Abscesses
Diabetes mellitus
Digestion
Endocrinology
Endocrinology, pediatric
Fetal tissue transplantation
Food biochemistry
Gastroenterology
Gastroenterology, pediatric
Gastrointestinal disorders
Gastrointestinal system
Glands
Hormones
Internal medicine
Malabsorption

Metabolism
Pancreas
Pancreatitis
Stomach, intestinal, and pancreatic cancers
Transplantation

PSYCHIC-EMOTIONAL SYSTEM

Addiction
Aging
Alcoholism
Alzheimer's disease
Amnesia
Anesthesia
Anesthesiology
Anorexia nervosa
Anxiety
Aphasia and dysphasia
Aromatherapy
Attention-deficit disorder (ADD)
Auras
Autism
Biofeedback
Bipolar disorder
Bonding
Brain
Brain disorders
Bulimia
Chronic fatigue syndrome
Club drugs
Cluster headaches
Cognitive development
Colic
Coma
Concussion
Death and dying
Delusions
Dementias
Depression
Developmental stages
Dizziness and fainting
Domestic violence
Down syndrome
Dyslexia
Eating disorders
Electroencephalography (EEG)
Emotions: Biomedical causes and effects
Endocrinology
Endocrinology, pediatric
Factitious disorders
Failure to thrive
Grief and guilt

Gulf War syndrome
Hallucinations
Headaches
Hormone replacement therapy
Hormones
Hydrocephalus
Hypnosis
Hypochondriasis
Kinesiology
Klinefelter syndrome
Lead poisoning
Learning disabilities
Light therapy
Memory loss
Menopause
Mental retardation
Midlife crisis
Migraine headaches
Miscarriage
Motor skill development
Narcolepsy
Narcotics
Neurology
Neurology, pediatric
Neurosis
Neurosurgery
Nightmares
Obesity
Obsessive-compulsive disorder
Palpitations
Panic attacks
Paranoia
Pharmacology
Pharmacy
Phobias
Postpartum depression
Post-traumatic stress disorder
Precocious puberty
Psychiatric disorders
Psychiatry
Psychiatry, child and adolescent
Psychiatry, geriatric
Psychoanalysis
Psychosis
Psychosomatic disorders
Puberty and adolescence
Rabies
Schizophrenia
Separation anxiety
Sexual dysfunction
Sexuality
Shock therapy
Sibling rivalry
Sleep disorders

Sleepwalking
Soiling
Speech disorders
Sperm banks
Stammering
Steroid abuse
Stillbirth
Stress
Strokes
Stuttering
Suicide
Tics
Toilet training
Tourette's syndrome
Weight loss and gain

REPRODUCTIVE SYSTEM

Abdomen
Abdominal disorders
Abortion
Acquired immunodeficiency syndrome (AIDS)
Amenorrhea
Amniocentesis
Anatomy
Anorexia nervosa
Breast-feeding
Breasts, female
Candidiasis
Catheterization
Cervical, ovarian, and uterine cancers
Cervical procedures
Cesarean section
Childbirth
Childbirth complications
Chlamydia
Chorionic villus sampling
Circumcision, female, and genital mutilation
Circumcision, male
Conception
Contraception
Culdocentesis
Cyst removal
Cysts
Dysmenorrhea
Eating disorders
Ectopic pregnancy
Electrocauterization
Endocrinology
Endometrial biopsy
Endometriosis
Episiotomy

Fetal alcohol syndrome
Fistula repair
Genetic counseling
Genital disorders, female
Genital disorders, male
Glands
Gonorrhea
Gynecology
Hermaphroditism and
  pseudohermaphroditism
Hernia
Herpes
Hormone replacement therapy
Hormones
Human immunodeficiency virus
  (HIV)
Hydrocelectomy
Hypospadias repair and
  urethroplasty
Hysterectomy
In vitro fertilization
Infertility in females
Infertility in males
Internal medicine
Klinefelter syndrome
Laparoscopy
Menopause
Menorrhagia
Menstruation
Miscarriage
Multiple births
Mumps
Myomectomy
Obstetrics
Orchitis
Ovarian cysts
Pelvic inflammatory disease (PID)
Penile implant surgery
Precocious puberty
Pregnancy and gestation
Premature birth
Premenstrual syndrome (PMS)
Prostate cancer
Prostate gland
Puberty and adolescence
Reproductive system
Sex change surgery
Sexual differentiation
Sexual dysfunction
Sexuality
Sexually transmitted diseases
Sperm banks
Sterilization
Steroid abuse

Stillbirth
Syphilis
Systems and organs
Testicles, undescended
Testicular surgery
Testicular torsion
Tubal ligation
Turner syndrome
Ultrasonography
Urology
Urology, pediatric
Vasectomy
Warts

RESPIRATORY SYSTEM
Abscess drainage
Abscesses
Altitude sickness
Amyotrophic lateral sclerosis
Apgar score
Apnea
Asphyxiation
Asthma
Bacterial infections
Bronchiolitis
Bronchitis
Chest
Chickenpox
Childhood infectious diseases
Choking
Common cold
Coughing
Croup
Cystic fibrosis
Diphtheria
Edema
Embolism
Emphysema
Epiglottitis
Exercise physiology
Fluids and electrolytes
Fungal infections
Halitosis
Hanta virus
Head and neck disorders
Heart transplantation
Hiccups
Influenza
Internal medicine
Interstitial pulmonary fibrosis
  (IPF)
Kinesiology
Laryngectomy
Laryngitis

Legionnaires' disease
Lung cancer
Lung surgery
Lungs
Measles
Mononucleosis
Multiple chemical sensitivity
  syndrome
Nasopharyngeal disorders
Otorhinolaryngology
Oxygen therapy
Pharyngitis
Plague
Pleurisy
Pneumonia
Poisoning
Pulmonary diseases
Pulmonary medicine
Pulmonary medicine, pediatric
Respiration
Resuscitation
Rheumatic fever
Rhinitis
Roundworm
Sinusitis
Smallpox
Sneezing
Sore throat
Strep throat
Systems and organs
Thoracic surgery
Thrombolytic therapy and TPA
Thrombosis and thrombus
Tonsillectomy and adenoid removal
Tonsillitis
Toxoplasmosis
Tracheostomy
Transplantation
Tuberculosis
Tumor removal
Tumors
Voice and vocal cord disorders
Whooping cough
Worms

SKIN
Abscess drainage
Abscesses
Acne
Acupressure
Acupuncture
Age spots
Albinos
Allergies

ENTRIES BY SPECIALTIES AND RELATED FIELDS

Bacteriology
Cholesterol
Digestion
Endocrinology
Endocrinology, pediatric
Enzymes
Fluids and electrolytes
Fluoride treatments
Food biochemistry
Genetic engineering
Glands
Glycolysis
Gram staining
Histology
Hormones
Human Genome Project
Leptin
Lipids
Malabsorption
Metabolism
Nephrology
Nephrology, pediatric
Nutrition
Pathology
Pharmacology
Pharmacy
Respiration
Stem cell research
Steroids
Toxicology
Urinalysis

BIOTECHNOLOGY
Bionics and biotechnology
Biophysics
Cloning
Computed tomography (CT) scanning
Dialysis
Electrocardiography (ECG or EKG)
Electroencephalography (EEG)
Gene therapy
Genetic engineering
Human Genome Project
In vitro fertilization
Magnetic resonance imaging (MRI)
Pacemaker implantation
Positron emission tomography (PET) scanning
Sperm banks
Stem cell research

CARDIOLOGY
Aging
Aging: Extended care
Aneurysmectomy
Aneurysms
Angina
Angiography
Angioplasty
Anxiety
Arrhythmias
Arteriosclerosis
Biofeedback
Blue baby syndrome
Bypass surgery
Cardiac rehabilitation
Cardiology
Cardiology, pediatric
Catheterization
Chest
Cholesterol
Circulation
Congenital heart disease
Critical care
Critical care, pediatric
Dizziness and fainting
Electrocardiography (ECG or EKG)
Emergency medicine
Endocarditis
Exercise physiology
Geriatrics and gerontology
Heart
Heart attack
Heart disease
Heart failure
Heart transplantation
Heart valve replacement
Hematology
Hypercholesterolemia
Hypertension
Internal medicine
Ischemia
Kinesiology
Leptin
Marfan syndrome
Mitral valve prolapse
Muscles
Neonatology
Noninvasive tests
Nuclear medicine
Pacemaker implantation
Palpitations
Paramedics
Physical examination
Progeria

Rheumatic fever
Sports medicine
Thoracic surgery
Thrombolytic therapy and TPA
Thrombosis and thrombus
Transplantation
Ultrasonography
Vascular medicine
Vascular system
Venous insufficiency

CRITICAL CARE
Accidents
Aging: Extended care
Amputation
Anesthesia
Anesthesiology
Apgar score
Burns and scalds
Catheterization
Club drugs
Coma
Critical care
Critical care, pediatric
Electrical shock
Electrocardiography (ECG or EKG)
Electroencephalography (EEG)
Emergency medicine
Emergency medicine, pediatric
Geriatrics and gerontology
Grafts and grafting
Hanta virus
Heart attack
Heart transplantation
Heat exhaustion and heat stroke
Hospitals
Hyperthermia and hypothermia
Necrotizing fasciitis
Neonatology
Nursing
Oncology
Osteopathic medicine
Pain management
Paramedics
Psychiatry
Psychiatry, child and adolescent
Psychiatry, geriatric
Pulmonary medicine
Pulmonary medicine, pediatric
Radiation sickness
Resuscitation
Safety issues for children
Safety issues for the elderly
Shock

Tattoo removal
Tattoos and body piercing
Touch
Warts
Wrinkles

EMBRYOLOGY
Abortion
Amniocentesis
Birth defects
Blue baby syndrome
Brain disorders
Cerebral palsy
Chorionic villus sampling
Cloning
Conception
Down syndrome
Embryology
Fetal alcohol syndrome
Genetic counseling
Genetic diseases
Genetics and inheritance
Growth
Hermaphroditism and
    pseudohermaphroditism
In vitro fertilization
Klinefelter syndrome
Miscarriage
Multiple births
Obstetrics
Pregnancy and gestation
Reproductive system
Rh factor
Rubella
Sexual differentiation
Spina bifida
Stem cell research
Toxoplasmosis
Ultrasonography

EMERGENCY MEDICINE
Abdominal disorders
Abscess drainage
Accidents
Aging
Altitude sickness
Amputation
Anesthesia
Anesthesiology
Aneurysms
Angiography
Appendectomy
Appendicitis
Asphyxiation

Bites and stings
Bleeding
Blurred vision
Botulism
Burns and scalds
Cardiology
Cardiology, pediatric
Catheterization
Cesarean section
Choking
Club drugs
Coma
Computed tomography (CT)
    scanning
Concussion
Critical care
Critical care, pediatric
Croup
Diphtheria
Dizziness and fainting
Domestic violence
Electrical shock
Electrocardiography (ECG
    or EKG)
Electroencephalography (EEG)
Emergency medicine
Emergency medicine, pediatric
Epiglottitis
Food poisoning
Fracture and dislocation
Frostbite
Grafts and grafting
Head and neck disorders
Heart attack
Heart transplantation
Heat exhaustion and heat stroke
Hospitals
Hyperthermia and hypothermia
Intoxication
Jaw wiring
Laceration repair
Lumbar puncture
Lung surgery
Meningitis
Necrotizing fasciitis
Noninvasive tests
Nosebleeds
Nursing
Osteopathic medicine
Oxygen therapy
Pain management
Paramedics
Peritonitis
Physician assistants

Plague
Plastic surgery
Pneumonia
Poisoning
Pulmonary diseases
Pulmonary medicine
Pulmonary medicine, pediatric
Radiation sickness
Resuscitation
Reye's syndrome
Safety issues for children
Safety issues for the elderly
Salmonella infection
Shock
Snakebites
Spinal cord disorders
Splenectomy
Sports medicine
Staphylococcal infections
Streptococcal infections
Strokes
Sunburn
Surgical technologists
Thrombolytic therapy and TPA
Tracheostomy
Transfusion
Transplantation
Typhoid fever and typhus
Unconsciousness
Wounds

ENDOCRINOLOGY
Addison's disease
Adrenalectomy
Anti-inflammatory drugs
Breasts, female
Chronobiology
Cretinism
Cushing's syndrome
Diabetes mellitus
Dwarfism
Endocrine disorders
Endocrinology
Endocrinology, pediatric
Enzymes
Estrogen replacement therapy
Failure to thrive
Galactosemia
Geriatrics and gerontology
Gigantism
Glands
Goiter
Growth
Gynecology

Gynecomastia
Hair loss and baldness
Hermaphroditism and
    pseudohermaphroditism
Hormone replacement therapy
Hormones
Hyperadiposis
Hyperparathyroidism and
    hypoparathyroidism
Hypertrophy
Hypoglycemia
Hysterectomy
Infertility in females
Infertility in males
Insulin resistance syndrome
Internal medicine
Klinefelter syndrome
Laboratory tests
Laparoscopy
Leptin
Liver
Melatonin
Menopause
Menstruation
Nephrology
Nephrology, pediatric
Neurology
Neurology, pediatric
Nuclear medicine
Obesity
Pancreas
Pancreatitis
Parathyroidectomy
Pharmacology
Pharmacy
Precocious puberty
Prostate gland
Puberty and adolescence
Radiopharmaceuticals
Sex change surgery
Sexual differentiation
Sexual dysfunction
Stem cell research
Steroids
Testicles, undescended
Thyroid disorders
Thyroid gland
Thyroidectomy
Toxicology
Tumors
Turner syndrome
Vitamins and minerals
Weight loss and gain
Weight loss medications

ENVIRONMENTAL HEALTH
Allergies
Arthropod-borne diseases
Asthma
Bacteriology
Blurred vision
Cholera
Cognitive development
Elephantiasis
Environmental diseases
Environmental health
Epidemiology
Food poisoning
Frostbite
Gulf War syndrome
Hanta virus
Heat exhaustion and heat stroke
Holistic medicine
Hyperthermia and hypothermia
Interstitial pulmonary fibrosis
    (IPF)
Lead poisoning
Legionnaires' disease
Lice, mites, and ticks
Lung cancer
Lungs
Lyme disease
Malaria
Microbiology
Mold and mildew
Multiple chemical sensitivity
    syndrome
Nasopharyngeal disorders
Occupational health
Parasitic diseases
Pigmentation
Plague
Poisoning
Poisonous plants
Pulmonary diseases
Pulmonary medicine
Pulmonary medicine, pediatric
Salmonella infection
Skin cancer
Snakebites
Stress
Stress reduction
Toxicology
Trachoma
Tropical medicine

EPIDEMIOLOGY
Acquired immunodeficiency
    syndrome (AIDS)

Anthrax
Arthropod-borne diseases
Bacterial infections
Bacteriology
Biostatistics
Childhood infectious diseases
Cholera
Creutzfeldt-Jakob disease and
    mad cow disease
Disease
E. coli infection
Ebola virus
Elephantiasis
Environmental diseases
Environmental health
Epidemiology
Food poisoning
Forensic pathology
Gulf War syndrome
Hanta virus
Hepatitis
Influenza
Laboratory tests
Legionnaires' disease
Leprosy
Lice, mites, and ticks
Malaria
Measles
Microbiology
Multiple chemical sensitivity
    syndrome
Necrotizing fasciitis
Occupational health
Parasitic diseases
Pathology
Plague
Pneumonia
Poisoning
Poliomyelitis
Prion diseases
Pulmonary diseases
Rabies
Salmonella infection
Sexually transmitted diseases
Stress
Tropical medicine
Viral infections
World Health Organization
Yellow fever
Zoonoses

ETHICS
Abortion
Animal rights vs. research

Liver cancer
Liver disorders
Liver transplantation
Malabsorption
Malnutrition
Metabolism
Nausea and vomiting
Nutrition
Obstruction
Pancreas
Pancreatitis
Peristalsis
Poisonous plants
Proctology
Pyloric stenosis
Roundworm
Salmonella infection
Shigellosis
Soiling
Stomach, intestinal, and pancreatic
    cancers
Stone removal
Stones
Tapeworm
Taste
Toilet training
Trichinosis
Ulcer surgery
Ulcers
Vagotomy
Weight loss and gain
Worms

GENERAL SURGERY
Abscess drainage
Adrenalectomy
Amputation
Anesthesia
Anesthesiology
Aneurysmectomy
Appendectomy
Biopsy
Bone marrow transplantation
Breast biopsy
Breast surgery
Bunions
Bypass surgery
Cataract surgery
Catheterization
Cervical procedures
Cesarean section
Cholecystectomy
Circumcision, female, and genital
    mutilation

Circumcision, male
Cleft lip and palate repair
Colon and rectal polyp removal
Colon and rectal surgery
Corneal transplantation
Craniotomy
Cryotherapy and cryosurgery
Cyst removal
Cystectomy
Disk removal
Ear surgery
Electrocauterization
Endarterectomy
Endometrial biopsy
Eye surgery
Face lift and blepharoplasty
Fistula repair
Ganglion removal
Gastrectomy
Grafts and grafting
Hair transplantation
Hammertoe correction
Heart transplantation
Heart valve replacement
Heel spur removal
Hemorrhoid banding and removal
Hernia repair
Hip replacement
Hydrocelectomy
Hypospadias repair and
    urethroplasty
Hysterectomy
Kidney transplantation
Kneecap removal
Laceration repair
Laminectomy and spinal fusion
Laparoscopy
Laryngectomy
Laser use in surgery
Liposuction
Liver transplantation
Lung surgery
Malignant melanoma removal
Mastectomy and lumpectomy
Myomectomy
Nail removal
Nasal polyp removal
Nephrectomy
Neurosurgery
Oncology
Ophthalmology
Orthopedic surgery
Otoplasty
Parathyroidectomy

Penile implant surgery
Periodontal surgery
Phlebitis
Plastic surgery
Prostate gland removal
Rhinoplasty and submucous
    resection
Sex change surgery
Shunts
Skin lesion removal
Sphincterectomy
Splenectomy
Sterilization
Stone removal
Surgery, general
Surgery, pediatric
Surgical procedures
Surgical technologists
Sympathectomy
Tattoo removal
Tendon repair
Testicular surgery
Thoracic surgery
Thyroidectomy
Tonsillectomy and adenoid removal
Tracheostomy
Transfusion
Transplantation
Tumor removal
Ulcer surgery
Vagotomy
Varicose vein removal
Vasectomy

GENETICS
Aging
Albinos
Alzheimer's disease
Amniocentesis
Attention-deficit disorder (ADD)
Autoimmune disorders
Bionics and biotechnology
Birth defects
Bone marrow transplantation
Breast cancer
Breast disorders
Chorionic villus sampling
Cloning
Cognitive development
Colon cancer
Color blindness
Cystic fibrosis
Diabetes mellitus
DNA and RNA

Down syndrome
Dwarfism
Embryology
Endocrinology
Endocrinology, pediatric
Enzymes
Failure to thrive
Fragile X syndrome
Galactosemia
Gene therapy
Genetic counseling
Genetic diseases
Genetic engineering
Genetics and inheritance
Grafts and grafting
Hematology
Hematology, pediatric
Hemophilia
Hermaphroditism and
    pseudohermaphroditism
Human Genome Project
Hyperadiposis
Immunodeficiency disorders
In vitro fertilization
Insulin resistance syndrome
Klinefelter syndrome
Laboratory tests
Leptin
Malabsorption
Marfan syndrome
Mental retardation
Motor skill development
Muscular dystrophy
Mutation
Neonatology
Nephrology
Nephrology, pediatric
Neurofibromatosis
Neurology
Neurology, pediatric
Obstetrics
Oncology
Osteogenesis imperfecta
Pediatrics
Phenylketonuria (PKU)
Porphyria
Precocious puberty
Reproductive system
Rh factor
Screening
Sexual differentiation
Sexuality
Sperm banks
Stem cell research

Tay-Sachs disease
Tourette's syndrome
Transplantation
Turner syndrome

**GERIATRICS AND
    GERONTOLOGY**
Age spots
Aging
Aging: Extended care
Alzheimer's disease
Arthritis
Bed-wetting
Blindness
Blurred vision
Bone disorders
Bones and the skeleton
Brain
Brain disorders
Cataract surgery
Cataracts
Corns and calluses
Critical care
Crowns and bridges
Death and dying
Dementias
Dentures
Depression
Domestic violence
Emergency medicine
Endocrinology
Estrogen replacement therapy
Euthanasia
Family practice
Fatigue
Fracture and dislocation
Fracture repair
Gray hair
Hearing aids
Hearing loss
Hip fracture repair
Hip replacement
Hormone replacement therapy
Hormones
Hospitals
Incontinence
Memory loss
Nursing
Nutrition
Ophthalmology
Orthopedics
Osteoporosis
Pain management
Paramedics

Parkinson's disease
Pharmacology
Psychiatry
Psychiatry, geriatric
Rheumatology
Safety issues for the elderly
Sarcopenia
Sleep disorders
Spinal cord disorders
Spine, vertebrae, and disks
Suicide
Visual disorders
Wrinkles

GYNECOLOGY
Abortion
Amenorrhea
Amniocentesis
Biopsy
Breast biopsy
Breast cancer
Breast disorders
Breast-feeding
Breasts, female
Cervical, ovarian, and uterine
    cancers
Cervical procedures
Cesarean section
Childbirth
Childbirth complications
Chlamydia
Circumcision, female, and genital
    mutilation
Conception
Contraception
Culdocentesis
Cyst removal
Cystectomy
Cystitis
Cysts
Dysmenorrhea
Electrocauterization
Endocrinology
Endometrial biopsy
Endometriosis
Endoscopy
Episiotomy
Estrogen replacement therapy
Genital disorders, female
Glands
Gonorrhea
Gynecology
Hermaphroditism and
    pseudohermaphroditism

Host-defense mechanisms
Human immunodeficiency virus (HIV)
Hypnosis
Immune system
Immunization and vaccination
Immunodeficiency disorders
Immunology
Immunopathology
Impetigo
Laboratory tests
Leprosy
Liver cancer
Lung cancer
Lupus erythematosus
Lymphatic system
Microbiology
Multiple chemical sensitivity syndrome
Oncology
Oxygen therapy
Pancreas
Prostate cancer
Pulmonary diseases
Pulmonary medicine
Pulmonary medicine, pediatric
Rheumatology
Sarcoma
Sarcopenia
Serology
Skin cancer
Stem cell research
Stomach, intestinal, and pancreatic cancers
Stress
Stress reduction
Thalidomide
Transfusion
Transplantation
Tropical medicine

INTERNAL MEDICINE
Abdomen
Abdominal disorders
Anatomy
Anemia
Angina
Anti-inflammatory drugs
Antioxidants
Anxiety
Arrhythmias
Arteriosclerosis
Autoimmune disorders
Bacterial infections

Beriberi
Biofeedback
Bleeding
Bronchiolitis
Bronchitis
Burping
Bursitis
Candidiasis
Chickenpox
Childhood infectious diseases
Cholecystitis
Cholesterol
Chronic fatigue syndrome
Cirrhosis
Claudication
Cluster headaches
Colitis
Colonoscopy
Common cold
Constipation
Coughing
Cretinism
Crohn's disease
Diabetes mellitus
Dialysis
Diarrhea and dysentery
Digestion
Diverticulitis and diverticulosis
Dizziness and fainting
Domestic violence
E. coli infection
Edema
Embolism
Emphysema
Endocarditis
Endoscopy
Factitious disorders
Family practice
Fatigue
Fever
Fungal infections
Gallbladder diseases
Gangrene
Gastroenterology
Gastroenterology, pediatric
Gastrointestinal disorders
Gastrointestinal system
Genetic diseases
Geriatrics and gerontology
Glomerulonephritis
Goiter
Gout
Guillain-Barré syndrome
Hanta virus

Headaches
Heart
Heart attack
Heart disease
Heart failure
Heartburn
Heat exhaustion and heat stroke
Hepatitis
Hernia
Histology
Hodgkin's disease
Human immunodeficiency virus (HIV)
Hypercholesterolemia
Hyperlipidemia
Hypertension
Hyperthermia and hypothermia
Hypertrophy
Hypoglycemia
Incontinence
Indigestion
Infection
Inflammation
Influenza
Insulin resistance syndrome
Internal medicine
Intestinal disorders
Intestines
Ischemia
Itching
Jaundice
Kaposi's sarcoma
Kidney disorders
Kidneys
Legionnaires' disease
Leprosy
Leukemia
Liver
Liver disorders
Lupus erythematosus
Lyme disease
Lymphadenopathy and lymphoma
Malignancy and metastasis
Mitral valve prolapse
Mononucleosis
Motion sickness
Multiple sclerosis
Nephritis
Nephrology
Nephrology, pediatric
Nosebleeds
Nuclear medicine
Nutrition
Obesity

Occupational health
Osteopathic medicine
Paget's disease
Pain
Palpitations
Pancreas
Pancreatitis
Parasitic diseases
Parkinson's disease
Peristalsis
Peritonitis
Pharyngitis
Phlebitis
Physical examination
Physician assistants
Physiology
Pneumonia
Proctology
Psoriasis
Puberty and adolescence
Pulmonary medicine
Pulmonary medicine, pediatric
Radiopharmaceuticals
Rashes
Renal failure
Reye's syndrome
Rheumatic fever
Rheumatoid arthritis
Roundworm
Rubella
Scarlet fever
Schistosomiasis
Sciatica
Scurvy
Septicemia
Sexuality
Sexually transmitted diseases
Shingles
Shock
Sickle-cell disease
Sneezing
Sports medicine
Staphylococcal infections
Stone removal
Stones
Streptococcal infections
Stress
Supplements
Tapeworm
Tetanus
Thrombosis and thrombus
Toxemia
Tumor removal
Tumors

Ulcer surgery
Ulcers
Ultrasonography
Viral infections
Vitamins and minerals
Weight loss medications
Whooping cough
Worms
Wounds

MICROBIOLOGY

Abscesses
Anthrax
Antibiotics
Autopsy
Bacterial infections
Bacteriology
Bionics and biotechnology
Drug resistance
E. coli infection
Epidemiology
Fluoride treatments
Fungal infections
Gangrene
Gastroenterology
Gastroenterology, pediatric
Gastrointestinal disorders
Gastrointestinal system
Genetic engineering
Gram staining
Immune system
Immunization and vaccination
Immunology
Impetigo
Laboratory tests
Microbiology
Microscopy
Pathology
Pharmacology
Pharmacy
Protozoan diseases
Serology
Smallpox
Toxicology
Tropical medicine
Tuberculosis
Urinalysis
Urology
Urology, pediatric
Viral infections

NEONATOLOGY

Apgar score
Birth defects

Blue baby syndrome
Bonding
Cardiology, pediatric
Cesarean section
Childbirth
Childbirth complications
Chlamydia
Cleft lip and palate
Cleft lip and palate repair
Congenital heart disease
Critical care, pediatric
Cystic fibrosis
Down syndrome
E. coli infection
Endocrinology, pediatric
Failure to thrive
Fetal alcohol syndrome
Gastroenterology, pediatric
Genetic diseases
Genetics and inheritance
Hematology, pediatric
Hemolytic disease of the
   newborn
Hydrocephalus
Jaundice
Jaundice, neonatal
Malabsorption
Motor skill development
Multiple births
Neonatology
Nephrology, pediatric
Neurology, pediatric
Nursing
Obstetrics
Orthopedics, pediatric
Pediatrics
Perinatology
Phenylketonuria (PKU)
Physician assistants
Premature birth
Pulmonary medicine, pediatric
Respiratory distress syndrome
Rh factor
Shunts
Sudden infant death syndrome
   (SIDS)
Surgery, pediatric
Tay-Sachs disease
Toxoplasmosis
Transfusion
Tropical medicine
Umbilical cord
Urology, pediatric
Well-baby examinations

Positron emission tomography (PET) scanning
Radiation therapy
Radiopharmaceuticals

NURSING
Aging: Extended care
Allied health
Anesthesiology
Cardiac rehabilitation
Critical care
Critical care, pediatric
Emergency medicine
Emergency medicine, pediatric
Geriatrics and gerontology
Holistic medicine
Hospitals
Immunization and vaccination
Neonatology
Noninvasive tests
Nursing
Nutrition
Pediatrics
Physical examination
Physician assistants
Surgery, general
Surgery, pediatric
Surgical procedures
Surgical technologists
Well-baby examinations

NUTRITION
Aging: Extended care
Anorexia nervosa
Antioxidants
Beriberi
Breast-feeding
Bulimia
Cardiac rehabilitation
Cholesterol
Digestion
Eating disorders
Enzyme therapy
Exercise physiology
Food biochemistry
Galactosemia
Gastroenterology
Gastroenterology, pediatric
Gastrointestinal disorders
Gastrointestinal system
Geriatrics and gerontology
Hyperadiposis
Hypercholesterolemia
Irritable bowel syndrome (IBS)

Jaw wiring
Kwashiorkor
Lactose intolerance
Leptin
Lipids
Malabsorption
Malnutrition
Metabolism
Nursing
Nutrition
Obesity
Osteoporosis
Scurvy
Sports medicine
Supplements
Taste
Tropical medicine
Ulcers
Vagotomy
Vitamins and minerals
Weaning
Weight loss and gain
Weight loss medications

OBSTETRICS
Amniocentesis
Apgar score
Birth defects
Breast-feeding
Breasts, female
Cervical, ovarian, and uterine cancers
Cesarean section
Childbirth
Childbirth complications
Chorionic villus sampling
Conception
Cytomegalovirus (CMV)
Down syndrome
Eclampsia
Ectopic pregnancy
Embryology
Emergency medicine
Episiotomy
Family practice
Fetal alcohol syndrome
Genetic counseling
Genetic diseases
Genetics and inheritance
Genital disorders, female
Gonorrhea
Growth
Gynecology
Hemolytic disease of the newborn
In vitro fertilization

Incontinence
Invasive tests
Miscarriage
Multiple births
Neonatology
Noninvasive tests
Obstetrics
Perinatology
Postpartum depression
Pregnancy and gestation
Premature birth
Reproductive system
Rh factor
Rubella
Sexuality
Sperm banks
Spina bifida
Stillbirth
Toxoplasmosis
Ultrasonography
Urology

OCCUPATIONAL HEALTH
Altitude sickness
Asphyxiation
Biofeedback
Blurred vision
Cardiac rehabilitation
Carpal tunnel syndrome
Environmental diseases
Environmental health
Gulf War syndrome
Hearing aids
Hearing loss
Interstitial pulmonary fibrosis (IPF)
Lead poisoning
Lung cancer
Lungs
Multiple chemical sensitivity syndrome
Nasopharyngeal disorders
Occupational health
Pneumonia
Pulmonary diseases
Pulmonary medicine
Pulmonary medicine, pediatric
Radiation sickness
Skin cancer
Skin disorders
Stress
Stress reduction
Tendon disorders
Tendon repair
Toxicology

ONCOLOGY
Aging
Aging: Extended care
Amputation
Antioxidants
Biopsy
Blood testing
Bone cancer
Bone disorders
Bone grafting
Bone marrow transplantation
Bones and the skeleton
Breast biopsy
Breast cancer
Breasts, female
Cancer
Carcinoma
Cells
Cervical, ovarian, and uterine cancers
Chemotherapy
Colon and rectal polyp removal
Colon cancer
Cryotherapy and cryosurgery
Cystectomy
Cytology
Cytopathology
Dermatology
Dermatopathology
Endometrial biopsy
Ewing's sarcoma
Gastrectomy
Gastroenterology
Gastrointestinal disorders
Gastrointestinal system
Gastrostomy
Gene therapy
Genital disorders, female
Genital disorders, male
Gynecology
Hematology
Histology
Hodgkin's disease
Hysterectomy
Imaging and radiology
Immunology
Immunopathology
Kaposi's sarcoma
Laboratory tests
Laryngectomy
Laser use in surgery
Liver cancer
Lung cancer
Lung surgery

Lungs
Lymphadenopathy and lymphoma
Malignancy and metastasis
Malignant melanoma removal
Mammography
Massage
Mastectomy and lumpectomy
Nephrectomy
Oncology
Pain management
Pathology
Pharmacology
Pharmacy
Plastic surgery
Proctology
Prostate cancer
Prostate gland
Prostate gland removal
Pulmonary diseases
Pulmonary medicine
Radiation sickness
Radiation therapy
Radiopharmaceuticals
Sarcoma
Sarcopenia
Serology
Skin
Skin cancer
Skin lesion removal
Smoking
Stem cell research
Stomach, intestinal, and pancreatic cancers
Stress
Sunburn
Thalidomide
Toxicology
Transplantation
Tumor removal
Tumors

OPHTHALMOLOGY
Aging: Extended care
Albinos
Anti-inflammatory drugs
Arthritis, juvenile rheumatoid
Astigmatism
Biophysics
Blindness
Blurred vision
Cataract surgery
Cataracts
Color blindness
Conjunctivitis

Corneal transplantation
Eye surgery
Eyes
Geriatrics and gerontology
Glaucoma
Laser use in surgery
Macular degeneration
Marfan syndrome
Microscopy, slitlamp
Myopia
Ophthalmology
Optometry
Optometry, pediatric
Ptosis
Sense organs
Strabismus
Styes
Trachoma
Visual disorders

OPTOMETRY
Aging: Extended care
Astigmatism
Biophysics
Blurred vision
Cataracts
Eyes
Geriatrics and gerontology
Glaucoma
Myopia
Ophthalmology
Optometry
Optometry, pediatric
Ptosis
Sense organs
Styes
Visual disorders

ORGANIZATIONS AND PROGRAMS
Allied health
American Medical Association
Blood banks
Centers for Disease Control and Prevention (CDC)
Clinical trials
Education, medical
Food and Drug Administration (FDA)
Health maintenance organizations (HMOs)
Hospice
Hospitals
Human Genome Project

Medicare
National Cancer Institute (NCI)
National Institutes of Health (NIH)
Sperm banks
Stem cell research
World Health Organization

ORTHODONTICS
Bones and the skeleton
Dental diseases
Dentistry
Dentistry, pediatric
Jaw wiring
Orthodontics
Periodontal surgery
Teeth
Teething
Tooth extraction
Wisdom teeth

ORTHOPEDICS
Amputation
Arthritis
Arthritis, juvenile rheumatoid
Arthroplasty
Arthroscopy
Bone cancer
Bone disorders
Bone grafting
Bones and the skeleton
Bowlegs
Bunions
Bursitis
Cancer
Chiropractic
Craniosynostosis
Disk removal
Dwarfism
Ewing's sarcoma
Feet
Flat feet
Foot disorders
Fracture and dislocation
Fracture repair
Geriatrics and gerontology
Growth
Hammertoe correction
Hammertoes
Heel spur removal
Hip fracture repair
Hip replacement
Jaw wiring
Kinesiology
Kneecap removal

Knock-knees
Kyphosis
Laminectomy and spinal fusion
Lower extremities
Marfan syndrome
Motor skill development
Muscle sprains, spasms, and
  disorders
Muscles
Neurofibromatosis
Orthopedic surgery
Orthopedics
Orthopedics, pediatric
Osgood-Schlatter disease
Osteoarthritis
Osteochondritis juvenilis
Osteogenesis imperfecta
Osteomyelitis
Osteopathic medicine
Osteoporosis
Paget's disease
Physical examination
Physical rehabilitation
Pigeon toes
Podiatry
Rheumatoid arthritis
Rheumatology
Scoliosis
Slipped disk
Spina bifida
Spinal cord disorders
Spine, vertebrae, and disks
Sports medicine
Tendon disorders
Tendon repair
Upper extremities

OSTEOPATHIC MEDICINE
Alternative medicine
Bones and the skeleton
Exercise physiology
Family practice
Holistic medicine
Muscle sprains, spasms, and
  disorders
Muscles
Nutrition
Osteopathic medicine
Physical rehabilitation

OTORHINOLARYNGOLOGY
Anti-inflammatory drugs
Aromatherapy
Audiology

Cleft lip and palate
Cleft lip and palate repair
Common cold
Croup
Ear infections and disorders
Ear surgery
Ears
Epiglottitis
Gastrointestinal system
Halitosis
Head and neck disorders
Hearing aids
Hearing loss
Hearing tests
Laryngectomy
Laryngitis
Ménière's disease
Motion sickness
Myringotomy
Nasal polyp removal
Nasopharyngeal disorders
Nausea and vomiting
Nosebleeds
Otorhinolaryngology
Pharyngitis
Pulmonary diseases
Pulmonary medicine
Pulmonary medicine, pediatric
Quinsy
Respiration
Rhinitis
Rhinoplasty and submucous
  resection
Sense organs
Sinusitis
Smell
Sore throat
Strep throat
Taste
Tonsillectomy and adenoid removal
Tonsillitis
Voice and vocal cord disorders

PATHOLOGY
Autopsy
Bacteriology
Biopsy
Blood testing
Cancer
Cytology
Cytopathology
Dermatopathology
Disease
Electroencephalography (EEG)

Whooping cough
Worms

PERINATOLOGY
Amniocentesis
Birth defects
Breast-feeding
Cesarean section
Childbirth
Childbirth complications
Chorionic villus sampling
Cretinism
Critical care, pediatric
Embryology
Fetal alcohol syndrome
Hematology, pediatric
Hydrocephalus
Motor skill development
Neonatology
Neurology, pediatric
Nursing
Obstetrics
Pediatrics
Perinatology
Pregnancy and gestation
Premature birth
Reflexes, primitive
Shunts
Stillbirth
Sudden infant death syndrome
    (SIDS)
Umbilical cord
Well-baby examinations

PHARMACOLOGY
Acid-base chemistry
Aging: Extended care
Anesthesia
Anesthesiology
Antibiotics
Anti-inflammatory drugs
Bacteriology
Blurred vision
Chemotherapy
Club drugs
Critical care
Critical care, pediatric
Digestion
Drug resistance
Emergency medicine
Emergency medicine, pediatric
Enzymes
Fluids and electrolytes
Food biochemistry

Genetic engineering
Geriatrics and gerontology
Glycolysis
Herbal medicine
Homeopathy
Hormones
Laboratory tests
Melatonin
Metabolism
Narcotics
Oncology
Pain management
Pharmacology
Pharmacy
Poisoning
Psychiatry
Psychiatry, child and adolescent
Psychiatry, geriatric
Rheumatology
Self-medication
Sports medicine
Steroid abuse
Steroids
Thrombolytic therapy and TPA
Toxicology
Tropical medicine

PHYSICAL THERAPY
Aging: Extended care
Amputation
Amyotrophic lateral sclerosis
Arthritis
Bell's palsy
Biofeedback
Bowlegs
Burns and scalds
Cardiac rehabilitation
Cerebral palsy
Disk removal
Exercise physiology
Grafts and grafting
Hemiplegia
Hip fracture repair
Hip replacement
Hydrotherapy
Kinesiology
Knock-knees
Lower extremities
Massage
Motor skill development
Muscle sprains, spasms, and
    disorders
Muscles
Muscular dystrophy

Neurology
Neurology, pediatric
Numbness and tingling
Orthopedic surgery
Orthopedics
Orthopedics, pediatric
Osteopathic medicine
Osteoporosis
Pain management
Palsy
Paralysis
Paraplegia
Parkinson's disease
Physical examination
Physical rehabilitation
Plastic surgery
Quadriplegia
Rickets
Scoliosis
Slipped disk
Spina bifida
Spinal cord disorders
Spine, vertebrae, and disks
Sports medicine
Tendon disorders
Torticollis
Upper extremities

PLASTIC SURGERY
Aging
Amputation
Birthmarks
Breast cancer
Breast disorders
Breast surgery
Breasts, female
Burns and scalds
Cancer
Carcinoma
Circumcision, female, and genital
    mutilation
Circumcision, male
Cleft lip and palate
Cleft lip and palate repair
Craniosynostosis
Cyst removal
Cysts
Dermatology
Dermatology, pediatric
Face lift and blepharoplasty
Grafts and grafting
Hair loss and baldness
Hair transplantation
Healing

Jaw wiring
Laceration repair
Liposuction
Malignancy and metastasis
Malignant melanoma removal
Moles
Necrotizing fasciitis
Neurofibromatosis
Obesity
Otoplasty
Otorhinolaryngology
Plastic surgery
Ptosis
Rhinoplasty and submucous
  resection
Sex change surgery
Skin
Skin lesion removal
Surgical procedures
Tattoo removal
Tattoos and body piercing
Varicose vein removal
Varicose veins
Wrinkles

PODIATRY
Athlete's foot
Bone disorders
Bones and the skeleton
Bunions
Corns and calluses
Feet
Flat feet
Foot disorders
Fungal infections
Hammertoe correction
Hammertoes
Heel spur removal
Lower extremities
Nail removal
Orthopedic surgery
Orthopedics
Physical examination
Pigeon toes
Podiatry
Tendon disorders
Tendon repair
Warts

PREVENTIVE MEDICINE
Acupressure
Acupuncture
Aging: Extended care
Alternative medicine

Aromatherapy
Biofeedback
Cardiology
Chiropractic
Cholesterol
Chronobiology
Disease
Electrocardiography (ECG or
  EKG)
Environmental health
Exercise physiology
Family practice
Genetic counseling
Geriatrics and gerontology
Holistic medicine
Host-defense mechanisms
Hypercholesterolemia
Immune system
Immunization and vaccination
Immunology
Mammography
Massage
Meditation
Melatonin
Noninvasive tests
Nursing
Nutrition
Occupational health
Osteopathic medicine
Pharmacology
Pharmacy
Physical examination
Preventive medicine
Psychiatry
Psychiatry, child and adolescent
Psychiatry, geriatric
Qi gong
Screening
Serology
Spine, vertebrae, and disks
Sports medicine
Stress
Stress reduction
Tai Chi Chuan
Tropical medicine
Yoga

PROCTOLOGY
Colon and rectal polyp removal
Colon and rectal surgery
Colon cancer
Colonoscopy
Crohn's disease
Cystectomy

Diverticulitis and diverticulosis
Endoscopy
Fistula repair
Gastroenterology
Gastrointestinal disorders
Gastrointestinal system
Genital disorders, male
Geriatrics and gerontology
Hemorrhoid banding and removal
Hemorrhoids
Hirschsprung's disease
Internal medicine
Intestinal disorders
Intestines
Irritable bowel syndrome (IBS)
Physical examination
Proctology
Prostate cancer
Prostate gland
Prostate gland removal
Reproductive system
Urology

PSYCHIATRY
Addiction
Aging
Aging: Extended care
Alcoholism
Alzheimer's disease
Amnesia
Amyotrophic lateral sclerosis
Anorexia nervosa
Anxiety
Attention-deficit disorder (ADD)
Auras
Autism
Bipolar disorder
Bonding
Brain
Brain disorders
Breast surgery
Bulimia
Chronic fatigue syndrome
Circumcision, female, and genital
  mutilation
Club drugs
Delusions
Dementias
Depression
Developmental stages
Domestic violence
Eating disorders
Electroencephalography (EEG)
Emergency medicine

Emotions: Biomedical causes and
  effects
Factitious disorders
Failure to thrive
Family practice
Fatigue
Grief and guilt
Gynecology
Hallucinations
Hypnosis
Hypochondriasis
Incontinence
Intoxication
Light therapy
Masturbation
Memory loss
Mental retardation
Midlife crisis
Münchausen syndrome by proxy
Neurosis
Neurosurgery
Nightmares
Obesity
Obsessive-compulsive disorder
Pain
Pain management
Panic attacks
Paranoia
Penile implant surgery
Phobias
Postpartum depression
Post-traumatic stress disorder
Psychiatric disorders
Psychiatry
Psychiatry, child and adolescent
Psychiatry, geriatric
Psychoanalysis
Psychosis
Psychosomatic disorders
Schizophrenia
Separation anxiety
Sex change surgery
Sexual dysfunction
Sexuality
Shock therapy
Sleep disorders
Speech disorders
Steroid abuse
Stress
Stress reduction
Sudden infant death syndrome (SIDS)
Suicide
Toilet training
Tourette's syndrome

PSYCHOLOGY
Addiction
Aging
Aging: Extended care
Alcoholism
Amnesia
Amyotrophic lateral sclerosis
Anorexia nervosa
Anxiety
Aromatherapy
Arthritis, juvenile rheumatoid
Attention-deficit disorder (ADD)
Auras
Bed-wetting
Biofeedback
Bipolar disorder
Bonding
Brain
Bulimia
Cardiac rehabilitation
Cirrhosis
Club drugs
Cognitive development
Death and dying
Delusions
Depression
Developmental stages
Domestic violence
Dyslexia
Eating disorders
Electroencephalography (EEG)
Emotions: Biomedical causes and
  effects
Environmental health
Factitious disorders
Failure to thrive
Family practice
Forensic pathology
Genetic counseling
Grief and guilt
Gulf War syndrome
Gynecology
Hallucinations
Holistic medicine
Hormone replacement therapy
Hypnosis
Hypochondriasis
Kinesiology
Klinefelter syndrome
Learning disabilities
Light therapy
Meditation
Memory loss
Mental retardation

Midlife crisis
Motor skill development
Münchausen syndrome by proxy
Neurosis
Nightmares
Nutrition
Obesity
Obsessive-compulsive disorder
Occupational health
Pain management
Panic attacks
Paranoia
Phobias
Plastic surgery
Postpartum depression
Post-traumatic stress disorder
Psychosomatic disorders
Puberty and adolescence
Separation anxiety
Sex change surgery
Sexual dysfunction
Sexuality
Sibling rivalry
Sleep disorders
Sleepwalking
Speech disorders
Sports medicine
Steroid abuse
Stillbirth
Stress
Stress reduction
Stuttering
Sudden infant death syndrome
  (SIDS)
Suicide
Temporomandibular joint (TMJ)
  syndrome
Tics
Toilet training
Tourette's syndrome
Weight loss and gain
Yoga

PUBLIC HEALTH
Acquired immunodeficiency
  syndrome (AIDS)
Aging: Extended care
Allied health
Alternative medicine
Anthrax
Arthropod-borne diseases
Bacteriology
Beriberi
Biostatistics

Emergency medicine
Environmental diseases
Environmental health
Enzyme therapy
Food poisoning
Forensic pathology
Hepatitis
Herbal medicine
Homeopathy
Intoxication
Itching
Laboratory tests
Lead poisoning
Liver
Mold and mildew
Multiple chemical sensitivity
 syndrome
Occupational health
Pathology
Pharmacology
Pharmacy
Poisoning
Poisonous plants
Rashes
Snakebites
Toxemia
Toxicology
Toxoplasmosis
Urinalysis

UROLOGY
Abdomen
Abdominal disorders
Bed-wetting
Catheterization
Chlamydia
Circumcision, male
Cystectomy
Cystitis
Cystoscopy
Dialysis
E. coli infection
Endoscopy
Fluids and electrolytes
Genital disorders, female
Genital disorders, male
Geriatrics and gerontology
Gonorrhea
Hermaphroditism and
 pseudohermaphroditism
Hydrocelectomy
Hypospadias repair and
 urethroplasty
Incontinence

Infertility in males
Kidney disorders
Kidney transplantation
Kidneys
Lithotripsy
Nephrectomy
Nephritis
Nephrology
Nephrology, pediatric
Pediatrics
Pelvic inflammatory disease (PID)
Penile implant surgery
Prostate cancer
Prostate gland
Prostate gland removal
Reproductive system
Schistosomiasis
Sex change surgery
Sexual differentiation
Sexual dysfunction
Sexually transmitted diseases
Sterilization
Stone removal
Stones
Syphilis
Testicles, undescended
Testicular surgery
Testicular torsion
Toilet training
Transplantation
Ultrasonography
Urethritis
Urinalysis
Urinary disorders
Urinary system
Urology
Urology, pediatric
Vasectomy

VASCULAR MEDICINE
Amputation
Aneurysmectomy
Aneurysms
Angiography
Angioplasty
Anti-inflammatory drugs
Arteriosclerosis
Biofeedback
Bleeding
Blood and blood disorders
Bypass surgery
Catheterization
Cholesterol
Circulation

Claudication
Dehydration
Diabetes mellitus
Dialysis
Embolism
Endarterectomy
Exercise physiology
Glands
Healing
Hematology
Hematology, pediatric
Hemorrhoid banding and removal
Hemorrhoids
Histology
Hypercholesterolemia
Hyperlipidemia
Ischemia
Lipids
Lymphatic system
Mitral valve prolapse
Necrotizing fasciitis
Osteochondritis juvenilis
Phlebitis
Podiatry
Progeria
Shunts
Smoking
Strokes
Thrombolytic therapy and TPA
Thrombosis and thrombus
Transfusion
Varicose vein removal
Varicose veins
Vascular medicine
Vascular system
Venous insufficiency

VIROLOGY
Acquired immunodeficiency
 syndrome (AIDS)
Chickenpox
Childhood infectious diseases
Chlamydia
Chronic fatigue syndrome
Common cold
Creutzfeldt-Jakob disease and mad
 cow disease
Croup
Cytomegalovirus (CMV)
Drug resistance
Ebola virus
Encephalitis
Fever
Glomerulonephritis

Hanta virus
Hepatitis
Herpes
Human immunodeficiency virus
  (HIV)
Infection
Influenza
Laboratory tests
Measles
Microbiology
Microscopy

Mononucleosis
Mumps
Parasitic diseases
Pelvic inflammatory disease (PID)
Poliomyelitis
Pulmonary diseases
Rabies
Rheumatic fever
Rhinitis
Roseola
Rubella

Serology
Sexually transmitted diseases
Shingles
Smallpox
Tonsillitis
Tropical medicine
Viral infections
Warts
Yellow fever
Zoonoses

INDEX

A page number or range in boldface type indicates that an entire entry devoted to that topic appears in the Guide; *italicized page numbers indicate illustrations appearing outside of the topic's primary entry.*

Anthropology, 2443

Antianxiety drugs, 1860

Antibiotics, 14, **133-138**, 207-208, *210*, 548-549, 623, 661, 664, 679, 738, 885, 1198, 1244, 1268, 1388, 1491, 1786, 1837, 1928, 2041, 2126, 2320, 2356, 2443; antitumor, 396; broad-spectrum, 134, 136, 662, 665; oral, 27; topical, 27

Antibodies, 265, 1147, 1212, 1214, 1225, 1242, 1976, 2043-2044, 2443

Anticancer drugs. *See* Chemotherapy

Anticholinergic drugs, 1759, 2444

Anticoagulants, 1064, 2377, 2444

Anticonvulsants, 2444

Antidepressants, 185, 194, 241, 586, 1654, 1760, 1860, 1900, 2192

Antidiuretic hormone. *See* Vasopressin

Antidote, 2444

Antiemetic drugs, 1579, 2444

Antifungal agents, 346, 886, 888, 2444

Antigens, 1211, 1225, 1976, 2043, 2304, 2444

Antihistamines, 68, 405, 493, 592-593, 1018, 1120

Anti-inflammatory drugs, **138-140**, 165, 484, 2444

Antimetabolites, 396, 2444

Antioxidants, **140-141**, 1462, 2197

Antipsychotic drugs, 1900

Antipyretic drugs, 843, 1170

Antisense therapy, 341

Antiserum, 2444

Antitoxins, 132, 897, 2246-2247, 2287

Antitrypsin, 778

Antitumor antibiotics, 396

Antivenin, 252

Anus, 767, 913, 1082, 1200, 1880

Anxiety, 55, **141-146**, 185, 653, 733, 827, 1183, 1497, 1615, 1652, 1799, 1901, 2107, 2444

Anxiety disorders, 2444

Aorta, 503

Aperistalsis, 1780

Apgar score, **146-147**

Aphasia, **147**, 2127-2128, 2181, 2444

Apheresis, 2444

Apicoectomy, 1776

Aplastic anemia. *See* Anemia, aplastic

Apnea, **147**, 828, 1557, 2104, 2188

Apogeusia, 2221

Apothecaries, 1788, 2444

Appendectomy, **148-149**, 2444

Appendicitis, 6, 8, 148, **149-151**, 1276, 2444

Appendix, *148*, 150

Appetite, 1350

Apraxia, 81

Aqueous fluid, 367, 965, 1672

Aqueous humor, 2444

Arch bar, 2444

Arches, 832

Areola, 2444

Ariboflavinosis, 1431

Aromatherapy, 78, **151-152**, 1029, 2444

Arrhythmias, **152**, 355, 358, 643, *709*, 1053, 1055, 1716, 1970, 2183, 2444

Artaeus of Cappadocia, 242

Arterial distension, 121-122

Arterial plaque. *See* Plaque, arterial

Arterial pressure points, 256

Arteries, 123, 152, *444*, 1165, 1385, 2212, 2350, 2375, 2379, 2444; chest, 400

Arteriography. *See* Angiography

Arteriosclerosis, 52, 121, **152-158**, 445, 610, 1045, 1048, 1052, 1119, 1158-1159, 1165, 1363, 1644, 1648, 2031, 2055, 2182, 2186, 2253, 2375, 2444

Arthritis, 50, 139, **158-164**, 166, 284-285, 976, 1108, 1227, 1308, 1401, 1687, 1691, 1981, 1983, 2144, 2150, 2233, 2444; juvenile rheumatoid, **164-166**

Arthroplasty, **166-168**, 1107, 1986, 2444

Arthropod-borne diseases, **168-174**, 251, 715, 740, 781, 1419, 1424, 1753, 1829, 2108, 2311, 2332

Arthroscopy, 18, **174-175**, *765*-766, 1690, 2444

Articulations, 292, 2444

Artificial insemination, 1249, 1252, 1254-1255, 2130

Artificial lens, *365*, 369

Artificial limbs. *See* Prostheses

Artificial respirator, 1926

Asbestosis, 769

Ascites, 453, 701, 908, 1377, 1380, 2343

Ascorbic acid. *See* Vitamin C

Aseptic techniques, 2200, 2444

Asian flu, 1260

Asperger's syndrome, 192-193

Aspergillosis, 887

Asphyxiants, 18

Asphyxiation, **175-176**, 2246, 2444

Aspiration, 233, 305, *554*, 893, 1283, 1889, 2323, 2444

Aspirin, 139, 1094, 1228, 1399, 1845, 1975, 2185, 2252, 2254, 2335, 2338

Assessment, 2444

Asthma, 68, **176-181**, 441, 589, 1180, 1268, 1394, 1502, 1925, 1929-1932, 1965, 2176, 2444

Astigmatism, **181-182**, 370, 815, 2038, 2399, 2444

Astrocytes, 301

Asymptomatic, 2444

Ataxia, **182**, 2444

Atherectomy, 1050

Atherosclerosis. *See* Arteriosclerosis

Athletes, 2157

Athlete's foot, **182-183**, 834, 886, 1491, 1554, 2444

Athletic injuries. *See* Sports injuries

Atom, 2444

Atopic dermatitis, 589-590, 592, 697

ATP. *See* Adenosine triphosphate (ATP)

Atresia, 1038

Atria, 1043

Atrial fibrillation, 152-153, 355, 570, *709*, 1046, 1053, 1724, 2254

Atrioventricular defects, 505

Atrioventricular (A-V) node, 354, 1044, 1535, 1716, 2444

Atrium, 2444

Atrophy, 1175, 1386, 1508, 1535, 1635, 1727, 2351, 2445; vaginal, 1470

Attention-deficit disorder (ADD), **183-186**, 1900, 2271

Attention-deficit hyperactivity disorder. *See* Attention-deficit disorder (ADD)

Attenuation, 2445

Audiology, 128, **186-191**, 2445

Audiometer, 2445

Gram staining, 204, 896, **983-988**, 1838, 2462
Grand mal seizure, 786, 2030, 2462
Granulocytes, 264, 1210, 2302, 2462
Granulomas, 2155, 2385, 2462
Granulomatosis, 1222
Graves' disease, 750, 754, 963, 2263, 2266, 2462
Gray hair, **988**
Gray matter, 297, 1117
Grief, 563, **988-993**, 2193
Groin pull, 2235
Gross pathology, 2462
Group therapy, 1860
Growth, 338, 666, 757, 836, **993-997**, 1174, 1177, 1688, 1768, 1803, 1918-1919, 2462
Growth hormone, 666, 668, 753, 957, 962-963, 997, 1177, 1189, 2214
Growth hormone-releasing hormone (GHRH), 753
Guillain-Barré syndrome, **997-1001**, 1606, 1741, 2462
Guilt, **988-993**, 1184, 1652, 2191, 2193
Gulf War syndrome, **1001-1003**
Gum bleeding, 257, 958
Gum disease, 2118. *See also* Periodontitis
Gums, 1776, 2229
Gustation, 2462
Gynecology, **1003-1007**, 1804, 2463
Gynecomastia, 403, **1008**

H & E. *See* Hematoxylin and eosin (H & E)
Hair, 988, *1014*, 1823, 2093, 2098, 2282
Hair color, 988, 1823
Hair implants, 1011, *1014*
Hair loss, **1009-1013**, 2100
Hair transplantation, 1011, **1013-1014**, 2463
Half-life, 2463
Halitosis, **1014-1015**, 1569-1570, 1777, 2463
Hallucinations, **1015**, 1556, 1749, 1849, 1914-1915, 2463
Hallucinogens, 42
Hallucis, 2463
Hammertoe correction, **1016**, 1841

Hammertoes, 867, **1016-1017**, 1841, 2463
Hamstring muscles, 1384
Hamstring pull, 2235
Hand-foot-and-mouth disease, **1017**
Hands, *2348*
Hansen's disease. *See* Leprosy
Hanta virus, **1017-1018**
Haploid, 2463
Hard palate, 2463
Hare lip. *See* Cleft palate
Harrington rod technique, 2021
Hashimoto's thyroiditis, 197, 962, 1226, 1229, 2263, 2463
Hay fever, 66, **1018-1019**. *See also* Allergies; Rhinitis
Hazardous wastes, 309, 769
HDLs. *See* High-density lipoproteins (HDLs)
Head disorders, **1019-1020**
Head trauma, 16, 18, 488, 569, 1019, 1464, 1480, 1745, 2031, 2128, 2221
Headaches, 217, 468, 741, **1020-1025**, 1500, 2090, 2463; cluster, 468; migraine, 468
Healing, **1025-1029**, 1130, 1156, 1257, 1807, 1935, 2253, 2430, 2463
Health, 1701, 1811, 2463
Health care reform, 795, 1437, 1813, 1815
Health care workers, 71, 2044
Health information, 380
Health insurance, 461, 1030, 1456, 2023
Health maintenance, 2463
Health maintenance organizations (HMOs), **1029-1033**, 1273, 1815, 2463
Hearing, 187, 677, 1035, 2037
Hearing aids, 190, **1033-1035**, 1039
Hearing loss, 49, 187, 457, 677, 679-681, 683, 685, 953, 1034, **1035-1040**, 1041, 1464, 1568, 1711, 2128, 2463; conductive, 681, 683, 1033, 1037; sensorineural, 682-683, 1033, 1038-1039
Hearing tests, **1040-1042**
Heart, 276, 336-*337*, 348, 354, 400, 444, 709, **1042-1047**, 1061, 1063, 1534, 1624, 1716, 1949, 1970, 2212, 2463; anatomy of the, 354,

400, 444, 503, 1042, *1043*, 1047, 1051
Heart attack, 52, 154, 218, 349, 355, 358, 632, 1045, **1047-1051**, 1052, 1119, 1165, 1718, 1785, 1875, 1972, 2071, 2118, 2254, 2258, 2381, 2463
Heart block, 152, 355, *709*, 1053, 1716, 2463
Heart defects, 356
Heart disease, 52, 124, 153, 348, 354, 359, 504, 747, **1051-1056**, 1165, 1267, 1501, 2176, 2343; congenital, 503
Heart disorders, 1176, 1501
Heart failure, 504, 699, 1045, 1053, **1056-1060**, 1176, 2072, 2463
Heart-lung machine, 506, 1046
Heart murmurs, 356, 505-506, 746, 1064, 1801, 1804, 2148
Heart rate, 807, 953, 2463
Heart transplantation, 1046, 1059, **1060-1062**, 2251, 2463
Heart valve replacement, **1062-1065**, 2251, 2463
Heart valves, 1043, *1063*-1064
Heartbeat, 152, 228, 354, 1053
Heartbeat, irregular. *See* Arrhythmias
Heartburn, 627, 908, 914, **1065-1066**, 1241, 1662, 2463
Heat, 2463; therapeutic use of, 1808
Heat exhaustion, 566, **1066-1067**, 2463
Heat rash, 1952
Heat stroke, 566, 631, **1066-1067**, 2463
Heat therapy, 162
Heel spur removal, **1067-1068**
Heel spurs, 867, 1068, 2463
Heels, 832, 1068, 1383
Heimlich maneuver, 424-425, 1965, 2000
Helicobacter pylori, 2339
Helminths, 2463
Hemangiomas, 249
Hemarthroses, 257
Hematocrit levels, 2300
Hematology, **1068-1073**, 1313, 2463; pediatric, **1073-1075**
Hematomas, 122, 257, 569, 684, 1079, 1119, 1740, 2385, 2463; epidural, 16; subdural, 16
Hematopoiesis, 2463

922, 927, 942, 1151, 2285, 2351.
See also Brain disorders
Hurler's syndrome, 839
Hutchinson-Gilford syndrome, 1882
Hydatid disease, 1754
Hydro-, 2465
Hydrocarbon, 2465
Hydrocelectomy, **1154**, 2465
Hydroceles, 951, 1154, 2465
Hydrocephalus, 303-304, 569, 923,
  1154-1156, 1480, 1767, 1770,
  2081, 2136, 2465
Hydrochloric acid, 625, 627, 914,
  2337, 2370, 2405
Hydrogenation, 1361
Hydrophilic, 2465
Hydrophobic, 2465
Hydrostatic pressure, 698, 700, 1410
Hydrotherapy, 77, **1156-1157**, 1810,
  2465
Hydroxymethylglutaryl coenzyme A,
  429
Hygiene, 2465
Hygienic Laboratory, 1573
Hymen, 1004
Hyper-, 2465
Hyperactivity, 183, 741, 2271. *See
  also* Attention-deficit disorder
  (ADD)
Hyperadiposis, **1157-1158**
Hyperalimentation, 690
Hyperbaric oxygen chamber, 897,
  1715
Hypercalcemia, 851, 2167
Hypercholesterolemia, **1158**, 2161;
  familial, 943
Hypericum perforatum, 587
Hyperinsulinemia, 1264
Hyperlipidemia, 154, 608, 927,
  1159-1160, 1735, 2465
Hypernatremia, 2465
Hyperopia, 277, 815, 2038, 2398,
  2465
Hyperparathyroidism, **1160-1163**,
  1755, 2167, 2465
Hyperplasia, 1174, 1374, 1471,
  1884, 2465; epithelial, 311
Hypersensitivity, 67, 2465
Hypersplenism, 2144
Hypertension, 49, 52, 121, 154-155,
  218, 304, 570, 695, 1045, 1053,
  1163-1169, 1176, 1269, 1648,
  1775, 2055, 2186, 2376, 2465;

portal, 453, 2081; renovascular,
  2376
Hyperthermia, **1169-1174**, 2189,
  2465
Hyperthyroidism, 2263, 2309. *See
  also* Graves' disease
Hypertrophy, 323, 1064, **1174-1178**,
  1539-1540, 2465
Hyperuricemia, 977
Hyperventilation, 1737
Hyphae, 885
Hypnosis, 90, **1178-1182**, 2179,
  2465
Hypo-, 2465
Hypocalcemia, 851
Hypochondriasis, **1182-1187**, 2465
Hypocretins, 1557
Hypodermis, 2465
Hypogammaglobulinemia,
  1221-1222
Hypoglycemia, 642-643, **1187-1191**,
  2030, 2165, 2465
Hypogonadotropic hypogonadism,
  1920
Hypokalemic paralysis, 1741
Hyponychium, 1552
Hypoparathyroidism, **1160-1163**,
  2465
Hypophysectomy, 1617
Hypospadias, 1192, 1959, 2465
Hypospadias repair, **1191-1192**
Hypotension, 2465
Hypothalamus, 298, 749, 752, 962,
  1066, 1648, 2115, 2263, 2465
Hypothermia, 616, 841, 880,
  1169-1174, 1809, 2466
Hypothyroidism, 521, 750, 962,
  1189, 1648, 2263, 2266, 2466
Hypovolemia, 642
Hypovolemic shock, 2071, 2073
Hypoxia, 175, 302, 417, 555, 631,
  880, 2189, 2466
Hypoxic anoxia, 175
Hysterectomy, 12, 389-390, 762,
  1192-1197, 1468, 1960,
  2154-2155, 2466; abdominal,
  1193, 1196; vaginal, 1193, 1196
Hysteria, 1615
Hysterotomy, 12

Iatrogenic, 2466
Iatrogenic disorders, **1198-1199**
IBD. *See* Inflammatory bowel
  disease (IBD)

IBS. *See* Irritable bowel syndrome
  (IBS)
Ichthyosis, 2100
ICU. *See* Intensive care unit (ICU)
Id, 1911
Ideal body weight, 1647
Identical twins, 1517
Idiopathic, 2466
Idiopathic thrombocytopenic purpura
  (ITP), 254, 258
IgE antibodies, 66, 69, 178, 589-590
Ileostomy, 478, 481, **1199-1204**,
  2466
Ileum, 901, 913, 1200, 2466
Illicit drugs, 2033, 2466
Illness; acute, 630; chronic, 380,
  630
Imaging, 495, *497*, 903, 915,
  1204-1209, 1417, 1439, 1801,
  1805, *1857*, 1949, 2343, 2466
Imaging magnets, *1416*
Immobilization, 877
Immune response, 2466
Immune system, 29, 178, 196, 206,
  252, 289, 340, 344, 436-437,
  632, 981, 1145, 1180,
  1209-1214, 1221, 1225, 1242,
  1301, 1409, 1762, 2043, 2176,
  2178, 2305, 2395, 2466
Immune thrombocytopenic purpura.
  See Idiopathic thrombocytopenic
  purpura (ITP)
Immunity, 2466
Immunization, 223, 382, 981, 1147,
  1214-1221, 1268, 1454, 1994,
  2045, 2466. *See also* Vaccination
Immunoassay, 1314, 2466
Immunocompromised, 2466
Immunocompromised patients, 344,
  346, 559, 887, 1102, 1223
Immunodeficiency disorders, 1219,
  1221-1225, 1762, 2466
Immunoglobulin E (IgE), 2466
Immunoglobulins, 314, 1219, 2466
Immunologic stains, 231
Immunology, 396, 1213, **1225-1229**,
  1230, 2466
Immunopathology, **1230**, 2466
Immunosuppression, 2466
Immunosuppressive drugs, 533,
  1079, 1213, 1228, 1301, 1373,
  1380, 1382, 2305
Impacted teeth, *578*, 2229, 2277
Impetigo, 618, **1230-1231**

Jaundice, 891-892, 908, 1075, 1087, 1091, **1288**, 1371, 1375, 1377, 1379, 2040, 2169, 2171, 2433, 2468; neonatal, **1288-1290**
Jaw, 1291, 1682, 2228, 2233
Jaw wiring, **1291-1294**
Jealousy, 2083
Jejunoileal bypass, 1158
Jejunum, 901, 913, 2468
Jenner, Edward, 1149, 1220, 1245, 1876, 2111
Jet lag, 441, 2468
Joint, 2468
Joint diseases, 158, 166, 335, 976, 1227-1228, 1396-1397, 1981, 1983, 2144, 2233. *See also* Arthritis
Joint replacement, *167*, 1687. *See also* Arthroplasty; Hip replacement
Joints, 158, 164, *167*, *174*, 1016, 1107-1108, 1227-1228, 1283, 1401, 1686-1687, 1690, 1982, 2233
Journal of the American Medical Association, 88
Jung, Carl, 1616

Kala-azar, 1344, 1754, 1893, 2312
Kaposi's sarcoma, 29, 1222, **1295-1296**, 2096
Karyotype, 923
Karyotyping, 95, 232, 659, 928, 1920, 2468
Kava, 1094
Kefauver-Harris Amendment, 856
Keratin, 517, 1551, 2468
Keratinocytes, 1552, 2091, 2468
Keratitis, 1673, 2468
Keratomileusis, 2401
Keratoplasty, 515
Keratoses, **1296**, 2102, 2468
Keratosis pilaris, 590
Keratotomy, 2468
Ketoacidosis, 860, 1569
Ketones, 2468
Ketonuria, 608
Kevorkian, Jack, 800
Kidney disorders, 4, 7, 50, 547, 610, 667, 942, 970, 1137, 1166, **1296-1299**, 1302-1303, 1588, 2170
Kidney failure. *See* Renal failure
Kidney removal. *See* Nephrectomy

Kidney stone removal. *See* Kidney stones; Stone removal
Kidney stones, 1161, 1297, 1299, 1304, 1320, *1368*-1369, 1590, *2168*-2170, 2361
Kidney transplantation, 4, 1299, **1300-1301**, 1589, 1597, 2215, 2468
Kidneys, 3, 22, 1192, *1300*, **1301-1306**, 1588-*1589*, 1591, 1596, 1630, 1950, 2170, 2213, 2215, 2358, 2363, 2468; anatomy of, 1302
Killer bees, 252
Killer T cells, 1212
Kilocalorie, 2468
Kinase, 2468
Kinesiology, 79, 806, **1306-1307**, 1537, 2468
Kinesthetic imprinting, 672
Kinsey, Alfred C., 2060
Klinefelter syndrome, 403, 721, **1307-1308**
Klumpke's palsy, 1727
Kluver-Bucy syndrome, 732, 2468
Knee replacement, *167*
Kneecap, 1308, 1383
Kneecap removal, **1308-1309**
Knees, 17-18, *167*, *174*, 1308, 1383, 1982, 2469
Knock-knees, **1309**, 1686
Knockout mouse, 2469
Koch, Robert, 133, 211, 427, 2321
Kocher, Emil Theodor, 2265
Kock pouch, 478, 1200
Koller, Carl, 370
Korsakoff's psychosis, 61, 90
Kraepelin, Emil, 243, 1902, 2014
Kübler-Ross, Elisabeth, 561, 1139
Kupffer cells, 2469
Kuru, 523, 1878
Kwashiorkor, **1309**, 1430, 1432-1433, 2312, 2469
Kyphosis, **1309-1310**, 1703, 2141

L-dopa, 1728, 1759-1760, 2469
Labia, 2469
Labia major, 1004
Labia minor, 1004
Labor, 407, 1865, 2469; induction of, 409
Laboratories, 1315
Laboratory tests, 134, 778, 906,

1267, **1311-1316**, 2288, 2353, 2364, 2368, 2469
Labyrinth, 2469
Labyrinthitis, 641, 685
Laceration repair, **1316-1317**
Lacerations, 1020, 1028, 1316, 2469
Lactase, 1317
Lactation, 322, 1959. *See also* Breast-feeding
Lacteals, 2469
Lactic acid, 973, 1485
Lactiferous duct, 2469
Lactose, 859, 985, 1317
Lactose intolerance, 859, **1317-1318**
Laetrile, 854
Lakhovsky, Georges, 1172
Lamellar keratoplasty, 2469
Lamina, 2469
Laminaria, 2469
Laminectomy, **1318-1319**, 1618, 2469
Landsteiner, Karl, 1976, 1978
Langerhans' cells, 2098
Language development, 471
Language disturbances, 147, 1808, 2127-2128
Laparoscopy, 426, 760, *765*, 891, **1319-1321**, 2154, 2316, 2469
Laparotomy, 2469
Large intestine. *See* Colon
Laryngectomy, **1321**, 1712, 2469
Laryngitis, **1321-1322**, 1566, 1569, 2407-2408, 2469
Larynx, 1321, 1392, 2469
Laser in-situ keratomileusis (LASIK), 1325, 2401
Lasers, 229, 262, 762, 968, 1085, 1322, 1619, 2469; use in surgery, 229, 580, 810, **1322-1327**, 1619, 2201, 2205, 2224, 2372, 2401
LASIK. *See* Laser in-situ keratomileusis (LASIK)
Latent, 2469
Lateral, 2469
Laughing gas. *See* Nitrous oxide
Law and medicine, 201, 800, 869, 1114, **1327-1332**, 1435, 2290
Law of Similars, 1128
Laxatives, 508, 620-621, 689
LDLs. *See* Low-density lipoproteins (LDLs)
Lead poisoning, 631, 768, **1332-1334**, 1336, 1479, 1846, 2001, 2031, 2469

Maillard reaction, 2399
Major histocompatibility complex, 940, 981
Major histocompatibility proteins, 1212
Malabsorption, 373, 900, **1418-1419**
Malaise, 2471
Malaria, 128, 169, 251, 843, **1419-1424**, 1491, 1546, 1754, 1892-1893, *2311*-2312, 2436, 2471
Male circumcision. *See* Circumcision, male
Male genital disorders. *See* Genital disorders, male
Male pattern baldness, 1009, 1013
Male reproductive system. *See* Reproductive system, male
Malignancy, 339, 388, **1424-1429**, 2471
Malignant cells, 556
Malignant melanoma, 596, 1429, 2093, 2102, 2471; removal, **1429**
Malleus, 2037
Malnutrition, 55, 315, 619, 632, 667, 700, 827, 859, 997, 1309, **1429-1434**, 1476, 2312, 2471
Malocclusion, 573-574, 1683, 2471
Malpractice, 1114, **1434-1438**, 2209, 2471
Malpractice insurance, 2471
Mammary glands, 322, 403
Mammography, 305, 307, **1438-1444**, 1448, 1625, 1669, 2027, 2471
Managed care, 1030
Mandible, 2471
Manic-depressive disorder. *See* Bipolar disorder
Manic episode, 239
Manicure, 1553
Manometry, 1781
Manson, Patrick, 717
MAOIs. *See* Monoamine oxidase inhibitors (MAOIs)
Marasmus, 667, 1430, 1433, 2312, 2471
Marburg virus, 693
March of Dimes, 1852
Marfan syndrome, 942, **1444-1445**
Marijuana, 42
Martial arts, 1935, 2217
Massage, 151, **1445-1446**, 1810
Mast cell inhibitors, 738

Mast cells, 1027, 2471
Mastalgia, 311
Mastectomy, 309, 325, **1446-1451**, 1944, 2471; preventive, 924
Mastication, 2471
Mastitis, 311, 323, **1451**, 2471
Mastoidectomy, 2471
Mastoiditis, 687, 1568
Masturbation, **1451-1452**
Materia Medica, 1130, 2471
Matrix, 2471
Maxilla, 2471
Maxillofacial surgery, 2471
Maximal oxygen uptake, 2471
Maximally tolerated dose, 461
Measles, 415, 418, 742-743, 782, 1218, **1452-1456**, 2045, 2471
Mechanoreceptors, 2471
Meconium ileus, 543
Medial, 2471
Median nerve, 362
Medical College Admission Test (MCAT), 2471
Medical experts, 1328
Medical schools, 410, 703
Medicare, **1456-1460**, 2240, 2471; hospice and, 1141
Medications. *See* Drugs; Pharmacology
Medicine, 2472
Meditation, 77, 1029, 1126, **1460-1461**, 2179, 2433, 2472
Medulla oblongata, 297
Megadose, 2472
Megaloblastic anemia, 2472. *See also* Anemia, megaloblastic
Meganblase syndrome, 334
Meiosis, 657-658, 940, 2472
Meissner's corpuscles, 2035, 2282, 2284, 2472
Melancholia, 242, 2014
Melanin, 988, *1822*-1823, 2091-2092, 2099, 2472
Melanocytes, 988, 1552, 1822-1823, 2091, 2096, 2098-2099
Melanoma, 596, 1429, 1504, 1824, 2096, 2101, 2327, 2472. *See also* Malignant melanoma removal; Skin cancer
Melasmas, 2099
Melatonin, 440, 748, 750, 961, **1461-1463**, 2472
Membranes, 1362, 1364, 2472
Memory cells, 1212

Memory loss, 90, 568, **1463-1464**, 1557, 2078
Menarche, 87, 307, 1005, 1473, 1919, 2472
Mendel, Gregor, 943
Ménière's disease, 641, 679-680, 685, 1038, **1464-1465**, 1712, 2472
Meninges, 1599
Meningitis, 416, 418, 741, 1219, 1388, **1465-1467**, 1599, 2136, 2425, 2472; bacterial, 1466
Menopause, 50, 307, 791, 1195, **1467-1472**, 1703, 2472
Menorrhagia, 257, **1473**, 1476, 2472
Menstrual extraction, 11
Menstruation, 87, 257, 315, 321, 500-501, 674, 689, 759, 791, 945, 1247, 1471, **1473-1478**, 1863, 1872, 1959, 2153, 2472
Menstruation, painful. *See* Dysmenorrhea
Mental distress, 1331
Mental illness. *See* Psychiatric disorders; *specific diseases*
Mental impairment, 2004
Mental incompetence, 571
Mental retardation, 521, 658, 836, 878, **1478-1483**, 1768, 2128, 2472
Mercury poisoning, 769
Mercy killing. *See* Euthanasia
Meridians, 34-35, 2472
Merkel's disks, 2282, 2284, 2472
Merozoites, 1421
Mesenchyme, 1117
Messenger ribonucleic acid (mRNA), 1151, 2472
Metabolic equivalent (MET), 2472
Metabolic rate, 2472
Metabolism, 21, 542, 805, 858, 928, 960, 973, 1169, 1190, 1370, **1483-1488**, 1647, 2009, 2118, 2472; errors in, 859, 1372
Metastasis, 339, 388, 1374, **1424-1429**, 2323, 2472. *See also* Cancer; Malignancy
Metastasize, 2472
Metatarsals, 832, 1383
Metformin, 1265
Methadone, 1888
Methamphetamine, 42
Methotrexate, 1897, 2472
Methylprednisolone, 1524

Myenteric plexus, 1778
Myocardial infarction. *See* Heart
attack
Myocardium, 356, 2474
Myoclonus, 2474
Myomas, 2327
Myomectomy, 1194, **1547-1548**,
2474
Myopia, 277, 815, **1548-1549**, 2038,
2398, 2474
Myosarcoma, 2327
Myringotomy, 682, 686, **1549-1550**,
2474

Nail bed, 1552
Nail plate, 1552
Nail polish, 1553
Nail removal, **1551**, *1552*
Nails, **1551-1555**, 2093
Naltrexone, 45
Nanobots, 224
Narcolepsy, **1555-1560**, 2105, 2107,
2474
Narcotics, 18, 112, 1023, 1140,
1561-1565, 2474
Nasal cavity, *1565*, 2114
Nasal polyp removal, **1565-1566**
Nasal polyps, *1565*, 1569
Nasal surgery, *1565*, 1987
Nasogastric tube, 899
Nasopharyngeal, 2474
Nasopharyngeal disorders,
1566-1571, 2090
National Cancer Institute (NCI),
461, **1571-1573**, 1574
National Center for Environmental
Health (NCEH), 380
National Center for Health Statistics
(NCHS), 380
National Center for Infectious
Diseases (NCID), 381
National Center for Injury
Prevention and Control (NCIPC),
381
National Hospice Organization, 1141
National Human Genome Research
Institute, 1152
National Institute for Occupational
Safety and Health (NIOSH), 382
National Institute of Neurological
Disorders and Stroke (NINDS),
386
National Institutes of Health (NIH),
839, 937, 1571, **1573-1576**

National Vaccine Plan, 382
Natural childbirth, 411
Nausea, 907, **1576-1581**, 2474
NCEH. *See* National Center for
Environmental Health (NCEH)
NCHS. *See* National Center for
Health Statistics (NCHS)
NCI. *See* National Cancer Institute
(NCI)
NCID. *See* National Center for
Infectious Diseases (NCID)
NCIPC. *See* National Center for
Injury Prevention and Control
(NCIPC)
Nearsightedness, 2474. *See also*
Myopia
Nebulizers, 737
Neck, 745, 1321
Neck disorders, **1019-1020**
Necropsy, 2474
Necrosis, 556, 560, 1118, 2474. *See
also* Frostbite; Gangrene
Necrotizing fasciitis, **1581-1582**
Needle biopsy, 233, 305, *554*, 1283,
1889, 2323, 2474
Negative feedback, 1818, 2214,
2474
Neglect, 651, 654
Negligence, 1435, 2209, 2474
Nematodes, 169, 1753, 1993
Neonatal intensive care unit (NICU),
2474
Neonatal period, 2474
Neonate, 2474
Neonatology, **1582-1588**, 1766,
1933, 2300, 2474
Neoplasm, 2474. *See also* Tumors
Nephrectomy, **1588-1590**, 2366,
2474
Nephritis, 1297, **1590**, 1592, 2276,
2361, 2474; interstitial, 1297
Nephrology, **1591-1595**, 2364, 2474;
pediatric, **1595-1597**
Nephrons, 1303, 2359, 2363, 2474
Nephrotic syndrome, 1297, 1593,
2474
Nephroureterectomy, 2474
Nerve block, 113
Nerve cells, 105, 296, 554, 731,
980, 1117, 1174, 1598, 1603,
1608, 1738, 2137, 2281
Nerve deafness, 1033
Nerve disorders, 362

Nerves, 112, 228, 362, *1598*, 2035,
2350, *2370*, 2475; lower
extremities, 1386
Nervous system, 49, 161, 228, 421,
731, 787, 995, 1117, 1522,
1597-1602, 1603, 1608, 1613,
1617, 1722, 1738, 1740, 1758,
1819, 2137, 2210-2211, 2475
Neural therapy, 79
Neural tube, 720, 2475
Neuralgia, **1602-1606**, 2475
Neuritic plaques, 81
Neuritis, **1602-1606**, 2475
Neurofibrillary tangles, 81, 85, 2475
Neurofibromas, 1607, 2327
Neurofibromatosis, 942, **1606-1607**,
2327
Neurogenic bladder, 2368
Neuroglia, 297, 1117, 1611
Neuroglial cell, 2475
Neurologic, 2475
Neurology, **1607-1612**, 1613, 2475;
pediatric, **1612-1615**
Neuromas, 2327
Neuromusculoskeletal, 2475
Neurons, 2475. *See also* Nerve cells
Neuropathy, **1602-1606**, 2475
Neuroscience, 2475
Neurosis, **1615-1616**, 2475
Neurosurgery, **1616-1621**, 1712,
2475
Neurotransmitters, 586, 731, 787,
1535, 1561, 1599, 1608, 1723,
1739, 1782, 2192, 2475
Neutrophils, 264, 1146, 1210,
1242-1243, 2475
Nevi, 249
Newborns, 146, 1583, 1774
Niacin, 1645, 2403
Nicotinamide adenine dinucleotide
(NAD), 2475
Nicotine, 42, 143, 316
Niemann-Pick disease, 1363
Night blindness, 1431
Night terrors, 1622, 2105
Nightmares, **1621-1623**
NIH. *See* National Institutes of
Health (NIH)
NINDS. *See* National Institute of
Neurological Disorders and
Stroke (NINDS)
NIOSH. *See* National Institute for
Occupational Safety and Health
(NIOSH)

Osteochondritis juvenilis, **1695-1696**
Osteoclasts, 292, 1117, 2477
Osteocytes, 290, 1116, 2477
Osteogenesis imperfecta, **1696-1697**
Osteomalacia, 284-285, 1431
Osteomas, 684
Osteomyelitis, 284, 873, **1697-1698**
Osteopathic medicine, 703,
   1698-1702, 2477
Osteopenia, 2010
Osteopetrosis, 292
Osteoporosis, 51, 284-285, 293-294,
   632, 792, 875, 953, 1107,
   1161-1162, 1195, 1310, 1431,
   1433, 1469, 1689, **1702-1708**,
   2139, 2477
Osteosarcoma, 281, 2327
Osteosclerosis, 685
Ostomy, 1200, 2477
Otitis, 2477
Otitis externa, 677, 684
Otitis media, 677-678, 682, 685,
   1038, 1041, 1549, 1568, 1570,
   2038, 2174; acute, 1567
Otoacoustic emissions, 189
Otologist, 2477
-otomy, 2477
Otoplasty, **1708-1709**, 1832
Otorhinolaryngology, 687, 1321,
   1709-1713, 2477
Otosclerosis, 678, 680, 682, 1033,
   1038, 1696, 2477
Otoscope, 686, 2477
Outer ear, 2477
Outpatient care, 2478
Ovarian cancer, **387-391**, 946-947
Ovarian cyst removal. *See* Cyst
   removal; Ovarian cysts
Ovarian cysts, 540, 945, 947,
   1713-1715, 2478
Ovariectomy, 2478
Ovaries, 540, 961, 1005, 1193,
   1195, 1247, 1474, 1713, 1959,
   2050, 2478
Over-the-counter drugs, 42, 1399,
   2033-2034, 2338, 2478
Overbite, 1683
Overdoses, 1844-1845, 1957
Overhydration, 850
Oviducts, 498-499, 501, 1248, 1959,
   2478
Ovulation, 498-500, 510, 791, 1232,
   1247, 1475, 1656, 1863, 2478

Ovum, 462, 499, 501, 659, 696,
   1232, 2478
Oxygen, 972, 1044, 1392, 1715,
   1964
Oxygen deprivation. *See*
   Asphyxiation
Oxygen therapy, 77, **1715**, 2478
Oxytocin, 313, 752, 962, 1658,
   1819, 2214, 2478
Ozone layer, 1824, 2097

Pacemaker implantation, **1716-1721**
Pacemakers, 152, 228, 1055, 1624,
   1716-*1717*, 1972, 2478
Pacifiers, 2414
Pacinian corpuscles, 2035, 2282,
   2284, 2478
Paget's disease, 1137, **1721**, 2478
Pain, 1561, 1617-1618, **1721-1723**,
   1724, 1785, 2017, 2478;
   abdominal, 6, 474, 532, 767, 956,
   1285, 2171; back, 633-634, 1310,
   1318, 1703, 2110; chest, 122,
   349, 710, 747, *1048*, 1066, 1165,
   1389, 1781, 1835, 1925; chronic,
   163, 1723; hip, 1108; stomach, 6
Pain management, 34, 37, 1157,
   1180, 1445, **1724**, 2478
Painkillers, 112, 409, 828, 1079,
   1140, 1561, 1723-1724, 1736,
   1785
Palatability, 2222
Palate, 455, 459, 911
Palliative care, 1141
Palliative treatments, 2478
Palpation, 1801, 2478
Palpitations, 1469, **1724-1725**, 2478
Palsy, 215, 385, **1725-1729**, 2478
Pancreas, 2, 543, 607, 610, 625,
   748, 774, 902, 909, 961, 1188,
   1729-1734, 2163, 2165, 2306,
   2343, 2478
Pancreatic cancer, 1732, **2163-2167**
Pancreatic insufficiency, 775
Pancreatin, 774
Pancreatitis, 7, 416, 615, 909, 1731,
   1734-1736, 2478
Pandemics, 780, 2478
Panic attacks, 142, 144, 733,
   1736-1738, 2478
Panic disorder, 142, 144, 733
Pap smear, 388, 390-391, 947, *1004*,
   1006, 1284, 1804, 2478
Papain, 775

Papillae, 2219
Papillomaviruses, 2409, 2412, 2478
Paracentesis, 1283
Paralysis, 215, 701, 998, 1020,
   1075, 1556, 1600, 1725,
   1738-1742, 1750, 1850-1851,
   1935, 1937, 2135, 2351, 2478;
   sleep, 1556, 2105; spastic, 2246
Paralytic ileus, 1277
Paramedical, 2478
Paramedics, 725, **1743-1748**, 1971,
   2478
Paranoia, 55, **1748-1750**, 2015,
   2478
Paraplegia, 1075, 1741, **1750**, 2478
Parasite, 2478
Parasitic diseases, 714, 716, 956,
   1277, 1419, 1424, **1750-1755**,
   1826, 1892, 1993, 2014, 2108,
   2428
Parasympathetic nervous system,
   1044, 1599, 1819, 2478
Parathyroid glands, 748, 961,
   1161-1162, 1755, 2214,
   2262-2263, 2268, 2478
Parathyroid hormone, 961,
   1161-1162, 1755, 2214
Parathyroidectomy, **1755-1756**, 2478
Parenting, 2083
Parkinsonism, 1757
Parkinson's disease, 51, 569, 741,
   838, 1600, 1617, 1726, 1728,
   1756-1761, 2055, 2309, 2478
Paroxysm, 2479
Paroxysmal hemoglobinuria, 1228
Partial dentures, 583
Partial pressure of a gas in a gas,
   2479
Parturition, 2479
Passive euthanasia, 2479
Passive immunity, 2479
Pasteur, Louis, 208, 211, 1940
Patella, 1308, 1383
Patent ductus, 504-506
Patents, 854
Pathogen, 2479
Pathogenesis, 200, 630, 1267, 1761
Pathogenicity, 2479
Pathologic, 2479
Pathology, 199, 232, 556, 560, 600,
   629, 1244, 1315, **1761-1766**,
   2479
Pathophysiology, 2479
Patient advocacy, 2479

Pilocarpine, 967
Pilosebaceous, 2481
Pimples, 24, 595, **1825-1826**, 2481
Pineal gland, 748, 750, 961, 1461
Pinel, Philippe, 1902
Pinkeye. *See* Conjunctivitis
Pinworm, 1753, **1826-1827**
Pituitary gland, 292, 666-667,
    748-749, 752, 755, 957, 961,
    996, 1474, 1617, 2115, 2214,
    2481
Pituitary tumors, 957
Pityriasis, 2100
Pityriasis alba, **1827**
Pityriasis rosea, **1827**
P-K test, 69
PKU. *See* Phenylketonuria (PKU)
Placebo, 237, 2481
Placenta, 408-409, 413, 434, 719,
    1517, 1775, 1863, 2481
Placenta abruptio, 413, 1775, 1870
Placenta previa, 393, 413, 1775,
    1870
Plague, **1827-1829**, 2436, 2481;
    bubonic, 780, 1828, 2312, 2436;
    pneumonic, 1828, 1926
Plaintiff, 2481
Plantar, 2481
Plantar warts, 834, 867, 2410-2411,
    2481
Plaque, 2481; arterial, 152, 153,
    354, 445, 718, *745*, 1045, 1048,
    1052, 1159, 1165, 2161, 2182,
    2253, 2375; dental, 23, 573, *578*,
    958, 1777, 2229
Plasma, 266, 270, 1069, 1078, 1228,
    2213, 2301, 2481
Plasma coagulation system, 258
Plasma exchange, 1525
Plasma proteins, 2481
Plasmapheresis, 1000, 1078, 1228,
    1531
Plasmids, 662, 918
Plasmin, 2253, 2481
Plasminogen, 2253
Plastic surgery, 48, 818, 1365, 1712,
    1829-1835, 2431, 2481. *See also*
    Cosmetic surgery; Reconstructive
    surgery
Plasticity, 2481
Platelets, 257-258, 260, *265*, 270,
    1069, 1077, 1351, 2252, 2257,
    2300, 2481
Platinum analogues, 397

Pleura, 401, 1391, 1393
Pleurisy, **1835**, 1837, 2481
Pluripotent, 2481
PMS. *See* Premenstrual syndrome
    (PMS)
Pneumococcal infections, 663, 1219
Pneumocystis carinii pneumonitis,
    29, 1837-1838
Pneumocystis pneumonia, 2482
Pneumonia, 206, 327, 491-492, 888,
    1218, 1261, 1268, 1310, 1340,
    1389, 1394, 1828, **1835-1839**,
    1924, 1931, 2144, 2150, 2174,
    2482
Pneumonic plague, 1828, 1926
Pneumothorax, 1391, 1393
Podiatry, 834, **1839-1843**, 2482
Point-of-service plans, 1031
Poison ivy, 1848
Poison oak, 1848
Poison sumac, 1848
Poisoning, 17-19, 202, 489, 528,
    631, 856, **1843-1847**, 1848, 2000,
    2038, 2120, 2289, 2482
Poisonous plants, **1847-1850**, 2482
Poisons, 17, 202, 251, 555, 1762,
    1846, 2038, 2291
Poliomyelitis, 416, 418, 1119,
    1216-1217, **1850-1855**, 2136,
    2394-2395, 2426, 2482
Pollution, 518, 772, 1394, 2290
Polycystic kidney disease, 942, 1304
Polycystic ovary syndrome, 1960
Polycythemia, 2482
Polydactyly, 245, 2482
Polygraph, 732
Polymerase chain reaction, 232, 273,
    275, 1138, 1152
Polymethylmethacrylate, 2482
Polyp removal. *See* Colon and rectal
    polyp removal; Nasal polyp
    removal; Polyps
Polypharmacy, 2482
Polyposis, familial, 1202
Polyps, 480, 482, 484, 486, 906,
    1277, 1321, *1565*, 1569, 1881,
    2407-2408, 2482
Polysaccharides, 857
Polyspermy, 1232, 2482
Pons, 298
Pontiac fever, 1340
Population, 2482
Porphyria, **1855-1856**, 2482

Port-wine stains, 249, 594, 1325,
    2096
Portacaval shunts, 2081, 2482
Portal system, 2482
Positive feedback, 1818, 2482
Positron emission tomography
    (PET) scanning, 1207, 1629,
    1856-1858, 1949, 2482
Positrons, 2482
Posterior, 2482
Postmaturity, 413
Postpartum depression, **1858-1859**,
    2482
Post-traumatic stress disorder, 90,
    143, **1859-1860**
Postural drainage, 738
Postural hypotension, 641-642
Posture, 1310
Potassium, 2404
Potency, 2482
Prader-Willi syndrome, 926
Precocious puberty, **1860-1862**,
    1921
Predisposition, 943
Preeclampsia, 695, 1867, 2482
Preferred provider, 1031
Pregnancy, 92, *246*, 322, *408*, 434,
    499, 500, 1081, 1083, 1176,
    1500, 1578-1579, 1656, 1775,
    1819, **1862-1868**, *1977*, 2162,
    2287, 2343, 2357, 2482; alcohol
    use and, 835; cervical cancer
    and, 389; ectopic, 538, 696-697,
    1006, 1865, 2155
Premature, 2482
Premature birth, 386, 413, 1585,
    1766, 1775, **1868-1872**, 1933
Premature infants, 1967
Premenstrual syndrome (PMS),
    1477, **1872**, 2482
Premolars, 2482
Preoperational stage, 470, 603
Prep, 2482
Presbycusis, 685, 953, 1033
Presbyopia, 277, 815, 953, 2038
Prescription drugs, 855, 2482
Presenilins, 82, 2482
Pressure, 2482
Pressure sores, 1310
Prevalence, 2482
Preventive medicine, 349, 634, 808,
    903, 924, 1049, 1055, 1699,
    1807, 1813, 1816, **1872-1877**,
    1972, 2255, 2482

Prevnar, 1219
Priapism, 950, 2055
Prima facie, 2482
Primary care, 2482
Primary infection, 2482
Primitive reflexes, 1954-1957
Primitive streak, 719
Prion diseases, 522, **1877-1879**
Prions, 522, 1877
Privacy, 2482
PRK. *See* Photorefractive
    keratectomy (PRK)
Probability, 2483
Procedure, 2483
Proctology, **1879-1882**, 2483
Professional licensing, 2483
Progeria, **1882-1883**
Progesterone, 321, 388, 390, 407,
    509, 791, 1177, 1247, 1474,
    1657, 2483
Progestins, 762
Prognosis, 2483
Prokaryotic cells, 204
Prolactin, 313, 322, 753-754, 1658,
    2483
Prolactinomas, 754
Prolapse; mitral valve, 356,
    1501-1502, 1736; rectal, 909,
    1880; uterine, 945, 947,
    1193-1194, 1960
Prone, 2483
Prophylactic treatment, 2483
Prostaglandins, 12, 407, 498, 1257,
    1475, 1985, 2337, 2483
Prostate cancer, 950, **1883-1886**,
    1889, 1891, 2161, 2385
Prostate gland, 949, 954, 1883,
    1886-1890, 1958, 2161, 2483
Prostate gland removal, **1890-1892**
Prostate specific antigen (PSA),
    1885
Prostatectomy, 1885
Prostatic hypertrophy, 954
Prostheses, 19, 97-98, 100, 166,
    1691, 1831, 2201, 2483; breast,
    317, 319; penile, 1772, 2056
Prosthetist, 2483
Prosthodontics, 2483
Prostoglandular carcinoma, 2483
Protease inhibitors, 32
Proteases, 774
Protein, 2009
Protein kinase, 2483
Proteins, 223, 270, 376, 625, 646,

775, 858, 917, 1135, 1280, 1362,
    1370, 1546, 1642, 2483
Proteinuria, 1594
Proton beam therapy, 1413
Protozoa, 136, 168, 1489, 1751,
    1754, 1892, 2483
Protozoan diseases, 1345, 1419,
    1424, 1489, **1892-1893**
Proving, 2483
Proximal, 2483
Pruritus. *See* Itching
PSA. *See* Prostate specific antigen
    (PSA)
Pseudohermaphroditism, **1095-1096**,
    2051, 2053
Pseudo-obstruction, 1662-1663
Psoralen, 1896, 2095
Psoriasis, 595, 1010, 1553,
    1893-1898, 2093, 2100, 2483
Psyche, 2483
Psychedelic drugs, 466, 2483
Psychiatric disorders, 529, 733,
    1898-1903, 1904, 1906, 1908,
    1911, 2076, 2176, 2192
Psychiatric evaluation, 1329
Psychiatry, **1903-1905**, 2483; child
    and adolescent, **1905-1907**;
    geriatric, **1907-1909**
Psychoanalysis, 1182, 1615, 1654,
    1909-1913, 2483
Psychoanalyst, 2483
Psychogenic, 2483
Psychophysiological disorders, 217
Psychosis, **1913-1915**, 2483
Psychosomatic disorders, 1615,
    1915-1917, 2483
Psychosurgery, 587, 1618, 1654,
    2483
Psychotherapy, 241-242, 587, 1499,
    1654, 1860, 1901, 1911, 2179,
    2483; behavioral, 588; cognitive,
    588
Psychotic, 2484
Psychotropic drugs, 2484
Pterygium, 809
Pterygium removal, 809
Ptosis, **1917-1918**, 2484
Puberty, 24-25, 87, 321, 961, 996,
    1350, 1769, 1861, 1886,
    1918-1923, 2115, 2484
Public health, 89, 379, 782, 1573,
    2315, 2425, 2484. *See also*
    Environmental health;
    Occupational health

Public Health Service, 1573
Pulled muscles, 1531, 1535
Pulmonary, 2484
Pulmonary artery, 503-504
Pulmonary diseases, 49, 177, 327,
    628, 736, 769, 1018, 1275, 1388,
    1390, 1394, 1835, *1836*,
    1923-1928, *1929*, 1933, 1965,
    2317
Pulmonary edema, 358, 699, 1054,
    1118, 1410, 2484
Pulmonary embolism, 2373
Pulmonary function tests, 1929,
    1933
Pulmonary medicine, 128,
    1928-1931, 2484; pediatric,
    1931-1934
Pulp, 2484
Pulse, 2484
Pulse rate, 1803
Pulsed laser, 2484
Puncture wounds, 1028
Pupil, 367-368, 1672, 1674, 2484
Pure Food and Drug Act, 855
Purging, 689
Pus, 14, 1210, 1243
Pyelonephritis, 547, 549, 1297,
    1590, 2356-2357
Pyloric stenosis, **1934**, 2335, 2484
Pyoderma, 590
Pyonephrosis, 1297
Pyorrhea, 573-574, 579, 2484
Pyridostigmine bromide, 2484
Pyrogens, 842-843, 1243, 2484
Pyruvic acid, 971

Qi gong, 78, **1935**, 2484
Quadriplegia, 385, 1075, 1726,
    1741, **1935**, 2484
Quantum theory, 2484
Quickening, 9, 1775, 2484
Quinine, 1423
Quinsy, 1567, 1569, **1935-1936**,
    2276
Quintuplets, 1519

Rabies, 251, **1937-1942**, 2436, 2484
Radial, 2484
Radial keratotomy (RK), 2401
Radiation, 245, 282, 368, 631, 722,
    770, 773, 1441, 1632, 1856,
    1942, 1944-1945, *1948*
Radiation dose, 2484
Radiation sickness, **1942**, 2484

Tooth decay, 852, 2493. *See also* Cavities
Tooth extraction, 579, 2229, **2277-2278**, 2494
Tooth loss, 536, 583; smoking and, 2118
Tooth pulp, 2494
Toothache, 572, 575, **2278**, 2494
Tophi, 976
Tophus, 2494
Topical anesthesia, 113
Torrey, E. Fuller, 2015
Torsion, 2241
Tort, 2494
Torticollis, **2278-2279**
Totipotence, 2494
Touch, 2035, **2279-2285**, 2494
Tourette's syndrome, 1653, 2270-2271, **2285-2287**
Toxemia, 1870, **2287**, 2494
Toxic shock syndrome, 206, 1475, 2150
Toxicokinetics, 2494
Toxicology, 202, 1128, **2287-2292**, 2494
Toxins, 78, 251, 774, 1282, 1336, 1372-1373, 1762, 1784, 1843, 2041, 2244, 2289, 2309, 2494
Toxoid, 2494
Toxoplasmosis, 129, 862, 1754, 1893, **2292-2293**, 2436-2437, 2494
TPA. *See* Tissue plasminogen activator (TPA or tPA)
Trabeculectomy, 968
Trace elements, 2494
Trace evidence, 2494
Tracer, 2494
Trachea, 764, 1390, 1393, 1963, *2293-2294*, 2494
Tracheostomy, 526, 2247, **2293-2294**, 2494
Trachoma, 262, 515, **2294-2295**, 2312, 2399, 2494
Tracking, 1272
Tract, 2494
Traction, 873-874, 878
Traffic accidents, 773, 2003
Trance, 1178
Tranquilizers, 1654
Transcranial magnetic stimulation (TMS), 2079
Transcription, 2494
Transducer (probe), 2494

Transference, 2494
Transfusion, 270-272, 1313, 1977, 2074, 2249, **2295-2304**, 2494
Transgenic animals, 935
Transient ischemic attacks (TIAs), 52, 153, 154, 302, 304, 2182, 2381, 2494. *See also* Strokes
Transitional cell carcinoma, 2494
Translation, 2494
Translocation, 658, 660
Transplantation, 128, 288, 464, 559, 941, 1062, 1213, *1300*, 2205, **2304-2309**, 2494; bone marrow, 287-289, 292, 309, 983, 1124-1125, 1223-1224, 1354, 1942, 2089; corneal, 515-517; hair, 1011, 1013-1014; heart, 1046, 1059-1062, 2251; kidney, 1299-1301, 1589, 1597; liver, 1373, 1380-1382, 2306
Transposition of the great arteries, 504, 506
Transposon, 662, 919
Transsexualism, *2047*-2048, 2053
Transsexuals, 2494
Transverse processes, 2494
Trauma, 90, 528, 631, 1019, 1107, 1745, 1762, 1807, 2135, 2494; emotional, 90, 1859
Travelers' diarrhea, 621, 623, 675, 914
Treatment, 2494
Trembling, **2309-2310**
Tremor, 1757, 2309
Trench mouth. *See* Vincent's infection
Trephination, 1620, 2495
Trephine, 2495
Tretinoin, 2181
Triage, 726, 729, 1143, 2495
Trichiasis, 2294
Trichinosis, 1753, **2310**, 2429
Trichomoniasis, 946-947, 2065-2066, 2068
Tricyclics, 2495
Triglycerides, 857, 1280, 1361-1362, 1370
Triiodothyronine, 960
Trimester, 2495
Triplets, 1518-1519
Trisomy 21. *See* Down syndrome
Troglitazone, 1265
Tropical diseases, 717, 784, 1419, 1424, 1753, 2310-*2311*, 2433

Tropical medicine, **2310-2316**, 2426, 2495
Trunk, 2495
Trust, 603-604
Tsetse fly, 2108
TSH. *See* Thyroid-stimulating hormone (TSH)
Tubal ligation, 1194, 1320, 2154, **2316-2317**, 2386, 2495
Tubercles, 2317
Tuberculin skin test, 2320
Tuberculosis, 206, 381, 569, 663, 1216, 1394, 1396, 1924, 1928, 1930, 2025, **2317-2322**, 2436, 2495; AIDS and, 29
Tubular reabsorption, 2495
Tubular secretion, 2495
Tularemia, 1357
Tumor removal, *483*, 1409, 1548, **2322-2325**
Tumor suppressor genes, 943, 1425
Tumors, 339, 482, 484, 556, 754, 802, 1189, 1277, 1321, 1374, 1424, 1630, 1667, 1712, 1732, 1888, 1960, 2322, **2325-2330**, 2343, 2495; nerve, 1606
Turbidity, 2353
Turbulence, 445
Turgor, 2495
Turner syndrome, 403, 667, 721, 757, 1519, 2050, **2330**
Twins, 462, 464, 923, 1515-*1516*, 2495. *See also* Multiple births
Tympanic membrane, 682, 2037, 2495
Tympanoplasty, 682, 686, 2495
Type A individuals, 2177
Type B individuals, 2177
Typhoid fever, 2006, **2330-2333**, 2495
Typhus, 1356, **2330-2333**, 2495
Tyrosine, 1822

Ulcer surgery, **2334-2336**
Ulcerative colitis, 2495. *See also* Colitis
Ulcers, 8, 846, 899, 902, 908, 914, 1269, 1280, 1325, *2334-2335*, **2336-2340**, 2370, 2387, 2495; corneal, 1673
Ulna, 2347, 2495
Ulnar, 2495
Ultrasonic, 2495
Ultrasonography, 903, 915, 923,

1369, 1624, 1658, 1774, 2168, **2340-2345**, 2495
Ultrasound, 156-157, 246, 890, 1379, 2184, 2186
Ultraviolet light, 1822, 1896, 2096
Ultraviolet radiation, 1822, 1824, 2495
Umbilical cord, 1863, 2244, **2345**
Umbilical hernias, 1100
Umbilicus, 2495
Unconsciousness, 1556, 1845, **2346**, 2495
Upper arm, 2495
Upper extremities, 98, **2346-2352**, 2495
Uprima, 2056
Urea, 2495
Uremia, 2495
Ureter, 2495
Ureterolithotomy, 2495
Ureters, 2170, 2360, 2364
Urethra, 765, 949, 1004, 1192, 1884, 1887, 1890, 1958, 2352, 2355, 2360, 2495
Urethritis, 2065, **2352**, 2355-2356, 2361, 2366, 2495
Urethroplasty, **1191-1192**, 2495
-uria, 2495
Uric acid, 976-977, 2169
Uricosuric drugs, 978
Urinalysis, 1311, 1593, 1596, **2352-2354**, 2364, 2369, 2495
Urinary bladder, 2496
Urinary disorders, 345, 547-548, 1236, 2172, 2352, **2354-2358**, 2361, 2365, 2368
Urinary system, 3, **2358-2363**, 2368, 2496
Urinary tract, 2172
Urinary tract infections, 450-451, 986, 1305, 2169, 2361, 2366, 2368, 2496
Urination, 2360
Urination, painful. *See* Dysuria
Urine, 3, 1311, 2170, 2213, 2353, 2359, 2363, 2368, 2496
Urine, bacteria in. *See* Bacteriuria
Urine, blood in. *See* Hematuria
Urine, protein in. *See* Proteinuria
Urolithiasis, 2496
Urology, **2363-2367**, 2496; pediatric, **2368-2369**
Uterine cancer, **387-391**, 946-947, 1470

Uterine fibroids, 945, 947, 1193, 1548
Uterine prolapse, 945, 947, 1193-1194, 1960
Uterus, 407, 758-759, 1005, 1176-1177, *1193*, 1247, 1959, 2496
Uvea, 2496
Uveitis, 1674, 2496

Vaccination, 208, 223, 382, 417, 494, 1090, 1147, 1149, **1214-1221**, 1245, 1261, 1454, 1528, 1770, 1852-1853, 1939, 1994, 2045, 2111, 2247, 2395, 2425; AIDS and, 33. *See also* Immunization
Vaccines, 935, 1147, 1149, *1215*, 1770, 2045, 2425, 2496
Vaccinia, 2496
Vacuum aspiration, 11
Vacuum tumescence therapy, 2057
Vagina, 510, 790, 1005, 1958, 2047, 2496
Vaginal cancer, 946
Vaginitis, 548, 945-946, 2065; atrophic, 1470
Vagotomy, **2370-2371**, 2496
Vagus nerve, 625, 902, 1020, *2370*, 2496
Valerian root, 1094
Valgus, 2496
Validity, selective, 2496
Vallate papillae, 2220, 2496
Valley fever, 886
Valsalva maneuver, 642-643
Valves, 2496
Vancomycin, 663
Variable, 2496
Varicella. *See* Chickenpox; Herpes zoster; Shingles
Varicella-zoster virus, 404
Varicocele removal. *See* Testicular surgery; Varicoceles
Varicoceles, 951, 1252, 1254, 1960, 2242, 2496
Varicose vein removal, **2371-2373**
Varicose veins, 446, 700, 915, 1081, 2254, 2371-*2372*, **2373-2375**, 2382, 2387
Varicosis, 2374, 2496
Varus, 2496
Vas deferens, 949, 1887, 1958, 2383-*2384*, 2496

Vascular, 2496
Vascular compartment, 698
Vascular dementia, 568, 570
Vascular medicine, **2375-2379**, 2382, 2496
Vascular system, 2343, 2375, **2379-2382**, 2496
Vascularized transplant, 2496
Vasculature, 2496
Vasectomy, 2154, **2383-2387**, 2496
Vasoconstriction, 445, 640, 1025, 1077, 1257, 1269, 2210, 2252, 2496
Vasodilation, 445, 640, 642, 1026, 1059, 1066, 1257, 2496
Vasodilator drugs, 1059, 1167
Vasopressin, 638, 752, 962, 1137, 2214, 2360
Vasospasm, 2183
Vectors, 168, 251, 918, 1421, 2496
Vegans, 1431
Vegetarians, 1431
Vegetations, 746-747
Veins, *444*-445, 1385, 1796, 2212, 2350, 2371-2373, 2377, 2379, 2387, 2497; chest, 400
Venereal diseases, 2497. *See also* Sexually transmitted diseases
Venipuncture, 1073, 2497
Venography, 1797
Venom, 251, 2121
Venous insufficiency, **2387-2388**, 2497
Venous thrombosis, 700, 1797, 2381, 2497
Venter, J. Craig, 1153
Ventricles, 1043, 2497
Ventricular fibrillation, 355, 707, *709*, 1046, 1053, 1972
Ventriculoperitoneal shunts, 2081, 2497
Vermiform appendix. *See* Appendix
Vertebrae, 399, 419, 422, 1309, 1618, **2138-2143**, 2497
Vertigo, 212, 641, 679, 1464, 2038, 2183
Vestibular, 2497
Vestibule, 1004
Veterans, 1001, 1860
Veterinary medicine, 127, **2388-2392**, 2497
Viability, 1330
Viagra, 2056
Vibrant Soundbridge, 1039